EXPERTddx™

MUSCULOSKELETAL

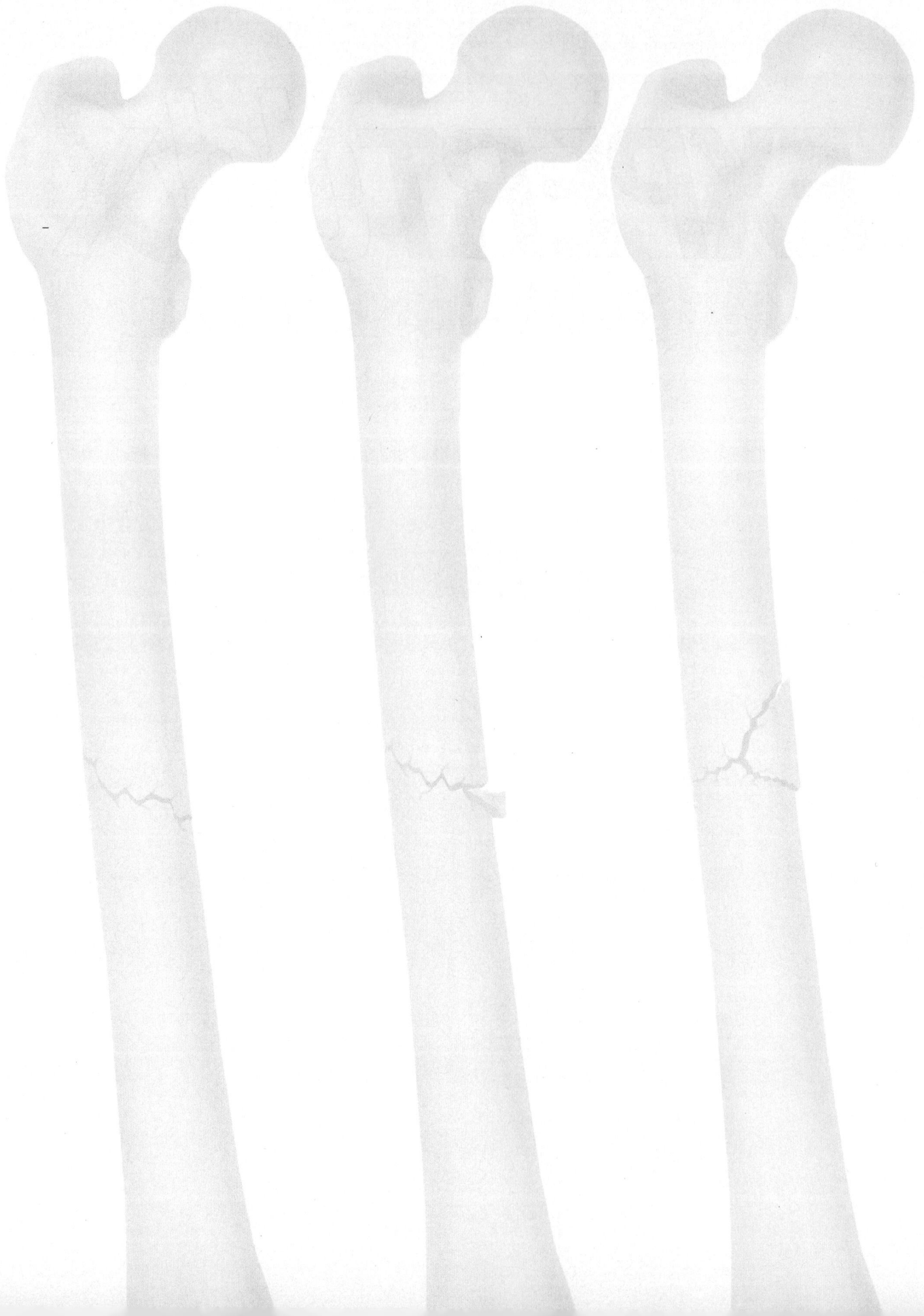

EXPERT*ddx*™
MUSCULOSKELETAL

B.J. Manaster, MD, PhD, FACR
Professor of Radiology
University of Utah School of Medicine
Salt Lake City, Utah

Carol L. Andrews, MD
Musculoskeletal Radiology
Mink Radiologic Imaging
Beverly Hills, California

Cheryl A. Petersilge, MD
Chair, Department of Radiology
Vice Chair, Regional Radiology
Marymount Hospital, Cleveland Clinic Health System
Cleveland, Ohio

Catherine C. Roberts, MD
Associate Dean, Mayo School of Health Sciences
Associate Professor of Radiology
Consultant Radiologist
Mayo Clinic
Scottsdale, Arizona

AMIRSYS®
Names you know. Content you trust.®

Composition by Amirsys, Inc., Salt Lake City, Utah

Printed in Canada by Friesens, Altona, Manitoba, Canada

ISBN: 978-1-9318-8403-7

Notice and Disclaimer

Library of Congress Cataloging-in-Publication Data

Manaster, B. J.
  Expertddx. Musculoskeletal / B.J. Manaster. -- 1st ed.
     p. ; cm.
  title: Musculoskeletal
  Includes index.
  ISBN 978-1-931884-03-7
  1. Musculoskeletal system--Diseases--Diagnosis--Atlases. 2. Diagnosis, Differential--Atlases. I. Title. II. Title: Musculoskeletal.
  [DNLM: 1. Musculoskeletal Diseases--diagnosis--Atlases. 2. Musculoskeletal System--Atlases. 3. Diagnosis, Differential--Atlases. WE 17 M267e 2008]
  RC925.7.M348 2008
  612.7022'2--dc22

                              2008039950

The authors wish to dedicate this book to our fellow musculoskeletal radiologists, past and present.

It was not so many decades ago that osseous neoplasms were not recognized as distinguishable entities, and arthritides were treated radiographically as a single process. Dedicated musculoskeletal radiologists were few and far between; however, these few individuals began to make important observations and share them with one another. This sharing process grew into two major societies, the Society of Skeletal Radiology and the International Skeletal Society, both of which continue to serve as excellent sounding boards and learning opportunities for musculoskeletal radiologists. Many of these individuals served as our mentors. As we conducted research for this book, we came to realize how significant their contributions were; we are truly standing on the shoulders of giants. We authors have also reinforced our affection for one another; throughout the process of producing this book, we have continued to learn from one another, enjoy one another's support, and feel inspired toward continued growth.

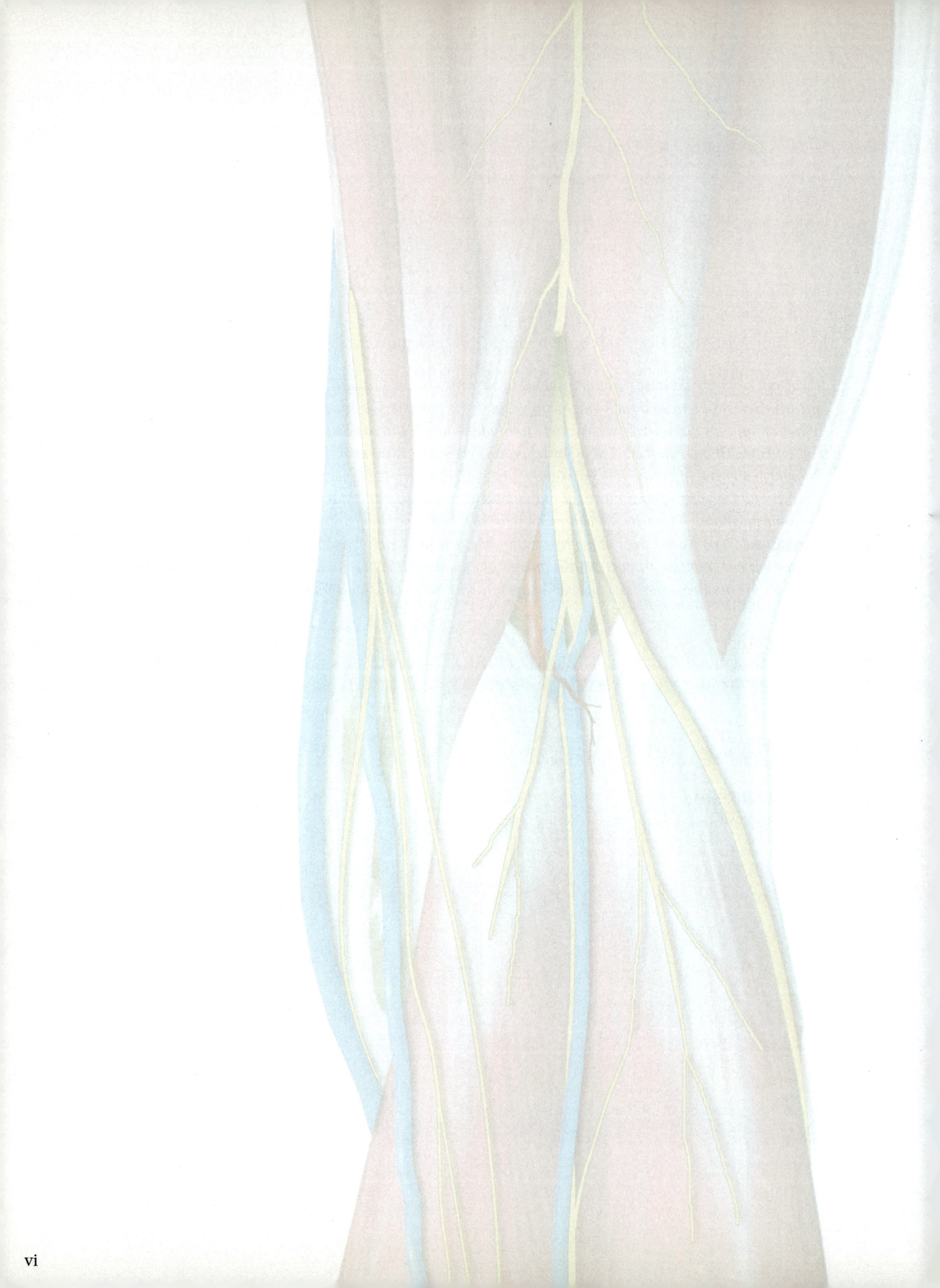

EXPERTddx™
MUSCULOSKELETAL

Once the appropriate technical protocols have been delineated, the best quality images obtained, and the cases queued up on PACS, the diagnostic responsibility reaches the radiology reading room. The radiologist must do more than simply "lay words on" but reach a real conclusion. If we cannot reach a definitive diagnosis, we must offer a reasonable differential diagnosis. A list that's too long is useless; a list that's too short may be misleading. To be useful, a differential must be more than a rote recitation from some dusty book or a mnemonic from a lecture way back when. Instead, we must take into account key imaging findings and relevant clinical information.

With these considerations in mind, we at Amirsys designed our Expert Differential Diagnoses series—EXPERTddx for short. Leading experts in every subspecialty of radiology identified the top differential diagnoses in their respective fields, encompassing specific anatomic locations, generic imaging findings, modality-specific findings, and clinically based indications. Our experts gathered multiple images, both typical and variant, for each EXPERTddx. Each features at least eight beautiful images that illustrate the possible diagnoses, accompanied by captions that highlight the pertinent imaging findings. Hundreds more are available in the eBook feature that accompanies every book. In classic Amirsys fashion, each EXPERTddx includes bulleted text that distills the available information to the essentials. You'll find helpful clues for diagnoses, ranked by prevalence as Common, Less Common, and Rare but Important.

Our EXPERTddx series is designed to help radiologists reach reliable—indeed, expert—conclusions. Whether you are a practicing radiologist or a resident/fellow in training, we think the EXPERTddx series will quickly become your practical "go-to" reference.

Anne G. Osborn, MD
Executive Vice President and Editor-in-Chief, Amirsys Inc.

Paula J. Woodward, MD
Executive Vice President and Medical Director, Amirsys Inc.

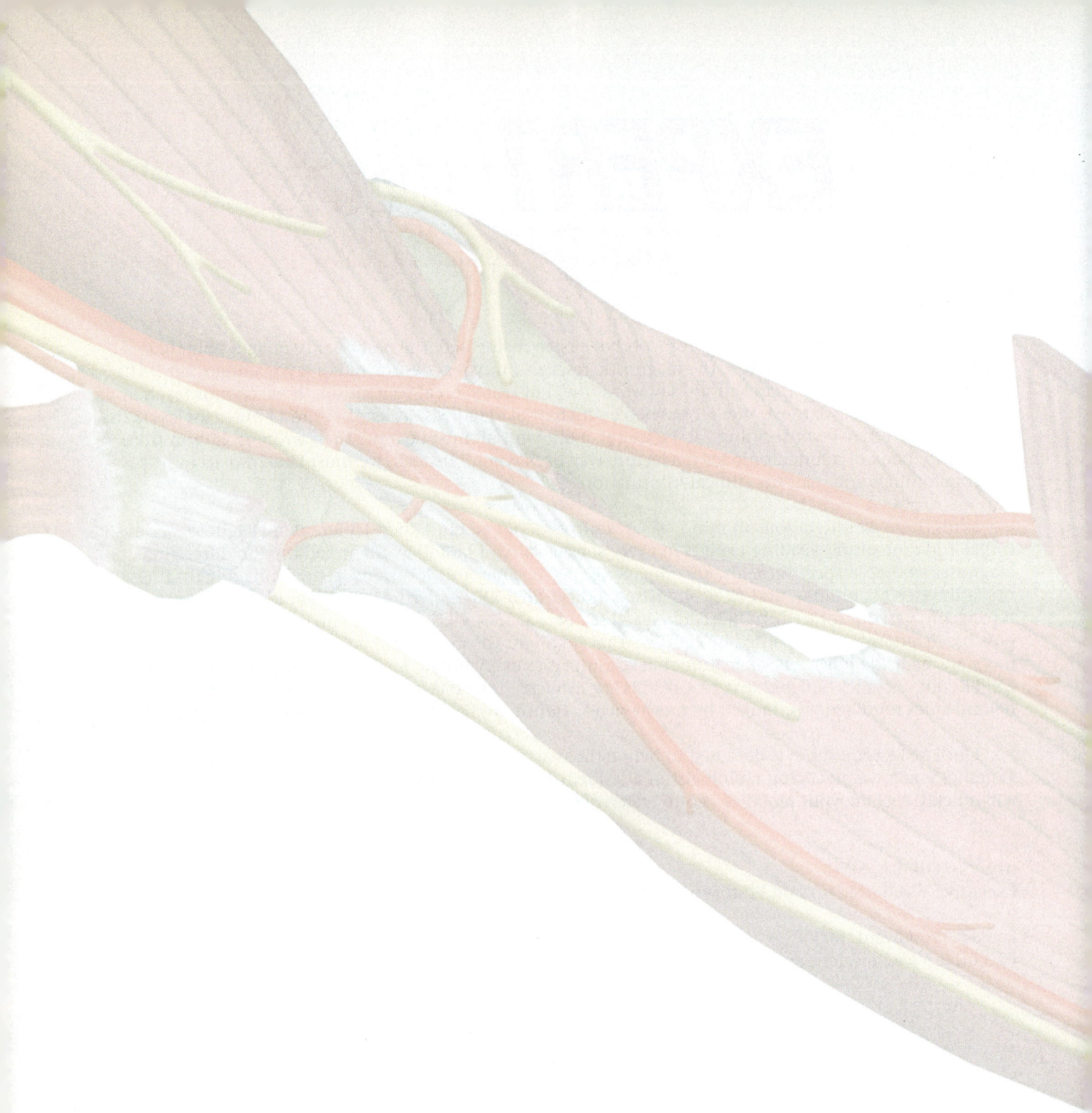

viii

PREFACE

The world of musculoskeletal radiology is becoming daunting, with a huge knowledge base required as we confront an exponentially expanding number of diagnoses and their associated imaging characteristics. We all continually attack the steep learning curve required to stay "on top" of the subspecialty, and we welcome reference material that can quickly address specific questions regarding an imaging finding or clinical presentation. Expert Differential Diagnosis: Musculoskeletal is a unique collection addressing this need; it offers over 200 expert differential diagnoses that cover a broad spectrum of musculoskeletal diseases, including trauma, arthritis, tumor, congenital, and metabolic disease. The lists are those our authors feel are most useful in our daily work. They are organized according to likelihood of occurrence, and there is both text and imaging provided to further differentiate among the differential possibilities.

The book has three major sections. The "Clinically Based" differentials will serve you best when you are given a general directive to determine the source of pain (for example, "lateral hip pain", "nerve entrapment of the lower extremity") or clinically observed abnormality (for example, "cavus foot deformity", "arthritis in a teenager", "hemihypertrophy"). The "Image Based" differentials will serve you best when you have a unique imaging appearance that has a relatively short differential (for example, "target lesions of bone", "nodular calcification", "lesion with bright T1 signal", "enlarged peripheral nerves"). The "Anatomy Based" differential list is necessarily long in this musculoskeletal text. Anatomic location of abnormalities is crucially important in the musculoskeletal system. Thus, there are lists of abnormalities involving some specific bone or joint locations (for example, "solitary rib lesion", "tibial bowing", "fluid collections about the knee"). There are also anatomic differential lists with more generic locations (for example, "flat bone, bubbly lesion", "long bone, undertubulation", "MCP-predominant arthritis"). Note that, among the long bone differential lists, there is a differentiation according to location along the length of the bone (epiphyseal/subchondral, metaphyseal, diaphyseal) as well as transversely across the bone (central, eccentric, cortically based, surface location).

Take a few moments to look at the table of contents and familiarize yourself with the layout of the book. You will then recognize that an abnormality you are seeking to define may be found in several lists. For example, an abnormality consisting of multiple aggressive lesions in the pelvic girdle of a child would be included in the "flat bones, permeative lesion" list in the anatomy based section, but also would be discussed in the "polyostotic lesions, child" list in the image based section. Another example might be of a hand radiograph showing acroosteolysis and DIP erosions. This would be included in the anatomically based list "acroosteolysis" found listed under "fingers and toes" as well as in the anatomically based list "IP-predominant arthritis" found under "joints". Perusal of the table of contents will be valuable in making best use of this reference.

We hope that you find this book useful in your daily practice of radiology and as a study guide if you are just entering our specialty. It should be useful to orthopedic surgeons, physiatrists, rheumatologists, and other practitioners as well. It is, of course, inevitable that we have neglected to discuss some differentials (remember, though, that most spine discussions are found in the Brain and Spine text). It is just as inevitable that we have left out some entities that belong in some of the lists or that the order we have chosen in a list is debatable. We would be happy to hear your comments and suggestions. The eBook companion allows us to add, alter, and update our lists. Email me at bjmanaster@amirsys.com and we will consider your suggestions.

B.J. Manaster, MD, PhD, FACR
Professor of Radiology
University of Utah School of Medicine
Salt Lake City, UT

ACKNOWLEDGMENTS

Text Editing

Douglas Grant Jackson

Ashley R. Renlund, MA

Kellie J. Heap

Image Editing

Jeffrey J. Marmorstone

Mitch D. Curinga

Medical Text Editing

Jay Johnson, MD

Art Direction and Design

Lane R. Bennion, MS

Richard Coombs, MS

Production Lead

Melissa A. Hoopes

Some images were previously published in Manaster BJ, May DA, Disler DG. Musculoskeletal Imaging: The Requisites. 2nd ed. Philadelphia, PA: Mosby, Elsevier; 2002. Each of these images is identified by "MSK Req" in the caption.

These images appear as follows: part.page.image; I.5.1; I.10.1; I.14.2; I.25.1; I.25.3; I.36.5; I.37.1; I.37.5; I.39.5; I.39.6; I.42.5; I.46.1; I.47.6; I.49.2; I.50.2; I.53.2; I.54.2; I.55.2; I.55.5; I.55.6; I.57.5; I.61.1; I.61.2; I.62.6; I.65.3; I.65.4; I.77.6; I.82.5; I.82.6; I.86.5; I.87.1; I.87.5; I.87.6; I.94.1; I.95.1; I.95.3; I.95.4; I.104.3; I.106.2; I.118.5; I.121.3; I.123.1; I.124.1; I.127.2; I.129.1; I.150.4; I.156.1; I.156.3; I.157.4; I.163.6; I.182.5; I.184.1; I.189.5; I.191.3; I.191.4; I.239.6; I.249.2; I.253.1; I.253.2; I.254.6; I.257.3; I.266.1; I.278.1; I.333.5; I.339.1; I.355.3; I.355.4; I.371.2; I.371.6; II.7.6; II.8.2; II.13.2; II.15.2; II.16.3; II.17.4; II.18.1; II.19.2; II.22.6; II.23.3; II.27.1; II.31.4; II.31.6; II.35.6; II.41.1; II.41.2; II.42.2; II.43.2; II.46.4; II.47.3; II.48.2; II.49.3; II.51.1; II.57.1; II.58.1; II.86.3; II.87.4; II.91.1; II.102.1; II.102.2; II.114.3; II.114.5; II.115.2; II.118.4; II.119.3; II.120.1; II.120. 5; II.121.5; II.123.2; II.129.6; II.142.5; II.144.1; II.145.1; II.145.4; II.158.1; II.188.6; III.17.1; III.75.1; III.112.4; III.137.6; III.151.5; III.159.6; III.177.3; III.181.2; and III.183.3.

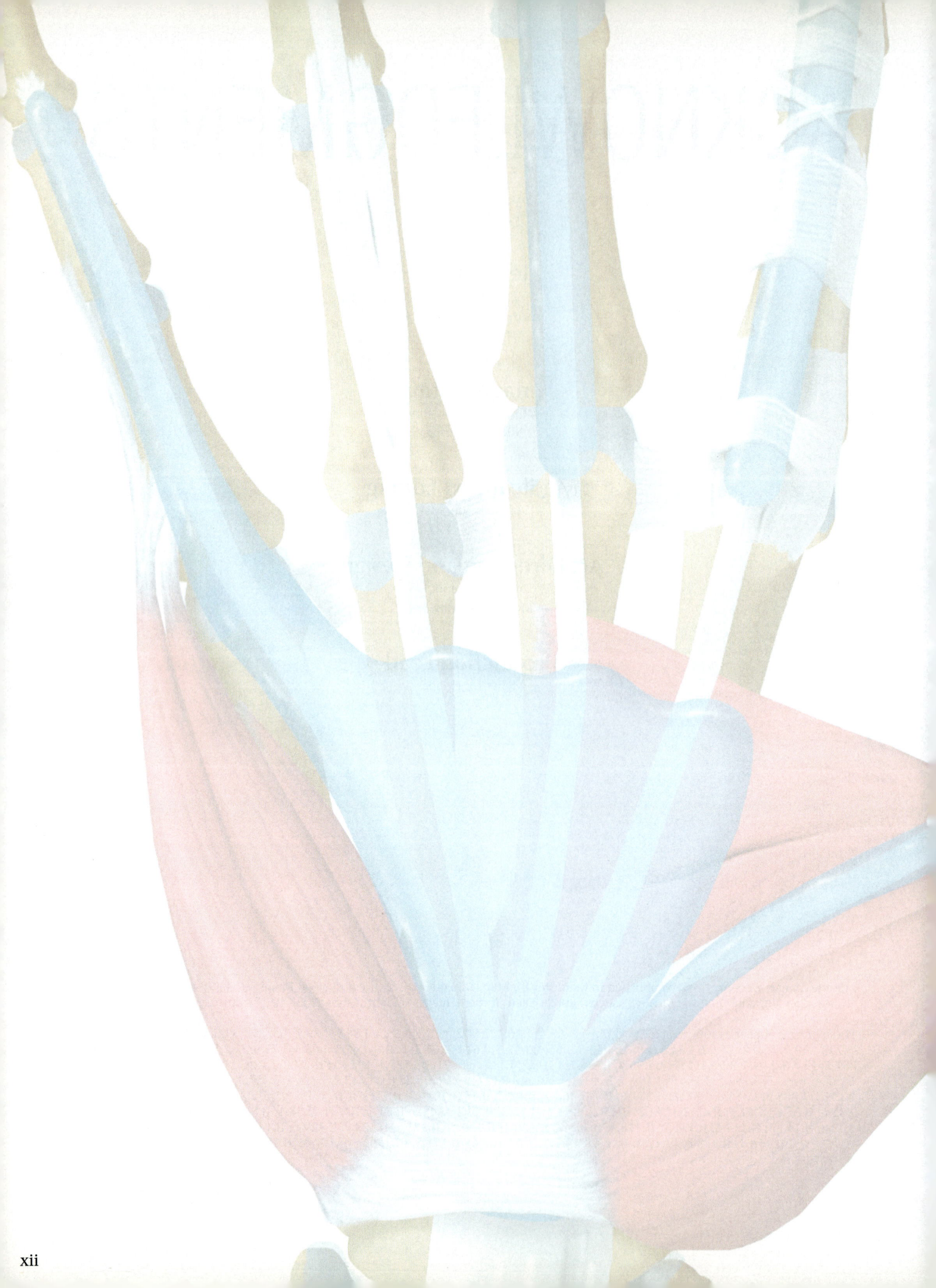

SECTIONS

PART I
Anatomy Based

Flat Bones
Long Bone, Epiphyseal
Long Bone, Metaphyseal
Long Bone, Meta-Diaphyseal
Long Bone, Growth Plate
Periosteum
Joint Based
Shoulder Girdle and Upper Arm
Elbow and Forearm
Wrist and Hand
Fingers and Toes
Intervertebral Disc
Paraspinal Abnormalities
Vertebral Shape
Vertebral Lesions
Ribs
Pelvis
Hip and Thigh
Knee and Lower Leg
Foot and Ankle

PART II
Image Based

Radiograph/CT, Osseous
Radiograph/CT, Soft Tissue
MR, Osseous
MR, Soft Tissue
MR, Joint
Ultrasound
Nuclear Medicine

PART III
Clinically Based

Shoulder Girdle and Upper Arm
Elbow and Forearm
Wrist and Hand
Pelvis, Hip, and Thigh
Knee and Leg
Ankle and Foot
Spine
Systemic Disease

TABLE OF CONTENTS

PART II
Image Based

Radiograph/CT, Osseous

PART III
Clinically Based

EXPERTddx™

MUSCULOSKELETAL

PART I
Anatomy Based

Flat Bones
Long Bone, Epiphyseal
Long Bone, Metaphyseal
Long Bone, Meta-Diaphyseal
Long Bone, Growth Plate
Periosteum
Joint Based
Shoulder Girdle and Upper Arm
Elbow and Forearm
Wrist and Hand
Fingers and Toes
Intervertebral Disc
Paraspinal Abnormalities
Vertebral Shape
Vertebral Lesions
Ribs
Pelvis
Hip and Thigh
Knee and Lower Leg
Foot and Ankle

FLAT BONES, FOCALLY EXPANDED OR BUBBLY LESION

DIFFERENTIAL DIAGNOSIS

Common
- Giant Cell Tumor (GCT)
- Plasmacytoma
- Fibrous Dysplasia (FD), Pelvis
- Metastases: Thyroid, Kidney

Less Common
- Aneurysmal Bone Cyst (ABC)
- Chondrosarcoma, Conventional
- Unicameral Bone Cyst (UBC)
- Hemophilia
- Hyperparathyroidism, Brown Tumor

Rare but Important
- Chondromyxoid Fibroma
- Chondroblastoma
- Osteoblastoma
- Langerhans Cell Histiocytosis (LCH)
- Cystic Angiomatosis

ESSENTIAL INFORMATION

Key Differential Diagnosis Issues
- Bubbly lesion in pelvis is usually a benign process
  - Exceptions: Metastatic, plasmacytoma, chondrosarcoma may appear relatively nonaggressive & should be considered
- **Hint**: Patient age can be a helpful differentiator among these lesions, though not always reliable
- **Hint**: Cartilage tumors are common in pelvis & scapula; remember to consider both benign & malignant varieties
- Note that list order is not the likelihood of the individual lesion occurring, but its occurring with this specific appearance
  - For example, LCH is common in pelvis, but only rarely appears bubbly, so is listed as "rare"

Helpful Clues for Common Diagnoses
- **Giant Cell Tumor (GCT)**
  - Lytic lesion which is usually only moderately expanded in long bones
  - Often large, highly expanded & even bubbly in pelvis
  - Prime age range: 30-60 years
  - MR usually contains some low signal within predominant high signal on T2; may have fluid levels

- **Plasmacytoma**
  - Pelvis & spine are most frequent locations
    - Though it develops into multiple myeloma, the lesion itself often appears relatively non-aggressive
  - Lytic & bubbly in pelvis; occasionally more aggressive with cortical breakthrough
  - Requires MR survey to determine whether it has advanced to more diffuse myeloma
- **Fibrous Dysplasia (FD), Pelvis**
  - FD has different manifestations in different types of bones
  - Pelvic FD is usually lytic & bubbly
    - Expanded lesion may be quite large
    - Occasionally, more mild expansion with ground-glass matrix, similar to lesion in long bone
  - Nonaggressive appearance
  - Often polyostotic, which suggests diagnosis
- **Metastases: Thyroid, Kidney**
  - Flat bones & axial skeleton most common sites for metastatic osseous lesions
    - Most metastases are focal or permeative, and multiple
  - Solitary expanded metastases less common
    - Tend to have either renal cell or thyroid as primary lesion
  - Note: Renal cell metastases may be extremely vascular
    - When renal cell metastasis is suspected & axial imaging is performed, include a look at kidneys
    - If kidney shows suspicious lesion, consider embolization of metastatic lesion prior to biopsy
    - Bleeding from biopsy can be excessive & even life-threatening if it is at a site which cannot be compressed

Helpful Clues for Less Common Diagnoses
- **Aneurysmal Bone Cyst (ABC)**
  - ABC is common lesion in patients < 30 years of age
  - More common in long than flat bones
  - When present in flat bones, has typical lytic bubbly expanded appearance
  - MR shows fluid levels except in small minority which are solid
- **Chondrosarcoma, Conventional**
  - Common lesion in adults (30-60 years age range most frequent), rare in teenagers

FLAT BONES, FOCALLY EXPANDED OR BUBBLY LESION

- Flat bones & metaphyses of long bones are most frequent locations
- Generally low grade at presentation, so may be mildly expanded, without cortical breakthrough
- Rarely will present as expanded or bubbly
- Chondroid matrix (but not invariably)
- **Hint**: Consider chondrosarcoma for any lesion in flat bone in patient in 30-60 year age range
  - Chondrosarcoma often underdiagnosed as a benign lesion
  - Inadequate resection at initial treatment is devastating; inevitable recurrence
- **Unicameral Bone Cyst (UBC)**
  - UBC most frequent in metaphyses of children (especially proximal humerus)
  - When UBC occurs in adult, tends to be in unusual location, particularly pelvis
  - Shows mild expansion of lytic lesion
  - No reactive change
  - MR confirms fluid centrally
- **Hemophilia**
  - Pelvis is frequent location for pseudotumor
  - Expanded lytic "lesion" arises from subperiosteal or intraosseous bleed
    - Focal destruction of bone due to pressure erosion
    - Development of large mass containing pools of blood
    - Though lesion may appear alarmingly aggressive, borders of osseous destruction often are well-marginated
- **Hyperparathyroidism, Brown Tumor**

- HPTH is common (along with Brown tumors) in pelvis
- Expanded bubbly appearance much less common for Brown tumor than lytic, focal, well-marginated destruction

Helpful Clues for Rare Diagnoses
- **Chondromyxoid Fibroma**
  - Rare lesions, but when in pelvis or scapula may be bubbly
- **Chondroblastoma**
  - Relatively common lesion in epiphyses
  - Pelvic presentation is rare
- **Osteoblastoma**
  - Rare lesion in non-axial location
- **Langerhans Cell Histiocytosis (LCH)**
  - Common childhood lesion; pelvis is frequent location
  - Presentation most commonly is minimally expanded; bubbly appearance is rare
- **Cystic Angiomatosis**
  - Rare vascular lesion
  - Location in pelvis is relatively common for all intraosseous vascular tumors, including this one
  - Slowly expanding lytic lesion which may become quite large
  - Other vascular tumors tend to be less expansile and more likely to be aggressive

Giant Cell Tumor (GCT)

AP radiograph shows a hugely expanded lytic lesion arising from the inferior pubic ramus, extending to the acetabulum ➡. It appears non-aggressive, despite its size. GCT may be highly expansile in the pelvis.

Plasmacytoma

AP radiograph shows an expanded lytic lesion occupying the superior pubic ramus ➡. It is moderately aggressive, without cortical breakthrough; plasmacytoma commonly presents in this way.

FLAT BONES, FOCALLY EXPANDED OR BUBBLY LESION

(Left) AP radiograph shows a bubbly, wildly expanded lesion arising from the iliac wing ➡. Despite its size, the lesion is non-aggressive. Fibrous dysplasia is bubbly when it arises in the pelvis; this is an extreme case.
(Right) AP radiograph shows a highly expanded lytic lesion of the distal clavicle ➡ with destruction of the acromion by contiguous extent ➡. This was a solitary expansile renal cell metastasis; a thin layer of bone actually encased the lesion.

Fibrous Dysplasia (FD), Pelvis

Metastases: Thyroid, Kidney

(Left) Anteroposterior radiograph shows an expanded lytic lesion occupying the iliac wing ➡ in a 2 year old. ABC is more frequently seen in long bones, but may be found in flat bones occasionally.
(Right) Anteroposterior radiograph shows a pathologic fracture into a lytic expanded acetabular lesion ➡ in a 60 year old. The lesion is well-circumscribed. Although it most resembles GCT, biopsy proved low grade chondrosarcoma.

Aneurysmal Bone Cyst (ABC)

Chondrosarcoma, Conventional

(Left) Anteroposterior radiograph shows a subtle lytic lesion in the iliac wing which contains pseudotrabeculations ➡. The lesion is not aggressive. This is a middle aged patient; UBC should be considered.
(Right) Axial bone CT in the same patient as previous image shows mild expansion of the lesion ➡, proved to be UBC. When this lesion arises in an adult, the location is frequently the pelvis.

Unicameral Bone Cyst (UBC)

Unicameral Bone Cyst (UBC)

FLAT BONES, FOCALLY EXPANDED OR BUBBLY LESION

Hemophilia

Hemophilia

(Left) AP radiograph shows an expanded lytic lesion of the pelvis with a sclerotic margin ➡. It appears moderately aggressive. In a patient with hemophilia, pseudotumor of the iliac wing can be highly destructive, yet maintain a sclerotic margin. (†MSK Req). *(Right)* Axial CECT in the same patient shows the expansion of the iliac wing from intraosseous bleeds ➡ as well as a sharp cut-off ➡ providing a sclerotic margin. The iliacus is distended by hematoma ➡.

Hyperparathyroidism, Brown Tumor

Chondromyxoid Fibroma

(Left) AP radiograph shows an expanded bubbly lesion ➡. The bones show generalized osteopenia, but in this case there are no other clues that this is a Brown tumor in a patient with hyperparathyroidism. *(Right)* Anteroposterior radiograph shows a lytic lesion of the iliac wing, expanded but with a densely sclerotic border ➡. Cartilage lesions should be considered in cases of non-aggressive pelvic tumors; this proved to be chondromyxoid fibroma.

Chondroblastoma

Cystic Angiomatosis

(Left) AP radiograph shows a lytic bubbly lesion in the iliac wing in this child ➡. Axial imaging proved mild expansion. This is a rare presentation of chondroblastoma in the pelvis; it is usually an epiphyseal lesion. *(Right)* AP radiograph shows highly expanded lytic lesions involving both pubic rami ➡ as well as the iliac wing ➡. They are large but non-aggressive; growth was documented over at least 10 years. This is a vascular tumor, cystic angiomatosis.

FLAT BONES, PERMEATIVE LESION

DIFFERENTIAL DIAGNOSIS

Common
- Metastases, Bone Marrow
- Osteomyelitis
- Ewing Sarcoma
- Osteosarcoma, Conventional
- Chondrosarcoma
- Malignant Fibrous Histiocytoma, Bone
- Langerhans Cell Histiocytosis (LCH)
- Lymphoma
- Multiple Myeloma (MM)
- Leukemia
- Hyperparathyroidism/Renal Osteodystrophy, Brown Tumor
- Fibrosarcoma
- Plasmacytoma

Less Common
- Angiosarcoma, Osseous
- Radiation Osteonecrosis

Rare but Important
- Radiation-Induced Sarcoma
- Paget Sarcoma
- Chronic Recurrent Multifocal Osteomyelitis

ESSENTIAL INFORMATION

Key Differential Diagnosis Issues
- Wide range of aggressive lesions arise in flat bones
- **Hint:** Watch for evidence of polyostotic lesions, which may narrow the differential

Helpful Clues for Common Diagnoses
- **Metastases, Bone Marrow**
  - Metastases most commonly involve axial skeleton & flat bones
  - Diagnosis may be difficult in pelvis & scapula
    - Thin bones, often in osteoporotic patients
    - Overlying soft tissues
- **Osteomyelitis**
  - Either from hematogenous seeding or direct trauma
  - Watch for air in sinus tract
  - Watch for dense reactive bone formation
  - Chronic recurrent multifocal osteomyelitis
    - Occurs in children with several months of vague pain
    - Often no systemic symptoms

  - Radiograph often normal; MR diagnosis
- **Ewing Sarcoma**
  - Wider age range (5-30 years) than osteosarcoma
  - Location tends to be different with age
    - Younger patients: Long bones
    - Teenagers & young adults: Flat bones
  - Highly aggressive permeative lesion
  - Large soft tissue mass
- **Osteosarcoma, Conventional**
  - Common location: Long bones, metaphyseal
  - Flat bones, especially pelvis, are less frequently involved
    - However, osteosarcoma is such a common lesion that pelvic osteosarcomas are seen not infrequently
  - Usually produce tumor osteoid: Amorphous, osseous density
  - Highly aggressive, with soft tissue mass
- **Chondrosarcoma**
  - Pelvis is common location of chondrosarcoma; scapula less so
  - May appear permeative & aggressive
    - Often is lower in grade than the other sarcomas listed above, which accounts for its lower position on this list
  - Chondroid matrix usually present
  - Because lesion often undetected for long period of time, may be large, with huge soft tissue mass extending intrapelvically
  - Watch for multiple hereditary exostosis, which predisposes to degeneration
    - Proximal sites in body are most likely to degenerate to chondrosarcoma
- **Malignant Fibrous Histiocytoma, Bone**
  - Flat bones are less common site of involvement than long bones
  - Nonspecific appearance: Lytic, permeative, cortical breakthrough with soft tissue mass
  - Fibrosarcoma: Similar appearance
- **Langerhans Cell Histiocytosis (LCH)**
  - Pelvis & scapula are common sites
  - Watch for polyostotic lesions in a child
  - Lesions are lytic; range of appearance from non-aggressive to highly aggressive
  - Aggressive lesions may show more rapid destruction than sarcomas
  - Aggressive lesions may have cortical breakthrough with soft tissue mass
- **Lymphoma**

FLAT BONES, PERMEATIVE LESION

- ○ Adults: Generally solitary bone lesion
  - ▪ Pelvis & scapula are common locations
  - ▪ Destructive lytic lesion with cortical breakthrough
  - ▪ Soft tissue mass often enormous, showing a more infiltrative character than sarcoma
- ○ Children: 50% present as polyostotic
  - ▪ Aggressive lesion with cortical breakthrough and soft tissue mass
- • **Multiple Myeloma (MM)**
  - ○ Both MM and plasmacytoma generally have well-defined lytic lesions
  - ○ Aggressive or permeative pattern is uncommon
  - ○ Exception for MM is a presentation without focality but with diffuse infiltration
    - ▪ Permeative pattern is so subtle that lesions not detected on radiograph; presents with osteoporosis
    - ▪ Diagnosis made on MR survey
- • **Leukemia**
  - ○ Often presents with such a subtle infiltrative pattern that only osteoporosis is detected by radiograph
  - ○ MR shows extent of lesions, which often include flat bones
- • **Hyperparathyroidism/Renal Osteodystrophy, Brown Tumor**
  - ○ Brown tumor is usually well-defined, but surrounding bone is so osteoporotic that overall appearance may be aggressive
  - ○ Watch for other signs of bone resorption

Helpful Clues for Less Common Diagnoses
- • **Angiosarcoma, Osseous**
  - ○ Rare tumor, but pelvic involvement frequent
  - ○ Often polyostotic; especially lower extremities
- • **Radiation Osteonecrosis**
  - ○ Common in sites frequently treated with radiation: Pelvis & scapula
  - ○ May become less common with more modern radiation treatment
    - ▪ Old cases will persist for many years
  - ○ Appearance: Mixed lytic & sclerotic; may be somewhat permeative; no mass
  - ○ Watch for distribution in a radiation port

Helpful Clues for Rare Diagnoses
- • **Radiation-Induced Sarcoma**
  - ○ Common locations same as those for radiation osteonecrosis: Pelvic, scapula
  - ○ Destructive change superimposed on radiation osteonecrosis; soft tissue mass
  - ○ Generally occurs 7-10 years following RT
- • **Paget Sarcoma**
  - ○ Rare degeneration of Paget bone lesion
  - ○ Only with extensive & long term disease
  - ○ Degeneration more frequently seen in axial & flat bones than long bones
  - ○ Acquires appearance of lesion it degenerates into
    - ▪ Osteosarcoma: Amorphous osteoid
    - ▪ Chondrosarcoma: Chondroid matrix
    - ▪ May be mixed types of sarcomas

Metastases, Bone Marrow

AP radiograph shows a diffuse permeative lytic lesion involving the entire scapula, destroying all osseous integrity of the bone. The patient had undergone arthroscopy 3 months earlier for shoulder pain.

Metastases, Bone Marrow

Coronal T1WI MR of the same patient shows the expanded lesion arising from the body of the scapula ➡. The patient was discovered to have renal cell carcinoma, which often results in solitary metastases.

FLAT BONES, PERMEATIVE LESION

Osteomyelitis

Osteomyelitis

(Left) Axial bone CT shows "multiple lytic lesions" ➡ in the scapula of a patient who has just arrived from Ethiopia. With this history & appearance, infection must be considered. *(Right)* Axial T1 C+ FS MR of the same patient shows multiple abscesses in the soft tissues on either side of the scapula ➡; they communicated through an osseous defect. This was a Staphylococcus osteomyelitis.

Ewing Sarcoma

Ewing Sarcoma

(Left) Lateral radiograph shows a highly aggressive lesion with destruction of the body of the scapula ➡ in a young adult. Axial imaging showed a very large associated soft tissue mass. In a patient of this age, Ewing sarcoma must be considered and was proven. *(Right)* Lateral bone scan of the same patient shows multiple osseous metastases at the time of diagnosis. Of all bone sarcomas, Ewing sarcoma is the most likely to present with osseous metastases.

Osteosarcoma, Conventional

Osteosarcoma, Conventional

(Left) AP radiograph shows a sclerotic lesion of the posterior iliac wing ➡, overlapping the sacral ala, in a teenager. The sclerosis is typical of dense osteoid matrix, and the lesion must be presumed to be osteosarcoma. *(Right)* Axial T2WI FS MR of the same patient confirms the highly destructive iliac wing lesion, with a soft tissue mass extending both anteriorly and posteriorly ➡. This was a high grade osteosarcoma, requiring an internal hemipelvectomy.

FLAT BONES, PERMEATIVE LESION

Chondrosarcoma

Chondrosarcoma

(Left) AP radiograph shows a lytic lesion in the iliac wing ➡ of a 35 year old. It contains a dense chondroid matrix; the diagnosis must be chondrosarcoma. Note, however, that the lesion does not appear particularly permeative; chondrosarcoma often presents with a lower grade than other sarcomas. *(Right)* Axial bone CT in a different patient shows destruction of the iliac wing ➡. There is a huge soft tissue mass arising from the bone that contains a chondroid matrix.

Malignant Fibrous Histiocytoma, Bone

Malignant Fibrous Histiocytoma, Bone

(Left) AP radiograph shows a "naked SI joint" on the right. Note how lucent the right SI joint appears ➡ compared with the left, where there is normal overlap of the posterior iliac wing & sacral ala. The naked SI joint indicates a lesion involving the right posterior iliac wing. *(Right)* Axial bone CT of the same patient shows the lytic lesion of the posterior iliac wing ➡ with cortical breakthrough. Biopsy proved MFH.

Langerhans Cell Histiocytosis (LCH)

Langerhans Cell Histiocytosis (LCH)

(Left) AP radiograph shows a lytic permeative lesion involving the acetabulum of this child ➡. Concern for Ewing sarcoma should be raised, but it should also be remembered that LCH is frequently found in the flat bones and occasionally appears highly aggressive. *(Right)* Axial PD FSE MR of the same patient shows the osseous destruction and confirms a large soft tissue mass ➡ deviating the rectum. At biopsy this proved to be a highly aggressive LCH.

FLAT BONES, PERMEATIVE LESION

(Left) Anteroposterior radiograph shows a highly permeative lesion in the pelvis of a young woman ➡. It could represent several malignant processes; this is lymphoma, with a large soft tissue mass. (†MSK Req). **(Right)** Anteroposterior radiograph shows permeative lytic lesions involving both right & left iliac wings ➡, as well as a femoral neck lesion ➡ in an African American child. 50% of lymphomas present as a polyostotic process in children.

Lymphoma

Lymphoma

(Left) AP radiograph shows diffuse osteoporosis, which is abnormal for a 50 year old man. This appearance is suspicious for a permeative infiltrative process; at this age, multiple myeloma or leukemia should be considered. **(Right)** Coronal STIR MR in the same patient, part of a myeloma survey, shows abnormal signal throughout the majority of the pelvis ➡, confirming infiltration. There is also a focal femoral neck lesion ➡. Biopsy showed multiple myeloma.

Multiple Myeloma (MM)

Multiple Myeloma (MM)

(Left) Axial STIR MR shows a diffuse infiltrative process involving the entire pelvis as well as sacrum. The 30 year old patient had diffuse bone pain but no focal abnormalities on radiograph (not shown), typical of leukemia. **(Right)** AP radiograph shows a poorly marginated, mildly aggressive lesion within the acetabulum ➡. There is also a well-circumscribed lesion in the femoral neck ➡, as well as osteopenia. This makes the diagnosis of Brown tumor.

Leukemia

Hyperparathyroidism/Renal Osteodystrophy, Brown Tumor

FLAT BONES, PERMEATIVE LESION

Fibrosarcoma

Plasmacytoma

(Left) Anteroposterior radiograph shows a lytic permeative lesion in the pubic bones ➡ with cortical breakthrough and a soft tissue mass. This is a nonspecific appearance; biopsy showed fibrosarcoma. *(Right)* AP radiograph shows a highly aggressive lytic lesion destroying the left iliac wing ➡, extending to the sacrum. Though plasmacytoma most frequently has a less aggressive appearance, that proved to be the diagnosis in this case.

Angiosarcoma, Osseous

Radiation Osteonecrosis

(Left) Anteroposterior radiograph shows a highly aggressive lytic lesion destroying the iliac wing in a young adult. The patient had other lesions in the lower extremity; the diagnosis is angiosarcoma. *(Right)* AP radiograph shows a mixed lytic and sclerotic lesion involving the scapula, clavicle, ribs, and proximal humerus. Though it appears somewhat aggressive, the port-like configuration of the abnormality helps make the diagnosis of radiation osteonecrosis.

Radiation-Induced Sarcoma

Paget Sarcoma

(Left) Lateral radiograph shows destructive change in the scapula, with osteoid formation within a large soft tissue mass ➡. The patient had radiation to the scapula 7 years earlier, and this is a radiation-induced osteosarcoma. *(Right)* AP radiograph shows an enlarged iliac wing with amorphous osteoid production ➡ replacing the underlying bone. Additionally, there is an enlarged, disordered, vertebral body ➡. Findings are of Paget osteosarcoma.

LONG BONE, EPIPHYSEAL: IRREGULAR OR STIPPLED

DIFFERENTIAL DIAGNOSIS

Common
- Normal Variant in Child (Mimic)
- Osteonecrosis
- Legg-Calvé-Perthes (LCP)
- Juvenile Idiopathic Arthritis (JIA)

Less Common
- Rickets
- Hypothyroidism
- Osteomyelitis
- Complications of Warfarin (Coumadin)
- Chondrodysplasia Punctata
- Trevor Fairbank (Dysplasia Epiphysealis Hemimelica)
- Spondyloepiphyseal Dysplasia
- Nail Patella Disease (Fong)

Rare but Important
- Thermal Injury, Frostbite
- Complications of Dilantin
- Hypoparathyroidism
- Hyperparathyroidism
- Hypopituitarism
- Acromegaly
- Trisomy 18
- Down Syndrome (Trisomy 21)
- Fetal Alcohol Syndrome
- Mucopolysaccharidoses
- Multiple Epiphyseal Dysplasia
- Pseudoachondroplasia
- Homocystinuria
- Ollier Disease/Maffucci (Mimic)

ESSENTIAL INFORMATION

Key Differential Diagnosis Issues
- May be able to separate into irregular versus stippled epiphyses
  - Common diagnoses for "irregular" epiphyses
    - Normal variant, knee
    - Osteonecrosis
    - Legg-Calvé-Perthes
    - Juvenile idiopathic arthritis
    - Rickets
    - Osteomyelitis
    - Trevor Fairbank
    - Spondyloepiphyseal dysplasia
  - Common diagnoses for "stippled" epiphyses
    - Hypothyroidism

- Warfarin embryopathy
- Chondrodysplasia punctata

Helpful Clues for Common Diagnoses
- **Normal Variant in Child (Mimic)**
  - Seen in adolescents
  - Located on posterior aspect of femoral condyles
    - Seen best on AP notch view which profiles posterior femoral condylar surface
    - Generally not visible on regular AP view
    - May be seen on lateral
  - MR shows overlying cartilage to be normal
  - Do not confuse with pathologic process such as osteochondral injury or JIA
- **Osteonecrosis**
  - Prior to significant flattening, may see punctate fragments in bed of site of necrosis
- **Legg-Calvé-Perthes (LCP)**
  - Femoral head osteonecrosis in child (usual age range 4-8 years)
  - Capital epiphyseal flattening, increased density, fragmentation
  - Results in coxa magna deformity
- **Juvenile Idiopathic Arthritis (JIA)**
  - "Crenulated" irregularity of carpal bones
  - Irregularity on femoral condylar articular surface

Helpful Clues for Less Common Diagnoses
- **Rickets**
  - True abnormality is metaphyseal/physeal widening & fraying
  - With weakened physis, epiphysis may slip, resulting in irregularity & fragmentation
- **Hypothyroidism**
  - Infant: Stippled epiphyses
  - Toddler: Severe delay in skeletal maturation
    - Fragmentation of femoral capital epiphysis
- **Osteomyelitis**
  - Prenatal or childhood infections may cross from metaphysis to involve epiphysis
    - Epiphysis may slip
    - Destructive change results in irregularity, fragmentation
- **Complications of Warfarin (Coumadin)**
  - Maternal ingestion during early pregnancy
  - Stippled epiphyses

○ Hypoplastic nose, eye malformations, mental retardation
- **Chondrodysplasia Punctata**
  ○ Stippled epiphyses
  ○ Non-rhizomelic type: Conradi Hunermann; nonlethal & autosomal dominant
  ○ Rhizomelic type: Lethal autosomal recessive; multiple other abnormalities
- **Trevor Fairbank (Dysplasia Epiphysealis Hemimelica)**
  ○ Cartilaginous proliferation at epiphysis
    ▪ Considered analogous to epiphyseal osteochondroma
  ○ Irregular lobulations superimposed on epiphyses
  ○ Lower limb (knee, ankle, hip) most frequently affected
  ○ May be polyarticular
  ○ Monomelic
- **Spondyloepiphyseal Dysplasia**
  ○ Group of disorders resulting in short trunk dwarfism
  ○ Congenita & tarda forms, with spectrum of abnormalities
  ○ Platyspondyly
  ○ Generalized delay in epiphyseal ossification
  ○ Once epiphysis forms, it is flattened & irregular
  ○ May have metaphyseal flaring
  ○ Develops coxa vara, genu valgum
  ○ Early osteoarthritis
- **Nail Patella Disease (Fong)**

○ a.k.a., Fong disease, osteo-onychodysplasia
○ Absent or small patellae
○ Posterior iliac "horns"
○ Nail dysplasia
○ Radial head hypoplasia, subluxation
○ Irregularity & flattening of epiphyses; less constant finding than nail & patella abnormalities

Helpful Clues for Rare Diagnoses
- **Thermal Injury, Frostbite**
  ○ Epiphyses at risk for vascular injury with vasoconstriction from cold temperature
  ○ May become dense, fragmented
  ○ Early fusion results in short phalanges
  ○ Thumb generally not involved (folded into palm in cold temperatures)
- **Multiple Epiphyseal Dysplasia**
  ○ Hereditary disease, usually autosomal dominant
  ○ Delayed & irregular mineralization of epiphyses
  ○ Results in coxa vara & genu vara or valgum
  ○ Early osteoarthritis
  ○ Vertebral involvement variable & generally mild
- **Pseudoachondroplasia**
  ○ Heterogeneous inherited skeletal dysplasia with dwarfism
  ○ Malformations not apparent until early childhood
  ○ Shortening of tubular bones
    ▪ Flaring of metaphyses
    ▪ Variable irregularity of epiphyses

Normal Variant in Child (Mimic)

AP notch view shows irregularity of the medial & lateral femoral condyles ➡ in a child. The notch view profiles the posterior portions of the femoral condyles, the expected location of this normal variant.

Normal Variant in Child (Mimic)

AP radiograph of the same knee shows smooth, normal femoral condyles. This, in combination of the notch view, localizes the epiphyseal irregularities to the posterior condyles.

LONG BONE, EPIPHYSEAL: IRREGULAR OR STIPPLED

Osteonecrosis

Legg-Calvé-Perthes (LCP)

(Left) Anteroposterior radiograph shows fragmentation of the humeral head ➡. This is in the weight-bearing portion and is typical of both the location and appearance of osteonecrosis. *(Right)* Anteroposterior radiograph shows irregularity, flattening, and increased density in the femoral capital epiphysis ➡. This child has typical Legg-Calvé-Perthes. (†MSK Req).

Juvenile Idiopathic Arthritis (JIA)

Rickets

(Left) Lateral radiograph shows irregularity involving the entire surface of the femoral condyles ➡ in this patient with JIA. Such "crenulation" may be seen involving carpal bones as well. *(Right)* AP radiograph shows irregularity of the femoral capital epiphysis ➡, along with fraying of the metaphysis ➡, widened zone of provisional calcification, and slipped epiphysis. These are typical changes of rickets in a patient with renal osteodystrophy.

Hypothyroidism

Hypothyroidism

(Left) Anteroposterior radiograph shows fragmentation of the femoral capital epiphysis ➡. This patient also had severely delayed skeletal maturation. This appearance suggests LCP, but it is also seen in hypothyroidism. *(Right)* Anteroposterior radiograph in an infant shows stippled epiphyses ➡ at the femoral head/greater trochanter. Hypothyroidism is one of several entities that may present with stippled epiphyses.

LONG BONE, EPIPHYSEAL: IRREGULAR OR STIPPLED

Osteomyelitis

Complications of Warfarin (Coumadin)

(Left) Lateral radiograph shows irregularity & fragmentation of the calcaneal apophysis ➡. This patient has osteomyelitis, with the associated destruction. *(Right)* AP radiographs show stippling of the epiphyses and apophyses ➡ of the acetabulum and femoral head. This infant's mother had been given Warfarin during pregnancy; stippled epiphyses are one manifestation of Warfarin embryopathy.

Chondrodysplasia Punctata

Trevor Fairbank (Dysplasia Epiphysealis Hemimelica)

(Left) Anteroposterior radiograph shows stippled epiphyses at the sacrum ➡ and femoral heads ➡. This finding is nonspecific, but this patient had other manifestations of chondrodysplasia punctata. *(Right)* Anteroposterior radiograph shows irregularity of the epiphyses of the tibiotalar joint ➡. This is actually an epiphyseal osteochondroma, termed Trevor Fairbank dysplasia. The irregular bone results in joint damage.

Spondyloepiphyseal Dysplasia

Nail Patella Disease (Fong)

(Left) Lateral radiograph shows irregularity of the femoral condyles ➡. This is the appearance of a relatively mild form of spondyloepiphyseal dysplasia. *(Right)* Anteroposterior radiograph shows irregularity and flattening of the femoral condyles of the left knee. There is also hypoplasia of the patellae. Both findings are seen in nail patella (Fong) disease.

LONG BONE, EPIPHYSEAL, OVERGROWTH/BALLOONING

DIFFERENTIAL DIAGNOSIS

Common
- Juvenile Idiopathic Arthritis (JIA)
- Hemophilia: MSK Complications

Less Common
- Septic Joint
- Epiphyseal Fracture, Pediatric
- Epiphyseal Dysplasia
- Hyperemia, Other Causes
- Turner Syndrome (Mimic)
- Blount Disease (Mimic)

Rare but Important
- Meningococcemia (Mimic)

ESSENTIAL INFORMATION

Key Differential Diagnosis Issues
- Hyperemia is the fundamental cause of overgrowth in several cases
  - In skeletally immature patient
    - Prolonged hyperemia adjacent to joint → overgrowth (ballooning) of epiphysis
    - In addition to enlarged epiphysis, hyperemia → early physeal fusion → short limb
  - Etiologies of overgrowth secondary to hyperemia include
    - Hemophilia
    - Juvenile idiopathic arthritis
    - Septic joint, particularly tuberculosis or fungal etiology
    - Epiphyseal or metaphyseal fracture

Helpful Clues for Common Diagnoses
- **Juvenile Idiopathic Arthritis (JIA)**
  - Hemophilia: Similar to JIA
  - Chronic hyperemia from synovitis (JIA) or recurrent intraarticular bleed (hemophilia)
  - Knee > elbow > ankle
  - Erosion of intercondylar or trochlear notch
  - Erosions, cartilage loss in both
    - JIA may be distinguished by carpal fusion
    - Hemophilia may be distinguished by dense effusion (hemosiderin deposition)

Helpful Clues for Less Common Diagnoses
- **Septic Joint**
  - Effusion, cartilage loss, erosions
  - Tuberculosis or fungal etiologies more likely to result in overgrowth than bacterial
    - Slower joint destruction, so occurs over a longer period of time, allowing chronic hyperemia
    - Less likely to have reactive osseous change than bacterial etiology
- **Epiphyseal Fracture, Pediatric**
  - Hyperemia with fracture healing results in overgrowth
  - Watch for malunion
- **Epiphyseal Dysplasia**
  - May be fragmented in severe cases or overgrown if less severe
- **Turner & Blount Disease (Mimics)**
  - Underdevelopment or collapse of medial tibial condyle results in relative overgrowth of medial femoral condyle

Juvenile Idiopathic Arthritis (JIA)

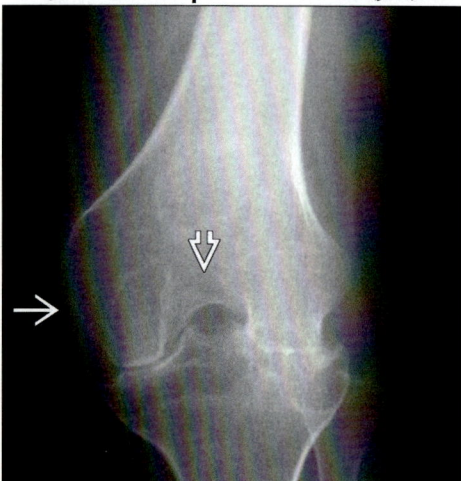

AP radiograph shows significant enlargement (overgrowth) of the femoral epiphyses ➡ relative to the diaphyses. There are severe erosions & widening of the intercondylar notch ➡ in this patient with JIA.

Hemophilia: MSK Complications

Lateral radiograph shows no erosions but a huge effusion ➡ in a hemophilic. There is a widened notch (displacement of Blumensaat line ➡). The epiphyses & patella are overgrown relative to the diaphyses.

LONG BONE, EPIPHYSEAL, OVERGROWTH/BALLOONING

Septic Joint

Epiphyseal Fracture, Pediatric

(Left) AP radiograph shows an enlarged left femoral head & neck ➡. This 12 year old had a septic joint treated 9 months earlier. The hyperemia from the process resulted in overgrowth in this child. *(Right)* AP radiograph demonstrates relative overgrowth of the left patella and epiphyses ➡ (compare to normal right side ➡). The patient had a patellar fracture as a child, resulting in hyperemia, enough to result in overgrowth of the patella and adjacent femoral epiphyses.

Epiphyseal Dysplasia

Turner Syndrome (Mimic)

(Left) AP radiograph shows symmetric enlarged femoral epiphyses, giving a "ballooned" appearance. Note also the morphologic flattening of the tibial plateaus. The patient is short; the diagnosis is spondyloepiphyseal dysplasia. *(Right)* AP radiograph shows relative flattening/underdevelopment of the medial tibial condyle ➡, which results in an overgrowth of the medial femoral condyle ➡. This appears as focal ballooning of the femoral epiphysis.

Blount Disease (Mimic)

Meningococcemia (Mimic)

(Left) AP radiograph shows collapse of the medial tibial metaphysis ➡ in Blount disease. There may be compensatory overgrowth of the medial femoral condyle ➡, but rarely enough to prevent a significant varus deformity. *(Right)* AP radiograph shows fragmentation & dysmorphic changes in the femoral capital epiphysis ➡ typical of meningococcemia. This mimics a ballooned epiphysis, but is due to ischemia from thrombotic episodes.

LONG BONE, EPIPHYSIS, SCLEROSIS/IVORY

DIFFERENTIAL DIAGNOSIS

Common
- Osteonecrosis (AVN)
- Renal Osteodystrophy

Less Common
- Cement & Bone Fillers, Normal
- Neoplasm
  - Chondroblastoma
  - Ewing Sarcoma
  - Osteosarcoma, Conventional
- Legg-Calvé-Perthes (LCP)
- Osteopoikilosis
- Osteopetrosis
- Pycnodysostosis

Rare but Important
- Down Syndrome (Trisomy 21)
- Hypopituitarism
- Hypothyroidism
- Turner Syndrome
- Morquio Syndrome
- Thiemann Disease
- Deprivation Dwarfism
- Multiple Epiphyseal Dysplasia
- Trichorhinophalangeal Dysplasia
- Seckel Syndrome
- Lesch-Nyhan
- Idiopathic Hypercalcemia
- Homocystinuria
- Complications of Fluoride

ESSENTIAL INFORMATION

Key Differential Diagnosis Issues
- Differentiate between extent of sclerosis
  - Focal, isolated to epiphysis
    - Osteonecrosis
    - Chondroblastoma
    - Legg-Calvé-Perthes
  - Epiphyseal/metaphyseal
    - Ewing sarcoma
    - Chondrosarcoma
    - Osteopoikilosis
  - Diffuse
    - Renal osteodystrophy
    - Osteopetrosis
    - Pycnodysostosis
    - All diagnoses listed as "rare but important"

Helpful Clues for Common Diagnoses
- **Osteonecrosis (AVN)**
  - Sclerosis is 1st radiographic sign of AVN, secondary to surrounding osteopenia (relative sclerosis)
    - Classic appearance is central sclerosis in femoral head
  - Later, sclerosis is secondary to osseous impaction from collapse
  - Even later, sclerosis is from reparative bone formation
- **Renal Osteodystrophy**
  - Diffuse sclerosis, including epiphyses
    - May be part of primary disease, due to activation of osteoblasts
    - More prominent, as neostosis, when undergoing effective treatment
  - Indistinct trabeculae
  - Other signs of renal osteodystrophy
    - Rickets: Widened zone of provisional calcification, frayed metaphyses
    - Hyperparathyroidism: Resorption patterns (subperiosteal, endosteal, subchondral, subligamentous)
    - Soft tissue calcification

Helpful Clues for Less Common Diagnoses
- **Cement & Bone Fillers, Normal**
  - Commonly used to fill lesion sites following curettage
    - Most common lesion in epiphyseal region treated this way is giant cell tumor
  - Cement: Homogeneous, more dense than cortical bone
  - Non-structural bone graft: Round or square pieces, same density as cortical bone
    - As it incorporates, approaches normal bone density
  - Rare use of coral as structure with haversian canal-like morphology to allow substitution by normal bone
- **Neoplasm**
  - **Chondroblastoma**
    - Most common epiphyseal neoplasm
    - Generally arise in skeletally immature (teenage, young adult) patients
    - Margin generally sclerotic
    - May contain chondroid matrix, resulting in greater sclerosis
    - Often elicits dense periosteal reaction
  - **Ewing Sarcoma**

- Generally metadiaphyseal lesion, but may cross into epiphysis (physis is only a relative barrier)
- Age range: 5-30 years
- Lesion generally is highly aggressive, with permeative destruction, cortical breakthrough, & soft tissue mass
- Rarely may be more indolent, remaining contained for a variable amount of time
- Elicits significant osseous reaction, in the form of new bone formation; this is the source of sclerosis
  ○ **Osteosarcoma, Conventional**
    - Generally metaphyseal in location, but may cross into epiphysis
    - Highly aggressive lesion, with permeative bone destruction, cortical breakthrough, soft tissue mass
    - Tumor osteoid results in amorphous sclerosis, both in the bone and in the soft tissue mass
- **Legg-Calvé-Perthes (LCP)**
  ○ Osteonecrosis of femoral head in child
    - Age 4-8 most common
  ○ Early sign: Sclerosis of femoral head
  ○ Later signs
    - Fragmentation of femoral head
    - Flattening of femoral head
  ○ Late appearance
    - Coxa magna deformity (short, broad femoral head and neck)
    - Early development of osteoarthritis
- **Osteopoikilosis**

  ○ Round, regular, generally subcentimeter sclerotic lesions
    - Bone islands (hamartoma)
  ○ Epiphyseal & metaphyseal
  ○ Generally bilaterally symmetric
  ○ One of the sclerosing dysplasias
  ○ Incidental finding
- **Osteopetrosis**
  ○ Severe sclerosing dysplasia, involving entire skeleton (axial & appendicular)
  ○ Homogeneously dense bones
  ○ Undertubulation of long bones
    - Due to poor function of osteoclasts; inhibiting remodeling
    - May also be manifest as "bone-in-bone" appearance
- **Pycnodysostosis**
  ○ Severe sclerosing dysplasia, involving entire skeleton (axial & appendicular)
  ○ Homogeneously dense bones
  ○ Undertubulation of long bones
  ○ Similar in appearance to osteopetrosis
  ○ Morphologic differentiating factors
    - Wormian bones
    - Acroosteolysis
    - Small angle of jaw

Helpful Clues for Rare Diagnoses
- Those listed under "rare but important" are extraordinarily uncommon
  ○ Disease process itself is rare
  ○ Manifestation of sclerotic epiphyses in these diagnoses is even more rare

Osteonecrosis (AVN)

AP radiograph shows sclerosis in the femoral head ➡, an early indication of osteonecrosis. An outline of a renal transplant is seen in the iliac fossa ➡, indicating steroids as the etiology of the osteonecrosis.

Osteonecrosis (AVN)

Anteroposterior radiograph shows sclerosis, flattening, and irregularity of the femoral head ➡ in a young adult. There are linear densities in the neck ➡, indicating pin tracks; the patient had SCFE resulting in AVN.

(Left) Anteroposterior radiograph shows diffuse increased density, including the humeral epiphysis. There is also subperiosteal resorption ➔ and a Brown tumor ➔; the patient has renal osteodystrophy. *(Right)* Posteroanterior radiograph shows sclerosis in the radial epiphysis ➔, but there is also generalized increased density as well as indistinctness of the trabeculae. Endosteal resorptive pattern adds to the findings of renal osteodystrophy.

Renal Osteodystrophy

Renal Osteodystrophy

(Left) Lateral radiograph shows sclerosis of the ring apophyses and endplates ➔ in a patient with renal osteodystrophy, termed "rugger jersey" sign. *(Right)* Posteroanterior radiograph shows an expanded lytic lesion of the distal radius which has been treated by curettage and bone grafting ➔. Non-structural bone graft may have rounded or square pieces & should be differentiated from chondroid or osteoid matrix.

Renal Osteodystrophy

Cement & Bone Fillers, Normal

(Left) Anteroposterior radiograph shows dense material placed at the MTP joint ➔ following resection of a failed arthroplasty ➔. The material has canals the width of Haversian canals; it is a coral graft. *(Right)* Frog lateral radiograph shows an epiphyseal lesion with a dense sclerotic margin ➔, containing a small amount of chondroid matrix. The appearance is typical of chondroblastoma.

Cement & Bone Fillers, Normal

Chondroblastoma

Chondroblastoma

Ewing Sarcoma

(Left) Lateral radiograph shows a lytic lesion with surrounding dense sclerosis ⮕. There is thick, dense periosteal reaction ⮕. The lesion is typical of chondroblastoma. (Right) Lateral radiograph shows uniform sclerosis of the epiphysis ⮕ without destructive changes. This patient had Ewing sarcoma that originated in the metaphysis & extended to involve the epiphysis; the density is due to reactive change.

Osteosarcoma, Conventional

Legg-Calvé-Perthes (LCP)

(Left) Anteroposterior radiograph shows a densely sclerotic metaphysis, extending to the epiphysis, with periosteal reaction and soft tissue mass ⮕, all typical of osteosarcoma. There is an ossified lymph node metastasis ⮕. (Right) Anteroposterior radiograph shows flattened and sclerotic femoral capital epiphysis ⮕. This is typical of advanced Legg-Calvé-Perthes disease and will develop into a coxa magna deformity.

Osteopoikilosis

Osteopetrosis

(Left) Axial NECT shows multiple small round sclerotic densities in both femoral epiphyses and both acetabulae. The appearance is typical of osteopoikilosis, a sclerosing dysplasia. (Right) Anteroposterior radiograph shows uniform density of the epiphyses ⮕ as well as the remainder of the bones in this child. Note also the undertubulation of the femora ⮕, indicating poor remodeling with growth. This is typical osteopetrosis.

LONG BONE, EPIPHYSEAL/APOPHYSEAL/SUBCHONDRAL LYTIC LESION

DIFFERENTIAL DIAGNOSIS

Common
- Giant Cell Tumor
- Chondroblastoma
- Pyrophosphate Arthropathy
- Osteomyelitis, Pediatric
- Lymphoma
- Langerhans Cell Histiocytosis
- Pigmented Villonodular Synovitis (PVNS)
- Metastases, Bone Marrow
- Osteoarthritis

Less Common
- Gout
- Giant Cell Tumor Tendon Sheath
- Osteomyelitis, Adult

Rare but Important
- Amyloid Deposition
- Soft Tissue Mass Erosion (Mimic)
- Chondrosarcoma, Clear Cell

ESSENTIAL INFORMATION

Key Differential Diagnosis Issues
- **Hint**: Consider patient age; only a limited number of lesions are epiphyseal/apophyseal in children
- **Hint**: In older adult, look for reasons to suspect an arthritic etiology, with subchondral cyst creating the "lytic lesion"

Helpful Clues for Common Diagnoses
- **Giant Cell Tumor**
  - GCT: Lytic lesion arising eccentrically in metaphysis; location is highly specific
    - By time of discovery, has usually extended to subchondral bone; this makes GCT fall into the subchondral bone lesion category
    - **Hint**: Narrow zone of transition but margin generally not sclerotic; this character is often a distinguishing feature
    - Occasionally may appear & behave aggressively
    - Most frequent age range: 30-60
  - Rarely arises in skeletally immature patient
    - Begins in metaphysis & crosses into epiphysis as physis fuses
    - Will not show the sclerotic margin of chondroblastoma
- **Chondroblastoma**
  - Lytic lesion arising eccentrically within the epiphysis
    - May extend into the metaphysis as the physis fuses, but origin is clearly epiphysis
    - Location of origin may be confusing at irregular physis in proximal humerus
  - Narrow zone of transition, but margin usually sclerotic; this helps to distinguish from GCT
  - May contain subtle chondroid matrix, but may be entirely lytic
- **Subchondral Cyst**: May become large, simulating a lytic subchondral lesion
  - **Pyrophosphate Arthropathy**
    - May develop particularly large subchondral cysts
    - **Hint**: Watch for subtle chondrocalcinosis to consider the diagnosis
    - Most frequent locations: Knee, wrist, hip
  - **Pigmented Villonodular Synovitis (PVNS)**
    - May develop large subchondral cysts/erosions
    - Monoarticular
    - Associated nodular or lining synovitis which contains mixed low & high MR signal on T2 and enhances
  - **Osteoarthritis**
    - Associated subchondral cysts are particularly large in acetabulum (termed "Egger cysts"); this is the site most likely to be confused with lytic lesion
    - In long bones, watch for associated osteophytes & cartilage loss
  - **Gout**
    - Occasionally develops large subchondral cysts without other signs of arthritis, which may be confusing
    - Watch for other sites of arthritis, may have more typical appearance of gout
  - **Amyloid Deposition**
    - Deposition in bone appears as subchondral lesion containing low signal material
    - Usually associated prominent thickening of tendons &/or capsule which remains low signal intensity on MR
- **Osteomyelitis, Pediatric**

LONG BONE, EPIPHYSEAL/APOPHYSEAL/SUBCHONDRAL LYTIC LESION

- Metaphyseal location is most common site of osteomyelitis in child, due to terminal vascular configuration
  - Young children have vessels crossing physis; they may develop osteomyelitis in epiphysis or both locations
- **Lymphoma**
  - In children, 50% of cases present as multifocal lesion
  - Most lesions are metadiaphyseal & are highly aggressive
  - When in epiphysis, lesions are aggressive
- **Langerhans Cell Histiocytosis**
  - Often polyostotic; most frequent location is flat bones and diaphyses
  - May also appear in epiphyses & apophyses
  - Range of appearance & behavior from non-aggressive to highly aggressive
- **Metastases, Bone Marrow**
  - May occur in long bones, subchondral or epiphyseal location: Femur and humerus
  - Age and history should be suggestive

Helpful Clues for Less Common Diagnoses
- **Giant Cell Tumor Tendon Sheath**
  - Not infrequently causes focal erosion of underlying bone, simulating a lytic lesion
  - Associated soft tissue swelling in path of a tendon; hands & feet are primary locations
- **Osteomyelitis, Adult**
  - More frequently diaphyseal, but may arise in subchondral region
  - Serpiginous pattern & reactive sclerosis

Helpful Clues for Rare Diagnoses
- **Soft Tissue Mass Erosion (Mimic)**
  - Erosion from adjacent soft tissue mass usually is only focal scalloping
  - Larger erosion may, if imaged en face, give the appearance of a lytic lesion
- **Chondrosarcoma, Clear Cell**
  - Rare chondrosarcoma arising in the epiphysis or subchondral region
  - Generally does not appear aggressive
  - **Hint**: Often misdiagnosed as chondroblastoma; if pathology not in agreement, consider this lesion

Alternative Differential Approaches
- True epiphyseal lesions (prior to skeletal maturation)
  - Chondroblastoma
  - Osteomyelitis, pediatric
  - Langerhans cell histiocytosis
  - Lymphoma
  - GCT (extending from metaphysis)
- Subchondral cysts/lytic lesions (following skeletal maturation)
  - Subchondral cysts, arthritis-related: Osteoarthritis, pyrophosphate arthropathy, gout
  - Giant cell tumor
  - Osteomyelitis, adult
  - Metastases, bone marrow
  - Pigmented villonodular synovitis (PVNS)
  - Soft tissue mass erosion (mimic)
  - Amyloid deposition
  - Chondrosarcoma, clear cell

Giant Cell Tumor

AP radiograph shows a lytic geographic lesion with non-sclerotic margin ➡. It arises in the metaphysis but extends to the subchondral cortex. The constellation of findings in this young adult is typical of GCT.

Chondroblastoma

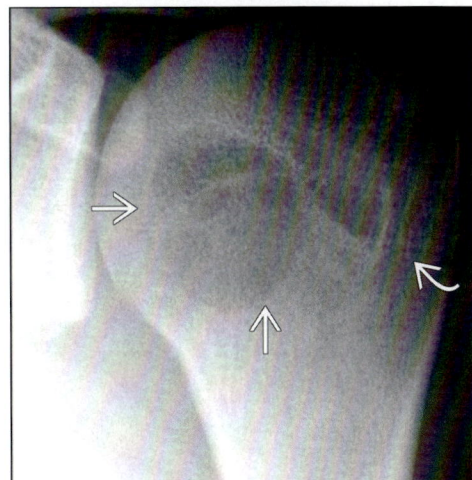

AP radiograph shows a lytic lesion arising in the epiphysis of the humerus ➡ in a teenager (note the nearly fused physis ➡). The margin is more sclerotic than in most GCTs but typical of chondroblastoma.

LONG BONE, EPIPHYSEAL/APOPHYSEAL/SUBCHONDRAL LYTIC LESION

Pyrophosphate Arthropathy

Osteomyelitis, Pediatric

(Left) Sagittal T2WI MR shows multiple subchondral cysts ➥, along with osteophytes in an older patient. The radiograph showed chondrocalcinosis. The diagnosis is pyrophosphate arthropathy, which may develop huge subchondral cysts. *(Right)* Sagittal T1WI MR shows low signal replacing Hoffa fat pad, extending into the tibial epiphysis ➥ in a 4 year old. This is typical of epiphyseal osteomyelitis, which may be seen in children. The radiograph was normal.

Lymphoma

Langerhans Cell Histiocytosis

(Left) AP radiograph shows a lytic lesion occupying the epiphysis ➥ with reactive bone sclerosis ➥. This 7 year old had multiple other permeative lesions, which proved to be lymphoma. This tumor presents as a polyostotic lesion 50% of the time in children. *(Right)* AP radiograph shows a lytic lesion within the greater trochanteric apophysis ➥ in a teenager. LCH most frequently is found in the diaphysis or flat bones but may be epiphyseal or apophyseal.

Pigmented Villonodular Synovitis (PVNS)

Metastases, Bone Marrow

(Left) Sagittal T1WI MR shows a lesion containing low signal material which has replaced Hoffa fat pad ➥. The lesion has also eroded into the tibial epiphysis ➥. PVNS frequently is found in the knee and may cause erosions, presenting as a lytic lesion on radiograph. *(Right)* AP radiograph shows a subtle lytic lesion occupying the trochlea ➥. This was painful & showed cortical breakthrough on MR; it proved to be a renal cell metastasis.

LONG BONE, EPIPHYSEAL/APOPHYSEAL/SUBCHONDRAL LYTIC LESION

Gout

Giant Cell Tumor Tendon Sheath

(Left) AP radiograph shows a lytic well-circumscribed lesion ➡ in a 45 year old woman. There was no other finding of knee arthropathy. However, there were classic findings of gout involving the 1st MTP; sodium urate crystals were seen on knee aspirate. (†MSK Req). *(Right)* Lateral radiograph shows lytic lesions involving the epiphysis & head of adjacent phalanges ➡. Volar soft tissue mass helps make the diagnosis of GCT tendon sheath, which may erode underlying bone.

Osteomyelitis, Adult

Amyloid Deposition

(Left) Axial bone CT shows a serpiginous lytic lesion ➡ within the femoral subchondral region. There is surrounding sclerotic osseous reaction. The pattern is typical of osteomyelitis. Subchondral location is unusual in absence of septic joint. (†MSK Req). *(Right)* Sagittal T2WI MR shows a subchondral erosion containing low signal material ➡, along with low signal thickening of the rotator cuff tendons ➡. Both findings are typical of amyloid deposition.

Soft Tissue Mass Erosion (Mimic)

Soft Tissue Mass Erosion (Mimic)

(Left) Anteroposterior radiograph shows a lytic lesion within the lateral humeral condyle ➡. The lesion appears well-marginated, though there are regions that appear slightly more aggressive ➡. *(Right)* Sagittal STIR MR of the same patient shows a large soft tissue lesion ➡ which proved to be schwannoma, with local invasion into the distal humerus ➡. It is unusual to have such extensive local osseous invasion.

LONG BONE, METAPHYSEAL BANDS & LINES

DIFFERENTIAL DIAGNOSIS

Common
- Growth Arrest Lines
- Chronic Illness
- Trauma
- Normal Variant
- Disuse Osteoporosis
- Chemotherapy
- Malnutrition or Prolonged Hyperalimentation
- Hyperemia
- Heavy Metal or Chemical Ingestion
- Rickets
- Radiation

Less Common
- Leukemia
- Juvenile Idiopathic Arthritis (JIA)
- Ankylosing Spondylitis
- Complications of High Dose Drug Therapy (Non-Chemotherapeutic)
- Metastases
- Osteoporosis

Rare but Important
- Complications of Vitamin D
- Osteopetrosis
- Hypothyroidism, Treated
- Complications of Fluoride
- Hypoparathyroidism
- Pseudohypoparathyroidism
- Idiopathic Hypercalcemia
- Scurvy
- Congenital Infection
- Aminopterin Fetopathy
- Hypophosphatasia
- Erythroblastosis Fetalis
- Osteopathia Striata
- Primary Oxalosis

ESSENTIAL INFORMATION

Key Differential Diagnosis Issues
- Manifestations include: Dense horizontal bands (DB), lucent bands (LB), alternating dense & lucent bands (AB), vertical dense bands (VB)
  - AB indicate multiple insults separated in time
- Most are systemic, involve multiple physes
  - Especially at knee, wrist (sites of greatest growth)

- Isolated physeal involvement: Trauma, radiation, metastatic disease, disuse osteoporosis, hyperemia

Helpful Clues for Common Diagnoses
- **Growth Arrest Lines**
  - DB, VB: Sharply defined, thin dense lines
  - Variable distance from metaphysis depending on age of insult
  - Underlying insult may not be identifiable
- **Chronic Illness**
  - LB, VB: Any illness including sickle cell anemia, rickets, osteogenesis imperfecta, neoplasm
  - LB: Nonspecific manifestation of illness
  - May develop DB during healing
- **Trauma**
  - LB: Acute injury, early healing
  - DB, VB: Healing Salter fractures, chronic injury, stress fracture
    - ± Metaphyseal cupping/fraying
- **Normal Variant**
  - DB, LB: Otherwise normal skeleton
  - Normal fibula helps differentiate from other conditions such as lead poisoning
- **Disuse Osteoporosis**
  - LB: Regional distribution
- **Chemotherapy**
  - LB, VB
- **Malnutrition or Prolonged Hyperalimentation**
  - LB
- **Hyperemia**
  - LB: Bone resorption leads to osteoporosis
  - Arthritis, infection
- **Heavy Metal or Chemical Ingestion**
  - DB, AB: Lead most common; lines are late manifestation
- **Rickets**
  - LB, VB (healing): Manifestation of bone resorption of hyperparathyroidism
- **Radiation**
  - VB, LB, DB; ± physeal widening, fraying
  - DB, AB during healing

Helpful Clues for Less Common Diagnoses
- **Leukemia**
  - LB: May also see osteolytic lesions, periostitis
  - DB, during healing
  - 2-5 years old
- **Juvenile Idiopathic Arthritis (JIA)**
  - LB due to hyperemia & chronic illness

- ○ Monoarticular to symmetric polyarticular
- ○ Uniform joint space narrowing, marginal erosions, periostitis
- **Ankylosing Spondylitis**
  - ○ LB due to osteoporosis, hyperemia
  - ○ Anterior & posterior spinal fusion
  - ○ Symmetric sacroiliitis
  - ○ Hip, shoulder arthritis; enthesopathy
- **Complications of High Dose Drug Therapy (Non-Chemotherapeutic)**
  - ○ DB
- **Metastases**
  - ○ LB, DB (during healing), especially neuroblastoma, lymphoma
    - Osteolytic lesions & periostitis from direct tumor invasion
- **Osteoporosis**
  - ○ LB: Juvenile idiopathic, Cushing disease

Helpful Clues for Rare Diagnoses
- **Complications of Vitamin D**
  - ○ DB, AB: Variable manifestations; osteoporosis, osteosclerosis, cortical thickening, soft tissue calcification
- **Osteopetrosis**
  - ○ DB, LB, AB: Generalized osteosclerosis
  - ○ Metaphyseal expansion
- **Hypothyroidism, Treated**
  - ○ DB: Abnormal epiphyses
- **Complications of Fluoride**
  - ○ DB: ↑ Bone density, osteophytes, ligament calcification
  - ○ Axial changes dominate
- **Hypoparathyroidism**

- ○ DB: Ligament & tendon ossification, axial & appendicular
- ○ Osteosclerosis, abnormal dentition, subcutaneous calcification
- **Pseudohypoparathyroidism**
  - ○ DB: Same as hypoparathyroidism
  - ○ Differentiating features
    - Short stature, developmental delay
    - Short metacarpals, especially 4 & 5
    - Subcutaneous calcification, ossification
- **Idiopathic Hypercalcemia**
  - ○ DB: Diffuse bone sclerosis
- **Scurvy**
  - ○ DB, LB: Orientation of growth plate:lucent line (scurvy line):dense line
  - ○ Metaphyseal beaks, periostitis
- **Congenital Infection**
  - ○ DB, VB, celery stalk
  - ○ Includes rubella, CMV, syphilis, herpes simplex, toxoplasmosis
- **Aminopterin Fetopathy**
  - ○ DB
- **Hypophosphatasia**
  - ○ LB, VB: Physis mimics rickets
- **Erythroblastosis Fetalis**
  - ○ LB: Diffuse soft tissue edema
- **Osteopathia Striata**
  - ○ VB: Mild metaphyseal expansion
  - ○ Asymptomatic
- **Primary Oxalosis**
  - ○ DB, AB ± renal osteodystrophy
  - ○ Drumstick metacarpals
  - ○ Renal calculi, parenchymal calcification
  - ○ Vascular calcification

Growth Arrest Lines

Lateral radiograph shows a single growth recovery line in the distal tibia ➡. *In many cases an underlying contributing cause is not known.*

Growth Arrest Lines

Anteroposterior radiograph shows diffuse osteopenia from osteogenesis imperfecta. Multiple metaphyseal lines ➡ *are present, corresponding to growth lines associated with bisphosphonate therapy.*

LONG BONE, METAPHYSEAL BANDS & LINES

Trauma

Trauma

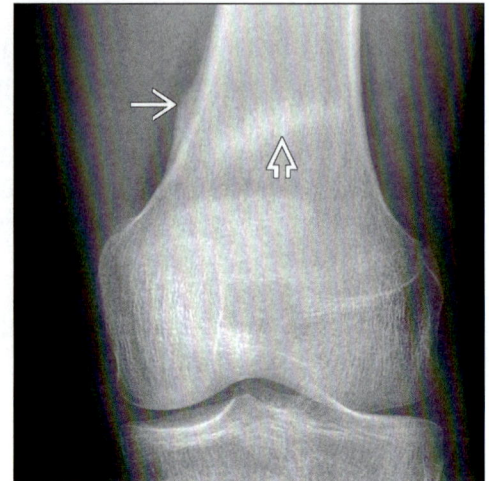

(Left) Anteroposterior radiograph shows irregularity of the physis with sclerosis along the metaphyseal margin ➡ in this Little League pitcher with a chronic repetitive injury. *(Right)* Anteroposterior radiograph shows a typical stress fracture with ill-defined sclerotic line ➡ and adjacent periosteal new bone formation ➡.

Normal Variant

Disuse Osteoporosis

(Left) Anteroposterior radiograph shows the appearance of normal physes ➡, mimicking dense metaphyseal bands. Differentiation from other entities such as lead poisoning can be difficult. *(Right)* Anteroposterior radiograph shows lucent metaphyseal band ➡, caused by disuse osteoporosis following immobilization after open reduction, internal fixation (ORIF) of a tibial diaphyseal fracture.

Heavy Metal or Chemical Ingestion

Rickets

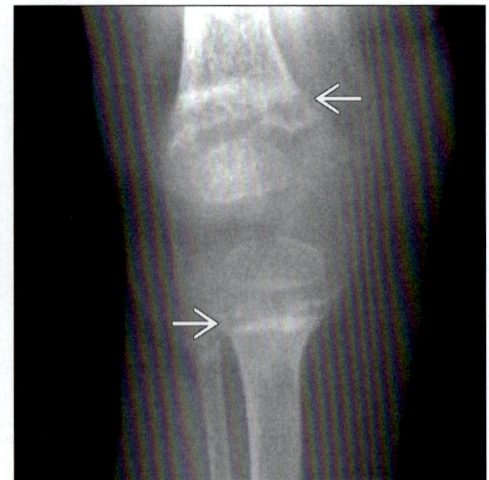

(Left) Anteroposterior radiograph shows the classic dense metaphyseal lines ➡ seen with lead poisoning. Involvement of the fibula helps distinguish this appearance from a normal variant. *(Right)* Anteroposterior radiograph shows markedly abnormal physis in this patient with renal rickets. The physes are cupped and frayed with lucent and sclerotic metaphyseal bands ➡.

LONG BONE, METAPHYSEAL BANDS & LINES

Leukemia

Leukemia

(Left) Anteroposterior radiograph shows diffuse osteopenia and subtle lucent metaphyseal bands ➡ in this patient with leukemia. *(Right)* Oblique radiograph shows typical appearance of leukemic metaphyseal lucent lines ➡ at the ankle.

Ankylosing Spondylitis

Scurvy

(Left) Anteroposterior radiograph shows lucent bands at the metaphyses ➡ as an early manifestation of osteoporosis in a patient with hyperemia from ankylosing spondylosis. *(Right)* Anteroposterior radiograph shows classic signs of scurvy including diffuse osteopenia and dense lines at the metaphyses and epiphyses. The dense metaphyseal line ➡ is known as the white line of Frankel.

Congenital Infection

Congenital Infection

(Left) Anteroposterior radiograph shows typical appearance of syphilis on radiographs. The tibias show Wimberger signs ➡ and generalized metaphyseal osteitis, which appears as lucent bands ➡. *(Right)* Anteroposterior radiograph shows a typical appearance of congenital syphilis with generalized metaphyseal osteitis manifesting as metaphyseal lucencies ➡.

LONG BONE, METAPHYSEAL CUPPING

DIFFERENTIAL DIAGNOSIS

Common
- Normal Variant
- Child Abuse, Metaphyseal Fx (Mimic)

Less Common
- Renal Osteodystrophy
- Rickets
- Pediatric Fracture
- Prolonged Immobilization
- Sickle Cell Anemia

Rare but Important
- Post Infection
- Radiation-Induced
- Scurvy
- Hypophosphatasia
- Achondroplasia
- Metaphyseal Dysplasias
- Polio (Prolonged Immobilization)
- Hypervitaminosis A

ESSENTIAL INFORMATION

Key Differential Diagnosis Issues
- Rickets, renal osteodystrophy & hypophosphatasia: Overgrowth of disorganized chondrocytes
  - Hint: Involves sites of rapid growth: Distal radius/ulna, distal femur, proximal tibia, costochondral articulations
- Other entities: Oligemia, thrombosis create central metaphyseal depression; causative insult need not be at growth plate

- May be isolated or involve random sites

Helpful Clues for Common Diagnoses
- **Child Abuse, Metaphyseal Fx (Mimic)**
  - Horizontal shear through growth plate; periostitis during healing

Helpful Clues for Less Common Diagnoses
- **Renal Osteodystrophy**
  - Combination of rickets & hyperparathyroidism (HPTH)
- **Pediatric Fracture**
  - Delayed complication
- **Prolonged Immobilization**
  - Associated disuse osteoporosis
- **Sickle Cell Anemia**
  - Metacarpals, metatarsals; AVN, infarcts, coarse trabecula, dactylitis, osteomyelitis

Helpful Clues for Rare Diagnoses
- **Radiation-Induced**
  - Regional mixed ↑ & ↓ bone density
- **Scurvy**
  - Subperiosteal hemorrhage, osteopenia
- **Hypophosphatasia**
  - Coarse trabecula, osteopenia
- **Achondroplasia**
  - Short femora & humeri; spine & pelvic anomalies
- **Metaphyseal Dysplasias**
  - Short stature, bowing of long bones
- **Polio (Prolonged Immobilization)**
  - Especially knees, metatarsals; muscle wasting, thin gracile osteoporotic bones
- **Hypervitaminosis A**
  - Hyperostosis, premature physeal fusion

Child Abuse, Metaphyseal Fx (Mimic)

Anteroposterior radiograph shows 2 metaphyseal corner fractures ➡ of the upper humerus in this victim of child abuse. The fractures mimic the appearance of a widened and cupped metaphysis.

Renal Osteodystrophy

Posteroanterior radiograph shows a widened zone of provisional calcification and cupping/fraying of the metaphyses of the radius and ulna ➡ in this child with chronic renal disease.

LONG BONE, METAPHYSEAL CUPPING

Rickets

Rickets

(Left) Anteroposterior radiograph shows changes of nutritional deficiency rickets including metaphyseal cupping and fraying of the distal radius and ulna ➡. *(Right)* Anteroposterior radiograph shows changes of rickets. The growth plate changes are due to an increase in the number of chondrocytes with loss of the normal columnar organization, leading to widening and cupping of the growth plate.

Scurvy

Hypophosphatasia

(Left) Anteroposterior radiograph shows classic signs of scurvy including osteopenia and dense lines at the metaphyses and epiphyses. Mild cupping is present at the proximal and distal metaphyses of both tibia and fibula ➡. *(Right)* Anteroposterior radiograph of a patient with hypophosphatasia shows osteopenia and a widened zone of provisional ossification of the growth plates ➡ with mild cupping of the distal femur ➡.

Achondroplasia

Metaphyseal Dysplasias

(Left) Anteroposterior radiograph shows flaring (cupping) of the metaphyses of the distal femora ➡ in this patient with achondroplasia. *(Right)* Lateral radiograph shows widening of the distal radial metaphysis ➡ with mild irregularity of the growth plate in this patient with metaphyseal dysplasia.

LONG BONE, METAPHYSEAL FRAYING

DIFFERENTIAL DIAGNOSIS

Common
- Chronic Repetitive Trauma
- Osteomyelitis, Pediatric
- Physeal Fractures, Pediatric
- Child Abuse, Metaphyseal Fracture

Less Common
- Rickets
- Thermal Injury
- Neuropathic Disease

Rare but Important
- Radiation
- Hypophosphatasia
- Copper Deficiency, Infantile
- Metaphyseal Chondrodysplasias

ESSENTIAL INFORMATION

Key Differential Diagnosis Issues
- **Hint**: Differentiate isolated/multisite from systemic involvement
  - Systemic: Sites of rapid growth = proximal & distal tibia/fibula, distal radius/ulna
  - Isolated/multisite: Chronic repetitive trauma, osteomyelitis, fracture, thermal injury, neuropathic disease, radiation
- Metaphyseal sclerosis common
- Periosteal new bone with fractures, trauma, osteomyelitis, neuropathic disease

Helpful Clues for Common Diagnoses
- **Chronic Repetitive Trauma**
  - Sport/situation & site specific

- **Osteomyelitis, Pediatric**
  - Focal metaphyseal osteopenia & destruction
- **Physeal Fractures, Pediatric**
  - Any healing fracture or avulsion
- **Child Abuse, Metaphyseal Fracture**
  - Corner fractures, cupping late

Helpful Clues for Less Common Diagnoses
- **Rickets**
  - Metaphyseal osteolysis & cupping, coarse ill-defined trabecula, rachitic rosary, enlarged knees, ankles, & wrists
  - Generalized osteopenia, delayed skeletal maturation, bowing
- **Thermal Injury**
  - Soft tissues changes including calcification
- **Neuropathic Disease**
  - Exaggerated changes including extensive fragmentation

Helpful Clues for Rare Diagnoses
- **Radiation**
  - Regional osteopenia
- **Hypophosphatasia**
  - **Hint**: Distinct finger-like lucent extension into metaphysis from growth plate
  - Osteopenia, cranial synostosis, bowing, fractures, metaphyseal spurs
- **Copper Deficiency, Infantile**
  - Metaphyseal cupping & spurs, hypotonia, seizures, mental retardation
- **Metaphyseal Chondrodysplasia**
  - Metaphyseal cupping, short stature, bowing

Chronic Repetitive Trauma

Anteroposterior radiograph shows osteolysis of the distal radius ➡ in a skeletally immature patient. This is a form of chronic Salter I injury that is seen particularly in young gymnasts.

Chronic Repetitive Trauma

Coronal oblique T1WI MR shows widening and irregularity of the physis ➡ in this Little League pitcher with chronic injury from throwing curve balls.

LONG BONE, METAPHYSEAL FRAYING

Osteomyelitis, Pediatric

Physeal Fractures, Pediatric

(Left) Lateral radiograph shows demineralization of the posterior calcaneus with irregularity of the central portion of the metaphyseal side of the growth plate ➡ in this patient with biopsy & culture-proven osteomyelitis. *(Right)* Anteroposterior radiograph shows changes of a healing ischial tuberosity avulsion. The growth plate is widened and irregular ➡ when compared to the opposite normal physis.

Child Abuse, Metaphyseal Fracture

Rickets

(Left) Anteroposterior radiograph shows 2 metaphyseal corner fractures ➡ of the upper humerus. Periosteal reaction is occurring along the shaft ➡. The metaphyseal margin of the growth plate has lost its normal sharp margin ➡, indicating injury throughout the physis. *(Right)* Anteroposterior radiograph shows typical bone changes in nutritional rickets. The metaphyses are widened (cupping) ➡, and the margins of the growth plate are irregular (fraying) ➡.

Rickets

Hypophosphatasia

(Left) Anteroposterior radiograph shows a widened zone of provisional calcification at all the physes of the knee ➡ in this patient with nutritional rickets. The weakened physes have allowed a valgus deformity to develop. *(Right)* Anteroposterior radiograph shows a widened zone of provisional ossification at the physes ➡ as well as diffuse osteopenia. Serological studies proved hypophosphatasia.

LONG BONE, CENTRAL METAPHYSEAL LESION, NON-AGGRESSIVE

DIFFERENTIAL DIAGNOSIS

Common
- Enchondroma
- Enostosis (Bone Island)
- Paget Disease
- Chronic Osteomyelitis
- Bone Infarct
- Hyperparathyroidism
- Chondrosarcoma, Conventional
- Desmoplastic Fibroma
- Intraosseous Lipoma
- Plasmacytoma
- Langerhans Cell Histiocytosis
- Fibrous Dysplasia
- Unicameral Bone Cyst
- Metastases, Bone Marrow
- Fibroxanthoma (NOF) (Thin Bone)
- Giant Cell Tumor (Large)
- Aneurysmal Bone Cyst (Thin Bone)

Less Common
- Liposclerosing Myxofibrous Tumor (LSMFT)
- Tuberculosis
- Fungal
- Osteoblastoma

Rare but Important
- Vascular Tumor
- Chondrosarcoma, Clear Cell
- Sarcoidosis
- Ollier Disease
- Maffucci Syndrome

ESSENTIAL INFORMATION

Key Differential Diagnosis Issues
- Metaphysis is most frequent site of osseous lesions in long bones; long differential, but somewhat limited in this list by central location & non-aggressive appearance
- Consider separating out those lesions generally restricted to patients < 30 years
  - Langerhans cell histiocytosis
  - Unicameral bone cyst
  - Fibroxanthoma (thin bone)
  - Aneurysmal bone cyst (thin bone)

Helpful Clues for Common Diagnoses
- **Enchondroma**
  - Geographic but without sclerotic margin
  - Usually contains punctate chondroid matrix; rarely completely lytic

  - May have small focal regions of endosteal scalloping; no periosteal reaction
- **Enostosis (Bone Island)**
  - Dense, regular hamartomatous cortical bone formation in marrow
  - Fades into normal bone at edges
  - May be large and continue to enlarge
  - Elicits no reaction; low signal on all MR sequences; does not enhance
- **Paget Disease**
  - Usually originates at subchondral bone and progresses through metaphysis towards diaphysis
  - Variably lytic, mixed lytic and sclerotic, depending on stage
  - Enlarges the involved bone
  - Sharp sclerotic margin ("blade of grass")
- **Chronic Osteomyelitis**
  - Applies to any variety (e.g., bacterial, tuberculosis, fungal)
  - Lytic, oval, well-marginated, metaphyseal lesion; not as permeative as acute bacterial osteomyelitis
  - Elicits surrounding reactive bone formation in marrow and thick periosteal/endosteal reaction
    - TB and fungal osteomyelitis generally elicit less prominent osseous reaction
  - MR may show chronic intraosseous abscess
- **Bone Infarct**
  - Central, metaphyseal, geographic, lytic lesion; often noted only after dystrophic calcification forms
    - Dystrophic calcification often serpiginous in pattern
  - When diffuse (as in sickle cell disease), may appear as a generalized ↑ density
- **Hyperparathyroidism**
  - Brown tumor is lytic and geographic, with subtle sclerotic margin
  - Often central metaphyseal, but not restricted to this location
  - Should see other signs of osseous resorption: Mixed increased & decreased bone density & various resorption patterns
  - Brown tumor often hyperossifies once treated, mimicking a sclerotic lesion
- **Chondrosarcoma, Conventional**
  - Location: Central metaphysis, particularly for chondrosarcoma arising in enchondroma

- o Chondroid matrix usually present, though it may be sparse or even absent
- o Most metaphyseal chondrosarcomas are low grade, appearing geographic & non-aggressive
  - ▪ Watch for change in character of lytic lesion or chondroid matrix to suggest degeneration of enchondroma to chondrosarcoma
  - ▪ Extensive endosteal scalloping suggests degeneration to chondrosarcoma, but is infrequently seen
  - ▪ Watch for thickening of endosteum: Good clue for degeneration to chondrosarcoma
- o This lesion is often underdiagnosed as a benign tumor
  - ▪ Curettage yields poor results, with almost inevitable recurrence, often with higher grade lesion
  - ▪ Suggest diagnosis of chondrosarcoma despite non-aggressive appearance
- **Desmoplastic Fibroma**
  - o Lytic non-aggressive osseous lesion
  - o Metadiaphyseal
  - o Predominantly low signal on T2 weighted MR images; enhances
    - ▪ Analogous to soft tissue fibromatosis
- **Intraosseous Lipoma**
  - o Central metaphyseal lytic lesion
  - o May contain dystrophic calcification
  - o Follows fat signal on all MR sequences
- **Plasmacytoma**

- o Initial plasma cell lesion, prior to dissemination as multiple myeloma
- o Generally non-aggressive to minimally aggressive in appearance
- o Pelvic, axial, or central metaphyseal
- o Lytic, geographic lesion, generally without cortical breakthrough or osseous reaction
  - ▪ Narrow zone of transition, but usually non-sclerotic margin
- **Langerhans Cell Histiocytosis**
  - o Common childhood lesion, ranges from non-aggressive to highly aggressive
  - o Lytic, metaphyseal or diaphyseal; long bones, skull, axial skeleton
- **Fibrous Dysplasia**
  - o Ground-glass matrix in long bones; mildly expansile
  - o Central, but located anywhere along length of bone, including metaphyses
  - o Frequent bowing deformities
- **Unicameral Bone Cyst**
  - o Lytic, expanded, cystic (may have "fallen fragment" sign)
  - o As it matures, "grows away" from metaphysis
- **Metastases, Bone Marrow**
  - o May be solitary & appear relatively non-aggressive
- **Fibroxanthoma (NOF) (Thin Bone) & Aneurysmal Bone Cyst (Thin Bone)**
  - o In thin bone, these normally eccentric lesions appear central
- **Giant Cell Tumor (Large)**
  - o Usually eccentric; if large, appears central

Enchondroma

Anteroposterior radiograph shows a geographic central metaphyseal lesion without sclerotic margin which contains punctate chondroid matrix. This is the most common location and appearance for enchondroma.

Enostosis (Bone Island)

Anteroposterior radiograph shows a uniformly dense central metaphyseal sclerotic lesion. The edges "fade" into normal bone and may appear almost spiculated ➜. *This appearance is typical of a giant bone island.*

Paget Disease

Chronic Osteomyelitis

(Left) Anteroposterior radiograph shows focal enlargement of the distal metaphysis of the humerus. The lesion occupies the bone from the subchondral cortex, moving proximally, with a sharp border with normal bone. It is mixed lytic & sclerotic and entirely typical of Paget disease. *(Right)* Anteroposterior radiograph shows mild expansion of the distal radius, containing a lytic, well-margined lesion ➡. Prominent surrounding osseous reaction ➡ is seen, typical of chronic infection.

Bone Infarct

Hyperparathyroidism

(Left) AP radiograph shows a central metaphyseal lesion containing dense dystrophic calcification which follows a somewhat serpiginous pattern ➡. The appearance is typical of bone infarct. *(Right)* AP radiograph shows a nonspecific, geographic, central, metaphyseal lesion ➡. However, the patient has generalized increased bone density, coarsened trabeculae, and subperiosteal resorption ➡, all typical of HPTH. The lesion is a Brown tumor.

Chondrosarcoma, Conventional

Desmoplastic Fibroma

(Left) AP radiograph shows a lytic central metaphyseal lesion, which causes minimal endosteal scalloping ➡. Note the endosteal thickening ➡. Despite the non-aggressive appearance, chondrosarcoma must be considered; it was proven at biopsy. (†MSK Req). *(Right)* Lateral radiograph shows a non-aggressive central metadiaphyseal lesion with distal pathologic fracture. In an adult, desmoplastic fibroma should be considered; it was proven at biopsy.

LONG BONE, CENTRAL METAPHYSEAL LESION, NON-AGGRESSIVE

Intraosseous Lipoma

Plasmacytoma

(Left) AP radiograph shows a faint lytic lesion in the central metaphysis ➡ which has no other defining features on radiograph. It has elicited no host reaction. MR proved fat signal within the entire lesion on all sequences. (†MSK Req). *(Right)* Anteroposterior radiograph shows a large central metaphyseal lytic lesion. It appears geographic, but with non-sclerotic margins ➡. This description applies to giant cell tumor as well as plasmacytoma; the latter was proven at biopsy.

Langerhans Cell Histiocytosis

Fibrous Dysplasia

(Left) AP radiograph shows a geographic lytic lesion in the central metadiaphysis of a child ➡. It has elicited dense periosteal thickening ➡, but itself does not appear aggressive. This is 1 typical appearance that may be seen in the range of LCH appearance. *(Right)* AP radiograph shows a central metaphyseal lesion which contains ground-glass density ➡. This is a typical appearance and location for fibrous dysplasia. The lesion has not yet caused bowing or thinning of the cortex.

Unicameral Bone Cyst

Metastases, Bone Marrow

(Left) AP radiograph shows a typical UBC in the central metaphysis of the radius of a child. The lytic geographic lesion has a pathologic fracture ➡ as well as a "fallen fragment" sign ➡, demonstrating its cystic nature. (†MSK Req). *(Right)* AP radiograph shows a solitary lytic lesion in a metaphyseal equivalent ➡. The lesion appears geographic and relatively non-aggressive, but proved to be metastatic breast carcinoma. Metastases may appear relatively benign.

LONG BONE, CENTRAL METAPHYSEAL LESION, NON-AGGRESSIVE

(Left) AP radiograph in this young child shows a large bubbly lesion occupying the central metadiaphysis. The humerus is thin at this age, and fibroxanthoma may occupy the entire width of the bone, rather than having its usual cortically based appearance. **(Right)** AP radiograph in a child shows a lytic lesion occupying the entire metaphysis of the fibula ⮕. Normally eccentric lesions like NOF may appear central in thin bones. Note the more typical lesion in the tibia ⮕.

Fibroxanthoma (NOF) (Thin Bone)

Fibroxanthoma (NOF) (Thin Bone)

(Left) Sagittal CT reformat shows a lytic central metaphyseal lesion causing endosteal scalloping. It is geographic but has a non-sclerotic margin. GCT, when this large, may occupy the entire width of the metaphysis and appear central rather than eccentric. **(Right)** Anteroposterior radiograph shows a lytic lesion occupying the entire metaphysis of the fibula, extending to the subchondral cortex. It proved to be GCT, appearing central in a small bone.

Giant Cell Tumor (Large)

Giant Cell Tumor (Large)

(Left) AP radiograph shows a highly expanded but geographic lytic lesion of the proximal fibular metaphysis ⮕ in a teenager. The cortex is thin but intact. This is an ABC; though this lesion is usually eccentric, it occupies the entire width of a small bone. **(Right)** AP radiograph shows a well-defined central metaphyseal lesion ⮕ which has mixed lytic and sclerotic regions. This is typical of LSMFT; this lesion is found almost exclusively in this proximal femoral location.

Aneurysmal Bone Cyst (Thin Bone)

Liposclerosing Myxofibrous Tumor (LSMFT)

LONG BONE, CENTRAL METAPHYSEAL LESION, NON-AGGRESSIVE

Tuberculosis

Osteoblastoma

(Left) PA radiograph shows a multiloculated central metaphyseal lytic lesion ➡. It has elicited a small amount of periosteal reaction ➡ but no osseous sclerosis. This is typical of TB or fungal osteomyelitis. The distal osteoporosis suggests the lesion has been present for a long period of time. *(Right)* AP radiograph shows a central lytic lesion in a metaphyseal equivalent ➡. It is non-aggressive. Osteoblastoma rarely occurs outside the axial skeleton, but this is one such case.

Vascular Tumor

Sarcoidosis

(Left) Anteroposterior radiograph shows a longstanding lytic lesion within the central metaphysis of the femur. It has elicited very regular periosteal and endosteal reaction. This was a case of lymphangiomatosis, present for > 10 years. *(Right)* Oblique radiograph shows central metaphyseal lytic lesions containing lacy trabeculae ➡, typical of phalangeal sarcoidosis.

Ollier Disease

Maffucci Syndrome

(Left) PA radiograph shows multiple central metaphyseal lytic lesions ➡. Chondroid matrix is seen in one lesion ➡, though it is not required for the diagnosis of Ollier disease. This patient also had the typical unilateral metaphyseal long bone lesions. (†MSK Req). *(Right)* PA radiograph shows central metaphyseal lytic lesions similar to the previous case. In addition there is a soft tissue hemangioma showing phleboliths ➡, securing the diagnosis of Maffucci syndrome. (†MSK Req).

LONG BONE, CENTRAL METAPHYSEAL LESION, AGGRESSIVE

DIFFERENTIAL DIAGNOSIS

Common
- Metastases, Bone Marrow
- Multiple Myeloma
- Osteosarcoma, Conventional
- Osteomyelitis, Adult
- Osteomyelitis, Pediatric
- Chondrosarcoma
- Malignant Fibrous Histiocytoma (MFH), Bone
- Fibrosarcoma
- Plasmacytoma
- Ewing Sarcoma
- Leukemia
- Langerhans Cell Histiocytosis

Less Common
- Giant Cell Tumor, Aggressive
- Angiosarcoma, Osseous
- Chronic Recurrent Multifocal Osteomyelitis

ESSENTIAL INFORMATION

Key Differential Diagnosis Issues
- Majority of osseous lesions occur predominantly in metaphysis, so list of metaphyseal lesions is lengthy; this differential deals with those that appear aggressive
- Lesions tend to preferentially occur centrally, eccentrically, cortically, or at osseous surface; this list covers those that are located centrally

Helpful Clues for Common Diagnoses
- **Metastases, Bone Marrow**
  - Metastases are most common aggressive osseous lesion
  - Aside from axial lesions, central metaphysis is a common location of metastases
  - Generally proximal to knees and elbows
  - Solitary metastasis is most likely renal or thyroid carcinoma
- **Multiple Myeloma**
  - Myeloma is a relatively common aggressive bone lesion
  - Generally presents with polyostotic lesions
  - May present with single axial or metaphyseal lesion, plus others that are not apparent (too small, or diffuse infiltration seen only as osteoporosis)

- **Osteosarcoma, Conventional**
  - Common sarcoma; metaphyseal location is most typical
  - Though location is more frequently eccentric within metaphysis, once lesion becomes large, it occupies entire metaphysis and appears central
  - May be lytic, but more frequently contains immature amorphous osteoid
  - Highly aggressive, with cortical breakthrough, periosteal reaction, soft tissue mass
- **Osteomyelitis, Adult**
  - Central metaphysis is a frequent location
  - Appearance may be highly permeative and aggressive, with periosteal reaction and soft tissue mass
  - Radiograph/CT may show typical serpiginous pattern of bone destruction
  - MR demonstrates abscesses
- **Osteomyelitis, Pediatric**
  - Central metaphysis is most frequent location of childhood osteomyelitis, through hematogenous spread
  - May appear highly aggressive, with permeative change, periosteal reaction, and abscesses
- **Chondrosarcoma**
  - Central proximal metaphysis is most frequent location of chondrosarcoma
  - Mirrors the most frequent location of enchondroma, a common precursor of chondrosarcoma
  - Often contains punctate chondroid matrix, but may be entirely lytic
  - Lesion often appears moderately aggressive or non-aggressive; may be geographic or may have only subtle regions which appear aggressive
  - May have endosteal scalloping; however, frequently has endosteal thickening
  - Cortical breakthrough and soft tissue mass are uncommon in low grade lesions
- **Malignant Fibrous Histiocytoma (MFH), Bone**
  - Central metaphyseal location is most common
  - Aggressive permeative lesion with periosteal reaction, cortical breakthrough, and soft tissue mass
  - Fibrosarcoma appears similar to MFH

- MFH may arise secondary to bone infarct
  - Central metaphysis is most frequent location of bone infarct
  - Lesions may contain central dystrophic calcification, residua of infarct
- **Plasmacytoma**
  - Most frequent location is pelvis, in a metaphyseal equivalent
  - May also arise in the central metaphysis
  - Characteristically appears fairly geographic
    - Narrow zone of transition
    - Non-sclerotic margin
    - Generally only moderately aggressive
- **Ewing Sarcoma**
  - Central aggressive lesion, with periosteal reaction, cortical breakthrough, and soft tissue mass
  - Most frequently diaphyseal, but not uncommonly is metadiaphyseal
  - May have prominent reactive bone formation within the osseous portion of the lesion
- **Leukemia**
  - Generally presents as diffuse osteopenia
  - Focal lytic metaphyseal lesion may rarely be seen
  - MR usually shows extensive metaphyseal lesions throughout skeleton
- **Langerhans Cell Histiocytosis**
  - Most frequent location is axial skeleton or central metadiaphyseal portion of long bone
  - Lytic lesion with wide range of appearances

- May be geographic, with sclerotic margin
- May be highly permeative, eliciting periosteal reaction, cortical breakthrough, and soft tissue mass

Helpful Clues for Less Common Diagnoses
- **Giant Cell Tumor, Aggressive**
  - GCT arises in the metaphysis, extending towards the subchondral bone
  - GCT generally is eccentric within the metaphysis, but as it grows to occupy the entire metaphysis it may appear central
  - Most GCT cases are geographic
    - Narrow zone of transition, but non-sclerotic margin
  - GCT may occasionally develop a more aggressive appearance and behavior, with rare malignant behavior
- **Angiosarcoma, Osseous**
  - Discussion includes other aggressive vascular lesions (hemangioendothelioma, hemangiopericytoma)
  - Located preferentially in lower extremities (including pelvis)
  - Lesions in long bones tend to be located centrally in metaphysis
  - May be solitary, but often polyostotic
  - Range of aggressiveness from geographic to highly permeative
- **Chronic Recurrent Multifocal Osteomyelitis**
  - Long term pain, but X-rays often normal
  - Metaphyseal & axial lesions seen optimally on MR, appearing aggressive & multifocal

Metastases, Bone Marrow

AP radiograph shows an aggressive permeative lesion located centrally in the metaphysis ➡, with pathologic fracture ➡. The patient is 38 years old; despite the young age, metastasis must be strongly considered.

Metastases, Bone Marrow

PA bone scan in the same patient shows the expected lesion ➡ & demonstrates it to be solitary. Note the morphologic abnormality of the left kidney ➡; this leads to the diagnosis of metastatic renal cell carcinoma.

LONG BONE, CENTRAL METAPHYSEAL LESION, AGGRESSIVE

(Left) Anteroposterior radiograph shows a lytic, slightly geographic lesion in the central metaphysis ➡. Careful observation suggests a similar lesion in the left femoral neck and another in the left inferior pubic ramus. Non-marginated multiple lesions suggest myeloma. *(Right)* Lateral radiograph shows a dense permeative lesion within the metaphysis, with large osteoid-producing soft tissue mass ➡. There is aggressive periosteal reaction; this is classic osteosarcoma.

Multiple Myeloma

Osteosarcoma, Conventional

(Left) Anteroposterior radiograph shows a highly permeative lytic lesion ➡ occupying the central metaphysis of the tibia. There is periosteal reaction ➡. This appearance could be an aggressive tumor, but in this case is osteomyelitis. *(Right)* Anteroposterior radiograph in a 13 year old shows a highly aggressive lytic metadiaphyseal lesion ➡. The diagnosis could easily be Ewing sarcoma, but biopsy proved staphylococcal osteomyelitis.

Osteomyelitis, Adult

Osteomyelitis, Pediatric

(Left) AP radiograph shows a lytic, moderately aggressive lesion in the central metaphysis ➡. The lesion changes character distally, where chondroid matrix is seen ➡, indicating enchondroma degenerating to chondrosarcoma. (†MSK Req). *(Right)* AP radiograph shows central metaphyseal bone infarct ➡. There is a highly permeative lesion extending from the infarct ➡. MFH may arise secondary to bone infarct; central metaphyseal location is typical.

Chondrosarcoma

Malignant Fibrous Histiocytoma (MFH), Bone

LONG BONE, CENTRAL METAPHYSEAL LESION, AGGRESSIVE

Plasmacytoma

Ewing Sarcoma

(Left) AP radiograph shows a lytic expanded lesion ➡ that has no sclerotic margin and has cortical breakthrough, located in a metaphyseal equivalent. This moderately aggressive appearance and location is typical of plasmacytoma. *(Right)* AP radiograph in an 8 year old shows a highly aggressive central metadiaphyseal lesion ➡. Though Ewing sarcoma is thought of as a diaphyseal lesion, it is not uncommon for it to arise in the metadiaphysis.

Leukemia

Langerhans Cell Histiocytosis

(Left) Coronal STIR MR shows a prominent metadiaphyseal lesion ➡ in this 30 year old, which proved to be acute leukemia. The radiograph was normal. This permeative lesion was not solitary; note lesions throughout the pelvis and left femur. *(Right)* AP radiograph shows an aggressive permeative lesion in the femoral neck ➡. This is a nonspecific appearance, but it should be remembered that LCH may appear highly aggressive, imitating Ewing sarcoma and osteomyelitis.

Giant Cell Tumor, Aggressive

Angiosarcoma, Osseous

(Left) AP radiograph shows a moderately aggressive lesion ➡ occupying the proximal femoral metaphysis. GCT can be quite aggressive in appearance & behavior. Though usually eccentric, a large GCT may appear central, as in this case. *(Right)* AP radiograph shows a moderately aggressive lesion in the central femoral neck metaphysis ➡. There are other subtle lesions in the femoral neck and ischium ➡. Angiosarcoma is often polyostotic.

LONG BONE, METAPHYSEAL LESION, BUBBLY

DIFFERENTIAL DIAGNOSIS

Common
- Fibroxanthoma (Non-Ossifying Fibroma)
- Giant Cell Tumor (GCT)
- Aneurysmal Bone Cyst (ABC)
- Metastases: Thyroid, Kidney
- Chondrosarcoma, Conventional

Less Common
- Chondromyxoid Fibroma (CMF)
- Chondroblastoma (CB)
- Unicameral Bone Cyst (UBC)
- Enchondroma, Phalanx
- Ollier Disease
- Maffucci Syndrome
- Osteosarcoma, Telangiectatic
- Osteoblastoma (OB)

Rare but Important
- Plasmacytoma

ESSENTIAL INFORMATION

Key Differential Diagnosis Issues
- **Hint**: Age is an important parameter in this differential
  - Bubbly metaphyseal lesion in child
    - Fibroxanthoma
    - Aneurysmal bone cyst
    - Less common: CMF, CB, UBC, telangiectatic osteosarcoma, OB
  - Bubbly metaphyseal lesion in teenager or young adult
    - Fibroxanthoma
    - Giant cell tumor
    - Aneurysmal bone cyst
    - Less common: CMF, CB, UBC, telangiectatic osteosarcoma, OB
  - Bubbly metaphyseal lesion in adult > 30 years
    - Giant cell tumor
    - Metastases (thyroid, kidney)
    - Chondrosarcoma
    - Plasmacytoma
- **Hint**: In older patient, be certain to consider chondrosarcoma
  - Common lesion in metaphysis that usually appears relatively non-aggressive, though not often truly bubbly
  - Underdiagnosis & undertreatment have serious consequences

- **Hint**: Enchondroma, Ollier disease, Maffucci syndrome usually bubbly only when located in small bones of hand & foot

Helpful Clues for Common Diagnoses
- **Fibroxanthoma (Non-Ossifying Fibroma)**
  - Common lesion in children
  - Eccentric (cortically based), metaphyseal is most common location
    - In thin bone, may occupy entire width
  - Generally has bubbly appearance; occasionally quite large
  - Sclerotic rim; natural history is to heal, increasing peripheral sclerosis & replacing with normal bone
- **Giant Cell Tumor (GCT)**
  - Common lesion in adults (30-60 most frequent age range)
  - Originates eccentrically in metaphysis
    - Usually extends to subchondral bone by time of discovery
  - As lesion increases in size, it expands & progresses towards bubbly appearance
  - Lesion is lytic; may acquire pseudotrabeculations in wall
    - Pseudotrabeculations add to "bubbly" appearance
  - Important differentiating feature is narrow zone of transition but non-sclerotic margin
  - Most frequent locations: Around knee, distal forearm bones, proximal femur
- **Aneurysmal Bone Cyst (ABC)**
  - Common lesion in children & up to age 30
  - Most common location: Eccentric metaphyseal
    - In thin bone, may occupy entire width
  - Expansion may be tremendous, but generally retains a thin rim of calcification (best seen on CT)
  - MR usually shows lesion full of fluid levels; rarely may be solid
- **Metastases: Thyroid, Kidney**
  - Metaphyses are common location for metastatic deposits
  - Most metastases cause only mild expansion
    - Exception: Thyroid & kidney metastases often are solitary & highly expanded
  - If kidney metastasis is suspected, consider embolization prior to biopsy
    - Highly vascular lesion may bleed significantly

LONG BONE, METAPHYSEAL LESION, BUBBLY

- **Chondrosarcoma, Conventional**
  - Most common location: Central metaphysis
    - Proximal long bones > distal
  - Potentially dangerous lesion since it may appear quite non-aggressive
    - Generally low grade (though may be large) when first discovered
    - May cause mild expansion, with pseudotrabeculation, appearing bubbly
    - Adjacent cortex generally thinned, but may cause endosteal thickening, especially immediately distal to lesion
    - Chondroid matrix, but may be lytic
  - Danger lies in underdiagnosis, leading to potentially catastrophic undertreatment
    - If treated as benign with curettage & bone grafting, lesion will recur, often with spread to local soft tissues
  - **Hint**: Always consider chondrosarcoma in following circumstances
    - Proximal femoral or humeral metaphyseal, PLUS
    - "Non-aggressive bubbly" lesion, PLUS
    - Patient falls in 30-60 year age range!

Helpful Clues for Less Common Diagnoses
- **Chondromyxoid Fibroma (CMF)**
  - Most frequent location is eccentric in proximal tibial metaphysis
  - Uncommon lesion seen mostly in children and young adults
  - Sclerotic margination & bubbly appearance
  - Usually lytic, though may have chondroid

- **Chondroblastoma (CB)**
  - Eccentric lesion originating in epiphysis, generally in teenager
    - As patient becomes skeletally mature, lesion often extends into metaphysis
    - However, "bubbly metaphyseal" is an unusual appearance for the lesion
  - If adjacent to cortex, expansion may lead to a mild bubbly appearance
  - Lytic or small amount of chondroid
- **Unicameral Bone Cyst (UBC)**
  - Common lesion of childhood
  - Central metaphyseal (especially proximal humerus) is most frequent location
  - Most common appearance is of central lucency with mild expansion of bone & thinning of endosteal cortex
    - With time, may develop pseudotrabeculations in wall, giving a "bubbly" appearance
    - Generally not truly significantly expanded or bubbly
- **Enchondroma, Phalanx**
  - Enchondroma in long bone is generally not expansile, except for mild focal scalloping of endosteal cortex
  - Exception: Small bones of hands & feet
    - Enchondroma may show significantly bubbly expansion
    - Appears more aggressive than it behaves
    - Often has punctate chondroid matrix, but may be entirely lytic
  - Ollier disease & Maffucci syndrome have similar bubbly appearance of phalangeals

Fibroxanthoma (Non-Ossifying Fibroma)

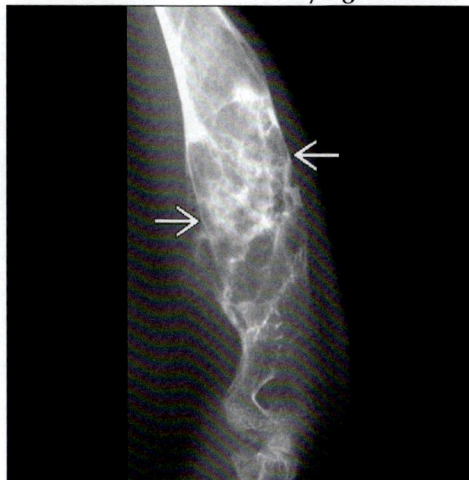

Lateral radiograph shows well-marginated bubbly lesion in the metadiaphysis ➡. The lesion is cortically based and is typical of fibroxanthoma. The natural history is to heal in with normal bone.

Fibroxanthoma (Non-Ossifying Fibroma)

Oblique radiograph shows bubbly lesion occupying entire width of the metadiaphysis ➡. When a fibroxanthoma becomes large in a thin bone (fibula, or humerus in a child), it may appear central in location.

LONG BONE, METAPHYSEAL LESION, BUBBLY

Giant Cell Tumor (GCT)

Giant Cell Tumor (GCT)

(Left) PA radiograph shows a bubbly lesion in distal radial metaphysis, a common location for GCT. Though these lesions are usually less bubbly in appearance than in this case, GCT may contain pseudotrabeculations that give such an appearance. (†MSK Req). *(Right)* AP radiograph shows a longstanding GCT that has expanded with a somewhat bubbly appearance. There are pseudotrabeculations; the location & appearance is typical of GCT.

Aneurysmal Bone Cyst (ABC)

Aneurysmal Bone Cyst (ABC)

(Left) Lateral radiograph shows an extremely expanded bubbly lesion arising eccentrically from the metaphysis of the ulna ➡. The location and appearance is typical of ABC. *(Right)* Lateral radiograph shows a bubbly expanded lesion occupying the entire width of the fibula ➡ with a thin cortical rim, in a teenager. The age and appearance are typical for ABC; when ABC arises in a thin bone such as the fibula, it may appear to be central in location.

Metastases: Thyroid, Kidney

Chondrosarcoma, Conventional

(Left) AP radiograph shows an expanded lesion of the metaphysis ➡ with thin rim of lesser trochanter remaining ➡. The patient is middle-aged; though the lesion could be a giant cell tumor, solitary metastasis must be considered (thyroid in this case). *(Right)* Lateral radiograph in a middle-aged patient shows a somewhat bubbly metaphyseal lesion. Few other bubbly metaphyseal lesions occur in this location or age. Chondrosarcoma must be suspected & was proven.

LONG BONE, METAPHYSEAL LESION, BUBBLY

Chondromyxoid Fibroma (CMF)

Chondroblastoma (CB)

(Left) Anteroposterior radiograph shows a mildly expanded and bubbly lesion located eccentrically in the tibial metaphysis ➡. The tibia is the most frequent location, and this is a typical appearance of CMF. (Right) Axial bone CT shows a small bubbly eccentric lesion ➡ at the junction of epiphysis & metaphysis in a young adult. There is a small focus of chondroid matrix ➡; this is chondroblastoma.

Unicameral Bone Cyst (UBC)

Enchondroma, Phalanx

(Left) AP radiograph in a child shows a mildly expanded metaphyseal lesion. Pseudotrabeculations may occasionally be seen in UBC ➡, particularly in the healing phase, making them appear bubbly. UBC more normally is more bland in appearance. (Right) PA radiograph shows a bubbly, highly expanded phalangeal lesion. Enchondroma in other locations does not appear bubbly but often does when located in the phalanx. Note the subtle chondroid matrix.

Ollier Disease

Maffucci Syndrome

(Left) Sagittal bone CT reformat shows bubbly lesions in several small bones of the foot ➡, with a normal adjacent metatarsal ➡, all typical of Ollier disease. Note the absence of chondroid matrix; it need not be present in enchondromas. (Right) PA radiograph shows multiple bubbly lesions in the small bones of the hand, along with phleboliths in a soft tissue hemangioma ➡. The constellation is typical of Maffucci syndrome. (†MSK Req).

LONG BONE, ECCENTRIC METAPHYSEAL LESION, NON-AGGRESSIVE

DIFFERENTIAL DIAGNOSIS

Common
- Enostosis (Bone Island)
- Fibroxanthoma (Non-Ossifying Fibroma)
- Stress Fracture, Adult
- Giant Cell Tumor (GCT)
- Aneurysmal Bone Cyst (ABC)
- Bone Infarct
- Metaphyseal Extension of Subchondral Cyst
- Arthroplasty Component Wear/Particle Disease
- Chronic Osteomyelitis
- Hyperparathyroidism, Brown Tumor
- Langerhans Cell Histiocytosis (LCH)

Less Common
- Liposclerosing Myxofibrous Tumor (LSMFT)
- Chondromyxoid Fibroma (CMF)
- Chondroblastoma (Mimic)
- Osteosarcoma, Telangiectatic

Rare but Important
- Tuberculosis
- Fungal
- Vascular Tumors
- Osteoblastoma

ESSENTIAL INFORMATION

Key Differential Diagnosis Issues
- Wide variety of lesions arise in an eccentric location in the metaphysis
- Most can be distinguished from one another with a high degree of confidence
  - **Hint**: Pay attention to details of lesion

Helpful Clues for Common Diagnoses
- **Enostosis (Bone Island)**
  - Normal hamartomatous bone formation within medullary space; metaphysis is most common location
  - Dense sclerotic bone with edges that "fade" into normal bone
  - Only significant differential is a sclerotic metastasis
    - MR or PET/CT helps to differentiate
- **Fibroxanthoma (Non-Ossifying Fibroma)**
  - Lesion of childhood and teenagers
  - Metaphysis is most common location (may become metadiaphyseal)
  - When eccentric (or cortically based, appearing eccentric), diagnosis is secure
  - Dense sclerotic border around a lytic, sometimes bubbly, lesion
  - Natural history is to heal, with sclerosis first, then remodeling to normal bone
- **Stress Fracture, Adult**
  - Typical location in long bones
    - Medial subcapital femur
    - Medial basicervical femur
    - Medial proximal tibial metaphysis
    - Distal tibial metaphysis
  - Linear sclerosis is diagnostic
  - If uncertain, MR is diagnostic
- **Giant Cell Tumor (GCT)**
  - Eccentric metaphysis is most frequent location
    - Though it usually reaches subchondral bone, origin is metaphyseal, NOT epiphyseal
  - Most common age range: 30-60 years
  - Distinct radiographic appearance: Narrow zone of transition but non-sclerotic margin
  - Usually non-aggressive, but may have aggressive or even malignant features
  - MR usually has some central low T2 signal
- **Aneurysmal Bone Cyst (ABC)**
  - Generally highly eccentric & metaphyseal
  - May be highly expanded, but generally retains thin cortical rim
    - Rim may not be visible on radiograph but seen on CT
    - Completely lytic
  - MR shows fluid levels in the vast majority
    - Remember that many other lesions may contain fluid levels
    - Remember that rarely ABC may be solid, without fluid levels
  - Age: Generally < 30 years
- **Bone Infarct**
  - Metaphysic most frequent location
    - When extensive, as in sickle cell, extends to diaphysis
  - When lytic, unlikely to be visible on radiograph
  - Visible with dystrophic calcification
    - May be globular or serpiginous
    - Calcification may enlarge over time
    - Beware of changing character of lesion; new permeative change suggests degeneration to malignant fibrous histiocytoma

LONG BONE, ECCENTRIC METAPHYSEAL LESION, NON-AGGRESSIVE

- **Metaphyseal Extension of Subchondral Cyst**
  - Some arthritic processes may develop particularly large subchondral cysts
    - May mimic metaphyseal tumor
    - Most frequent mimics: Pyrophosphate arthropathy, gout, pigmented villonodular synovitis
  - Watch for chondrocalcinosis, other evidence of arthritis
- **Arthroplasty Component Wear/Particle Disease**
  - Lytic lesions around prosthesis should stimulate search for source of particles producing osteolysis
    - Polyethylene, cement, metallic beads, bone
    - Patients generally also of age typical for metastatic disease/myeloma
- **Chronic Osteomyelitis**
  - Metaphysis is most frequent location of osteomyelitis
  - If chronic, lytic lesion is well-marginated
  - Sclerotic reactive bone surrounds lesion; also endosteal sclerosis
- **Hyperparathyroidism, Brown Tumor**
  - Brown tumor is lytic & generally geographic but without sclerotic margin
  - Location not specific to either metaphysis or diaphysis
  - Diffusely abnormal bone density & other resorptive patterns should suggest HPTH
- **Langerhans Cell Histiocytosis (LCH)**
  - Location not specific: May be metaphyseal, diaphyseal, or epiphyseal
    - May be central or eccentric
  - Degree of aggressiveness unreliable; has wide range of appearance

Helpful Clues for Less Common Diagnoses
- **Liposclerosing Myxofibrous Tumor (LSMFT)**
  - Highly location-specific: Eccentric proximal femoral metaphysis
  - Generally contains some degree of sclerosis; may have lipomatous portions
- **Chondromyxoid Fibroma (CMF)**
  - Rare tumor which has high degree of location specificity: Eccentric metaphyseal in tibia
  - Sclerotic margin, may be bubbly
  - Either chondroid matrix or lytic
- **Chondroblastoma (Mimic)**
  - Generally not confusing; if lesion extends from epiphysis into metaphysis following physeal fusion, may appear metaphyseal
    - Most common potential site of confusion: Proximal humerus
- **Osteosarcoma, Telangiectatic**
  - Most frequent site: Eccentric metaphyseal
  - Dangerous lesion: Much of lesion appears non-aggressive (narrow sclerotic margin)
    - Lytic; no osteoid produced
    - Contains fluid levels; easily misdiagnosed as ABC
  - Despite appearance, behavior & prognosis same as conventional osteosarcoma

Enostosis (Bone Island)

Anteroposterior radiograph shows a slightly eccentric densely sclerotic giant bone island. Note the dense regular matrix fading off into normal bone, an expected finding in enostosis.

Fibroxanthoma (Non-Ossifying Fibroma)

AP radiograph shows a well-marginated lytic lesion located eccentrically in the metaphysis ➡. Though NOF is usually cortically based, it may appear eccentric. This lesion is beginning to heal, with peripheral sclerosis.

LONG BONE, ECCENTRIC METAPHYSEAL LESION, NON-AGGRESSIVE

Stress Fracture, Adult

Giant Cell Tumor (GCT)

(Left) AP radiograph shows a slightly linear sclerotic "lesion" ➡ located eccentrically in the medial metaphysis of the femur. This is a stress fracture, located in the typical medial basicervical location. *(Right)* AP radiograph shows a lytic lesion located eccentrically within the metaphysis ➡. The lesion has a narrow zone of transition but no sclerotic margin and reaches the subchondral cortex; this is the classic location and appearance of a giant cell tumor. (†MSK Req).

Aneurysmal Bone Cyst (ABC)

Bone Infarct

(Left) Anteroposterior radiograph shows a lytic eccentric lesion in the metaphysis of the great toe ➡. Lesion is geographic. Appearance is typical, though not pathognomonic, of ABC. Multiple fluid levels were shown on MR. *(Right)* AP radiograph shows a sclerotic, angularly shaped focus, located eccentrically in the metaphysis ➡. The shape & character of the dystrophic calcification is typical of bone infarct; location may be either central or eccentric.

Metaphyseal Extension of Subchondral Cyst

Arthroplasty Component Wear/Particle Disease

(Left) AP radiograph shows an eccentric, subchondral, metaphyseal lesion ➡ that appears non-aggressive. Note that there is chondrocalcinosis present as well ➡. This is a large subchondral cyst in a patient with pyrophosphate arthropathy. *(Right)* Anteroposterior radiograph shows an eccentric metaphyseal lytic lesion surrounding a screw ➡ in a knee arthroplasty. This is osteolysis resulting from particle disease secondary to wear of the polyethylene.

LONG BONE, ECCENTRIC METAPHYSEAL LESION, NON-AGGRESSIVE

Chronic Osteomyelitis

Hyperparathyroidism, Brown Tumor

(Left) AP radiograph shows an eccentric, lytic, geographic lesion within the metaphysis ➡. There is a fairly dense surrounding osseous reaction. The appearance is typical of chronic osteomyelitis, or Brodie abscess. *(Right)* Lateral radiograph shows a lytic lesion located eccentrically in metaphysis ➡. There is generalized abnormal bone density with abnormal trabeculae; this is a brown tumor in a patient with hyperparathyroidism & renal osteodystrophy.

Langerhans Cell Histiocytosis (LCH)

Liposclerosing Myxofibrous Tumor (LSMFT)

(Left) AP radiograph shows a lytic, fairly geographic lesion located eccentrically in the metaphysis ➡ of an infant. It does not appear aggressive, though there is a small amount of periosteal reaction ➡. LCH may be eccentric, as in this case, but is more frequently central. *(Right)* AP radiograph shows an eccentric metaphyseal, lytic lesion containing a sclerotic focus ➡. LSMFT is highly location-specific, being found almost exclusively in the proximal femoral metaphysis.

Chondromyxoid Fibroma (CMF)

Chondroblastoma (Mimic)

(Left) AP radiograph shows a slightly bubbly lytic lesion with a sclerotic border located eccentrically within the tibial metaphysis. The appearance & location are typical for a CMF. *(Right)* Lateral radiograph shows an eccentric lytic lesion in the humerus arising in the epiphysis of a teenager ➡. Though the majority of the lesion is within the epiphysis, it extends slightly into the metaphysis ➡ once the physis fuses, possibly misleading one as to its origin.

LONG BONE, ECCENTRIC METAPHYSEAL LESION, AGGRESSIVE

DIFFERENTIAL DIAGNOSIS

Common
- Osteosarcoma, Conventional
- Osteomyelitis
- Giant Cell Tumor
- Metastases, Bone Marrow

Less Common
- Langerhans Cell Histiocytosis
- Aneurysmal Bone Cyst
- Malignant Fibrous Histiocytoma, Bone
- Lymphoma
- Osteosarcoma, Telangiectatic
- Fibrosarcoma
- Radiation-Induced Sarcoma

Rare but Important
- Angiosarcoma, Osseous
- Hemangioendothelioma, Osseous
- Hemangiopericytoma, Osseous

ESSENTIAL INFORMATION

Key Differential Diagnosis Issues
- Differential includes a variety of malignant & benign lesions
  - Malignant lesions which appear aggressive
    - Osteosarcoma, conventional
    - Metastases
    - Malignant fibrous histiocytoma
    - Lymphoma
    - Fibrosarcoma
    - Radiation-induced sarcoma
    - Vascular sarcomas
  - Outlier: Benign lesions appearing aggressive
    - Osteomyelitis
    - Giant cell tumor
    - Langerhans cell histiocytosis
    - Aneurysmal bone cyst
  - Outlier: Malignant lesions which may have only subtle signs of aggressiveness
    - Metastases
    - Osteosarcoma, telangiectatic
    - Vascular sarcomas
- **Hint:** Remember to keep the outliers in mind for this differential

Helpful Clues for Common Diagnoses
- **Osteosarcoma, Conventional**
  - Eccentric metaphyseal is most common location

- Most common aggressive metaphyseal tumor in children & teenagers
    - Uncommon in adults 25-70 years of age
    - Second peak of cases in patients > 70 years of age 2° to radiation, Paget degeneration, chondrosarcoma dedifferentiation
  - Almost invariably highly aggressive
  - Tumor osteoid in majority of cases
    - Amorphous; may be extremely subtle in soft tissue mass
    - Disorganized, less dense than bone
    - When tumor osteoid is in bone, may appear densely sclerotic
    - Matrix may be absent altogether
  - MR shows variable regions of low signal relating to osteoid
- **Osteomyelitis**
  - Metaphyseal site is common 2° to blood supply to that site, especially in children
  - May be central or eccentric
  - Permeative with periosteal reaction
    - May follow a serpiginous pattern
  - With bacterial infections (the most common), often have adjacent sclerotic bone reaction
  - Cortical breakthrough with soft tissue mass (abscess), fascial fluid
    - On radiograph, fat planes obliterated rather than distorted (as with tumors)
  - Watch for sequestrum (dense isolated devascularized bone fragment)
- **Giant Cell Tumor**
  - Eccentric site within metaphysis is most common location
  - Most frequent appearance is geographic, but without sclerotic margin
  - Not rarely, appearance & behavior is more aggressive or even metastatic
    - Wide zone of transition
    - Cortical breakthrough, soft tissue mass
  - MR usually has areas of low T2 signal within mass, though majority are high SI
- **Metastases, Bone Marrow**
  - Metastases frequent in long bones, especially metaphyseal locations
  - Metastases may be only subtly aggressive
    - Usually do not have large soft tissue mass

Helpful Clues for Less Common Diagnoses
- **Langerhans Cell Histiocytosis**
  - Common lesion in children

LONG BONE, ECCENTRIC METAPHYSEAL LESION, AGGRESSIVE

○ Lesions may be metaphyseal, diaphyseal, or epiphyseal
○ Most lesions are central, but metaphyseal lesions may be eccentric (especially in proximal humerus)
○ Range of appearances from nonaggressive to highly aggressive
○ Frequently polyostotic
• **Aneurysmal Bone Cyst**
  ○ Benign lesion that may appear highly aggressive
    ▪ Aggressive expansion with ballooning of cortex
    ▪ May be aggressive within metaphysis, with less sclerotic margin than usual
  ○ Most frequent location is eccentric in metaphysis
  ○ Usually has very thin surrounding cortex, even with aggressive lesion
  ○ MR shows fluid levels in vast majority, though solid ABC does occur
• **Malignant Fibrous Histiocytoma, Bone**
  ○ Aggressive lesion that may be metaphyseal or diaphyseal
  ○ Cortical breakthrough, soft tissue mass
  ○ Often central, but may be eccentric
  ○ Generally adult, but rarely seen in children
  ○ Usually not specific in appearance
    ▪ Exception is MFH arising in bone infarct, where dystrophic calcification of infarct may be distinguishing factor
    ▪ Fibrosarcoma appears similar to MFH
• **Lymphoma**
  ○ Generally central diaphyseal lesion

○ May occur eccentrically in metaphysis
○ Early lesions may not appear aggressive; watch for any signs pointing towards aggressiveness
○ Advanced lesion is highly permeative, often with large soft tissue mass
○ Rapidly advancing tumor may contain a sequestrum
• **Osteosarcoma, Telangiectatic**
  ○ Uncommon variety of osteosarcoma
  ○ Most frequently eccentric in metaphysis
  ○ Generally is lytic, without tumor osteoid
  ○ Dangerous lesion since majority of lesion may appear non-aggressive on radiograph
    ▪ Much of lesion may be geographic, even with sclerotic margin
    ▪ Watch for any red flag suggesting a permeative portion or any small sign of cortical breakthrough
  ○ Also dangerous on MR since the majority of lesion is filled with fluid levels
    ▪ Watch for nodularity in periphery of lesion which enhances
  ○ **Hint**: This is a lesion one must watch for carefully
    ▪ Undertreatment as "ABC" is devastating
    ▪ Small tumor nodules may be missed by pathologist
    ▪ Same metastatic potential & poor prognosis as conventional osteosarcoma
• **Radiation-Induced Sarcoma**
  ○ Watch for radiation osteonecrosis with changing (aggressive) behavior

Osteosarcoma, Conventional

AP radiograph shows an aggressive permeative metaphyseal lesion ➡ that has tumor osteoid formation both within the bone and within the soft tissue mass ➡. This is a classic osteosarcoma.

Osteosarcoma, Conventional

AP radiograph shows an eccentric lesion with a sclerotic margin ➡ about much of the circumference. However, there is subtle cortical breakthrough ➡, an indication of aggressiveness in this osteosarcoma. (†MSK Req).

LONG BONE, ECCENTRIC METAPHYSEAL LESION, AGGRESSIVE

Osteosarcoma, Conventional

Osteomyelitis

(Left) Anteroposterior radiograph shows a highly aggressive eccentric lesion in the metaphysis of a child ➡. Even though there is no osteoid matrix, osteosarcoma is the most likely diagnosis and was subsequently proven. (Right) Anteroposterior radiograph shows an eccentric, rather permeative lesion ➡ within the metaphysis of a child. Osteomyelitis most frequently arises in the metaphysis in this age group due to hematogenous spread. (†MSK Req).

Giant Cell Tumor

Giant Cell Tumor

(Left) Lateral radiograph of the hip shows a large, lytic, metaphyseal lesion that is eccentrically located, with absent cortex anteriorly ➡. The remainder of the lesion shows a non-sclerotic but geographic margin, typical of giant cell tumor (GCT). (Right) Axial bone CT of the same case shows the destruction of the anterior cortex ➡ and suggests that the remaining borders are irregular. This is a typical appearance and location for an aggressive GCT.

Metastases, Bone Marrow

Langerhans Cell Histiocytosis

(Left) AP radiograph shows an aggressive-appearing eccentric lytic lesion in the metaphysis of the femur ➡, with avulsion fracture of the lesser trochanter ➡. This is a typical expanded solitary metastasis; the primary was thyroid. (Right) AP radiograph shows a highly permeative & aggressive lesion ➡ located eccentrically in the metaphysis of an infant. This could represent osteomyelitis or a neuroblastoma metastasis, but LCH must be considered & was proven.

LONG BONE, ECCENTRIC METAPHYSEAL LESION, AGGRESSIVE

Aneurysmal Bone Cyst

Aneurysmal Bone Cyst

(Left) AP radiograph shows a lytic eccentric lesion in the metaphysis ➡. It is so permeative that it almost cannot be seen, but there is a subtle margin present. Though osteosarcoma is the most likely lesion to present in this way, other lesions might be considered. *(Right)* Axial T2WI MR of the same case shows fluid levels throughout the lesion ➡. ABC was proven after a careful pathologic search proved no evidence of telangiectatic osteosarcoma. (†MSK Req).

Malignant Fibrous Histiocytoma, Bone

Lymphoma

(Left) Anteroposterior radiograph shows a highly aggressive eccentric metaphyseal lesion, with permeative change & cortical breakthrough. This appearance is best for a diagnosis of osteosarcoma in this teenager, but biopsy proved MFH. *(Right)* Anteroposterior radiograph shows an eccentric lytic lesion in the femoral neck ➡ that appears of intermediate aggressiveness, with a moderately narrow zone of transition. This proved to be lymphoma.

Osteosarcoma, Telangiectatic

Osteosarcoma, Telangiectatic

(Left) AP radiograph shows a lytic, eccentric, metaphyseal lesion that, in places, appears geographic ➡. Other regions show a wider zone of transition ➡, and there is cortical breakthrough ➡. Concern for telangiectatic osteosarcoma must be raised. (†MSK Req). *(Right)* Axial T2WI MR in the same patient shows the osseous lesion ➡ with a large soft tissue mass ➡. A few fluid levels are present ➡, along with solid tumor in this telangiectatic OS. (†MSK Req).

LONG BONE, CORTICALLY BASED METAPHYSEAL LESION

DIFFERENTIAL DIAGNOSIS

Common
- Insufficiency Fractures, Appendicular
- Stress Fracture, Adult
- Osteoid Osteoma
- Osteochondroma
- Fibrous Dysplasia
- Fibroxanthoma (Non-Ossifying Fibroma)
- Aneurysmal Bone Cyst

Less Common
- Adamantinoma
- Soft Tissue Tumor Excavation (Mimic)

Rare but Important
- Langerhans Cell Histiocytosis
- Osteofibrous Dysplasia

ESSENTIAL INFORMATION

Key Differential Diagnosis Issues
- Cortically based metaphyseal lesions require special attention
  - May put patient at risk for fracture
  - May actually be a fracture
  - In either case, patient needs protection against completion of fracture
  - **Hint**: Include insufficiency or stress fractures of the metaphyses in your search pattern
- **Hint**: In child or teenager with hip pain, search femoral neck for osteoid osteoma
  - Relatively common location
  - May result in morphologic changes which obscure the actual diagnosis

Helpful Clues for Common Diagnoses
- **Insufficiency Fractures, Appendicular**
  - Insufficiency fractures of long bones often occur in metaphyseal region
    - Surgical neck humerus
    - Femoral neck (subcapital, intertrochanteric)
    - Medial proximal tibia
  - On radiograph, watch for subtle changes
    - Cortical buckle
    - Focal linear sclerosis at expected site
  - If insufficiency fracture is suspected clinically or radiographically, MR should be performed
    - Linear low signal fracture line seen on either T1 or fluid sensitive sequences
    - Edema may obscure fracture line
  - Have a high degree of suspicion for these fractures in elderly or osteoporotic patients
- **Stress Fracture, Adult**
  - Stress fractures of long bones often occur in metaphyseal region
    - Femoral neck (basicervical)
    - Medial proximal tibia
  - On radiograph, watch for subtle abnormalities
    - Focal linear sclerosis
    - Periosteal reaction
  - If suspected, MR should be performed
    - May show only stress reaction (high signal in cortex on fluid sequences, low on T1, with surrounding edema but no fracture line)
    - If fractured, linear low signal fracture line with surrounding edema
    - Edema rarely may obscure fracture line
- **Osteoid Osteoma**
  - Most osteoid osteoma (OO) are cortically based in the diaphysis
  - Next most frequent location is intraarticular, particularly at femoral neck
  - Femoral neck OO generally are in the mid-cervical region
    - OO itself is cortically based; on axial imaging, either anterior, medial, or posterior cortex
    - Axial imaging used to localize lesion, generally for radiofrequency ablation
  - Femoral neck OO is within hip joint
    - Elicits long-term joint effusion
    - Large effusion may result in long-term lateral subluxation of femoral head
  - Lateral subluxation of femoral head, over several months, results in morphologic changes
    - Calcar buttressing
    - Osteophyte formation, femoral head
    - Femoral neck valgus
    - Widening of radiographic teardrop (overgrowth of medial acetabular wall)
  - Morphologic changes may divert attention towards a dysplasia or arthritis
  - Intraarticular OO elicits densely sclerotic reactive osseous formation
    - Unlike diaphyseal OO, reactive bone may not surround OO; generally is distal to OO, in subtrochanteric region

LONG BONE, CORTICALLY BASED METAPHYSEAL LESION

- Reactive bone may divert attention away from the OO nidus
- Between the morphologic changes & reactive sclerosis, lesion itself may be difficult to visualize
  - **Hint:** In correct age group, search for this lesion in femoral neck
- **Osteochondroma**
  - Usually metaphyseal in location, arising from cortex
  - Exophytic (cauliflower) variety
    - Normal cortex and marrow from underlying metaphysis seen extending into stalk of lesion
    - Periphery of lesion may have less well organized bone
    - Cartilage cap should not be greater than 1.5 cm in thickness
  - Sessile variety
    - Seen frequently in multiple hereditary exostosis (MHE)
    - Broad base extending along the metaphysis
    - Normal marrow and cortex in this base
    - Results in a morphologic change at the metaphyses which is often symmetric
    - Morphologic change gives the appearance of broadened metaphyses & undertubulation
    - Often mistakenly called a dysplasia
    - **Hint**: MHE is far more frequent than metaphyseal dysplasias; with broad metaphyses, look for a way to diagnose sessile exostoses

- **Fibrous Dysplasia**
  - Generally central, but may arise in cortex
  - Common lesion, so a cortical location should not be surprising
  - Ground-glass matrix is helpful in the diagnosis, but not always present
  - Generally polyostotic
- **Fibroxanthoma (Non-Ossifying Fibroma)**
  - Usually more metadiaphyseal than purely metaphyseal
  - Cortically based, but may become large enough that the cortical origin is obscured
  - Lytic, with sclerotic margin in children
  - Natural history is to heal, with sclerosis, then remodeling to normal bone
- **Aneurysmal Bone Cyst**
  - ABC generally arises eccentrically within metaphysis; true cortical origin uncommon

Helpful Clues for Less Common Diagnoses
- **Adamantinoma**
  - Cortical, generally anterior tibia metadiaphysis
- **Soft Tissue Tumor Excavation (Mimic)**
  - Cortical invasion by soft tissue mass may mimic lytic cortical lesion on radiograph

Helpful Clues for Rare Diagnoses
- **Langerhans Cell Histiocytosis**
  - Common lesion; cortical origin is rare
- **Osteofibrous Dysplasia**
  - Rare cortical lesion; generally proximal anterior tibial metadiaphysis rather than metaphysis

Insufficiency Fractures, Appendicular

AP radiograph shows a faint linear sclerosis at the cortical aspect of the metaphysis ➡. There is significant osteoporosis in this patient with rheumatoid arthritis; the radiograph is diagnostic of insufficiency fracture.

Insufficiency Fractures, Appendicular

Coronal T2WI MR of the same patient shows the fracture, with impacted fragments ➡ and fluid at fracture site ➡. Proximal tibia, along with proximal femur, is a frequent site for an insufficiency fracture.

LONG BONE, CORTICALLY BASED METAPHYSEAL LESION

Stress Fracture, Adult

Stress Fracture, Adult

(Left) Coronal T1WI MR shows a basicervical stress fracture in a runner ➡. This is the classic location of a stress fracture, as opposed to an insufficiency fracture at the subcapital or intertrochanteric locations. *(Right)* AP radiograph shows sclerosis at the medial basicervical site expected for a stress fracture ➡. This patient is a marathon runner who ignored advice to rest and "ran through the pain". This led to completion of the fracture ➡.

Osteoid Osteoma

Osteoid Osteoma

(Left) AP radiograph shows a small round lytic lesion in the femoral neck metaphysis ➡. There is reactive sclerosis extending distal to the lesion ➡. The appearance is typical of intraarticular osteoid osteoma. *(Right)* Axial CT obtained during ablative procedure shows the needle entering the osteoid osteoma, which is localized at the cortex ➡. Localization of intraarticular osteoid osteoma is virtually always at the cortex. Note the adjacent thick cortical reaction.

Osteochondroma

Osteochondroma

(Left) Lateral radiograph shows normal bone extending from the metaphysis as a stalk ➡ into the exostosis. More peripherally the bone is not as organized into regular trabeculae. This continuation of marrow and cortex into the mass is the hallmark of osteochondroma. (†MSK Req). *(Right)* AP radiograph shows a patient with multiple hereditary exostoses, with the typical exophytic type ➡ as well as the sessile forms ➡, broadly based at the cortex.

LONG BONE, CORTICALLY BASED METAPHYSEAL LESION

Fibrous Dysplasia

Fibroxanthoma (Non-Ossifying Fibroma)

(Left) Axial NECT shows a cortically based metaphyseal lesion which has a ground-glass matrix ➡. The appearance of the matrix is typical of fibrous dysplasia. Although the lesion is usually located centrally, it may arise eccentrically or cortically. (Right) Lateral radiograph shows a large lytic lesion with sclerotic margins, located in the cortex of the metadiaphysis ➡. The lesion is beginning to heal, with peripheral sclerosis. Despite the size, the appearance & location are typical of NOF.

Aneurysmal Bone Cyst

Adamantinoma

(Left) AP radiograph shows a cortically based metaphyseal lytic lesion that is expanded but retains a thin cortical rim ➡. This is an ABC; these lesions usually arise eccentrically within the marrow but occasionally may arise within the cortex. (Right) AP radiograph shows a lytic lesion arising from the cortex of the distal tibial metaphysis ➡. Though the lesion appears well-marginated, it enlarged rapidly & behaved aggressively. This is an adamantinoma.

Soft Tissue Tumor Excavation (Mimic)

Langerhans Cell Histiocytosis

(Left) Axial T1 C+ MR shows a soft tissue lesion ➡ (MFH) that is adjacent to the distal femoral metaphysis, resulting in local invasion ➡. This cortical excavation results in an apparent, cortically based, lytic lesion on the radiograph. (Right) Lateral radiograph shows a lytic, cortically based lesion in the distal tibial metaphysis ➡. Although by location this lesion is most likely adamantinoma, at biopsy it proved to be LCH with an unusual presentation.

LONG BONE, SURFACE (JUXTACORTICAL) LESION

DIFFERENTIAL DIAGNOSIS

Common
- Osteosarcoma, Parosteal
- Periosteal Chondroma
- Myositis Ossificans (Mimic)

Less Common
- Osteochondroma (Mimic)
- Aneurysmal Bone Cyst (Mimic)
- Osteosarcoma, Periosteal
- Tug Lesion (Mimic)
- Avulsion Fractures (Mimic)
- Florid Reactive Periostitis & Bizarre Osteochondromatous Proliferation
- High Grade Surface Osteosarcoma
- Subperiosteal Ganglion
- Subperiosteal Abscess

Rare but Important
- Parosteal Lipoma
- Osteoma
- Osteoid Osteoma, Periosteal
- Parosteal Chondrosarcoma

ESSENTIAL INFORMATION

Key Differential Diagnosis Issues
- **Hint**: Limited number of true surface lesions
  - Mimics may be cortically based or highly expanded eccentric lesions
  - Mimics may relate to local trauma
- **Hint**: Be careful not to confuse early myositis ossificans with periosteal osteosarcoma
  - Both radiograph and biopsy may be confusing, depending on stage of lesion
  - Axial imaging & attention to zoning of ossification helps to differentiate
  - **Hint**: Myositis is much more frequently seen than periosteal osteosarcoma

Helpful Clues for Common Diagnoses
- **Osteosarcoma, Parosteal**
  - Most common surface lesion of bone
  - Mature bone formation at surface
    - When it is large, appears to "wrap around" the cortex, often with a cleft between most of the mass & the underlying bone
    - Zoning: More mature centrally than peripherally

  - **Hint**: Most extend to intramedullary space; must include this observation to ensure adequate resection
  - Location: Distal femur > proximal tibia > proximal femur > proximal humerus
- **Periosteal Chondroma**
  - a.k.a., juxtacortical chondroma
  - Matrix arising at surface of bone, extending into soft tissues; often difficult to differentiate between chondroid & osteoid
  - Scallops underlying cortex but does not involve medullary space
  - May be impossible to differentiate from periosteal osteosarcoma by imaging
    - **Hint**: Periosteal chondroma is much more common than periosteal osteosarcoma
- **Myositis Ossificans (Mimic)**
  - Mature myositis ossificans (MO) not difficult to diagnose
  - Immature myositis forms amorphous osteoid (6-8 weeks following trauma)
    - If it is adjacent to bone, may mimic periosteal or surface osteosarcoma
    - May elicit periosteal reaction & even abnormal marrow signal on MR
    - Watch for zoning of more mature bone peripherally, which is the opposite of the growing pattern of osteosarcoma

Helpful Clues for Less Common Diagnoses
- **Osteochondroma (Mimic)**
  - Usually not difficult to differentiate, but a small exostosis may mimic parosteal osteosarcoma
  - Continuation of cortex and marrow into stalk-like lesion makes the diagnosis
- **Aneurysmal Bone Cyst (Mimic)**
  - Arises from cortex or highly eccentrically in bone, so is not a true surface lesion
  - May balloon so extensively that it has an appearance of arising from the surface
  - Watch for thin rim of cortex continuing around lesion & fluid levels
- **Osteosarcoma, Periosteal**
  - Rare form of surface osteosarcoma, with low grade appearance & behavior
  - Generally produces matrix (though may not) at surface of cortex, extending into soft tissues

LONG BONE, SURFACE (JUXTACORTICAL) LESION

○ Often scallops underlying cortex, but generally does not invade marrow
- **Tug Lesion (Mimic)**
  ○ Tendinous insertion may "tug" its attachment, resulting in mimic of surface mass
    - Underlying cortex may resorb
    - Reactive soft tissue forms "mass", sometimes with reactive calcification
    - "Cortical desmoid" at posteromedial corner of distal femoral metaphysis is best known site
    - Avulsion fracture may mimic surface lesion of bone in same way
- **Florid Reactive Periostitis & Bizarre Osteochondromatous Proliferation**
  ○ Very similar appearing to mature myositis or parosteal osteosarcoma
  ○ Involves small bones of hands > feet
  ○ Likely related to trauma
- **High Grade Surface Osteosarcoma**
  ○ Tumor osteoid formation surface lesion
  ○ Osteoid is amorphous & disordered; no strong zoning to periphery is seen
  ○ Soft tissue mass, evaluated on MR, is more extensive than osteoid
  ○ Histology: Same as conventional osteosarcoma; higher grade & degree of aggressiveness than parosteal or periosteal osteosarcoma
- **Subperiosteal Ganglion**
  ○ Rare location of ganglion
  ○ Lifts the periosteum, may result in horizontal periosteal reaction formation

○ May scallop underlying cortex but is not invasive
○ Mass follows fluid signal on all sequences
- **Subperiosteal Abscess**
  ○ Raises the periosteum, soft tissue abscess
  ○ Obliterates soft tissue fat planes
  ○ Initially adjacent cortex becomes less distinct; eventually may extend into medullary space as osteomyelitis

Helpful Clues for Rare Diagnoses
- **Parosteal Lipoma**
  ○ Rare appearance of deep soft tissue lipoma
  ○ Lipoma is classic in appearance but arises immediately adjacent to surface of bone
  ○ Elicits a prominent periosteal reaction, often horizontal in relation to cortex
- **Osteoma**
  ○ Rarely occurs in long bones; generally part of a polyposis syndrome (Gardner)
  ○ Sclerotic "bumps" of dense bone arising from cortex: Hamartomatous bone
- **Osteoid Osteoma, Periosteal**
  ○ Least common site of osteoid osteoma
  ○ Soft tissue mass adjacent to & scalloping bone
  ○ Little host reactive bone formation
- **Parosteal Chondrosarcoma**
  ○ Identical to conventional chondrosarcoma, but arising on surface of bone with fibrous pseudocapsule connecting to periosteum
  ○ May cause scalloping of cortex, but generally no medullary invasion

Osteosarcoma, Parosteal

Lateral radiograph shows posterior cortical thickening ➡ without other features. Location & appearance are typical of stress fracture, for which this young man was treated, with no improvement. (†MSK Req).

Osteosarcoma, Parosteal

Axial T2WI MR on the same patient shows the cortical thickening ➡, but there is also an associated soft tissue mass ➡. The mass contains punctate ossification ➡. This is an early parosteal osteosarcoma. (†MSK Req).

LONG BONE, SURFACE (JUXTACORTICAL) LESION

Osteosarcoma, Parosteal

Periosteal Chondroma

(Left) Lateral radiograph shows an advanced parosteal osteosarcoma, with mature bone appearing to wrap around the cortex ➡, leaving a cleft where the lesion is not attached to the surface ➡. The tumor bone is more mature centrally than peripherally. *(Right)* AP radiograph shows the typical appearance of periosteal chondroma, with matrix arising from the osseous surface ➡. There is mild scalloping of the underlying cortex ➡ but not overt destruction.

Periosteal Chondroma

Periosteal Chondroma

(Left) Lateral radiograph shows a surface lesion containing faint matrix ➡ and causing minimal scalloping of the underlying cortex ➡. This is a surface lesion, without marrow involvement. *(Right)* Axial bone CT confirms the faint matrix and surface mass ➡, as well as minimal cortical scalloping ➡. Periosteal chondroma & periosteal osteosarcoma cannot be differentiated by the imaging; statistics favor the former, which was biopsy proven.

Myositis Ossificans (Mimic)

Myositis Ossificans (Mimic)

(Left) AP radiograph shows periosteal reaction ➡ & soft tissue mass containing faint matrix ➡ in a teenager. Though this could represent a surface sarcoma, it must be remembered that myositis can also elicit reaction from adjacent bone. *(Right)* Coronal T2WI FS MR of the same patient shows the high signal soft tissue "mass" that surrounds a halo of low signal material ➡. This halo is the maturing periphery of myositis; the surrounding high signal is edema. (†MSK Req).

LONG BONE, SURFACE (JUXTACORTICAL) LESION

Osteochondroma (Mimic)

Osteochondroma (Mimic)

(Left) Lateral radiograph shows an ossific mass ➡ in a position suggestive of parosteal osteosarcoma. The character of the mass, including zoning, must be assessed, usually by axial imaging, before final diagnosis is made. *(Right)* Axial bone CT of the same patient shows that the mass in fact arises from the femur, with continuous cortex and marrow extending from the bone into the mass ➡. This feature is diagnostic of osteochondroma rather than parosteal osteosarcoma.

Aneurysmal Bone Cyst (Mimic)

Aneurysmal Bone Cyst (Mimic)

(Left) Lateral radiograph shows a large lesion that appears to be surface in origin. There is apparent mild scalloping of the cortex ➡, with large soft tissue mass extending posteriorly ➡. Axial imaging is needed for further definition. *(Right)* Axial bone CT in the same patient shows that the mass arises eccentrically or from the cortex, but not the surface ➡ of the bone. There is a thin osseous rim surrounding the mass ➡. Other imaging showed fluid levels in this ABC.

Osteosarcoma, Periosteal

Osteosarcoma, Periosteal

(Left) Anteroposterior radiograph shows definite tumor osteoid formation at the osseous surface ➡ that is less mature at the surface than centrally. There is no disturbance of the underlying bone. *(Right)* Axial bone CT confirms the immature osteoid forming at the osseous surface ➡, without invasion of the underlying bone. The appearance is typical of periosteal osteosarcoma.

LONG BONE, SURFACE (JUXTACORTICAL) LESION

(Left) Axillary lateral shows heterotopic bone formation ➡ & cortical resorption at the site of the deltoid insertion ➡. This represents a "tug" lesion of the deltoid but could be mistaken for a surface lesion of bone. *(Right)* Oblique radiograph shows bone formation adjacent to & surrounding the third metatarsal ➡. Florid reactive periostitis or bizarre osteochondromatous proliferation likely arise secondary to trauma and result in surface bone formation.

Tug Lesion (Mimic)

Florid Reactive Periostitis & Bizarre Osteochondromatous Proliferation

(Left) AP radiograph shows a soft tissue tumor located immediately adjacent to the surface of the humerus ➡. It contains an osteoid matrix that appears moderately amorphous & aggressive. Differentiating between surface osteosarcoma and periosteal/parosteal osteosarcoma is difficult on the radiograph. *(Right)* Coronal T1 C+ FS MR shows the lesion ➡ to be larger than suspected by radiograph. By location & appearance, it is a high grade surface osteosarcoma.

High Grade Surface Osteosarcoma

High Grade Surface Osteosarcoma

(Left) Anteroposterior radiograph shows a surface lesion that does not contain matrix but has elicited horizontal periosteal reaction ➡. There is subtle and non-aggressive scalloping of the underlying cortex ➡. *(Right)* Axial T2WI MR confirms the surface origins and shows the lesion to be fluid signal ➡. It confirms the surface origins and the subtle cortical scalloping ➡. This proved to be an unusual surface lesion, a subperiosteal ganglion.

Subperiosteal Ganglion

Subperiosteal Ganglion

LONG BONE, SURFACE (JUXTACORTICAL) LESION

Subperiosteal Abscess

Subperiosteal Abscess

(Left) Lateral radiograph shows subtle loss of posterior cortical bone integrity ➡. There is no other overt destruction. The soft tissues show obliteration of the fat planes ➡ that would normally be expected to be present. (Right) Sagittal T1 C+ MR in the same patient confirms cortical loss ➡. There is also a large abscess arising from the subperiosteal location ➡. Yersinia pestis was cultured; plague had been reported in the region where this teenager had been camping.

Parosteal Lipoma

Parosteal Lipoma

(Left) Lateral radiograph shows fluffy bone formation arising from posterior cortex ➡ that appears to be reactive rather than tumor bone. There is a faint suggestion of fat density surrounding it ➡. (†MSK Req). (Right) Axial bone CT in the same patient shows the reactive bone formation ➡ and the surrounding lipoma ➡. Occasionally when a lipoma arises adjacent to a long bone, it elicits this type of reaction. It is termed parosteal lipoma. (†MSK Req).

Osteoma

Osteoma

(Left) AP radiograph shows sclerotic, rounded, normal bone arising from the cortex ➡; these are osteomas. An osteoma involving a long bone should raise the question of a polyposis syndrome. This patient had "hundreds" of colonic polyps. (Right) Axial T1 C+ FS MR from the same patient shows a small osteoma ➡ but also shows a huge soft tissue mass ➡. The mass was low signal on all sequences and shows minimal enhancement; this is a classic desmoid tumor.

LONG BONE, CENTRAL DIAPHYSEAL LESION, NON-AGGRESSIVE

DIFFERENTIAL DIAGNOSIS

Common
- Enchondroma
- Paget Disease
- Langerhans Cell Histiocytosis (LCH)
- Fibrous Dysplasia
- Unicameral Bone Cyst (UBC)
- Fibroxanthoma (Non-Ossifying Fibroma)
- Aneurysmal Bone Cyst, Thin Bones
- Chronic Osteomyelitis

Less Common
- Sickle Cell Anemia
- Bone Infarct
- Radiation Osteonecrosis
- Hyperparathyroidism, Brown Tumor
- Tuberculosis
- Fungal Osteomyelitis

Rare but Important
- Vascular Tumors
- Neurofibromatosis
- Desmoplastic Fibroma
- Tuberous Sclerosis
- Mastocytosis

ESSENTIAL INFORMATION

Key Differential Diagnosis Issues
- Non-aggressive central diaphyseal lesions are much more common in 1st three decades
- **Hint**: "Common" lesions are MUCH more common than others
  - Very few choices of diagnoses in adults
    - Enchondroma, Paget disease, chronic osteomyelitis
  - Relatively few choices in children
    - LCH, Fibrous dysplasia, UBC, chronic osteomyelitis
- Many of the other lesions in the differential require special circumstances
  - Gigantic NOF
  - Thin bone location of NOF or ABC
  - Underlying abnormality: Radiation, renal osteodystrophy

Helpful Clues for Common Diagnoses
- **Enchondroma**
  - Adult lesion, generally in metaphysis
  - Common lesion, so diaphyseal location is also relatively common
  - Usually some chondroid matrix is present, but may be lytic
  - May scallop endosteum, but otherwise is or appears non-aggressive
  - Often an incidental finding; usually asymptomatic
- **Paget Disease**
  - Common in adults
  - Lesion usually originates at subchondral bone and proceeds into diaphysis
    - May be extensive, involving the majority of diaphysis
  - Lesion may originate at mid-diaphysis (usually tibia) and extend proximally or distally
    - With diaphyseal origin, lesion usually begins in anterior cortex
  - Lesion always results in bone enlargement
  - Appearance ranges from lytic to mixed lytic/sclerotic
    - Trabeculae appear coarsened & disordered, but usually overall appearance is not aggressive
    - Leading edge of lesion has straight sclerotic line
- **Langerhans Cell Histiocytosis (LCH)**
  - Lesion of childhood
  - Often polyostotic, with axial & flat bones involved as well as long bones
  - Long bone lesions may be metaphyseal or epiphyseal, but diaphyseal is common
  - Appearance ranges from lytic geographic (non-aggressive) to extremely aggressive
- **Fibrous Dysplasia**
  - Lesion of childhood and young adults
  - Often polyostotic, with flat bones & skull frequently involved
  - Long bone lesions usually central & diaphyseal
    - Metaphyseal & epiphyseal extension is common
    - Central location is most common, but cortical lesions occur as well
  - Mild expansion of bone with thinning of endosteal cortex
  - Subtle "ground-glass" matrix is most common, though lesion may be lytic
  - Bone is soft, resulting in bowing deformities
- **Unicameral Bone Cyst (UBC)**
  - Common; generally a lesion of childhood

LONG BONE, CENTRAL DIAPHYSEAL LESION, NON-AGGRESSIVE

- Adult lesions tend to be pelvic or humeral
  - Lesion begins in metaphysis
    - As it becomes less active, metaphysis grows away, leaving it in diaphyseal position
  - Lytic lesion with mild expansion of bone & thinning of endosteal cortex
  - Usually asymptomatic unless develops pathologic fracture
    - Fracture may result in a "floating fragment", pathognomonic for UBC
- **Fibroxanthoma (Non-Ossifying Fibroma)**
  - Common lesion of childhood and young adulthood
  - Generally metaphyseal & cortically based lesion
  - It is the exceptional cases that fit into the central diaphyseal differential
    - Giant NOF may occupy the entire width of a long bone & extend well into diaphysis
    - NOF in a thin bone (ulna, fibula) may occupy entire width of bone
  - Lytic & well-circumscribed when active
  - Natural history is to heal in with sclerosis, then remodel to normal bone
- **Aneurysmal Bone Cyst, Thin Bones**
  - Common lesion of childhood & young adults
  - Generally eccentric & metadiaphyseal
  - Exception is in thin bones (ulna, fibula) where it occupies entire width
- **Chronic Osteomyelitis**

  - May be diaphyseal in either child or adult, usually from direct trauma
  - Chronicity results in sclerotic margin & surrounding reactive bone formation

Helpful Clues for Less Common Diagnoses
- **Sickle Cell Anemia**
  - Bone infarcts may appear lytic and non-aggressive, though often not visualized on radiograph
- **Radiation Osteonecrosis**
  - Mixed lytic & sclerotic disordered bone
  - No soft tissue mass or cortical disruptions
- **Hyperparathyroidism, Brown Tumor**
  - Brown tumor may occupy central diaphysis
  - Generally well-marginated, though not sclerotic
  - Surrounding bone is osteopenic & trabeculae are coarsened
- **Tuberculosis**
  - Destruction tends to be slower & less aggressive than bacterial osteomyelitis
    - Lesion may appear well-defined & have little reactive change in host bone
    - Fungal osteomyelitis appears similar

Helpful Clues for Rare Diagnoses
- **Vascular Tumors**
  - Range from non-aggressive to aggressive
  - Lower extremities predominate
- **Neurofibromatosis**
  - Bone dysplasia results in pseudarthroses & deformities

Enchondroma

Lateral radiograph shows typical enchondroma with punctate chondroid matrix located centrally within the femoral diaphysis. There is a small region of endosteal scalloping ➡ but no other suggestion of aggressiveness.

Paget Disease

Lateral radiograph shows an expanded lytic/sclerotic lesion arising in the diaphysis of the tibia with a sharply marginated leading edge ➡. Once Paget disease fully expands, it may appear central.

LONG BONE, CENTRAL DIAPHYSEAL LESION, NON-AGGRESSIVE

(Left) Anteroposterior radiograph shows a central lytic lesion with narrow zone of transition ➡. It is mildly expanded and has slight endosteal scalloping. LCH has a range of presentations but often is less aggressive. **(Right)** Anteroposterior radiograph shows a lytic & ground-glass density mildly expanded central lesion of the diaphysis which significantly thins the cortex ➡. There is a daughter lesion seen proximally ➡. This is typical fibrous dysplasia.

Langerhans Cell Histiocytosis (LCH)

Fibrous Dysplasia

(Left) Anteroposterior radiograph shows a central lytic lesion in the diaphysis of the humerus which has mild endosteal scalloping ➡. UBC often is metadiaphyseal; purely diaphyseal location such as this is somewhat unusual. **(Right)** Anteroposterior radiograph shows a lytic, well-marginated lesion located slightly eccentrically within the diaphysis. NOF may appear to be more central when it is large and be more difficult to diagnose.

Unicameral Bone Cyst (UBC)

Fibroxanthoma (Non-Ossifying Fibroma)

(Left) Anteroposterior radiograph shows a lytic lesion in the fibular diaphysis that is expanded but not aggressive. This is an ABC, which may become centrally located when expanding the width of a thin bone such as the fibula. **(Right)** AP radiograph shows mild expansion of the fibula, with endosteal thickening nearly obliterating the marrow space ➡, as well as thick cortical reactive bone. The patient had hit the leg 1 year earlier & developed chronic osteomyelitis.

Aneurysmal Bone Cyst, Thin Bones

Chronic Osteomyelitis

LONG BONE, CENTRAL DIAPHYSEAL LESION, NON-AGGRESSIVE

Sickle Cell Anemia

Bone Infarct

(Left) Lateral radiograph shows extensive chronic bone infarct involving the tibial diaphysis in a sickle cell patient. There is mixed lytic & sclerotic bone which has a disordered appearance. *(Right)* AP radiograph shows a non-aggressive lytic lesion ➡ containing pseudotrabeculations ➡. This is a nonspecific appearance that proved to be bone infarct. When dystrophic calcification is present, the diagnosis of infarct is more straightforward.

Radiation Osteonecrosis

Hyperparathyroidism, Brown Tumor

(Left) Anteroposterior radiograph shows mixed lytic/sclerotic disordered bone throughout the entire humerus ➡ in a patient who received whole bone RT. This is typical of radiation osteonecrosis, along with the radiation-induced osteosarcoma ➡. *(Right)* Lateral radiograph shows diffusely abnormal bone density, with coarsened trabeculae (HPTH). There is abnormal bowing, as well as several hyperossified round lesions ➡, which are Brown tumors.

Tuberculosis

Desmoplastic Fibroma

(Left) AP radiograph shows a lytic diaphyseal lesion with a narrow zone of transition and regular periosteal reaction ➡. There is no other host reaction. This is TB osteomyelitis in a patient who also had pulmonary disease. *(Right)* Lateral radiograph shows a non-aggressive lytic expanded lesion in the fibular diaphysis. There is pseudotrabeculation ➡ & a pathologic fracture ➡. Lesion is predominantly low signal on MR but enhances, typical of desmoid.

LONG BONE, DIAPHYSEAL LESION, AGGRESSIVE: ADULT

DIFFERENTIAL DIAGNOSIS

Common
- Osteomyelitis
- Metastases, Bone Marrow
- Multiple Myeloma (MM)
- Lymphoma
- Ewing Sarcoma
- Plasmacytoma
- Hyperparathyroidism, Brown Tumor

Less Common
- Chondrosarcoma, Conventional
- Malignant Fibrous Histiocytoma, Bone
- Fibrosarcoma
- Osteosarcoma, Conventional
- Fibrous Dysplasia
- Angiosarcoma, Osseous

Rare but Important
- Adamantinoma
- Hemophilia: MSK Complications
- Radiation-Induced Sarcoma
- Tertiary Syphilis

ESSENTIAL INFORMATION

Key Differential Diagnosis Issues
- **Hint**: Most common diagnoses in this differential have been called "small round blue cell" lesions
  - All have similar appearance on radiograph: Permeative, lytic, with periosteal reaction, cortical breakthrough, & soft tissue mass
  - These lesions include both benign & malignant entities
    - Osteomyelitis
    - Metastases
    - Myeloma lymphoma
    - Ewing sarcoma
  - MR may help differentiate by showing abscess, but tumor necrosis may appear similar
- **Hint**: Most infiltrative lesions may initially be so permeative that radiograph appears normal
  - MR or PET/CT makes diagnosis

Helpful Clues for Common Diagnoses
- **Osteomyelitis**
  - Diaphyseal location seen more frequently in adults than children, particularly following trauma

  - Permeative change may be highly aggressive, with aggressive-appearing periosteal reaction
  - May not be able to differentiate from aggressive tumor
  - May elicit reactive bone formation, including endosteal thickening
  - MR demonstrates abscess & fascial fluid
- **Metastases, Bone Marrow**
  - May be highly permeative & therefore extremely subtle
  - Often more apparent with MR or PET/CT
- **Multiple Myeloma (MM)**
  - MM may be so highly infiltrative that it is inapparent on radiograph
    - May appear as osteoporosis
    - Usually discovered on MR or PET/CT
    - Eventually develops lytic lesion that appears more focal than permeative
  - Plasmacytoma generally arises in pelvis, spine, or metaphyses
    - Rarely may be diaphyseal, particularly if pubic ramus is considered a diaphyseal equivalent
- **Lymphoma**
  - Frequently found in long bone diaphyses
  - Highly permeative; may have cortical breakthrough with large & infiltrative soft tissue mass
  - May elicit prominent bone reaction, including endosteal thickening
  - May have a bony sequestrum
- **Ewing Sarcoma**
  - Age range is 5-30, so Ewing sarcoma may be seen in young adults as well as children
  - Involvement of long bones is generally in the younger portion of age range, but diaphyseal involvement may still be found in adults
  - Generally arises in mid-diaphysis, with an aggressive permeative pattern
  - Aggressive periosteal reaction, cortical breakthrough, often large soft tissue mass
  - May elicit prominent reactive bone formation, located within osseous margins but not soft tissues
    - May elicit dense endosteal thickening
- **Hyperparathyroidism, Brown Tumor**
  - Brown tumor is generally geographic rather than permeative

LONG BONE, DIAPHYSEAL LESION, AGGRESSIVE: ADULT

- Surrounding bone may appear so abnormal as to mimic aggressive process
- Watch for other resorptive patterns to verify HPTH

Helpful Clues for Less Common Diagnoses
- **Chondrosarcoma, Conventional**
  - Common lesion, but most frequently metaphyseal or meta-diaphyseal
    - Diaphyseal chondrosarcoma is unusual
  - If permeative or aggressive, likely higher grade lesion than is usually seen
  - Chondroid matrix suggests diagnosis, but lesion may be entirely lytic
- **Malignant Fibrous Histiocytoma, Bone**
  - Primary MFH metaphyseal/diaphyseal
    - Secondary MFH usually metaphyseal, associated with bone infarcts
  - Lytic, permeative, periosteal reaction, cortical breakthrough
- **Fibrosarcoma**
  - Unusual lesion in diaphysis of long bone
  - Rarely fibrous dysplasia may degenerate into fibrosarcoma
    - Appearance is of fibrous dysplasia (ground-glass matrix, central diaphysis) with superimposed destructive change
- **Osteosarcoma, Conventional**
  - Common lesion, but usually metaphyseal or meta-diaphyseal
    - Diaphyseal osteosarcoma is unusual
  - Permeative, aggressive, with cortical breakthrough & soft tissue mass

- Generally has amorphous osteoid matrix in bone & soft tissues, though may be lytic
- **Fibrous Dysplasia**
  - Long bone lesions may be lytic or have ground-glass matrix
  - Expanded, thin cortex but no reaction
  - Rarely will degenerate to fibrosarcoma
  - Pathologic fracture may make the lesion appear more aggressive
- **Angiosarcoma, Osseous**
  - Lytic permeative aggressive lesion
  - Predilection for lower extremities
  - Often polyostotic

Helpful Clues for Rare Diagnoses
- **Adamantinoma**
  - Diaphyseal/meta-diaphyseal, tibia
  - Lesion originates in cortex, may be aggressive but usually not permeative
  - May become malignant with associated increase in degree of aggressiveness
- **Hemophilia: MSK Complications**
  - Pseudotumor may appear highly aggressive, with periosteal reaction & cortical scalloping
    - Subperiosteal or cortical bleeds
    - Femur frequently involved long bone
- **Radiation-Induced Sarcoma**
  - Whole long bone radiation may result in radiation osteonecrosis
    - Radiation-induced sarcoma may arise (average 10-14 years post treatment)

Osteomyelitis

Oblique radiograph shows a highly permeative lytic lesion of the fibula, with periosteal reaction ➡ and cortical breakthrough ➡. Radiograph cannot differentiate between aggressive tumor & osteomyelitis.

Metastases, Bone Marrow

Anteroposterior radiograph shows a subtle permeative mid-humeral lesion with endosteal scalloping ➡. The extent of the lesion cannot be determined on this image. It proved to be metastatic fibrosarcoma.

LONG BONE, DIAPHYSEAL LESION, AGGRESSIVE: ADULT

(Left) Sagittal STIR and AP radiograph of the humerus shows a large humeral diaphyseal lesion detected on MR that is not visible on radiograph. The marrow infiltration in myeloma may be so subtle & permeative as to be detected only on MR or PET/CT. *(Right)* Lateral radiograph of the femur shows a large diaphyseal permeative lesion, eliciting reactive bone in the form of endosteal thickening ➡, while thinning the endosteum in another region ➡. This lesion is lymphoma.

Multiple Myeloma (MM)

Lymphoma

(Left) Lateral radiograph shows an aggressive permeative lesion with associated periosteal reaction ➡ in a 23 year old. The radiograph does not differentiate between osteomyelitis, lymphoma, Ewing sarcoma, and other such diaphyseal lesions. *(Right)* Axial T2WI MR in the same patient shows the diaphyseal lesion to have a huge soft tissue mass ➡ with associated edema. No abscess was shown post-contrast. The lesion proved to be Ewing sarcoma.

Ewing Sarcoma

Ewing Sarcoma

(Left) AP radiograph shows a lytic expanded moderately aggressive lesion occupying the entire superior pubic ramus ➡, a diaphyseal equivalent. Appearance is typical for plasmacytoma, which frequently arises in the pelvis. *(Right)* Oblique radiograph shows a lytic, expanded, diaphyseal lesion that has thinned the endosteum and appears moderately aggressive ➡. The bone density is abnormal and patchy; the findings are typical of a brown tumor of HPTH.

Plasmacytoma

Hyperparathyroidism, Brown Tumor

LONG BONE, DIAPHYSEAL LESION, AGGRESSIVE: ADULT

Chondrosarcoma, Conventional

Malignant Fibrous Histiocytoma, Bone

(Left) AP radiograph shows a large, lytic, expanded, permeative lesion occupying the diaphysis. There is a pathologic fracture, with matrix extruded into the soft tissues. The matrix is chondroid, typical of chondrosarcoma. *(Right)* AP radiograph shows a highly aggressive mid-diaphyseal lesion, with cortical breakthrough, soft tissue mass, and periosteal reaction. The diagnosis is MFH, surprising only because it occurred in a teenager.

Fibrosarcoma

Osteosarcoma, Conventional

(Left) Lateral radiograph shows underlying fibrous dysplasia (FD), with correction of bowing deformity. A highly aggressive fibrosarcoma is superimposed ➡. FD will rarely degenerate into this malignant tumor. *(Right)* AP radiograph shows an aggressive, permeative, diaphyseal lesion that has cortical breakthrough & is producing a tumor osteoid ➡. Though it is unusual for an osteosarcoma to arise in the mid-diaphysis, there is no other possible diagnosis.

Fibrous Dysplasia

Radiation-Induced Sarcoma

(Left) AP radiograph shows long-term fibrous dysplasia with ground-glass matrix, involving the entire humeral diaphysis. There is focal expansion that makes this case of fibrous dysplasia appear more aggressive ➡. This proved to be a healing fx. *(Right)* AP radiograph shows a short humerus with abnormal marrow: Radiation osteonecrosis. The mid-diaphysis shows an aggressive radiation-induced osteosarcoma containing tumor bone in the soft tissue mass ➡.

LONG BONE, DIAPHYSEAL LESION, AGGRESSIVE: CHILD

DIFFERENTIAL DIAGNOSIS

Common
- Osteomyelitis, Pediatric
- Ewing Sarcoma
- Langerhans Cell Histiocytosis (LCH)
- Leukemia
- Osteosarcoma
- Metastases, Bone Marrow
- Lymphoma

Less Common
- Sickle Cell Anemia
- Malignant Fibrous Histiocytoma, Bone
- Chondrosarcoma, Conventional
- Adamantinoma
- Radiation-Induced Sarcoma

Rare but Important
- Hemophilia
- Congenital Syphilis

ESSENTIAL INFORMATION

Key Differential Diagnosis Issues
- **Hint**: Most common of these lesions fall into the small, round, blue cell category
  - All have an appearance that may be indistinguishable from one another
  - Must consider each of these diagnoses with this aggressive appearance
    - Osteomyelitis
    - Ewing sarcoma
    - Langerhans cell histiocytosis
    - Leukemia
    - Metastases
    - Lymphoma
  - **Hint**: Note that in each of these cases, lesion may be polyostotic
- **Hint**: Ewing sarcoma & osteosarcoma usually have a distinct appearance from one another
  - Occasionally they can be indistinguishable, if
    - Osteosarcoma is diaphyseal & lytic
    - Ewing sarcoma is metadiaphyseal & has sclerotic reactive bone formation
    - **Hint**: In these cases, watch for tumor osteoid formation in soft tissue mass; this can only occur in osteosarcoma
- **Hint**: Rarely, four of these lesions may be aggressive, yet induce endosteal & cortical thickening

- Osteomyelitis
- Ewing sarcoma
- Lymphoma
- Chondrosarcoma

Helpful Clues for Common Diagnoses
- **Osteomyelitis, Pediatric**
  - Usually metaphyseal in children, but diaphyseal with direct trauma
  - Highly aggressive & permeative, often with reactive sclerosis & periosteal reaction
- **Ewing Sarcoma**
  - Common in long bones in children
  - Highly aggressive permeative lesion, cortical breakthrough & soft tissue mass
  - Elicits reactive bone formation
    - May have appearance of tumor osteoid & mimic osteosarcoma
    - Reactive bone NOT in soft tissue mass in Ewing, but present in osteosarcoma
  - May appear polyostotic since it may present with osseous metastases
- **Langerhans Cell Histiocytosis (LCH)**
  - Ranges in appearance between geographic non-aggressive and highly aggressive
    - When aggressive, is permeative & may have soft tissue mass
    - May be indistinguishable from the malignant lesions in the differential
  - Often polyostotic
  - Beveled edge of skull lesion may help distinguish
- **Leukemia**
  - Usually polyostotic
  - May be so highly infiltrative that it is not visible on radiograph; MR makes diagnosis
- **Osteosarcoma**
  - Common lesion, but usually is metaphyseal
  - Less frequently is diaphyseal; if it is lytic in this location, may not be distinguished from other lesions in the differential
  - Usually some tumor osteoid is visible
- **Metastases, Bone Marrow**
  - Usually polyostotic in children
  - Metaphyseal is more frequent, but may be diaphyseal
  - Neuroblastoma is most frequent in children
- **Lymphoma**
  - 50% of childhood lymphomas are polyostotic at presentation

○ Highly aggressive; metaphyseal more frequent than diaphyseal

Helpful Clues for Less Common Diagnoses

- **Sickle Cell Anemia**
  - ○ Early bone infarcts (particularly dactylitis) present with periosteal reaction
  - ○ With evolution of infarct, will see mixed lytic & sclerotic pattern
    - Often longitudinal, involving entire diaphysis
    - Remember that bone infarct need not be serpiginous and subchondral, especially in sickle cell patients
- **Malignant Fibrous Histiocytoma, Bone**
  - ○ Unusual lesion in children, may be seen in teenager
  - ○ Aggressive, may be metaphyseal or diaphyseal
  - ○ No other distinguishing characteristics
- **Chondrosarcoma, Conventional**
  - ○ Uncommon in children
  - ○ Should be considered if subtle matrix is seen in diaphyseal lesion of teenager
  - ○ May induce endosteal thickening rather than showing cortical breakthrough
- **Adamantinoma**
  - ○ Almost invariably tibial metadiaphysis; cortically based
  - ○ Generally only moderately aggressive initially
    - May become aggressive & malignant
- **Radiation-Induced Sarcoma**

○ Generally at least 7 years post radiation (RT), so seen in teenagers
○ Highly aggressive region in bone that shows underlying radiation-related abnormality
  - Usually osteosarcoma; tumor osteoid
○ Consider locations likely to be radiated in childhood
  - Long bones (Ewing sarcoma, lymphoma)
  - Spine (Wilms tumor, leukemia)
○ Watch for underlying signs of radiation osteonecrosis
  - Mixed lytic & sclerotic, disordered bone
○ Watch for growth deformities associated with radiation
  - Long bone may be short if subjected to whole bone radiation (physes at risk for vascular injury in RT)
  - Spine may develop scoliosis if spine not completely included in radiation field
○ Watch for port-like distribution of osseous abnormalities, indicating RT

Helpful Clues for Rare Diagnoses

- **Hemophilia**
  - ○ Pseudotumor appears aggressive: Soft tissue, intraosseous, & subperiosteal bleeds
  - ○ Femur most commonly involved long bone
- **Congenital Syphilis**
  - ○ Periosteal reaction, infiltrative appearance

Osteomyelitis, Pediatric

AP radiograph shows a highly aggressive lesion in the radial diaphysis ➡ in a 7 year old. There is prominent periosteal reaction and cortical breakthrough. The fat planes are obliterated, indicating osteomyelitis.

Osteomyelitis, Pediatric

Axial T1 C+ MR on the same patient shows infiltration of the marrow of the radius ➡ and a large soft tissue abscess ➡, confirming the diagnosis of osteomyelitis. This child had direct trauma to the forearm.

LONG BONE, DIAPHYSEAL LESION, AGGRESSIVE: CHILD

Ewing Sarcoma

Langerhans Cell Histiocytosis (LCH)

(Left) Lateral radiograph shows a permeative mid-diaphyseal lesion in a 10 year old. There is periosteal reaction ➡ and a large soft tissue mass ➡; this is a classic age & appearance for Ewing sarcoma. *(Right)* Lateral radiograph shows a highly permeative diaphyseal lesion with prominent periosteal reaction ➡, cortical breakthrough, & soft tissue mass ➡ in an 8 year old. This case appears as aggressive as the previous case of Ewing sarcoma but proved to be LCH.

Leukemia

Osteosarcoma

(Left) AP radiograph shows diffuse osteopenia in both femoral diaphyses ➡ along lucent metaphyseal lines ➡ in a 5 year old. Though no periosteal reaction is seen, this must be interpreted as aggressive; leukemia was proven. *(Right)* Lateral radiograph shows a highly aggressive mid-diaphyseal humeral lesion with Codman triangle ➡, an aggressive periosteal reaction. There is tumor osteoid forming in the soft tissue mass ➡, diagnostic of osteosarcoma.

Metastases, Bone Marrow

Lymphoma

(Left) Lateral radiograph shows a permeative lesion occupying the entire length of the ulna, with extensive periosteal reaction ➡. This 6 month old patient has medulloblastoma metastases. *(Right)* AP radiograph shows a lytic lesion with reactive sclerosis occupying the entire diaphysis and metaphysis of the femur in a 7 year old African American child ➡. There is periosteal reaction and soft tissue mass. The lesion is polyostotic; it proved to be lymphoma.

LONG BONE, DIAPHYSEAL LESION, AGGRESSIVE: CHILD

Sickle Cell Anemia

Malignant Fibrous Histiocytoma, Bone

(Left) AP radiograph shows periosteal reaction ➡ and a permeative appearance in most of the metacarpals and phalanges in the hand of this 1 year old African American child. This is sickle cell dactylitis. *(Right)* AP radiograph shows a lytic permeative lesion occupying the mid-diaphysis in a 13 year old. The lesion is aggressive, with cortical breakthrough and soft tissue mass and prominent periosteal reaction. MFH is rare in children but certainly does occur.

Chondrosarcoma, Conventional

Chondrosarcoma, Conventional

(Left) Lateral radiograph shows mild expansion of the diaphysis ➡, with endosteal thickening ➡ in a 17 year old. This is suggestive of osteomyelitis or Ewing sarcoma, but chondrosarcoma must also be considered. *(Right)* Axial NECT of the same patient shows endosteal thickening, with a central chondroid matrix ➡. This matrix makes the diagnosis of chondrosarcoma. It is an unusual diagnosis in teenagers but must be considered.

Adamantinoma

Adamantinoma

(Left) AP radiograph shows a lytic lesion in the diaphysis of the tibia of a 17 year old. The lesion proved to be entirely restricted to the cortex ➡, which is typical of adamantinoma. Note the pathologic fracture ➡. *(Right)* Axial T1WI MR of the same patient shows that the tibial lesion is indeed based entirely in the cortex ➡. The marrow is not entirely normal, suggesting involvement, which contributes to the aggressive appearance and behavior of this lesion. (†MSK Req).

LONG BONE, AGGRESSIVE DIAPHYSEAL LESION WITH ENDOSTEAL THICKENING

DIFFERENTIAL DIAGNOSIS

Common
- Osteomyelitis
- Chondrosarcoma

Less Common
- Lymphoma
- Ewing Sarcoma

ESSENTIAL INFORMATION

Key Differential Diagnosis Issues
- Note: This discussion of endosteal thickening does **not** include non-aggressive lesions
  - Stress fracture, stress reaction, & osteoid osteoma will show focal diaphyseal endosteal thickening
    - Thickening should not be circumferential, as it is listed in diagnoses of this differential
- Note: All lesions in this differential diagnosis may appear much more aggressive than shown in this discussion
  - All may show permeative osseous destruction, aggressive periosteal reaction, cortical breakthrough, and soft tissue mass
- Purpose of the differential is to remind us that each of these lesions in the differential may have a non-aggressive appearance as one of their manifestations
- **Hint**: Dense endosteal thickening should force at least a consideration of these diagnoses

- If not considered, endosteal thickening in one of these lesions may lull the reader into thinking it is a benign process
- MR should be performed to further define lesion

Helpful Clues for Common Diagnoses
- **Osteomyelitis**
  - Dense reactive bone formation, located both at the periosteum & endosteum
  - Underlying lytic lesion may show serpiginous tracking, proving the diagnosis
- **Chondrosarcoma**
  - Most are low grade & metaphyseal at presentation
  - Need not have radiographically evident chondroid matrix
  - Underlying lesion may not appear alarming
    - May appear rather geographic
    - May be so permeative as to not be visible radiographically
  - Endosteal thickening is common in these metadiaphyseal lesions
    - In correct age group (30-60 years), must alert reader to possibility of chondrosarcoma

Helpful Clues for Less Common Diagnoses
- **Lymphoma & Ewing Sarcoma**
  - Most frequently has aggressive appearance
  - Permeative change may be extremely subtle, with only diaphyseal endosteal thickening seen
  - Sequestrum suggests lymphoma

Osteomyelitis

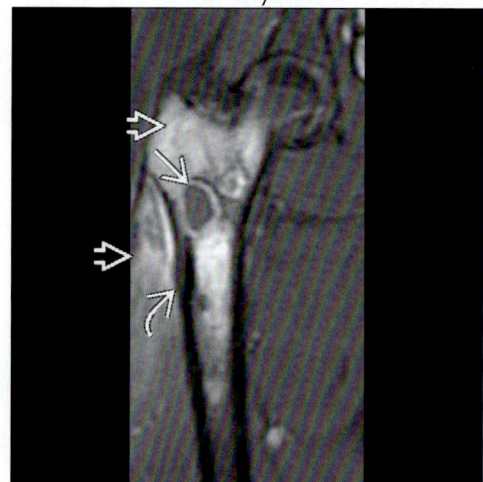

Lateral radiograph shows permeative change throughout the proximal femur ➡, along with a focal marginated lytic lesion ⬂. There is dense periosteal & endosteal reaction ➡, all typical of osteomyelitis.

Osteomyelitis

Coronal T1 C+ FS MR in the same patient shows a focal fluid collection ➡, diffuse marrow, & soft tissue edema ⬂ and confirms the thick cortical reactive bone formation ➡. Staphylococcus was cultured.

LONG BONE, AGGRESSIVE DIAPHYSEAL LESION WITH ENDOSTEAL THICKENING

Chondrosarcoma

Chondrosarcoma

(Left) AP radiograph shows chondroid matrix ➡ with a surrounding permeative lytic lesion ➡, indicating chondrosarcoma. Note the associated dense endosteal & periosteal reaction ➡. *(Right)* AP radiograph shows dense, regular endosteal & periosteal reaction ➡. There is an extremely subtle permeative change in the adjacent marrow. No matrix is seen. The diagnosis of chondrosarcoma is difficult to make here, but age, location, & reaction should be suggestive.

Lymphoma

Lymphoma

(Left) Anteroposterior radiograph shows a permeative lytic lesion centrally within the marrow, associated with dense thick endosteal & periosteal reaction ➡. *(Right)* Lateral radiograph of the same patient shows not only the cortical reaction ➡, but also endosteal scalloping ➡. The permeative central lesion is obvious. There is also a small sequestrum ➡ present; this is a finding that has been described in primary lymphoma of bone, though it is also seen in osteomyelitis.

Ewing Sarcoma

Ewing Sarcoma

(Left) AP radiograph shows a lytic permeative lesion in the meta-diaphysis ➡ that has elicited dense periosteal and endosteal reaction ➡. This is a child, and the diagnosis should be either Ewing sarcoma or osteomyelitis; the former was proven at biopsy. *(Right)* Lateral radiograph shows thick, regular endosteal and periosteal bone formation ➡. There is no obvious marrow lesion, and this might be dismissed as stress reaction. However, Ewing sarcoma must be considered and was proven.

LONG BONE, CORTICALLY BASED DIAPHYSEAL LESION, SCLEROTIC

DIFFERENTIAL DIAGNOSIS

Common
- Stress Fracture, Adult
- Tibial Stress Syndrome
- Adductor Insertion Avulsion Syndrome
- Stress Fracture, Pediatric
- Osteoid Osteoma
- Fibroxanthoma (Non-Ossifying Fibroma)
- Metastases, Bone Marrow
- Chronic Osteomyelitis (Brodie Abscess)
- Stress Fracture Related to Bisphosphonate Use

Less Common
- Melorheostosis
- Fibrous Dysplasia

Rare but Important
- Osteoma
- Paget Disease

ESSENTIAL INFORMATION

Key Differential Diagnosis Issues
- Most urgent diagnoses on this list relate to those at risk for fracture completion
  - Stress reaction needs to be evaluated by MR for fracture; must be protected
  - Stress fracture needs MR evaluation for extent & to determine treatment
- **Hint**: Maintain a high index of suspicion of stress reaction/fracture in subtrochanteric region in patients on bisphosphonates
- **Hint**: Remember the classic differential for focal diaphyseal cortical sclerosis: Osteoid osteoma, stress fracture (reaction), Brodie abscess

Helpful Clues for Common Diagnoses
- **Stress Fracture, Adult or Pediatric**
  - Common, especially in tibia
  - Results from increased or unaccustomed activities leading to abnormal stresses on bone
    - Repetitive axial loading
    - Abnormal biomechanics
    - Excessive muscular forces
  - Stress reaction is first abnormality seen
    - Cortical sclerotic focus of bone remodeling
  - If not protected at stage of stress reaction, develops stress fracture

- Radiographs have range of appearance, depending on stage
  - Initially, focus of sclerotic cortical thickening →
  - Linear fracture line sclerosis
- MR
  - Edema in marrow, cortex, and tissues adjacent to cortex
  - Fracture line usually seen well as linear low signal on T1 or fluid sensitive sequences, surrounded by edema
- **Tibial Stress Syndrome/Adductor Insertion Avulsion Syndrome**
  - Results from repetitive stress at periosteal insertion of tendons
  - → Traction periostitis
    - Site of medial soleus insertion at posteromedial tibia → "shin splints"
    - Site of adductor insertion at medial femoral diaphysis → "thigh splints"
  - Radiographs show a spectrum of abnormalities, depending on stage & longevity of injury
    - Normal
    - Subtle periostitis
    - Focal sclerosis
  - MR shows marrow edema & linear fluid signal along the outer cortex
    - Evaluate MR carefully for evidence of fracture
    - As long as no fracture line is shown, recovery is made with rest
    - In continuum with stress fracture, which may require more aggressive therapy; differentiating the two is crucial
- **Osteoid Osteoma**
  - Diaphyseal osteoid osteomas occur in the cortex
    - May be at the surface of cortex or deep, at junction of cortex & marrow
    - Those that are deep are often closely associated with a nutrient vessel; do not confuse the vessel with the nidus
  - Lytic nidus may contain a small sclerotic central focus
  - Lesion elicits tremendous cortical reaction, both periosteal and endosteal
    - Reaction may obscure the nidus completely, making it impossible to differentiate on radiograph

LONG BONE, CORTICALLY BASED DIAPHYSEAL LESION, SCLEROTIC

- Axial imaging differentiates osteoid osteoma from stress fracture & Brodie abscess
- **Fibroxanthoma (Non-Ossifying Fibroma)**
  - Common lesion in children, generally metadiaphyseal
  - Cortically based except in small-diameter bones such as fibula
  - With skeletal maturation, natural history is for NOF to heal, sclerosing from peripheral to central
  - Eventually most revert to completely normal bone
- **Metastases, Bone Marrow**
  - Rare cortical metastases are usually due to either lung or breast primaries
  - Either may be lytic or sclerotic
  - Weakens the bone, even when sclerotic; at risk for fracture
- **Chronic Osteomyelitis (Brodie Abscess)**
  - May be within cortex; generally well-defined borders
  - Elicit prominent cortical reaction; may be difficult to differentiate from stress reaction or osteoid osteoma
- **Stress Fracture Related to Bisphosphonate Use**
  - Bisphosphonates inhibit osteoclasts, slowing osteoporosis
    - Also inhibit bone turnover; it is suspected that this weakens bone
  - Fractures distinctively located in the subtrochanteric femur
    - Initial appearance: Focus of cortical sclerosis lateral cortex at junction of proximal & middle 3rd of femur
    - Generally bilateral, though may develop at different rates
    - With minor trauma, develops a transverse fracture
  - Patients have prodromal pain (groin, thigh)
    - **Hint**: Watch for lateral cortical abnormality on pelvic imaging (usually at base of image)
    - Need MR to determine risk of fracture
  - Patients need protection against fracture & probable termination of drug

Helpful Clues for Less Common Diagnoses
- **Melorheostosis**
  - Cortical & endosteal sclerosis; "dripping candle wax" pattern
  - Generally monomelic & may follow sclerotomal distribution
- **Fibrous Dysplasia**
  - May be cortically based, but generally not sclerotic with that presentation

Helpful Clues for Rare Diagnoses
- **Osteoma**
  - Rare involvement of long bones; when present, suspect polyposis (Gardner syndrome)
- **Paget Disease**
  - Rare initial lesion at tibial cortex, mid-diaphyseal; generally not sclerotic since it is an early lesion

Stress Fracture, Adult

Lateral radiograph shows subtle cortical sclerosis ➡ at the proximal tibial diaphysis. There is no other characterizing finding, and the diagnosis is most likely stress reaction or early stress fracture.

Stress Fracture, Adult

Lateral radiograph obtained one week later in the same patient proves stress fracture, with the sclerosis now crossing the bone in a linear fashion ➡. MR proved the linear fracture line with surrounding edema.

LONG BONE, CORTICALLY BASED DIAPHYSEAL LESION, SCLEROTIC

Tibial Stress Syndrome

Tibial Stress Syndrome

(Left) Lateral radiograph shows subtle periosteal reaction at the tibial diaphysis ➔; this is an early finding of tibial stress syndrome in a young adult runner. *(Right)* Sagittal PD FSE FS MR obtained at the same time as the previous image shows edema within the marrow ➔ and in the soft tissues at the cortical surface ➔, but no fracture line; this confirms tibial stress syndrome and the patient would be well-advised to protect the leg.

Adductor Insertion Avulsion Syndrome

Stress Fracture, Pediatric

(Left) Anteroposterior radiograph shows cortical thickening at the medial aspect of the mid-femoral diaphysis ➔. This is typical of adductor insertion avulsion syndrome, proven by MR. *(Right)* Lateral radiograph shows dense cortical reaction of a healing stress fracture ➔ in a 9 year old who began an unaccustomed exercise activity. The fracture has robust reaction and, with protection, healed before becoming complete.

Osteoid Osteoma

Osteoid Osteoma

(Left) Lateral radiograph shows prominent cortical reaction ➔ in a child, seen over a more extensive length of the diaphysis than is usually present with stress fx. One must suspect osteoid osteoma, with the lytic nidus being obscured by the reactive bone formation. (†MSK Req). *(Right)* Axial NECT (same patient) proves osteoid osteoma, a small lytic nidus ➔ adjacent to a nutrient vessel ➔, located deep beneath the dense cortical reactive bone ➔. (†MSK Req).

Fibroxanthoma (Non-Ossifying Fibroma)

Chronic Osteomyelitis (Brodie Abscess)

(Left) AP radiograph shows metadiaphyseal ➡ NOFs, most frequently multiple in neurofibromatosis. With skeletal maturation, the lytic lesions heal, with sclerotic ossification. (Right) Lateral radiograph of the femur shows an irregular lytic lesion containing a sclerotic center ➡, both located within a cortex which is thickened with reactive bone formation. This is typical of osteomyelitis; the central sclerotic body is a sequestrum.

Stress Fracture Related to Bisphosphonate Use

Stress Fracture Related to Bisphosphonate Use

(Left) AP radiograph shows dense cortical and endosteal reaction in the subtrochanteric region of the femur ➡ in a 70 year old woman placed on bisphosphonate therapy for osteoporosis. (Right) Frog lateral view shows linear sclerosis in the same patient, indicating fracture ➡. The femur was not protected, & the patient went on to a displaced fracture. The process occurred bilaterally. Subtrochanteric fractures are now recognized as a complication of this therapy.

Melorheostosis

Osteoma

(Left) Sagittal PD FSE FS MR shows a lobulated mass ➡ arising from the ulnar cortex which was densely sclerotic. At resection, it was consistent with the dense bone formation of melorheostosis. (Right) AP radiograph shows multiple osteomas ➡ projecting from the femoral cortex in this patient with Gardner syndrome. The contralateral femur was involved as well. In the absence of polyposis syndromes it is distinctly unusual to find an osteoma involving the long bones.

LONG BONE, CORTICALLY BASED DIAPHYSEAL LESION, LYTIC

DIFFERENTIAL DIAGNOSIS

Common
- Fibroxanthoma (Non-Ossifying Fibroma)
- Metastases, Bone Marrow
- Paget Disease
- Osteomyelitis
- Osteoid Osteoma
- Fibrous Dysplasia
- Aneurysmal Bone Cyst

Less Common
- Adamantinoma
- Tendon Injury (Tug Lesion)
- Osteofibrous Dysplasia
- Soft Tissue Mass Invasion (Mimic)
- Langerhans Cell Histiocytosis
- Hyperparathyroidism

Rare but Important
- Bacillary Angiomatosis
- Hemophilia: MSK Complications
- Hardware, Reactive Changes

ESSENTIAL INFORMATION

Key Differential Diagnosis Issues
- Cortically based lesions within the tibia present a special circumstance
  - Three lesions have a remarkably similar appearance & propensity to occupy the anterior cortex of tibia
    - Cortically based fibrous dysplasia
    - Osteofibrous dysplasia
    - Adamantinoma
  - These lesions have subtle pathologic differences
    - May be considered to be in a spectrum of pathology
    - Behavior may differ, since adamantinoma may have malignant behavior
  - **Hint**: Statistically, fibrous dysplasia is far more frequent than the other two lesions

Helpful Clues for Common Diagnoses
- **Fibroxanthoma (Non-Ossifying Fibroma)**
  - Extremely common lesion in children, especially about the knees
  - Cortically based, but generally originates in metaphysis
    - With skeletal growth, the metaphysis migrates away from lesion
    - Generally ends up in metadiaphysis; mid-diaphyseal location is rare
  - Natural history is to fill in with normal bone (from periphery to center) and disappear in adulthood
- **Metastases, Bone Marrow**
  - Most frequently located in marrow of metaphysis
  - Diaphyseal & cortical location of metastases is most suggestive of either breast or lung primary lesion
- **Paget Disease**
  - Lesion usually originates in subchondral region of bone & advances through metadiaphysis to diaphysis
  - Occasionally long bone lesion will originate in diaphysis
    - Most frequent bone for this occurrence: Tibia, anterior cortex
    - Earliest lesion is lytic; has defined margin as leading edge of lesion
    - Eventually extends to subchondral bone
- **Osteomyelitis**
  - May originate in cortex, especially if related to direct inoculation
  - Watch for serpiginous pattern
  - Generally will also see periosteal reaction
  - MR likely to show associated soft tissue fluid & abscess
- **Osteoid Osteoma**
  - Mid-diaphyseal lesion located in cortex
    - Often deep within the cortex, at margin with marrow
    - Often associated with nutrient vessel
  - Lesion is lytic, oval with regular margins
    - Lesion may have central ossific density
  - Elicits significant reactive bone formation surrounding it; reactive bone may obscure the lytic nidus
- **Fibrous Dysplasia**
  - Most frequently, FD is central and expansile within long bone
  - Occasionally, FD originates in cortex
    - FD is such a common lesion that this presentation is not considered rare
    - May expand and extend around the cortex, surrounding normal marrow
    - Cortical FD in the differential with osteofibrous dysplasia & adamantinoma
  - Watch for additional lesions; FD is often polyostotic, which may help distinguish it

LONG BONE, CORTICALLY BASED DIAPHYSEAL LESION, LYTIC

- **Aneurysmal Bone Cyst**
  - Usual location eccentrically within bone
    - May expand so significantly that it appears to arise within the cortex
    - Rarely may actually arise within the cortex; this is shown on axial imaging
  - Generally retains a thin cortical rim; fluid levels are commonly seen on axial imaging

Helpful Clues for Less Common Diagnoses
- **Adamantinoma**
  - Infrequently seen lesion
  - Generally quite location-specific
    - Anterior tibia, cortically based
    - Distal tibia more common than proximal
  - In the spectrum with cortical fibrous dysplasia & osteofibrous dysplasia
    - Cannot reliably distinguish by imaging
    - Treated with wide excision, since its behavior may be malignant (unlike the other lesions in its differential)
- **Tendon Injury (Tug Lesion)**
  - Any tug lesion may result in resorption of adjacent cortex
  - Most recognized site is posteromedial distal femoral metadiaphysis
    - Site of insertion of adductor fibers
    - Cortical resorption may have associated periosteal reaction & small mass
    - Termed cortical desmoid; location helps differentiate from a more ominous lesion
- **Osteofibrous Dysplasia**
  - Infrequently seen lesion, generally in child or young adult

- In the radiographic & pathologic spectrum of cortical fibrous dysplasia/osteofibrous dysplasia/adamantinoma
  - Most frequent location is anterior tibial cortex; generally proximal tibia
  - May be fully lytic, or may contain a small amount of osteoid
- **Soft Tissue Mass Invasion (Mimic)**
  - Soft tissue mass adjacent to cortex may cause focal erosion, mimicking mass originating within cortex
- **Langerhans Cell Histiocytosis**
  - Location is usually central diaphyseal
  - Common lesion in children; rarely may originate in unusual cortical location
  - Range of behavior from aggressive to indolent
- **Hyperparathyroidism**
  - Brown tumor usually arises centrally in marrow but may also be a cortical lesion
  - Watch for other abnormalities in bone density, trabecular coarsening, and resorption patterns

Helpful Clues for Rare Diagnoses
- **Bacillary Angiomatosis**
  - May be cortical
- **Hemophilia: MSK Complications**
  - Pseudotumor may arise from intracortical or subperiosteal bleed
- **Hardware, Reactive Changes**
  - Usually inert, but old hardware occasionally causes adjacent cortical reactive change

Fibroxanthoma (Non-Ossifying Fibroma)

AP radiograph shows a cortically based lytic lesion ⮕ that proved to be NOF. These lesions are more frequently based in the metadiaphysis but are extremely common; diaphyseal location should not be surprising.

Metastases, Bone Marrow

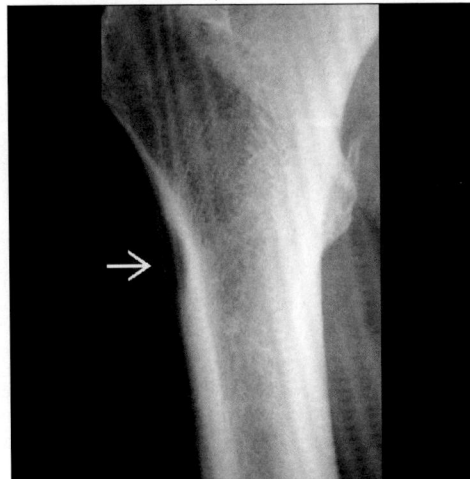

AP radiograph shows a cortically based non-aggressive lesion ⮕ in an elderly patient. Metastatic disease must be suspected; lung and breast are the most common metastases to be located within the cortex.

LONG BONE, CORTICALLY BASED DIAPHYSEAL LESION, LYTIC

Paget Disease

Paget Disease

(Left) Lateral radiograph shows a cortically based lytic lesion in the tibial diaphysis ➡. This is an early manifestation of Paget disease. Although lesions of Paget disease usually originate at the ends of long bones, the tibia is an exception and a diaphyseal origin is not uncommon. *(Right)* Lateral radiograph obtained 2 years later on the same patient shows classic Paget disease, now with mixed lytic & sclerotic lesions, extending to the subchondral bone.

Osteomyelitis

Osteoid Osteoma

(Left) Lateral radiograph shows a mildly expanded lytic cortically based diaphyseal lesion ➡. This 20 year old had normal lab values, but this proved to be Staphylococcal osteomyelitis. *(Right)* Anteroposterior radiograph shows a cortically based lytic lesion ➡ in the diaphysis. The appearance is typical of an osteoid osteoma, with dense surrounding sclerosis ➡. This sclerosis occasionally is so dense as to obscure the lytic lesion.

Fibrous Dysplasia

Fibrous Dysplasia

(Left) Lateral radiograph shows a lytic, mildly expanded, cortical lesion in the diaphysis of the tibia ➡ as well as a "daughter" lesion in the fibula ➡. The tibial lesion is so large that one cannot be certain that it is entirely cortical in location. (†MSK Req). *(Right)* Axial bone CT of the same patient shows that the lesion is entirely cortical and mildly expanded with a ground-glass matrix ➡. Findings are typical of cortically based fibrous dysplasia.

LONG BONE, CORTICALLY BASED DIAPHYSEAL LESION, LYTIC

Fibrous Dysplasia

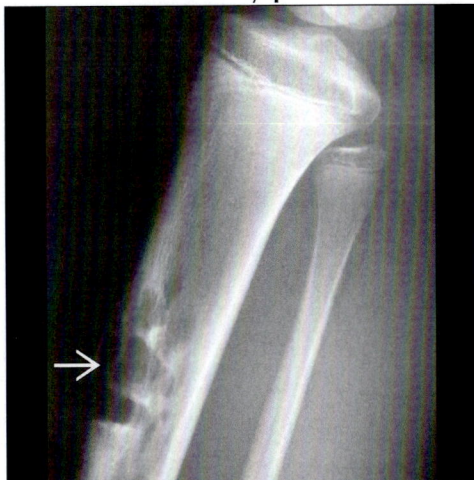

Fibrous Dysplasia

(Left) Lateral radiograph shows a rather complex lytic lesion originating in the anterior cortex of the tibia ➡. There appear to be several "daughter" lesions. Though fibrous dysplasia most frequently arises within the central portion of a long bone, it is not rare for it to occupy the cortex. (†MSK Req). (Right) Sagittal T1WI MR of the same lesion shows the lesion to be based entirely within the anterior cortex of the tibia ➡. FD was proven at excisional biopsy.

Aneurysmal Bone Cyst

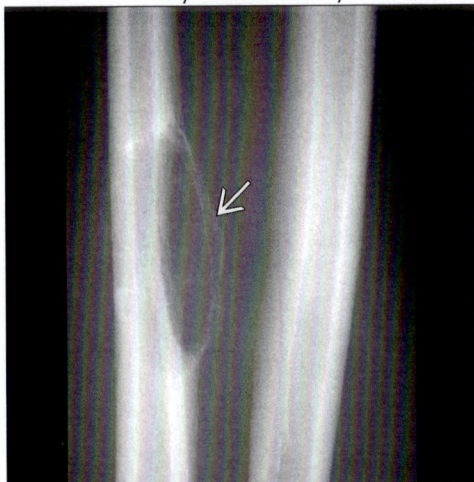

Aneurysmal Bone Cyst

(Left) AP radiograph shows a lytic expansile diaphyseal lesion that is based in the cortex ➡. This proved to be an ABC, though it is unusual for this lesion to be diaphyseal, rather than metaphyseal, and truly cortically based, rather than eccentric and expansile. (Right) Axial T2WI MR of the same lesion shows the true cortical origin of the lesion within the radius ➡. There are a few fluid levels, but the majority of the lesion was solid, unusual for ABC.

Adamantinoma

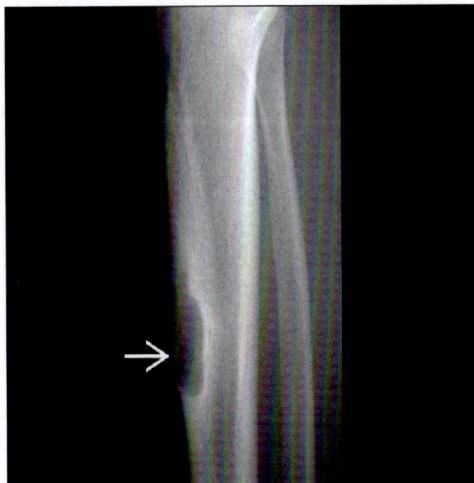

Adamantinoma

(Left) Lateral radiograph shows a lytic lesion arising within the anterior cortex of the tibia ➡. This lesion is an adamantinoma, though statistically a cortically based fibrous dysplasia is more likely. (†MSK Req). (Right) Axial T2WI MR of the same patient shows the lesion to be based entirely within the anterior cortex ➡. This adamantinoma is not distinguishable from cortically based FD or osteofibrous dysplasia by imaging. (†MSK Req).

LONG BONE, CORTICALLY BASED DIAPHYSEAL LESION, LYTIC

Tendon Injury (Tug Lesion)

Tendon Injury (Tug Lesion)

(Left) Axillary lateral radiograph shows ossification of one of the slips of the deltoid tendon ➡, along with apparent lytic lesion in the cortex ➡. This cortical "lesion" is resorption due to the avulsive injury. *(Right)* Axial bone CT shows an apparent cortically based lytic lesion in the distal femoral metadiaphysis ➡. This medial "lesion" has also been termed a cortical desmoid and is secondary to tug injury of the adductor tendon.

Osteofibrous Dysplasia

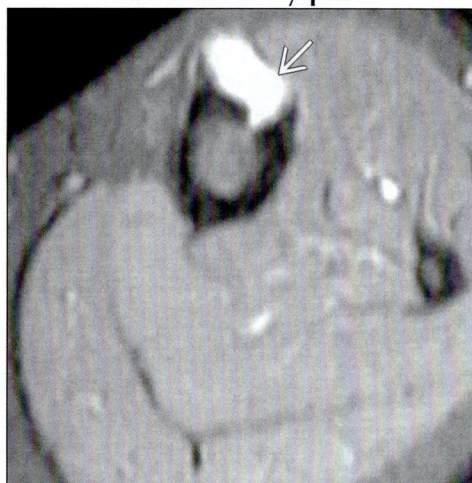

Osteofibrous Dysplasia

(Left) Lateral radiograph shows a nonspecific anterior tibial cortical lesion ➡, falling into the differential of cortical fibrous dysplasia, osteofibrous dysplasia, and adamantinoma. *(Right)* Axial STIR MR of the same case shows the cortical nature of the lesion ➡. Biopsy proved osteofibrous dysplasia. This lesion is usually seen in children or teenagers and is distinctly unusual.

Soft Tissue Mass Invasion (Mimic)

Soft Tissue Mass Invasion (Mimic)

(Left) Lateral radiograph shows a lytic lesion that appears to be cortically based ➡. Location is not proven in this image, which is not in tangent to the lesion. *(Right)* Axial T1 C+ MR of the same lesion shows a soft tissue lesion that is focally invading and eroding the cortical bone ➡. This proved not to be actually cortically based but rather a mimic. The lesion has a target sign of low central signal ➡ and proved to be a schwannoma.

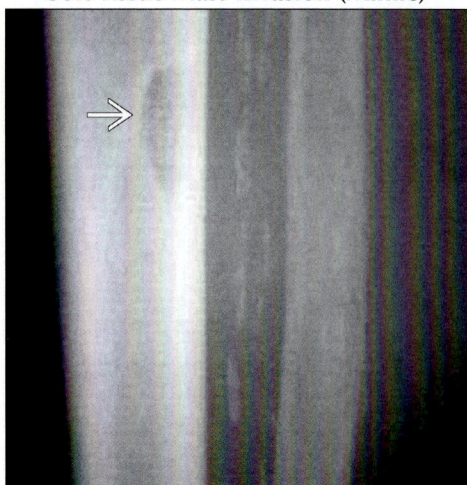

LONG BONE, CORTICALLY BASED DIAPHYSEAL LESION, LYTIC

Langerhans Cell Histiocytosis

Langerhans Cell Histiocytosis

(Left) Lateral radiograph shows a cortically based lytic lesion within the anterior tibial metadiaphysis ➡. This appearance and location are typical of adamantinoma. However, biopsy proved the lesion to be Langerhans cell histiocytosis. (Right) Lateral radiograph from the same patient obtained 3 months later shows significant interval growth of the lesion ➡. Rapid growth can be seen with LCH, as in this case.

Hyperparathyroidism

Bacillary Angiomatosis

(Left) Anteroposterior radiograph shows a cortically based lytic lesion ➡ within the bone that is extremely osteoporotic, with coarsened trabeculae. The patient has a parathyroid adenoma; the focal lesion is a brown tumor. Although a brown tumor is a common lesion, it is most frequently located within the marrow rather than cortex. (Right) Lateral radiograph shows a subtle cortically based lytic lesion ➡, which proved to be bacillary angiomatosis in a patient with HIV-AIDS.

Hemophilia: MSK Complications

Hardware, Reactive Changes

(Left) Anteroposterior radiograph shows cortically based and surface excavations ➡, with prominent periosteal change in this patient with hemophilia. Intraosseous and subperiosteal bleeds result in this bizarre appearance of cortical destruction, termed pseudotumor. (Right) Lateral radiograph shows a grossly loose plate & screws ➡ and scalloped destructive change of the cortex. This proved to be a granulomatous reaction to the metal, a form of particle disease.

LONG BONE, DIFFUSE CORTICAL/ENDOSTEAL THICKENING

DIFFERENTIAL DIAGNOSIS

Common
- Paget Disease
- Venous Stasis
- Chronic Recurrent Multifocal Osteomyelitis (CRMO)
- Hypertrophic Osteoarthropathy

Less Common
- Melorheostosis
- Sickle Cell Anemia: MSK Complications
- Renal Osteodystrophy
- Juvenile Idiopathic Arthritis (JIA)

Rare but Important
- Complications of Prostaglandins
- Engelmann-Camurati Disease
- Ribbing Disease
- Acromegaly
- Intramedullary Osteosclerosis
- Complications of Fluoride
- Caffey Disease (Infantile Cortical Hyperostosis)
- Pachydermoperiostosis
- Thyroid Acropachy
- Ewing Sarcoma

ESSENTIAL INFORMATION

Key Differential Diagnosis Issues
- Many of the differential diagnosis entities have an overlapping appearance
- Patient age, history & additional skeletal findings can help differentiate

Helpful Clues for Common Diagnoses
- **Paget Disease**
  - Location: Long bones most common, pelvis, skull
  - Early lytic lesions originate at the subchondral cortex of long bone
    - Tibia is the exception, often originating in diaphysis
  - Sclerotic phase is less common than mixed lytic & sclerotic phase
  - Cortical & trabecular thickening results in overall enlargement of bone
  - Bowing deformities, pathologic fractures
- **Venous Stasis**
  - Cortical thickening from solid periosteal reaction usually mild

- Additional findings: Subcutaneous edema, phleboliths, varicose veins
- **Chronic Recurrent Multifocal Osteomyelitis (CRMO)**
  - Location: Long bone metaphysis
  - Findings range from radiographically occult to exuberant new bone formation causing dense sclerosis of the majority of the involved bone
- **Hypertrophic Osteoarthropathy**
  - Symmetric, solid periosteal reaction thickens cortex
  - Evaluate for underlying malignancy or chronic pulmonary, cardiac or gastrointestinal disease

Helpful Clues for Less Common Diagnoses
- **Melorheostosis**
  - Begins as linear hyperostosis in proximal end of tubular bone
  - Distal progression with progressive cortical thickening
  - Usually limited to single extremity
  - Typically follows sclerotome distribution
- **Sickle Cell Anemia: MSK Complications**
  - Diffuse cortical infarction in the long bones
  - Diametaphysis may be widened by infarction &/or chronic infection
  - Endosteal splitting = linear increased densities paralleling the cortices
    - May produce a bone-in-bone appearance
- **Renal Osteodystrophy**
  - Location: Tubular bones most common, pubic rami, spine
  - Neostosis = rapid new bone formation in patients undergoing treatment
  - Additional findings include generalized skeletal sclerosis, subperiosteal resorption, joint erosions, vertebral endplate sclerosis
  - Rare in primary hyperparathyroidism
- **Juvenile Idiopathic Arthritis (JIA)**
  - Location: Periarticular
  - Distribution: Localized or generalized

Helpful Clues for Rare Diagnoses
- **Complications of Prostaglandins**
  - Location: Long bone diaphysis
  - Distribution: Generalized
  - Correlate with drug therapy
- **Engelmann-Camurati Disease**
  - Location: Long bone diaphysis, skull
  - Distribution: Bilateral, symmetric

LONG BONE, DIFFUSE CORTICAL/ENDOSTEAL THICKENING

- ○ Exuberant endosteal new bone
- ○ Presents in childhood
- ○ Autosomal dominant (differentiate from Ribbing disease)
- **Ribbing Disease**
  - ○ Location: Long bone diaphysis
  - ○ Unilateral or bilaterally asymmetric
  - ○ Radiographically identical to Engelmann disease & intramedullary osteosclerosis
  - ○ Eventual obliteration of marrow space & circumferential bone growth
  - ○ Presents after puberty
  - ○ Autosomal recessive (differentiate from Engelmann & intramedullary osteosclerosis)
  - ○ Can have similar appearance to stress fracture, chronic osteomyelitis, metabolic disorder, endocrine disorder, bone-forming malignancy
- **Acromegaly**
  - ○ Bone enlargement & flared long bone ends
  - ○ Clinically differentiated from other entities by elevated growth hormone & IGF-1
  - ○ Additional findings: Thick skull, large frontal sinuses, enlarged mandible, spade-like finger tufts, wide phalangeal bases, wide MCP joints, thick heel pad, posterior vertebral body scalloping
- **Intramedullary Osteosclerosis**
  - ○ Similar appearance to Engelmann & Ribbing disease but is nonhereditary
    - ▪ Adult female is most commonly affected demographic

- ○ Location: Tibia diaphysis; femur & tibial metaphysis less common
- ○ Distribution: Unilateral or asymmetric bilateral endosteal thickening
- ○ Minimal cortical thickening & lacks periosteal reaction
- **Complications of Fluoride**
  - ○ Location: Tubular bones, symmetric
  - ○ Additional findings of tendon & ligament calcification
- **Caffey Disease (Infantile Cortical Hyperostosis)**
  - ○ Ossification begins in soft tissues and progresses to join cortex of underlying bone
  - ○ One or more long bones, mandible, scapula, ribs may be involved
  - ○ Onset less than six months of age
  - ○ Spontaneous resolution; residual bowing uncommon
- **Pachydermoperiostosis**
  - ○ Primary hypertrophic osteoarthropathy
  - ○ Thick, shaggy periosteal reaction produces cortical thickening
- **Thyroid Acropachy**
  - ○ Location: Tubular bones of hands & feet; long bones rare
  - ○ Correlate with hyperthyroidism treatment
- **Ewing Sarcoma**
  - ○ Exceptionally rare to have dense, solid periosteal reaction obscure permeative destruction of tumor
  - ○ MR can evaluate for underlying malignancy

Paget Disease

Anteroposterior radiograph shows the tibia shaft to be significantly expanded ➡ with a mixed sclerotic and lytic appearance. The lesion extends distally with a blade of grass or flame-shaped pattern ➡.

Venous Stasis

Oblique radiograph shows a thickened appearance to the distal tibial cortex ➡. This is due to smooth periosteal reaction. Additional signs of venous stasis include phleboliths ➡ and subcutaneous edema ➡.

LONG BONE, DIFFUSE CORTICAL/ENDOSTEAL THICKENING

(Left) Coronal T1WI MR shows massive thickening of the proximal left femoral cortex ➡. The endosteal bone has similarly extensive regions of sclerosis ➡. Marked edema in the bone, soft tissues and a joint effusion suggested osteosarcoma. CRMO was proven on biopsy. **(Right)** Anteroposterior radiograph shows periosteal reaction of the tibia that is so dense it presents as extremely thick cortex ➡. More typical solid periosteal reaction involves the fibula ➡.

Chronic Recurrent Multifocal Osteomyelitis (CRMO)

Hypertrophic Osteoarthropathy

(Left) Anteroposterior radiograph shows abnormal endosteal sclerosis involving the medial aspect of the tibia ➡. The dense sclerotic bone seems to "flow" down the long bone in a manner that has been described as dripping candle wax. **(Right)** Lateral radiograph shows cortical thickening ➡ of the distal femoral diaphysis and metaphysis. Linear increased densities parallel to the endosteal cortex ➡ are due to diffuse osteonecrosis in sickle cell disease.

Melorheostosis

Sickle Cell Anemia: MSK Complications

(Left) Lateral radiograph shows a dense linear periosteal reaction ➡ that thickens the femoral cortex. The underlying bone density is abnormal for a young adult, with mixed lucency and sclerosis, typical of renal osteodystrophy/neostosis. **(Right)** Lateral radiograph shows dense, thick, new bone formation involving this infant's humerus ➡ and forearm bones ➡. One should also consider diffuse osteomyelitis or nutritional deficiency in an infant with long-term hospitalization.

Renal Osteodystrophy

Complications of Prostaglandins

LONG BONE, DIFFUSE CORTICAL/ENDOSTEAL THICKENING

Engelmann-Camurati Disease

Engelmann-Camurati Disease

(Left) Anteroposterior radiograph shows disordered cortical and endosteal bone, resulting in a cortical thickening which is restricted to the diaphyses ➡. Note the normal epiphyses and metaphyses ➡. *(Right)* Anteroposterior radiograph shows marked endosteal and periosteal cortical thickening ➡. This was bilaterally symmetric and involved the entire length of the diaphyses, leaving the metaphyses and epiphyses unaffected.

Intramedullary Osteosclerosis

Intramedullary Osteosclerosis

(Left) Lateral radiograph shows typical changes of diffuse sclerosis in the tibial diaphysis ➡. This finding was bilateral, which is a consistent feature of this process. In some cases the distal tibial metaphysis may also be involved. *(Right)* Coronal T1WI MR in the same patient confirms the sclerotic process with diffuse low signal within the medullary canal ➡. There is some sparing of the central most area of the medullary cavity ➡.

Caffey Disease (Infantile Cortical Hyperostosis)

Ewing Sarcoma

(Left) Lateral radiograph shows marked new bone formation thickening the cortex of the tibia ➡. Ossification began in the soft tissues. *(Right)* Lateral radiograph shows nonspecific endosteal & periosteal thickening ➡. Although rare, one should consider a permeative tumor, masked by intense bone reaction. Possibilities include Ewing sarcoma, lymphoma, and chondrosarcoma. MR would differentiate stress fracture from underlying malignancy.

TIBIAL METADIAPHYSEAL CORTICALLY BASED LESION

DIFFERENTIAL DIAGNOSIS

Common
- Fibrous Dysplasia (FD)
- Osteosarcoma, Parosteal (Mimic)

Less Common
- Osteofibrous Dysplasia
- Adamantinoma

Rare but Important
- Osteosarcoma, Periosteal (Mimic)

ESSENTIAL INFORMATION

Key Differential Diagnosis Issues
- Classic differential diagnosis
  - **Hint**: Generally cannot reliably differentiate cortically based FD, osteofibrous dysplasia, & adamantinoma from one another
    - Imaging characteristics are usually indistinguishable
    - Must offer all 3 diagnoses as a differential
  - **Hint**: Cortically based FD is uncommon form of FD, but is far more common than either osteofibrous dysplasia or adamantinoma
  - **Hint**: Osteofibrous dysplasia rarely is seen beyond 3rd decade
- The 2 surface lesions (mimics) on this list can usually be recognized as such
  - Generally are identified as surface lesions
  - Generally have identifiable matrix

Helpful Clues for Common Diagnoses
- **Fibrous Dysplasia (FD)**
  - May be either central or cortically based when involving tibial metadiaphysis
    - Tibia is the exception; in other bones, FD is only central in location
  - Cortically based lesions are lytic & expansile, appearing moderately aggressive
  - May "wrap around", involving cortex circumferentially
- **Osteosarcoma, Parosteal (Mimic)**
  - Surface osteoid-producing lesion; may involve marrow
  - Early lesions may mimic a cortically based lesion, but matrix differentiates it

Helpful Clues for Less Common Diagnoses
- **Osteofibrous Dysplasia**
  - Lytic cortically based lesion seen reliably most frequently in tibial metadiaphysis
  - Generally proximal 1/3; anterior bowing
  - Patients generally < 30 years old
- **Adamantinoma**
  - Lytic cortically based lesion, generally anterior tibia
  - Often appears non-aggressive initially but may progress to a more destructive lesion
    - May become malignant

Helpful Clues for Rare Diagnoses
- **Osteosarcoma, Periosteal (Mimic)**
  - Rare surface lesion, produces osteoid
  - May mimic cortically based lesion if underlying bone is significantly scalloped

Fibrous Dysplasia (FD)

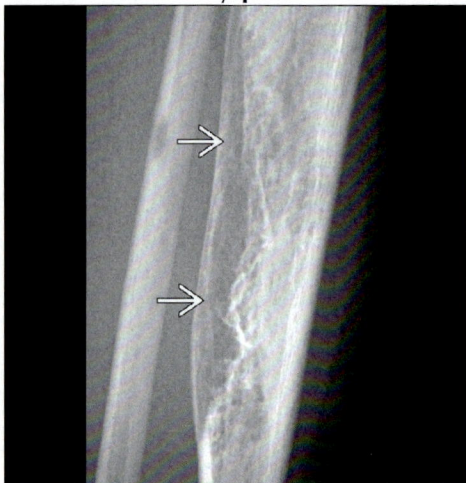

Lateral radiograph shows an extensive lytic cortically based lesion of the tibia ➡. The lesion is so large that it may be difficult to confirm that it is restricted to the cortex. (†MSK Req).

Fibrous Dysplasia (FD)

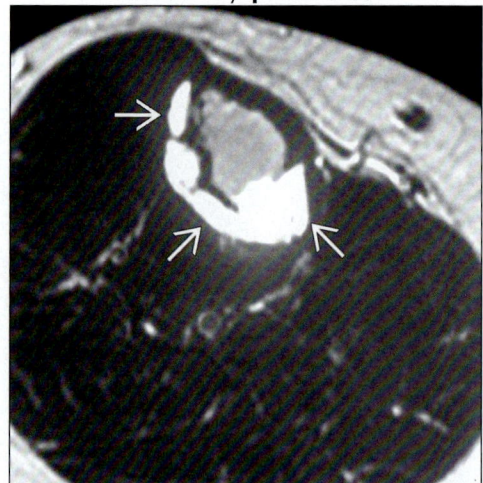

Axial T2WI MR in the same patient shows high signal intensity within the lesion ➡, which is restricted to the cortex. Though FD usually is located within the marrow, it occasionally arises in the cortex of the tibia.

TIBIAL METADIAPHYSEAL CORTICALLY BASED LESION

Osteosarcoma, Parosteal (Mimic)

Osteofibrous Dysplasia

(Left) Axial bone CT shows a surface lesion consisting of mature bone ➡, with less mature tumor bone formed peripherally ➡. This is the typical appearance of parosteal osteosarcoma. This lesion may involve the cortex and extend into the marrow, thus mimicking a cortically based lesion. (†MSK Req). *(Right)* Axial bone CT shows a lytic lesion arising in the anterior cortex of the tibia ➡ in a 23 year old. The appearance is nonspecific but proved to be osteofibrous dysplasia.

Adamantinoma

Adamantinoma

(Left) Lateral radiograph shows a lytic lesion arising from the cortex of the tibial metadiaphysis ➡. The lesion does not appear to involve the underlying marrow and does not appear highly aggressive. (†MSK Req). *(Right)* Axial T2WI FS MR in the same patient shows the lesion to arise from the cortex ➡ but to extend into the adjacent soft tissue ➡. There is no marrow involvement. Adamantinoma can be locally aggressive and even malignant. (†MSK Req).

Osteosarcoma, Periosteal (Mimic)

Osteosarcoma, Periosteal (Mimic)

(Left) Anteroposterior radiograph shows a bone-forming tumor arising from the surface of the tibia ➡. There is no suggestion of a permeative bone lesion involving the cortex or marrow. *(Right)* Axial bone CT in the same patient shows the lesion to be arising from the surface of the bone ➡. There is no involvement of the marrow or cortex. Therefore it is a surface lesion, though it mimics a cortically based lesion.

LONG BONE, UNDERTUBULATION

DIFFERENTIAL DIAGNOSIS

Common
- Multiple Hereditary Exostoses (MHE)
- Fibrous Dysplasia (FD)
- Unicameral Bone Cyst (Mimic)
- Paget Disease (Mimic)
- Storage Diseases
  - Gaucher Disease
  - Niemann Pick
  - Mucopolysaccharidoses
- Thalassemia
- Sickle Cell Anemia
- Chronic Osteomyelitis

Less Common
- Achondroplasia
- Ollier Disease
- Rickets (Healing)
- Osteogenesis Imperfecta (OI)
- Osteopetrosis
- Engelmann-Camurati Disease

Rare but Important
- Maffucci Syndrome
- Pycnodysostosis
- Hypophosphatasia
- Scurvy (Healing)
- Caffey Disease
- Pyle Dysplasia

ESSENTIAL INFORMATION

Key Differential Diagnosis Issues
- Undertubulation: Widening of long bone
- Distinguish between solitary & polyostotic
  - Solitary: FD, unicameral bone cyst, Paget disease, chronic osteomyelitis
  - Polyostotic but generally monomelic: Ollier disease, Maffucci syndrome
  - Remainder are polyostotic & symmetric

Helpful Clues for Common Diagnoses
- **Multiple Hereditary Exostoses (MHE)**
  - Most exostoses in MHE are elongated & sessile, along metaphyses
    - Mimics actual metaphyseal widening
  - ± Cauliflower-like exostoses
  - Easily misinterpreted as a metaphyseal dysplasia or storage disorder!
- **Fibrous Dysplasia (FD)**
  - Lesion is usually central, metadiaphyseal, or diaphyseal

- Widens bone, while thinning endosteum
- May not have geographic border
  - Polyostotic lesions could be misinterpreted as undertubulation; ground-glass density
- **Unicameral Bone Cyst (Mimic)**
  - Metaphyseal or metadiaphyseal
  - Central, with osseous expansion, thinning the endosteal cortex
  - Solitary lesion; watch for mildly sclerotic geographic margin; ± fallen fragment
- **Paget Disease (Mimic)**
  - Expands the involved bone
  - Generally easily distinguished by means of the distinct border between normal & abnormal bone ("blade of grass")
    - Involvement of entire bone may mimic undertubulation; mixed lytic/sclerotic
- **Gaucher Disease**
  - Storage disease resulting in expansion of metadiaphyses, especially of distal femora
    - "Erlenmeyer flask" sign
  - Hepatosplenomegaly, osteonecrosis
- **Niemann Pick**
  - Lipid storage disorder
  - Accumulates in bone marrow, leading to undertubulation
  - Accumulates in lungs (Kerley B lines), liver & spleen (hepatosplenomegaly), & brain (learning problems)
- **Mucopolysaccharidoses**
  - Family of storage disorders with similar morphologic abnormalities of the skeleton
  - Long bones may be short & broad, particularly metacarpals
    - Constricted proximal ends of metacarpals gives a "fan-like" appearance
- **Thalassemia**
  - Severe anemia → marrow hyperplasia
  - Long bones lose all distinguishing morphology ("squared")
  - Severe osteoporosis
- **Sickle Cell Anemia**
  - Osteonecrosis, bone infarcts are predominant features
  - Rarely results in significant marrow hyperplasia
  - May see mild widening of the metadiaphyses, with patchy bone sclerosis indicating widespread infarcts
- **Chronic Osteomyelitis**

LONG BONE, UNDERTUBULATION

○ Chronic disease may show little destructive change (permeative destruction, periosteal reaction)
○ Sclerosis & endosteal bone formation may predominate, resulting in widening of the bone around the focus of infection
○ May not have associated soft tissue abscess

Helpful Clues for Less Common Diagnoses

- **Achondroplasia**
  ○ Dysplastic metaphyses may reduce tubulation
  ○ Short bones make normal width of diaphyses appear undertubulated
- **Ollier Disease**
  ○ Dysplasia that affects metadiaphyses
    ▪ Widening & abnormal growth metaphyses
    ▪ Vertical striations, ± chondroid matrix
  ○ Usually unilateral, → limb length discrepancy
- **Rickets (Healing)**
  ○ Widened, frayed metaphyses may heal with a widened morphology
  ○ Watch for abnormal bone density, hyperossified brown tumors, neostosis
- **Osteogenesis Imperfecta (OI)**
  ○ OI congenita: Multiple intrauterine fx → short, broad, bowed long bones
  ○ OI tarda: Severe form results in overtubulation; less severe forms show fewer fractures, but undertubulation at the metadiaphyses
  ○ Severity of osteoporosis varies

- **Osteopetrosis**
  ○ Uniformly dense bones, axial, & appendicular skeleton
  ○ Abnormality is in osteoclastic activity; with skeletal growth, ↓ remodeling
    ▪ → Undertubulation of metadiaphyses
    ▪ → Bone-in-bone appearance
- **Engelmann-Camurati Disease**
  ○ Dense sclerosis & bone accretion, endosteum and cortical bone
  ○ Only diaphyses affected; abrupt change to normal-appearing metaphyses
  ○ Bilaterally symmetric

Helpful Clues for Rare Diagnoses

- **Maffucci Syndrome**
  ○ Ollier disease + soft tissue hemangiomas
- **Pycnodysostosis**
  ○ Osteopetrosis + acroosteolysis
- **Hypophosphatasia**
  ○ Osteopenic, bowed bones; similar appearance to rickets
- **Scurvy (Healing)**
  ○ Collagen abnormality → periosteal elevation from metaphyseal corner fx
  ○ → Dense, thick periosteal healing bone mimics undertubulation
- **Caffey Disease**
  ○ Dense periosteal reaction → undertubulation
  ○ Self-limited; returns to normal by 2 years
- **Pyle Dysplasia**
  ○ a.k.a., craniometaphyseal dysplasia; failure of modeling of long bones

Multiple Hereditary Exostoses (MHE)

AP radiograph shows apparent widening of the metadiaphyses of the femora & tibiae →. While this is suggestive of a storage disease, it in fact represents multiple sessile osteochondromas in MHE.

Multiple Hereditary Exostoses (MHE)

Anteroposterior radiograph shows widening & loss of normal modeling of the femoral metaphyses →. Note also the widening of the pubic rami. These all represent sessile osteochondromas in a patient with MHE.

LONG BONE, UNDERTUBULATION

Fibrous Dysplasia (FD)

Unicameral Bone Cyst (Mimic)

(Left) AP radiograph shows widening of the proximal metadiaphysis ➡, with normal distal metadiaphysis ➡ of the tibia. The fibula shows similar features. The cortices are thinned, & there is ground-glass matrix in the affected areas, typical of FD. *(Right)* AP radiograph shows widening of the proximal metaphysis with thinning of the cortices ➡ in a child with a solitary lesion. There is a fallen fragment sign ➡, typical of a unicameral bone cyst.

Paget Disease (Mimic)

Paget Disease (Mimic)

(Left) AP radiograph shows widening of the proximal metadiaphysis ➡, with abrupt change to normal appearance distally ➡. The cortices are thick, and there is a mixed lytic/sclerotic pattern, typical of Paget disease. *(Right)* AP radiograph shows apparent undertubulation, with widening of the femur along its entire length ➡. A normal tibia is seen at the edge of the image. Mixed lytic & sclerotic change is typical of Paget disease.

Gaucher Disease

Mucopolysaccharidoses

(Left) Anteroposterior radiograph shows gradual widening of the distal metadiaphysis, without thinning of cortex or osseous destruction ➡. This flaring gives the appearance of an "Erlenmeyer flask" and is typical of Gaucher disease. *(Right)* Posteroanterior radiograph shows widening of the metacarpals, with proximal constriction giving the fan appearance ➡ that is typical of the mucopolysaccharidoses storage diseases.

LONG BONE, UNDERTUBULATION

Thalassemia

Thalassemia

(Left) PA radiograph shows diffuse abnormal modeling of the bones, with widening of the diaphyses and loss of the expected metaphyseal morphology. Cortices are thin, & trabeculae are abnormal. This is typical marrow hyperplasia in thalassemia. *(Right)* AP radiograph shows widening of the metaphyses ➡, extending to include much of the diaphysis. This widening results from marrow hyperplasia in a patient with thalassemia.

Sickle Cell Anemia

Chronic Osteomyelitis

(Left) Lateral radiograph shows patchy sclerosis throughout the tibia, representing extensive bone infarction in a patient with sickle cell disease. There is minimal widening of the proximal tibial metaphysis, likely related to marrow hyperplasia. This is less extensive in sickle cell disease than thalassemia. *(Right)* AP radiograph shows widening of the metaphysis ➡, with sclerosis surrounding a lytic lesion. This is typical chronic osteomyelitis in a child.

Chronic Osteomyelitis

Achondroplasia

(Left) AP radiograph shows widening of the diaphysis of the fibula ➡ (compare with adjacent tibia), with extensive sclerosis and cortical thickening. This teenager had leg pain for 1 year; this proved to be chronic staphylococcal osteomyelitis. *(Right)* Anteroposterior radiograph shows short, broad bones in this case of achondroplastic dwarfism. Undertubulation is a prominent feature in this process.

LONG BONE, UNDERTUBULATION

(Left) AP radiograph shows broadening of the metaphysis, with vertical striations within it ➡. All the metaphyses of the right lower limb showed similar undertubulation and the limb was short; findings are typical of Ollier disease. *(Right)* AP radiograph shows bowing & undertubulation of the distal femoral metaphyses ➡ in a case of healing rickets, where the widened and frayed metaphyses are becoming ossified. Remodeling may occur with further treatment.

Ollier Disease

Rickets (Healing)

(Left) Anteroposterior radiograph shows bowing & undertubulation of the femur in a case of OI tarda ➡, along with pathologic fracture. While more severe cases of OI tarda show overtubulation, less severe cases show fewer fractures and metadiaphyseal widening. *(Right)* AP radiograph shows severe shortening, osteoporosis, & undertubulation ➡ in the long bones of a patient with OI congenita, resulting from multiple intrauterine fractures.

Osteogenesis Imperfecta (OI)

Osteogenesis Imperfecta (OI)

(Left) AP radiograph shows dense (marble) bones and severe undertubulation of the metadiaphyses ➡. Osteopetrosis results from osteoclastic abnormality; with skeletal growth, remodeling cannot occur normally. *(Right)* AP radiograph shows diffuse widening (undertubulation) of the diaphyses of both tibiae & fibulae. There is increased density. Note that the metaphyses are normal. This is an early manifestation of Engelmann-Camurati disease.

Osteopetrosis

Engelmann-Camurati Disease

Engelmann-Camurati Disease

Maffucci Syndrome

(Left) AP radiograph shows severe undertubulation of the diaphysis ➡, along with cortical and endosteal thickening. The metaphysis is normal ➡, and the findings were bilateral, all typical of Engelmann-Camurati disease. *(Right)* AP radiograph shows undertubulation of the metadiaphysis, with chondroid matrix within the lesion ➡. There were hemangiomas elsewhere in this patient's soft tissues, making the diagnosis of Maffucci syndrome.

Pycnodysostosis

Hypophosphatasia

(Left) AP radiograph shows undertubulation of the long bones, along with diffuse increased density. This appearance is typical of either osteopetrosis or pycnodysostosis; the patient also had acroosteolysis, making the latter the diagnosis. *(Right)* AP radiograph shows severe osteoporosis, bowing, & undertubulation ➡ of the upper extremity. There is also widening of the physis ➡, typical of hypophosphatasia.

Scurvy (Healing)

Caffey Disease

(Left) AP radiograph shows a metaphyseal fracture ➡ and severely elevated periosteum ➡, along with osteoporosis & the dense lines typical of scurvy. As the injury heals, the elevated periosteum will form bone, resulting in undertubulation. *(Right)* Lateral radiograph shows thick, dense periosteal reaction involving all the long bones. This infant also had clavicle and mandibular involvement, helping to confirm the diagnosis of Caffey disease.

LONG BONE, OVERTUBULATION

DIFFERENTIAL DIAGNOSIS

Common
- Paralysis/Disuse
  - Polio
  - Cerebral Palsy
- Neurofibromatosis
- Juvenile Idiopathic Arthritis (JIA)

Less Common
- Hemophilia
- Marfan Syndrome (Phalanges)
- Muscular Disorders
  - Arthrogryposis
  - Muscular Dystrophy
- Osteogenesis Imperfecta (OI)

Rare but Important
- Homocystinuria (Phalanges)
- Achondroplasia (Mimic)
- Hypophosphatasia
- Radiation
- Caudal Regression Syndrome
- Epidermolysis Bullosa
- Progeria
- Polymyositis/Dermatomyositis
- Restrictive Dermopathy
- Hypopituitarism
- Stickler Syndrome

ESSENTIAL INFORMATION

Key Differential Diagnosis Issues
- Abnormality in long bone modeling, resulting in a relatively narrow diaphysis
  - Concentric narrowing of the shaft
  - Typically related to chronic disease that affects a growing skeleton
- Most of listed processes involve all bones
- Those diseases that may have single or nonsymmetric involvement (site may be predictable)
  - Polio
  - Neurofibromatosis
  - Hemophilia
  - Arthrogryposis
  - Muscular dystrophy
  - Caudal regression syndrome
  - Radiation
  - Epidermolysis bullosa

Helpful Clues for Common Diagnoses
- Polio
  - Muscular atrophy → insufficient muscle pull to promote normal growth of bones
  - Usually unilateral; limb length discrepancy
- Cerebral Palsy
  - Spasticity with disuse atrophy of muscles → insufficient muscle pull to promote normal growth of long bones
  - Patella alta common, with C-shaped patella
- Neurofibromatosis
  - Long bone abnormality generally restricted to tibia/fibula
  - Dysplasia of tibia, rather than neurofibromas causing the abnormality
  - Bone may be bowed in any direction
  - Often thin diaphysis; dysplastic bone at risk for pathologic (transverse) fractures
  - May result in pseudarthrosis of either tibia or fibula at mid-diaphysis
  - Multiple fibroxanthomas (nonossifying fibromas) may be present, especially around knee
- Juvenile Idiopathic Arthritis (JIA)
  - Systemic variety of JIA results in prolonged chronic illness
  - Chronic illness & muscle atrophy slows growth of long bones
  - Ends of long bones (metaphyses & epiphyses) show overgrowth (ballooning) due to chronic hyperemia at involved joints
    - Overgrowth of ends of bones emphasizes gracile nature of diaphyses, giving overall impression of overtubulation

Helpful Clues for Less Common Diagnoses
- Hemophilia
  - Chronic illness delays growth, resulting in gracile (thin) long bones
  - Ends of long bones (metaphyses & epiphyses) show overgrowth (ballooning) due to chronic hyperemia at involved joints
    - Overgrowth of ends of bones emphasizes gracile nature of diaphyses, giving overall impression of overtubulation
  - Knee, elbow, ankle most frequently involved with arthropathy
    - Overtubulation therefore seen most frequently in femur, tibia, & humerus
  - Gender specific (male)

LONG BONE, OVERTUBULATION

- ○ Watch for dense effusions (deposition of hemosiderin from chronic joint bleeding) & destructive arthropathy
- **Marfan Syndrome (Phalanges)**
  - ○ Arachnodactyly emphasizes the thin diaphyses of hands & feet
  - ○ Associated dural ectasia & posterior vertebral body scalloping
- **Arthrogryposis**
  - ○ Congenital persistent contracture of multiple joints
    - ▪ → Muscle atrophy, disuse → delayed growth & gracile long bones
  - ○ Lower extremity may predominate
  - ○ Often associated congenital hip dislocation & congenital foot deformities (club foot, congenital vertical talus)
- **Muscular Dystrophy**
  - ○ Muscle atrophy → disuse → delayed growth & gracile long bones if occurs at young age
- **Osteogenesis Imperfecta (OI)**
  - ○ Tarda form of OI develops excessively thin long bones
  - ○ Severe osteoporosis
  - ○ Bones are fragile, develop multiple fractures
    - ▪ Bowing may be severe
    - ▪ Fracture callus may be prominent

Helpful Clues for Rare Diagnoses
- **Homocystinuria (Phalanges)**
  - ○ Arachnodactyly emphasizes the thin diaphyses of hands & feet
  - ○ Severe osteoporosis

- **Achondroplasia (Mimic)**
  - ○ Broadened, dysplastic metaphyses may make diaphyses appear relatively thin
    - ▪ Bones are not truly gracile but are short & of normal breadth
- **Hypophosphatasia**
  - ○ Tarda form results in thin, fragile diaphyses of long bones
    - ▪ Multiple fractures result in bowing
  - ○ Growth abnormalities at physis resembling those of rickets
    - ▪ Wide zone of provisional calcification
    - ▪ Fraying of metaphyses
- **Radiation**
  - ○ Overtubulation extremely rare
    - ▪ Requires a radiation field encompassing majority of diaphysis to cease growth across width of a tubular bone
    - ▪ Whole-bone radiation, such as for Ewing sarcoma or lymphoma
  - ○ Widening, fraying epiphysis/metaphysis with early fusion & subsequent shortening of bone is more common
- **Caudal Regression Syndrome**
  - ○ Variable degree of absence of sacrum, lumbar spine, & femoral heads
  - ○ Muscle atrophy; nonambulatory → gracile lower extremities
  - ○ Often infant of diabetic mother
- **Epidermolysis Bullosa**
  - ○ Contractures, muscle atrophy → overtubulation
  - ○ Esophageal strictures, digital webbing

Polio

Anteroposterior radiograph shows asymmetry of the soft tissues, pelvis, & femora, with a gracile, undertubulated femur ⇒ and hypoplastic iliac wing ⇒ on the right, compared with a normal left side.

Cerebral Palsy

Lateral radiograph shows a gracile femoral diaphysis ⇒, along with a C-shaped patella ⇒. Note the patella alta. The combination is typical of cerebral palsy, in which overtubulation of the long bones is common.

LONG BONE, OVERTUBULATION

(Left) Anteroposterior radiograph shows severe bowing and overtubulation of a dysplastic tibia ➡ in a patient with neurofibromatosis. Note the pseudarthrosis of the fibula ➡, not corrected with surgery. **(Right)** Anteroposterior radiograph shows erosive change with protrusio of the right hip ➡, along with a severely gracile right femur ➡. The left side is less significantly involved in this chronically ill patient with JIA. Note the hypoplastic iliac wings.

(Left) Lateral radiograph shows an extremely thin femoral diaphysis ➡, along with an overgrown epiphysis ➡. Along with the destructive joint changes and dense effusion, the findings are typical of hemophilia. Chronic illness contributes to the overtubulation of the long bones, which is exaggerated by the distal ballooning. († MSK Req). **(Right)** Posteroanterior radiograph shows long, thin diaphyses of the metacarpals and phalanges in this patient with Marfan syndrome.

(Left) Frontal radiograph shows the extremely thin, overtubulated forearm bones ➡ in a patient with arthrogryposis. Note the apparent "webbing" at the contracted elbow ➡, as well as lack of musculature. **(Right)** Anteroposterior radiograph shows severely thinned and bowed forearm bones, with a similar appearance of the humerus. There are pathologic fractures ➡ along with bowing in this patient with OI tarda.

Neurofibromatosis

Juvenile Idiopathic Arthritis (JIA)

Hemophilia

Marfan Syndrome (Phalanges)

Arthrogryposis

Osteogenesis Imperfecta (OI)

LONG BONE, OVERTUBULATION

Osteogenesis Imperfecta (OI)

Homocystinuria (Phalanges)

(Left) Anteroposterior radiograph shows protrusio ⟹, along with severe osteoporosis. The femora are overtubulated ⟹; bowing deformities have been treated with osteotomy and intramedullary rodding. (Right) Posteroanterior radiograph shows thin diaphyses of the metacarpals and phalanges in this patient with arachnodactyly and osteopenia. The combination is seen in homocystinuria.

Achondroplasia (Mimic)

Hypophosphatasia

(Left) Anteroposterior radiograph shows short bones of the limbs. The metaphyses are broad and flat, giving the impression of overtubulation. However, the diaphyses are not truly thinned in this patient with achondroplasia. (Right) Anteroposterior radiograph shows thinning, bowing, and deformity of the femora ⟹. There is severe osteopenia, which has worsened with time. Protrusio and widened, irregular physes contribute to the diagnosis of hypophosphatasia.

Radiation

Caudal Regression Syndrome

(Left) Anteroposterior radiograph shows a short humerus, with thinning of the distal diaphysis ⟹ (compare size with the normal thorax). This patient had whole bone radiation as a child for Ewing sarcoma, resulting in growth abnormalities. Radiation sarcoma is also seen ⟹. (Right) Anteroposterior radiograph shows absence of lumbar spine ⟹ and hypoplastic iliac wings with absent sacrum ⟹, typical of caudal regression. Note the thin, ill-formed femora ⟹.

GROWTH PLATE, PREMATURE PHYSEAL CLOSURE

DIFFERENTIAL DIAGNOSIS

Common
- Fracture

Less Common
- Osteomyelitis
- Septic Joint
- Iatrogenic (Surgical)
- Juvenile Idiopathic Arthritis (JIA)
- Ollier/Maffucci Syndrome (Mimic)
- Radiation-Induced Growth Deformities
- Thermal Injury

Rare but Important
- Complications of Vitamin A
- Hemophilia: MSK Complications
- Meningococcemia

ESSENTIAL INFORMATION

Key Differential Diagnosis Issues
- # & distribution of physes may be diagnostic

Helpful Clues for Common Diagnoses
- **Fracture**
  - Hyperemia in metadiaphyseal fracture may result in early fusion of physis
  - Salter injury (usually III, IV, or V) may result in focal early bony bridging

Helpful Clues for Less Common Diagnoses
- **Osteomyelitis**
  - Usually located in metaphysis in child
    - Occasionally, process will cross physis to involve epiphysis → early fusion
  - Hyperemia from chronic infection may result in early fusion of entire physis
- **Septic Joint**
  - Early fusion: Chronic hyperemia or direct extension to physis if intracapsular (hip)
- **Iatrogenic (Surgical)**
  - Epiphysiodesis performed for angular deformity or short contralateral limb
- **Juvenile Idiopathic Arthritis (JIA)**
  - Chronic hyperemia at involved joints has 2 growth-related consequences
    - Epiphyseal/metaphyseal overgrowth
    - Early fusion of physis → short limb
  - Knee > elbow > ankle, not symmetric
- **Ollier/Maffucci Syndrome (Mimic)**
  - Short, broad, abnormally tubulated metaphyses; often chondroid matrix
- **Radiation-Induced Growth Deformities**
  - Vasculitis from radiation puts physis at risk
  - Nonviable physis → fusion & hypoplasia
  - Watch for port-like distribution
- **Thermal Injury**
  - Vessels supplying physes at risk, particularly in hands or feet
    - → Short, stubby fingers in adults
  - Burn: Contractures & calcification
  - Frostbite: Abnormality spares the thumb

Helpful Clues for Rare Diagnoses
- **Complications of Vitamin A**
  - Focal bony bridging across physis
  - Diffuse periostitis, coned epiphyses
- **Hemophilia: MSK Complications**
  - Same as JIA, with dense effusions

Fracture

Sagittal bone CT shows premature bony bridge (physeal bar) formed at site of physeal fracture ➡. This partial early fusion will result in relative overgrowth anteriorly & posteriorly, deforming the distal tibia.

Osteomyelitis

Coronal T2WI MR shows a metaphyseal focus of osteomyelitis crossing the physis ➡ and involving the epiphysis in an 8 yo. This involvement of the physis may result in early focal bridging of the physis. (†MSK Req).

GROWTH PLATE, PREMATURE PHYSEAL CLOSURE

Iatrogenic (Surgical)

Juvenile Idiopathic Arthritis (JIA)

(Left) Anteroposterior radiograph shows typical Blount disease ➡ involving the medial tibia. Since this results in tibia vara, prophylactic epiphysiodesis is performed laterally ➡, now showing closure of this portion of the physis. *(Right)* Anteroposterior radiograph shows early physeal closure in this 16 year old with JIA. This joint shows severe involvement, with overgrowth of the epiphyses, joint destruction, and widening of the intercondylar notch.

Ollier/Maffucci Syndrome (Mimic)

Radiation-Induced Growth Deformities

(Left) Lateral radiograph shows short ulna in a patient with Ollier disease ➡, mimicking early physeal closure. Short bone results from metaphyseal dysplasia rather than true early fusion. *(Right)* AP radiograph shows hypoplastic left iliac wing ➡ in 20 year old who had radiation therapy to left hemipelvis as a child. Vascular damage results in early fusion of epiphyses & apophyses, with cessation of growth. Exostosis ➡ is also a complication of radiation.

Thermal Injury

Meningococcemia

(Left) Posteroanterior radiograph shows premature closure of the physes of the distal phalanges of digits 2-5 ➡, resulting in short, stubby digits. This is due to vascular damage from frostbite. Note the normal physis and distal phalanx of the thumb ➡, typical of frostbite. *(Right)* Anteroposterior radiograph shows early bony bridging of a portion of the physis of the left hip ➡ in a patient with meningococcemia. Short limbs are often a consequence of this process.

GROWTH PLATE, WIDENED PHYSIS

DIFFERENTIAL DIAGNOSIS

Common
- Physeal Fracture
- Chronic Repetitive Trauma
- Slipped Capital Femoral Epiphysis (SCFE)
- Renal Osteodystrophy (Renal OD)
- Rickets

Less Common
- Osteomyelitis
- Legg-Calvé-Perthes (LCP)
- Blount Disease
- Total Parenteral Nutrition
- Gigantism
- Mucopolysaccharidoses
- Osteogenesis Imperfecta (OI)
- Hypophosphatasia

Rare but Important
- Hypothyroidism
- Scurvy
- Copper Deficiency (Menkes Kinky-Hair Syndrome)
- Metaphyseal Dysplasias

ESSENTIAL INFORMATION

Key Differential Diagnosis Issues
- Involvement of all physes rather than a single or few sites seen in several processes
  - Rickets & renal OD
  - Total parenteral nutrition
  - Gigantism
  - Mucopolysaccharidoses
  - Osteogenesis imperfecta
  - Hypophosphatasia
  - Hypothyroidism
  - Copper deficiency
  - Metaphyseal dysplasias

Helpful Clues for Common Diagnoses
- **Physeal Fracture**
  - Salter I: Fracture through physis; difficult to visualize unless displaced
  - Salter II: Fracture through physis, extending through metaphysis
    - Metaphyseal portion may be subtle; easier to visualize if displaced
  - Salter III: Fracture through physis, extending through epiphysis

- Salter IV: Fracture through epiphysis, physis, & metaphysis; generally does not result in physeal widening
- Salter V: Crush fracture of physis; does not result in widening
- **Chronic Repetitive Trauma**
  - In child, repeated microtrauma to a physis results in resorption & appearance of widening
  - Analogous to Salter I injury
  - Associated with competitive athletes
    - Distal radius/ulna: Gymnasts
    - Distal tibia/fibula: Runners
    - Proximal humerus: Baseball pitchers
- **Slipped Capital Femoral Epiphysis (SCFE)**
  - Slip direction generally posterior and medial
  - Results in appearance of widened physis & "short" capital epiphysis
  - Bilateral in 20-25%, but need not be synchronous
  - Optimal age range: 8-14
- **Renal Osteodystrophy (Renal OD)**
  - Combined findings of rickets & hyperparathyroidism (HPTH)
  - Rickets results in widening of physis
  - Watch for HPTH as well
    - Subperiosteal resorption
    - Subchondral resorption with collapse (particularly sacroiliac joints)
- **Rickets**
  - Similar appearance, whether renal or nutritional etiology
  - Results from lack of mineralization of osteoid laid down at metaphyseal zone of provisional calcification
  - Widened physis, often with fraying of metaphyses
  - Decreased bone density, smudgy trabeculae

Helpful Clues for Less Common Diagnoses
- **Osteomyelitis**
  - If metaphyseal osteomyelitis crosses physis, may result in slip of physis & appearance of widening
  - Watch for osseous destruction, periosteal reaction
- **Legg-Calvé-Perthes (LCP)**
  - Osteonecrosis of femoral capital epiphysis
  - Increased density, flattening, fragmentation of epiphysis

- ○ Associated appearance of widened physis
- ○ Optimal age range: 4-8
- **Blount Disease**
  - ○ Fragmentation & abnormal ossification of medial tibial metaphysis
  - ○ Focal "widening" of physis medially
  - ○ Usually bilateral; results in tibia vara
- **Total Parenteral Nutrition**
  - ○ Premature infant dependent on total parenteral nutrition for a long period of time
  - ○ Diffuse widening of physes, thought to be due to nutritional deficiency of copper
  - ○ Indistinguishable from rickets, though true rickets does not appear prior to 6 months of age
- **Gigantism**
  - ○ With overgrowth of gigantism, physes may appear mildly widened diffusely
- **Mucopolysaccharidoses**
  - ○ Delay in epiphyseal ossification may give the appearance of a relatively widened physis
  - ○ Other manifestations: Fan-shaped carpus, oar-shaped ribs, narrow inferior ilium with steep acetabular roof
- **Osteogenesis Imperfecta (OI)**
  - ○ OI tarda may show physeal widening and mild slip of epiphyses
  - ○ Other manifestations: Osteoporosis & more fractures than normally expected in a child
- **Hypophosphatasia**
  - ○ Nearly indistinguishable from rickets

- ○ Diffuse widening of physes
- ○ Osteopenia
- ○ Ranges from mild tarda form to severe destructive form
- ○ Bowing of long bones with excrescences may help differentiate from rickets
- ○ May have "button sequestra" in skull

Helpful Clues for Rare Diagnoses
- **Hypothyroidism**
  - ○ Severe retardation of skeletal maturation
  - ○ Widened physes, short broad phalanges
  - ○ Hip may show fragmentation of femoral capital epiphysis
    - Appearance may be similar to Legg-Calvé-Perthes; watch for abnormal bone age to differentiate
  - ○ Infant shows stippled epiphyses
- **Scurvy**
  - ○ Osteopenia, with sclerotic metaphyseal line (white line of Frankel) and sclerotic rim of epiphysis (Wimberger sign)
  - ○ Corner metaphyseal fracture may cause a slip & mild physeal widening
    - Wide periosteal "reaction" due to subperiosteal hemorrhage
- **Copper Deficiency (Menkes Kinky-Hair Syndrome)**
  - ○ Rare disorder resulting in physeal widening
  - ○ Myeloneuropathy
- **Metaphyseal Dysplasias**
  - ○ Metaphyses flared & irregular with apparent physeal widening

Physeal Fracture

Frog lateral radiograph shows widening of the physis ➡ due to a Salter II fracture. The fracture line extends on through the metaphysis ➡. Salter II fractures are rarely subtle; Salter I is more difficult to recognize.

Chronic Repetitive Trauma

Anteroposterior radiograph shows osteolysis at the distal radial epiphyseal plate ➡, a type of Salter I injury occurring in gymnasts due to chronic repetitive trauma. Note the similar abnormality involving the ulna.

GROWTH PLATE, WIDENED PHYSIS

Slipped Capital Femoral Epiphysis (SCFE)

Renal Osteodystrophy (Renal OD)

(Left) Frog lateral radiograph shows a left SCFE (compare with normal right side). With the posteromedial slip of the head ➡, the physis appears to widen ➡. (Right) AP radiograph shows severe renal OD, manifest in the hips as rickets, with widening of the zone of provisional calcification ➡ and slip of the capital epiphyses ➡. There is also typical hyperparathyroidism, with widened sacroiliac joints ➡ due to subchondral resorption and collapse on the iliac side.

Rickets

Osteomyelitis

(Left) Anteroposterior radiograph shows a widened physis ➡ at both the tibia and femur due to nutritional rickets. The abnormality is secondary to the formation of osteoid which is not mineralized; the appearance is identical in rickets due to renal OD. (Right) Anteroposterior radiograph shows metaphyseal destruction ➡ and periosteal reaction secondary to osteomyelitis. Infection has crossed the physis, resulting in widening ➡ and slip of the epiphysis ➡.

Legg-Calvé-Perthes (LCP)

Blount Disease

(Left) AP radiograph shows a dense, flattened femoral capital epiphysis ➡ in a young child; this is LCP or osteonecrosis. The abnormality may result in widening and fraying of the metaphysis, as in this case ➡. (Right) Anteroposterior radiograph shows beaking & underdevelopment of the medial metaphysis of the left tibia. This results in an appearance of physeal widening ➡. The patient has undergone epiphysiodesis laterally to address the growth inequity.

GROWTH PLATE, WIDENED PHYSIS

Total Parenteral Nutrition

Mucopolysaccharidoses

(Left) Lateral radiograph shows widening of the physis and fraying of the metaphyses ➡ in a case of neonatal rickets; the patient was a 26 week premature infant, now 3 months old. Infants nourished for long periods with total parenteral nutrition may develop the appearance of rickets. *(Right)* AP radiograph shows typical skeletal findings of dysostosis multiplex, with inferior tapering of ilia, steep acetabular roofs, & coxa valga. The physes may appear widened ➡.

Osteogenesis Imperfecta (OI)

Hypophosphatasia

(Left) Anteroposterior radiograph shows osteopenia and multiple healed fractures typical of OI tarda. The physes are mildly widened and slipped ➡. *(Right)* Lateral radiograph shows widening of the physis ➡ that is reminiscent of rickets. This is a mild case of hypophosphatasia. In severe cases, the bone density is significantly reduced and the physes show more significant widening, with fraying of the metaphyses.

Hypothyroidism

Scurvy

(Left) AP radiograph shows widening of the physes ➡ & severe growth retardation in this 4 year old with hypothyroidism. There is also fragmentation of the right femoral capital epiphysis ➡, which has been termed the "cretinoid" hip. *(Right)* AP radiograph shows typical findings of scurvy, with a metaphyseal corner ➡ fracture. With such a fracture, the physis may be displaced & appear widened. Note the wide periosteal reaction ➡, related to subperiosteal hemorrhage.

PERIOSTEUM: AGGRESSIVE PERIOSTITIS

DIFFERENTIAL DIAGNOSIS

Common
- Osteosarcoma, Conventional
- Ewing Sarcoma
- Malignant Fibrous Histiocytoma
- Metastasis
- Fracture Healing Process

Less Common
- Osteomyelitis
- Leukemia
- Osteosarcoma, Periosteal (Mimic)
- Lymphoma

Rare but Important
- Fibrosarcoma
- Angiosarcoma, Osseous

ESSENTIAL INFORMATION

Key Differential Diagnosis Issues
- Periosteal reaction or periostitis is the reaction of cortical bone to an insult
- Differential diagnosis is aided by the pattern & location of periosteal reaction, although the presence is nonspecific
- Periosteal reaction is visible on radiographs 10 days to 3 weeks post insult
  - Periosteum is more active in childhood & thus more likely to show osteoblastic activity than in adults
- Aggressive periosteal reaction is also termed "interrupted"
  - Indicates a rapidly progressing process, benign or malignant
  - Is in contrast to solid (more benign-appearing) periosteal reaction
- Main interrupted periosteal reaction patterns
  - Lamellated
  - Spiculated
  - Disorganized
- Lamellated
  - a.k.a., "onion skin"
  - Multiple parallel layers
  - Seen most commonly with hyperemic entities
- Spiculated
  - a.k.a., "sunburst", "hair on end", "velvet"
  - Linear spicules of new bone radiate from the bone cortex
    - Divergent, perpendicular or sloping
- Disorganized
  - a.k.a., amorphous or complex
  - Irregular collection of reactive bone
  - Complex pattern can be due to rapid tumor growth, infection, or fracture
- Codman triangle
  - Focal triangular elevation of calcified periosteum at site of bone insertion
  - Classically associated with malignancy, but also seen with infection and trauma
- Thin periosteal reaction, < 1 mm, is equivocal for an aggressive process
  - May progress to either interrupted or solid periosteal reaction

Helpful Clues for Common Diagnoses
- **Osteosarcoma, Conventional**
  - Location: Femur, tibia, humerus most common
  - Periosteal reactions: "Sunburst", "hair on end", lamellated, solid thin, disorganized
  - Codman triangle common
  - Osteoid matrix visible in 80%
  - Wide zone of transition
  - Cortical breakthrough & soft tissue mass
- **Ewing Sarcoma**
  - Location: Tubular bones predominate if < 20 years old; flat bones if > 20 years old
  - Periosteal reactions: Lamellated, "hair on end", solid thin
  - Codman triangle common
  - Tumor permeates through cortex
  - Large soft tissue mass is common
  - Lacks metaphyseal lucent lines
- **Malignant Fibrous Histiocytoma**
  - Location: Long bone metaphysis, pelvis
  - Periosteal reactions: Thin or disorganized; lamellated with pathologic fracture
  - Codman triangle uncommon
  - Ill-defined, permeative lesion
  - May arise secondarily in abnormal bone
- **Metastasis**
  - Location: Multifocal
  - Periosteal reactions: Thin, disorganized
  - Lamellated & perpendicular periosteal reactions are less common
    - Sunburst-type periosteal reaction with metastatic neuroblastoma
  - Osteoblastic, osteolytic or mixed density underlying lesions
    - Axial & proximal appendicular skeleton most common

PERIOSTEUM: AGGRESSIVE PERIOSTITIS

○ Metastases 25x more common than primary bone malignancy
• **Fracture Healing Process**
  ○ Location: Region of trauma
  ○ Periosteal reactions: Thin, disorganized
  ○ If soft tissue mass present, follow to confirm resolving hematoma
    ▪ Tumor will not resolve
  ○ Transverse long bone fracture without significant trauma should increase vigilance for underlying pathologic lesion

Helpful Clues for Less Common Diagnoses
• **Osteomyelitis**
  ○ Location: Localized; long bones
    ▪ Multifocal uncommon
  ○ Periosteal reaction: Disorganized, thin, lamellated, spiculated
  ○ Codman triangle relatively common
  ○ Lytic destruction of bone in acute phase most common
    ▪ Geographic with sclerotic margin possible but rare
  ○ Look for associated air, sinus tract, sequestrum
  ○ Can mimic Ewing sarcoma, lymphoma, leukemia
• **Leukemia**
  ○ Location: Long bones in children, axial skeleton in adults
  ○ Periosteal reactions: Thin or lamellated; "hair on end" in skull
  ○ Radiolucent transverse metaphyseal bands
    ▪ "Leukemic lines"

▪ Also seen in metastatic neuroblastoma & rhabdomyosarcoma
○ Radiographs can be normal
• **Osteosarcoma, Periosteal (Mimic)**
  ○ Location: Surface of bone diaphysis
  ○ Periosteal reactions: Not periostitis
    ▪ Ossified tumor matrix produces similar appearance to periosteal reaction
  ○ Rare subtype, 1%, of osteosarcoma
  ○ Underlying medullary canal uninvolved
• **Lymphoma**
  ○ Location: Long or flat bones
  ○ Periosteal reactions: Thin or disorganized
  ○ Codman triangle unusual
  ○ Moth-eaten lytic lesion
    ▪ Soft tissue mass larger than bone destruction
  ○ Cortical destruction late in disease

Helpful Clues for Rare Diagnoses
• **Fibrosarcoma**
  ○ Location: Eccentric metaphysis of long tubular bones
  ○ Periosteal reactions: Thin or disorganized
  ○ Codman triangle unusual
  ○ Wide range of appearances: Circumscribed to permeative
• **Angiosarcoma, Osseous**
  ○ Location: Long bones
  ○ Periosteal reactions: Thin or disorganized
  ○ Codman triangle unusual

Osteosarcoma, Conventional

Anteroposterior radiograph shows a "sunburst" periosteal reaction ➡. Note the permeative destruction of the radius, with tumor osteoid formed in both the bone and soft tissue mass.

Osteosarcoma, Conventional

Anteroposterior radiograph shows a large, permeative lesion with osteoid matrix and a wide zone of transition. There is extensive periosteal reaction ➡ and a large soft tissue mass ➡.

PERIOSTEUM: AGGRESSIVE PERIOSTITIS

(Left) Anteroposterior radiograph shows a highly aggressive lytic lesion ⇨ of the proximal fibular metaphysis that has traversed the cortex. There is a wide zone of transition, a large soft tissue mass, and aggressive appearing periosteal reaction ➡. *(Right)* Lateral radiograph shows Codman triangle of aggressive periosteal reaction ➡ along the anterior cortex of the mid-femoral diaphysis. There is underlying permeative medullary lesion and a subtle soft tissue mass.

(Left) Lateral radiograph shows a highly aggressive lytic lesion ⇨ arising in the central diaphysis. There is a wide zone of transition, cortical breakthrough, interrupted periosteal reaction ➡, and a soft tissue mass. *(Right)* Lateral radiograph shows a medulloblastoma metastasis ⇨ in the proximal ulna with a mixed lytic and sclerotic appearance. Note the marked aggressive, perpendicular periosteal reaction ➡.

(Left) Lateral radiograph shows a transverse supracondylar distal humerus fracture ➡. Extensive disorganized periosteal new bone surrounds the fracture ➡ due to the lack of proper fracture immobilization. *(Right)* Lateral radiograph shows a nightstick fracture site complicated by osteomyelitis. There is permeative bone destruction ⇨, a dense central bone sequestrum ➡, and disorganized surrounding periosteal reaction ➡.

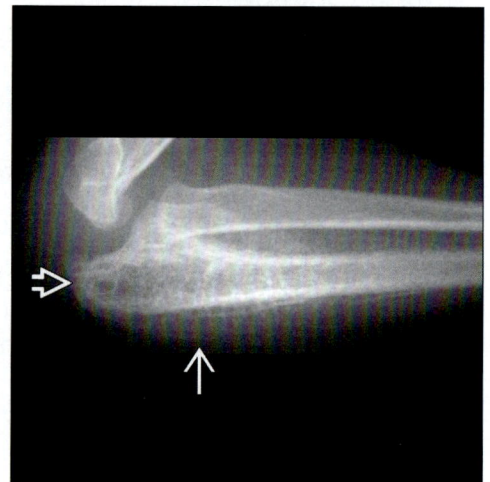

Ewing Sarcoma

Ewing Sarcoma

Malignant Fibrous Histiocytoma

Metastasis

Fracture Healing Process

Osteomyelitis

PERIOSTEUM: AGGRESSIVE PERIOSTITIS

Osteomyelitis

Osteosarcoma, Periosteal (Mimic)

(Left) Anteroposterior radiograph shows severe permeative destructive change of the proximal radius ➡, along with disorganized periosteal reaction ➡. This could represent either osteomyelitis or an aggressive tumor. This was found to be staphylococcus osteomyelitis. *(Right)* Axial NECT shows a lesion on the surface of the tibia which produces fairly mature-appearing bone ➡. It does not involve the marrow space.

Osteosarcoma, Periosteal (Mimic)

Lymphoma

(Left) Lateral radiograph shows spiculated osteoid matrix ➡ along the surface of the bone. An MR showed no involvement of the marrow. This is a mimic of a periosteal reaction since the radiodense material is tumor osteoid. *(Right)* Oblique radiograph shows mildly disorganized periosteal reaction ➡ at the distal tibia. Hypertrophic osteoarthropathy or osteomyelitis could be considered, but MR documented an extensive underlying medullary lesion.

Fibrosarcoma

Angiosarcoma, Osseous

(Left) Lateral radiograph shows only a "smudginess" of the bone trabeculae ➡, as well as subtle interrupted periosteal reaction ➡. These findings represent an extremely permeative and aggressive underlying lesion. *(Right)* Coronal NECT shows a destructive mass ➡ in the proximal tibia. There is breech of the cortex ➡ and a small amount of disorganized periosteal reaction ➡. Both infection and malignancy were initially considered in the differential diagnosis.

PERIOSTEUM: SOLID PERIOSTITIS

DIFFERENTIAL DIAGNOSIS

Common
- Fracture Healing Process
- Venous Stasis
- Psoriatic Arthritis
- Chronic Osteomyelitis
- Hypertrophic Osteoarthropathy
- Stress Fracture
- Chondroblastoma
- Osteoid Osteoma

Less Common
- Renal Osteodystrophy, Neostosis
- Juvenile Idiopathic Arthritis (JIA)
- Chronic Reactive Arthritis
- Sickle Cell Anemia: MSK Complications
- Metastases, Treated
- Melorheostosis (Mimic)

Rare but Important
- Complications of Vitamin A
- Osteitis Condensans of Clavicle
- Chronic Recurrent Multifocal Osteomyelitis
- Complications of Vitamin D
- Complications of Fluoride
- Thyroid Acropachy
- Pachydermoperiostosis
- Engelmann Disease (Engelmann-Camurati)
- Physiologic Periostitis, Lower Extremity
- Caffey Disease (Infantile Cortical Hyperostosis)
- Scurvy
- Secondary Syphilis

ESSENTIAL INFORMATION

Key Differential Diagnosis Issues
- Thick, solid periosteal reactions typically reflect a nonmalignant underlying process
  - Exception: Hypertrophic osteoarthropathy
  - Very rarely seen in osteosarcoma, Ewing sarcoma, and untreated metastases

Helpful Clues for Common Diagnoses
- **Fracture Healing Process**
  - Periosteal reaction: Wide range depending on motion at fracture site during healing
    - Greater motion = greater disorganization
  - Periosteal reaction from traumatic and pathologic fractures can be similar
- **Venous Stasis**
  - Location: Lower extremity
  - Distribution: Localized or generalized
  - Associated findings: Phleboliths, cellulitis
- **Psoriatic Arthritis**
  - Location: Periarticular, peripheral ligament, and tendon insertions
  - Distribution: Localized or generalized
  - Periosteal reaction: Solid, irregular
- **Chronic Osteomyelitis**
  - Location: Any location is possible
  - Distribution: Localized
  - Periosteal reaction: Thick, dense
  - Underlying mixed sclerotic and lytic lesion ± sequestrum
- **Hypertrophic Osteoarthropathy**
  - Location: Long bone diaphyses
  - Distribution: Symmetric, generalized
  - Evaluate for underlying carcinoma or chronic disease (thoracic or abdominal)
- **Stress Fracture**
  - Location: Tibia, metatarsals, long bones, pelvis, calcaneus
  - Distribution: Localized
  - Periosteal reaction: Linear, ovoid, or concentric
- **Chondroblastoma**
  - Location: Along metadiaphysis adjacent to epiphyseal chondroblastoma
  - Periosteal reaction: Thick, solid, or layered
  - Lytic epiphyseal lesion with variable chondroid matrix and variably sclerotic border
- **Osteoid Osteoma**
  - Location: Femur, tibia, fibula, humerus
  - Periosteal reaction: Thick & dense; blends with thickened cortex
  - Central lucent nidus
  - Intraarticular location has paucity of periosteal new bone

Helpful Clues for Less Common Diagnoses
- **Renal Osteodystrophy, Neostosis**
  - Location: Phalanges, metatarsals, metacarpals
  - Seen in healing phase
- **Juvenile Idiopathic Arthritis (JIA)**
  - Location: Periarticular, ligament and tendon insertions
  - Distribution: Localized or generalized
- **Chronic Reactive Arthritis**
  - Location: Calcaneus, metatarsals, lower leg
  - Distribution: Localized
- **Sickle Cell Anemia: MSK Complications**

PERIOSTEUM: SOLID PERIOSTITIS

○ Location: Tubular bones of hands & feet (dactylitis), long bones
○ Distribution: Generalized
• **Metastases, Treated**
○ Solid periosteal reaction most common in treated metastases
• **Melorheostosis (Mimic)**
○ Sclerosing bone dysplasia produces endosteal &/or cortical ossification, not true periosteal reaction
○ Sclerotomal distribution common

Helpful Clues for Rare Diagnoses
• **Complications of Vitamin A**
○ Location: Ulna, lower leg, metatarsals, clavicle
○ Retinoid drug administration in teens
• **Osteitis Condensans of Clavicle**
○ Location: Medial end of clavicle
○ Sclerosis of normal-sized bone with solid periosteal reaction
• **Chronic Recurrent Multifocal Osteomyelitis**
○ Location: Long bone metaphysis, clavicle, spine
○ Radiographically ranges from occult to mimicking osteosarcoma
• **Complications of Vitamin D**
○ Rickets = wide physes; cupped, frayed epiphyses
○ Periosteal elevation from unmineralized osteoid or occult fracture
• **Complications of Fluoride**
○ Location: Tubular bones, symmetric

○ Calcified ligaments and tendons
  ▪ Ossified posterior longitudinal ligament common
○ Osteosclerosis
• **Thyroid Acropachy**
○ Location: Metacarpals, metatarsals
○ Periosteal reaction: Solid, "fluffy" border
○ History of treatment for hyperthyroidism
• **Pachydermoperiostosis**
○ Primary form of hypertrophic osteoarthropathy
○ Periosteal reaction: Thick, shaggy
○ Male predominance with onset at puberty
• **Engelmann Disease (Engelmann-Camurati)**
○ Diaphyseal broadening of long bones
• **Physiologic Periostitis, Lower Extremity**
○ Location: Long bones, symmetric
○ Infants up to 6 months of age
  ▪ More common in premature infants
• **Caffey Disease (Infantile Cortical Hyperostosis)**
○ Location: Jaw, long bone diaphysis, clavicle, scapula, ribs
○ 1st seen in infants < 6 months of age
• **Scurvy**
○ Location: Long bones
○ Follows location of subperiosteal bleed & subsequent calcification
• **Secondary Syphilis**
○ Location: Long bones, skull
○ Periosteal reaction: Solid with short spicules

Fracture Healing Process

Anteroposterior radiograph shows a healing fracture ▶ of the distal femoral diaphysis. Smooth, solid periosteal reaction ▶ is present along the medial cortex due to the fracture and placement of locking screws.

Venous Stasis

Anteroposterior radiograph shows solid periosteal reaction ▶ along both sides of the fibula. These findings were present bilaterally and are associated with subcutaneous edema ▶ from venous insufficiency.

PERIOSTEUM: SOLID PERIOSTITIS

(Left) Anteroposterior radiograph shows subtle, solid periostitis ➡ and cartilage narrowing at several joints ➡. The presence of periostitis makes rheumatoid arthritis unlikely. *(Right)* Anteroposterior radiograph shows solid to perpendicular periostitis ➡ along the medial edge of the distal phalanx of the great toe. The productive changes seen here are typical of both psoriatic arthritis and chronic reactive arthritis.

Psoriatic Arthritis

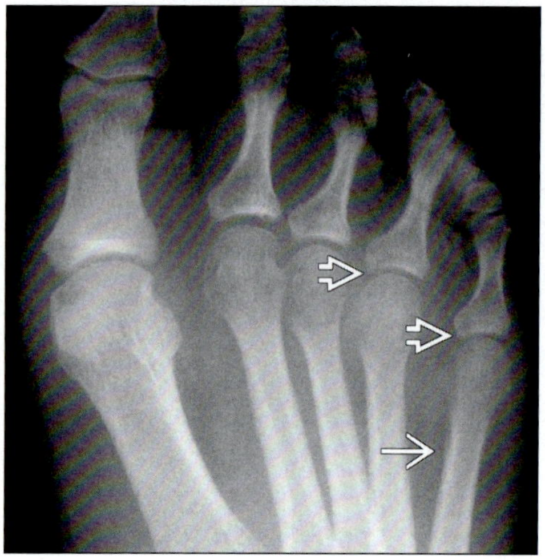

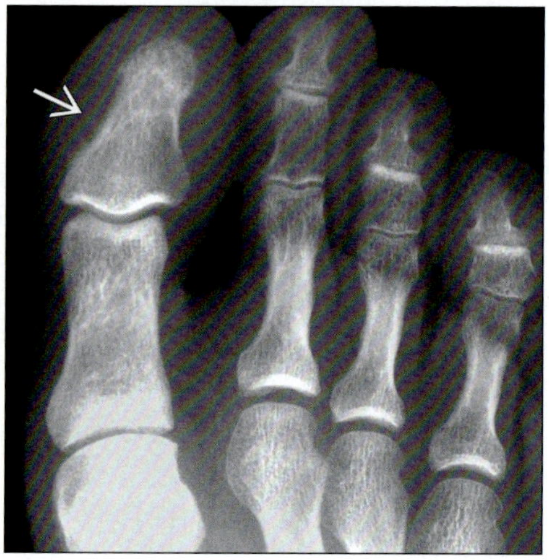

Psoriatic Arthritis

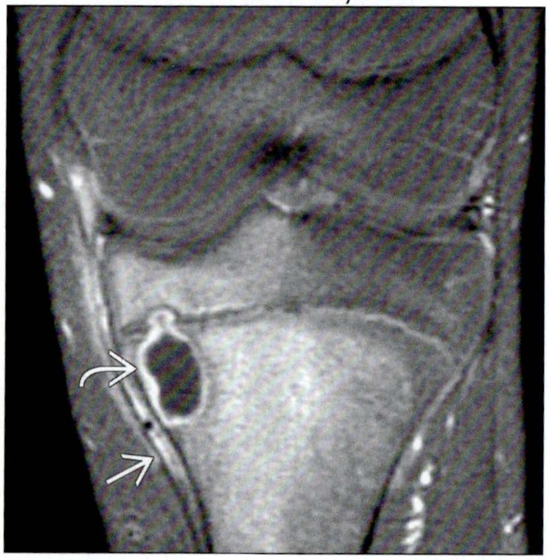

(Left) Radiograph of the forearm shows solid, mature periosteal reaction ➡ along the radius. Early in the course of the disease, permeative destructive changes of the underlying bone were visible. *(Right)* Coronal T1 C+ MR shows a proximal medial metaphyseal lesion ➡ crossing the physis into the epiphysis, with extensive marrow edema, a well-defined rim of enhancement, and periosteal elevation ➡. A Brodie abscess was found at surgery.

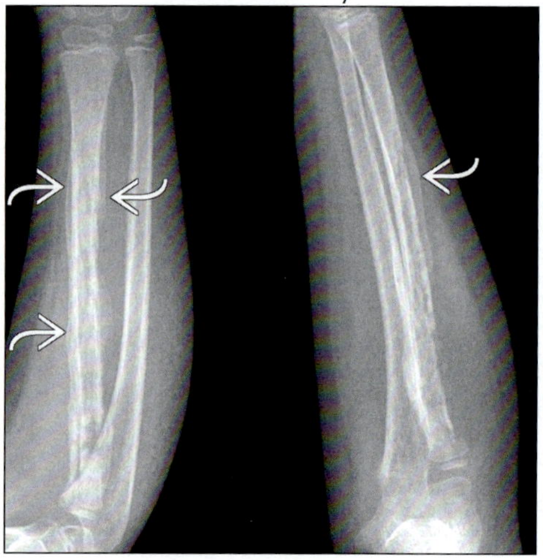

Chronic Osteomyelitis

Chronic Osteomyelitis

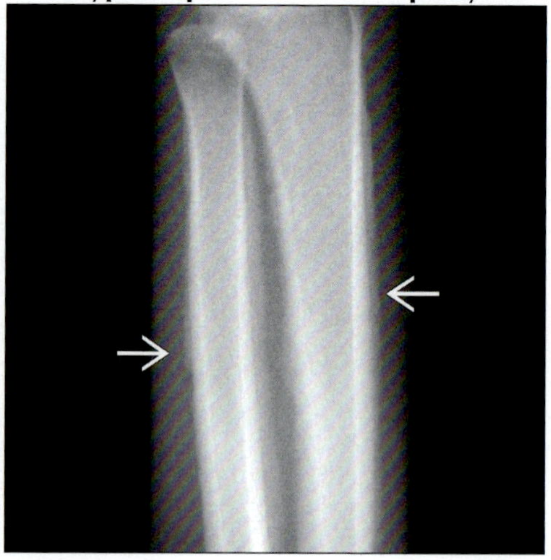

(Left) Anteroposterior radiograph shows exuberant periosteal reaction at the proximal tibia ➡ and a less prominent reaction involving the distal femur ➡ and fibula ➡. These changes were secondary to lung cancer. (†MSK Req). *(Right)* Oblique radiograph shows symmetric, solid periosteal reaction ➡ along the radius and ulna. Secondary causes are far more common than primary; thus occult malignancy should be excluded when these findings are encountered.

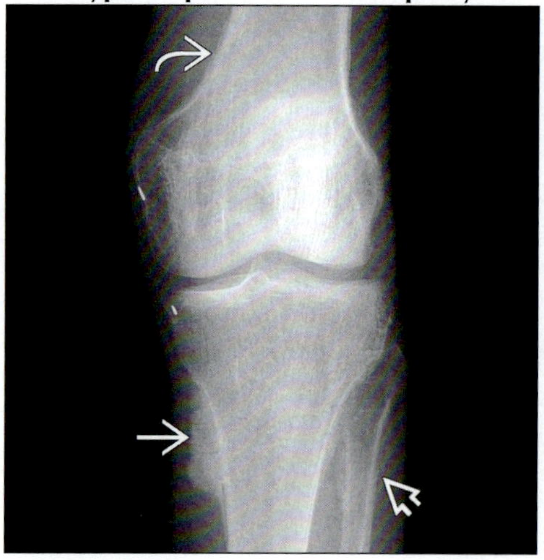

Hypertrophic Osteoarthropathy

Hypertrophic Osteoarthropathy

PERIOSTEUM: SOLID PERIOSTITIS

Stress Fracture

Stress Fracture

(Left) Coronal TSE TRIM MR shows bone marrow edema ➡ in the area of stress and increased signal in the muscles ➡ and periosteum ➡. Radiographs were normal at this time. (Right) Anteroposterior radiograph in the same patient ten weeks later shows dense circumferential periosteal new bone formation ➡ in the area of the stress fracture.

Chondroblastoma

Osteoid Osteoma

(Left) Anteroposterior radiograph shows a lytic epiphyseal lesion of the humerus ➡. The lesion contains a faint calcific matrix ➡ and has a dense periosteal reaction in the metaphyseal region ➡, typical for this diagnosis. (Right) Axial NECT shows a cortically based osteoid osteoma with a typical lucent nidus ➡. It is surrounded by densely sclerotic cortical thickening and periosteal new bone ➡.

Renal Osteodystrophy, Neostosis

Juvenile Idiopathic Arthritis (JIA)

(Left) Posteroanterior radiograph shows an exuberant healing response in this patient being treated for renal disease. The finger shows conventional neostosis, with dense periosteal new bone formation along the phalanges ➡. (Right) Lateral radiograph shows solid periosteal reaction along the phalanges ➡ with soft tissue swelling, but normal joints. The differential diagnosis includes juvenile idiopathic arthritis, sickle cell dactylitis, and tuberculosis dactylitis.

PERIOSTEUM: SOLID PERIOSTITIS

Chronic Reactive Arthritis

Sickle Cell Anemia: MSK Complications

(Left) Posteroanterior radiograph shows soft tissue swelling of the index finger, as well as cartilage narrowing in the DIP ➡. Additionally, there is prominent periostitis at the middle phalanx ➡. *(Right)* Anteroposterior radiograph shows a typical instance of sickle cell dactylitis in a baby. Solid periosteal reaction ➡ surrounds several metacarpals. These findings were present bilaterally.

Metastases, Treated

Melorheostosis (Mimic)

(Left) Anteroposterior radiograph shows a treated lung carcinoma metastasis ➡. The lesion was initially lytic with an aggressive periosteal reaction. After radiation therapy, it became sclerotic with a solid periosteal reaction ➡. *(Right)* Anteroposterior radiograph shows sclerosis involving endosteal ➡ and periosteal ➡ portions of the cortex. The tibia was also involved. A sclerotomal distribution is often present but is not seen in this case.

Complications of Vitamin A

Osteitis Condensans of Clavicle

(Left) Posteroanterior radiograph shows dense solid periostitis at the ulna ➡ in this patient who was overdosed with vitamin A by his zealous mother. Several other bones showed similar solid periostitis. *(Right)* Axial NECT shows dense sclerosis ➡ and solid periosteal new bone ➡ involving the medial right clavicle. The opposite clavicle is normal ➡. This can be due to chronic recurrent osteomyelitis or SAPHO syndrome.

PERIOSTEUM: SOLID PERIOSTITIS

Chronic Recurrent Multifocal Osteomyelitis

Thyroid Acropachy

(Left) Lateral radiograph shows a mixed sclerotic and lytic lesion ➜ with prominent solid periosteal reaction ➜. A similar lesion was present in the sacrum. Diagnosis required open biopsy after a percutaneous biopsy specimen was inconclusive. *(Right)* Posteroanterior radiograph shows fluffy periosteal reaction and soft tissue swelling involving multiple phalanges ➜. There is also clubbing of the digits ➜ in this patient treated for hyperthyroidism.

Pachydermoperiostosis

Engelmann Disease (Engelmann-Camurati)

(Left) Anteroposterior radiograph shows solid periosteal reaction ➜ along the metacarpals and phalanges. There were no joint changes, underlying lesions, or metabolic disease. Solid periosteal reaction was present throughout the body. (†MSK Req). *(Right)* Anteroposterior radiograph shows marked endosteal and periosteal cortical thickening ➜. The process was bilaterally symmetric and involved the entire length of the diaphyses but spared the metaphyses and epiphyses.

Physiologic Periostitis, Lower Extremity

Scurvy

(Left) Anteroposterior radiograph shows subtle diffuse increased density of the lower extremity long bones, resulting from subtle solid periostitis ➜. Findings are particularly prominent along the diaphyses and were bilaterally symmetric. *(Right)* Anteroposterior radiograph shows diffuse osteopenia with metaphyseal corner fractures ➜, termed Pelken fractures. With these fractures, the patient may develop an extensive subperiosteal bleed, elevating the periosteum ➜.

PERIOSTEUM: BIZARRE HORIZONTAL PERIOSTEAL REACTION

DIFFERENTIAL DIAGNOSIS

Common
- Hypertrophic Osteoarthropathy (HOA)
- Renal Osteodystrophy, Neostosis

Less Common
- Parosteal Lipoma
- Hemophilic Pseudotumor
- Fibromatosis
- Juvenile Aponeurotic Fibroma
- Osteosarcoma (Mimic)
- Skull Hemangioma (Mimic)
- Thalassemia (Mimic)
- Aneurysmal Bone Cyst (Mimic)

Rare but Important
- Soft Tissue Tumor Adjacent To Bone
- Subperiosteal Ganglion

ESSENTIAL INFORMATION

Key Differential Diagnosis Issues
- True bizarre horizontal periosteal reaction is uncommon
  - Most of the entities generally present with linear, regular periosteal bone formation
  - Occasional bizarre appearance may be confusing; this list addresses these uncommon instances

Helpful Clues for Common Diagnoses
- **Hypertrophic Osteoarthropathy (HOA)**
  - Periosteal reaction in the appendicular skeleton, with either 1° or 2° etiology
  - Primary HOA (pachydermoperiostosis)
    - Dense periosteal reaction along diaphyses of long bones
    - Associated clubbing of fingers
    - Associated thickening of skin on forehead and dorsum of hands
  - Secondary HOA
    - Dense periosteal reaction along diaphyses of long bones
    - Associated clubbing of fingers
    - Associated thoracic (lung cancer) or abdominal abnormalities
  - Though the periosteal reaction is usually thick & linear (whether primary or secondary etiology), it may occasionally project horizontally
    - Horizontal projection, if localized, might mimic a surface osteosarcoma

- **Hint**: In presence of a focus of odd, horizontal periosteal reaction, look for other bones showing more normal-appearing periosteal reaction
- **Renal Osteodystrophy, Neostosis**
  - Renal osteodystrophy, when active, shows subperiosteal resorption along metaphyses of long bones
  - When in a healing phase, shows new bone formation
    - Most prominent appearance when renal osteodystrophy was severe and adequate treatment is first instituted
    - New bone formation along periosteum gives an appearance of dense linear periosteal reaction, but is neostosis
    - Neostosis rarely has an exuberant horizontal extension
    - New bone is also seen in a round pattern, filling in and healing brown tumors
    - New bone is also seen as a diffuse density within long bones
  - **Hint**: When suspecting neostosis, watch for coarsened trabeculae, brown tumors (perhaps hyperossified), & patterns of residual resorption

Helpful Clues for Less Common Diagnoses
- **Parosteal Lipoma**
  - Soft tissue lipoma, adjacent to long bone
    - Most do not elicit a reaction
    - Occasionally, juxta-osseous lipoma elicits extensive horizontal periosteal reaction
    - **Hint**: The adjacent lipoma has all characteristics typical of lipoma
- **Hemophilic Pseudotumor**
  - Pseudotumor arises from recurrent bleeding episodes affecting bone
    - Soft tissue
    - Subperiosteal
    - Intraosseous
  - Several effects on bone, depending on source of bleeding
    - Expansion, with thinning of endosteum
    - Extrinsic scalloping of cortex
    - May have long horizontal spicules of bone, either as reaction or from the extrinsic scalloping
  - Most common sites: Iliac wing, femur, calcaneus
  - **Hint**: Gender specific; often has oligoarticular disease (knee, elbow, ankle)

PERIOSTEUM: BIZARRE HORIZONTAL PERIOSTEAL REACTION

- **Fibromatosis**
  - Soft tissue fibrous mass; benign but locally invasive, not respecting compartments
  - **Hint**: MR is suggestive of diagnosis
    - Infiltrative rather than having the pseudocapsule seen with sarcomas
    - Fluid-sensitive sequences often have low signal & are inhomogeneous
    - Intense enhancement
  - Adjacent osseous structures
    - Generally not affected
    - May cause destruction, especially in hand/foot: Pressure erosion
    - Rarely elicit horizontal periosteal reaction
- **Juvenile Aponeurotic Fibroma**
  - Child with soft tissue mass, generally in forearm or hand
  - With growth, often causes bowing or extrinsic erosion of adjacent bones
    - Generally no osseous reaction to the adjacent slow-growing mass
    - Rarely, bizarre horizontal periosteal reaction is seen
  - May develop dystrophic calcification
  - **Hint**: Location, patient age, & MR suggest the diagnosis
    - Local infiltration
    - Fluid-sensitive sequences often have low signal areas & are inhomogeneous
    - Intense enhancement
- **Osteosarcoma (Mimic)**
  - Osteosarcoma generally elicits an aggressive periosteal reaction
    - Parallel to long bone, but interrupted
    - Codman triangle
  - Uncommonly, tumor osteoid extends horizontally from underlying long bone, giving the appearance of horizontal periosteal reaction
  - **Hint**: Underlying bone shows highly permeative destruction, usually with tumor osteoid formation
- **Skull Hemangioma (Mimic) & Thalassemia (Mimic)**
  - Hemangioma (focal) & thalassemia (diffuse) skull disease
  - Expands the diploic space
  - Trabeculae extending between inner & outer tables give the appearance of sunburst periosteal reaction
- **Aneurysmal Bone Cyst (Mimic)**
  - Eccentric metaphyseal lytic lesion, usually with thin cortical rim
  - MR usually distinctive, showing fluid-fluid levels; not specific
  - Lesion usually completely lytic, but may contain pseudotrabeculations
    - If cortical rim is so thin as to not be visible, pseudotrabeculations may mimic horizontal periosteal reaction

Helpful Clues for Rare Diagnoses

- **Soft Tissue Tumor Adjacent To Bone**
  - Rarely elicits horizontal periosteal reaction; nonspecific
- **Subperiosteal Ganglion**
  - Rare location of lesion; horizontal reaction

Hypertrophic Osteoarthropathy (HOA)

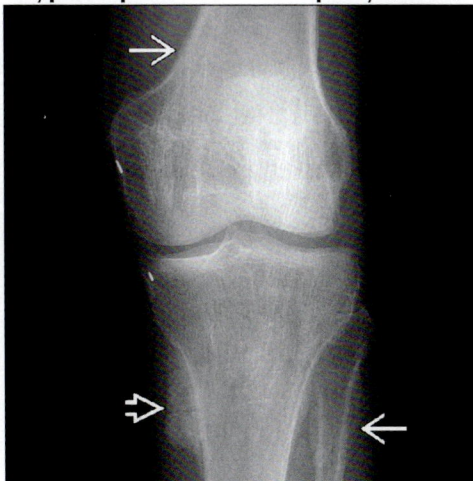

AP radiograph shows bizarre tibial periosteal reaction ➡. Surface tumor might be considered, except for the more regular periosteal reaction seen at the fibula & femur ➡. Diagnosis: Lung cancer. (†MSK Req).

Renal Osteodystrophy, Neostosis

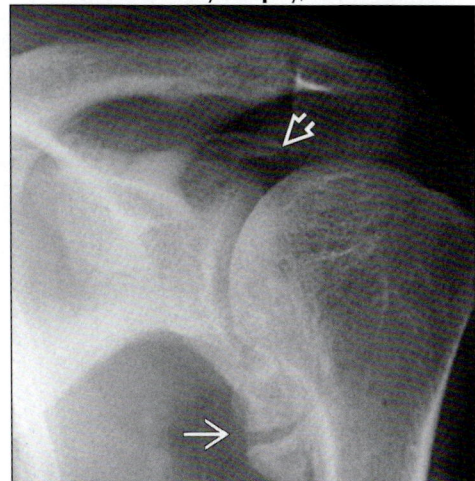

AP radiograph shows exuberant new bone formation arising from the glenoid ➡ and humeral metaphysis ➡ in this patient with renal disease, treated by dialysis. Treatment may result in new bone formation.

PERIOSTEUM: BIZARRE HORIZONTAL PERIOSTEAL REACTION

Parosteal Lipoma

Parosteal Lipoma

(Left) Lateral radiograph shows horizontal periosteal reaction arising from the posterior femoral shaft ➡ with adjacent fat density in the soft tissues ➡. (†MSK Req). *(Right)* Axial bone CT in the same patient shows the horizontal periosteal reaction arising from the osseous surface ➡, again with the surrounding fat density ➡. The fat is typical of lipoma; when it is in close proximity to bone, it may elicit bizarre periosteal reaction; the combination is termed parosteal lipoma.

Hemophilic Pseudotumor

Fibromatosis

(Left) Anteroposterior radiograph shows several sites of horizontal periosteal reaction arising from the femoral shaft ➡ in a young man with hemophilia. There is also cortical scalloping. The changes are due to subperiosteal bleeds. *(Right)* Oblique radiograph shows bizarre horizontal periosteal reaction ➡ to a soft tissue aggressive fibromatosis lesion that causes local scalloping of the bone. This reaction is a rare manifestation of fibromatosis.

Juvenile Aponeurotic Fibroma

Osteosarcoma (Mimic)

(Left) Oblique radiograph shows a juvenile aponeurotic fibroma, that has caused scalloping of both the forearm bones. The ulna shows tremendous periosteal reaction ➡, occasionally seen in this disease. *(Right)* AP radiograph shows severe horizontal (sunburst) osteoid formation in a soft tissue mass arising from the distal radius in a child. There is permeative change & osteoid tumor bone formation in this osteosarcoma. The horizontal bone is osteoid rather than reactive bone.

PERIOSTEUM: BIZARRE HORIZONTAL PERIOSTEAL REACTION

Skull Hemangioma (Mimic)

Thalassemia (Mimic)

(Left) Lateral radiograph shows a large hemangioma of the skull, expanding the outer table ➡, with a honeycomb appearance of the trabeculations ➡. This is not a true periosteal reaction. *(Right)* Lateral radiograph shows the "hair on end" appearance of the skull ➡ in a patient with thalassemia. This in fact is not a periosteal reactive process but represents the widened diploic space required for the erythropoietic needs in this severe anemia.

Aneurysmal Bone Cyst (Mimic)

Soft Tissue Tumor Adjacent To Bone

(Left) AP radiograph shows what appears to be dense horizontal periosteal reaction ➡. In reality, these are pseudotrabeculations within the wall of an ABC; the thin outer rim is faintly seen superimposed on the radius ➡. *(Right)* Axial NECT shows normal underlying bone but prominent horizontal periosteal reaction ➡, related to a large adjacent soft tissue mass ➡. This is a rare osseous reaction, in this case to a malignant fibrous histiocytoma.

Subperiosteal Ganglion

Subperiosteal Ganglion

(Left) Oblique radiograph shows a surface lesion of bone, slightly scalloping the cortex and containing horizontal osseous projections ➡ that could represent either reaction or pseudotrabeculations. *(Right)* Axial T2WI MR of the same lesion as previous image shows the fairly thick osseous projections ➡ within the cystic lesion. This proved to be a subperiosteal ganglion cyst with dense cortical reaction.

PERIOSTEUM: PERIOSTITIS MULTIPLE BONES/ACROPACHY, ADULT

DIFFERENTIAL DIAGNOSIS

Common
- Hypertrophic Pulmonary Osteoarthropathy (HPOA)
- Extrathoracic Hypertrophic Osteoarthropathy
- Vascular Insufficiency

Less Common
- Subperiosteal Resorption (Mimic)
- Renal Osteodystrophy, Neostosis
- Psoriatic Arthritis
- Pachydermoperiostosis
- Chronic Reactive Arthritis
- Thyroid Acropachy

Rare but Important
- Tuberous Sclerosis
- Hypervitaminosis A
- Hypervitaminosis D
- Complications of Retinoids
- Fluorosis
- Osteogenesis Imperfecta (OI) Tarda
- Leukemia

ESSENTIAL INFORMATION

Key Differential Diagnosis Issues
- Multiple sites of periosteal reaction: Much more limited differential than solitary bone involvement
- **Hint**: Most important diagnosis is HPOA
  - Radiologist must direct clinician to look for lung pathology
  - May allow early detection of lung cancer in a situation where there is no clinical suspicion of the disease

Helpful Clues for Common Diagnoses
- **Hypertrophic Pulmonary Osteoarthropathy (HPOA)**
  - Multiple intrathoracic etiologies, including infection, pleural disease, & congestive heart failure, but most frequent is lung cancer
  - Elicits dense periosteal reaction in long bones without underlying osseous abnormality
    - Periosteal reaction usually linear & regular
    - Occasionally it is exuberant, mimicking a surface bone-forming tumor
  - Clubbing of fingers
  - Patients complain of joint pain
    - Because of site of pain, radiograph is often of wrist/hand or ankle/foot
    - Periosteal reaction is often seen only on the corner of the radiograph, involving the diaphysis of long bone
    - Small bones of hand or foot may be involved, less frequently than long bones
- **Extrathoracic Hypertrophic Osteoarthropathy**
  - Less common etiology of hypertrophic osteoarthropathy than HPOA
  - May be associated with biliary disease, cirrhosis, inflammatory bowel disease
  - Radiographically identical to HPOA
- **Vascular Insufficiency**
  - Periosteal reaction in lower extremity, particularly tibia & fibula
  - Varicosities, cellulitis, & phleboliths

Helpful Clues for Less Common Diagnoses
- **Subperiosteal Resorption (Mimic)**
  - Hyperparathyroidism or renal osteodystrophy
  - Subperiosteal resorption may be aggressive, mimicking fluffy periosteal reaction
  - Most common locations
    - Radial aspect of middle phalanges (with severe disease, involves all phalanges, both radial & ulnar sides)
    - Proximal medial humerus, tibia, femur
  - Watch for suggestion that it is resorption rather than added bony reaction
    - No solid cortex will be seen underlying the abnormality
    - Bone density is abnormal, with smudginess of trabeculae
    - May have other sites of resorption (subchondral, subligamentous)
    - May have brown tumors &/or soft tissue calcification
- **Renal Osteodystrophy, Neostosis**
  - When severe renal osteodystrophy is newly & adequately treated, it results in new bone formation
    - May take the form of periosteal new bone, termed neostosis
  - Watch for other new bone formation
    - Hyperossification of brown tumors
    - Increased bone formation on trabeculae leads to overall increased density

PERIOSTEUM: PERIOSTITIS MULTIPLE BONES/ACROPACHY, ADULT

○ Watch for underlying signs of renal osteodystrophy
  ▪ Various patterns of resorption
  ▪ Bowing deformities
- **Psoriatic Arthritis**
  ○ Early changes, even pre-erosive, include
    ▪ Sausage digit: Swelling of entire digit
    ▪ Periostitis: Fluffy bone formation along shaft and metaphyses
  ○ Later changes include aggressive erosive change; pencil-in-cup, arthritis mutilans
  ○ Hand involvement with interphalangeal joint predominance
- **Pachydermoperiostosis**
  ○ a.k.a., 1° hypertrophic osteoarthropathy
  ○ Inherited condition, male > female
  ○ Dense periosteal reaction along long bones without underlying osseous abnormality
  ○ Associated thickening of skin of forehead & dorsum of hand
  ○ Pain & periostitis tend to be self-limited, resolving in adulthood
- **Chronic Reactive Arthritis**
  ○ As with psoriatic arthritis, early changes
    ▪ Sausage digit: Swelling of entire digit
    ▪ Periostitis: Fluffy bone formation along shaft and metaphyses
  ○ Later changes mixed erosive & productive
  ○ Lower extremity predominates (ankle, forefoot, & calcaneus)
- **Thyroid Acropachy**
  ○ Fluffy periostitis of phalanges
  ○ Patient is usually euthyroid, having been treated for thyroid disease

○ May have thyrotoxicosis
○ May have clubbing of fingers

Helpful Clues for Rare Diagnoses
- **Tuberous Sclerosis**
  ○ Uncommon disease; periosteal reaction is rare manifestation
- **Hypervitaminosis A**
  ○ May have undulating periosteal reaction
  ○ Soft tissue nodularity
  ○ Intracranial hypertension
- **Hypervitaminosis D**
  ○ Enthesopathy, rare periostitis
- **Complications of Retinoids**
  ○ Usually productive change is in the form of spinal anterior bridging osteophytes
  ○ Periosteal bone formation is uncommon
- **Fluorosis**
  ○ May have sacrospinous or sacrotuberous ligament calcification
  ○ Periosteal reaction less common than enthesopathy
  ○ Osteoporotic or osteosclerotic; metaphyseal dense lines
- **Osteogenesis Imperfecta (OI) Tarda**
  ○ Prominent callus formation at fracture sites & other sites of injury
- **Leukemia**
  ○ Periosteal reaction is uncommon
  ○ Generally seen as osteoporosis on radiograph
  ○ Radiography is often normal
    ▪ Lesions demonstrated by MR

Hypertrophic Pulmonary Osteoarthropathy (HPOA)

Anteroposterior radiograph shows dense periosteal reaction along the femoral shaft ➔. There were other long bones similarly involved, all with normal underlying bone. This is HPOA; the patient had lung cancer.

Hypertrophic Pulmonary Osteoarthropathy (HPOA)

Anteroposterior radiograph shows dense periosteal reaction along the femur ➔, fibula ➔, and particularly exuberant reaction along the tibia ➔. This proved to be HPOA; the patient had lung cancer. (†MSK Req).

Extrathoracic Hypertrophic Osteoarthropathy

Vascular Insufficiency

(Left) Anteroposterior radiograph shows very regular periosteal reaction involving all metacarpals ➔. Although one should primarily suspect lung cancer with HPOA, in this case the hypertrophic osteoarthropathy was related to liver cirrhosis. *(Right)* AP radiograph shows dense periosteal reaction ➔ along the tibia. This was a bilateral finding but only involved the legs. This exclusive lower extremity distribution favors vascular insufficiency as the etiology.

Subperiosteal Resorption (Mimic)

Renal Osteodystrophy, Neostosis

(Left) PA radiograph shows severe subperiosteal resorption involving both the radial ➔ and ulnar ➔ side of the phalanges. Occasionally the resorption is so severe that it mimics periosteal reaction. *(Right)* Posteroanterior radiograph shows dense regular neostosis ➔, new bone formed in this patient with end-stage renal disease, placed on dialysis approximately 6 months earlier.

Psoriatic Arthritis

Psoriatic Arthritis

(Left) PA radiograph shows soft tissue swelling of the third ray, an appearance termed a "sausage digit" ➔, as well as prominent periosteal reaction along the shaft of the proximal phalanx ➔. This appearance is one of the typical manifestations of early psoriatic arthritis. *(Right)* PA radiograph shows soft tissue swelling of adjacent digits, with prominent periostitis ➔. There is some articular damage as well, involving interphalangeal joints, typical of psoriatic arthritis.

Pachydermoperiostosis

Pachydermoperiostosis

(Left) Anteroposterior radiograph shows prominent periosteal reaction involving all metacarpals & phalanges ➡. All the long bones had a similar appearance, & the skin of the patient's forehead & dorsal hand was thickened. The combination makes the diagnosis of pachydermoperiostosis. (†MSK Req). *(Right)* Frontal Tc99m bone scan in the same patient shows diffuse periosteal uptake in all long bones, indicating extent of periosteal reaction in this patient with 1° HOA.

Chronic Reactive Arthritis

Thyroid Acropachy

(Left) PA radiograph shows diffuse soft tissue swelling along the 2nd ray, periostitis ➡, and cartilage loss ➡. This is HIV-AIDS-related arthritis, a variant of chronic reactive arthritis. *(Right)* PA radiograph shows fluffy periostitis involving many of the phalanges ➡ in this patient treated successfully for hyperthyroidism eight months earlier. There is clubbing of the fingers ➡ as well.

Tuberous Sclerosis

Osteogenesis Imperfecta (OI) Tarda

(Left) Anteroposterior radiograph shows dense wavy periosteal reaction along all the metatarsals ➡ in a patient with tuberous sclerosis. The appearance is not specific; the history gives the etiology in this case. *(Right)* Anteroposterior radiograph shows thick periosteal reaction along the iliac wing ➡ in this patient with OI tarda. This mild form of the disease often results in hypertrophic fracture callus & subperiosteal bleeds & associated periosteal bone formation.

PERIOSTEUM: PERIOSTITIS MULTIPLE BONES, CHILD

DIFFERENTIAL DIAGNOSIS

Common
- Physiologic Periostitis
- Child Abuse
- Multifocal Osteomyelitis
- Juvenile Idiopathic Arthritis (JIA)
- Hypervitaminosis A
- Polyostotic Aggressive Bone Tumor

Less Common
- Prostaglandin Periostitis
- Sickle Cell Dactylitis

Rare but Important
- Caffey Disease
- Renal Osteodystrophy (Mimic)
- Leukemia
- Scurvy
- Complications of Chemotherapeutic Drugs, Methotrexate
- Hypertrophic Osteoarthropathy, Cystic Fibrosis
- Complications of Retinoids

ESSENTIAL INFORMATION

Key Differential Diagnosis Issues
- Periosteal reaction is common in a single bone, with a multitude of etiologies
- Polyostotic periostitis is much less common; the polyostotic nature and patient age helps to limit the diagnosis
- **Hint**: Some etiologies are limited by patient age
  - First appearance BEFORE 6 months of age
    - Physiologic (should disappear by age 6 months)
    - Congenital osteomyelitis
    - Caffey disease
    - Prostaglandin periostitis
  - First appearance AFTER 6 months of age
    - Juvenile idiopathic arthritis
    - Hypervitaminosis A
    - Sickle cell dactylitis
    - Renal osteodystrophy
    - Scurvy
- **Hint**: ALWAYS consider the possibility of child abuse/nonaccidental trauma

Helpful Clues for Common Diagnoses
- **Physiologic Periostitis**
  - Normal growth may be so rapid during first 6 months that new periosteal bone is produced
    - Symmetric, regular
    - Resolves by 6 months of age
- **Child Abuse**
  - Always consider this diagnosis when periosteal reaction is seen in a child!
  - Often not symmetric
  - Often 2° to metaphyseal corner fracture
    - Fracture causes subperiosteal bleeding & lifting of periosteum
  - May occur without fracture 2° to normally loose periosteum and a twisting injury
- **Multifocal Osteomyelitis**
  - Congenital infections
    - TORCH infections
    - Congenital syphilis (may have "celery stalking" at metaphyses as well)
  - Infections from newborn ICU: Generally Streptococcus
  - Multifocal osteomyelitis later in childhood
    - Hematogenous spread (metaphyseal)
    - Consider underlying disease: HIV/AIDS or sickle cell anemia
  - Tuberculosis (TB) involvement in hands: Dactylitis is termed spina ventosa
- **Juvenile Idiopathic Arthritis (JIA)**
  - First osseous manifestation may be periostitis of hand or foot phalanges
  - Later, joints will be involved
  - Differential is sickle cell & TB dactylitis
- **Hypervitaminosis A**
  - Excessive intake of vitamin A results initially in periosteal reaction
    - Subtle at first but may become quite dense & thick
    - Painful
  - Continued use of excessive vitamin A may lead to coned epiphyses
- **Polyostotic Aggressive Bone Tumor**
  - Bone metastases
    - Ewing sarcoma presents with osseous metastases as frequently as lung mets
    - Others to consider: Medulloblastoma, neuroblastoma, osteosarcoma
  - Leukemia: Common but usually presents with lucent metaphyseal bands or diffuse osteoporosis
    - Periostitis is a rare manifestation

○ Langerhans cell histiocytosis: Often polyostotic; may be aggressive enough to elicit periosteal reaction

Helpful Clues for Less Common Diagnoses

- **Prostaglandin Periostitis**
  ○ Prostaglandins used for congenital heart disease in infancy to keep ductus open
  ○ Dense, nonspecific periosteal reaction on long bones
- **Sickle Cell Dactylitis**
  ○ Generally young children (< 7 years of age)
  ○ Cold temperature → vasoconstriction of terminal vessels in phalanges → sludging of sickled red blood cells → bone infarct
  ○ Bone infarct may initially elicit periostitis; eventually has mixed lytic & sclerotic appearance

Helpful Clues for Rare Diagnoses

- **Caffey Disease**
  ○ Rare disease manifests at birth
  ○ Painful periostitis of long bones
  ○ Involvement of clavicle & mandible is suggestive of diagnosis since not usually seen with other diagnoses
  ○ Self-limited; spontaneously resolves over first 2 years of life
- **Renal Osteodystrophy (Mimic)**
  ○ Severe subperiosteal resorption, especially at the proximal humeral, tibial, or femoral metaphysis or at the radial aspect of middle phalanx may mimic fluffy periostitis

- Watch for underlying abnormal bone density, signs of rickets (widening at zone of provisional calcification)
  ○ Severe renal osteodystrophy may result in bone accretion when effective treatment is initiated; mimics periosteal reaction
- **Scurvy**
  ○ Rare metabolic disease affecting collagen
  ○ Osseous manifestations
    - Osteopenia
    - Sclerotic ring around epiphyses (Wimberger sign)
    - Sclerotic metaphyseal line (white line of Frankel)
    - Corner fractures at metaphyses
    - Subperiosteal bleed (especially with corner fracture) → elevates periosteum → reparative bone formation which mimics periosteal reaction
- **Complications of Chemotherapeutic Drugs, Methotrexate**
  ○ Rare periosteal reaction, nonspecific
- **Hypertrophic Osteoarthropathy, Cystic Fibrosis**
  ○ Lung disease may elicit hypertrophic osteoarthropathy, just as in adults
  ○ Periosteal reaction that is painful, referred to joints
- **Complications of Retinoids**
  ○ May induce productive bone changes
    - Most frequently, large syndesmophytes at anterior vertebral bodies
    - Rarely, periostitis

Physiologic Periostitis

Lateral radiograph shows dense, regular periosteal reaction ➡ in a 6 week old which was symmetric. There were no other abnormalities. Under the age of 6 months, rapid growth results in this normal appearance.

Child Abuse

AP radiograph shows dense periosteal reaction ➡ representing healing following subperiosteal bleed from a proximal metaphyseal corner fracture. The child had other sites of periosteal reaction & fractures.

PERIOSTEUM: PERIOSTITIS MULTIPLE BONES, CHILD

(Left) Anteroposterior radiograph shows periosteal reaction ➡ related to a metaphyseal corner fracture seen only on the lateral view; fracture occurred 19 days earlier. Periosteal reaction should alert radiologist to seek other signs of nonaccidental trauma. *(Right)* Anteroposterior radiograph shows periosteal reaction along tibia ➡ of an infant. Other bones were similarly involved. Finding is nonspecific but can be seen with congenital infections such as syphilis in this case.

(Left) Lateral radiograph shows thin regular periosteal reaction along many of the phalanges ➡ in this child, along with soft tissue swelling. *(Right)* Posteroanterior radiograph in the same patient also demonstrates the periosteal reaction ➡. The findings are not specific but in this case were the first manifestation of JIA. In this age group, sickle cell dactylitis would be considered if the child was black.

(Left) Posteroanterior radiograph shows dense periosteal accretion along the ulnar diaphysis ➡. This was seen on other bones, including both legs. This 1 year old was being given large doses of vitamin A. *(Right)* Lateral radiograph shows thick & prominent periosteal reaction along the ulna ➡. Other bones showed lytic lesions and others showed simply periosteal reaction in this child with metastatic medulloblastoma.

Child Abuse

Multifocal Osteomyelitis

Juvenile Idiopathic Arthritis (JIA)

Juvenile Idiopathic Arthritis (JIA)

Hypervitaminosis A

Polyostotic Aggressive Bone Tumor

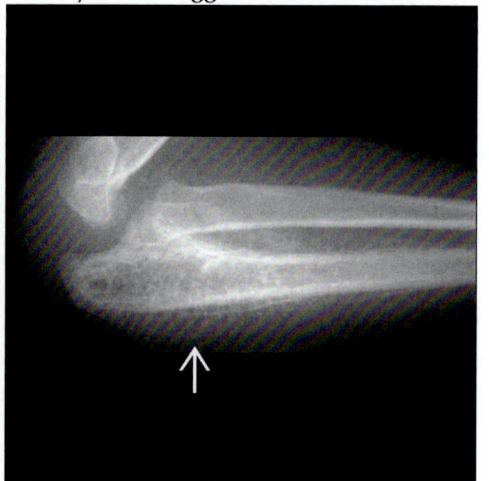

PERIOSTEUM: PERIOSTITIS MULTIPLE BONES, CHILD

Prostaglandin Periostitis

Sickle Cell Dactylitis

(Left) Lateral radiograph shows thick, dense periosteal reaction in the humerus ➡ as well as the bones of the forearm ➡. This infant had been treated with prostaglandins for a cardiac defect. *(Right)* Anteroposterior radiograph shows subtle periosteal reaction ➡ and underlying bone abnormality in this African-American child who developed hand pain on the first cold day of winter. This represents a bone infarct in sickle cell disease.

Caffey Disease

Caffey Disease

(Left) Lateral radiograph shows dense periosteal new bone formation along the humerus as well as the radius in this child. The child also had mandibular periosteal bone change, which is considered highly suggestive of Caffey disease. *(Right)* Lateral radiograph shows thick, dense periosteal new bone formation along all long bones in a severe case of Caffey disease. The process is painful but self-limited; this patient returned to normal by 3 years of age.

Renal Osteodystrophy (Mimic)

Scurvy

(Left) AP radiograph shows what might be mistaken for fluffy periostitis ➡ along the proximal humerus. This is aggressive subperiosteal resorption in a patient with renal disease; note the rickets and slipped humeral epiphysis ➡. *(Right)* AP radiograph shows dense metaphyseal lines of Frankel as well as a metaphyseal corner fracture ➡ in this patient with scurvy. There was a subperiosteal bleed, and periosteal bone formation is developing ➡ along the tibia.

ARTHRITIS WITH NORMAL BONE DENSITY

DIFFERENTIAL DIAGNOSIS

Common
- Osteoarthritis (OA)
- Erosive Osteoarthritis (EOA)
- Gout
- Synovial Osteochondromatosis
- Psoriatic Arthritis (PSA)
- Pyrophosphate Arthropathy
- DISH & OPLL (Mimics)
- Pigmented Villonodular Synovitis (PVNS)
- Neuropathic Arthropathy (Not Diabetic)

Less Common
- Hemochromatosis
- Chronic Reactive Arthritis (CRA)

Rare but Important
- Robust Rheumatoid Arthritis
- Multicentric Reticulohistiocytosis

ESSENTIAL INFORMATION

Key Differential Diagnosis Issues
- In all cases, discussion is not of end-stage arthritis
  - If joint is immobilized, by end-stage of process bones will become osteopenic
  - Inflammatory processes, at end stage, will develop osteoporosis; this includes psoriatic arthritis, chronic reactive arthritis, gout, & robust RA
- Patient may have the listed arthritides superimposed on other processes which may make them osteopenic
  - Age & gender (senile, postmenopausal osteoporosis)
  - Metabolic bone disease
  - Immobility (stroke, paraplegia: Disuse osteoporosis)
  - Collagen vascular disease (systemic lupus erythematosus, dermatomyositis)
  - Use of steroids or other drugs causing osteopenia; alcohol abuse

Helpful Clues for Common Diagnoses
- **Osteoarthritis (OA)**
  - OA is completely productive
    - Subchondral sclerosis, osteophytes
  - Predictable sites of involvement
    - Hip: 80% superolateral subluxation, 20% protrusio
    - Knee: Varus > valgus deformity
    - Hand: 1st carpometacarpal (CMC), scapho-trapezoid-trapezium (STT), interphalangeal (IP) joints
    - Distribution fairly symmetric
  - Density remains normal for the individual
- **Erosive Osteoarthritis (EOA)**
  - a.k.a., inflammatory osteoarthritis
  - Retain normal density for the individual
    - Focal periarticular osteopenia may occur during active inflammatory phase
  - Majority of joint involvement is productive (osteophyte-forming)
  - IP joints (occasionally others) are erosive
    - Classic "gull-wing" appearance of direct subchondral erosion is often seen
    - May have marginal & other erosive patterns
  - Sites of involvement identical to OA
    - Difference is the erosive character of the IP joints
    - Distribution is fairly symmetric
  - Diagnosis of IP erosive disease depends on other sites of involvement
    - Productive or mixed erosive-productive involvement of CMC or STT joints yields diagnosis of EOA
    - Lack of involvement of other carpal joints or metacarpal phalangeal (MCP) joints eliminates psoriatic or other inflammatory arthritides
- **Gout**
  - Normal bone density retained unless other patient factors are superimposed
  - Characterized by dense tophi, erosions with sclerotic margins
  - Relatively late cartilage destruction
  - Distribution
    - Rarely symmetric
    - 1st metatarsophalangeal joint is classic
    - Otherwise, remember that gout may be seen anywhere!
- **Synovial Osteochondromatosis**
  - Normal bone density retained unless other patient factors are superimposed
  - Often (not exclusively) monoarticular
  - Multiple round bodies of similar size
    - May not be visible on radiograph; diagnosed on MR
- **Psoriatic Arthritis (PSA)**
  - Normal bone density retained unless other patient factors are superimposed

- Exception may be periarticular osteoporosis seen during active inflammatory process
  ○ May initially present as "sausage digit"
    ▪ Ray distribution of soft tissue swelling and periostitis
  ○ May initially present as joint disease
    ▪ Initially erosive; may become mixed erosive-productive
  ○ Distribution
    ▪ Peripheral: Upper > lower extremity
    ▪ IP joints > MCP joints
    ▪ Carpus: Not as predictable; pericapitate
    ▪ If spondyloarthropathy, bilateral but asymmetric sacroiliac joint involvement, bulky non-contiguous syndesmophytes
- **Pyrophosphate Arthropathy**
  ○ Hemachromatosis has similar appearance radiographically to pyrophosphate arthropathy
    ▪ Hemochromatosis seen in males, younger age than pyrophosphate
  ○ Early phase erosive; mixed erosive-productive or purely productive seen at end phase
    ▪ Chondrocalcinosis frequently associated, but may not be present
    ▪ Retention of normal bone density in absence of other patient factors
  ○ Distribution
    ▪ Hand: MCP (especially 2nd & 3rd), radiocarpal (may also involve intercarpals with SLAC wrist deformity as end result)

- Knee: Patellofemoral compartment has earlier & more severe involvement than medial or lateral
- **DISH & OPLL (Mimics)**
  ○ Mimic since joints not generally involved
  ○ Bulky bridging anterior vertebral body syndesmophytes (DISH > > OPLL)
  ○ Both may have ossification of posterior longitudinal ligament (OPLL > > DISH)
- **Pigmented Villonodular Synovitis (PVNS)**
  ○ Monoarticular; younger patient retains normal bone density
- **Neuropathic Arthropathy (Not Diabetic)**
  ○ One of features is retention of normal bone density (except diabetic)
  ○ Others: Fragmentation, large effusion, disorder of joint

Helpful Clues for Less Common Diagnoses
- **Chronic Reactive Arthritis (CRA)**
  ○ Retains normal bone density; generally young adult males
  ○ Peripheral: Lower > upper extremity
  ○ Spondyloarthropathy: Same as PSA

Helpful Clues for Rare Diagnoses
- **Robust Rheumatoid Arthritis**
  ○ Continued use of joints in adult RA
  ○ Retention of bone density & large subchondral cyst formation
- **Multicentric Reticulohistiocytosis**
  ○ Nodularity soft tissues
  ○ Well-marginated erosions, especially IP joints
  ○ Occasional acroosteolysis

Osteoarthritis (OA)

Anteroposterior radiograph shows large subchondral cyst ➔, complete cartilage loss on the weight-bearing surface, and osteophyte formation ➔, all typical of OA. Note the normal bone density.

Erosive Osteoarthritis (EOA)

Anteroposterior radiograph shows prominent erosions at the 1st carpometacarpal joint ➔ as well as an IP joint ➔. Findings are of erosive osteoarthritis. Patient retains normal bone density.

ARTHRITIS WITH NORMAL BONE DENSITY

(Left) *Oblique radiograph shows a prominent dense gouty tophus ⇨, along with an osseous erosion with overhanging edge ⇨. The bone density remains normal, as is typical of gout.* **(Right)** *Anteroposterior radiograph shows several round osseous bodies ⇨ within the elbow joint. The bone density is normal, as is expected with synovial osteochondromatosis.*

Gout

Synovial Osteochondromatosis

(Left) *Posteroanterior radiograph shows IP erosive disease, fusion of a DIP ⇨, and enthesopathy ⇨. Findings are typical of psoriatic arthritis. Bone density remains normal, despite fairly advanced disease.* **(Right)** *Posteroanterior radiograph shows advanced pyrophosphate arthropathy, with SLAC wrist deformity ⇨, large subchondral cysts, and chondrocalcinosis ⇨. Despite the advanced wrist disease, bone density remains normal.*

Psoriatic Arthritis (PSA)

Pyrophosphate Arthropathy

(Left) *Lateral radiograph shows large anterior bridging osteophytes ⇨ but otherwise normal vertebral bodies. The concavity of the anterior body is retained ⇨, typical of DISH. Unlike ankylosing spondylitis, DISH retains normal bone density.* **(Right)** *Lateral radiograph shows ossification of the posterior longitudinal ligament ⇨ & an anterior osteophyte ⇨, typical of OPLL. Bone density is normal (process is not inflammatory & normal motion is retained).*

DISH & OPLL (Mimics)

DISH & OPLL (Mimics)

ARTHRITIS WITH NORMAL BONE DENSITY

Pigmented Villonodular Synovitis (PVNS)

Neuropathic Arthropathy (Not Diabetic)

(Left) Anteroposterior radiograph shows huge subchondral cysts on both acetabular and femoral sides of the joint in a patient with PVNS. Note that normal bone density is retained. *(Right)* AP radiograph shows destructive changes in the joint ➤ resulting in subluxation & fragmentation. There are small osseous fragments dissecting down the leg ➤, secondary to overdistension of the joint. Despite the severity of this tabetic Charcot joint, bone density remains normal.

Hemochromatosis

Chronic Reactive Arthritis (CRA)

(Left) PA radiograph shows decreased cartilage width & hooked osteophytes ➤ in a young adult male with hemochromatosis. As is expected, bone density remains normal. *(Right)* Lateral radiograph shows a large erosion, with associated mild productive change, at the posterior calcaneus. This is typical, but not pathognomonic of, chronic reactive arthritis. The normal bone density helps differentiate it from rheumatoid arthritis.

Robust Rheumatoid Arthritis

Multicentric Reticulohistiocytosis

(Left) PA radiograph shows ulnar capping ➤, large subchondral cysts ➤, and normal bone density in a patient who has robust rheumatoid arthritis. Note the slight ulnar translocation of the carpus. *(Right)* PA radiograph shows soft tissue nodules ➤, acroosteolysis ➤, and well-defined IP erosions ➤. Normal bone density is retained. Findings are typical of a rare disorder, multicentric reticulohistiocytosis.

ARTHRITIS WITH OSTEOPENIA

DIFFERENTIAL DIAGNOSIS

Common
- Rheumatoid Arthritis (RA)
- Diabetic Charcot Joint
- Septic Joint
- Ankylosing Spondylitis (AS)

Less Common
- Systemic Lupus Erythematosus (SLE)
- Juvenile Idiopathic Arthritis (JIA)
- Progressive Systemic Sclerosis (PSS)
- Chronic Reactive Arthritis (CRA)
- Transient Osteoporosis (Mimic)
- Hemophilia
- Inflammatory Bowel Disease Arthritis

Rare but Important
- Amyloid Deposition
- Adult Still Disease
- Ochronosis
- Wilson Disease
- Mixed Connective Tissue Disease
- HIV-Associated Arthritis
- Tuberculosis Septic Joint
- Fungal Septic Joint
- Familial Mediterranean Fever

ESSENTIAL INFORMATION

Key Differential Diagnosis Issues
- Any highly inflammatory process will present with FOCAL osteopenia
  - This includes diagnoses that are typically considered to retain normal bone density, including gout & psoriatic arthritis
- Any end-stage arthritis that results in DISUSE will develop diffuse osteopenia
- This list represents those arthritic diseases that most commonly PRESENT with osteopenia
  - The distinction in this list is not whether the processes present with osteopenia commonly or rarely, but the frequency with which the arthritis with osteopenia occurs

Helpful Clues for Common Diagnoses
- **Rheumatoid Arthritis (RA)**
  - Osteopenia is the hallmark of RA
    - Initially, with early inflammatory change, location is juxtaarticular
    - Later, with disuse, osteopenia is diffuse

- Purely erosive process; erosions are not well-marginated
- Symmetric, typical distribution
  - MCP, distal radioulnar, radiocarpal joint
  - Uniform throughout knee
  - Uniform narrowing hip, with protrusio
- **Diabetic Charcot Joint**
  - Charcot joints retain whatever bone density was present prior to joint destruction
  - Diabetic hands & feet are osteoporotic; neuropathic changes are atrophic
- **Septic Joint**
  - Effusion & subchondral/cortical osteopenia are earliest changes
- **Ankylosing Spondylitis (AS)**
  - Osteopenia is hallmark of AS & occurs diffusely and early in disease
    - Other spondyloarthritides (psoriatic or CRA) do not have as early or widespread osteopenia
  - Combination of osteopenia & spine fusion puts spine at risk for fracture from minor trauma

Helpful Clues for Less Common Diagnoses
- **Systemic Lupus Erythematosus (SLE)**
  - Osteopenia typical & widespread in SLE
    - Due both to disease process & common use of steroids
  - Non-erosive deformities of hands & feet
    - Simulates RA, but would expect erosions with the degree of deformity seen
    - Late in disease, mechanical erosions
- **Juvenile Idiopathic Arthritis (JIA)**
  - Hyperemia from synovitis results in two typical features
    - Osteoporosis at involved joints
    - Overgrowth of epiphyses, but often early physeal closure → short limb
  - Destructive arthritic process continues, with erosions & cartilage loss
  - Systemic JIA may eventually show diffuse osteoporosis
  - Hemophilia has similar appearance to JIA
  - Hemophilia may show "dense" effusions
    - Hemosiderin deposition in synovium
    - Low signal which "blooms" on MR
- **Progressive Systemic Sclerosis (PSS)**
  - Diffuse osteoporosis
  - Acroosteolysis with soft tissue calcification
  - Eventual mixed erosive/productive disease

ARTHRITIS WITH OSTEOPENIA

- 1st carpometacarpal joint most severely affected, with subluxation
- **Chronic Reactive Arthritis (CRA)**
  - During inflammatory phase of arthritis, develops juxtaarticular osteopenia
  - Osteopenia is usually not widespread
  - CRA features
    - Bilateral asymmetric SI joint disease; bulky asymmetric syndesmophytes
    - Peripheral disease favors lower extremity, especially calcaneus
    - Associated features: Urethritis (cervicitis) & conjunctivitis
- **Transient Osteoporosis (Mimic)**
  - Effusion & osteoporosis around a joint
    - Usually large joint (hip, knee)
    - MR shows effusion & marrow edema
  - Differential is septic joint; must aspirate
  - Self-limited; does not affect cartilage
- **Inflammatory Bowel Disease Arthritis**
  - Osteopenia is diffuse, usually related to steroid treatment of bowel disease
  - Arthritis pattern identical to that of AS
    - Symmetric SI disease, thin vertical spine syndesmophytes
    - Large proximal joint involvement

Helpful Clues for Rare Diagnoses

- **Amyloid Deposition**
  - Amyloid usually occurs in patients with primary diseases resulting in osteopenia
    - End-stage renal disease, myeloma, RA
  - Pain & disuse → focal osteopenia
- **Adult Still Disease**

- As in RA and JIA, juxtaarticular & eventual diffuse osteopenia develops
- Distribution of disease
  - Identical to adult RA
  - DIP and pericapitate predominance
- **Ochronosis**
  - Osteoporosis is hallmark of disease
  - Usually extensive disk calcification
  - Long-standing disease results in cartilage breakdown and true arthritis
- **Wilson Disease**
  - Osteopenia in majority
  - Excrescences, cortical irregularity, or small ossicles adjacent to bones
  - Focal fragmentation → arthropathy
- **Mixed Connective Tissue Disease**
  - Overlap (clinically & radiographically) of SLE, PSS, dermatomyositis, & RA
  - Osteopenia plus various manifestations of the above diseases
- **HIV-Associated Arthritis**
  - Usually incomplete clinical features of CRA, but osseous features are same
- **Tuberculosis & Fungal Septic Joint**
  - Osteopenia is a routine feature
  - Slow but progressive destruction
  - Little host reactive change
- **Familial Mediterranean Fever**
  - May develop arthropathy (usually hip)
  - Initial osteoporosis & cartilage damage; eventual degenerative change

Rheumatoid Arthritis (RA)

AP radiograph shows uniform cartilage narrowing & ligamentous laxity, with medial translation of the tibia ➡, typical of RA. The bones are so osteoporotic as to have a moth-eaten appearance, a hallmark of RA.

Diabetic Charcot Joint

Oblique radiograph shows neuropathic joints at the talonavicular ➡ & calcaneocuboid ➡. Note the large air collection in a lateral & plantar ulcer ➡, along with diffuse osteopenia in this diabetic foot.

ARTHRITIS WITH OSTEOPENIA

(Left) AP radiograph shows erosions & cartilage destruction at the 5th MCP ➡. Both the 4th & 5th MCPs show severe osteopenia, due to hyperemia. This 25 year old man punched an opponent in the mouth & lacerated his knuckle. *(Right)* Lateral radiograph shows syndesmophytes ➡, ankylosis, & osteoporosis, typical of AS. The combination of limited motion & osteoporosis increases the risk of fracture from minor injury, seen here at the odontoid ➡.

Septic Joint

Ankylosing Spondylitis (AS)

(Left) PA radiograph shows diffuse osteopenia in a young woman. There are severe deformities that are not erosive. Combination is typical of SLE. True arthropathy with mechanical erosions develops late in disease. *(Right)* PA radiograph shows diffuse osteopenia, MCP erosions ➡, and carpal fusion ➡ in a 22 year old. There is overgrowth at the MCPs. Findings are typical of JIA; fusion would not be expected in adult RA.

Systemic Lupus Erythematosus (SLE)

Juvenile Idiopathic Arthritis (JIA)

(Left) PA radiograph shows prominent acroosteolysis with soft tissue calcification ➡, typical of PSS (scleroderma). Bones are typically osteopenic. Arthritis develops late in the disease, most frequently involving the 1st carpometacarpal joint ➡. *(Right)* Lateral radiograph shows effusion & osteoporosis, secondary to hyperemia in this young man with chronic reactive arthritis. CRA shows osteopenia with active inflammation, & has normal density otherwise.

Progressive Systemic Sclerosis (PSS)

Chronic Reactive Arthritis (CRA)

ARTHRITIS WITH OSTEOPENIA

Transient Osteoporosis (Mimic)

Hemophilia

(Left) AP radiograph shows diffuse osteopenia of the femoral head and, to a lesser extent, the acetabulum in a 25 year old male. Note that the cartilage width is normal ➡. Septic hip was disproved, leaving transient osteoporosis as a diagnosis of exclusion. *(Right)* AP radiograph shows severe osteoporosis, radial head overgrowth ➡, widening of the intercondylar notch ➡, and erosive articular disease. This is all typical of hemophilic arthropathy in this 25 year old male.

Inflammatory Bowel Disease Arthritis

Amyloid Deposition

(Left) AP radiograph shows sacroiliitis ➡ and a bowel staple line ➡ in this patient with inflammatory bowel disease arthritis. The osteopenia is related to steroid use as well as the inflammatory process. *(Right)* PA radiograph shows diffuse osteoporosis along with erosive disease in the MCP and carpal joints. The patient does not have RA, but rather amyloidosis, related to underlying multiple myeloma. Osteoporosis is expected in amyloidosis.

Adult Still Disease

Ochronosis

(Left) PA radiograph shows diffuse osteoporosis. There is fusion of a DIP joint ➡ as well as erosions of the PIP joints ➡; the MCP joints are relatively normal. The appearance is typical of adult Still disease. *(Right)* Anteroposterior radiograph shows diffuse osteopenia, typical of the disease process in ochronosis. Late in the disease, cartilage damage and arthritis may occur ➡.

ARTHRITIS WITH PRODUCTIVE CHANGES

DIFFERENTIAL DIAGNOSIS

Common
- Osteoarthritis (OA)
- Gout
- Pyrophosphate Arthropathy
- Abutment Processes
- Ankylosing Spondylitis (AS)
- Psoriatic Arthritis (PSA)
- DISH (Mimic)
- Chronic Reactive Arthritis (CRA)
- Inflammatory Bowel Disease Arthritis (IBD)
- Osteonecrosis (Mimic, with Secondary Osteoarthritis)

Less Common
- SAPHO (Mimic)
- Retinoid Spondyloarthropathy (Mimic)
- Hemochromatosis
- OPLL (Mimic)

Rare but Important
- Wilson Disease

ESSENTIAL INFORMATION

Key Differential Diagnosis Issues
- **Hint**: Very few diseases are purely productive
  - Osteoarthritis
  - DISH, OPLL, retinoid spondyloarthropathy, SAPHO, abutment processes
- **Hint**: Many processes may show coexistent erosive and productive changes
  - Spondyloarthropathies (AS, PSA, IBD, CRA)
  - Deposition arthropathies (gout, pyrophosphate, hemochromatosis, Wilson)
  - One site may be predominantly productive, another erosive
- **Hint**: Processes that result in abnormal alignment may result in mechanical erosions & productive changes
  - "Burned out" or inactive rheumatoid arthritis
    - May appear confusing, with distribution of RA but productive changes superimposed on inactive erosive disease
    - Usually these have a mixed pattern, with erosions seen as well as osteophytes
  - Systemic lupus erythematosus
  - Progressive systemic sclerosis

Helpful Clues for Common Diagnoses
- **Osteoarthritis (OA)**
  - OA is the classic purely productive arthropathy
  - Do not expect to see any erosions
    - Exception: Mechanical erosion if joint is significantly malaligned
    - Exception: Erosive (inflammatory) OA
  - Location is useful adjunct in diagnosis
    - Hand: IP joints > > MCP; 1st carpometacarpal, scapho-trapezoid-trapezium
    - Knee: Medial compartment often more significantly involved, though may be tri-compartmental
    - Hip: Inferomedial osteophyte is most prominent; usually superolateral subluxation femoral head
- **Gout**
  - Osteophyte formation is common, along with normal bone density
  - Focal erosions tend to be well-marginated, often with productive change at edge (overhanging edge)
  - Location may be classic, but also may be polyostotic with unusual locations
- **Pyrophosphate Arthropathy**
  - Earliest disease is erosive, then mixed
  - End stage may be purely productive, with large osteophytes
    - Has been described as "OA in an unusual distribution"
  - Location is particularly useful for diagnosis
    - Carpus: Radiocarpal, often with excavation of radius by scaphoid; may result in SLAC (scapholunate advanced collapse) deformity
    - Hand: 2nd & 3rd MCP most commonly involved; other MCPs with advanced disease
    - Knee: Patellofemoral joint most prominently involved
  - Large subchondral cysts; normal density
  - Chondrocalcinosis often present
  - **Hemochromatosis**
    - Same appearance as pyrophosphate arthropathy, but in younger male patient
- **Abutment Processes**
  - Most frequent is ulnar impaction due to ulnar positive variance

ARTHRITIS WITH PRODUCTIVE CHANGES

○ Hamate & lunate may develop productive changes with SLAC wrist deformity
○ Impacted structure develops sclerosis, osteophytes, subchondral cysts

• **Ankylosing Spondylitis (AS)**
○ Disease begins as erosive (inflammatory)
○ SI joints eventually fuse & spine develops productive changes (syndesmophytes & fusion)
○ Large proximal joints (hips, shoulders); erosive, mixed, or productive changes
○ May have synchronous erosive change at one site & productive change at another
○ Diffuse osteopenia early in disease process
○ IBD arthropathy, similar appearance

• **Psoriatic Arthritis (PSA)**
○ Disease begins as erosive (inflammatory)
○ SI joints may eventually fuse & spine develops bulky syndesmophytes & may fuse at facets
○ Normal bone density usually retained
○ PSA: Small peripheral joint involvement
  ▪ Hands > feet
  ▪ IP joints > MCP

• **Chronic Reactive Arthritis (CRA)**
○ Lower extremity peripheral joints
○ Calcaneus > midfoot & forefoot > ankle

• **DISH (Mimic) & OPLL (Mimic)**
○ Both may show large anterior bridging osteophytes at spine (DISH > OPLL)
○ Both may ossify posterior longitudinal ligament (OPLL > DISH)
○ Neither generally involves facets & therefore is not a true arthritis

○ DISH: Thoracic > cervical spine
○ OPLL: Cervical > thoracic spine

• **Osteonecrosis (Mimic, with Secondary Osteoarthritis)**
○ Severe & chronic AVN with flattening of femoral head may develop secondary OA
  ▪ Osteophytes, eventual cartilage involvement (late)
  ▪ Calcar buttressing along femoral neck

Helpful Clues for Less Common Diagnoses

• **SAPHO (Mimic)**
○ Sclerosis of anterior chest wall osseous structures
  ▪ Clavicle, manubrium, ribs, costochondral cartilage
○ Not articular process; joints remain intact

• **Retinoid Spondyloarthropathy (Mimic)**
○ Use of retinoids may result in prominent anterior syndesmophyte formation
○ Entire spine may be involved
○ Generally facets are uninvolved & it is not a true arthropathy
○ Suggestive of DISH, but in younger patient

Helpful Clues for Rare Diagnoses

• **Wilson Disease**
○ May produce "excrescences" of bone that mimic osteophytes
○ May produce ossicles that mimic osteophytes separated from underlying bone
○ Generalized osteoporosis
○ Eventually may develop true arthritis with mixed erosive/productive change

Osteoarthritis (OA)

PA radiograph shows typical DIP involvement with OA. There is loss of cartilage & osteophyte formation ➡ which broadens the base of the distal phalanges. On lateral view, these are especially prominent dorsally.

Gout

PA radiograph shows productive changes in gout, with osteophytes ➡ and overhanging edge ➡. The disease is active, with large dense tophi and adjacent erosion.

ARTHRITIS WITH PRODUCTIVE CHANGES

(Left) PA radiograph shows classic pyrophosphate arthropathy, with SLAC deformity & radiocarpal productive changes ➡ as well as hook-like osteophyte formation at the MCP heads ➡. No erosive changes are seen at this advanced stage. **(Right)** PA radiograph shows ulnar positive variance ➡ that has resulted in abnormal load and abutment on the lunate & triquetrum. The lunate shows sclerosis and osteophytes are seen at both the lunate & triquetrum ➡.

Pyrophosphate Arthropathy

Abutment Processes

(Left) AP radiograph shows what appears to be typical OA, with osteophyte formation ➡, subchondral cyst ➡, and calcar buttressing ➡. However, this male is only 25 years old, and another source for these abnormalities must be considered. **(Right)** AP radiograph in the same patient shows bilateral SI joint sclerosis and advanced erosive ➡ disease. The patient has AS; note that the manifestations are erosive in the SI joint but productive in the hip at this time.

Ankylosing Spondylitis (AS)

Ankylosing Spondylitis (AS)

(Left) AP radiograph shows tremendous productive change in the form of enthesopathy at the tips of the malleoli ➡ in this patient with psoriatic arthritis. Though articular changes almost always appear erosive, early findings may be productive, with periostitis. **(Right)** Lateral radiograph shows bulky bridging anterior syndesmophytes typical of DISH ➡. Note that the anterior concavity of the vertebral bodies is retained ➡ & bone density is normal.

Psoriatic Arthritis (PSA)

DISH (Mimic)

ARTHRITIS WITH PRODUCTIVE CHANGES

Chronic Reactive Arthritis (CRA)

Inflammatory Bowel Disease Arthritis (IBD)

(Left) Lateral radiograph shows fluffy osseous productive change at the posterior tubercle of the calcaneus ⮡ as well as the plantar aponeurosis insertion site ➡. This dense bone production is seen about the calcaneus with CRA. *(Right)* Anteroposterior radiograph shows a large osteophyte ringing the left femoral head ⮥ in a patient with inflammatory bowel disease. Note the mixed erosive/productive change at the SI joints ➡; the patient has spondyloarthropathy.

Osteonecrosis (Mimic, with Secondary Osteoarthritis)

SAPHO (Mimic)

(Left) Anteroposterior radiograph shows severe flattening of the femoral head from AVN ➡. This is a chronic process, which has resulted in secondary OA. Note the ring osteophyte at the femoral head ➡ as well as calcar buttressing ⮥. *(Right)* Coronal NECT shows dense sclerosis of the left manubrium ➡. Note that the clavicle and joint are normal; this is not a true arthritis, but the sclerosis may mimic this process.

Hemochromatosis

Wilson Disease

(Left) PA radiograph shows cartilage loss particularly involving the 2nd & 3rd MCP joints, with osteophyte formation ➡. A large hook-like osteophyte is seen at the 3rd MC head ➡. Findings in this young male are typical of hemochromatosis. *(Right)* PA radiograph shows bony excrescences arising from the lunate ➡ and radius ➡ in a patient showing diffuse osteoporosis. This productive change is one of the manifestations of Wilson disease.

EROSIVE ARTHRITIS

DIFFERENTIAL DIAGNOSIS

Common
- Rheumatoid Arthritis (RA)
- Erosive Osteoarthritis (EOA)
- Gout
- Pigmented Villonodular Synovitis (PVNS)
- Synovial Osteochondromatosis
- Ankylosing Spondylitis (AS)
- Psoriatic Arthritis (PSA)
- Pyrophosphate Arthropathy
- Juvenile Idiopathic Arthritis (JIA)
- Septic Joint
- Charcot, Neuropathic (Mimic)
- Hyperparathyroidism (HPTH) (Mimic)

Less Common
- Arthroplasty Component Wear/Particle Disease (Mimic)
- Chronic Reactive Arthritis (CRA)
- HIV-Related Arthritis
- Inflammatory Bowel Disease Arthritis (IBD)
- Hemophilia
- Amyloid Deposition
- Systemic Lupus Erythematosus, Late (SLE)
- Progressive Systemic Sclerosis, Late (PSS)
- Ochronosis (Alkaptonuria)
- Tuberculosis & Fungal Septic Arthritis

Rare but Important
- Adult Still Disease
- Robust Rheumatoid Arthritis
- Multicentric Reticulohistiocytosis

ESSENTIAL INFORMATION

Key Differential Diagnosis Issues
- Erosions may have different basic etiologies
  - Inflammatory: Majority of processes
  - Mechanical: Neuropathic, SLE
  - Direct invasion: PVNS, synovial osteochondromatosis
  - Subchondral collapse: HPTH

Helpful Clues for Common Diagnoses
- **Rheumatoid Arthritis (RA)**
  - The most classic solely erosive arthropathy
    - Exceptions: Ulnar "capping" in active RA; OA may develop in inactive RA
  - Location is symmetric & constant
    - MCP, distal radioulnar joint, radiocarpal joint; eventually intercarpal joints and IP
    - MTPs, particularly 5th

- Uniform involvement hip, knee, shoulder, elbow
- **Erosive Osteoarthritis (EOA)**
  - Erosive or mixed erosive/productive change IP joints
  - Involvement of 1st carpometacarpal (CMC) & scapho-trapezium-trapezoid
    - Usually productive as in typical OA, but may be erosive
  - No other findings to suggest PSA
- **Gout**
  - Erosions prominent when active; later show sclerotic margins
  - Dense tophi, overhanging edges help suggest diagnosis
- **Pigmented Villonodular Synovitis (PVNS)**
  - Nodular synovitis directly invades bone
  - Monostotic; normal bone density
  - Low signal masses which enhance on MR
- **Synovial Osteochondromatosis**
  - Multiple round bodies, ± ossified
  - Usually monostotic, with bodies entirely intraarticular; occasionally extraarticular
  - May focally invade bone, causing erosion
- **Ankylosing Spondylitis (AS)**
  - Early SI joint arthritis tends to be symmetric & is erosive, often → fusion
  - Large proximal joints (hips, shoulders)
    - Erosive initially, may become mixed or purely productive
  - With long-standing disease, small peripheral joints may become involved
  - Osteoporosis develops early in disease
  - IBD arthritis: Similar appearance
- **Psoriatic Arthritis (PSA)**
  - Peripheral disease favors hands (especially IP joints), but may involve feet as well
    - May initially be seen as sausage digit, with periostitis
    - Early joint disease is erosive; may become mixed or rarely productive
  - SI joints generally bilaterally asymmetric
    - Early SI joint disease is erosive, but may progress to fusion
    - Syndesmophytes are productive, but facet disease begins as erosions, sometimes progressing to fusion
- **Pyrophosphate Arthropathy**
  - Begins as erosive disease, often becomes mixed erosive/productive & may eventually appear purely productive

EROSIVE ARTHRITIS

- Location-specific
  - Hands: Radiocarpal, 2nd & 3rd metacarpals (MC)
  - Knee: Patellofemoral compartment involved earlier & more severely than medial or lateral compartments
- ± Chondrocalcinosis
- Large subchondral cysts often present
- **Juvenile Idiopathic Arthritis (JIA)**
  - Hemophilia
  - Both diseases arise during childhood, resulting in overgrowth of epiphyses
  - Both result in erosive joint disease
  - Location similar for both diseases: Knee > elbow > ankle > hip
  - JIA often has ankylosis of carpal or IPs
  - Hemophilia is gender-specific & may have dense effusions due to hemosiderin deposition in synovium
- **Septic Joint (Including TB & Fungal)**
  - Early changes: Effusion, hyperemia → osteopenia
  - → Cartilage destruction & focal erosions
- **Charcot, Neuropathic (Mimic)**
  - Cycle of unprotected abnormal motion → bone fragmentation & ligament instability → subluxation, dislocation → further fragmentation
  - "Erosions" mimicked by fragmentation donor sites
- **Hyperparathyroidism (HPTH) (Mimic)**
  - One of the many types of bone resorption is subchondral
  - Resorption & weight-bearing → collapse

- Since at joint surface, collapse mimics an erosion
- Locations are typical
  - IP joints, occasional carpal bones (mimics PSA)
  - SI joints (mimics widening of early spondyloarthropathy)
  - Distal clavicle (mimics erosions of RA or traumatic osteolysis)

Helpful Clues for Less Common Diagnoses
- **Arthroplasty Component Wear/Particle Disease (Mimic)**
  - Osteolysis from particle disease may mimic erosion or subchondral cyst
- **Chronic Reactive Arthritis (CRA)**
  - HIV-related arthritis: Similar appearance
  - Peripheral disease favors lower extremity (especially foot & calcaneus)
  - Sacroiliitis bilateral & asymmetric
- **Amyloid Deposition**
  - Deposition in cartilage, bone, synovium may → erosion
- **Systemic Lupus Erythematosus, Late (SLE)**
  - Deforming, generally nonerosive
  - Subchondral cysts, very rarely erosions
- **Progressive Systemic Sclerosis, Late (PSS)**
  - Most patients eventually develop erosions
  - Acroosteolysis, soft tissue calcification
- **Ochronosis (Alkaptonuria)**
  - Late in disease cartilage may fragment, leading to destructive disease

Helpful Clues for Rare Diagnoses
- **Adult Still Disease:** Erosive, as RA

Rheumatoid Arthritis (RA)

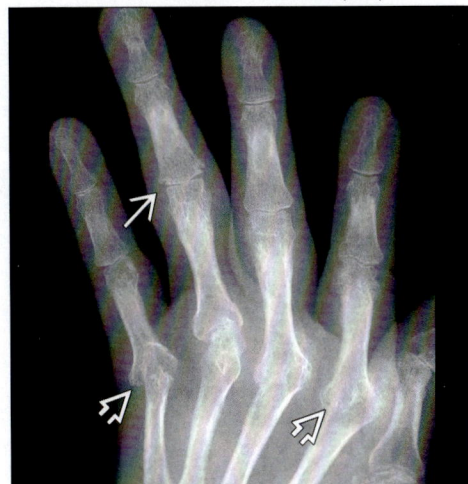

PA radiograph shows soft tissue swelling and marginal erosions ➡ at the PIP joint. A marginal location (within the joint capsule but where bone is not protected by cartilage) is typical for early erosive change.

Rheumatoid Arthritis (RA)

PA radiograph in the same patient shows the marginal erosions ➡ but also much more advanced subchondral erosions in the MCP joints ➡. The osteoporosis & ulnar deviation is classic as well.

EROSIVE ARTHRITIS

Erosive Osteoarthritis (EOA)

Gout

(Left) PA radiograph shows erosive disease involving the IP joint ➡. This is not specific, but when combined with arthritis at the 1st carpometacarpal joint ➡ and scapho-trapezium-trapezoid joint ➡, the diagnosis is confirmed as EOA. *(Right)* Anteroposterior radiograph shows severe erosive disease of the digits of the feet ➡ of this elderly male. Additionally, there is dense tophaceous material, as well as an overhanging edge ➡, all characteristic of gout.

Pigmented Villonodular Synovitis (PVNS)

Synovial Osteochondromatosis

(Left) Coronal T2WI MR shows a huge glenoid erosion ➡ and smaller humeral head erosion ➡. There is low signal material lining the synovium ➡ as well as the erosions. This is a teenager; the findings are typical of PVNS. *(Right)* Axial bone CT shows multiple tiny ossified bodies ➡ scattered throughout the knee joint and extending into the extraarticular soft tissues. There are large pressure erosions ➡ in this patient with aggressive synovial chondromatosis.

Ankylosing Spondylitis (AS)

Psoriatic Arthritis (PSA)

(Left) Anteroposterior radiograph shows erosive disease in moderately early AS. SI joint shows widening & mild sclerosis ➡; hip shows cartilage loss & erosions ➡. Later in the process, productive changes & fusion will occur. *(Right)* PA radiograph shows DIP erosive disease ➡ that is so severe that it has been termed "pencil-in-cup" deformity & results in "telescoping digits". Psoriatic arthritis certainly may show more mild disease, but this is the end stage.

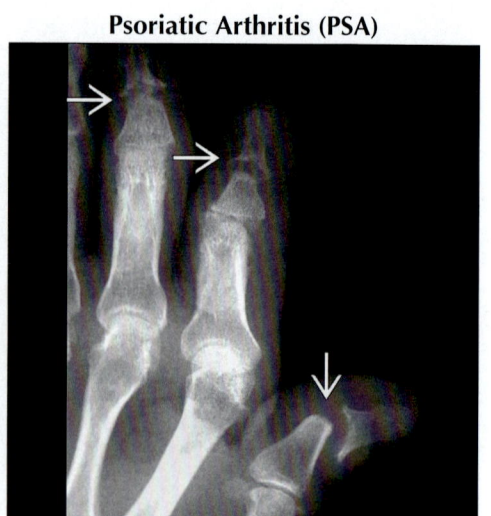

EROSIVE ARTHRITIS

Pyrophosphate Arthropathy

Juvenile Idiopathic Arthritis (JIA)

(Left) PA radiograph shows erosions ➡, along with large subchondral cysts ⮞ and chondrocalcinosis in the TFCC ➡. The predominance of radiocarpal disease is also typical of pyrophosphate arthropathy. *(Right)* Anteroposterior radiograph shows severe thinning of the femoral neck from erosive disease ➡ (remember the neck is intracapsular) as well as a direct subchondral erosion of the femoral head ⮞ in a patient with advanced JIA. There is cartilage destruction as well.

Septic Joint

Charcot, Neuropathic (Mimic)

(Left) AP radiograph shows contrast injected into a hip joint following aspiration for septic hip. The contrast outlines severely thinned cartilage & enters erosions in the acetabulum ➡, showing the erosive nature of the process. *(Right)* Oblique radiograph shows "erosive" disease at the Lisfranc joints ➡ in this diabetic neuropathic joint. Note the offset of the metatarsals relative to the tarsals. The "erosions" are due to fragmentation, followed by resorption of the debris.

Hyperparathyroidism (HPTH) (Mimic)

Arthroplasty Component Wear/Particle Disease (Mimic)

(Left) PA radiograph shows what appears to be marginal ➡ and subchondral ⮞ erosions in the DIPs of a patient with HPTH. The disease causes subchondral resorption, followed by collapse which mimics erosions. *(Right)* AP radiograph shows a large lytic lesion ➡ that might be mistaken for erosion or subchondral cyst related to the underlying arthropathy. However, this acetabular component has "shed" several metallic microspheres ➡, resulting in osteolysis.

EROSIVE ARTHRITIS

(Left) *Lateral radiograph shows a large erosion of the posterior tubercle of the calcaneus ➡. This location is typical of involvement by CRA, which may be erosive initially. Later productive disease will yield fluffy periostitis.* **(Right)** *PA radiograph shows swelling of the index finger (sausage digit) with narrowing of the DIP ➡ and periostitis ➡. This patient has HIV-AIDS; such patients may develop an arthropathy similar to chronic reactive arthritis.*

Chronic Reactive Arthritis (CRA)

HIV-Related Arthritis

(Left) *Anteroposterior radiograph shows sclerotic & eroded, but not yet fused, SI joints ➡. The patient has staple lines indicating ileoanal pull-through ➡ for IBD. The left hip has AVN with collapse ➡, secondary to steroid use.* **(Right)** *Lateral radiograph shows multiple erosions ➡ in the setting of a large dense effusion ➡, typical of hemophilia. Note the overgrowth of the patella & femoral condyles relative to the gracile diaphyses. (†MSK Req).*

Inflammatory Bowel Disease Arthritis (IBD)

Hemophilia

(Left) *Posteroanterior radiograph shows erosions in the DIP joints ➡. There is nothing specific about the erosion, but the patient also had large soft tissue masses over the dorsum of the wrist; biopsy proved amyloid.* **(Right)** *Oblique radiograph shows severe subluxation and swan neck deformities of the digits, typical of the deformities found in SLE. This is late disease, and mechanical erosions have formed at the DIP ➡ and MCP ➡.*

Amyloid Deposition

Systemic Lupus Erythematosus, Late (SLE)

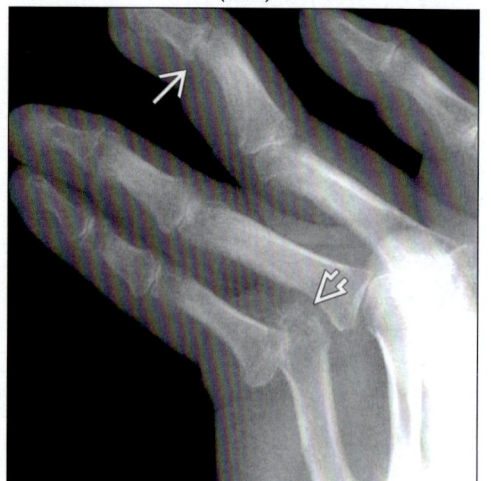

EROSIVE ARTHRITIS

Progressive Systemic Sclerosis, Late (PSS)

Ochronosis (Alkaptonuria)

(Left) PA radiograph shows the acroosteolysis ➡ and soft tissue calcifications ➡ typical of progressive systemic sclerosis. This is late disease, and the patient has developed erosions ➡. The 1st CMC joint was subluxated (not shown), as is typical in late PSS. *(Right)* Anteroposterior radiograph shows diffuse osteoporosis and severe erosive disease of the hip ➡. Ochronosis may develop cartilage fragmentation and erosive disease late in the disease process.

Tuberculosis & Fungal Septic Arthritis

Adult Still Disease

(Left) PA radiograph shows osteoporosis, cartilage destruction, and erosive disease of the triquetrum, ulna, radius, and lunate ➡. This is a septic radiocarpal joint; aspirate proved a fungal etiology: Sporotrichosis. *(Right)* PA radiograph shows IP erosive disease ➡ in a patient who also has ankylosis of a DIP joint ➡. The findings could be seen in either psoriatic or adult Still disease; the osteoporosis favors the latter, which was proven.

Robust Rheumatoid Arthritis

Multicentric Reticulohistiocytosis

(Left) PA radiograph shows severe erosive disease at the MCPs ➡ and the intercarpal joints, in the distribution of RA. There are large subchondral cysts ➡, making the diagnosis of robust rheumatoid arthritis. *(Right)* PA radiograph shows a combination of findings typical of multicentric reticulohistiocytosis. These include nodular soft tissue swelling ➡, acroosteolysis ➡, and erosions at the DIP joints ➡. The soft tissue nodules differentiate it from psoriatic arthritis.

MIXED EROSIVE/PRODUCTIVE ARTHRITIS

DIFFERENTIAL DIAGNOSIS

Common
- Pyrophosphate Arthropathy
- Erosive Osteoarthritis (EOA)
- Gout
- Ankylosing Spondylitis (AS)
- Psoriatic Arthritis (PSA)

Less Common
- Chronic Reactive Arthritis (CRA)
- Inflammatory Bowel Disease Arthritis (IBD)
- Hemochromatosis

Rare but Important
- SAPHO

ESSENTIAL INFORMATION

Key Differential Diagnosis Issues
- Purely erosive arthritis (RA) drops off list
- Purely productive arthritis (classic OA) and mimics (DISH, OPLL) drop off this list
- **Hint**: Most of the diagnoses on this list show erosive disease early, then progress to mixed & may end as purely productive

Helpful Clues for Common Diagnoses
- **Pyrophosphate Arthropathy**
  - Erosions early (particularly articular surface patella, radiocarpal joint)
  - Followed by osteophyte formation (particularly hook-like osteophytes at MCPs, patellofemoral joint)
  - ± Chondrocalcinosis
  - **Hemachromatosis**
    - Appears identical to pyrophosphate arthropathy; occurs in younger males
- **Erosive Osteoarthritis (EOA)**
  - IP joints show early erosions, may be mixed with osteophytes later
  - 1st carpometacarpal (CMC) joint & scapho-trapezium-trapezoid (STT) involvement confirms EOA as diagnosis
    - May be erosive, but usually productive
- **Gout**
  - Early erosions develop sclerotic margins later, associated osteophytes
- **Ankylosing Spondylitis (AS)**
  - Early erosions SI joints, generally bilaterally symmetric, followed by fusion
  - Large proximal joints (hip, shoulder) may show both erosions & osteophytes
  - Smaller peripheral joints show mixed disease, but involved only late in process
  - IBD arthritis appears similar
- **Psoriatic Arthritis (PSA) & Chronic Reactive Arthritis (CRA)**
  - Peripheral joints (hands predominate in PSA, foot/ankle predominate in CRA)
    - May have early periostitis, sausage digit
  - SI joint disease bilateral but asymmetric
  - SI & peripheral joint disease begin erosive but progress to productive

Helpful Clues for Rare Diagnoses
- **SAPHO**
  - Sclerosis (particularly anterior chest wall) defines productive change
  - Synovitis uncommon, actual erosions rare

Pyrophosphate Arthropathy

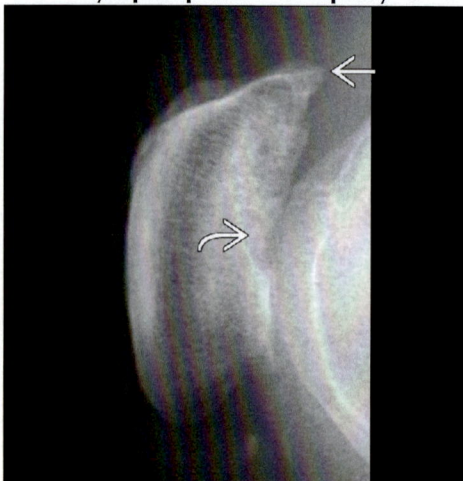

Lateral radiograph shows a mid-patellar erosion ➡ mixed with osteophytes ➡ in the patellofemoral joint of a middle-aged patient with meniscal chondrocalcinosis; the diagnosis is pyrophosphate arthropathy.

Erosive Osteoarthritis (EOA)

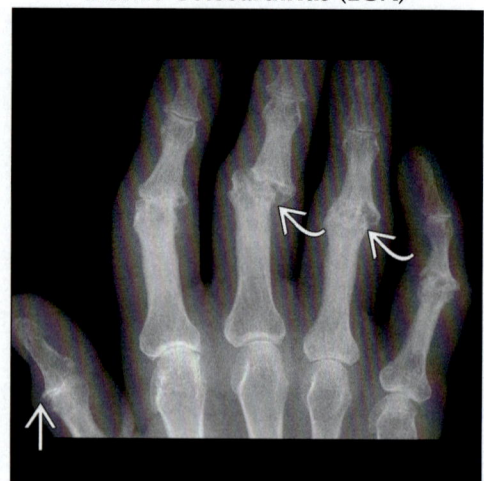

PA radiograph shows mixed disease, with osteophyte seen at the IP of the thumb ➡ and predominantly erosive disease at the PIP joints ➡. The CMC and STT joints showed productive change; this is EOA.

MIXED EROSIVE/PRODUCTIVE ARTHRITIS

Gout

Ankylosing Spondylitis (AS)

(Left) Lateral radiograph shows a large dense tophus, indicating gout in this elderly woman. There is osteophyte formation ⮕ seen simultaneously with active erosive disease ⮕, a typical pattern for gout. *(Right)* Axial bone CT shows mixed erosive/productive disease in the axial skeleton, with prominent erosions at the sternoclavicular joints ⮕ at the same time that the axial skeleton is fused; this image shows fusion at the costovertebral joints ⮕.

Psoriatic Arthritis (PSA)

Chronic Reactive Arthritis (CRA)

(Left) PA radiograph shows productive disease in the form of periostitis and osteophytes ⮕, along with erosions predominantly at the DIP joints ⮕. There is normal bone density; the appearance is typical of psoriatic arthritis. *(Right)* AP radiograph shows complete bilateral SI joint fusion ⮕ as well as primarily erosive disease in the left hip ⮕. This may be a typical appearance for AS, but the patient has advanced CRA, involving the more proximal joints.

Inflammatory Bowel Disease Arthritis (IBD)

Hemochromatosis

(Left) AP radiograph in a 21 year old woman with Crohn disease shows erosive change at the SI joint ⮕, indicating spondyloarthropathy. The hip shows cartilage loss and osteophyte formation ⮕. The patient has IBD spondyloarthropathy. *(Right)* PA radiograph shows mixed erosive ⮕ and productive ⮕ disease in a man with hemochromatosis. The same location and appearance may be seen with pyrophosphate arthropathy.

ARTHRITIS WITH LARGE SUBCHONDRAL CYSTS

DIFFERENTIAL DIAGNOSIS

Common
- Osteoarthritis (OA)
- Pyrophosphate Arthropathy
- Rheumatoid Arthritis (RA)
- Gout
- Massive Osteolysis/Particle Disease
- Pigmented Villonodular Synovitis (PVNS)
- Cysts, Chronic Repetitive Trauma

Less Common
- Giant Cell Tumor Tendon Sheath (Mimic)
- Hemophilia
- Juvenile Idiopathic Arthritis (JIA)
- Amyloid Deposition
- Hemochromatosis

Rare but Important
- Robust Rheumatoid Arthritis
- Ankylosing Spondylitis (AS)
- Psoriatic Arthritis (PSA)
- Chronic Reactive Arthritis (CRA)

ESSENTIAL INFORMATION

Key Differential Diagnosis Issues
- Subchondral cysts may occur with any arthropathy
  - Some diseases are particularly prone to large cyst formation
  - This feature may be useful in suggesting a diagnosis
- Subchondral cysts may be so large that they mimic neoplasm
  - **Hint**: In diagnosing a subchondral neoplasm, always look for a suggestion of arthropathy
- In weight-bearing bones, large subchondral cysts may result in pathologic fracture
  - Particularly in knee, secondary to pyrophosphate arthropathy or gout

Helpful Clues for Common Diagnoses
- **Osteoarthritis (OA)**
  - Large subchondral cysts seen particularly in acetabulum
    - Termed "Egger cyst"
  - Cyst often is initial finding in OA of hip
    - **Hint**: Be careful not to misdiagnose Egger cyst as neoplasm
  - Watch for other subtle signs of hip OA

- Calcar buttressing (thickening of medial femoral neck)
- Superolateral subluxation femoral head
- Sclerosis
- Cartilage narrowing in weight-bearing region
- Subtle osteophytes

- **Pyrophosphate Arthropathy**
  - Subchondral cysts are a prominent part of the arthropathy
  - Those in tibial condyle are not infrequently misdiagnosed as neoplasm
    - Knee pyrophosphate arthropathy often shows initial subtle erosive change at the patellofemoral compartment
    - Chondrocalcinosis in meniscus or hyaline cartilage may be subtle or absent
  - Those in carpal bones are multiple & prominent
    - Often have associated radiocarpal disease
    - Chondrocalcinosis in TFCC or hyaline cartilage may be obvious, subtle, or absent
    - May have associated SLAC (scapholunate advanced collapse) deformity
- **Rheumatoid Arthritis (RA)**
  - Subchondral cysts may be huge
  - Size tends not to be appreciated on radiograph due to diffuse osteoporosis
  - MR shows extent of cyst formation, along with other abnormalities
- **Gout**
  - Subchondral cysts tend to be well-marginated unless active
  - May be mistaken for neoplasm
  - Watch for associated findings
    - Dense soft tissue tophi
    - Overhanging edge at osseous erosion
- **Massive Osteolysis/Particle Disease**
  - Generally 4 considerations for lytic lesion adjacent to arthroplasty
    - Cyst related to underlying arthropathy, residual from arthroplasty placement
    - Metastasis or myeloma (patients are in the age group for these lesions & they must be considered)
    - Stress shielding (region of metaphysis that no longer carries significant weight, resulting in osseous resorption)
    - Massive osteolysis, relating to particle disease

ARTHRITIS WITH LARGE SUBCHONDRAL CYSTS

- ○ Sources of particles: Breakdown of bone, polyethylene, metallic beads, cement
  - ▪ Watch particularly for asymmetry of acetabular cup liner or tibial tray liner to indicate polyethylene wear
- ○ Osteolysis may be far greater in extent than suggested on radiograph
  - ▪ CT with reformats demonstrates extent of lysis & any pathologic fracture
- • **Pigmented Villonodular Synovitis (PVNS)**
  - ○ Cyst formation may be large, or else entirely absent
  - ○ On radiograph tend to be well-marginated
  - ○ Monoarticular lesion, generally teenager or young adult
  - ○ MR shows characteristic intraarticular low signal mass, either nodular or lining synovium
- • **Cysts, Chronic Repetitive Trauma**
  - ○ Fairly location-specific

Helpful Clues for Less Common Diagnoses
- • **Giant Cell Tumor Tendon Sheath (Mimic)**
  - ○ Extraarticular mass within tendon sheath
  - ○ Most frequent site: Digits, especially hand
  - ○ May cause focal osseous erosion, even on both sides of a joint, simulating articular process with cyst formation
  - ○ Watch for soft tissue mass location, often not centered over joint in question
- • **Hemophilia**
  - ○ Male, usually teenager or young adult
  - ○ Subchondral cysts can be large, along with erosions & cartilage damage

- ○ Overgrowth of epiphyses/metaphyses, dense effusion may suggest diagnosis
- • **Juvenile Idiopathic Arthritis (JIA)**
  - ○ Females more frequent; usually teenager or young adult
  - ○ Subchondral cysts can be large, along with erosions & cartilage damage
  - ○ Overgrowth of epiphyses/metaphyses (ballooned epiphyses) may suggest diagnosis
  - ○ Cervical spine fusion suggests diagnosis
- • **Amyloid Deposition**
  - ○ Deposits in bone may result in large subchondral cysts
  - ○ Associated thickening & low MR signal of tendons & joint capsule
  - ○ Generally secondary: Myeloma or end stage renal disease predispose to amyloid
- • **Hemochromatosis**
  - ○ Younger male patient, similar to pyrophosphate arthropathy

Helpful Clues for Rare Diagnoses
- • **Robust Rheumatoid Arthritis**
  - ○ Continued use of involved joint during active disease results in synovial fluid being forced into subchondral bone
    - ▪ May result in large subchondral cyst formation
  - ○ Distribution similar to adult RA; bone density retained
- • **Spondyloarthropathies (AS, PSA, CRA)**
  - ○ Small, but rarely large subchondral cysts are seen

Osteoarthritis (OA)

Anteroposterior radiograph shows a large subchondral cyst ➔, termed Egger cyst at this location. There is also a loss of cartilage, superolateral subluxation, & osteophyte formation, all typical of osteoarthritis.

Pyrophosphate Arthropathy

Anteroposterior radiograph shows a large subchondral cyst ➔ in a knee that also demonstrates chondrocalcinosis ➔. The combination is typical of pyrophosphate arthropathy.

ARTHRITIS WITH LARGE SUBCHONDRAL CYSTS

Pyrophosphate Arthropathy

Rheumatoid Arthritis (RA)

(Left) Posteroanterior radiograph shows large subchondral cysts within the scaphoid, capitate, & hamate, typical of pyrophosphate arthropathy. There is chondrocalcinosis in the hyaline cartilage ➔ as well as the TFCC ➔, confirming the diagnosis. (†MSK Req). *(Right)* Sagittal T2WI FS MR shows large subchondral cysts ➔ extending down the humeral shaft. Rotator cuff tear is seen, with fluid in the subdeltoid bursa ➔, common in RA.

Gout

Massive Osteolysis/Particle Disease

(Left) Axial CECT shows a subchondral cyst occupying the entire lateral femoral condyle ➔. The cyst is so large that it simulates a neoplasm. The patient had gout of the first MTP, & this "lesion" proved to be gout as well. (†MSK Req). *(Right)* Coronal bone CT shows massive osteolysis in the acetabulum ➔, developing from particle disease. The source of the particles is wear of the polyethylene cup, demonstrated by the asymmetric position of the head within the cup ➔.

Pigmented Villonodular Synovitis (PVNS)

Cysts, Chronic Repetitive Trauma

(Left) Coronal T2WI MR shows a large subchondral cyst occupying nearly the entire glenoid ➔. This is a monoarticular process in a 15 year old. There is low signal nodular material lining the synovium ➔, typical of PVNS. *(Right)* Axial PD FSE MR shows subchondral cysts ➔ in a patient with osteolysis of the distal clavicle, related to chronic repetitive trauma (a male cheerleader who lifted "stocky" cheerleaders). The patient developed a fracture through the cysts.

ARTHRITIS WITH LARGE SUBCHONDRAL CYSTS

Giant Cell Tumor Tendon Sheath (Mimic)

Hemophilia

(Left) PA radiograph shows large "cystic" lesions occupying the head of the 1st MC and base of the adjacent phalanx ⇒, mimicking an arthritic process. However, the soft tissue mass is not associated with the joint ➡. This proved to be a giant cell tumor of the tendon sheath with local invasion. *(Right)* Lateral radiograph shows large subchondral cysts occupying most of the talus ➡, with an erosive process of the tibiotalar joint in this hemophilic patient.

Juvenile Idiopathic Arthritis (JIA)

Amyloid Deposition

(Left) AP radiograph shows an end-stage elbow in a patient with JIA. There is widening of the trochlear notch, complete loss of cartilage with severe erosive change ➡, and a large subchondral cyst ➡. *(Right)* Sagittal T2WI MR shows a large subchondral cyst containing low signal material ➡, along with thickening of the rotator cuff tendons ➡. This patient had amyloid deposition involving the shoulder, which may result in formation of large cysts. (†MSK Req).

Hemochromatosis

Robust Rheumatoid Arthritis

(Left) PA radiograph shows large hook-like osteophytes at the MCP joints ➡, along with prominent subchondral cysts ➡. This is hemochromatosis; it is sometimes forgotten that the disease may have erosive characteristics. *(Right)* PA radiograph shows huge subchondral cysts ➡ in the MCPs of a patient who has erosive disease in the distribution of rheumatoid arthritis. With robust disease, synovial fluid is forced into the subchondral bone, forming large cysts.

ATROPHIC JOINT DESTRUCTION

DIFFERENTIAL DIAGNOSIS

Common
- Rheumatoid Arthritis
- Septic Joint
- Diabetic Foot: Charcot
- Syringomyelia: Charcot

Less Common
- Hemophilia: MSK Complications
- Tuberculosis Arthritis
- Fungal Arthritis

Rare but Important
- Rapidly Destructive Osteoarthritis of Hip
- Chondrolysis, Post-Traumatic

ESSENTIAL INFORMATION

Key Differential Diagnosis Issues
- "Atrophic": Joint destruction with resorption of most debris & a relative paucity of reactive sclerosis

Helpful Clues for Common Diagnoses
- **Rheumatoid Arthritis**
  - Location: Metacarpophalangeal, proximal interphalangeal, carpal joints, & similar locations in feet are most common
  - Distribution: Polyarticular, bilateral, symmetric
  - Periarticular erosions, progress centrally
  - Destruction may result in arthritis mutilans
  - Demineralization
  - Ligamentous laxity → subluxation, dislocation
  - Edematous synovium with effusion
  - Intraarticular rice bodies
  - Rheumatoid nodules along extensor surfaces or bony prominences
  - Shoulder involvement associated with rotator cuff tear & erosion of acromion and distal clavicle
- **Septic Joint**
  - Location: Knee, hip, shoulder, spine
  - Distribution: Monoarticular; polyarticular less common
  - Rapid cartilage & bone destruction
  - Involves entire joint
  - Large effusion, displaced fat pads
  - Demineralization on both sides of joint

- Differentiate from rheumatoid arthritis by rapidity of destructive changes
- **Diabetic Foot: Charcot**
  - Location: Lisfranc, talonavicular, intertarsal, hindfoot-midfoot (Chopart)
  - Distribution: Unilateral, asymmetric
  - Bone resorption & fragmentation
  - Amount of debris varies; often resorbed, resulting in atrophic destruction
  - Variable degree of reactive sclerosis
  - Large joint effusion
  - Joint subluxation or dislocation
  - Can be difficult to distinguish neuropathic joint from osteomyelitis
    - Sinus tract to bone favors osteomyelitis
    - Confluent low signal on T1WI favors osteomyelitis
    - Abscess next to bone favors osteomyelitis
- **Syringomyelia: Charcot**
  - Location: Shoulder, elbow, cervical spine
  - Distribution: Unilateral
  - Bone fragmentation that mimics erosions
    - Mild intraarticular bone debris common
    - Debris should not be confused with tumor matrix (chondrosarcoma mimic)
    - Extensive resorption of bone mimics surgical resection
  - Large joint effusion
    - Clinically often mistaken for soft tissue mass
    - Fluid can dissect away from joint
  - No reactive change in the bone
  - Joint often subluxed or dislocated
  - Image cervical spinal cord for syrinx
  - Rapid destruction mimics septic arthritis

Helpful Clues for Less Common Diagnoses
- **Hemophilia: MSK Complications**
  - Location: Knee, elbow, ankle
  - Distribution: Polyarticular, asymmetric
  - Dense effusion from hemorrhage
  - Synovitis & periarticular erosions
    - Can mimic Hill-Sachs deformity
  - Subchondral cysts
  - Growth deformities
    - Overgrown epiphyses & metaphyses from hyperemia
    - Wide intercondylar notch of knee
    - Premature growth plate closure
  - Blooming signal on gradient echo MR sequences from hemosiderin in joint
  - Secondary osteoarthritis late

ATROPHIC JOINT DESTRUCTION

- **Tuberculosis Arthritis**
  - Location: Spine, hip, knee
  - Distribution: Monoarticular
  - Slow clinical course compared with pyogenic septic joint; little debris
  - Extensive marginal erosions
    - More sclerotic rim than hemophilia
  - Severe demineralization
  - Preservation of joint space until late
  - Growth disturbance if skeletally immature
  - Spine involvement shows preservation of disc space & paravertebral abscess
- **Fungal Arthritis**
  - Location: Distal extremities
  - Distribution: Monoarticular
  - Indolent course
  - Marked osteoporosis
  - Destruction of joint space late
  - Similar appearance to tuberculous arthritis

Helpful Clues for Rare Diagnoses
- **Rapidly Destructive Osteoarthritis of Hip**
  - Location: Hip
  - Distribution: Unilateral
  - Rapid onset of clinical symptoms
  - Rapid chondrolysis followed by osseous destruction
  - "Hatchet deformity": Absent femoral head with well-defined border of femoral neck
    - Neoplasm or avascular necrosis would appear as a poorly marginated process
  - May represent insufficiency fracture of the femoral head

  - Low signal intensity lines on MR parallel the subchondral bone
  - Lacks demineralization
  - Normal acetabulum excludes inflammatory or infectious arthritis
- **Chondrolysis, Post-Traumatic**
  - Location: Hip, shoulder
  - Distribution: Monoarticular
  - History of trauma, surgery, burns or immobilization
  - Synovitis present
  - Bone scan shows increased tracer uptake on both sides of joint

Alternative Differential Approaches
- Monoarticular joint destruction & demineralization
  - Pyogenic infectious arthritis
  - Charcot joint
  - Tuberculous infectious arthritis
  - Fungal infectious arthritis
  - Chondrolysis, post-traumatic
  - Rheumatoid arthritis, monarticular
  - Chronic reactive arthritis
- Polyarticular joint destruction & demineralization
  - Rheumatoid arthritis
  - Progressive systemic sclerosis
  - Hemophilia
  - Chronic reactive arthritis
  - Lupus erythematosus, late
  - Ankylosing spondylitis

Rheumatoid Arthritis

Lateral radiograph shows severe destructive arthritis producing uniform cartilage loss ➡ with erosions involving all bones of the elbow. There is diffuse osteoporosis and a large joint effusion.

Rheumatoid Arthritis

Anteroposterior radiograph shows destruction of the shoulder joint ➡. Charcot from syringomyelia could be considered but involvement was symmetric, which virtually never happens with Charcot joints.

ATROPHIC JOINT DESTRUCTION

Rheumatoid Arthritis

Septic Joint

(Left) *Anteroposterior radiograph shows carpal collapse with probable fusion of some of the carpal bones. Note the marked narrowing of the intercarpal spaces* ➡ *and radiocarpal joint* ➡. *Degenerative changes are minimal compared to the degree of joint space narrowing.* (Right) *Oblique radiograph shows severe narrowing of the interphalangeal joint of the great toe* ➡. *Osseous destruction of the articular surfaces has occurred along both sides of the joint* ➡.

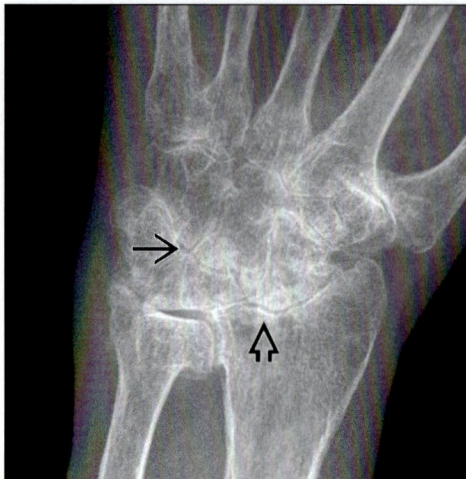

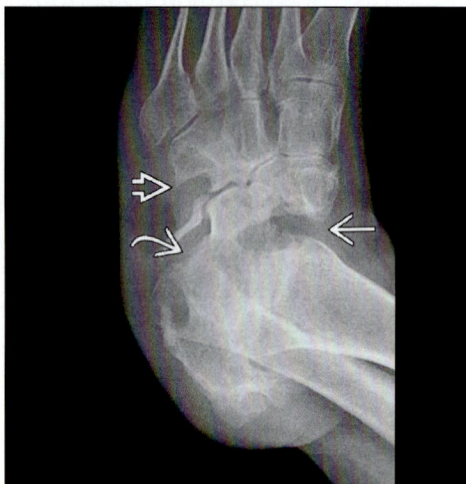

Diabetic Foot: Charcot

Diabetic Foot: Charcot

(Left) *Anteroposterior radiograph shows resorption of the talus, leaving the tibia articulating with the morphologically abnormal calcaneus* ➡ *and leaving the navicular without proximal articulation* ➡. *The calcaneocuboid joint is disrupted* ➡. (Right) *Lateral radiograph shows dislocation and erosive change of the talonavicular joint* ➡. *There is also subluxation with debris formation at the calcaneocuboid joint* ➡ *and a hypertrophic nonunion of a fibular fracture* ➡.

Syringomyelia: Charcot

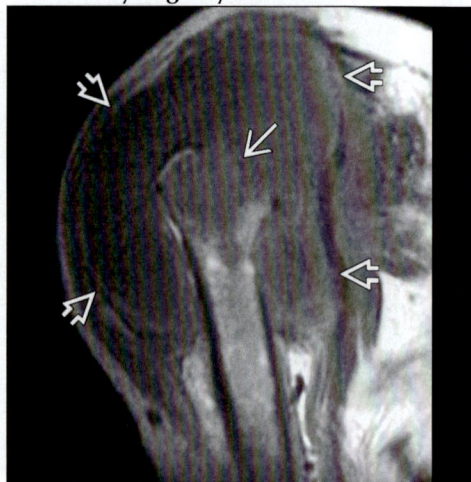

Syringomyelia: Charcot

(Left) *Anteroposterior radiograph shows abrupt cut-off of the humeral head* ➡, *almost a surgical appearance. Given the extent of the osseous destruction, the amount of bony debris is small. This is typical of Charcot shoulder due to syringomyelia.* (Right) *Coronal T1WI MR shows a destroyed humeral head* ➡, *surrounded by fluid in the distended joint* ➡. *The fluid communicates between the glenohumeral joint and subdeltoid bursa through a rotator cuff tear.*

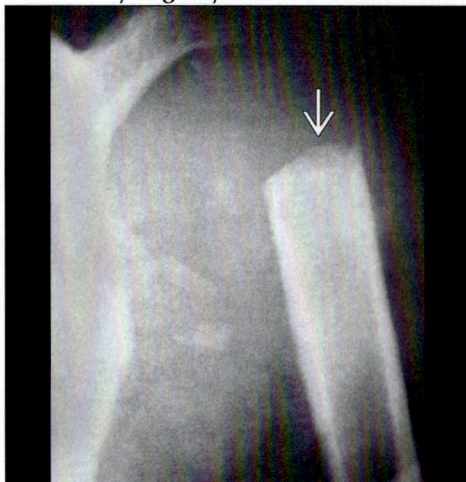

ATROPHIC JOINT DESTRUCTION

Hemophilia: MSK Complications

Hemophilia: MSK Complications

(Left) Anteroposterior radiograph shows significant erosive change ➡, as well as subchondral cyst formation. Note the relative overgrowth of the distal femur and proximal tibia and the widened intercondylar notch ⊳. *(Right)* Lateral radiograph shows complete loss of cartilage width ➡, an effusion and subchondral cyst formation in the elbow. The prominently overgrown radial head ⊳ is due to the hyperemia resulting from the repetitive bleeding episodes.

Tuberculosis Arthritis

Fungal Arthritis

(Left) Anteroposterior radiograph shows significant destruction of the glenohumeral joint ➡. While one might consider neuropathic joint as a diagnosis, it is important to note the densely calcified mass in the right upper lobe ➡ due to tuberculosis. *(Right)* Anteroposterior radiograph shows erosion and demineralization ➡ of the 2nd through 5th tarsometatarsal joints. This indolent fungal infection was due to Coccidioides immitis.

Rapidly Destructive Osteoarthritis of Hip

Chondrolysis, Post-Traumatic

(Left) Anteroposterior radiograph shows absence of the femoral head. The remaining femoral neck is sharply marginated without aggressive features ➡, known as the hatchet deformity. *(Right)* Anteroposterior radiograph shows complete loss of cartilage ➡ involving the left hip. The femoral head is medially displaced indicating slipped capital femoral epiphysis which was previously stabilized, seen by pin tracts ➡. Chondrolysis is a known complication.

ARTHRITIS MUTILANS

DIFFERENTIAL DIAGNOSIS

Common
- Rheumatoid Arthritis
- Psoriatic Arthritis
- Charcot, Neuropathic
- Juvenile Idiopathic Arthritis (JIA)

Less Common
- Gout
- Hyperparathyroidism (Mimic)
- Diabetes: MSK Complications
- Chronic Reactive Arthritis
- Mixed Connective Tissue Disease

Rare but Important
- Congenital Insensitivity/Indifference to Pain
- Leprosy
- Cutaneous T Cell Lymphoma

ESSENTIAL INFORMATION

Key Differential Diagnosis Issues
- a.k.a., "la main en lorgnette", opera glass hand, or resorptive arthropathy
- Destructive form of arthritis involving the hands and feet
- Resorption of bone ends with collapse of the soft tissues
- Produces "telescoping joints" and "pencil-in-cup" deformities; **hint:** This does not always indicate psoriatic arthritis
- Involvement is usually bilateral, regardless of underlying cause
- Spontaneous joint fusion is common

- Scoring systems to grade joint mutilation are rarely used except for research
- Due to end-stage joint destruction, differentiating between the differential diagnosis entities is often not possible without clinical information

Helpful Clues for Common Diagnoses
- **Rheumatoid Arthritis**
  - 5% of cases lead to arthritis mutilans
  - MCP & PIP joints most severely affected
  - Decreased bone mineralization
- **Psoriatic Arthritis**
  - 5% of cases lead to arthritis mutilans
  - Interphalangeal joints severely affected
  - Erosions & periostitis
  - Normal bone mineralization
- **Charcot, Neuropathic**
  - Joint destruction, distention, disorganization, debris
  - Mixed erosive & productive bone changes
  - MR to help differentiate neuropathic from septic joint changes

Helpful Clues for Less Common Diagnoses
- **Diabetes: MSK Complications**
  - Due to neuropathic joint changes
  - Most commonly in foot & wrist

Helpful Clues for Rare Diagnoses
- **Congenital Insensitivity/Indifference to Pain**
  - Rare cause of neuropathic joint
  - More likely to be polyarticular than classic Charcot joints

Rheumatoid Arthritis

Oblique radiograph shows typical changes of arthritis mutilans. The joints are severely eroded, producing pencil-in-cup deformities ➡, subluxations ➡, dislocations ➡, and resultant shortening of the digits.

Psoriatic Arthritis

Oblique radiograph shows diffuse erosive change of the metatarsophalangeal joints, with early pencil-in-cup erosions ➡. The patient also had sacroiliitis & enthesopathy, typical of psoriatic arthritis.

ARTHRITIS MUTILANS

Juvenile Idiopathic Arthritis (JIA)

Gout

(Left) PA radiograph shows carpal fusion ⊵ and extensive erosive change. The metacarpophalangeal ⊵ and carpal ➡ joint spaces are narrowed and deformed in this young adult patient with JIA. *(Right)* AP radiograph shows erosions involving nearly every joint of the foot, resulting in overall shortening of the digits. They are large and somewhat bizarre in appearance. One of the larger erosions is juxtaarticular in location ⊵, suggesting gout.

Hyperparathyroidism (Mimic)

Chronic Reactive Arthritis

(Left) Posteroanterior radiograph shows distal interphalangeal joint destruction ➡, approaching a pencil-in-cup appearance. This patient had no true arthropathy; she had hyperparathyroidism, resulting in subchondral resorption & collapse. *(Right)* Anteroposterior radiograph shows predominantly erosive change at the MTP ➡ and great toe IP joint ⊵. The spondyloarthropathies may exhibit erosive, productive, or mixed patterns of arthritic disease.

Congenital Insensitivity/Indifference to Pain

Leprosy

(Left) Lateral radiograph shows severe deformity of the ankle and hindfoot, with destruction of the tibiotalar, subtalar, talonavicular, and calcaneocuboid joints ➡. The remaining joints in this limb were normal. *(Right)* Posteroanterior radiograph shows marked destruction of most of the phalanges. Additionally, there is linear calcification in the location of a digital nerve ➡. This combination of findings is pathognomonic for leprosy. (†MSK Req).

NEUROPATHIC OSTEOARTHROPATHY

DIFFERENTIAL DIAGNOSIS

Common
- Diabetes: MSK Complications
- Charcot, Syringomyelia
- Charcot Spine, Paraplegia

Less Common
- Charcot, Congenital Insensitivity to Pain
- Charcot, Congenital Indifference to Pain
- Charcot, Alcoholic
- Charcot, Syphilis
- "Tall Man" Insensate Neuropathy

Rare but Important
- Charcot, Intraarticular Steroid Use
- Charcot, Multiple Sclerosis
- Charcot-Marie-Tooth Disease
- Riley-Day Syndrome
- Spinal Cord Compression
- Peripheral Nerve Tumors
- Meningomyelocele
- Polio
- Leprosy

ESSENTIAL INFORMATION

Key Differential Diagnosis Issues
- Charcot joints usually classic & similar
  - Disorganization of joint
  - Osseous debris (though may be atrophic)
  - Distension of joint (huge effusion)
  - Normal bone density (for the patient)
- Location may differentiate among etiologies
  - Diabetes: Foot > > hand

  - Syringomyelia: Shoulder > > elbow, hand
  - Paraplegia: Spine, below level of injury
  - Alcohol: Hip
  - Syphilis: Knee > hip > spine
  - Congenital insensitivity or indifference to pain: Knee > ankle

Helpful Clues for Common Diagnoses
- **Diabetes: MSK Complications**
  - Generally atrophic & osteoporotic
  - Lisfranc > Chopart > talonavicular
  - Early malalignment & fragmentation
  - Later loss of integrity of arches & associated ulceration/infection
- **Charcot, Syringomyelia**
  - Clinical signs of "mass" (due to distended joint) mislead to diagnosis of tumor
    - Destruction & debris in joint may mislead to diagnosis of chondrosarcoma
- **Charcot Spine, Paraplegia**
  - Generally stabilized at level of injury
  - Uncontrolled motion & insensate distal to stabilization lead to Charcot spine
  - Differential is disk space infection (patient population is prone to this as well)

Helpful Clues for Less Common Diagnoses
- **Charcot, Congenital Insensitivity to Pain**
  - Fragmentation multiple joints in child
  - Normal bone density; corneal & skin scars
- **Charcot, Congenital Indifference to Pain**
  - Same as congenital insensitivity to pain
- **"Tall Man" Insensate Neuropathy**
  - No other etiology found but tall stature noted in this population

Diabetes: MSK Complications

Sagittal radiograph shows disruption of the Chopart joint ➡, with little debris but distension at the dorsum of the joint. There is also a fracture of the fibula ➡, not noticed by the patient, who is diabetic.

Charcot, Syringomyelia

Anteroposterior radiograph shows destruction of the humeral head, with cut-off appearance. Osseous debris lines a distended axillary & subscapularis bursa ➡. Findings are typical of Charcot from syringomyelia.

NEUROPATHIC OSTEOARTHROPATHY

Charcot Spine, Paraplegia

Charcot, Congenital Insensitivity to Pain

(Left) Lateral radiograph shows disruption at several thoracic vertebral bodies, with osseous debris ➡. MR confirmed absence of abscess. This paraplegic patient has an unstable spine below his level of injury, resulting in Charcot changes. *(Right)* Sagittal T2WI FS MR shows a large effusion and osseous fragmentation at the posterior lateral femoral condyle ➡. The contralateral knee appeared similar. This teenager proved to have congenital insensitivity to pain.

Charcot, Congenital Indifference to Pain

Charcot, Syphilis

(Left) Lateral radiograph shows complete destruction of the distal tibia, fibula, talus, calcaneus, and midfoot. This teenager had a similar appearing contralateral knee. He has congenital indifference to pain. *(Right)* AP radiograph shows fracture and dislocation of the hip, along with abundant debris within a distended joint. The combination represents Charcot joint; the patient had tertiary syphilis. Typical sites of syphilis Charcot joint are hip, knee, & spine.

"Tall Man" Insensate Neuropathy

Charcot, Intraarticular Steroid Use

(Left) Anteroposterior radiograph shows neuropathic Chopart (hindfoot/midfoot) joint ➡. The patient had a peripheral neuropathy but no explanation for it other than his tall stature. *(Right)* Lateral radiograph shows large effusion ➡ as well as fragmentation at the tibial plateau ➡. This patient had a long history of intraarticular steroid injections, resulting in neuropathic joint.

ARTHRITIS WITH PRESERVED CARTILAGE SPACE

DIFFERENTIAL DIAGNOSIS

Common
- Any Arthritis in Early Stages
  - Rheumatoid Arthritis (Early)
  - Osteoarthritis (Early)
  - Septic Joint (Early)
  - Psoriatic Arthritis (PSA) (Early)
  - Pyrophosphate Arthropathy (Early)
  - Ankylosing Spondylitis (AS) (Early)
  - Juvenile Idiopathic Arthritis (JIA) (Early)
  - Hemophilia (Early)
  - Chronic Reactive Arthritis (CRA) (Early)
- Gout
- Femoral Acetabular Impingement (FAI)
- Osteonecrosis (Mimic)
- Systemic Lupus Erythematosus
- Pigmented Villonodular Synovitis (PVNS)
- Synovial Osteochondromatosis

Less Common
- Infection with Low Virulence Organisms
  - Tuberculosis
  - Fungal
- Silastic Arthropathy (Mimic)

Rare but Important
- Amyloid Deposition

ESSENTIAL INFORMATION

Key Differential Diagnosis Issues
- **Hint**: Condition of cartilage is dependent on stage in which it is evaluated
  - Initial stages of inflammatory arthritides retain normal cartilage width
  - All arthritides, even those classically stated to retain cartilage, eventually may result in cartilage destruction
- **Hint**: Even if cartilage width appears normal on radiograph, MR with contrast may show fraying, focal defects, or delamination

Helpful Clues for Common Diagnoses
- Arthritides that normally involve cartilage, presenting at early stage
  - **Rheumatoid Arthritis (Early)**
    - With very early disease, synovitis may result in distension of joint & apparent increase in cartilage width on radiograph
    - Early MR shows bone edema, synovitis, tenosynovitis
    - Disease progression results in relatively early marginal erosions & cartilage damage
  - **Osteoarthritis (Early)**
    - Early disease, especially in hip, may show subchondral cyst (Egger cyst) without other findings
    - Other early features: Osteophytes, subchondral sclerosis
    - Though radiographs show normal "joint space", may have cartilage damage
  - **Septic Joint (Early)**
    - May see distension of joint (effusion) prior to cartilage damage
    - May have early deossification of articular cortex secondary to hyperemia
  - **Spondyloarthropathies (PSA, AS, CRA)**
    - Early sacroiliac (SI) joint disease is erosive, with apparent "joint widening"
    - Even if joint space appears preserved, cartilage damage is present once erosive disease is established
    - Peripheral joints may show early preservation of cartilage with deossification secondary to hyperemia & synovitis
  - **Pyrophosphate Arthropathy (Early)**
    - Cartilage space retained in early disease, despite cartilage damage
    - Disease begins with erosions, progresses to mixed or productive
    - Highly location-specific: Radiocarpal, MCP joints, patellofemoral compartment of knee
  - **Juvenile Idiopathic Arthritis (JIA) (Early)**
    - Early stages of hyperemia show epiphyseal overgrowth & osteoporosis
    - Cartilage damage occurs later
  - **Hemophilia (Early)**
    - Early stages of hyperemia from recurrent joint bleeds show epiphyseal overgrowth & osteoporosis
    - Cartilage damage & erosions occur later
    - Watch for dense erosions (hemosiderin deposition in synovium)
- **Gout**
  - Classic arthropathy said to preserve the cartilage over a relatively long term
  - Even in presence of large tophi, erosions, overhanging edges, cartilage may remain intact

ARTHRITIS WITH PRESERVED CARTILAGE SPACE

- **Femoral Acetabular Impingement (FAI)**
  - FAI (cam or pincer mechanism), if not addressed, results in OA at a young age
    - Cam mechanism: Decrease in femoral head/neck cutback (usually lateral femoral neck "bump")
    - Pincer mechanism: Increase in anterior or lateral femoral head coverage by acetabulum
  - Early stage may show only the morphologic abnormalities, with preserved cartilage space
    - MR arthrogram may show cartilage thinning, defect, or delamination, along with labral tear
- **Osteonecrosis (Mimic)**
  - AVN is not an arthritis; occurs on only one side of joint
    - Preserved cartilage is a hallmark of AVN
  - Cartilage not affected until secondary OA develops, late in process
- **Systemic Lupus Erythematosus**
  - Noted for deformities without erosions or cartilage damage
    - Particularly hand & foot deformities: MCP, MTP, IP deviation/subluxation
    - Appears similar to RA, but severity of deformities would have associated erosions in RA
  - Noted for avascular necrosis
- **Pigmented Villonodular Synovitis (PVNS)**
  - Erosions are direct, related to sites of nodular masses

- Cartilage damage is uncommon & late in disease process
- **Synovial Osteochondromatosis**
  - Synovial metaplasia does not affect cartilage until late in process

Helpful Clues for Less Common Diagnoses
- **Infection with Low Virulence Organisms**
  - TB, fungal
  - Noted for slow joint destruction
  - Osteopenia, late cartilage damage, little host reaction
- **Silastic Arthropathy (Mimic)**
  - Careful observation required to identify relatively radiolucent silastic implant
  - Generally no metal associated with device
  - Rectangular implant may appear to "preserve" the joint space
  - Most common locations: MCP, MTP, IP joints, carpal bone replacements
  - As implant breaks down, osteolysis may become prominent
    - Implants & bone around them break down due to underlying osteoporosis & ligamentous imbalance

Helpful Clues for Rare Diagnoses
- **Amyloid Deposition**
  - MR shows low signal deposits in subchondral bone, tendons, capsule
  - Cartilage damage tends to be late
  - Diagnosis generally secured by MR
  - Association with multiple myeloma, end-stage renal disease, RA

Rheumatoid Arthritis (Early)

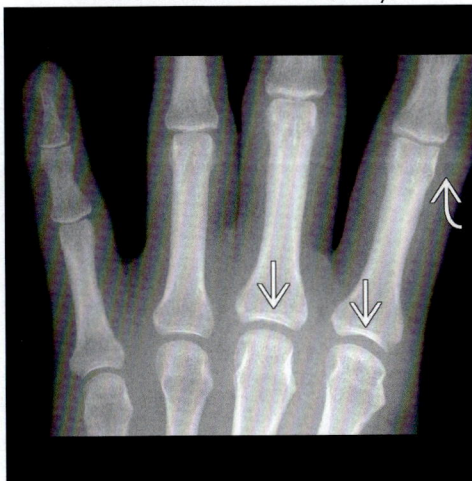

PA radiograph shows early RA with soft tissue swelling about the MCP joints & 2nd PIP joint ➡. No erosive change is seen, but there is modest widening, rather than narrowing of MCP joints ➡ related to synovitis.

Osteoarthritis (Early)

AP radiograph shows one of the earliest signs of OA of the hip, an Egger cyst ➡. At this early stage there is no cartilage narrowing, osteophyte formation, or change in alignment.

ARTHRITIS WITH PRESERVED CARTILAGE SPACE

(Left) Anteroposterior radiograph shows an early septic hip (Staphylococcus) in a 29 year old diabetic. There is an effusion, and the cortex of the femoral head has become indistinct ➡ due to hyperemia. No cartilage narrowing is seen. *(Right)* PA radiograph shows soft tissue swelling in a ray distribution along the 3rd digit ➡. Dense periostitis is noted along the proximal phalanx ➡. The apparent cartilage narrowing at the PIP is due to flexion of the joint.

Septic Joint (Early)

Psoriatic Arthritis (PSA) (Early)

(Left) PA radiograph shows subchondral cysts ➡ and early hook-like osteophytes ➡ in the 2nd and 3rd MCPs. This is typical of either pyrophosphate arthropathy or hemochromatosis. Cartilage is preserved early in the disease. *(Right)* AP radiograph shows bilateral widening of the SI joints ➡ from erosive change in this 18 year old with AS. There is a small osteophyte at the hip ➡. Neither joint shows radiographic evidence of cartilage space narrowing.

Pyrophosphate Arthropathy (Early)

Ankylosing Spondylitis (AS) (Early)

(Left) PA radiograph shows early JIA, with soft tissue swelling at the MCPs and overgrowth of the metacarpal head ➡ secondary to hyperemia. There is no cartilage narrowing at this point. *(Right)* Lateral radiograph shows a huge joint effusion ➡ as well as overgrowth of the femoral condyles relative to the diaphyses in this teenaged male hemophilic. The overgrowth is secondary to hyperemia from repeated bleeding episodes; cartilage narrowing is not yet seen.

Juvenile Idiopathic Arthritis (JIA) (Early)

Hemophilia (Early)

ARTHRITIS WITH PRESERVED CARTILAGE SPACE

Chronic Reactive Arthritis (CRA) (Early)

Gout

(Left) Lateral radiograph shows osteopenia but no cartilage narrowing in this patient with chronic reactive arthritis. Joints of the foot showed more advanced disease, but this early disease of the knee shows no true erosive or cartilage change. *(Right)* PA radiograph shows a large dense gouty tophus ➡ with prominent erosive change and overhanging edge ➡ typical of fairly advanced gout. Despite the advanced disease, the cartilage width ➡ remains normal.

Femoral Acetabular Impingement (FAI)

Osteonecrosis (Mimic)

(Left) AP radiograph shows lateral femoral neck bump ➡ & retroversion of the acetabulum ➡, resulting in FAI from the cam & pincer mechanisms, respectively. MR arthrogram showed a large bucket-handle labral tear, but cartilage was intact. *(Right)* Anteroposterior radiograph shows end-stage AVN of the femoral head with collapse ➡. Despite the severity of collapse, the cartilage width is intact ➡. AVN does not affect the cartilage until secondary OA develops.

Systemic Lupus Erythematosus

Silastic Arthropathy (Mimic)

(Left) PA radiograph shows a deforming arthritis, with significant subluxation of the MCPs. The alignment suggests RA, but in the absence of cartilage narrowing or erosions (as in this case) SLE should be the diagnosis. *(Right)* Oblique radiograph shows, at first glance, normal cartilage width. However, the cartilage space is occupied by a rectangular silastic implant ➡, which has a flange anchoring it in the phalanx ➡.

WIDENED JOINT SPACE

Common
- Muscle Atony
- Ligament Injury
- Hemarthrosis
- Septic Joint
- Rheumatoid Arthritis
- Retained Fracture Fragment
- Subluxation/Dislocation
- Entrapped Soft Tissue within Fracture
- Pigmented Villonodular Synovitis
- Viral (Toxic) Synovitis
- Joint Effusion, Unspecified

Less Common
- Developmental Dysplasia of the Hip
- Nerve Injury, Unspecified
- Synovial Osteochondromatosis
- Gout
- Tuberculosis
- Legg-Calvé-Perthes

Rare but Important
- Marfan Syndrome
- Ehlers-Danlos
- Acromegaly
- Lipoma Arborescens, Knee

ESSENTIAL INFORMATION

Key Differential Diagnosis Issues
- Numerous etiologies produce widening of the joint space of varying severity
  - Effusion, injury, cartilage thickening, bone destruction
- May be entirely nonspecific on radiographs

Helpful Clues for Common Diagnoses
- **Muscle Atony**
  - Wide joint space due to laxity of surrounding musculature
  - Commonly seen as inferior subluxation of humeral head after stroke or fracture
    - With fracture, can be misinterpreted as indicating brachial plexus injury or hematoma
- **Ligament Injury**
  - Wide joint space from damage to supporting soft tissues
  - Common in distal tibiofibular joint
- **Hemarthrosis**
  - Wide joint space from effusion

- Layering fat, serum, & cells on cross-table lateral radiograph or cross-sectional imaging
- **Septic Joint**
  - Wide joint space from effusion
    - Patellofemoral joint of knee most common in adults
    - Hip most common in children
  - Sacroiliac & sternoclavicular joints at risk in debilitated or immunosuppressed patients
  - Periarticular osteopenia progresses to cartilage & bone destruction
  - Reactive marrow & soft tissue edema
- **Rheumatoid Arthritis**
  - Distribution: Bilateral, polyarticular, symmetric
  - Early joint space widening and periarticular osteopenia
  - Late joint space widening due to synovitis & joint effusion, uncommon
    - Narrowed joint spaces more common
- **Retained Fracture Fragment**
  - Wide joint space from displaced bone fragment preventing reduction
  - Hip from posterior dislocation and acetabular fracture in adults
  - Elbow from displacement of epicondyle in children
  - Joint hemarthrosis
- **Subluxation/Dislocation**
  - Wide joint space from joint incongruence
  - Posterior dislocation of shoulder & hip can produce widened appearance
- **Entrapped Soft Tissue within Fracture**
  - Wide joint space from displaced soft tissue preventing reduction
- **Pigmented Villonodular Synovitis**
  - Wide joint space from effusion & intraarticular deposits
  - Distribution: Monarticular
  - Nodules with low signal T1WI & T2WI and gradient echo "blooming"
  - Underlying bone erosion may occur
  - Knee > ankle > hip > shoulder
- **Viral (Toxic) Synovitis**
  - Wide joint space from effusion & synovitis
  - Correlate with history of viral illness, usually respiratory
  - Differentiation from a bacterial septic joint can be challenging & require aspiration

WIDENED JOINT SPACE

- **Joint Effusion, Unspecified**
  - Infectious, inflammatory, neoplastic, & metabolic entities may all cause effusion
  - Pediatric hip effusion differential diagnosis
    - Hemarthrosis (trauma), septic hip, juvenile idiopathic arthritis, & viral (toxic) synovitis

Helpful Clues for Less Common Diagnoses
- **Developmental Dysplasia of the Hip**
  - Wide joint space from joint capsule laxity & other factors
  - Shallow acetabulum with laterally subluxed femoral head
  - Female newborns most common
- **Nerve Injury, Unspecified**
  - Wide joint space from effusion & bone destruction
  - Joint disorganization, dislocation or deformity
  - Neuropathic changes most common
    - Syringomyelia in shoulder
    - Diabetes in ankle & foot
- **Synovial Osteochondromatosis**
  - Wide joint space from effusion & intraarticular bodies
    - Osseous or cartilaginous bodies are usually visible on radiographs
  - Distribution: Monoarticular, large joints most common
- **Gout**
  - Wide joint space from effusion & tophi
- **Tuberculosis**

- Wide joint space from effusion & bone destruction
  - Distribution: Monoarticular
    - Spine > hip > knee
  - Slower clinical course than septic joint
- **Legg-Calvé-Perthes**
  - Wide joint space from bone destruction or subluxation
  - Preadolescent male children most common

Helpful Clues for Rare Diagnoses
- **Marfan Syndrome**
  - Wide joint space from ligamentous laxity
  - Tall stature, scoliosis, rib notching
  - Sternoclavicular & hip joint dislocation
- **Ehlers-Danlos**
  - Wide joint space from ligamentous laxity
  - Triphalangeal thumbs
  - Radioulnar synostosis
- **Acromegaly**
  - Wide joint space from cartilage hypertrophy
    - Metacarpophalangeal most common
  - Wide bones with normal cortex
  - Spade-like phalangeal tufts
  - Thick heel pad
- **Lipoma Arborescens, Knee**
  - Wide patellofemoral joint from intraarticular lipoma
  - Mass follows fat signal intensity on all sequences

Muscle Atony

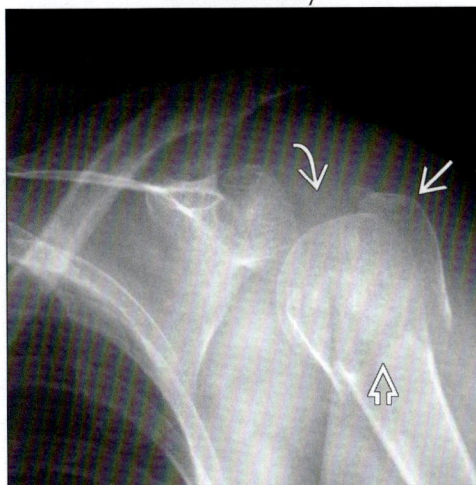

Anteroposterior radiograph shows greater tuberosity ➡ and surgical neck ➡ fractures. Inferior subluxation ➡ of the humeral head is due to muscle atony and is a common finding after humeral neck fracture.

Ligament Injury

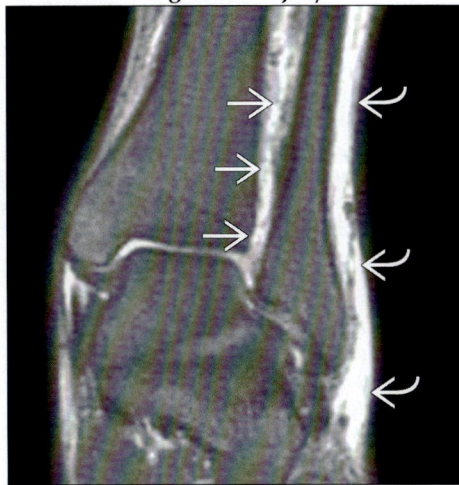

Coronal STIR MR shows disruption of the interosseous membrane ➡ in an acute syndesmotic sprain. There is extensive soft tissue edema ➡ without fracture. The anterior tibiofibular ligament was torn.

WIDENED JOINT SPACE

Hemarthrosis

Septic Joint

(Left) Lateral radiograph shows a large effusion ➔ that widens the patellofemoral joint. A small fat-fluid level is present ➔. A vertical lateral tibial plateau fracture was visible on additional views. *(Right)* Sagittal T2WI FS MR shows osteomyelitis of the distal humerus secondary to septic arthritis of the elbow. There is a significant joint effusion ➔ and diffuse soft tissue edema ➔. The effusion has resulted in widening of the radiocapitellar joint space.

Rheumatoid Arthritis

Rheumatoid Arthritis

(Left) PA radiograph shows widening of the MCP joint spaces ➔ but no erosive change or other indication of arthropathy. This may be the earliest manifestation of rheumatoid arthritis, due to synovitis. This patient was rheumatoid factor positive & later developed erosions. *(Right)* Axial T2WI FS MR shows an effusion and synovitis widening the distal radioulnar joint ➔. Extensive tenosynovitis ➔ is also present. Erosions in the hand and wrist were typical of rheumatoid arthritis.

Retained Fracture Fragment

Retained Fracture Fragment

(Left) Anteroposterior radiograph shows an entrapped medial epicondyle ➔. An avulsed medial epicondyle may displace into the elbow joint due to contraction of the common flexor muscles. *(Right)* Coronal bone CT shows fracture of a large portion of the anteroinferior femoral head, leaving behind a large donor site ➔. A small fracture fragment produces mild widening ➔ of the joint space. These injuries were due to a posterior hip dislocation.

WIDENED JOINT SPACE

Subluxation/Dislocation

Subluxation/Dislocation

(Left) Anteroposterior, internal rotation radiograph shows joint space widening →, suggesting a posterior shoulder dislocation. The fact that external rotation AP & standard axillary views could not be obtained supports the diagnosis, which was confirmed on a lateral axillary view. *(Right)* Axial bone CT shows the right clavicle is both superior and posterior in location → relative to the normal left clavicle →. This represents a posterior dislocation of the right sternoclavicular joint.

Pigmented Villonodular Synovitis

Viral (Toxic) Synovitis

(Left) Axial T1 C+ FS MR shows a distended distal radioulnar joint →. The joint is filled by a complex effusion containing multiple nodular low signal abnormalities, which appeared to "bloom" on gradient echo imaging. *(Right)* Anteroposterior radiograph shows the "teardrop distance" (space between proximal femoral metaphysis & radiographic teardrop) is slightly larger on the right → than the left →. This indicates the presence of an effusion.

Joint Effusion, Unspecified

Developmental Dysplasia of the Hip

(Left) Sagittal PD FSE MR shows a large joint effusion → widening the patellofemoral joint and a thickened medial plica →. The medial plica is usually present in knees, but when it is thickened, it may contribute to chondromalacia. *(Right)* Anteroposterior radiograph shows a developmental dysplasia with superior and lateral dislocation of the left femur → and a shallow acetabular roof →. Compare with the normally positioned right hip joint →.

WIDENED JOINT SPACE

(Left) Frogleg lateral radiograph shows a shallow left acetabular roof ➡ and subluxation of the left femur laterally ➡. The right hip is in normal position. *(Right)* Coronal T2WI MR shows a destroyed humeral head ➡, surrounded by fluid in the distended joint ➡. The fluid communicates between the glenohumeral joint and subdeltoid bursa through a full thickness rotator cuff tear. The findings are typical of Charcot shoulder. As expected, the etiology was syringomyelia.

Developmental Dysplasia of the Hip

Nerve Injury, Unspecified

(Left) Coronal STIR MR shows axillary nerve hyperintensity ➡ related to injury from a luxatio erecta shoulder dislocation (now reduced). Though not shown on the supine MR, in the upright position the shoulder "drooped", giving the appearance of a widened joint space & related to the nerve injury. *(Right)* Lateral radiograph shows multiple tiny ossified bodies, too numerous to count, distending the elbow joint & located in the anterior ➡ & posterior joint space ➡.

Nerve Injury, Unspecified

Synovial Osteochondromatosis

(Left) Axial T2WI MR shows a heterogeneous mass in the distal radioulnar joint. It had low signal intensity on both T1WI and T2WI ➡. This mass had caused an erosion in the ulna, typical of gout. *(Right)* Coronal NECT shows destruction of the glenohumeral joint ➡, with prominent surrounding osseous debris. The presence of superior hilar retraction ➡ and a calcified lung mass favored tuberculosis over neuropathic change from syringomyelia.

Gout

Tuberculosis

WIDENED JOINT SPACE

Tuberculosis

Legg-Calvé-Perthes

(Left) Axial NECT in the same patient as prior image shows destruction of the glenohumeral joint ➡, effusion, and bony debris. *(Right)* Anteroposterior radiograph shows an abnormal femoral head ➡ causing the superior joint space to appear widened. The femoral head is reduced in height with apparent loss of the lateral aspect of the head. Rather than a true defect, this lateral loss of femoral head bone is due to the loss of ossification within the cartilage of the head.

Legg-Calvé-Perthes

Marfan Syndrome

(Left) Anteroposterior radiograph shows the sequelae of Legg-Calvé-Perthes including flattening and broadening of the femoral head (coxa plana and coxa magna) ➡. The medial joint space of the hip appears widened ➡ due to subluxation. *(Right)* Posteroanterior radiograph shows arachnodactyly with mildly widened joint spaces but no other abnormality. The feet also showed arachnodactyly, along with a planovalgus deformity, typical of Marfan syndrome.

Acromegaly

Lipoma Arborescens, Knee

(Left) PA radiograph shows enlarged, "spade-like" distal phalangeal tufts ➡ & widened joint spaces ➡ at metacarpophalangeal joints due to cartilage overgrowth in patient with acromegaly. *(Right)* Sagittal PD FSE MR shows a very large lobulated intraarticular mass ➡ that widens the patellofemoral joint and has signal intensity identical to that of subcutaneus fat. Mass is located in both the suprapatellar bursa and the posterior joint space ➡.

ANKYLOSIS

DIFFERENTIAL DIAGNOSIS

Common
- Psoriatic Arthritis (PSA)
- Juvenile Idiopathic Arthritis (JIA)
- Surgical Ankylosis
- DISH (Mimic)
- Ankylosing Spondylitis (AS)

Less Common
- Tarsal Coalition
- Carpal Coalition
- Chronic Reactive Arthritis (CRA)
- Septic Joint

Rare but Important
- Rheumatoid Arthritis (RA)
- Adult Still Disease
- OPLL (Mimic)
- Fluorosis
- Ochronosis

ESSENTIAL INFORMATION

Key Differential Diagnosis Issues
- Note: Interphalangeal joints may appear fused on AP view if digits are flexed
  - Be certain to evaluate on lateral view before presuming IP joint fusion
- Spondyloarthropathies generally ankylose only in axial skeleton
  - Sacroiliac joints (SIJ) and spine facet joints
  - Peripheral joint fusion is rare in these diseases
- **Hint**: RA, JIA, & adult Still disease have different propensities to ankylose
  - Adult RA almost never fuses
  - JIA shows spinal & carpal fusion frequently
  - Adult Still disease shows carpal fusion occasionally
- **Hint**: Psoriatic arthritis is so predominant relative to the other nonsurgical etiologies of fusion of IP joints that it must be considered in every case

Helpful Clues for Common Diagnoses
- **Psoriatic Arthritis (PSA)**
  - Penetrance of psoriatic arthritis in patients with skin psoriasis not clear
    - Reported 0.5-25%
  - May present with sausage digit & periostitis

- Erosive disease affects hands more than other peripheral joints; feet also frequently affected
  - DIP > PIP > > MCP or MTP joints
  - Any joint may be affected in carpus; pericapitate distribution slightly predominates
- Mixed erosive & productive disease
- Two possible end-stage appearances
  - Fusion, especially at IP joints
  - Severe mutilating erosive disease; pencil-in-cup or telescoping fingers
- 30-50% patients with psoriatic arthritis develop spondyloarthropathy
  - Bilateral but asymmetric SI joint disease
  - Mixed erosive/productive
  - Bulky lateral spine syndesmophytes, noncontiguous
  - May fuse facet joints
- **Juvenile Idiopathic Arthritis (JIA)**
  - Multiple presentations, some with systemic symptomatology
  - Earliest signs not erosive
    - Periostitis of digits
    - Hyperemia results in asymmetric growth of ossification centers
  - Knee, elbow, ankle findings feature erosive disease & overgrowth (balloon joints)
  - Carpus features irregularity of bones & frequent fusion
  - Cervical spine
    - Frequent fusion of bodies & posterior elements
    - Fused bodies limited in growth potential; small relative to adjacent nonfused bodies
- **Surgical Ankylosis**
  - Surgical fusion is an option to treat a painful joint
  - Surgical fusion considered under circumstances of pain limiting function
    - If fusion will allow function of limb
    - If arthroplasty is not a viable choice (particularly carpal, tarsal IP joints)
  - Most frequently fused joints
    - Carpal (especially 4-corner ulnar column fusion for radiocarpal OA)
    - MCP of thumb, IP of digits
    - Tibiotalar, subtalar, hindfoot-midfoot
- **DISH (Mimic)**

ANKYLOSIS

- o Bulky anterior bridging osteophytes may mimic vertebral body fusion
  - ▪ Body & facet joint fusion are not a part of this process
- o Fusion of nonsynovial superior portion of SI joint is not a true ankylosis
  - ▪ Synovial portion of SI joint not affected
- **Ankylosing Spondylitis (AS)**
  - o Prominent axial distribution of fusion
    - ▪ Bilateral symmetric SI joint disease
    - ▪ Vertebral body & facet fusion; tends to be contiguous
    - ▪ Costovertebral & costosternal fusion
  - o Peripheral joint disease
    - ▪ Mixed erosive/productive
    - ▪ Fusion in peripheral joints rare
    - ▪ Proximal large joints predominate
    - ▪ With long-standing disease, smaller more peripheral joint disease is seen

Helpful Clues for Less Common Diagnoses
- **Tarsal Coalition**
  - o Usually due to congenital lack of segmentation
  - o Calcaneonavicular & subtalar (medial facet) most frequent locations
  - o Occasionally more widespread hindfoot fusion → ball & socket joint
- **Carpal Coalition**
  - o Usually congenital: Lunate-triquetral
- **Chronic Reactive Arthritis (CRA)**
  - o Most rare of spondyloarthropathies
    - ▪ Bilaterally asymmetric SI joint disease

- ▪ Bulky asymmetric vertebral body syndesmophytes
- ▪ May fuse facet joints
- o Peripheral arthritis generally lower extremity
  - ▪ Mixed erosive & productive
  - ▪ Foot & ankle, particularly posterior tubercle calcaneus
- **Septic Joint**
  - o Ankylosis is rare end-stage result of septic arthritis, especially if untreated

Helpful Clues for Rare Diagnoses
- **Rheumatoid Arthritis (RA)**
  - o Fusion extremely rare
    - ▪ Even surgical arthrodesis may be difficult to accomplish
    - ▪ Rare partial bony bridging may be seen
- **Adult Still Disease**
  - o Occasional DIP fusion & carpal fusion (particularly pericapitate)
- **OPLL (Mimic)**
  - o May have bulky anterior bony bridging in cervical spine
  - o Body & facet fusion not a part of the process
- **Fluorosis**
  - o Productive process rarely results in fusion
- **Ochronosis**
  - o Osteoporosis & eventual late cartilage breakdown rarely result in ankylosis

Psoriatic Arthritis (PSA)

PA radiograph shows fusion of a DIP joint ➤. Various PIP joints show marginal erosions ➤. The pattern of IP inflammatory disease with erosions leading to fusion is typical of psoriatic arthritis.

Psoriatic Arthritis (PSA)

Lateral radiograph shows a single vertical syndesmophyte ➤, along with complete fusion of the facet joints of the cervical spine ➤. Bone density is normal. This pattern may be seen in PSA.

ANKYLOSIS

Juvenile Idiopathic Arthritis (JIA)

Juvenile Idiopathic Arthritis (JIA)

(Left) PA radiograph shows fusion at the trapezium-trapezoid ⇨ as well as ankylosis at the trapezoid-capitate-2nd metacarpal ⇨ in a child with irregularity of the carpal bones. JIA frequently results in carpal fusion. (Right) Lateral radiograph shows fusion of the facets of cervical vertebrae 2-6 ⇨. There is also fusion of vertebral bodies 2-6 ⇨ which occurred at a young age, evidenced by the small size of these bodies compared with C7 ⇨.

Surgical Ankylosis

DISH (Mimic)

(Left) PA radiograph shows a "4 corner" fusion of the ulnar column (lunate, triquetrum, hamate, & capitate) ⇨. This is performed, along with scaphoidectomy, for radiocarpal OA ⇨. Even without hardware, this procedure should be recognized. (Right) AP radiograph shows fusion in the nonsynovial portions of the SI joints ⇨ but no fusion in the synovial porions ⇨. This is a feature that helps to differentiate DISH from spondyloarthropathies.

Ankylosing Spondylitis (AS)

Ankylosing Spondylitis (AS)

(Left) Axial bone CT shows osseous fusion between the anterior 1st ribs & manubrium ⇨ but severe erosions without fusion at the sternoclavicular joints ⇨. There is also ankylosis at the articulations of ribs with vertebral bodies & transverse processes ⇨ in this patient with AS. (Right) Lateral radiograph shows a case of advanced AS with severe erosive disease as well as complete subtalar fusion ⇨. Axial is more common than peripheral involvement in AS.

ANKYLOSIS

Tarsal Coalition

Carpal Coalition

(Left) Lateral radiograph shows tarsal coalition of the subtalar ➔, talonavicular ➔, and calcaneocuboid ➔ joints. The patient is otherwise normal; coalition is most commonly due to failure of segmentation at the embryologic stage. *(Right)* Oblique radiograph shows this patient has a carpal coalition, considered a normal variant. This is a failure of segmentation of the lunate and triquetrum ➔, the most frequent site of carpal coalition.

Chronic Reactive Arthritis (CRA)

Septic Joint

(Left) Lateral radiograph shows fusion of the facet joints of the cervical spine ➔ in a patient with chronic reactive arthritis. Fusion in this spondyloarthropathy is not as common as in ankylosing spondylitis. *(Right)* AP radiograph shows the sequelae of chronic osteomyelitis. The patient fractured his femur 25 years earlier & was treated with intramedullary rod. He developed chronic osteomyelitis, which extended to the hip joint, resulting in ankylosis ➔.

Rheumatoid Arthritis (RA)

Adult Still Disease

(Left) Lateral radiograph shows a small site of fusion in the cuboid-MT joint ➔ of a patient with RA. Non-surgical fusion is rare in patients with RA; when it occurs, it is generally in the hands or feet. An insufficiency fracture of the posterior calcaneal facet ➔ is also seen. *(Right)* PA radiograph shows fusion at the carpometacarpal joint & lunocapitate joint ➔. Adult Still disease often results in pericapitate erosions which may progress to fusion.

CALCIFIED INTRAARTICULAR BODY/BODIES

DIFFERENTIAL DIAGNOSIS

Common
- Loose Bodies/Impaction Fracture Fragments
- Intraarticular Avulsion Fractures
- Synovial Osteochondromatosis
- Chondrocalcinosis
- Charcot, Neuropathic

Less Common
- Intraarticular Chondroma
- Meniscal Ossicle
- Steroid Injection

Rare but Important
- Trevor Fairbank (Dysplasia Epiphysealis Hemimelica)
- Synovial Chondrosarcoma

ESSENTIAL INFORMATION

Key Differential Diagnosis Issues
- **Hint**: Do not mistake extraarticular avulsion fracture or sesamoid bones for intraarticular bodies
  - Fabella: Constant location posterior & lateral (lateral head gastrocnemius)
  - Common extraarticular avulsions around knee
    - Segond fracture (lateral capsular avulsion)
    - Avulsion of PCL extraarticular insertion on tibia
    - Reverse Segond fracture (medial coronary ligament avulsion)
    - Arcuate (fibular styloid) or fibular neck avulsion
    - Gerdy tubercle avulsion
    - Patellar sleeve avulsion
    - Tibial tuberosity avulsion (or Osgood Schlatter disease)
- **Hint**: Do not mistake calcific tendinitis or bursitis for intraarticular body
  - Shoulder is most common site of confusion
    - Calcific tendinitis in supraspinatus, infraspinatus, subscapularis, or biceps
    - Calcific bursitis in subacromial/subdeltoid bursa

Helpful Clues for Common Diagnoses
- **Loose Bodies/Impaction Fracture Fragments**
  - Location-specific in knee
    - Lateral femoral condylar recess: Associated with ACL injury
    - Anterior tibial plateau: Hyperextension or direct injury, associated with PCL & posterolateral corner injury
  - Shoulder: Bankart or reverse Bankart, associated with dislocations
  - Hip: Intraarticular fracture fragments following reduction of hip dislocation
  - Loose bodies from osteochondral injuries: Especially knee, ankle, & shoulder
- **Intraarticular Avulsion Fractures**
  - Location-specific in knee
    - Tibial spine: Anterior cruciate ligament (ACL)
    - Intracondylar notch, posterolateral at femoral condyle: ACL
    - Intracondylar notch, anteromedial at femoral condyle: PCL
- **Synovial Osteochondromatosis**
  - Cartilaginous or ossific bodies, arising from synovial metaplasia
  - May be large (> 1 cm) or tiny, but all tend to be similar in size within a joint
  - May be entirely lucent by radiograph and CT, seen only on MR
    - May be more prominently seen on either T1 or T2, depending on body composition
  - Generally monostotic
  - Large effusion
  - May cause mechanical erosions
  - Three different presentations
    - Most common: Multiple bodies, scattered freely throughout the joint
    - Less common: Conglomerate intraarticular mass containing hundreds of tiny bodies
    - Least common: Aggressive mass that begins intraarticularly but extends into extraarticular tissues
- **Chondrocalcinosis**
  - Most common sites are in fibrocartilage
    - Triangular fibrocartilage complex (TFCC) in wrist
    - Scapholunate or lunotriquetral ligaments of wrist
    - Menisci of knee
    - Labrum of hip

CALCIFIED INTRAARTICULAR BODY/BODIES

○ Also seen in hyaline cartilage, appearing to "line" the cortex
  ▪ Knee, hip, pubic symphysis, elbow, wrist
• **Charcot, Neuropathic**
  ○ Neuropathic joints may be hypertrophic or atrophic
  ○ Hypertrophic variety contains all the osseous debris of the breakdown of the joint & consequent appearance of loose bodies
    ▪ Fragments of various size
    ▪ Contained within a large effusion (may present clinically as a "mass")
    ▪ If effusion decompresses, the fragments are carried with the fluid into extraarticular positions
    ▪ Decompression of shoulder usually carries fragments into subscapularis region
    ▪ Decompression of hip usually carries fragments into iliopsoas bursa
    ▪ Decompression of knee usually carries fragments distally along fascial planes
  ○ Hypertrophic types
    ▪ Shoulder (fragments seen in enlarged axillary bursa & often extend through ruptured rotator cuff into subdeltoid bursa)
    ▪ Knee (fragments seen in hugely distended suprapatellar bursa; may decompress down fascial planes of leg)
    ▪ Hip (capsule is constricted; fragments extend around mid-cervical region; may decompress into iliopsoas bursa)

  ○ Atrophic variety
    ▪ Usually diabetic etiology (foot, hand)
    ▪ Osseous fragments are resorbed
    ▪ Occasionally fragments are seen in large effusions about the involved joint

Helpful Clues for Less Common Diagnoses
• **Intraarticular Chondroma**
  ○ Rarely seen in any location other than Hoffa fat pad
  ○ Calcification is common; punctate, popcorn, chondroid in appearance
  ○ May cause focal mechanical erosion
• **Meniscal Ossicle**
  ○ Ossicle within meniscus assumes triangular shape of meniscus
  ○ Usually posterior horn medial meniscus
  ○ Follows marrow signal on all MR sequences
• **Steroid Injection**
  ○ Chronic intraarticular steroid injections rarely result in calcification lining synovium

Helpful Clues for Rare Diagnoses
• **Trevor Fairbank (Dysplasia Epiphysealis Hemimelica)**
  ○ Intraarticular osteochondroma
  ○ Follows appearance of mature bone on all imaging
  ○ May be polyarticular but usually monomelic
  ○ Causes growth deformity
• **Synovial Chondrosarcoma**
  ○ Rare intraarticular cartilage lesion

Loose Bodies/Impaction Fracture Fragments

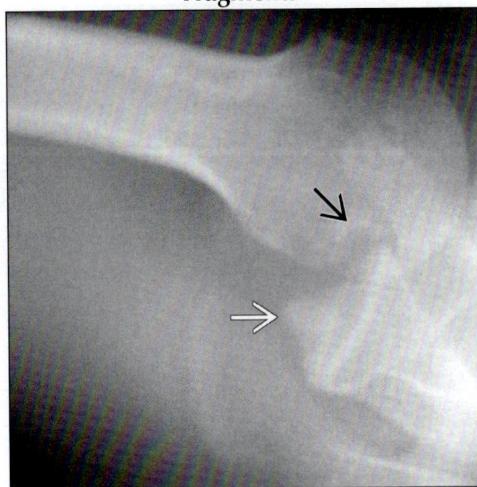

Lateral radiograph shows anterior shoulder dislocation with Hill Sachs impaction at the posterolateral humeral head ⇨ and loose body representing a Bankart fracture fragment ⇨ arising from the anterior glenoid.

Loose Bodies/Impaction Fracture Fragments

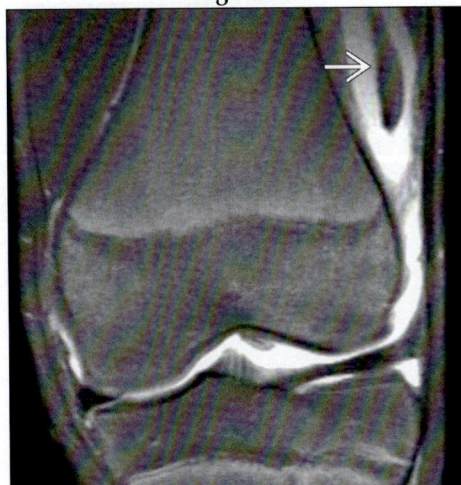

Coronal oblique T2WI FS MR shows a large loose body ⇨ arising from an impaction at the femoral trochlea. The body consists mostly of cartilage, with a thin edge of cortex. On radiograph it is only faintly seen.

CALCIFIED INTRAARTICULAR BODY/BODIES

(Left) *Lateral radiograph shows osseous body located adjacent to the tibial spines ➡. This is a large tibial spine avulsion, slightly retracted by the ACL, but without change in alignment.* **(Right)** *Anteroposterior radiograph shows a large ossified body within the intercondylar notch ➡. Based on location on both AP and lateral views, it can be determined that this is a PCL avulsion of the medial femoral condyle from the intercondylar notch.*

Intraarticular Avulsion Fractures

Intraarticular Avulsion Fractures

(Left) *Lateral radiograph shows several large rounded bodies within the elbow joint ➡. The fat pad is distended ➡, demonstrating the intraarticular location of the bodies. This is typical synovial chondromatosis.* **(Right)** *Axial bone CT shows an aggressive form of synovial chondromatosis, with multiple small calcified bodies within the joint ➡. There are also multiple similar bodies ➡ posterior to the knee that erode the femoral condyle but also extend extraarticularly.*

Synovial Osteochondromatosis

Synovial Osteochondromatosis

(Left) *PA radiograph shows chondrocalcinosis in the cartilage at the scapholunate joint ➡ & scapholunate ligament ➡ as well as within the TFCC ➡ in a patient with pyrophosphate arthropathy. (†MSK Req).* **(Right)** *AP radiograph shows a dislocated & destroyed humeral head. There are clouds of tiny osseous fragments located within a distended axillary bursa of the glenohumeral joint ➡. This Charcot shoulder resulted from cervical cord syringomyelia.*

Chondrocalcinosis

Charcot, Neuropathic

CALCIFIED INTRAARTICULAR BODY/BODIES

Charcot, Neuropathic

Intraarticular Chondroma

(Left) Anteroposterior radiograph shows a neuropathic joint in a patient with tabes. There is intraarticular fragmentation ➡ as well as dissection of several small fragments down the leg ➡ from overdistension of the joint by the large effusion. *(Right)* Lateral radiograph shows calcification within Hoffa fat pad ➡ which has caused a small erosion on the tibial plateau ➡. This appearance in this location is almost invariably due to intraarticular chondroma.

Meniscal Ossicle

Meniscal Ossicle

(Left) Lateral radiograph shows a faint triangular-shaped ossification located posteriorly within the joint ➡. Although the finding is nonspecific, the triangular shape mimics that of the meniscus and should make one consider the diagnosis of meniscal ossicle. *(Right)* Coronal T1WI MR of the same case shows the ossification to follow marrow signal and to be located in the posterior horn of the medial meniscus ➡. This proves the diagnosis of meniscal ossicle.

Trevor Fairbank (Dysplasia Epiphysealis Hemimelica)

Trevor Fairbank (Dysplasia Epiphysealis Hemimelica)

(Left) Anteroposterior radiograph shows fairly mature ossific density ➡ which is shown to be intraarticular on orthogonal images. The bone arises from the epiphysis, as is expected in Trevor Fairbank disease. *(Right)* Anteroposterior radiograph shows mature bone formation arising from the talus ➡, ending in an intraarticular position. This is a typical appearance for Trevor Fairbank disease. It may be polyarticular but is usually monomelic.

CHONDROCALCINOSIS

DIFFERENTIAL DIAGNOSIS

Common
- Pyrophosphate Arthropathy
- Osteoarthritis
- Chronic Repetitive Trauma
- Idiopathic
- Gout
- Hyperparathyroidism/Renal OD
- Progressive Systemic Sclerosis

Rare but Important
- Paraneoplastic Syndrome
- Hemochromatosis
- Amyloid Deposition
- Acromegaly
- Wilson Disease
- Hemophilia
- Hypothyroidism
- Hypophosphatasia
- Diabetes
- Ochronosis (Alkaptonuria)
- Oxalosis

ESSENTIAL INFORMATION

Key Differential Diagnosis Issues
- Chondrocalcinosis results from deposition of material in cartilage
  - May be deposited in fibrocartilage
    - Menisci, TFCC, labrum
  - May be deposited in hyaline cartilage
  - May be deposited in surrounding soft tissues as well: Ligaments, joint capsule

- **Hint**: Chondrocalcinosis seen in many arthritic processes, but does not imply any one arthropathy; etiology may be "idiopathic"
- **Hint**: Chondrocalcinosis can nearly always be attributed to those entities listed as "common"; remainder rare

Helpful Clues for Common Diagnoses
- **Pyrophosphate Arthropathy**
  - Most frequent arthritis associated with chondrocalcinosis
  - Distribution is diagnostic
    - Hand: Radiocarpal → SLAC wrist deformity; 2nd & 3rd MCP
    - Knee: Patellofemoral compartment
  - Early erosions, followed by mixed & productive disease
- **Osteoarthritis**
  - Frequently seen in association with chondrocalcinosis
  - Watch distribution: In hand, IP joints and 1st carpometacarpal (CMC)
- **Chronic Repetitive Trauma**
  - Most frequent site is ulnocarpal abutment due to positive ulnar variance
- **Gout**: Sodium urate deposits
- **Hyperparathyroidism/Renal OD**
  - Soft tissue calcification common, including chondrocalcinosis
- **Progressive Systemic Sclerosis**
  - Soft tissue calcification common, including chondrocalcinosis
  - Associated acroosteolysis

Pyrophosphate Arthropathy

PA radiograph shows extensive chondrocalcinosis in the TFCC ➡ as well as the scapholunate ligament ⇉ and hyaline cartilage ⇲. There are large subchondral cysts & a SLAC wrist deformity is developing. (†MSK Req).

Osteoarthritis

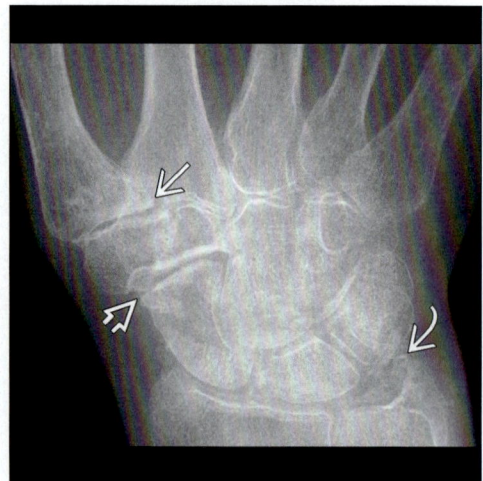

PA radiograph shows chondrocalcinosis involving the TFCC ➡. There are typical findings of OA involving the 1st CMC ➡ and scapho-trapezoid-trapezium ⇉ joints, with sclerosis & early osteophyte formation.

CHONDROCALCINOSIS

Chronic Repetitive Trauma

Idiopathic

(Left) PA radiograph shows chondrocalcinosis in the TFCC ➔ as well as the scapholunate ligament ➔. Note that there is ulnar positive variance; altered weight bearing through the TFCC & lunate creates chronic repetitive trauma. *(Right)* AP radiograph shows chondrocalcinosis in the hyaline cartilage ➔ as well as the joint capsule ➔ in this patient with generalized foot pain. There was no associated arthropathy or discernible cause of the deposition.

Gout

Hyperparathyroidism/Renal OD

(Left) PA radiograph shows calcific density within and around the TFCC and distal radioulnar joint ➔ in a young Polynesian male. This is gout, with sodium urate crystal deposition. *(Right)* PA radiograph shows chondrocalcinosis in the TFCC ➔. The bones are diffusely abnormal in density, with loss of trabecular distinctness in this patient with hyperparathyroidism. No other resorptive patterns are seen in the wrist.

Progressive Systemic Sclerosis

Paraneoplastic Syndrome

(Left) PA radiograph shows typical acroosteolysis ➔ with soft tissue calcification and chondrocalcinosis ➔ of the TFCC in this patient with scleroderma. The dislocated 1st carpometacarpal joint ➔ indicates chronicity. *(Right)* Anteroposterior radiograph shows chondrocalcinosis within the pubic symphysis & hip joint ➔ as well as juxtaarticular calcification ➔. This patient has known lung adenocarcinoma & paraneoplastic syndrome, resulting in hypercalcemia.

PERIARTICULAR CALCIFICATION

DIFFERENTIAL DIAGNOSIS

Common
- Calcific Tendinitis
- Calcific Bursitis
- Gout
- Pyrophosphate Arthropathy (Mimic)
- Myositis Ossificans
- Progressive Systemic Sclerosis
- Hyperparathyroidism
- Renal Osteodystrophy
- Chronic Repetitive Trauma/Ligamentous

Less Common
- Polymyositis/Dermatomyositis
- Thermal Injury, Burns
- Calcific Myonecrosis
- Periosteal Chondroma
- Hemangioma, Soft Tissue
- Synovial Sarcoma
- Dystrophic Calcification, Soft Tissue Tumor
- Soft Tissue Chondroma
- Charcot, Neuropathic
- Paraneoplastic Syndrome

Rare but Important
- Systemic Lupus Erythematosus
- Synovial Osteochondromatosis, Extraarticular
- Maffucci Syndrome
- Leprosy
- Pseudohypoparathyroidism
- Tumoral (Idiopathic) Calcinosis
- Mesenchymal Chondrosarcoma
- Extraskeletal Osteosarcoma
- Ochronosis
- Wilson Disease

ESSENTIAL INFORMATION

Key Differential Diagnosis Issues
- Radiograph is essential to differentiate types of calcification, which often have a distinct appearance (may limit the differential)
  - Mineralized osseous matrix: Ranges from faint & amorphous to distinct trabeculae surrounded by dense cortex
  - Mineralized cartilaginous matrix: Punctate density, termed "popcorn" or "rings & arcs"
  - Dystrophic calcification: Ranges from amorphous & cloudy, to linear or rounded, globular distinct calcification

Helpful Clues for Common Diagnoses
- **Calcific Tendinitis vs. Calcific Bursitis**
  - Character of calcification: Dense, globular, smooth "toothpaste" appearance
  - Calcific tendinitis located within tendon
    - Usually within 1-3 cm of insertion
    - Follows the tendinous insertion throughout range of motion of adjacent joint; rarely changes shape
  - Calcific bursitis located in position of bursa (often adjacent to tendon)
    - Shape of calcific density often changes from globular to more dispersed pattern with range of motion of adjacent joint
- **Gout**
  - Extraarticular calcification within soft tissue mass: Tophus
  - Character of calcification
    - Usually subtle amorphous increased density within mass
    - Rarely has focal, dense calcification
  - ± Adjacent juxta/intraarticular erosions
- **Pyrophosphate Arthropathy (Mimic)**
  - Calcification is intraarticular & rarely capsular
  - Linear calcification located in either fibrocartilage or hyaline cartilage
  - Watch for typical associated arthropathy
- **Myositis Ossificans**
  - Character changes over time
    - Calcification first seen 4-6 weeks following trauma
    - Initial calcification is faint & amorphous immature osteoid
    - With time, ossification matures, with more mature bone formation seen peripherally & circumferentially
- **Progressive Systemic Sclerosis**
  - Calcification: Globular or sheet-like
  - Watch for attenuated soft tissues and acroosteolysis
- **Hyperparathyroidism/Renal Osteodystrophy**
  - Calcification: Focal, dense, or amorphous
  - Character & location of calcification may change with treatment
    - May completely resolve
    - Renal osteodystrophy on dialysis: May develop fluffy large soft tissue deposits
  - **Hint:** Watch for the various resorption patterns of osseous structures

PERIARTICULAR CALCIFICATION

Helpful Clues for Less Common Diagnoses

- **Polymyositis/Dermatomyositis**
  - Calcification occurs after muscle inflammation, degeneration, & atrophy
  - Proximal thigh muscles predominate
  - Character of calcification
    - Dense sheet-like calcification is classic
    - Less than 50% of cases show this classic appearance; may be globular/amorphous
  - Watch for complications of steroid use (avascular necrosis, osteopenia)
- **Thermal Injury, Burns**
  - Character of calcification: Globular
  - Contractures, acroosteolysis are associated
- **Periosteal Chondroma**
  - Surface lesion may cause scalloping of underlying bone
  - Calcification: Punctate, chondroid
- **Hemangioma, Soft Tissue**
  - Tangled vessels, usually in fatty stroma
  - Character of calcification: Round calcific densities with lucent center (phleboliths)
- **Synovial Sarcoma vs. Dystrophic Calcification in Soft Tissue Sarcomas**
  - Any soft tissue tumor may develop dystrophic calcification
  - Character of calcification: Generally dense & dystrophic, either linear or globular
  - Synovial sarcoma contains dystrophic calcification 20-30% more frequently than other tumors
  - Factors that may help differentiate synovial sarcoma

- Patients generally younger adults than with other sarcomas
- Lower extremity, particularly about the knee (but extraarticular), is most frequent location of synovial sarcoma
- **Charcot, Neuropathic**
  - Intraarticular debris may dissect down fascial planes when joint is distended
  - Intraarticular debris may dissect into adjacent bursa, particularly in shoulder
  - Character of calcification: Bone fragments

Helpful Clues for Rare Diagnoses

- **Systemic Lupus Erythematosus**
  - Rarely seen globular calcification
  - Most frequent in lower extremities
- **Synovial Osteochondromatosis, Extraarticular**
  - Confluent mass may extend into soft tissues adjacent to joint
- **Maffucci Syndrome**
  - Phleboliths in hemangiomas associated with multiple enchondromatosis
- **Leprosy**
  - Calcification: Linear, in digital nerve
  - Associated acroosteolysis
- **Pseudohypoparathyroidism**
  - Calcification: Globular, dystrophic
  - Associated findings: Short, obese individuals with brachydactyly (especially 1st, 4th, & 5th metatarsal/metacarpals)
- **Tumoral (Idiopathic) Calcinosis**
  - Paraarticular cloudy, toothpaste-like calcification with normal underlying bone

Calcific Tendinitis

Anteroposterior radiograph shows a globular calcification ➡ superimposed over the glenohumeral joint in an internally rotated shoulder radiograph. This is nonspecific, but location suggests calcific tendinitis.

Calcific Tendinitis

Sagittal PD FSE MR of the same patient as previous image shows tendon sheath fluid ➡ and the calcification ➡ associated with biceps tendon ➡, confirming calcific tendinitis.

PERIARTICULAR CALCIFICATION

Calcific Bursitis

Calcific Bursitis

(Left) AP external rotation radiograph shows fairly dense calcification ➡ in a position that could either be supraspinatus calcific tendinitis or subdeltoid bursitis. *(Right)* AP internal rotation of the same shoulder demonstrates the density to spread out in a thinner line ➡ & to remain in the location of subdeltoid bursa. Since it does not follow the supraspinatus, the diagnosis of calcific bursitis is confirmed. Location of calcification confirms specific diagnosis.

Gout

Gout

(Left) Lateral radiograph shows distinct calcific densities within the olecranon bursa in a patient with gout. Tophi more frequently have amorphous calcific density, but this appearance is rarely seen. *(Right)* Lateral radiograph shows mild and amorphous increased density within a gouty tophus ➡ in the olecranon bursa. This is a more typical appearance of gouty tophus than the dense calcification seen in the previous image.

Pyrophosphate Arthropathy (Mimic)

Myositis Ossificans

(Left) Anteroposterior radiograph shows joint capsule chondrocalcinosis ➡. Although usually seen within the hyaline or fibrocartilage, it may mimic periarticular calcification when it is capsular. *(Right)* Posteroanterior radiograph shows mature bone adjacent to the 5th MCP after crush injury without fracture 5 months prior. Mature peripheral bone ➡ surrounding a less organized center is typical of myositis ossificans (fibroosseous pseudotumor of digits).

PERIARTICULAR CALCIFICATION

Progressive Systemic Sclerosis

Hyperparathyroidism

(Left) Lateral radiograph shows dense sheet-like calcification in the subcutaneous tissues, a pattern seen in PSS (scleroderma) as well as dermatomyositis. *(Right)* Posteroanterior radiograph shows periarticular calcifications ➡ in a patient with hyperparathyroidism. These are not sesamoids, as they do not have an ossific character.

Renal Osteodystrophy

Polymyositis/Dermatomyositis

(Left) Anteroposterior radiograph shows abnormal bone density, subchondral resorption at the SIJ ➡, and cloudy amorphous periarticular calcification ➡. This type of calcification not infrequently develops in patients on dialysis. *(Right)* Lateral radiograph shows sheet-like calcification in the subcutaneous and fascial tissue planes ➡. This appearance is classic for dermatomyositis, though the calcification may also be globular in this disease.

Periosteal Chondroma

Hemangioma, Soft Tissue

(Left) Oblique radiograph shows a surface lesion containing chondroid matrix which originated at the proximal phalanx ➡ and extends to the distal phalanx ➡. It excavates the underlying bone, typical for a periosteal chondroma. (†MSK Req). *(Right)* Anteroposterior radiograph shows phleboliths ➡ typical of those found in soft tissue hemangioma.

PERIARTICULAR CALCIFICATION

(Left) Lateral radiograph shows a soft tissue mass ➡ containing dystrophic calcification. Any soft tissue tumor may calcify, but synovial sarcoma is the most frequent; consider especially when seen in the lower extremity of young adults. **(Right)** Anteroposterior radiograph shows dense dystrophic calcification within a soft tissue mass ➡. Although synovial sarcoma should be considered, any tumor (such as this schwannoma) may calcify.

Synovial Sarcoma

Dystrophic Calcification, Soft Tissue Tumor

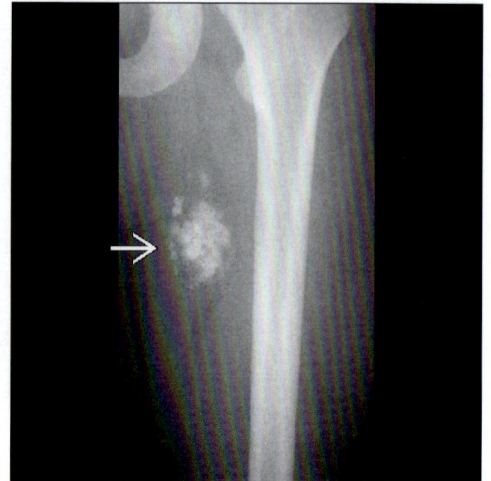

(Left) Anteroposterior radiograph shows osseous debris ➡ contained within the distended glenohumeral joint. Though this is typical for a Charcot shoulder, it is often mistaken for extraarticular calcification. **(Right)** Anteroposterior radiograph shows osseous debris ➡ dissecting down fascial planes in a knee showing destructive changes of a Charcot joint. When the effusion is large, it may decompress distally like this.

Charcot, Neuropathic

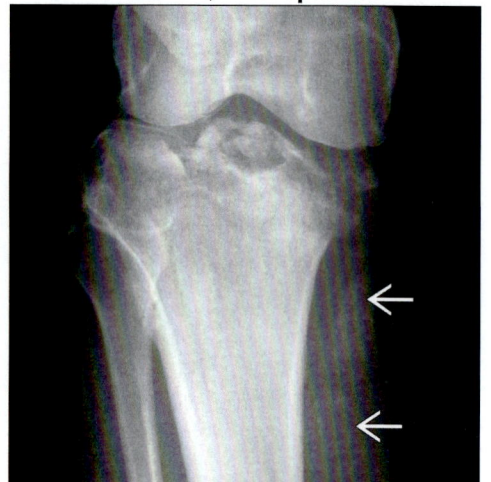

Charcot, Neuropathic

(Left) Anteroposterior radiograph shows chondrocalcinosis ➡ & juxtaarticular calcification ➡ resulting from hypercalcemia in this patient with adenocarcinoma of the lung and paraneoplastic syndrome. **(Right)** Anteroposterior radiograph shows dense globular soft tissue calcification ➡, along with avascular necrosis ➡. Occasionally SLE patients develop dystrophic calcification, predominantly in the lower extremities.

Paraneoplastic Syndrome

Systemic Lupus Erythematosus

PERIARTICULAR CALCIFICATION

Synovial Osteochondromatosis, Extraarticular

Synovial Osteochondromatosis, Extraarticular

(Left) Lateral radiograph shows hundreds of tiny ossified bodies, both intraarticular and periarticular. This is conglomerate synovial osteochondromatosis, extending into surrounding soft tissues. *(Right)* Axial bone CT shows typical round bodies within the suprapatellar bursa ➡, but there is extraarticular extension of the conglomerate mass extending into biceps & surrounding the neurovascular bundle ➡.

Maffucci Syndrome

Leprosy

(Left) PA radiograph shows multiple enchondromas within the phalanges, metacarpals, and an associated soft tissue mass ➡. The mass contains phleboliths; the constellation of findings is Maffucci syndrome. (†MSK Req). *(Right)* PA radiograph shows acroosteolysis, which has destroyed most of the phalanges. Additionally, there is linear calcification in the location of a digital nerve ➡. This combination of findings is pathognomonic for leprosy. (†MSK Req).

Pseudohypoparathyroidism

Tumoral (Idiopathic) Calcinosis

(Left) Anteroposterior radiograph shows subtle soft tissue calcification adjacent to the midfoot ➡. Note the short first metatarsal ➡. This combination of findings is typical for pseudohypoparathyroidism. *(Right)* Anteroposterior radiograph shows dense cloud-like periarticular calcification. The appearance is typical of, and proved to be, tumoral calcinosis.

MCP-PREDOMINANT ARTHRITIS

DIFFERENTIAL DIAGNOSIS

Common
- Rheumatoid Arthritis (RA)
- Pyrophosphate Arthropathy

Less Common
- Hemochromatosis
- Robust Rheumatoid Arthritis (Robust RA)
- Juvenile Idiopathic Arthritis (JIA)
- Systemic Lupus Erythematosus (Mimic)

Rare but Important
- Jaccoud Arthritis (Mimic)

ESSENTIAL INFORMATION

Key Differential Diagnosis Issues
- **Hint**: Character of MCP involvement may help differentiate
  - Erosive: RA, robust RA, JIA, SLE, & occasionally pyrophosphate & hemochromatosis arthropathy
  - Productive or mixed: Pyrophosphate & hemochromatosis arthropathy
- **Hint**: Location of carpal involvement may help differentiate

Helpful Clues for Common Diagnoses
- **Rheumatoid Arthritis (RA)**
  - MCP > > IP involvement
    - Both earlier and more severe
  - Purely erosive disease
  - Osteopenia (juxtaarticular; diffuse later)
  - Carpal involvement

- Earliest: Radiocarpal, often with ulnar translocation of carpus
- Later: Midcarpal, intercarpal
- **Pyrophosphate Arthropathy**
  - MCP involvement is hallmark
    - 2nd and 3rd MCPs earliest & most frequently involved
    - IPs not involved
  - Hook-like osteophytes are classic
    - May begin as erosive or mixed
  - Normal bone density
  - Carpal involvement
    - Radiocarpal, often with S-L dissociation
    - May evolve to SLAC deformity

Helpful Clues for Less Common Diagnoses
- **Hemochromatosis**
  - Same appearance & distribution as pyrophosphate arthropathy
  - Younger adult male population
- **Robust Rheumatoid Arthritis (Robust RA)**
  - Same appearance & distribution as RA, with large subchondral cysts
- **Juvenile Idiopathic Arthritis (JIA)**
  - MCP > IP involvement; may have fusion
  - Carpal involvement variable
- **Systemic Lupus Erythematosus (Mimic)**
  - Generally a nonerosive deformity
    - Hand deformities much more prominent than erosive change
    - Late erosions seen, MCP > IP

Helpful Clues for Rare Diagnoses
- **Jaccoud Arthritis (Mimic)**
  - Same appearance as SLE

Rheumatoid Arthritis (RA)

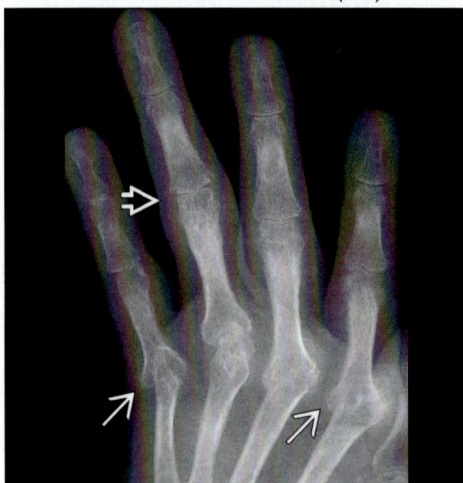

PA radiograph shows predominant MCP erosive disease ➡, with large erosions & subluxation. There is minimal IP disease, with only one site showing marginal erosions ➡. The MCP-predominant disease is typical of RA.

Rheumatoid Arthritis (RA)

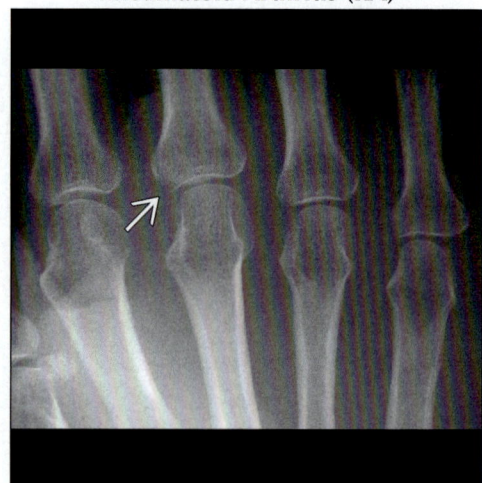

PA radiograph shows early RA, with MCPs showing uniform decrease in cartilage width. There is a small marginal erosion at a single MCP ➡. The patient had no involvement of the IP joints or the carpus.

MCP-PREDOMINANT ARTHRITIS

Pyrophosphate Arthropathy

Hemochromatosis

(Left) Posteroanterior radiograph shows cartilage narrowing at the 2nd and 3rd MCPs, along with a large hook-like osteophyte at the 3rd MCP ➡. The IP joints were normal. This pattern is typical of pyrophosphate arthropathy. *(Right)* Posteroanterior radiograph shows cartilage narrowing throughout the MCPs. There are associated erosions ➘ as well as hook-like osteophytes ➡. The IP joints were normal. The pattern is typical of hemochromatosis in this middle-aged male.

Robust Rheumatoid Arthritis (Robust RA)

Juvenile Idiopathic Arthritis (JIA)

(Left) Posteroanterior radiograph shows MCP-predominant erosions with large subchondral cysts ➡. IPs show minimal involvement. There is erosive change seen throughout the carpus. Cysts & normal bone density are typical of robust RA. *(Right)* Posteroanterior radiograph shows MCP erosive disease ➡. IPs are not well seen but were relatively normal. Erosions & fusion are seen involving the carpus in this teenager. This MCP-predominate arthritis is juvenile idiopathic arthritis.

Juvenile Idiopathic Arthritis (JIA)

Systemic Lupus Erythematosus (Mimic)

(Left) Posteroanterior radiograph shows overgrowth of the epiphysis as well as an erosion ➡ at the 3rd MCP. This was an early isolated site of involvement in a patient with JIA. *(Right)* Posteroanterior radiograph shows subluxation and mild erosive disease at the MCPs ➡. The IPs and carpus are normal. When the degree of subluxation and deformity is far greater than the erosive change, SLE should be considered rather than rheumatoid arthritis.

IP-PREDOMINANT ARTHRITIS

DIFFERENTIAL DIAGNOSIS

Common
- Osteoarthritis (OA)
- Psoriatic Arthritis (PSA)
- Erosive Osteoarthritis (EOA)

Less Common
- Hyperparathyroidism (HPTH) (Mimic)

Rare but Important
- Chronic Reactive Arthritis (CRA)
- HIV-AIDS Related Arthritis
- Adult Still Disease
- Amyloid Deposition
- Multicentric Reticulohistiocytosis

ESSENTIAL INFORMATION

Key Differential Diagnosis Issues
- **Hint**: Character of involvement may help differentiate among these processes
  - Erosive: All but OA may be purely erosive
  - Productive: OA is purely productive
  - Mixed erosive/productive: PSA, CRA, HIV, EOA
- **Hint**: Site of carpal involvement may help differentiate among these
- **Hint**: Skin changes rarely may help with diagnosis
  - Psoriatic rash
  - Nodules in multicentric reticulohistiocytosis

Helpful Clues for Common Diagnoses
- **Osteoarthritis (OA)**
  - Purely productive (osteophyte-forming)
  - DIP > PIP joints, but all may be involved
  - MCPs not involved unless prior trauma
  - Carpal location: 1st carpometacarpal (CMC), scapho-trapezoid-trapezium (STT)
    - These carpal locations are not involved in other arthridities & are a reliable differentiating feature
- **Psoriatic Arthritis (PSA)**
  - Erosive > productive changes, but may be mixed
  - DIP > PIP, but all may be involved
  - MCPs not involved until late in disease
  - Carpal location variable in proximal & distal carpal rows; may be peri-capitate
  - May present with a "sausage digit"
    - Swelling of entire digit

- Periostitis, especially along shaft
  - Late stages: Arthritis mutilans
    - Severe erosions → pencil-in-cup
    - Severe erosions → telescoping digits
  - May have spondyloarthropathy
    - Bilateral asymmetric sacroiliitis
    - Bulky, non-contiguous syndesmophytes
  - Psoriatic skin rash generally present, but arthritis may predate skin findings in 20%
- **Erosive Osteoarthritis (EOA)**
  - Same distribution as OA
  - Mixed erosive & productive disease, often resulting in "gull wing" deformity
    - Deep central subchondral erosion of middle phalanx, with more marginal erosions base of distal phalanx
    - Marginal osteophytes
  - DIP > PIP, but all may be involved
  - MCPs not involved in absence of trauma
  - Carpal location: 1st carpometacarpal, scapho-trapezoid-trapezium
    - Generally productive, but may be erosive
    - **Hint**: This location of carpal disease may serve as a differentiating factor from psoriatic arthritis

Helpful Clues for Less Common Diagnoses
- **Hyperparathyroidism (HPTH) (Mimic)**
  - Subchondral resorption at phalanges is not an uncommon form of resorption
    - Analogous to subchondral resorption at distal clavicle or iliac side of sacroiliac joint
    - With use, subchondral bone may collapse; this may mimic an erosive pattern
    - Critical evaluation shows the collapse is not always as rounded as an erosion & has a fairly distinct cortex
  - Seen with either HPTH or renal osteodystrophy
  - DIP is most frequent site, though seen in PIP & even in carpals
  - **Hint**: Watch for other suggestions of HPTH in the hand
    - Most common: Overtubulation of middle phalanges from subperiosteal resorption (may not be active)
    - Brown tumors
    - Tuft resorption

Helpful Clues for Rare Diagnoses
- **Chronic Reactive Arthritis (CRA)**

IP-PREDOMINANT ARTHRITIS

- Erosive > productive changes, but may be mixed
- Feet > hands
- DIP > PIP, but all may be involved
- Tarsal involvement variable; may see enthesopathy
- Calcaneal involvement common (erosive change plus periostitis posterior tubercle)
- May present with a "sausage digit"
  - Swelling of entire digit
  - Periostitis, especially along shaft
- Late stages: Arthritis mutilans
- May have spondyloarthropathy
  - Bilateral asymmetric sacroiliitis
  - Bulky, non-contiguous syndesmophytes
- Other components of syndrome: Urethritis (cervicitis), uveitis
- **HIV-AIDS Related Arthritis**
  - Similar manifestations to chronic reactive arthritis
  - Hands = feet
  - IP > MCP/MTP
  - Erosive > productive changes, but may be mixed
  - May present with a "sausage digit"
    - Swelling of entire digit
    - Periostitis, especially along shaft
  - May have incomplete syndrome of CRA
- **Adult Still Disease**
  - Systemic symptoms similar to juvenile idiopathic arthritis
  - Rheumatoid factor negative
  - Two arthritic manifestations
    - Similar distribution to RA (MCP > IP)

- Similar distribution to PSA (IP > MCP); fusion
- Carpal involvement: Variable, but may be pericapitate
- **Amyloid Deposition**
  - Deposition in soft tissues, synovium, cartilage, bone
  - Often have large soft tissue masses
    - Shoulders, wrists, ankles
    - Masses described as "lumpy"
  - MR fairly distinctive, but not specific
    - Low signal (may be heterogeneous) on T2
    - Gout may have a similar MR appearance
  - Articular deposition results in erosive change; DIP is common site
  - Diagnosis proven by biopsy
  - Most cases are secondary, with patients affected by
    - Rheumatoid arthritis
    - Multiple myeloma
    - Renal osteodystrophy
- **Multicentric Reticulohistiocytosis**
  - Rare disease with combination of
    - IP erosions
    - Acroosteolysis
    - Nodules on the digits

Osteoarthritis (OA)

PA radiograph shows normal bone density & osteophytes involving the DIP joints ➡. The PIP joints are not yet involved. MCPs are normal. As expected, carpal involvement was at the 1st CMC & STT joints.

Psoriatic Arthritis (PSA)

PA radiograph shows severe erosive change at the DIP joints ➡, with cartilage narrowing of the PIP joints. The IP joint of the thumb has eroded to a pencil-in-cup deformity ➡, with a clinically evident telescoping digit.

IP-PREDOMINANT ARTHRITIS

(Left) PA radiograph shows subchondral central erosion on the middle phalanx ➡ with marginal erosions and osteophytes on the distal phalanx ➡, which result in the "gull wing" deformity. The appearance is typical of EOA, which preferentially affects the IP joints. **(Right)** PA radiograph shows mixed erosive & productive change at the PIP joints ➡, some showing a gull wing deformity. DIPs show only cartilage narrowing. Carpus showed 1st CMC disease, diagnostic of EOA.

Erosive Osteoarthritis (EOA)

Erosive Osteoarthritis (EOA)

(Left) PA radiograph shows subchondral resorption & collapse at the DIPs ➡ resulting from HPTH. The hint in this case is the overtubulation of the middle phalanx ➡, resulting from prior subperiosteal resorption. **(Right)** PA radiograph shows severe deformity at the DIPs ➡, resulting from subchondral resorption & collapse in HPTH. The frequent location of subperiosteal resorption of the middle phalanges ➡ results in overtubulation & helps secure the diagnosis.

Hyperparathyroidism (HPTH) (Mimic)

Hyperparathyroidism (HPTH) (Mimic)

(Left) AP radiograph shows severe erosive disease in the IP joints of the foot ➡. The MCPs are less severely involved. The calcaneus (not shown) had significant erosions at the posterior tubercle; all findings are typical of CRA. **(Right)** Posteroanterior radiograph shows soft tissue swelling, periostitis ➡, and erosive change at the DIP joint ➡ in this HIV-positive patient. Locations and appearance of arthritic changes are similar to those of chronic reactive arthritis.

Chronic Reactive Arthritis (CRA)

HIV-AIDS Related Arthritis

IP-PREDOMINANT ARTHRITIS

Adult Still Disease

Adult Still Disease

(Left) Posteroanterior radiograph shows a fused DIP ➡, cartilage narrowing at other DIPs, and erosive change at the PIP joints ➡. The MCPs are relatively normal. This patient had systemic symptoms typical of adult Still disease. *(Right)* Posteroanterior radiograph shows DIP disease ➡; the PIP and MCP joints were normal. Pericapitate disease in the wrist and systemic symptoms helped confirm the diagnosis of adult Still disease.

Amyloid Deposition

Amyloid Deposition

(Left) PA radiograph shows cartilage loss and erosive change isolated to the DIPs ➡. This patient had prominent soft tissue nodularity around the wrist. Synovial biopsy of the DIP proved amyloid deposition. *(Right)* PA radiograph of the same patient shows nodular soft tissue swelling about the wrist and forearm ➡. The carpus shows no arthritic change. With underlying renal osteodystrophy, it is not surprising that this is secondary amyloid deposition.

Multicentric Reticulohistiocytosis

Multicentric Reticulohistiocytosis

(Left) PA radiograph shows erosions involving most joints of this hand, but it predominates at the DIP joints ➡. Note also that there is acroosteolysis ➡. This combination might suggest PSA, but the presence of nodularity suggests multicentric reticulohistiocytosis. *(Right)* PA radiograph shows acroosteolysis ➡ along with DIP erosions ➡. Note the nodularity along the digits. The combination yields the rare diagnosis of multicentric reticulohistiocytosis.

MONOARTHRITIS

DIFFERENTIAL DIAGNOSIS

Common
- Septic Joint
- Osteoarthritis, Post-Traumatic
- Gout
- Charcot, Neuropathic
- Pigmented Villonodular Synovitis (PVNS)
- Synovial Osteochondromatosis
- Viral (Toxic) Synovitis

Less Common
- Hemophilia
- Giant Cell Tumor Tendon Sheath (Mimic)
- Chondrolysis, Post-Traumatic

Rare but Important
- Tuberculosis
- Fungal

ESSENTIAL INFORMATION

Key Differential Diagnosis Issues
- Some processes are virtually always monoarticular
  ○ Pigmented villonodular synovitis
  ○ Synovial osteochondromatosis
  ○ Viral (toxic) synovitis
  ○ Giant cell tumor of tendon sheath (mimic)
  ○ Chondrolysis, post-traumatic
- Some processes may be monoarticular or polyarticular
  ○ Septic joint, whatever etiology
  ○ Gout
  ○ Charcot
  ○ Hemophilia

Helpful Clues for Common Diagnoses
- **Septic Joint**
  ○ Effusion may be first clue
  ○ Subchondral cortex may loose distinct "crispness" on radiograph
  ○ MR generally not necessary
    ▪ Confirms effusion
    ▪ May show cortical & marrow edema
    ▪ Nonspecific
  ○ Blood studies may be normal (white cell count, erythrocyte sedimentation rate)
  ○ Must maintain high index of suspicion
    ▪ Diagnosis is confirmed by aspiration
    ▪ Aspiration should be considered urgent, particularly in hip
- **Osteoarthritis, Post-Traumatic**

  ○ Osteoarthritis (OA) is generally polyarticular
  ○ Osteoarthritis generally is specific in location
  ○ Trauma may result in abnormalities predisposing a joint to osteoarthritis
    ▪ Fracture malunion
    ▪ Osteochondral defect
    ▪ Ligament laxity
  ○ If osteoarthritis is seen in an unusual location, consider trauma as the etiology
    ▪ OA is usually monoarticular in this case
- **Gout**
  ○ Often is monoarticular initially
  ○ Most common location: 1st metatarsal joint
  ○ When monoarticular, appearance is generally classic
    ▪ Well-defined erosions, both intraarticular & juxtaarticular
    ▪ Dense tophus
    ▪ MR shows largely low signal mass which enhances
  ○ Once gout is long-standing & untreated, it may be more difficult to diagnose
    ▪ Polyarticular, often involving unusual joints
    ▪ May appear severely erosive
    ▪ Absence of tophi may complicate diagnosis
- **Charcot, Neuropathic**
  ○ Some etiologies tend to be monoarticular
    ▪ Syringomyelia
    ▪ Diabetes (though occasionally polyarticular)
  ○ Some etiologies tend to be polyarticular
    ▪ Tabes
    ▪ Congenital insensitivity or indifference to pain
  ○ Classic locations of Charcot joint, related to etiology
    ▪ Diabetes: Ankle/foot, wrist
    ▪ Syringomyelia: Shoulder
    ▪ Tabes: Knee, spine
    ▪ Congenital insensitivity/indifference to pain: Knee, ankle
    ▪ Paraplegia: Spine, distal to stabilized site of injury
  ○ Classic appearance
    ▪ Osseous debris (though may be resorbed in atrophic variety)

MONOARTHRITIS

- Distension of joint (large effusion, often presents as "mass", especially shoulder)
- Disruption of joint
- **Pigmented Villonodular Synovitis (PVNS)**
  - Always monoarticular
  - Intraarticular nodular mass, either lining synovium or conglomerate
  - Nodularity low signal to inhomogeneous mixed signal on T2; blooms on gradient echo, enhances with contrast
  - May result in large subchondral cysts, direct erosions
- **Synovial Osteochondromatosis**
  - Generally monoarticular
  - Multiple round bodies of similar size
    - May be free within effusion
    - May be conglomerate mass
    - Bodies usually visible on radiograph, but may not be calcified enough to be seen
  - May cause erosions
  - Rarely may extend extraarticularly
- **Viral (Toxic) Synovitis**
  - Usually hip in child
  - Effusion seen by radiograph or ultrasound
  - No destructive osseous change
  - Must differentiate from septic joint
    - Usually requires aspiration, which will yield normal synovial fluid

Helpful Clues for Less Common Diagnoses
- **Hemophilia**
  - Usually monoarticular, though may involve more than one joint
  - Results from repeated intraarticular bleeds

- Hyperemia from bleeds in child result in epiphyseal/metaphyseal overgrowth
- Inflammatory change may cause erosion, cartilage damage
- Iron deposition in synovium following repeated bleeds may appear typical
  - Radiograph may show "dense" effusion
  - MR may show low signal deposits which bloom on gradient echo
- Knee > elbow > ankle
- May not be distinguishable by imaging from juvenile idiopathic arthritis (JIA)
  - JIA more frequently polyarticular
- **Giant Cell Tumor Tendon Sheath (Mimic)**
  - Usually seen along tendon sheath of digit
  - May cause extrinsic osseous erosion on both sides of a joint, mimicking erosions & arthritic process
  - Hint: Soft tissue mass is usually not centered on the joint
- **Chondrolysis, Post-Traumatic**
  - Most frequently seen following pinning of hip for slipped capital femoral epiphysis
  - Rapid chondrolysis, must be distinguished from septic hip

Helpful Clues for Rare Diagnoses
- **Tuberculosis & Fungal**
  - Major distinguishing feature from bacterial septic arthritis is lack of host reaction
  - Osteopenia generally prominent
  - Cartilage destruction & erosions generally develop late in process
  - May progress indolently

Septic Joint

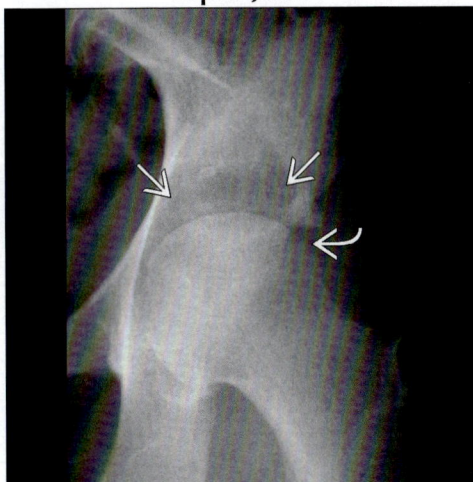

AP radiograph shows complete loss of cartilage ➔ as well as extensive erosive disease within the acetabulum ➔ and femoral head. Septic hip can develop destructive changes rapidly & is a clinical emergency.

Septic Joint

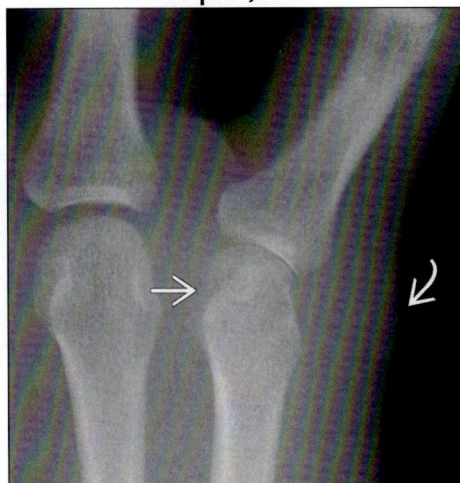

PA radiograph shows complete cartilage loss, erosive destruction ➔, & soft tissue swelling ➔. Septic joint must be considered at this location since it is a common site of injury from punching an opponent in the mouth.

MONOARTHRITIS

(Left) PA radiograph shows osteophytes at the junction of the lunate & triquetrum ➡. This is associated with ulnar positive variance ➡. Trauma from the overly-long ulna results in focal osteoarthritis, termed ulnar abutment syndrome. *(Right)* Anteroposterior radiograph shows a single juxtaarticular erosion ➡ at the 1st MTP joint. There is associated soft tissue swelling. This is an early radiographic finding of gout, diagnosed by type of erosion & location.

Osteoarthritis, Post-Traumatic

Gout

(Left) Anteroposterior radiograph shows cut-off destruction of the humeral head ➡ and a large amount of debris within a distended axillary bursa ➡ of the glenohumeral joint. The appearance is that of a neuropathic joint. *(Right)* Anteroposterior radiograph shows very large subchondral cysts on both sides of the hip joint. The bone density is normal, and this is a monostotic process. PVNS should be considered in such a case and was proven.

Charcot, Neuropathic

Pigmented Villonodular Synovitis (PVNS)

(Left) Sagittal T2WI MR shows a single posterior femoral metaphyseal erosion ➡ adjacent to a nodular low signal mass ➡. This is a monoarticular process and typical for PVNS. *(Right)* Lateral radiograph shows multiple round bodies within the elbow joint of a child, distending the posterior ➡ and anterior ➡ recesses of the joint. This is typical synovial osteochondromatosis, which is generally a monoarthritic process.

Pigmented Villonodular Synovitis (PVNS)

Synovial Osteochondromatosis

Viral (Toxic) Synovitis

Hemophilia

(Left) Anteroposterior radiograph shows a slightly widened "teardrop distance" of right hip compared with left (compare at ➡). This indicates effusion; aspiration of the right hip showed clear synovial fluid that proved to be uninfected. *(Right)* Lateral radiograph shows huge knee effusion ➡. Though there is no cartilage destruction or erosive change at this point, overgrown femoral epiphyses & patella in this young male suggest hemophilic arthritis.

Giant Cell Tumor Tendon Sheath (Mimic)

Chondrolysis, Post-Traumatic

(Left) Lateral radiograph shows erosions of the head of the middle phalanx & base of proximal phalanx ➡, mimicking an arthritic process. There is a soft tissue mass, not centered on the joint ➡. Mass is the primary process, giant cell tumor of tendon sheath, resulting in extrinsic erosions of the underlying bone. *(Right)* Anteroposterior radiograph shows cartilage narrowing ➡ along with evidence of old slipped capital femoral epiphysis (medial slip ➡)& pin tracks ➡.

Tuberculosis

Fungal

(Left) PA radiograph shows erosive change involving the entire midcarpal joint, extending between the scaphoid & lunate as well as the bases of the metacarpals, but sparing the radiocarpal joint. There is cartilage loss and osseous destruction, without reactive change. *(Right)* PA radiograph shows cartilage loss in the radiocarpal joint, with erosions involving both the radiocarpal and distal radioulnar joints ➡, extending across a ruptured TFCC, due to Sporotrichosis.

INTRAARTICULAR MASS

DIFFERENTIAL DIAGNOSIS

Common
- Loose Bodies
- Synovial Osteochondromatosis
- Pigmented Villonodular Synovitis (PVNS)
- Cyclops Lesion, ACL Reconstruction
- Meniscal Fragments
- Gout

Less Common
- Nodular Synovitis
- Lipoma Arborescens, Knee
- Intraarticular Chondroma

Rare but Important
- Trevor Fairbank (Dysplasia Epiphysealis Hemimelica)
- Synovial Chondrosarcoma
- Synovial Hemangioma

ESSENTIAL INFORMATION

Key Differential Diagnosis Issues
- Radiograph is essential to search for calcification within mass
- Specific location of mass within joint (particularly knee) helps to differentiate

Helpful Clues for Common Diagnoses
- **Loose Bodies**
  - Osseous loose bodies
    - Generally seen on radiograph
    - If large enough, bodies may follow bone signal centrally, with cortex, on MR
    - Smaller osseous loose bodies will be low signal on all sequences
  - Cartilaginous loose bodies
    - Not visualized on radiograph
    - Well-demonstrated on MR by surrounding effusion if > 5 mm in size
    - Watch for the osteochondral defects along the articular surface!
- **Synovial Osteochondromatosis**
  - Multinodular synovial membrane proliferation
  - Usually monoarticular, but may be polyarticular
  - Location: Intraarticular, bursal, or within tendon sheaths
    - Very rarely, extends extraarticularly
  - Usually seen as multiple round bodies, within an effusion

- Bodies range in size from tiny speckled calcifications to large bodies > 1 cm in size (may appear lamellated), but each case has bodies of a single similar size
  - Rarely, bodies may form a conglomerate mass, making diagnosis difficult
  - Occasional associated erosions
  - Bodies occasionally are radiolucent; only effusion seen on radiograph
  - MR: Signal varies with sequence & type of body (osseous or cartilage)
  - Most frequent differentiating feature: Multiple round, similar-sized bodies
- **Pigmented Villonodular Synovitis (PVNS)**
  - Proliferation of hemorrhagic synovium
  - Monoarticular, with large effusion
  - Does not calcify except very rarely & very late; this serves to differentiate PVNS from several items in this list
  - May have large subchondral cysts/erosions
  - MR appearance
    - Synovial-based mass may be solitary
    - Synovium may be thickened throughout the joint, with nodularity
    - Nodularity may extend through capsular defects along juxtaarticular ligaments
    - T1: Low signal, homogeneous (rare foci of high signal lipid laden macrophages)
    - T2: Variably low signal/inhomogeneous
    - Moderate to intense enhancement
    - Gradient echo sequence: "Blooming" low signal due to hemosiderin deposition
  - Most frequent differentiating feature: Blooming on gradient echo
  - If not a nodular mass, the diffuse synovial thickening may be indistinguishable from diffuse inflammatory synovitis, gouty synovitis, amyloid deposits, & hemophilic arthropathy
- **Cyclops Lesion, ACL Reconstruction**
  - Complication post ACL reconstruction with very specific appearance
    - Rarely seen following ACL injury without surgery
  - Location-specific: Intercondylar notch, anterior to ACL, usually encroaching on Hoffa fat pad
  - Variable low signal on T1 MR, variable low to high signal on T2 MR
- **Meniscal Fragments**

INTRAARTICULAR MASS

- Medial meniscal fragment generally seen in intracondylar notch
- Lateral meniscal fragment generally seen superior/anterior to its own anterior horn
- Meniscal fragment large enough to mimic a mass generally arises from a bucket-handle tear
- Fragment is low signal on all sequences, following normal meniscus signal
- Watch for absence or significant decrease in size of involved meniscus, particularly posterior horn & body

- **Gout**
  - Intraarticular deposits: Low signal on T1, variable low to high signal on T2, intense enhancement
    - May have adjacent erosions
    - May not be distinguishable from diffuse PVNS or synovitis
  - Possible amorphous calcific density on radiograph, potential distinguishing feature
  - Watch for juxtaarticular erosions &/or extraarticular tophi to aid in diagnosis

Helpful Clues for Less Common Diagnoses
- **Nodular Synovitis**
  - Benign proliferative synovitis arising from a single focal point of synovium
  - May arise anywhere in joint, but infrapatellar fat pad is most common site
  - Does not calcify
  - Variable T1 signal, but usually low
  - Variable T2 signal; intense enhancement

- May be indistinguishable from PVNS; generally less hemosiderin
- **Lipoma Arborescens, Knee**
  - Small to large mass within knee joint
  - May be nodular or may have frond-like extensions laden with lipid
  - MR signal follows fat on all sequences, high on T1 MR & low with fat suppression
  - Location and lipid signal is specific
- **Intraarticular Chondroma**
  - Most frequently located in Hoffa fat pad
  - Usually calcified; may mimic conglomerate synovial chondromatosis or the rare synovial chondrosarcoma

Helpful Clues for Rare Diagnoses
- **Trevor Fairbank (Dysplasia Epiphysealis Hemimelica)**
  - Usually joints of lower extremity; may be polyarticular; unilateral
  - Multiple cartilage & bone bodies attached to adjacent bone as an intraarticular exostosis; this is distinguishing factor
- **Synovial Chondrosarcoma**
  - Very rarely causes intraarticular mass
  - Calcified chondroid may not be distinguishable from conglomerate synovial chondromatosis or from intraarticular chondroma
- **Synovial Hemangioma**
  - Very rarely causes intraarticular mass
  - Phleboliths may help distinguish; otherwise MR signal not useful
  - Large draining veins, large erosions

Loose Bodies

Coronal oblique T2WI FS MR shows a large osteochondral loose body ➡ arising from a delamination injury of the femoral trochlea. Loose bodies are sometimes overlooked on MR examination.

Synovial Osteochondromatosis

Coronal T2WI FS MR shows bodies, too numerous to count, within the subdeltoid bursa, communicating with the glenohumeral joint. The bodies are similar in size, typical of primary synovial osteochondromatosis.

INTRAARTICULAR MASS

Synovial Osteochondromatosis

Pigmented Villonodular Synovitis (PVNS)

(Left) Sagittal T1WI MR shows a conglomerate mass within the suprapatellar bursa which follows bone signal on MR ➡. This proved to be synovial osteochondromatosis, which occasionally presents as a single mass rather than multiple bodies. *(Right)* Sagittal T2* GRE MR shows large effusion and synovial thickening with nodularity lining the entire joint ➡. Note that the nodules "bloom" on this gradient echo sequence due to the hemosiderin deposits.

Cyclops Lesion, ACL Reconstruction

Meniscal Fragments

(Left) Sagittal T2WI FS MR shows an intraarticular mass ➡ containing mixed low & high signal intensity, anterior to the ACL reconstruction, and encroaching on Hoffa fat pad. Location & morphology is typical of cyclops lesion. *(Right)* Axial T2WI FS MR shows a mass ➡ located anterior to the native anterior horn lateral meniscus ➡. There is absence of the posterior horn & body of the meniscus; the "mass" is the flipped fragment of the bucket-handle tear.

Gout

Nodular Synovitis

(Left) Sagittal T1WI MR shows a low signal mass in the medial gutter of the tibiotalar joint ➡. This mass remains mostly low signal on all sequences, & there are small associated erosions. Biopsy proved gout. *(Right)* Sagittal PD FSE MR shows low signal nodular density within Hoffa fat pad ➡. T2 signal was moderately high, & the lesion enhanced intensely. Differential diagnosis is PVNS vs. nodular synovitis. Location in Hoffa fat pad favors the latter.

INTRAARTICULAR MASS

Lipoma Arborescens, Knee

Lipoma Arborescens, Knee

(Left) Sagittal PD FSE MR shows a large mass located within the suprapatellar bursa and knee joint ➡. The mass follows the signal of subcutaneous fat on all sequences. Lipoma arborescens may either be mass-like or have frond-like projections. *(Right)* Coronal T1WI MR shows the frond-like character of the lesion ➡ in a different patient with lipoma arborescens. Again, note the signal of a lipomatous lesion, contained within the knee.

Intraarticular Chondroma

Intraarticular Chondroma

(Left) Lateral radiograph shows multiple calcific densities within Hoffa fat pad ➡. The location and appearance are typical of intraarticular chondroma. *(Right)* Sagittal T2WI FSE MR of the same patient as previous image shows the mass to have virtually replaced Hoffa fat pad ➡. The low signal regions within the mass stayed low on all sequences and represent the calcified portions of the lesion.

Trevor Fairbank (Dysplasia Epiphysealis Hemimelica)

Synovial Hemangioma

(Left) Sagittal T2* GRE MR shows posterior distension of the joint capsule ➡, containing multiple bodies ➡. Other sequences confirmed the bodies follow both bone & cartilage signal. This is an intraarticular exostosis (Trevor Fairbank disease). *(Right)* Axial T1 C+ MR shows a large mass occupying the knee joint ➡, causing significant tibial erosion. Other images demonstrated large associated draining veins, yielding the diagnosis of synovial hemangioma.

ARTHROPLASTY WITH LYTIC/CYSTIC LESIONS

DIFFERENTIAL DIAGNOSIS

Common
- Massive Osteolysis/Particle Disease
- Arthroplasty Loosening
- Stress Shielding (Mimic)
- Subchondral Cyst, Pre-Operative

Less Common
- Arthroplasty Infection
- Prior Lucencies in Revision

Rare but Important
- Adjacent Metastasis/Primary Neoplasm

ESSENTIAL INFORMATION

Key Differential Diagnosis Issues
- Lytic or cystic lesions are frequently seen around arthroplasties, including total hip (THA), total knee (TKA), total shoulder, & total ankle
- Some may be safely ignored; others need attention or may explain symptoms
- **Hint**: Remember to compare with prior imaging to help determine acuity of lesions

Helpful Clues for Common Diagnoses
- **Massive Osteolysis/Particle Disease**
  - Osteolysis resulting from inflammatory reaction to particles of a specific size
  - Source of particles variable: Polyethylene, metal, cement, osseous debris
    - Polyethylene wear is most frequent
- **Arthroplasty Loosening**
  - With loosening, component may subside (change position) within bone
  - Region of original placement may appear as a cystic or lucent lesion
- **Stress Shielding (Mimic)**
  - With placement of arthroplasty, line of force through joint may alter
  - Regions with less weight-bearing may resorb bone, becoming more lucent
    - Greater trochanter region in THA
    - Distal anterior femur in TKA
- **Subchondral Cyst, Pre-Operative**
  - Residual large subchondral cysts appear as lytic lesions
    - Acetabular most frequent in THA
    - Tibial most frequent in TKA
  - Cysts often, but not always, curetted and bone grafted at time of surgery

Helpful Clues for Less Common Diagnoses
- **Arthroplasty Infection**
  - Infection is not uncommon, but lytic lesion related to infection is uncommon
  - May be serpiginous
  - Dense linear periosteal reaction
- **Prior Lucencies in Revision**
  - Lytic regions from loosening or osteolysis may or may not be curetted & bone grafted at time of revision
    - Residual lucency mimics acute lesion

Helpful Clues for Rare Diagnoses
- **Adjacent Metastasis/Primary Neoplasm**
  - Patient age group for arthroplasties is same as that at greatest risk for metastases

Massive Osteolysis/Particle Disease

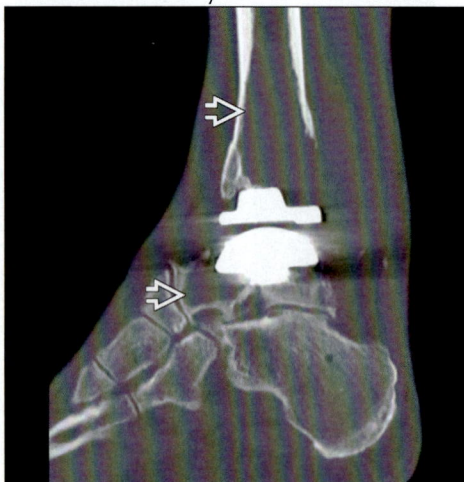

Sagittal bone CT shows massive osteolysis involving the tibia & talus ➡ following total ankle arthroplasty. There was no polyethylene wear, but a chronic fracture at the site of tibial placement contributes osseous particles.

Arthroplasty Loosening

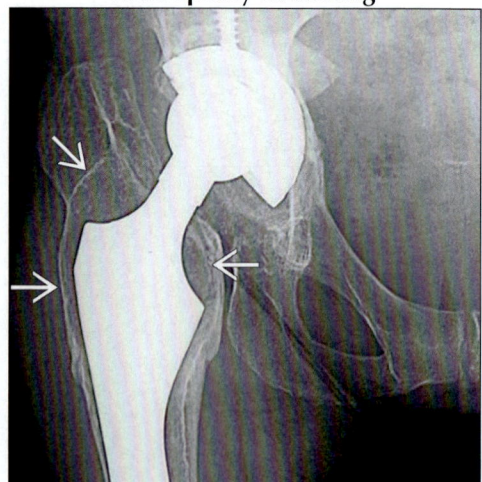

AP radiograph shows femoral component loosening with subsidence (distal displacement of component) by 2 cm. This results in an apparent lytic lesion ➡ surrounding the proximal portion of the component.

ARTHROPLASTY WITH LYTIC/CYSTIC LESIONS

Stress Shielding (Mimic)

Stress Shielding (Mimic)

(Left) Anteroposterior radiograph shows lucency within the greater trochanter ➡ of a THA. This is a typical location for stress shielding in a hip and should not be mistaken for a lytic lesion. Note the pathologic fracture ➡ at this site of weakened bone. *(Right)* Lateral radiograph shows lucency at the distal anterior femur ➡, the typical location for stress shielding in a TKA. The diagnosis is confirmed by the "streaming" of increased density posteriorly ➡.

Subchondral Cyst, Pre-Operative

Arthroplasty Infection

(Left) AP radiograph shows a well-marginated lucency in the subchondral region ➡. There was no evidence of component failure of polyethylene wear; this is simply a subchondral cyst that was present prior to arthroplasty placement. *(Right)* AP radiograph shows a rounded lucency surrounding the tip of the femoral component ➡ which does not continue proximally. There is tremendous dense periosteal reaction ➡; the findings are of infection.

Prior Lucencies in Revision

Adjacent Metastasis/Primary Neoplasm

(Left) AP radiograph shows lucency along lateral aspect of the femoral component ➡. While this may be concerning for pathology, comparison with pre-revision radiograph shows the same lucency; it was due to loosening of the prior arthroplasty. *(Right)* AP radiograph shows lytic lesion superior to a THA ➡. This patient has breast cancer; if lesion was not present on prior images (indicating residual subchondral cyst), metastatic disease must be considered.

CLAVICLE LESIONS, NONARTICULAR

DIFFERENTIAL DIAGNOSIS

Common
- Clavicle Fracture
- Metastatic Disease
- Rhomboid Fossa (Mimic)
- Multiple Myeloma

Less Common
- Radiation Osteonecrosis
- Paget Disease
- Aneurysmal Bone Cyst
- SAPHO
- Osteitis Condensans of Clavicle
- Ewing Sarcoma
- Leukemia & Lymphoma
- Cleidocranial Dysplasia

Rare but Important
- Caffey Disease (Infantile Cortical Hyperostosis)
- Congenital Pseudoarthrosis
- Friedrich Disease
- Fibromatosis Colli
- Holt Oram Syndrome
- Oxalosis
- Mucopolysaccharidoses
- Hypervitaminosis A
- Asphyxiating Thoracic Dystrophy

ESSENTIAL INFORMATION

Key Differential Diagnosis Issues
- List specifically excludes joint-based processes & resorption of distal end of clavicle
- List includes tumors with predilection for clavicle and is not fully inclusive

Helpful Clues for Common Diagnoses
- **Clavicle Fracture**
  - Most common pediatric fracture
  - Fall on outstretched hand or direct blow
  - Middle 1/3 most common
    - Proximal fragment overrides distal fragment, 1-2 cm shortening, ± butterfly fragment inferiorly
  - Distal fractures 2nd most common, high incidence of nonunion, site of stress-related fractures
  - Medial fractures least common, usually associated polytrauma
- **Metastatic Disease**
  - Most common neoplasm in clavicle
  - Most common: Breast, lung, prostate
  - Osteolytic or osteoblastic
  - ± Lesions in other bones
- **Rhomboid Fossa (Mimic)**
  - Notch with sclerotic margins along inferior surface of medial clavicle
  - Attachment site of costoclavicular ligament
- **Multiple Myeloma**
  - Multiple well-defined "punched out" lytic lesions, endosteal scalloping
  - Solitary expansile lesion (plasmacytoma) uncommon in clavicle
  - Multiple other bones involved, including ribs

Helpful Clues for Less Common Diagnoses
- **Radiation Osteonecrosis**
  - Most typical following radiation for breast cancer
    - Reduced incidence with newer delivery techniques
  - Regional osteoporosis involving ribs, scapula, humeral head
    - Progresses to patchy lysis, sclerosis, fragmentation, destruction
  - Osteochondroma following radiation in childhood
- **Paget Disease**
  - Older patients
  - Characteristic finding: Generalized enlargement of bone
    - Cortical thickening is early finding
    - Associated coarse trabecula
- **Aneurysmal Bone Cyst**
  - Children, teenagers
  - Lytic expansile lesion ± septations at the ends of bone
  - MR: Fluid-fluid levels
- **SAPHO**
  - Synovitis, Acne, Pustulosis, Hyperostosis, Osteitis
    - Wide spectrum of manifestations
    - Commonly involves clavicle
  - Chronic recurrent multifocal osteomyelitis (CRMO)
    - Early: Ill-defined destruction, immature often aggressive periosteal new bone
    - Late: Irregular sclerosis, hyperostosis, mature periosteal new bone

CLAVICLE LESIONS, NONARTICULAR

- Involves 2 or more bones, either synchronous or metachronous
- Usually seen in children but wide age range
  - Sternoclavicular hyperostosis
    - Older teenagers & adults, primarily men
    - Unilateral or bilateral sclerosis & enthesitis of clavicle, sternum or both, ± involvement of manubriosternal, 1st, 2nd costochondral articulations
- **Osteitis Condensans of Clavicle**
  - Pain & swelling, middle-aged women
  - Related to chronic stress
  - Unilateral sclerosis inferior medial clavicle, inferomedial osteophyte
- **Ewing Sarcoma**
  - Adolescents & young adults
  - Permeative destruction, aggressive periosteal new bone, soft tissue mass
- **Leukemia & Lymphoma**
  - Wide age range, especially lymphoma
  - Aggressive destruction, periosteal new bone formation, soft tissue mass
- **Cleidocranial Dysplasia**
  - Bilateral involvement ranges from complete absence to varying degrees of hypoplasia involving the distal ends
  - Associated wormian bones, symphyseal anomalies, facial deformities, abnormal dentition, short stature, scoliosis

Helpful Clues for Rare Diagnoses
- **Caffey Disease (Infantile Cortical Hyperostosis)**

- Manifests by 6 months of age
- Irritability, swelling, bone lesions
- Progresses from cortical thickening & lamellar new bone to diffuse cortical thickening, eventually remodels to normal
- **Congential Pseudoarthrosis**
  - Right clavicle, midportion
  - Atrophic with tapered sclerotic margins
  - Angulated, apex points cephalad
- **Friedrich Disease**
  - Clavicular head sclerosis in children 2° trauma or emboli
- **Fibromatosis Colli**
  - Well-defined notch along superior medial clavicle at insertion of sternocleidomastoid muscle (SCM), SCM enlarged
- **Holt Oram Syndrome**
  - Clavicles hypoplastic, upturned creating "handle bar" appearance
- **Oxalosis**
  - Sclerosis with bulbous enlargement medial clavicle creating "drumstick" appearance
- **Mucopolysaccharidoses**
  - Clavicles thick, short, widened
  - Thick ribs, small intercostal spaces
  - Abnormal epiphyses & vertebra
- **Hypervitaminosis A**
  - Children only, cortical thickening, non-aggressive periostitis
- **Asphyxiating Thoracic Dystrophy**
  - Horizontal clavicles create "handle bar" appearance
  - Short ribs, narrow thorax create "bell-shaped" chest

Clavicle Fracture

Anteroposterior radiograph shows fracture of the medial head of the clavicle ➡. This location is much less frequent than middle or distal and often has associated polytrauma.

Clavicle Fracture

Anteroposterior radiograph shows an extraarticular fracture of the distal clavicle ➡ located just lateral to the coracoclavicular ligaments ➡. (Courtesy S. Hatem, MD).

209

CLAVICLE LESIONS, NONARTICULAR

(Left) Anteroposterior radiograph shows typical midshaft clavicle fracture ➡ with a small inferior butterfly fragment ⇨. The proximal fragment is pulled upward by the sternocleidomastoid muscle, and the lateral fragment is anchored by the coracoclavicular ligaments. **(Right)** Anteroposterior radiograph shows a sclerotic lesion of the distal 1/3 of the clavicle ➡ in this patient with metastatic prostate carcinoma.

Clavicle Fracture

Metastatic Disease

(Left) Anteroposterior radiograph shows a defect with well-defined sclerotic margins along the inferior medial clavicle ➡. This is the typical appearance and location of a rhomboid fossa at the attachment of the costoclavicular ligament. **(Right)** Anteroposterior radiograph shows mixed lytic and sclerotic lesions within the scapula, clavicle, humeral head, and adjacent ribs ➡. The regional distribution is a clue to the diagnosis of radiation osteonecrosis.

Rhomboid Fossa (Mimic)

Radiation Osteonecrosis

(Left) Anteroposterior radiograph shows thickening and enlargement throughout the medial clavicle ➡ and marked cortical thickening of the lateral border of the scapula ⇨ in this patient with polyostotic Paget disease. **(Right)** Anteroposterior radiograph shows an expanded lytic lesion at the distal end of the clavicle ➡ surgically proven to be an aneurysmal bone cyst.

Paget Disease

Aneurysmal Bone Cyst

CLAVICLE LESIONS, NONARTICULAR

Osteitis Condensans of Clavicle

Ewing Sarcoma

(Left) Axial NECT shows typical case of osteitis condensans of the clavicle. There is dense sclerosis and mature periosteal new bone involving the medial right clavicle ➡. The medial left clavicle is normal ➡. *(Right)* Anteroposterior radiograph shows permeative destruction with aggressive periostitis involving the midclavicle in this 11 year old with a large palpable soft tissue mass. Biopsy confirmed Ewing sarcoma.

Leukemia & Lymphoma

Cleidocranial Dysplasia

(Left) Coronal T1WI MR shows low signal intensity marrow within the left clavicle ➡ and large associated soft tissue mass without significant cortical destruction ➡. Lymphoma is one tumor that may show marrow involvement and a soft tissue mass without associated cortical destruction. *(Right)* AP radiograph shows absence of both clavicles as well as hypoplastic glenoid fossae ➡ in this patient with cleidocranial dysplasia (or dysostosis).

Mucopolysaccharidoses

Asphyxiating Thoracic Dystrophy

(Left) Anteroposterior radiograph shows thick clavicles, wide ribs, and narrow intercostal spaces in this patient with a mucopolysaccharidosis storage disorder. *(Right)* Anteroposterior radiograph shows classic findings of asphyxiating thoracic dystrophy including high riding clavicles creating a "handle bar" appearance. Notice the short ribs creating a bell-shaped chest.

DISTAL CLAVICULAR RESORPTION

DIFFERENTIAL DIAGNOSIS

Common
- Chronic Rotator Cuff Tear
- Post-Operative
- Acromioclavicular Separation (Mimic)
- Rheumatoid Arthritis
- Post-Traumatic Osteolysis

Less Common
- Hyperparathyroidism (HPTH)
- Renal Osteodystrophy
- Progressive Systemic Sclerosis

Rare but Important
- Septic Joint

ESSENTIAL INFORMATION

Key Differential Diagnosis Issues
- **Hint**: Unilateral vs. bilateral involvement helpful in narrowing differential

Helpful Clues for Common Diagnoses
- **Chronic Rotator Cuff Tear**
  - Unilateral or bilateral asymmetric
  - Decreased acromiohumeral distance
  - Pressure erosion of clavicle & acromion
- **Post-Operative**
  - Unilateral or bilateral resection of distal clavicle in association with subacromial decompression of rotator cuff tendons
  - Clavicle margin flared, sclerotic, no periostitis
- **Acromioclavicular Separation (Mimic)**
  - Unilateral following fall onto shoulder

- Compare views of both shoulders with and without weights; asymmetric AC joint ± abnormal coracoclavicular distance
- **Rheumatoid Arthritis**
  - Synovitis leads to bilateral symmetric resorption distal clavicles ± acromion
  - Associated bilateral symmetric inflammatory arthritis hands, feet, wrists
- **Post-Traumatic Osteolysis**
  - Unilateral or bilateral depending on cause
    - Bilateral common in weight lifters
  - May see periostitis
  - MR: Marrow edema, fracture or cysts

Helpful Clues for Less Common Diagnoses
- **Hyperparathyroidismm (HPTH)**
  - Bilateral symmetric resorption distal clavicle & other sites
  - Other findings: Soft tissue calcific deposits
- **Renal Osteodystrophy**
  - Underlying mechanism is HPTH
  - Associated ill-defined coarse trabeculae, Looser's zones, pseudofractures
- **Progressive Systemic Sclerosis**
  - Bilateral symmetric resorption of distal clavicle ± acromion & other sites
  - Other findings: Soft tissue calcification, IP joint erosions (pencil-in-cup), loss of soft tissues over distal phalanges in hand

Helpful Clues for Rare Diagnoses
- **Septic Joint**
  - IV drug abusers; unilateral destruction clavicle & acromion, periostitis, effusion

Chronic Rotator Cuff Tear

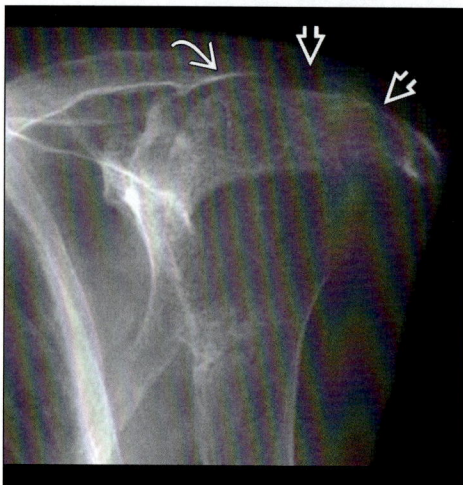

AP radiograph shows a high riding humeral head due to chronic rotator cuff tear. The humerus has eroded the distal clavicle ➡. AC joint widening & acromial erosion ➨ are due to underlying rheumatoid arthritis.

Post-Operative

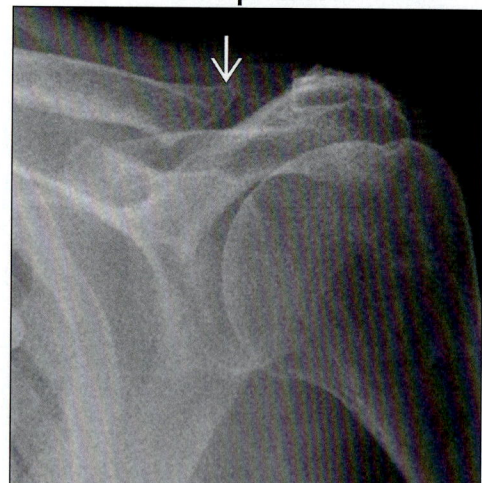

AP radiograph shows blunting of the distal end of the clavicle with a well-defined sclerotic margin ➡. The appearance is typical for a distal clavicle resection performed with a subacromial decompression.

DISTAL CLAVICULAR RESORPTION

Acromioclavicular Separation (Mimic)

Rheumatoid Arthritis

(Left) Coronal T1WI MR shows a large acromioclavicular joint effusion ➡. The clavicle is superiorly displaced relative to the acromion ➡, and the joint is widened in this patient with a type III acromioclavicular separation. *(Right)* Anteroposterior radiograph shows a typical case of long term RA with severe destruction of the humeral head ➡, glenoid, distal clavicle ➡, and acromion. Similar findings were present in the left shoulder.

Post-Traumatic Osteolysis

Post-Traumatic Osteolysis

(Left) Anteroposterior radiograph shows resorption of the distal clavicle ➡. The end of the clavicle is sharply marginated, & there is no destruction in the remaining bone. Periosteal new bone formation is present ➡. The acromion is unremarkable, which helps to exclude a joint-based process such as infection or arthritis. *(Right)* Axial PD FSE MR shows the presence of subchondral cysts within the distal clavicle ➡ in this person with post-traumatic osteolysis.

Hyperparathyroidism (HPTH)

Renal Osteodystrophy

(Left) Anteroposterior radiograph shows significant subchondral resorption of the distal clavicle ➡ simulating widening of the AC joint in this patient with hyperparathyroidism. *(Right)* Anteroposterior radiograph shows multiple sites of bone resorption in this patient with renal osteodystrophy. Changes include subchondral resorption of the distal clavicle ➡ as well as subligamentous resorption at the attachments of the coracoclavicular ligaments ➡.

PROXIMAL HUMERUS, EROSION MEDIAL METAPHYSIS

DIFFERENTIAL DIAGNOSIS

Common
- Rheumatoid Arthritis (RA)
- Chronic Rotator Cuff Tear
- Hyperparathyroidism (HPTH)
- Renal Osteodystrophy
- Shoulder Arthroplasty Impingement

Less Common
- Normal Variant ("Upper Humeral Notch")
- Hydroxyapatite Deposition Disease
- Metastases, Bone Marrow
- Leukemia
- Periosteal Chondroma

Rare but Important
- Sickle Cell Anemia: MSK Complications
- Hurler Syndrome
- Gaucher Disease
- Syphilis
- Niemann Pick

ESSENTIAL INFORMATION

Key Differential Diagnosis Issues
- Generally due either to mechanical erosion, resorption, or neoplasm

Helpful Clues for Common Diagnoses
- **Rheumatoid Arthritis (RA)**
  - Altered shoulder biomechanics places the medial humeral metaphysis in direct contact with the inferior glenoid, resulting in a mechanical erosion
    - Concentric joint space narrowing, chronic rotator cuff tear, osteopenia
  - Predisposes to surgical neck fracture of the humerus due to fulcrum effect of glenoid
- **Chronic Rotator Cuff Tear**
  - Similar mechanism as rheumatoid arthritis without concentric joint space narrowing
- **Hyperparathyroidism (HPTH)**
  - Subperiosteal resorption of the medial humeral metaphysis is one of many resorptive patterns in HPTH
  - Other findings: Brown tumors, abnormal bone density with smudgy trabeculae
- **Renal Osteodystrophy**
  - Similar to hyperparathyroidism
- **Shoulder Arthroplasty Impingement**
  - Mechanical impingement of the native proximal humeral metaphysis with the prosthetic glenoid component

Helpful Clues for Less Common Diagnoses
- **Normal Variant ("Upper Humeral Notch")**
  - Exaggerated convexity at the medial humeral head-neck junction without underlying abnormality
  - Smooth, intact cortex
- **Metastases, Bone Marrow**
  - Lytic metastases may erode the cortex
- **Leukemia**
  - Subcortical demineralization of the medial metaphyseal humeral cortex may be the initial radiographic finding of leukemia
    - Region is commonly visible on standard chest radiographs

Rheumatoid Arthritis (RA)

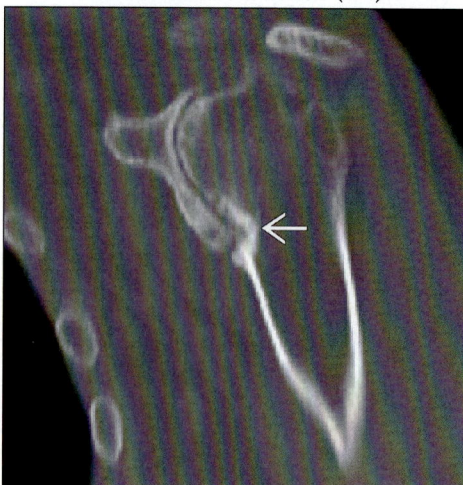

Coronal NECT shows an erosion ➡ in the medial humeral metaphysis, due to chronic rotator cuff tear & elevation of the humeral head. Joint space narrowing & osteoporosis confirm the diagnosis of RA.

Chronic Rotator Cuff Tear

AP radiograph shows a chronic rotator cuff tear, with erosion of the acromion and clavicle ➡, severe osteoporosis, and mechanical erosion of the medial humeral metaphysis ⇨. The patient has severe RA.

PROXIMAL HUMERUS, EROSION MEDIAL METAPHYSIS

Hyperparathyroidism (HPTH)

Renal Osteodystrophy

(Left) Anteroposterior radiograph shows abnormal general bone density with indistinct trabeculae. There is subperiosteal resorption at the proximal humerus ➡ as well as severe subchondral resorption at the distal clavicle ➡ and a Brown tumor in the rib ➡. *(Right)* Anteroposterior radiograph shows subtle subperiosteal resorption at the medial humeral metaphysis ➡ and a lytic lesion within the humeral metaphysis ➡, consistent with a Brown tumor.

Metastases, Bone Marrow

Leukemia

(Left) Anteroposterior radiograph shows a lytic medulloblastoma metastasis ➡ in the medial metaphysis of the proximal humerus. The bone cortex is destroyed by the tumor. *(Right)* Anteroposterior radiograph shows typical leukemic bone changes of lucent metaphyseal bands and erosion of the medial metaphysis within the proximal humeri ➡. These may be the initial radiographic findings of leukemia.

Periosteal Chondroma

Syphilis

(Left) Anteroposterior radiograph shows a lytic metadiaphyseal lesion ➡ that does not have obvious matrix or soft tissue mass. Differential dx would include periosteal chondroma, periosteal osteosarcoma, and a cortically based lesion with a very thin rim, such as fibrous dysplasia or aneurysmal bone cyst. *(Right)* AP radiograph shows subtle medial metaphyseal erosion ➡ due to congenital syphilis; there is also an acromial fracture ➡ from non-accidental trauma.

GLENOHUMERAL MALALIGNMENT

DIFFERENTIAL DIAGNOSIS

Common
- Rotator Cuff Tear (RCT) or Atrophy
- Humeral Head Rotation (Mimic)
- Surgical Neck Fracture
- Hanging Cast
- Osteoarthritis

Less Common
- Instability
- Intraarticular Fluid
- Neurologic Injury

Rare but Important
- Intraarticular Mass

ESSENTIAL INFORMATION

Key Differential Diagnosis Issues
- Shoulder joint capacious & highly mobile
  - Stability mainly from soft tissue support
  - Any soft tissue insult can produce malalignment
- Drooping shoulder: Inferior pseudosubluxation

Helpful Clues for Common Diagnoses
- **Rotator Cuff Tear (RCT) or Atrophy**
  - Superior migration 2° loss of soft tissues between acromion & humeral head
- **Humeral Head Rotation (Mimic)**
  - Maintain normal relationship between long axis scapula & center humeral head
- **Surgical Neck Fracture**
  - Inferior pseudosubluxation
  - Atony of rotator cuff muscles
- **Hanging Cast**
  - Inferior pseudosubluxation
    - Weight of cast pulls humerus inferiorly
- **Osteoarthritis**
  - Posterior translation 2° glenoid remodeling
  - Superior migration if associated RCT

Helpful Clues for Less Common Diagnoses
- **Instability**
  - Anterior or posterior translation
  - Labral, glenohumeral ligament, RCT
  - Multidirectional instability
- **Intraarticular Fluid**
  - Inferior, anterior, or posterior translation or joint space widening
  - Effusion, hemarthrosis
    - Trauma, infection, arthritis
  - Overdistention by intraarticular contrast
    - Exacerbates pre-existing instabilities
    - May predispose to dislocation
    - Contrast volume should not exceed 20 cc, typically 8-14 cc
- **Neurologic Injury**
  - Inferior pseudosubluxation
  - Leads to weakness of rotator cuff muscles
    - Especially axillary nerve injury

Helpful Clues for Rare Diagnoses
- **Intraarticular Mass**
  - Joint space widening, anterior or posterior translation
  - Capacity of joint means alignment rarely altered by mass or intraarticular body

Rotator Cuff Tear (RCT) or Atrophy

Anteroposterior radiograph shows humeral head abutting the acromion ➡ due to tear and retraction of the intervening rotator cuff tendons. The humeral head is superiorly migrated relative to the glenoid.

Rotator Cuff Tear (RCT) or Atrophy

Coronal oblique PD FSE MR shows extensive disruption of the supraspinatus tendon, leading to loss of distance between the humeral head and acromion and superior migration of the humeral head.

GLENOHUMERAL MALALIGNMENT

Humeral Head Rotation (Mimic)

Surgical Neck Fracture

(Left) Axial T1WI FS MR shows an anterior labral tear ➡. The humeral head is internally rotated, creating the appearance of posterior subluxation. Note that the center of the humeral head remains along the long axis of the glenoid. *(Right)* AP radiograph shows a drooping shoulder & inferior subluxation of the humeral head, accompanying a surgical neck fracture of the proximal humerus. With humeral neck fracture, the droop most frequently results from muscle atony.

Instability

Instability

(Left) Axial T1WI FS MR shows posterior subluxation of the humeral head, creating narrowing of the joint posteriorly relative to anterior ➡. There is loss of the discrete triangular contour of the posterior labrum ➡, which is torn. *(Right)* ABER T1WI FS MR shows an anterior labral tear to good advantage ➡, accompanied by significant subluxation of the humeral head.

Intraarticular Fluid

Intraarticular Mass

(Left) Axial T2WI MR shows widening of the glenohumeral joint ➡ in this patient with a massive rotator cuff tear and a large effusion. Normally only a thin layer of fluid separates the two articular surfaces. *(Right)* Axial T1WI MR shows osteosarcoma arising in the proximal humerus. A large soft tissue mass is present ➡, displacing the humeral head anteriorly relative to the glenoid ➡.

ANTEROSUPERIOR LABRAL VARIATIONS/PATHOLOGY

DIFFERENTIAL DIAGNOSIS

Common
- Superior Sublabral Recess (Sulcus)
- Sublabral Foramen
- SLAP Lesions I-IV
- SLAP Lesions V-X
- Biceps Labral Complex, Type 1
- Biceps Labral Complex, Type 2
- Biceps Labral Complex, Type 3

Less Common
- Sublabral Foramen with Superior Sublabral Recess (Sulcus)
- Buford Complex
- Pseudo-SLAP Lesion
- Thin Anterior Labrum with Thick Inferior Glenohumeral Ligament

ESSENTIAL INFORMATION

Key Differential Diagnosis Issues
- Normal labrum has wide variety of normal shapes, sizes, & attachments
  - Labral normal variants are most common in 11 to 3 o'clock positions
  - Variants typically do not extend posterior to biceps tendon attachment
  - Uncommon cases of normal variants have been reported below 3 o'clock position & posterior to biceps
- SLAP lesion = superior labral anteroposterior lesion
  - Features favoring tear over normal variant = irregular margin, lateral orientation of abnormal signal, extension posterior to biceps tendon, presence of perilabral cyst & > 2 mm separation from glenoid
  - Tears often centered at biceps tendon attachment
  - Anterosuperior labral tears are less common than anteroinferior tears
  - Causes include repetitive motion (throwing & swimming), trauma, degeneration
- Chronically inflamed folds of synovial tissue may mimic labral tear or fraying

Helpful Clues for Common Diagnoses
- **Superior Sublabral Recess (Sulcus)**
  - Most common normal variant in superior labrum, seen in up to 73% of population
    - Prevalence increases with increasing patient age
  - Space between labrum & glenoid cartilage confined to 11 to 1 o'clock position
    - In region of biceps attachment where the labrum is most loosely attached
  - Parallel course to glenoid cartilage
  - Classically described as not extending behind biceps anchor, but exceptions have been documented
  - Smooth free edge of labrum & width < 2 mm helps differentiate from tear
  - May be continuous with a sublabral foramen
- **Sublabral Foramen**
  - a.k.a., sublabral hole
  - Normal variant in 11-15% of population
  - Focal detachment of labrum from glenoid at 12 to 2 o'clock position
    - Anterior to biceps attachment
  - Smooth border of labrum
  - Has medial slip coursing posteromedially to glenoid
    - Differentiate from tears, which are typically oriented laterally, away from glenoid
- **SLAP Lesions I-IV**
  - Type I
    - Fraying of superior labrum without biceps involvement
    - Traumatic injury in young patients
    - May be degenerative in elderly patients
  - Type II
    - Labrum & biceps torn from superior glenoid
    - Most common type of SLAP lesion
    - Type IIA = anterosuperior labral tear
    - Type IIB = posterosuperior labral tear
    - Type IIC = anterior & posterior labral tear
    - Types IIB & IIC associated with infraspinatus tears
    - Differentiate from superior sublabral recess by irregular labral edge
  - Type III
    - Superior labrum bucket handle tear
    - May be displaced into joint space
    - Biceps tendon remains attached to glenoid
    - Associated with fall on outstretched arm
  - Type IV

ANTEROSUPERIOR LABRAL VARIATIONS/PATHOLOGY

- Bucket-handle tear + lateral extension into biceps tendon
- Similar to a type III with involvement of biceps
- May be seen along with type II tear
- Associated with fall on outstretched arm
- **SLAP Lesions V-X**
  - Type V
    - Anterior inferior glenoid/labral injury + superior extension to superior labrum & biceps
    - Associated with fall on outstretched arm & glenohumeral instability
  - Type VI
    - Anterior or posterior flap tear of labrum with biceps tendon separation
  - Type VII
    - Superior labrum & biceps tear extending into middle glenohumeral ligament
    - Associated with acute injury & glenohumeral instability
  - Type VIII
    - Superior labrum tear with posterior extension
    - More extensive than type IIB
    - Associated with posterior dislocation
  - Type IX
    - Complete or near complete detachment of the labrum circumferentially
    - Associated with traumatic injury
  - Type X
    - Superior labrum tear extending into rotator interval or structures that cross the interval

- **Biceps Labral Complex, Type 1**
  - No space between glenoid rim and biceps tendon insertion & superior labrum
- **Biceps Labral Complex, Type 2**
  - Small sulcus between glenoid rim and biceps tendon insertion & superior labrum
- **Biceps Labral Complex, Type 3**
  - Large sulcus between glenoid rim and biceps tendon insertion & superior labrum
  - Meniscoid projection into joint space
  - Can mimic a SLAP type II lesion

Helpful Clues for Less Common Diagnoses
- **Sublabral Foramen with Superior Sublabral Recess (Sulcus)**
  - a.k.a., "double Oreo cookie" sign
  - Mimics of this sign = superior labral tear in place of the superior sublabral recess or volume averaging with superior glenohumeral ligament
- **Buford Complex**
  - Normal variant in 1.5% of population
  - Absent anterosuperior labrum
  - Thick, cord-like middle glenohumeral ligament
    - Ligament attaches directly on anterosuperior glenoid
    - Can mimic a displaced labral tear or a sublabral foramen
- **Pseudo-SLAP Lesion**
  - Sulcus between biceps tendon origin & superior labrum
  - Variable depth of sulcus: Deep sulcus can mimic SLAP lesion

Superior Sublabral Recess (Sulcus)

Coronal oblique T1 C+ FS MR arthrogram shows contrast in a smooth bordered recess ➜ between the labrum and glenoid. The contour follows the curvature of the glenoid.

SLAP Lesions I-IV

Coronal oblique T1WI FS MR arthrogram shows a SLAP type I tear ➜. There is also a supraspinatus tendon tear ➜, with 1 cm of retraction.

ANTEROSUPERIOR LABRAL VARIATIONS/PATHOLOGY

(Left) Coronal oblique T1WI FS MR arthrogram shows a SLAP type II tear. Abnormal high signal in the labrum ➡ extends anteriorly to posteriorly and involves the biceps anchor ➡. (Right) Coronal oblique T1WI FS MR arthrogram shows a SLAP type IV lesion, with a bucket-handle tear ➡ extending into the biceps tendon ➡. The labral tear is extensive, but most important for classification is extension into the biceps tendon.

SLAP Lesions I-IV

SLAP Lesions I-IV

(Left) Coronal oblique T1WI FS MR arthrogram shows a tear involving the entire anterior labrum ➡. This is an extensive SLAP injury. Abnormal signal extending anteroinferior to anterosuperior classifies it as type V. (Right) Axial T1WI FS MR arthrogram shows a SLAP type VII lesion, with anterior to posterior extent ➡ in the labrum with maceration of the biceps tendon ➡. Extension into the middle glenohumeral ligament makes it a more extensive injury.

SLAP Lesions V-X

SLAP Lesions V-X

(Left) Axial T1WI FS MR shows an almost circumferential SLAP type VIII tear. This SLAP lesion continues both anteriorly and posteriorly ➡. If the tear had been completely circumferential, it would have been classified as type IX. (Right) Axial T1WI FS MR arthrogram shows a SLAP type IX lesion, consisting of a circumferential tear ➡ of the labrum along with an associated longitudinal tear of the superior glenohumeral ligament ➡.

SLAP Lesions V-X

SLAP Lesions V-X

Biceps Labral Complex, Type 1

Biceps Labral Complex, Type 2

(Left) Coronal oblique T1 C+ FS MR arthrogram shows the biceps tendon ➡ firmly adherent to the labrum and superior glenoid. This is a type 1 or slab type biceps labral complex. *(Right)* Coronal oblique T1WI MR shows a relatively shallow sulcus ➡ lying between the biceps labral complex and glenoid. This is a type 2 or intermediate type biceps labral complex. Note the smooth border of the sulcus and parallel orientation to glenoid cartilage.

Biceps Labral Complex, Type 3

Sublabral Foramen with Superior Sublabral Recess (Sulcus)

(Left) Coronal oblique T1 C+ FS MR arthrogram shows a deep sulcus ➡ lying between the biceps labral complex and glenoid. This is a type 3 or meniscoid type biceps labral complex. *(Right)* Coronal oblique T2WI FS MR arthrogram shows the "double Oreo cookie" sign. From medial to lateral, the layers of the cookie correspond to the glenoid cortex ➡ + sublabral recess ➡ + labrum ➡ + biceps/superior labrum sulcus ➡ + biceps tendon ➡.

Buford Complex

Buford Complex

(Left) Axial T1 C+ MR arthrogram image of the right shoulder shows the anterior superior glenoid labrum is absent ➡. The middle glenohumeral ligament is thickened ➡. The posterior labrum ➡ has abnormal size and shape due to a tear. This tear is unrelated to the Buford complex. *(Right)* Sagittal oblique T1 C+ MR arthrogram in the same patient as prior image best demonstrates the thickened middle glenohumeral ligament ➡.

FLUID COLLECTIONS ABOUT THE SHOULDER

DIFFERENTIAL DIAGNOSIS

Common
- Effusion
  - Osteoarthritis
  - Inflammatory Arthritis
  - Crystalline Arthropathy
  - Charcot, Neuropathic
- Bursitis
- Tendon Tear
- Labral Cyst

Less Common
- Bicipital Tenosynovitis
- Hemarthrosis
- Hematoma
- Muscle Injury
- Ganglion Cyst
- Synovial Cyst
- Iatrogenic
- Infection
  - Septic Joint
  - Soft Tissue Abscess

Rare but Important
- Venous Distension (Mimic)
- Neoplasm
- Synovial Osteochondromatosis
- Amyloid Deposition

ESSENTIAL INFORMATION

Key Differential Diagnosis Issues
- Fluid may be blood, inflammatory transudate, purulent exudate, iatrogenic
- **Hint:** Evaluate in ALL 3 planes to locate
- **Hint:** Consider surrounding tissues to further characterize

Helpful Clues for Common Diagnoses
- **Effusion**
  - Synovial transudate due to arthropathy
  - Intraarticular (glenohumeral, acromioclavicular)
  - **Osteoarthritis**
    - Osteophytes, joint space loss, normal bone mineralization, subchondral sclerosis & cysts; ± loose bodies of varying sizes
  - **Inflammatory Arthritis**
    - Rheumatoid arthritis, SLE, psoriatic, ankylosing spondylitis, juvenile idiopathic arthritis
    - Rheumatoid arthritis: Osteopenia, erosions, joint space loss, synovial hypertrophy, ± rice bodies
    - Psoriatic: Bilateral involvement, normal mineralization, bone proliferation
  - **Crystalline Arthropathy**
    - Gout, pyrophosphate (CPPD), hydroxyapatite (HADD)
    - Gout: Prefers acromioclavicular joint, difficult to distinguish from osteoarthritis
    - Pyrophosphate: Normal mineralization, bilateral involvement, chondrocalcinosis
    - Milwaukee shoulder: Mixed crystals (HADD, CPPD, etc.) with rapid glenohumeral & rotator cuff (RC) destruction
  - **Charcot, Neuropathic**
    - Osteolysis, joint dissolution, subluxation, ± debris; due to cervical syringomyelia, diabetes
- **Bursitis**
  - Bursae: Subacromial/subdeltoid, subcoracoid, coracoclavicular, supraacromial
  - Inflammation due to subacromial impingement, RC tear, arthropathy including HADD, etc.
  - Calcific bursitis: Focal ↓ SI nodules due to HADD, particularly near RC
- **Tendon Tear**
  - ↑ SI within tendon substance with complete or partial tendon fiber disruption
  - Look for tendon retraction
- **Labral Cyst**
  - Thin-walled fluid collection, ± multilobulated, ± direct connection to labral tear; posterior location most common
  - **Hint:** Cyst location helps reader find the associated labral tear; posteroinferior & posterosuperior are most common

Helpful Clues for Less Common Diagnoses
- **Bicipital Tenosynovitis**
  - Tendon sheath inflammation
  - Look for accompanying long head biceps tendinopathy, subluxation, dislocation
- **Hemarthrosis**
  - Typically related to acute trauma, look for surrounding osseous, soft tissue injury

FLUID COLLECTIONS ABOUT THE SHOULDER

- In absence of injury, consider vascular malformations, hemophilia
- Look for fluid/fluid level (hematocrit effect)
- **Hematoma**
  - Intramuscular or along fascial planes
  - Acute (< 48 hrs): T1 isointense to muscle
  - Subacute (< 30 days): ↑ SI on T1 & T2 (methemoglobin)
  - Chronic: Heterogeneous; ↓ SI if hemosiderin
- **Muscle Injury**
  - Related to acute or subacute muscle fiber disruption (grade 2, 3 muscle strain)
  - Associated hematoma
- **Ganglion Cyst**
  - Thin-walled fluid collection, ± multiple septations, no visible connection to joint
  - May be seen anywhere around shoulder girdle
- **Synovial Cyst**
  - Thin-walled fluid collection, ± multiple septations, connected to joint
  - Typically related to acromioclavicular joint
  - May result in large soft tissue "mass"
- **Iatrogenic**
  - Intramuscular, intraarticular, postsurgical effusion or seroma
  - History is key to diagnosis
  - Intraarticular fluid on T2/STIR imaging may be native or injected; look at T1 for ↑ SI if fluid results from dilute gadolinium injection
- **Infection**
  - **Septic Joint**
    - Effusion, synovial hypertrophy, avid enhancement; ± marrow edema; diagnosis by aspiration
  - **Soft Tissue Abscess**
    - Focal fluid collection with thickened, irregular, enhancing wall

Helpful Clues for Rare Diagnoses
- **Venous Distension (Mimic)**
  - Tubular structure becomes evident when evaluated in 3 planes; typically seen in spinoglenoid notch
- **Neoplasm**
  - May incite shoulder effusion
    - Pigmented villonodular synovitis: Effusion; heterogeneous nodular mass may be subtle
- **Synovial Osteochondromatosis**
  - Multiple relatively similar sized filling defects within joint effusion
    - Typically in glenohumeral joint
    - May be bursal
  - Synovial lining metaplasia, multiple cartilaginous nodules, ± calcification (may appear as fluid if not calcified)
- **Amyloid Deposition**
  - History of chronic hemodialysis
  - Effusion, synovial thickening, bulky erosions, rotator cuff tear
  - Look for intermediate to ↓ SI masses in periarticular soft tissues = "shoulder pad" sign

Osteoarthritis

Coronal oblique T2WI FS MR shows acromioclavicular osteoarthritis with joint effusion ⤵ & osteophytes ➡. Note glenohumeral joint effusion ⧩ & small soft tissue ganglion ⧩ as well.

Inflammatory Arthritis

Axial T1 C+ FS MR shows a glenohumeral effusion (↓ SI) ⤵ with enhancing hypertrophic synovium ⧩ in rheumatoid arthritis. There is bicipital tenosynovitis ➡ with similar enhancement ⧩.

FLUID COLLECTIONS ABOUT THE SHOULDER

(Left) Coronal oblique T2WI MR shows destruction of the humeral head ⇨ & glenoid ⇨, disruption of rotator cuff, & debris & distension of the glenohumeral ⇨ & subdeltoid ⇨ spaces, all typical of Charcot joint. *(Right)* Coronal oblique PD FSE FS MR shows a large subacromial/subdeltoid bursal effusion ⇨ in a patient with osteoarthritis of the glenohumeral ⇨ & acromioclavicular ⇨ joints. The chronic effusion contains thin septations ⇨.

Charcot, Neuropathic

Bursitis

(Left) Coronal oblique PD FSE FS MR shows a partial undersurface supraspinatus tendon tear as a small focal fluid (↑ SI) ⇨ collection along the tendon articular surface. *(Right)* Coronal oblique T2WI FS MR shows a massive rotator cuff tear ⇨ with retraction to the glenoid rim with extensive effusion in the glenohumeral ⇨ & acromioclavicular ⇨ joints as well as the subacromial bursa with superior subluxation ⇨ of the humeral head.

Tendon Tear

Tendon Tear

(Left) Axial PD FSE FS MR shows a thin-walled multiseptate cyst ⇨ arising from a small posterior labral tear ⇨. There is effusion in subdeltoid bursa ⇨ as well as the subcoracoid recess of the glenohumeral joint ⇨. *(Right)* Coronal oblique PD FSE FS MR shows heterogeneous (↑ to ↓ SI) subdeltoid ⇨ & intraarticular ⇨ mass representing chronic hematoma & a focal ↑ SI area of acute hemorrhage ⇨ due to recent fall in this patient taking Coumadin.

Labral Cyst

Hematoma

FLUID COLLECTIONS ABOUT THE SHOULDER

Muscle Injury

Ganglion Cyst

(Left) Axial PD FSE FS MR shows a large fluid collection ➡ representing acute hemorrhage in a patient who sustained a pectoralis major muscle tear ⊳ with retraction. (Right) Sagittal PD FSE FS MR shows a thin-walled multilobulated cyst ➡ just distal to the spinoglenoid notch ➡. It does not arise from glenoid labrum & therefore represents a ganglion rather than a paralabral cyst.

Synovial Cyst

Soft Tissue Abscess

(Left) AP fluoroscopic spot radiograph obtained during arthrography shows glenohumeral contrast flowing through a massive RC tear ➡, into & through the acromioclavicular joint, ➡ & into ⊳ the large synovial cyst ➡ arising from the superior surface of the joint. (Right) Axial T2WI MR shows a septic shoulder joint ➡ as well as abscesses ➡ in the anterior soft tissues that have resulted in rupture of the pectoralis major muscle ➡.

Neoplasm

Synovial Osteochondromatosis

(Left) Coronal oblique T2WI FS MR shows a subacromial/subdeltoid effusion ➡ as ↑ SI with a focal nodule of intermediate SI ➡ in the subdeltoid bursa. Note the slight heterogeneous ↓ SI focus ➡ in the pigmented villonodular synovitis. (Right) Coronal oblique T2WI FS MR shows multiple loose bodies ➡ within the subdeltoid bursa effusion ➡, all of uniform size, typical of synovial osteochondromatosis.

RADIAL DYSPLASIAS/APLASIA

DIFFERENTIAL DIAGNOSIS

Common
- Fanconi Anemia
- Holt-Oram Syndrome
- Thrombocytopenia-Absent Radius (TAR) Syndrome

Less Common
- Klippel Feil
- VATER Association
- Trisomy 18
- Trisomy 13-15
- Radioulnar Synostosis
- Dyschondrosteosis

Rare but Important
- Pseudothalidomide Syndrome
- Thalidomide Embryopathy
- Fetal Varicella Syndrome
- Fetal Valproic Acid Exposure
- Cornelia de Lange Syndrome
- Radial Clubhand
- Ulnar Clubhand
- Mesomelic Dysplasias
- Oculo-Auriculo-Vertebral Spectrum
- Nail Patella Disease (Fong)

ESSENTIAL INFORMATION

Key Differential Diagnosis Issues
- Radial hypoplasia, dysplasia, & aplasia are associated with many congenital syndromes and skeletal dysplasias
  - Forearm radiographs are often nonspecific

Helpful Clues for Diagnoses
- **Fanconi Anemia**
  - Thumb aplasia or short metacarpal
  - Absent or malformed navicular
  - Brachydactyly, clinodactyly
- **Holt-Oram Syndrome**
  - Brachydactyly, camptodactyly, & clinodactyly
  - Thumb aplasia or malformation ± triphalangeal thumb
  - Abnormal navicular ± fusion
  - Os centrale
- **Trisomy 18**
  - Thumb aplasia or short metacarpal
  - Ulnar deviation of MCP joints
  - Clinodactyly, syndactyly
- **Trisomy 13-15**
  - Polydactyly, clinodactyly
  - Triphalangeal thumb
  - Broad thumb distal phalanx
- **Dyschondrosteosis**
  - Decreased carpal angle
  - Carpal fusion
  - Cone-shaped epiphyses
- **Cornelia de Lange Syndrome**
  - Short, wide thumb metacarpal
  - Clinodactyly, brachydactyly
  - Volar-radial curvature of fifth digit distal phalanx (Kirner deformity)
- **Ulnar Clubhand**
  - Aplasia or hypoplasia of the ulna with radius deformity
  - Thumb present, absent 4th and 5th digits

Fanconi Anemia

Anteroposterior radiograph shows a dysplastic radius ➡ that is fused to the ulna. The thumb is absent ➡, as are the trapezium and scaphoid bones. The distal carpal row is dysplastic.

Fanconi Anemia

Posteroanterior radiograph shows an absence of the radius and thumb. There is clinodactyly of the fifth digit ➡. Skeletal changes in this entity range from nonexistent to major congenital malformations.

RADIAL DYSPLASIAS/APLASIA

Holt-Oram Syndrome

VATER Association

(Left) AP radiograph shows an absence of the radius, trapezium, and scaphoid. The thumb is severely dysplastic ➔. A small triangular bone proximal and radial to the capitate likely represents an os centrale ➔ anatomic variant. *(Right)* PA radiograph shows phocomelia with near complete aplasia of the radius, a short curved ulna ➔, and absent scaphoid and thumb. The findings were bilateral, and the patient also had renal abnormalities.

Trisomy 18

Radioulnar Synostosis

(Left) AP radiograph shows aplasia of the radius and hypoplastic thumb. Overlapping fingers ➔ and ulnar deviation of the metacarpophalangeal joints are common findings. *(Right)* Lateral radiograph shows fusion of the proximal radius to the ulna ➔. The degree of fusion and location in the forearm is variable. This bony fusion can be congenital, due to lack of segmentation, or post-traumatic, due to fracture or heterotopic ossification most commonly.

Ulnar Clubhand

Nail Patella Disease (Fong)

(Left) Anteroposterior radiograph shows absence of the ulna. The radius ➔ is dysplastic and bowed. The thumb and index finger are absent, which is unusual. This infant is too young to definitively assess for carpal abnormalities. *(Right)* Oblique radiograph shows a hypoplastic radial head ➔, which results in osteoarthritis of the elbow and an increased carrying angle. This also causes relative elongation of the ulna, with subluxation of the distal radioulnar joint.

FOREARM DEFORMITY

DIFFERENTIAL DIAGNOSIS

Common
- Fracture, Malunion
- Post-Operative
- Osteomyelitis

Less Common
- Multiple Hereditary Exostosis
- Madelung Deformity
- Ollier Disease
- Radioulnar Synostosis
- Osteogenesis Imperfecta
- Maffucci Syndrome

Rare but Important
- Fanconi Syndrome
- Holt-Oram Syndrome
- Thrombocytopenia Absent Radius Syndrome
- VATER Association
- Paget Disease
- Trisomy 18
- Trisomy 13-15
- Dyschondrosteosis
- Thalidomide Embryopathy
- Cornelia de Lange Syndrome
- Ulnar/Radial Clubhand
- Mesomelic Dysplasia
- Nail Patella Disease (Fong)
- Klinefelter Syndrome
- Camptomelic Dysplasia

ESSENTIAL INFORMATION

Helpful Clues for Common Diagnoses
- **Fracture, Malunion**
  - History of trauma most helpful
  - Focal deformity or deformities with sclerosis and lack of additional findings
  - Bowing fracture in young children
- **Post-Operative**
  - Joint replacement after trauma, infection, inflammatory or degenerative disease
  - Amputation after neoplasm, trauma, or severe infection
- **Osteomyelitis**
  - Deformity or bowing of affected bone
    - More common in lower extremities
  - Bony sequestrum, sinus tract

Helpful Clues for Less Common Diagnoses
- **Multiple Hereditary Exostosis**
  - Short ulna due to exostoses

- Bowing ± radial head dislocation
- **Madelung Deformity**
  - Ulnar, volar distal radius angulation
  - Decreased carpal angle
  - Distal ulna dorsally subluxated
  - Unilateral or bilateral
- **Ollier Disease**
  - Multiple enchondromas preferentially involving extremity long bones & phalanges
    - Cartilaginous dysplasia involving the metaphyses
    - Endosteal scalloping, chondroid matrix
  - Skull involvement ± mild platyspondyly
  - Up to 30% will develop bone malignancy
    - Pelvis > shoulder > femur > proximal tibia
- **Radioulnar Synostosis**
  - Developmental or post-traumatic
  - Bones are small with developmental causes due to lack of muscular stress
- **Osteogenesis Imperfecta**
  - Multiple healed fractures
  - Wide metaphyses with thin cortices
  - Bowing deformities
- **Maffucci Syndrome**
  - Multiple enchondromas, as in Ollier
  - Soft tissue cavernous hemangiomas with phleboliths
  - Be vigilant for malignant transformation

Helpful Clues for Rare Diagnoses
- **Fanconi Syndrome**
  - Thumb aplasia or short metacarpal
  - Absent or malformed navicular
  - Brachydactyly, clinodactyly
  - Renal abnormalities
- **Holt-Oram Syndrome**
  - Brachydactyly, camptodactyly, & clinodactyly
  - Thumb aplasia or malformation ± triphalangeal thumb
  - Abnormal navicular ± fusion
  - Os centrale
- **Thrombocytopenia Absent Radius Syndrome**
  - Radius absent with thumb present
  - Malformed ulna
  - Carpal bone hypoplasia or fusion
  - Humerus may be absent
  - 5th digit middle phalanx hypoplastic/absent

FOREARM DEFORMITY

- **VATER Association**
  - a.k.a., VACTEL, VACTERL, VACTER
  - Multiple birth defects
    - Vertebral anomalies
    - Anal atresia
    - Cardiac defect
    - Tracheoesophageal fistula
    - Renal abnormalities
    - Limb abnormalities
  - Radial dysplasia or aplasia
  - Thumb hypoplasia or triphalangeal thumb
  - Hypoplastic fifth digit middle phalanx
- **Paget Disease**
  - Enlargement of bone
  - Thick cortex
  - Coarse trabeculae
  - Bowing more common in lower extremities
- **Trisomy 18**
  - Thumb aplasia or short metacarpal
  - Ulnar deviation of MCP joints
  - Clinodactyly, syndactyly
- **Trisomy 13-15**
  - Polydactyly, clinodactyly
  - Triphalangeal thumb
  - Broad thumb distal phalanx
- **Dyschondrosteosis**
  - Decreased carpal angle
  - Carpal fusion
  - Cone-shaped epiphyses
  - Bowed tibia, short fibula, valgus knee
- **Thalidomide Embryopathy**
  - Radial malformation or aplasia
  - Thumbs usually are present

- Hips dislocated
- Cardiac, renal, & intestinal abnormalities
- **Cornelia de Lange Syndrome**
  - Short, wide thumb metacarpal
  - Clinodactyly, brachydactyly
  - Volar-radial curvature of fifth digit distal phalanx (Kirner deformity)
- **Ulnar/Radial Clubhand**
  - Absence of the ulna/ulnar ray or radius/radial ray is associated with numerous different syndromes & dysplasias
- **Mesomelic Dysplasia**
  - Short, curved radius
  - Madelung deformity
  - Short metacarpals
- **Nail Patella Disease (Fong)**
  - Hypoplastic radial head & capitellum
    - Asymmetric joint development
    - Degenerative arthritis
    - Limited elbow extension
    - Increased carrying angle
  - Lax finger joints
  - Absent or hypoplastic patella
  - Iliac horns
- **Klinefelter Syndrome**
  - Radioulnar synostosis
  - Short metacarpals
  - Capitate malformation
- **Camptomelic Dysplasia**
  - Short, angulated upper extremities
  - Radial head dislocation
  - Squared distal phalanges
  - Fifth digit clinodactyly

Fracture, Malunion

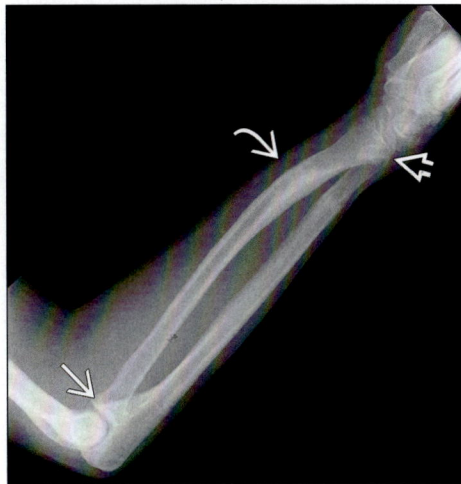

Anteroposterior radiograph shows a severe lateral condylar fracture malunion. The capitellum is significantly displaced proximally ➡ with a normally articulated radial head ➡. The ulna ➡ is subluxated.

Fracture, Malunion

Lateral radiograph shows a healed bone fracture with volar bowing of the radius ➡. One method to assess for malrotation is to identify the coronoid process ➡ on the opposite side from the ulnar styloid process ➡.

FOREARM DEFORMITY

(Left) *Oblique radiograph shows placement of a total elbow arthroplasty. The ulna is dorsally subluxated ➡ at the distal radioulnar joint. The radial head is dislocated ➡, and the radial neck is eroded.* **(Right)** *Oblique radiograph shows a focal deformity of the radius ➡. There is an expanded lytic lesion present in the proximal shaft. A pathologic fracture has healed. The remainder of the radius and the ulna are normal. The infecting agent was blastomycosis.*

Post-Operative

Osteomyelitis

(Left) *Posteroanterior radiograph shows a sessile exostosis ➡ bridging between the forearm bones, resulting in synostosis and growth deformities. There is a Madelung deformity of the wrist. Additional exostoses involve the phalanges ➡.* **(Right)** *AP radiograph shows deformities of both the radius and ulna. Bony excrescences ➡ from multiple hereditary exostoses have caused the deformities, including decreased carpal angle and growth disturbance.*

Multiple Hereditary Exostosis

Multiple Hereditary Exostosis

(Left) *Posteroanterior radiograph shows a medially angulated distal radial articular surface ➡ and a long distal ulna ➡. The radiocarpal joint spaces ➡ are severely narrowed due to advanced secondary degenerative change.* **(Right)** *Lateral radiograph in the same patient as the prior image shows dorsal subluxation/dislocation of the ulna ➡. This subluxation occurs because the sigmoid notch on the medial side of the distal radius has not formed.*

Madelung Deformity

Madelung Deformity

FOREARM DEFORMITY

Ollier Disease

Osteogenesis Imperfecta

(Left) Lateral radiograph shows a short, malformed ulna and dislocated radial head ➡. Lesions with chondroid matrix, representing enchondromas, are seen in the distal ulna ➡ and the metacarpals ➡. *(Right)* Anteroposterior radiograph shows extremely thin and osteoporotic bones. There are multiple new and old fractures with bowing of the bones ➡. This autosomal recessive subtype of osteogenesis imperfecta usually results in death soon after birth.

Maffucci Syndrome

VATER Association

(Left) Anteroposterior radiograph shows a severely foreshortened forearm, with metaphyseal deformities due to multiple enchondromas ➡. Soft tissue hemangiomas were present elsewhere, making the diagnosis of Maffucci syndrome. *(Right)* Posteroanterior radiograph shows a very short forearm. The ulna ➡ is short and bowed, but the radius ➡ is nearly completely absent. The scaphoid is absent, as is the thumb. The patient also had significant renal abnormalities.

Paget Disease

Nail Patella Disease (Fong)

(Left) Oblique radiograph shows the radius to be bowed ➡ and enlarged. The osseous cortex is thickened ➡ and the trabeculae are coarse, typical of Paget disease. *(Right)* Anteroposterior radiograph shows characteristic congenital radial head dislocation, with morphologic distortion of both the radial head ➡ and capitellum ➡. The knee showed absence of an ossified patella, typical of nail patella disease.

CARPAL CYSTIC/LYTIC LESIONS

DIFFERENTIAL DIAGNOSIS

Common
- Osteoarthritis
- Pyrophosphate Arthropathy
- Chronic Repetitive Trauma
- Gout
- Ganglion, Intraosseous
- Ulnar Abutment Syndrome

Less Common
- Brown Tumor
- Rheumatoid Arthritis
- Hemochromatosis

Rare but Important
- Pigmented Villonodular Synovitis (PVNS)
- Amyloid Deposition
- Sarcoidosis

ESSENTIAL INFORMATION

Helpful Clues for Common Diagnoses
- **Osteoarthritis**
  - 1st carpal-metacarpal & scaphomultangular joints, normal bone mineralization, joint space narrowing, subchondral sclerosis, osteophytes, subluxation, loose bodies
- **Pyrophosphate Arthropathy**
  - Chondrocalcinosis (TFCC, lunotriquetral & scapholunate ligaments, articular cartilage), bilateral asymmetric radiocarpal involvement
- **Chronic Repetitive Trauma**

- Normal joints or 2° osteoarthritis
- **Gout**
  - Bilateral asymmetric erosions, overhanging edges, soft tissue nodules, joint space narrowing occurs late
- **Ganglion, Intraosseous**
  - Solitary, communicates with joint
- **Ulnar Abutment Syndrome**
  - Ulna positive deformity, ulna abuts lunate; subchondral sclerosis, cysts

Helpful Clues for Less Common Diagnoses
- **Brown Tumor**
  - Often single lesion, bone resorption of HPTH, periarticular calcium deposits
- **Rheumatoid Arthritis**
  - Bilateral symmetric, periarticular osteoporosis, uniform joint space narrowing, erosions/cysts, soft tissue
- **Hemochromatosis**
  - Osteoporosis, chondrocalcinosis, large subchondral cysts, uniform joint space narrowing, subchondral sclerosis, osteophytes; mimics pyrophosphate

Helpful Clues for Rare Diagnoses
- **Pigmented Villonodular Synovitis (PVNS)**
  - Single compartment distribution, multiple cystic lesions, MR with low T1 & T2 signal
- **Amyloid Deposition**
  - Osteopenia, cysts & erosions, joint space normal or widened, bulky soft tissue masses, intermediate T2WI signal
- **Sarcoidosis**
  - Well-defined cystic lesions

Osteoarthritis

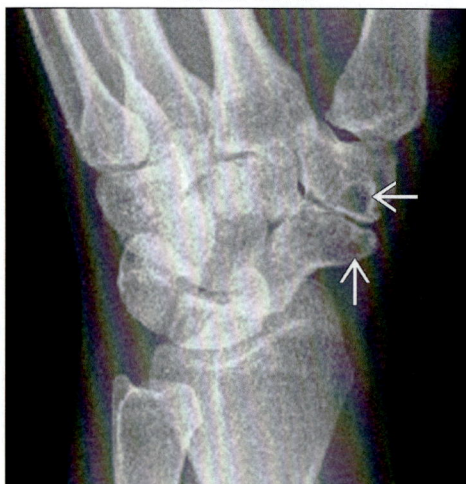

Oblique radiograph shows scaphomultangular joint space narrowing with associated subchondral cysts ➡. Isolated involvement of this joint may be seen with osteoarthritis or CPPD deposition disease.

Pyrophosphate Arthropathy

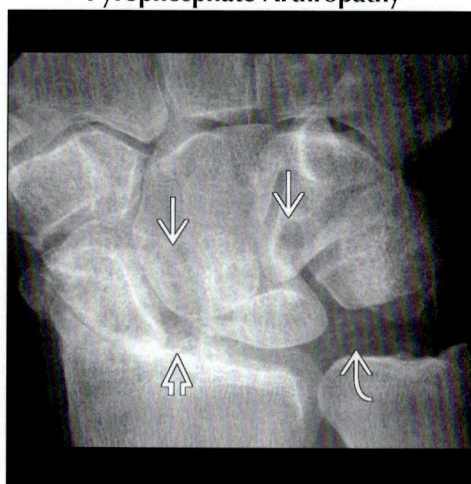

PA radiograph shows subchondral cysts in the capitate & hamate ➡, scapholunate ligament tear ➡, TFCC chondrocalcinosis ➡, & radioscaphoid narrowing, all common findings in pyrophosphate arthropathy.

CARPAL CYSTIC/LYTIC LESIONS

Chronic Repetitive Trauma

Gout

(Left) Sagittal T2WI FS MR shows cystic lesions within the volar and dorsal surfaces of the lunate ➡ attributable to chronic repetitive trauma in the dominant hand of this carpenter. *(Right)* Posteroanterior radiograph shows multiple cysts and erosions involving the distal ulna, triquetrum, lunate, capitate ➡ with accompanying radiocarpal and mid-carpal joint space narrowing. A large soft tissue tophus is characteristic of gout ⇨.

Ulnar Abutment Syndrome

Rheumatoid Arthritis

(Left) Posteroanterior radiograph shows an ulnar plus variance (the ulna is longer than the radius). This variance results in impaction on the lunate. In this case there is a cyst and sclerosis in the lunate at the point of impaction ➡. *(Right)* Coronal T1 C+ FS MR shows erosive changes in the carpal bones ➡ as well as extensive synovial pannus formation penetrating into the osseous erosions ⇨ in this patient with rheumatoid arthritis.

Pigmented Villonodular Synovitis (PVNS)

Amyloid Deposition

(Left) Oblique radiograph shows cysts in the lunate, capitate, and hamate ➡. The cysts are well-defined and are all within the mid-carpal joint space. Localization to one compartment is typical of PVNS of the carpus. *(Right)* Posteroanterior radiograph shows diffuse osteopenia of the carpus. Large, well-defined cysts with sclerotic margins are present in the distal radius, lunate, scaphoid and trapezium ➡ in this patient with biopsy proven amyloidosis.

DIFFERENTIAL DIAGNOSIS

Common
- Fracture, Malunion
- Madelung Deformity
- Turner Syndrome
- Multiple Hereditary Exostosis

Less Common
- Ollier Disease
- Marfan Syndrome
- Maffucci Syndrome
- Cleidocranial Dysplasia
- Multiple Epiphyseal Dysplasia
- Down Syndrome (Trisomy 21)

Rare but Important
- Arthrogryposis
- Mucopolysaccharidoses
- Hurler Syndrome
- Morquio Syndrome
- Mesomelic Dysplasia
- Dyschondrosteosis (Leri-Weill)
- Otopalatodigital Syndrome
- Frontometaphyseal Dysplasia
- Arthroophthalmopathy Syndrome
- Chondroectodermal Dysplasia (Ellis-van Creveld)
- Larsen Syndrome
- LEOPARD Syndrome

ESSENTIAL INFORMATION

Helpful Clues for Common Diagnoses
- **Fracture, Malunion**
  - Malunion may result in increased or decreased carpal angle
  - Post-traumatic decreased carpal angle may be differentiated from Madelung deformity by lack of volar radial tilt
- **Madelung Deformity**
  - V-shaped, steep radiocarpal joint producing a decreased carpal angle
    - Short radius with volar bowing
    - Triangular distal radial epiphysis
    - Carpal bones wedged together with lunate at apex
    - Dorsal subluxation or dislocation of ulna
  - Numerous potential etiologies of this deformity
- **Turner Syndrome**
  - Madelung deformity
  - Short fourth metacarpal/metatarsal
  - Carpal bone fusion
  - Drumstick phalanges
  - Delayed bone age
- **Multiple Hereditary Exostosis**
  - Madelung deformity
  - Short ulna & fibula
  - Metaphyseal exostoses with exostosis apex "dripping" away from joint
  - Cortex and marrow space of exostosis is contiguous with underlying bone
  - Onset in infancy and early childhood
  - Watch for malignant degeneration, usually chondrosarcoma

Helpful Clues for Less Common Diagnoses
- **Ollier Disease**
  - Multiple enchondromas: Lytic lesions with cartilaginous matrix
  - Longitudinal steaks of alternating lucency & sclerosis in metaphyses
  - Resultant bone deformity
    - Madelung deformity
    - Long bones, tubular bones of hands/feet, pelvis, ribs
  - Increased risk of malignant transformation
- **Marfan Syndrome**
  - Long fingers (arachnodactyly)
    - Third finger > 1.5x metacarpal length
  - Clinodactyly
  - Vertical talus, flatfoot
  - Protrusio deformity of hips
  - Enlarged paranasal sinuses
- **Maffucci Syndrome**
  - Madelung deformity
  - Same as Ollier Disease + cutaneous hemangiomas (phleboliths)
  - Increased risk of malignant degeneration
- **Cleidocranial Dysplasia**
  - Increased carpal angle
  - Long second & fifth metacarpals
  - Short middle phalanges
  - Cone-shaped epiphyses
  - Delayed bone age
- **Multiple Epiphyseal Dysplasia**
  - Flat epiphyses cause increased carpal angle
  - Small, irregular, fragmented epiphyses
  - Short tubular bones of hands & feet
  - Delayed bone age
- **Down Syndrome (Trisomy 21)**
  - Increased carpal angle
  - Dislocated radial head
  - Dysplastic fifth digit middle phalanx

ABNORMAL RADIOCARPAL ANGLE

- ○ Pseudoepiphysis of hands
- ○ Variable skeletal maturation

Helpful Clues for Rare Diagnoses

- **Dyschondrosteosis (Leri-Weill)**
  - ○ Madelung deformity
  - ○ Mesomelic dwarfism
  - ○ Short, curved tibia
  - ○ Short metacarpals & metatarsals
- **Chondroectodermal Dysplasia (Ellis-van Creveld)**
  - ○ Enlarged distal radius causing increased carpal angle
  - ○ Bony spike at distal humeral metaphysis medially
  - ○ Short, heavy tubular bones
  - ○ Ninth carpal bone
  - ○ Delayed skeletal maturation
- **Larsen Syndrome**
  - ○ Increased carpal angle
  - ○ Short metacarpals & distal phalanges
  - ○ Spatulate thumbs
  - ○ Multiple accessory ossicles
- **LEOPARD Syndrome**
  - ○ Lentigines, EKG conduction abnormalities, Ocular hypertelorism, Pulmonary stenosis, Abnormal genitalia, Retardation of growth, Deafness (LEOPARD)
  - ○ Madelung deformity
  - ○ Decreased bone age
  - ○ Hypoplastic fifth digit
  - ○ Syndactyly or soft tissue webbing

Alternative Differential Approaches

- Decreased carpal angle (< 125 degrees)
  - ○ Madelung deformity
  - ○ Turner syndrome
  - ○ Fracture, malunion
  - ○ Multiple hereditary exostosis
  - ○ Ollier disease
  - ○ Maffucci syndrome
  - ○ Mucopolysaccharidoses
  - ○ Hurler syndrome
  - ○ Morquio syndrome
  - ○ Mesomelic dysplasia
  - ○ Dyschondrosteosis (Leri-Weill)
- Madelung deformity
  - ○ Trauma
  - ○ Turner syndrome
  - ○ Multiple hereditary exostosis
  - ○ Ollier disease
  - ○ Maffucci syndrome
  - ○ Dyschondrosteosis (Leri-Weill)
  - ○ LEOPARD syndrome
- Increased carpal angle (> 135 degrees)
  - ○ Fracture, malunion
  - ○ Marfan syndrome
  - ○ Cleidocranial dysplasia
  - ○ Multiple epiphyseal dysplasia
  - ○ Down syndrome (trisomy 21)
  - ○ Arthrogryposis
  - ○ Otopalatodigital syndrome
  - ○ Frontometaphyseal dysplasia
  - ○ Arthroophthalmopathy syndrome
  - ○ Chondroectodermal dysplasia (Ellis-van Creveld)
  - ○ Larsen syndrome

Fracture, Malunion

Posteroanterior radiograph shows a V-shaped radiocarpal joint ➡, decreasing the normal radiocarpal angle. The patient had a remote distal radius fracture and resultant malunion.

Madelung Deformity

Posteroanterior radiograph shows a developmentally steep distal radius articular surface ➡ and a dorsally dislocated ulna ➡, as confirmed on the lateral view.

ABNORMAL RADIOCARPAL ANGLE

(Left) Posteroanterior radiograph shows a short, curved radius ➡ and a dislocated ulna ➡ with resultant decreased carpal angle. Carpal bone fusion and a short fourth metacarpal are not seen in this case but are often also present. (Right) Posteroanterior radiograph shows a sessile exostosis ➡ resulting in synostosis and decreased forearm growth, including a decreased carpal angle. The rounded densities on the phalanges ➡ are exostoses protruding volarly.

Turner Syndrome

Multiple Hereditary Exostosis

(Left) PA radiograph shows an abnormally short ulna with cartilage type matrix ➡ distally. Several similar lesions involve the metaphyseal regions of multiple metacarpals and phalanges ➡. The polyostotic nature and cartilaginous matrix suggest enchondromatosis. (Right) PA radiograph shows a flattened (increased) radiocarpal angle ➡ and long fingers ➡ relative to the metacarpal length. The appearance of the hands is otherwise normal.

Ollier Disease

Marfan Syndrome

(Left) Posteroanterior radiograph shows abnormal epiphyses ➡ causing an increased carpal angle. Note the excrescences ➡ arising from the metaphyses. This epiphyseal abnormality results in short, stubby bones, particularly in the hands and feet. (Right) Oblique radiograph shows a flattened radiocarpal angle ➡. Several of the carpal bones are fused ➡. Note the gracile radius & ulna and atrophy of the musculature, typical of arthrogryposis.

Multiple Epiphyseal Dysplasia

Arthrogryposis

ABNORMAL RADIOCARPAL ANGLE

Mucopolysaccharidoses

Morquio Syndrome

(Left) Posteroanterior radiograph shows a decreased radiocarpal angle ➡. The metacarpals are short, broad, and constricted proximally. This "fan-shaped" appearance ➡ is classic for mucopolysaccharidoses. (Right) PA radiograph shows findings similar to the prior image. There is a decreased radiocarpal angle ➡, and the metacarpals are short & constricted proximally ➡. The middle and distal phalanges ➡ have pointed ends.

Mesomelic Dysplasia

Dyschondrosteosis (Leri-Weill)

(Left) AP radiograph shows a V-shaped (decreased) radiocarpal angle ➡. Both the radius and ulna are short in this patient with mesomelic dysplasia. The radius is curved ➡. (Right) Oblique radiograph shows a severely narrowed radiocarpal angle ➡. The radius is short and bowed ➡. The distal ulna is dorsally subluxed, although difficult to appreciate on this image. The widened distance ➡ between the radius and ulna is typical of dyschondrosteosis.

Chondroectodermal Dysplasia (Ellis-van Creveld)

Larsen Syndrome

(Left) Anteroposterior radiograph shows the beginnings of a flat (increased) radiocarpal angle ➡. The metacarpal ➡ and forearm ➡ bones are short. Skeletal maturation is delayed in this patient. (Right) Posteroanterior radiograph shows a flat (increased) radiocarpal angle ➡. Multiple accessory ossicles ➡ in the wrist are typical. The third through fifth metacarpals are short ➡. Note the thick soft tissues of the thumb ➡, typical of Larsen syndrome.

ARACHNODACTYLY

DIFFERENTIAL DIAGNOSIS

Common
- Marfan Syndrome
- Ehlers-Danlos
- Localized Giantism (Mimic)

Less Common
- Homocystinuria
- Congenital Contractural Arachnodactyly

Rare but Important
- Myotonic Dystrophy
- Multiple Endocrine Neoplasia Type IIB
- Frontometaphyseal Dysplasia
- Stickler Disease
- Chromosome XYY (Klinefelter) Syndrome
- Ichthyosis Syndrome
- Cleidocranial Dysplasia

ESSENTIAL INFORMATION

Key Differential Diagnosis Issues
- Arachnodactyly is a rare condition, so the list of "common" diagnoses is relative
- Arachnodactyly itself is nonspecific; clinical or rarely other radiographic features may differentiate the diagnoses
- Metacarpal index > 8.8 (male) or 9.4 (female)
  - Obtained by dividing the sum of the lengths of 2nd through 5th metacarpals by the sum of their respective widths

Helpful Clues for Common Diagnoses
- **Marfan Syndrome**
  - Dural ectasia with lumbar vertebral body scalloping
  - Spondylolisthesis, ± spondylolysis
  - Aortic root dilatation; may dissect ascending aorta
  - Lens dislocation, myopia
  - Pectus carinatum or excavatum
  - Hypermobility of joints
- **Ehlers-Danlos**
  - Dural ectasia with lumbar vertebral body scalloping
  - Hypermobility of joints
  - Skin hyperextensibility
  - Multiple aneurysms (friable vessels)
- **Localized Giantism (Mimic)**
  - Vascular malformations, macrodystrophia lipomatosa, Klippel Trenaunay Weber

Helpful Clues for Less Common Diagnoses
- **Homocystinuria**
  - Arachnodactyly plus osteopenia
  - May have joint laxity
    - More frequently develop joint contractures
  - Pectus carinatum or excavatum
  - Lens subluxation, myopia
  - Mental deficiency
  - Thromboembolic episodes
- **Congenital Contractural Arachnodactyly**
  - Long thin limbs, scoliosis, joint contractures
  - No eye or cardiac abnormalities

Marfan Syndrome

Posteroanterior radiograph shows fairly uniform elongation of the metacarpals, and especially proximal phalanges, in a patient with Marfan syndrome.

Marfan Syndrome

Lateral radiograph from the same patient shown in the previous image shows posterior scalloping and tall vertebral bodies ➡, typical of and helping to confirm the diagnosis of Marfan syndrome.

ARACHNODACTYLY

Localized Giantism (Mimic)

Localized Giantism (Mimic)

(Left) Posteroanterior radiograph shows overgrowth of the 2nd and 3rd digits contributing to a focal "arachnodactyly". This patient had Klippel Trenaunay Weber syndrome. (Right) AP radiograph shows focal overgrowth of the 1st, 2nd, and 3rd digits of the foot (compare with 4th and 5th toes). This may mimic arachnodactyly, though it is not as uniform as would be expected for true arachnodactyly. In this case, the patient had macrodystrophia lipomatosa.

Homocystinuria

Homocystinuria

(Left) PA radiograph shows fairly uniform elongation of the metacarpals and especially proximal phalanges, allowing the nonspecific diagnosis of arachnodactyly. The bones are osteopenic. (Right) Lateral radiograph in the same patient as previous image shows the bones are diffusely osteoporotic. There is mild platyspondyly from multiple compression fractures. The combination of arachnodactyly and osteopenia is seen with homocystinuria.

Ichthyosis Syndrome

Ichthyosis Syndrome

(Left) Posteroanterior radiograph shows mild arachnodactyly. There is also irregularity along the skin surface ➡; clinically the skin disease was proven ichthyosis. (Right) Lateral radiograph obtained 8 years later in the same patient as the previous image shows prominent spondylosis ➡. This was present throughout the spine in this 22 year old and resulted from use of retinoids for the skin disease. (†MSK Req).

SOFT TISSUE MASS IN A FINGER

DIFFERENTIAL DIAGNOSIS

Common
- Mucoid Cysts
- Giant Cell Tumor Tendon Sheath
- Hematoma
- Gout
- Soft Tissue Abscess
- Infectious Tenosynovitis
- Foreign Body
  - Paint Gun Injury
- Granulation Tissue
- Fibroma of Tendon Sheath
- Glomus Tumor
- Epidermal Inclusion Cyst
- Rheumatoid Nodule

Less Common
- Progressive Systemic Sclerosis
- Tumoral (Idiopathic) Calcinosis
- Heterotopic Ossification
- Soft Tissue Chondroma
- Hemangioma, Soft Tissue
- Arteriovenous Malformation
- Pyrophosphate Arthropathy

Rare but Important
- Malignant Fibrous Histiocytoma
- Chondrosarcoma
- Metastasis, Subcutaneous
- Lipoma, Soft Tissue
- Tenosynovial Chondromatosis
- Klippel Trenaunay Weber Syndrome
- Acral Myxoinflammatory Fibroblastic Sarcoma

ESSENTIAL INFORMATION

Helpful Clues for Common Diagnoses
- **Mucoid Cysts**
  - a.k.a., ganglion cyst
  - Follows fluid signal intensity on all sequences
  - Thin peripheral rim of enhancement
    - Lacks central enhancement
  - Located near joint or tendon sheath
  - May have loculations or internal septations
- **Giant Cell Tumor Tendon Sheath**
  - Low to intermediate signal mass on T1WI & T2WI MR
    - Preferential location along volar aspect of finger

- Enhances more intensely than fibroma of tendon sheath
- Lacks surrounding soft tissue edema
- **Hematoma**
  - Absence of central enhancement helps differentiate from hemorrhagic tumor
  - Surrounding soft tissue edema
- **Gout**
  - Multiple gouty tophi often present
    - Tophi may show mild, irregular enhancement
  - Bone erosions with overhanging edges
- **Soft Tissue Abscess**
  - Thick, irregularly enhancing border
  - Central nonenhancing necrosis or debris
- **Infectious Tenosynovitis**
  - Fluid & debris in tendon sheath
  - More prominent enhancement than inflammatory tenosynovitis
- **Foreign Body**
  - Wide variety of embedded material can produce an inflammatory response
  - Tends to have superficial location
  - **Paint Gun Injury**
    - Lead in paint is visible on radiographs
- **Fibroma of Tendon Sheath**
  - Mass is isointense or hypointense to skeletal muscle on T1WI & T2WI MR
  - May have very low signal regions of collagen within mass
  - Enhancement variable
    - 50% moderate to marked enhancement
    - 50% little to no enhancement
- **Glomus Tumor**
  - Soft tissue mass centered in nail bed
  - Pressure erosion of distal phalanx
  - No matrix
- **Rheumatoid Nodule**
  - Soft tissue mass associated with changes of rheumatoid arthritis
  - Pressure erosion of underlying bone

Helpful Clues for Less Common Diagnoses
- **Progressive Systemic Sclerosis**
  - Lobulated soft tissue calcifications
  - Additional findings of soft tissue atrophy & acroosteolysis
- **Tumoral (Idiopathic) Calcinosis**
  - Calcified masses around joints
  - Associated with chronic renal disease
  - More common around large joints
- **Heterotopic Ossification**

SOFT TISSUE MASS IN A FINGER

- ○ Ossified mass in soft tissues
- ○ Cleavage plane between mass & bone
- ○ Matures peripheral to central
- **Soft Tissue Chondroma**
  - ○ Mass with chondroid matrix
  - ○ Adjacent to bone surface
- **Hemangioma, Soft Tissue**
  - ○ Slightly higher signal than muscle on T1WI MR
  - ○ Very high signal on T2WI MR
  - ○ Internal septa, lobulated borders
  - ○ Fat & fibrous tissue may be visible in addition to vascular channels
  - ○ Can be difficult to differentiate arteries from veins
    - ▪ Cavernous hemangioma is most common subtype
- **Arteriovenous Malformation**
  - ○ Enlarged vascular channels
  - ○ Marked vascular enhancement
  - ○ May contain fat
- **Pyrophosphate Arthropathy**
  - ○ Lobulated calcified mass
  - ○ Additional findings of chondrocalcinosis & narrowing of radiocarpal and metacarpophalangeal joint spaces

Helpful Clues for Rare Diagnoses
- **Malignant Fibrous Histiocytoma**
  - ○ Soft tissue mass with heterogeneous signal + enhancement on MR
  - ○ May have well-defined borders
  - ○ Hemorrhage & edema can obscure underlying mass

- **Chondrosarcoma**
  - ○ Soft tissue mass originating from a destructive bone lesion
  - ○ Chondroid matrix usually present
  - ○ Most common site in hand is proximal phalanx
- **Metastasis, Subcutaneous**
  - ○ Nonspecific, heterogeneously enhancing mass most common
  - ○ History of malignant melanoma or high grade adenocarcinoma
- **Lipoma, Soft Tissue**
  - ○ Fat signal intensity on all MR sequences
  - ○ Thin septations without solid soft tissue nodules
  - ○ May produce mass effect on neurovascular structures in confined spaces, e.g., carpal tunnel
- **Tenosynovial Chondromatosis**
  - ○ Multiple round to oval cartilaginous or osseous bodies of similar size within tendon sheath
    - ▪ Commonly visible on radiographs
  - ○ May cause pressure erosion of adjacent bone
- **Klippel Trenaunay Weber Syndrome**
  - ○ Bone and soft tissue hypertrophy
  - ○ Capillary hemangiomas & varicose veins
  - ○ Arteriovenous fistulas are rarely found in enlarged regions
- **Acral Myxoinflammatory Fibroblastic Sarcoma**
  - ○ Ill-defined mass in distal extremity
  - ○ Can mimic an inflammatory process

Giant Cell Tumor Tendon Sheath

Posteroanterior radiograph shows a soft tissue mass ➡ causing smooth, extrinsic erosion ⇨ around the thumb metacarpophalangeal joint.

Giant Cell Tumor Tendon Sheath

Oblique T2WI MR shows a large intermediate signal intensity soft tissue mass ➡, which erodes the adjacent bones and surrounds the flexor tendon of the thumb.

SOFT TISSUE MASS IN A FINGER

Gout

Infectious Tenosynovitis

(Left) Posteroanterior radiograph shows an impressive soft tissue tophus ⇨, with density typical of sodium urate deposition. There is a large erosion at the PIP that has resulted in a classic overhanging edge ⇨. *(Right)* Axial T1 C+ FS MR of the second finger shows abnormal enhancing soft tissue ⇨ around and particularly deep to the superficialis ➔ and profunda ⇨ flexor tendons of the digit. This was caused by a puncture wound with secondary infection.

Foreign Body

Foreign Body

(Left) Sagittal T1WI MR demonstrates an ill-defined, ovoid nodular lesion ➔ in the volar soft tissues of the distal aspect of the fifth finger. This collection is isointense to muscle and abuts the skin surface. *(Right)* Sagittal T2WI FS MR in the same patient as the previous image again shows the nodular lesion ➔, which has high signal on T2WI. There was moderate enhancement, except for a 2 mm focus that likely was the clinically-reported rose thorn fragment.

Paint Gun Injury

Granulation Tissue

(Left) Lateral radiograph shows radiodense foreign material ➔ in the soft tissues of the index finger. Paint gun injuries in which there is skin penetration have this typical appearance due to the lead in the paint. *(Right)* Axial T2WI MR shows an ill-defined enhancing lesion ➔ along the dorsal aspect of the proximal interphalangeal joint of the index finger. The extensor tendon ➔ is visualized within this enhancing lesion. The patient had a history of finger laceration.

SOFT TISSUE MASS IN A FINGER

Fibroma of Tendon Sheath

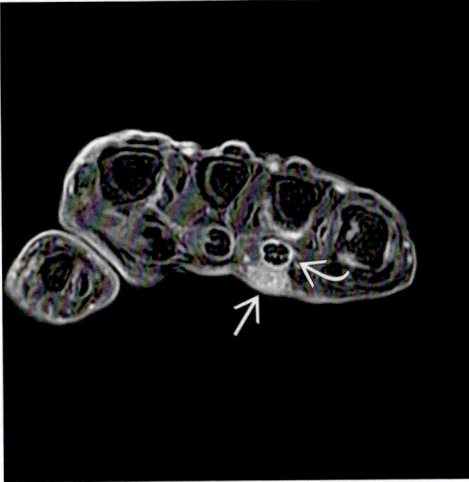

Glomus Tumor

(Left) Axial T1 C+ FS MR with subtraction shows an inhomogeneously enhancing mass ➡ abutting the mildly enhancing flexor tendon sheath ➡. The mass had intermediate to low signal on T1WI and T2WI. A giant cell tumor of tendon sheath could have a similar appearance. *(Right)* Axial T2WI MR demonstrates a well-defined, solid, subungual tumor ➡ that extends radially and ulnarly to almost surround the shaft of the distal phalanx. The lesion moderately enhanced.

Glomus Tumor

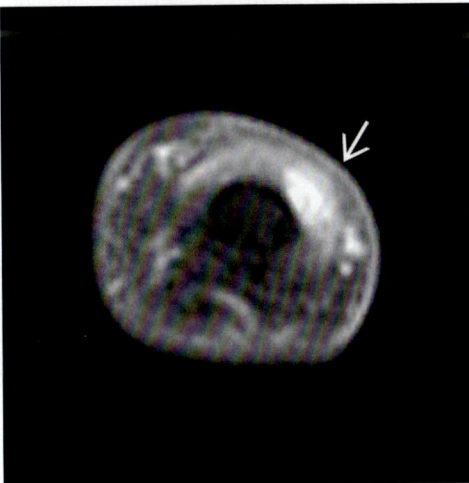

Epidermal Inclusion Cyst

(Left) Axial T1 C+ FS MR demonstrates a mass ➡ involving subungual space of the distal long finger. It is well-defined, solid, and moderately enhancing. *(Right)* Oblique radiograph shows a lytic lesion involving the terminal phalanx ➡. There is circumferential soft tissue swelling and suggestion of invasion from the soft tissues beneath the nail bed. This makes either glomus tumor or epidermal inclusion cyst the most likely diagnosis; the latter was proven.

Rheumatoid Nodule

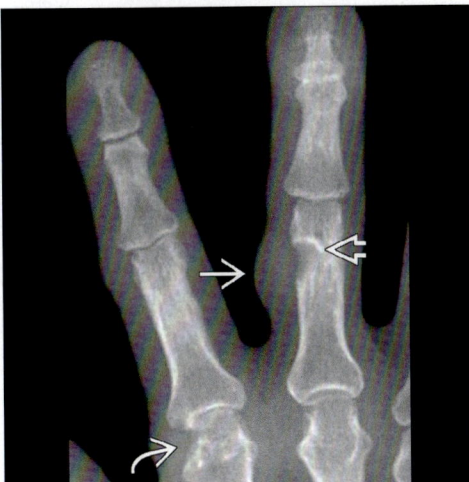

Progressive Systemic Sclerosis

(Left) Posteroanterior radiograph shows a focal soft tissue nodule ➡ with scalloping of the underlying bone ➡. There is second metacarpophalangeal joint space narrowing, along with marginal erosions along the radial side of the metacarpal head ➡, all typical of rheumatoid arthritis. *(Right)* Posteroanterior radiograph shows multiple lobular calcifications ➡, which have a predominantly periarticular location. The calcifications produce palpable soft tissue masses.

SOFT TISSUE MASS IN A FINGER

(Left) Posteroanterior radiograph shows several foci of soft tissue dystrophic calcification ➡, most notably seen around the base of the first metacarpal ⇨. The terminal phalanges show acroosteolysis ➡, with tapered soft tissues. **(Right)** Oblique radiograph shows tumoral calcinosis ➡ involving the soft tissues of the thumb. Soft tissue calcification is particularly prominent in patients with renal osteodystrophy once they are treated with dialysis.

Progressive Systemic Sclerosis

Tumoral (Idiopathic) Calcinosis

(Left) Posteroanterior radiograph shows soft tissue calcification ➡ in a patient with end-stage renal disease, now on dialysis. There are no other abnormalities to suggest renal osteodystrophy. **(Right)** Posteroanterior radiograph shows calcified soft tissue masses ➡ and vascular calcifications ⇨. Findings are consistent with osteomalacia and dystrophic calcification due to chronic renal disease.

Tumoral (Idiopathic) Calcinosis

Tumoral (Idiopathic) Calcinosis

(Left) Oblique radiograph shows an ossified mass ➡ in the soft tissues dorsal and ulnar to the third digit middle phalanx. There is a cleavage plane between the bone and ossification in the soft tissue. **(Right)** Posteroanterior radiograph demonstrates a nonspecific, irregular soft tissue calcification ➡. This was presumed to represent post-traumatic soft tissue calcification due to instability in this manual laborer.

Heterotopic Ossification

Heterotopic Ossification

SOFT TISSUE MASS IN A FINGER

Soft Tissue Chondroma

Hemangioma, Soft Tissue

(Left) Posteroanterior radiograph shows a nonspecific mass ➔ in the soft tissues adjacent to the distal interphalangeal joint. The mass contains faint calcification. On excision, this was identified as a periosteal chondroma. (Right) Lateral radiograph shows bulky soft tissues, with fatty stroma of the forearm and hand ➔. Although no phleboliths are present, this proved to be a hemangioma.

Arteriovenous Malformation

Metastasis, Subcutaneous

(Left) MRA shows a large arteriovenous malformation ➔ in the circumferential subcutaneous soft tissues of the ring finger, predominantly at the level of the middle and proximal phalanges. There was no involvement of the underlying bone except for overgrowth. (Right) Axial T1 C+ FS MR shows a moderately enhancing mass ➔ with a 2 mm hypo-enhancing area, which is nonspecific. Metastatic adenocarcinoma was found on biopsy.

Tenosynovial Chondromatosis

Klippel Trenaunay Weber Syndrome

(Left) Lateral T2WI FS MR shows a large soft tissue mass ➔ at the dorsal aspect of the hand which extended into the base of the third digit. Numerous oval bodies are highly suggestive of chondromatosis. (Right) Posteroanterior radiograph shows diffuse hypertrophy ➔ of the second and third digits and metacarpals involving both the bony structures and subcutaneous fat ➔, which is markedly thickened and can be mass-like clinically.

ACROOSTEOLYSIS

DIFFERENTIAL DIAGNOSIS

Common
- Trauma: Amputation
- Hyperparathyroidism (HPTH)
- Progressive Systemic Sclerosis (PSS)
- Thermal Injury
  - Thermal Injury, Frostbite
  - Thermal Injury, Burns

Less Common
- Psoriatic Arthritis (PSA)
- Vasculitis
  - Raynaud Disease
- Diabetes (Neuropathic)
- Congenital Indifference/Insensitivity to Pain
- Meningococcemia

Rare but Important
- Leprosy
- Lesch-Nyhan
- Hajdu-Cheney Acroosteolysis Syndrome
- Polyvinyl Chloride (PVC)
- Occupational Acroosteolysis
- Pycnodysostosis
- Multicentric Reticulohistiocytosis
- Amniotic Band Syndrome
- Progeria
- Pachydermoperiostosis
- Sarcoidosis
- Epidermolysis Bullosa
- Venom Induced Complications
- Complications of Dilantin

ESSENTIAL INFORMATION

Key Differential Diagnosis Issues
- **Hint:** Presence & character of soft tissue calcification may help make diagnosis
  - HPTH: Globular soft tissue calcification & small vessel calcification
  - PSS (a.k.a., scleroderma): Globular calcification very often present
  - Thermal injury (burns): Globular calcification, infrequently present
  - Leprosy: Linear calcification in digital nerve
- **Hint:** First 6 diagnoses on list are far, far more prevalent than others

Helpful Clues for Common Diagnoses
- **Trauma: Amputation**
  - Generally a clean transverse or oblique osseous edge
  - 2-3 adjacent: Snowblower or lawn mower injury
- **Hyperparathyroidism (HPTH)**
  - Resorption of the tufts of distal phalanges is one of the resorptive processes in HPTH
    - May be subtle, or severe, with dissolution of entire tuft
    - Overlying soft tissues remain normal in size (no tapering)
  - **Hint:** Watch for other signs of HPTH
    - Subperiosteal, subligamentous, subchondral resorption
    - Soft tissue or vascular calcification
    - Brown tumors
- **Progressive Systemic Sclerosis (PSS)**
  - Resorption of tufts is common
  - Associated tapering of distal soft tissues, matching that of osseous resorption
  - May have globular soft tissue calcification
  - Systemic abnormality: Involvement of lungs, GI system (particularly esophagus)
- **Thermal Injury, Frostbite**
  - Frostbite in adult may result in tuft resorption
  - Frostbite in child results in injury to epiphyses of distal phalanges
    - Resorption of epiphyses & cessation of growth → short distal phalanges
  - Usually have normal thumb
    - When cold, thumb is usually curled into palm and protected
- **Thermal Injury, Burns**
  - Soft tissue contractures
  - Acroosteolysis, involves both bone and soft tissues
  - May have associated globular soft tissue calcification

Helpful Clues for Less Common Diagnoses
- **Psoriatic Arthritis (PSA)**
  - Distal tuft resorption may be absent, subtle, or severe
  - Distal tuft may be sclerotic ("ivory tuft")
  - **Hint:** Watch for other signs of PSA
    - "Sausage digit" type of soft tissue swelling
    - Periostitis
    - Erosive or mixed erosive/productive articular disease, particular interphalangeal joints

- End stage: Arthritis mutilans, with telescoping digits and pencil-in-cup deformities
- **Vasculitis**
  - Any type of vasculitis may affect small terminal vessels in digits
  - Raynaud and systemic lupus erythematosus are typical
  - Results in acroosteolysis & loss of soft tissues, often with ulceration
- **Diabetes (Neuropathic)**
  - Neuropathic osseous destruction of terminal digits not as common as neuropathic joint disease
  - Fragmentation of bone
  - **Hint**: Watch for other signs of diabetes
    - Charcot joints, especially Lisfranc
    - Small vessel calcification
- **Congenital Indifference/Insensitivity to Pain**
  - Neuropathic fragmentation & destruction of terminal digits
  - Often associated scarring of soft tissues (particularly from burns on stove, but any trauma may be causative)
  - **Hint**: Patient also may have corneal scarring & Charcot joints involving lower extremity
- **Meningococcemia**
  - Usually involves epiphyses, with coning; true acroosteolysis is rare

Helpful Clues for Rare Diagnoses
- **Leprosy**

- Acroosteolysis may be severe, involving all phalanges as well as metacarpals
- Linear calcification of digital nerve
- **Lesch-Nyhan**
  - X-linked disorder of male children
  - Compulsive self-mutilation by biting fingers & lips
  - Both soft tissue & osseous destruction
- **Hajdu-Cheney Acroosteolysis Syndrome**
  - Osteolysis, particularly of distal phalanges hands & feet
  - May have skull abnormalities (Wormian bones, dolichocephalic skull with basilar impression, delayed suture closure)
- **Polyvinyl Chloride (PVC)**
  - Fairly distinct form of acroosteolysis, with lucency crossing the neck of distal phalanx & consequent shortening
  - Tuft & soft tissues usually intact
- **Occupational Acroosteolysis**
  - Guitar players rarely develop acroosteolysis, with lucency crossing neck of distal phalanx (mimicking PVC)
- **Pycnodysostosis**
  - Combination of diffuse osseous density & acroosteolysis
- **Multicentric Reticulohistiocytosis**
  - Combination of acroosteolysis, DIP erosions, & nodules on fingers
- **Amniotic Band Syndrome**
  - Band may cause necrosis & amputation of fingers in any pattern, depending on entrapment

Hyperparathyroidism (HPTH)

PA radiograph shows severe acroosteolysis involving all the digits ➡. The bones are osteoporotic, and there is prominent subperiosteal resorption at the radial aspect of the phalanges ➡ in this patient with HPTH.

Progressive Systemic Sclerosis (PSS)

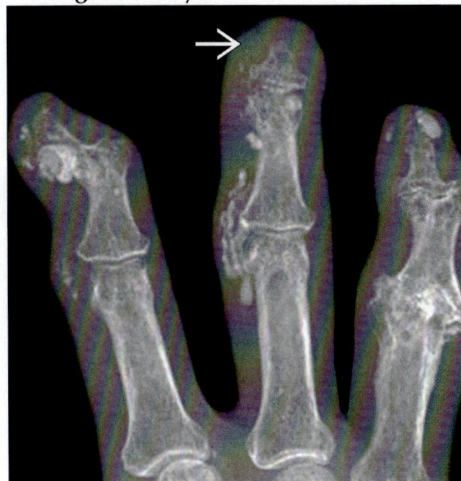

PA radiograph shows acroosteolysis, most severe at the 3rd terminal phalanx ➡. The patient has significant soft tissue calcification as well; the findings are typical of progressive systemic sclerosis (a.k.a., scleroderma).

ACROOSTEOLYSIS

Thermal Injury, Frostbite

Thermal Injury, Frostbite

(Left) Posteroanterior radiograph shows absence of epiphyses of terminal digits 2-5 ➡, indicating injury. This results in shortening of the terminal digit, a form of acroosteolysis. The epiphysis is at greater risk than the tuft for thermal injury. Note the thumb is normal ➡, typical of frostbite. *(Right)* Lateral radiograph shows short terminal phalanges of digits 2-5 ➡ & normal length of terminal phalanx of the thumb ➡, sequela of frostbite during childhood.

Thermal Injury, Burns

Psoriatic Arthritis (PSA)

(Left) Lateral radiograph shows severe contractures of digits 1 & 2, with more mild contractures of the other digits. There is significant acroosteolysis at all the terminal phalanges ➡. The combination is typical of burn injury. *(Right)* Oblique radiograph of both thumbs shows acroosteolysis of the tufts ➡ in a patient with psoriatic arthritis. Note the erosive changes involving the interphalangeal joints. Acroosteolysis is seen with moderate frequency in psoriatic arthritis.

Psoriatic Arthritis (PSA)

Vasculitis

(Left) Anteroposterior radiograph shows severe changes of end-stage psoriatic arthritis, including erosive change and ankylosis at the great toe ➡. These patients may develop prominent acroosteolysis ➡, as in this case. *(Right)* Posteroanterior radiograph shows early acroosteolysis ➡ and soft tissue tapering with ulceration ➡ in a patient with lupus vasculitis and dry gangrene.

ACROOSTEOLYSIS

Raynaud Disease

Leprosy

(Left) Posteroanterior radiograph shows tapering of the soft tissues of the terminal phalanges ➡ with osteolysis involving the right thumb and both index fingers. The findings are nonspecific, but this patient had Raynaud disease. *(Right)* Posteroanterior radiograph shows severe acroosteolysis involving all the fingers, most significantly the 4th & 5th digits ➡. Additionally, there is linear calcification of a digital nerve ➡; this is pathognomonic for leprosy. (†MSK Req).

Polyvinyl Chloride (PVC)

Pycnodysostosis

(Left) Posteroanterior radiograph shows shortening of the terminal phalanges of digits 1-3, with lucent lines crossing the tufts ➡. This is a typical acroosteolysis pattern for polyvinyl chloride workers. It is also rarely seen in guitar players. *(Right)* AP radiograph shows dense bones & acroosteolysis of the terminal phalanges ➡. There is also a transverse fracture through the 5th metatarsal ➡ & other bones (not shown). This combination is typical of pycnodysostosis.

Multicentric Reticulohistiocytosis

Amniotic Band Syndrome

(Left) Posteroanterior radiograph shows mild acroosteolysis ➡ associated with nodularity and erosive change at the interphalangeal joint ➡. The combination of features is typical of a rare diagnosis, multicentric reticulohistiocytosis. *(Right)* PA radiograph shows severe acroosteolysis of the 2nd and 3rd fingers ➡ along with a pressure erosion on the proximal phalanx of the thumb. This was the only site of abnormality in this patient with amniotic bands.

ACROOSTEOSCLEROSIS

DIFFERENTIAL DIAGNOSIS

Common
- Normal Variant
- Psoriatic Arthritis
- Rheumatoid Arthritis
- Enostosis (Bone Island)
- Osteopoikilosis
- Progressive Systemic Sclerosis
- Sarcoidosis

Less Common
- Fracture Healing Process
- Chronic Osteomyelitis
- Osteopetrosis
- Systemic Lupus Erythematosus
- Lymphoma, Hodgkin
- Hepatitis
- Osteonecrosis

Rare but Important
- Paget Disease
- Hyperparathyroidism
- Hyperparathyroidism, Healed Brown Tumors
- Thermal Injury, Frostbite
- Melorheostosis
- Metastasis, Osteoblastic
- POEMS
- Foreign Body
- Tuberous Sclerosis

ESSENTIAL INFORMATION

Key Differential Diagnosis Issues
- Increased density of the terminal phalanges

- o Very uncommon finding, even for "common" diagnoses
- o Sclerosis is typically subtle

Helpful Clues for Common Diagnoses
- **Normal Variant**
  - o Endosteal thickening
  - o Young adult female predominant
- **Psoriatic Arthritis**
  - o Asymmetric polyarthritis, distal interphalangeal joint involvement
- **Rheumatoid Arthritis**
  - o Bilateral, symmetric joint changes
  - o Marginal erosions & MCP ulnar deviation
- **Osteopoikilosis**
  - o Multiple bone islands
  - o Clustered around joints
  - o Differentiate from sclerotic metastases
- **Sarcoidosis**
  - o Lacy appearance of phalanges

Helpful Clues for Less Common Diagnoses
- **Chronic Osteomyelitis**
  - o Permeative destruction early with late sclerotic changes ± sequestrum
- **Osteopetrosis**
  - o Diffuse bone sclerosis that lacks definition between medulla & cortex

Helpful Clues for Rare Diagnoses
- **Thermal Injury, Frostbite**
  - o Focal or asymmetric distribution with adjacent normal digits possible
- **Tuberous Sclerosis**
  - o Irregular sclerotic & lytic lesions throughout skeleton

Psoriatic Arthritis

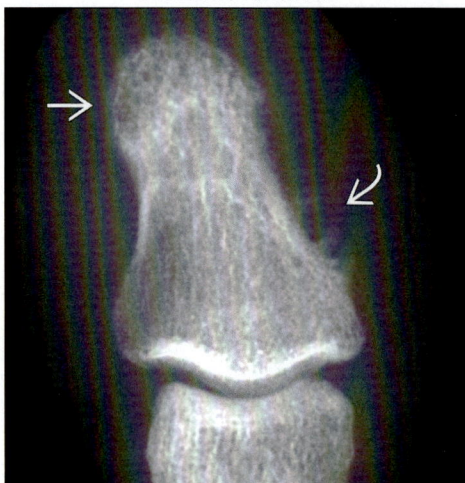

Posteroanterior radiograph shows faint sclerosis ➡ of the distal tuft of the digit. The presence of periosteal new bone ➡ suggests the diagnosis of psoriatic arthritis.

Progressive Systemic Sclerosis

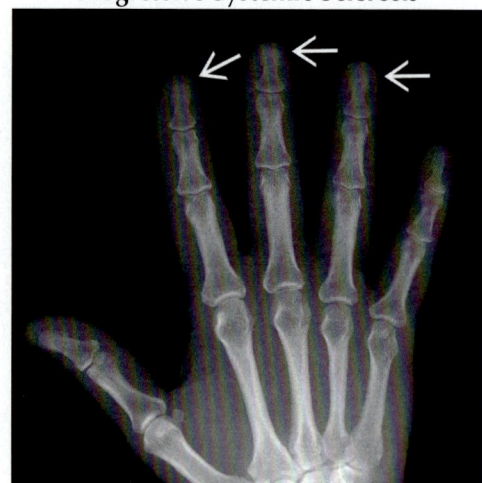

Posteroanterior radiograph shows increased density of the distal phalangeal tufts ➡, a nonspecific finding that is reflective of scleroderma in this case.

ACROOSTEOSCLEROSIS

Chronic Osteomyelitis

Hyperparathyroidism, Healed Brown Tumors

(Left) PA radiograph shows sclerosis of the index finger distal phalanx in this diabetic patient with treated osteomyelitis ➡. Note the prior amputation ➡ of the third digit and severe atherosclerotic disease ➡. *(Right)* Posteroanterior radiograph shows a round sclerotic focus ➡ in the tuft of the index finger. This finding developed after the patient was treated for hyperparathyroidism, increasing the likelihood that it represents a healed Brown tumor.

Thermal Injury, Frostbite

Melorheostosis

(Left) Oblique radiograph shows the terminal phalanges of the second through fifth digits to be short and faintly sclerotic ➡. Note that the terminal phalanx of the thumb is normal in size ➡. This represents the sequela of frostbite during childhood. *(Right)* Oblique radiograph shows sclerosis of the index finger distal tuft ➡. Sclerosis of the proximal and middle phalanges of the second and third digits ➡ is also due to melorheostosis.

Foreign Body

Tuberous Sclerosis

(Left) Posteroanterior radiograph shows two dense foci ➡ surrounded by a lucent region in the distal tuft of the index finger. The patient had embedded sewing needle fragments with a surrounding epidermoid inclusion cyst. *(Right)* Posteroanterior radiograph shows a sclerotic appearance of the ring finger distal tuft ➡. This may be partially artifactual due to multiple lytic lesions. A soft tissue mass adjacent to the sclerotic area was due to a periungual fibroma.

PHALANGEAL CYSTIC/LYTIC LESIONS

DIFFERENTIAL DIAGNOSIS

Common
- Enchondroma
- Osteoarthritis (OA)
- Gout
- Aneurysmal Bone Cyst (ABC)
- Giant Cell Tumor (GCT)
- Osteomyelitis
- Hyperparathyroidism, Brown Tumor (HPTH)
- Arthroplasty Component Wear/Particle Disease
- Giant Cell Tumor Tendon Sheath (Mimic)

Less Common
- Unicameral Bone Cyst (UBC)
- Glomus Tumor
- Epidermal Inclusion Cyst
- Sarcoidosis
- Robust Rheumatoid Arthritis

Rare but Important
- Langerhans Cell Histiocytosis (LCH)
- Ollier Disease
- Maffucci Syndrome
- Vascular Tumors, Osseous
- Fibrous Dysplasia (FD)
- Amyloid Deposition
- Tuberous Sclerosis

ESSENTIAL INFORMATION

Key Differential Diagnosis Issues
- **Hint**: Watch for associated arthritic process
- **Hint**: True non-aggressive lytic phalangeal lesions most commonly are one of the following
  - Enchondroma > > ABC, GCT, UBC
  - If there is no matrix present in an enchondroma, may not be able to differentiate by radiograph; MR is useful

Helpful Clues for Common Diagnoses
- **Enchondroma**
  - Most common true lesion of phalanges
  - Lytic ± chondroid matrix
  - May be expansile/bubbly, appearing more aggressive than it acts
- **Osteoarthritis (OA)**
  - Subchondral cyst formation occasionally predominates relative to osteophyte formation, especially in erosive OA
  - Watch for loss of cartilage width & pattern of DIP joints predominating
- **Gout**
  - Inactive erosions are well-marginated & may give appearance of lytic lesion
  - Juxtacortical erosions may distract from the arthritic appearance
  - Cartilage destruction is late in process; may not appear to be an arthritis
  - Watch for dense soft tissue tophi
- **Aneurysmal Bone Cyst (ABC)**
  - Lytic, expansile
  - Generally < 30 years of age
  - Usually have fluid-fluid levels
- **Giant Cell Tumor (GCT)**
  - Lytic, expansile
  - Unlike GCT in other bones, may occur prior to skeletal maturation
  - MR: Generally solid lesion with some focal low signal regions on T2; occasional fluid-fluid levels
- **Osteomyelitis**
  - Digits at risk for direct inoculation via trauma
  - Great toe distal phalanx particularly at risk
    - Nail bed base is directly adjacent to periosteum of distal phalanx
    - "Stubbed toe" may result in nail bed hematoma & subsequent infection
  - Lytic destruction, periosteal reaction
- **Hyperparathyroidism, Brown Tumor (HPTH)**
  - Often multiple
  - Lytic, generally geographic
  - Watch for other signs of bone resorption
    - Subperiosteal (generally radial side, middle phalanx), endosteal
    - Tuft acroosteolysis
- **Arthroplasty Component Wear/Particle Disease**
  - Silastic & similar arthroplasties used in hand & foot
  - Breakdown is common due to instability, malalignment
  - Particles elicit synovitis & particle disease, resulting in massive osteolysis
  - Osteolysis can be so prominent that the prosthesis may be overlooked
- **Giant Cell Tumor Tendon Sheath (Mimic)**
  - Soft tissue mass arising in tendon sheath

○ Focal extrinsic bone erosion may appear as lytic lesion
○ Watch for soft tissue mass adjacent to lesion
○ MR: Mass mostly low signal on T2; enhances

Helpful Clues for Less Common Diagnoses
• **Unicameral Bone Cyst (UBC)**
  ○ Less common but radiographically indistinguishable from lytic enchondroma, ABC, GCT
  ○ Most commonly seen in skeletally immature patient
• **Glomus Tumor**
  ○ Dermal hemangiopericytoma, commonly located beneath nail bed
  ○ Causes extrinsic scalloping of dorsal cortex distal phalanx; if large, appears on radiograph as lytic lesion
  ○ Nonspecific MR low signal T1, high signal T2, enhancing lesion
  ○ Diagnosis suggested by location
• **Epidermal Inclusion Cyst**
  ○ Benign lesion of cutis or subcutis
  ○ May result in local invasion of phalanx, usually terminal
• **Sarcoidosis**
  ○ Lytic, often "lacy" pattern in phalanges
• **Robust Rheumatoid Arthritis**
  ○ Large subchondral cysts develop in RA patient with continued activity
  ○ Watch for multiple digit involvement, particularly MCP disease

Helpful Clues for Rare Diagnoses
• **Langerhans Cell Histiocytosis (LCH)**
  ○ Rare lytic lesion, usually in young child
  ○ May be geographic or more aggressive, with rapid growth
  ○ Often polyostotic
• **Ollier Disease**
  ○ Multiple enchondromas in phalanges, usually with chondroid matrix
  ○ Usually other long bones affected as well
  ○ Often unilateral limb involvement
• **Maffucci Syndrome**
  ○ Similar to Ollier, but with soft tissue hemangiomas
  ○ Watch for phleboliths
• **Vascular Tumors, Osseous**
  ○ Range of benign to malignant vascular tumors may involve phalanges
  ○ Similar range of appearance from benign to aggressive
  ○ Often polyostotic
  ○ Lower extremity > upper extremity
• **Fibrous Dysplasia (FD)**
  ○ Rare involvement of digits, similar to FD elsewhere
• **Amyloid Deposition**
  ○ Subchondral cysts, erosions may mimic lytic lesion, especially DIP
  ○ Watch for lumpy soft tissue masses
  ○ Low T2 signal on MR
• **Tuberous Sclerosis**
  ○ Rare lytic lesion, non-aggressive
  ○ May have dense periosteal reaction

Enchondroma

PA radiograph shows lytic phalangeal lesion containing chondroid matrix. There is a pathologic fracture. Appearance is classic for enchondroma, the most common osseous lesion of the phalanges. (†MSK Req).

Enchondroma

PA radiograph shows a large lytic geographic lesion. There is no chondroid matrix present. Even without matrix, enchondroma is the most likely diagnosis, though other lesions are not excluded. (†MSK Req).

PHALANGEAL CYSTIC/LYTIC LESIONS

Osteoarthritis (OA)

Gout

(Left) PA radiograph shows lytic "lesions" within subchondral bone of middle phalanx ➡. Note that the process is articular; there is cartilage loss & marginal erosions are present. This is erosive osteoarthritis; subchondral cysts may give the appearance of lesions. *(Right)* AP radiograph shows a lytic lesion in the proximal phalanx ➡ of a young adult with end-stage renal disease. Lesion proved to be a gouty deposit, which is not uncommon in such patients.

Gout

Aneurysmal Bone Cyst (ABC)

(Left) Posteroanterior radiograph shows multiple well-circumscribed lytic lesions located on either side of the distal IP joint ➡. There is joint space narrowing as well, suggesting an arthritic process. Note the soft tissue tophus ➡. The findings are typical of gout. *(Right)* Oblique radiograph shows a lytic lesion at the distal end of the bone ➡ in a young adult. Without matrix, ABC or GCT should be considered, in addition to enchondroma. Biopsy proved the lesion to be ABC.

Aneurysmal Bone Cyst (ABC)

Aneurysmal Bone Cyst (ABC)

(Left) AP radiograph shows a lytic lesion expanding and occupying the entirety of the distal phalanx ➡. The appearance is nonspecific; it could represent enchondroma, ABC, GCT, or several other lesions. *(Right)* Sagittal T2WI FS MR of the same patient shows multiple fluid levels occupying the entire lesion ➡. Although fluid levels can occur in other lesions, their presence makes ABC the most likely diagnosis; this was proven at surgery. (†MSK Req).

PHALANGEAL CYSTIC/LYTIC LESIONS

Giant Cell Tumor (GCT)

Giant Cell Tumor (GCT)

(Left) PA radiograph shows expanded lytic lesion in subchondral aspect of a phalanx ➡. Image shows no differentiating features between ABC, GCT, or lytic enchondroma; at biopsy this was GCT. *(Right)* PA radiograph shows a lytic, moderately aggressive lesion in subchondral region of a phalanx. There is no sclerotic margin, & there is cortical breakthrough ➡. This is more aggressive than expected for lytic enchondroma, but not for GCT.

Osteomyelitis

Hyperparathyroidism, Brown Tumor (HPTH)

(Left) Oblique radiograph shows moderately aggressive lytic lesion of bone adjacent to nail bed in a child's great toe ➡. Trauma from stubbing the toe may result in infection due to intimate relationship of nail bed to periosteum. *(Right)* PA radiograph shows multiple lytic lesions of phalanges ➡ which are non-aggressive but otherwise nonspecific. Multiplicity should make one consider Brown tumor of HPTH. In addition, there is endosteal resorption ➡, confirming diagnosis.

Hyperparathyroidism, Brown Tumor (HPTH)

Arthroplasty Component Wear/Particle Disease

(Left) Posteroanterior radiograph shows lytic lesion in a phalanx ➡, itself otherwise nonspecific. However, there is also prominent subperiosteal resorption ➡ & tuft resorption ➡, making diagnosis of HPTH. *(Right)* Anteroposterior radiograph shows lytic lesions involving both metatarsal & proximal phalanx of great toe ➡. There is fractured silastic arthroplasty ➡; this has resulted in silastic particles inducing particle disease & associated osteolysis.

255

PHALANGEAL CYSTIC/LYTIC LESIONS

Giant Cell Tumor Tendon Sheath (Mimic)

Giant Cell Tumor Tendon Sheath (Mimic)

(Left) PA radiograph shows soft tissue swelling that is massive, surrounding much of the thumb ➡. There are also lytic lesions involving the metacarpal and phalanx ➡. Note that there is no cartilage loss; this is not an articular process. (Right) Oblique T1WI MR on the same patient shows a large low signal soft tissue mass ➡ with extension into the bone ➡. It is this focal invasion by GCT of the tendon sheath which causes osseous lesions.

Unicameral Bone Cyst (UBC)

Glomus Tumor

(Left) PA radiograph shows a lytic lesion in the metaphysis ➡. Note that the patient is skeletally immature. Although enchondroma, ABC, or GCT may have a similar appearance, patient's age is more suggestive for UBC. (Right) Axial T1WI MR shows a soft tissue mass beneath the nail bed ➡ that causes extrinsic scalloping on the underlying terminal phalanx ➡. Note typical location & appearance for glomus tumor. Radiograph would show scalloping or a lytic lesion.

Epidermal Inclusion Cyst

Sarcoidosis

(Left) Posteroanterior radiograph shows extrinsic invasion of the terminal phalanx from a soft tissue mass ➡. It results in a well-defined lytic lesion. The appearance and location are typical for either glomus tumor or epidermal inclusion cyst; the latter was proven. (Right) Oblique radiograph shows non-aggressive lacy trabeculated lytic lesions of phalanges ➡, typical for osseous sarcoidosis.

PHALANGEAL CYSTIC/LYTIC LESIONS

Robust Rheumatoid Arthritis

Langerhans Cell Histiocytosis (LCH)

(Left) PA radiograph shows subchondral cysts so large as to appear as lytic lesions ➡. The fact that they are multiple & all adjacent to a destroyed joint makes diagnosis of arthropathy; RA in patients who continue activity results in this appearance. *(Right)* PA radiograph shows a nonspecific lytic lesion in the phalanx ➡. History is of extremely rapid growth of the lesion in a very young patient, which helps suggest the unusual diagnosis of LCH in a phalanx.

Ollier Disease

Maffucci Syndrome

(Left) Posteroanterior radiograph shows multiple lytic lesions, some expanded & containing a chondroid matrix ➡. Appearance & multiplicity = multiple enchondromatosis or Ollier disease. (†MSK Req). *(Right)* Posteroanterior radiograph shows multiple lytic lesions that have significantly distorted the phalanges. There are also several calcified phleboliths ➡, indicating the presence of a soft tissue hemangioma. This combination = Maffucci syndrome.

Vascular Tumors, Osseous

Amyloid Deposition

(Left) PA radiograph shows an expanded & destructive lesion ➡ associated with a large soft tissue mass. The lesion is aggressive & nonspecific. Vascular tumors may occur in distal bones & feet more commonly than hands. *(Right)* Oblique radiograph shows lytic lesions in the digits ➡ as well as lumpy soft tissue swelling about the wrist ➡. Lesions have the nonspecific appearance of subchondral cysts, but the character of the soft tissue masses suggests amyloid deposits.

SESAMOIDITIS

DIFFERENTIAL DIAGNOSIS

Common
- Osteoarthritis
- Stress Reaction
- Fracture

Less Common
- Osteonecrosis
- Arthritis
- Plantar Plate Tear
- Tendon Injury

Rare but Important
- Infection
- Neoplasm

ESSENTIAL INFORMATION

Key Differential Diagnosis Issues
- Typically refers to 1st toe medial & lateral sesamoids, though any sesamoid can be involved

Helpful Clues for Common Diagnoses
- **Osteoarthritis**
  - Joint space narrowing, osteophytes, subchondral edema/cysts, sclerosis
  - Look for hallux valgus or rigidus
- **Stress Reaction**
  - Repetitive injury
  - Presents as ↑ SI on fluid-sensitive sequences; ± ↓ SI on T1; may progress to fracture
- **Fracture**
  - Acute: Sharp irregular margins, intense marrow edema; CT often useful to define osseous detail
  - Chronic: Fracture nonunion similar to bipartite sesamoid with smooth, rounded, well-corticated margins

Helpful Clues for Less Common Diagnoses
- **Osteonecrosis**
  - Initially marrow edema; evolves to sclerosis, ↓ SI on T1 & T2; may fragment
- **Arthritis**
  - Arthritides involving hallux may recruit sesamoids
    - Gout: Erosions, overhanging edges
    - Rheumatoid: Osteopenia, erosions
    - Psoriatic: Mixed erosive-productive; periostitis
- **Plantar Plate Tear**
  - Hyperextension injury; fibrocartilaginous disruption, partial or complete
- **Tendon Injury**
  - Ranges from tendinosis (↑ SI & thickening) to complete disruption

Helpful Clues for Rare Diagnoses
- **Infection**
  - Soft tissue infection: Swelling; ± abscess
  - Osteomyelitis: Cortical disruption, ± periostitis
- **Neoplasm**
  - Soft tissue: Giant cell tumor of tendon sheath; pigmented villonodular synovitis
  - Osseous: Extremely rare

Osteoarthritis

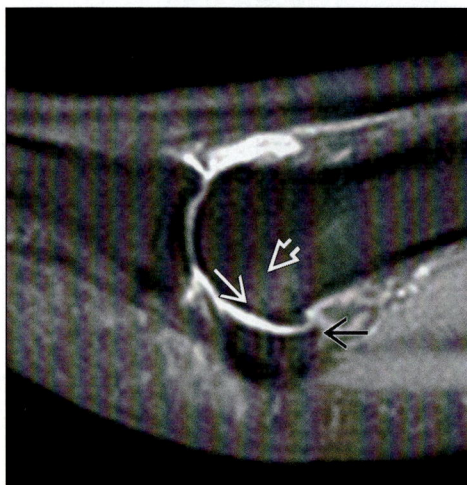

Sagittal PD FSE FS MR shows cartilage loss ➡, subchondral marrow edema ➡, & osteophytes ➡ in this metatarsal-sesamoid joint with early osteoarthritis. There is a small joint effusion.

Osteoarthritis

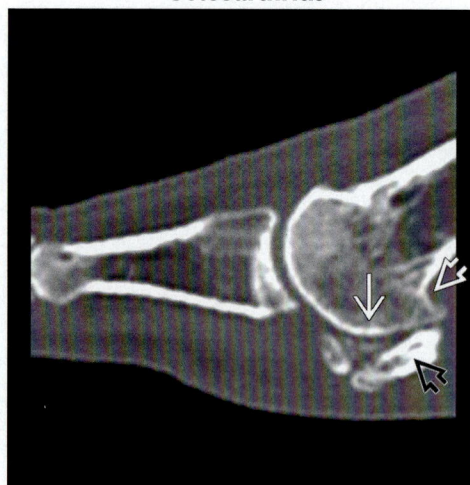

Sagittal bone CT reformation shows osteoarthritis of multipartite sesamoid articulating with the metatarsal head. Note joint space narrowing ➡, subchondral sclerosis ➡, & osteophyte ➡.

SESAMOIDITIS

Stress Reaction

Fracture

(Left) Coronal PD FSE FS MR shows intense lateral sesamoid edema (↑ SI) ⮕ & a small joint effusion ⮕ in this runner with stress response of the sesamoid, related to ill-fitting shoes. *(Right)* Sagittal T2* GRE MR shows the sharp, irregular margins ⮕ of a mid-body sesamoid fracture. A bipartite sesamoid has regular, rounded borders; this differentiates it from a fracture.

Osteonecrosis

Arthritis

(Left) Axial T1WI MR shows lateral sesamoid sclerosis (↓ SI) ⮕ due to chronic osteonecrosis. The sesamoid was ↓ SI on all sequences including STIR imaging (not shown). Note the normal bipartite medial sesamoid ⮕. *(Right)* Sagittal T1WI MR shows a ↓ SI intracapsular process eroding the 1st metatarsal neck ⮕, sesamoid ⮕, & proximal phalangeal base ⮕. This also showed ↓ SI on T2 (not shown). This is aspiration-proven gout.

Plantar Plate Tear

Infection

(Left) Coronal NECT shows abnormal widening between the medial sesamoid & 1st metatarsal head ⮕ due to tear of medial collateral ligament & plantar plate ⮕. This football player presented with "turf" toe due to extreme dorsiflexion with simultaneous varus misalignment. *(Right)* Lateral radiograph shows medial sesamoid osteomyelitis in a diabetic with cortical destruction ⮕, soft tissue swelling, & an air-filled sinus tract ⮕ extending to the bone.

SHORT METACARPAL/METATARSAL

DIFFERENTIAL DIAGNOSIS

Common
- Idiopathic (Normal Variant)
- Trauma

Less Common
- Osteonecrosis
- Juvenile Idiopathic Arthritis (JIA)
- Turner Syndrome
- Noonan Syndrome
- Hypothyroidism
- Hypoparathyroidism

Rare but Important
- Fetal Alcohol Syndrome
- Mucopolysaccharidoses
- Multiple Hereditary Exostoses
- Ollier Disease
- Maffucci Syndrome
- Achondroplasia
- Hypochondroplasia
- Chondrodysplasia Punctata
- Poland Syndrome
- Pseudohypoparathyroidism / Pseudo-Pseudohypoparathyroidism
- Fanconi Anemia
- VATER Association
- Basal-Cell Nevus Syndrome
- Multiple Epiphyseal Dysplasia
- Diastrophic Dysplasia

ESSENTIAL INFORMATION

Key Differential Diagnosis Issues
- Short metacarpal (MC) or metatarsal (MT) is usually nonspecific
  - Uncommonly, other features may be present which lead to a diagnosis
- Consider whether all digits are involved; if this is the case, differential is more limited
  - Hypothyroidism
  - Mucopolysaccharidoses
  - Achondroplasia
  - Hypochondroplasia
  - Noonan syndrome
  - Hypoparathyroidism
  - Chondrodysplasia punctata

Helpful Clues for Common Diagnoses
- **Idiopathic (Normal Variant)**
  - Far and away the most common reason for a solitary short MC or MT

- **Trauma**
  - Crush injury, bayonet apposition of fracture fragments may result in shortening

Helpful Clues for Less Common Diagnoses
- **Osteonecrosis**
  - Freiberg necrosis: Fragmentation & collapse of MT heads
    - Usually 2nd MT; collapse leads to shortening
  - Sickle cell: Bone infarct rarely results in cessation of growth
    - May see dactylitis (periosteal reaction)
  - Thalassemia
    - Short broad MCs and MTs generally due to marrow hyperplasia; osteonecrosis rarely may contribute
- **Juvenile Idiopathic Arthritis (JIA)**
  - Involvement of joint in child causes hyperemia
    - Initially causes overgrowth of epiphyses & metaphyses
    - Chronic hyperemia may result in early fusion & resultant shortening of bone
  - Generally not uniform or symmetric involvement
- **Turner Syndrome**
  - 4th MC most common; may involve 3rd & 5th
  - Often have Madelung deformity of carpus
  - May have metaphyseal excrescences
- **Noonan Syndrome**
  - Short stature, kyphoscoliosis
  - Short fingers, syndactyly
  - Klippel Feil
- **Hypothyroidism**
  - Severely delayed bone age
  - Uniformly short MC, MT, phalanges
  - Fragmented ("cretinoid") femoral capital epiphysis
- **Hypoparathyroidism**
  - Osteoporosis, calvarial thickening
  - Subcutaneous & basal ganglion calcification
  - Premature fusion of physes results in shortened bones, 4th & 5th MC & MT most frequent; 1st may be involved

Helpful Clues for Rare Diagnoses
- **Fetal Alcohol Syndrome**
  - Growth retardation, scoliosis
  - Renal hypoplasia & anomalies

SHORT METACARPAL/METATARSAL

- ○ Microcephaly & malformations of brain
- **Mucopolysaccharidoses**
  - ○ Short MC with proximal constriction, results in "fan-shaped" carpus
  - ○ Oar-shaped ribs, J-shaped sella
- **Multiple Hereditary Exostoses**
  - ○ Osseous exostoses arising from metaphyseal portions of bones
  - ○ May result in shortening & distortion of involved bone; mechanical distortion of adjacent bone
- **Ollier Disease**
  - ○ Multiple enchondromas; dysplasia of metaphyses results in disturbed growth & shortened bone
  - ○ Tends to be monomelic but not all bones of the limb may be affected
  - ○ Increased risk of degeneration to chondrosarcoma
- **Maffucci Syndrome**
  - ○ Same as Ollier disease, but with soft tissue hemangiomas (phleboliths may be seen)
  - ○ Bones of hand may be distorted grotesquely
- **Achondroplasia**
  - ○ Uniform shortening of MC, MT, phalanges
  - ○ Decreased interpediculate distance & short pedicles in lumbar spine
    - ▪ Spinal stenosis
    - ▪ Posterior vertebral body scalloping
- **Hypochondroplasia**
  - ○ Metaphyseal dysplasia → short stature

- ○ Lumbar spine similar to achondroplasia, with short pedicles & narrowing interpediculate distance
- **Chondrodysplasia Punctata**
  - ○ Multiple epiphyseal dysplasia; epiphyses become calcified in first year of life
  - ○ Short-limbed dwarfism
- **Poland Syndrome**
  - ○ Unilateral aplasia of chest wall musculature
  - ○ May have short MC and syndactyly
- **Pseudohypoparathyroidism / Pseudo-Pseudohypoparathyroidism**
  - ○ Phenotypic features of hypoparathyroidism
    - ▪ 4th & 5th MC or MT shortening is most common, followed by 1st
    - ▪ Soft tissue & basal ganglia dystrophic calcification often present
  - ○ Due to end organ resistance to parathyroid hormone, so levels of parathormone are ↑
    - ▪ Osteopenia; variable radiographic features of hyperparathyroidism
- **Fanconi Anemia**
  - ○ Growth retardation
  - ○ Skeletal anomalies, usually thumb
  - ○ Renal anomalies, microcephaly
- **VATER Association**
  - ○ Multisystem (vertebral, anorectal, tracheal, esophageal, renal)
  - ○ Radial side anomalies
    - ▪ Hypoplastic radius
    - ▪ Variable shortening to absence of radial-sided metacarpal & digits

Trauma

PA radiograph shows a patient who had a crush injury when she was 8 years of age. In addition to carpal and distal forearm fusion, the growth plates of metacarpals 3 & 4 were affected, resulting in early fusion.

Osteonecrosis

Anteroposterior radiograph shows flattening & fragmentation of the heads of metatarsals 2 and 3 ➡. This is typically secondary to Freiberg osteonecrosis. With collapse, the metatarsals become short.

SHORT METACARPAL/METATARSAL

(Left) Oblique radiograph shows diffuse shortening of the metacarpals. With involvement of joints by JIA, there is hyperemia. This chronic hyperemia may result in initial overgrowth, followed by early fusion and relative shortening. **(Right)** PA radiograph shows shortening of the 3rd through 5th metacarpals. Though this may be seen in several syndromes, in this case it is due to Turner syndrome. Madelung deformity is often present as well, though it is not in this case.

Juvenile Idiopathic Arthritis (JIA)

Turner Syndrome

(Left) Posteroanterior radiograph shows short metacarpals and phalanges. None of the epiphyses are ossified, yet the patient is 4 years of age. Severely delayed bone age resulting in short metacarpals and digits is typical of hypothyroidism. **(Right)** Posteroanterior radiograph shows short metacarpals with constricted proximal ends ➡. This results in a "fan-shaped" wrist that is typical of the mucopolysaccharidoses.

Hypothyroidism

Mucopolysaccharidoses

(Left) PA radiograph shows short metacarpals 3 and 4 (compare with metacarpal 2). Osseous excrescences are seen extending from the metaphyses of involved metacarpals ➡. These are exostoses, which may interfere with normal growth. **(Right)** AP radiograph shows a short 4th metatarsal with an expanded lytic lesion involving both metatarsal ➡ & adjacent phalanx. This is a patient with Ollier dz; the metaphyseal dysplasia results in arrested growth & consequent short bones.

Multiple Hereditary Exostoses

Ollier Disease

SHORT METACARPAL/METATARSAL

Maffucci Syndrome

Achondroplasia

(Left) Posteroanterior radiograph shows short metacarpals, along with severe distortion of all the bones. Each bone shows an expanded lesion resulting in shortening. Note also the phleboliths in the soft tissues; the complex is Maffucci syndrome. *(Right)* Anteroposterior radiograph shows short, broad metacarpals and phalanges. This is typical in this infant with achondroplasia, who will continue to have short bones through skeletal maturity.

Pseudohypoparathyroidism / Pseudo-Pseudohypoparathyroidism

Pseudohypoparathyroidism / Pseudo-Pseudohypoparathyroidism

(Left) Anteroposterior radiograph shows subtle soft tissue calcification ➡, as well as a short first metatarsal ➡. These illustrate the combination of findings which make the diagnosis of pseudohypoparathyroidism or pseudo-pseudohypoparathyroidism. *(Right)* Posteroanterior radiograph shows all the metacarpals to be short (most significantly, the first, fourth, and fifth); there is evidence of previous coning of the epiphyses, now fused and resulting in short digits.

Fanconi Anemia

VATER Association

(Left) AP radiograph shows an absent radius as well as short, bowed ulna. The entire ray of the thumb is absent. This is an extreme example of radial dysplasia seen in Fanconi anemia. Other cases may show just shortened bones. *(Right)* AP radiograph shows hypoplastic radius & absent thumb, part of the VATER syndrome. The patient had renal anomalies as well. This is an extreme example; other cases may show shortened bones on the radial side of the extremity.

ULNAR DEVIATION (MCP JOINTS)

DIFFERENTIAL DIAGNOSIS

Common
- Rheumatoid Arthritis
- Systemic Lupus Erythematosus (SLE)
- Psoriatic Arthritis
- Juvenile Idiopathic Arthritis (JIA)
- Mixed Connective Tissue Disease

Less Common
- Septic Joint
- Charcot, Neuropathic
- Jaccoud Arthropathy
- Ehlers-Danlos

Rare but Important
- Multicentric Reticulohistiocytosis
- Mass, Unspecified
- Pigmented Villonodular Synovitis (PVNS)
- Trisomy 18
- Exotic Infection
- Frontometaphyseal Dysplasia

ESSENTIAL INFORMATION

Key Differential Diagnosis Issues
- Ligamentous laxity or damage → joint deviation to subluxation

Helpful Clues for Common Diagnoses
- **Rheumatoid Arthritis**
  - Polyarticular, bilateral, symmetric
  - MCP & PIP joints most severely affected
  - Decreased bone mineralization
- **Systemic Lupus Erythematosus (SLE)**
  - Predisposition to osteonecrosis
  - Erosions & soft tissue calcification are uncommon; deformities are reducible
- **Psoriatic Arthritis**
  - Interphalangeal joints severely affected
  - Erosions & periostitis
  - Normal bone mineralization
- **Juvenile Idiopathic Arthritis (JIA)**
  - Juvenile onset of oligoarthritis or polyarthritis
  - Marginal erosions with joint space narrowing
  - ± Ankylosis
- **Mixed Connective Tissue Disease**
  - Globular or sheet-like periarticular calcification

Helpful Clues for Less Common Diagnoses
- **Septic Joint**
  - Bone & joint destruction
- **Charcot, Neuropathic**
  - Fragmented bone debris common
  - Indolent course
- **Jaccoud Arthropathy**
  - Subluxation & ulnar deviation of 2nd through 5th MCP joints
  - Reducible deformities
- **Ehlers-Danlos**
  - Hypermobile joints often with normal radiographs

Helpful Clues for Rare Diagnoses
- **Pigmented Villonodular Synovitis (PVNS)**
  - Typically monoarticular; polyarticular is exceptionally rare
  - Hemosiderin deposition

Rheumatoid Arthritis

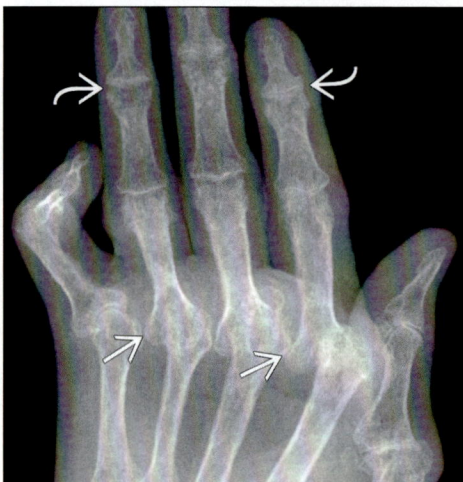

Posteroanterior radiograph shows metacarpophalangeal joint dislocation/subluxation with ulnar deviation ➡ and severe narrowing of the interphalangeal joints ➡.

Rheumatoid Arthritis

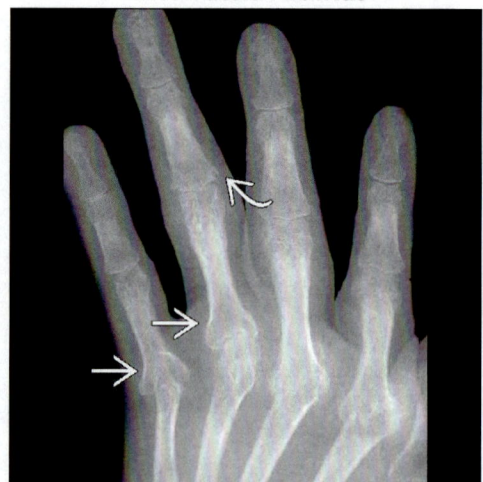

Posteroanterior radiograph shows erosive changes of the metacarpophalangeal joints with ulnar deviation ➡. There is a marginal erosion ➡ at the 4th digit PIP joint.

ULNAR DEVIATION (MCP JOINTS)

Systemic Lupus Erythematosus (SLE)

Systemic Lupus Erythematosus (SLE)

(Left) *"Open book" radiograph shows severe subluxation at the MCP joints ➡. The reducible deformities are more severe when the hand is not supported (as in this position, as opposed to the PA view, where the hand is placed on the cassette).* *(Right)* *Posteroanterior radiograph shows ulnar deviation ➡ of the 2nd through 5th MCP joints. This joint subluxation was reducible. The interphalangeal joints are diffusely narrowed ➡.*

Psoriatic Arthritis

Multicentric Reticulohistiocytosis

(Left) *Posteroanterior radiograph shows volar and ulnar subluxation of the metacarpophalangeal joints ➡. There is severe erosive disease of the interphalangeal joints ➡, more prominent than of the MCPs. These findings are typical of psoriatic arthritis.* *(Right)* *Posteroanterior radiograph shows severe erosions of the distal interphalangeal joints ➡ and thumb interphalangeal joint ➡, as well as ulnar deviation ➡ of the 5th MCP joint.*

Mass, Unspecified

Trisomy 18

(Left) *Posteroanterior radiograph shows ulnar deviation of the 5th metacarpophalangeal joint secondary to osseous mass ➡. The mass developed secondary to trauma and has been termed fibroosseous pseudotumor of the digit. Any mass in the web space may result in ulnar deviation.* *(Right)* *Lateral radiograph shows ulnar deviation ➡ of the metacarpophalangeal joints in an infant with radial aplasia ➡ and a short ulna ➡. The patient has a known chromosomal abnormality.*

SWELLING & PERIOSTITIS OF DIGIT (DACTYLITIS)

DIFFERENTIAL DIAGNOSIS

Common
- Psoriatic Arthritis, "Sausage Digit"
- Osteomyelitis
- Juvenile Idiopathic Arthritis (JIA)

Less Common
- Chronic Reactive Arthritis, "Sausage Digit"
- HIV-AIDS Related Arthritis
- Sickle Cell Disease, "Hand-Foot"

Rare but Important
- Fibroosseous Pseudotumor of Digits
- Tuberculosis, "Spina Ventosa"
- Sarcoidosis
- Secondary Syphilis
- Mycobacterium Marinum

ESSENTIAL INFORMATION

Key Differential Diagnosis Issues
- Periostitis may be the earliest manifestation of 4 forms of arthritis
  - Psoriatic arthritis, JIA, chronic reactive arthritis, HIV-AIDS related arthritis
  - May not have cartilage narrowing or erosions at this early stage
- Periostitis may be reactive
  - Infection, various sources
  - Infarction, granulomatous, trauma

Helpful Clues for Common Diagnoses
- **Psoriatic Arthritis, "Sausage Digit"**
  - Swelling along ray, not at single joint
  - Periostitis, especially along shafts of digits
  - ± Erosions and cartilage narrowing
- **Osteomyelitis**
  - Swelling, periosteal reaction
  - Osseous destruction, ± sequestrum
- **Juvenile Idiopathic Arthritis (JIA)**
  - Swelling and periostitis of multiple digits may be initial sign of JIA
  - Seen in younger children; may not have developed joint or overgrowth symptoms

Helpful Clues for Less Common Diagnoses
- **Chronic Reactive Arthritis, "Sausage Digit"**
  - Swelling along ray, not at single joint
  - Periostitis, especially along shafts of digits
  - ± Erosions & cartilage narrowing
- **HIV-AIDS Related Arthritis**
  - Same as chronic reactive arthritis
  - Do not overlook possibility of infection
- **Sickle Cell Disease, "Hand-Foot"**
  - Periosteal reaction to osseous infarct

Helpful Clues for Rare Diagnoses
- **Fibroosseous Pseudotumor of Digits**
  - Similar appearance to myositis ossificans
- **Tuberculosis, "Spina Ventosa"**
  - Fusiform swelling & periostitis; eventual expanded lytic lesion; children > adults
- **Sarcoidosis**
  - Subtle periostitis seen with MR
- **Secondary Syphilis**
  - Periosteal reaction, bone destruction
- **Mycobacterium Marinum**
  - Contact with fish spines
  - Nonspecific swelling & periostitis

Psoriatic Arthritis, "Sausage Digit"

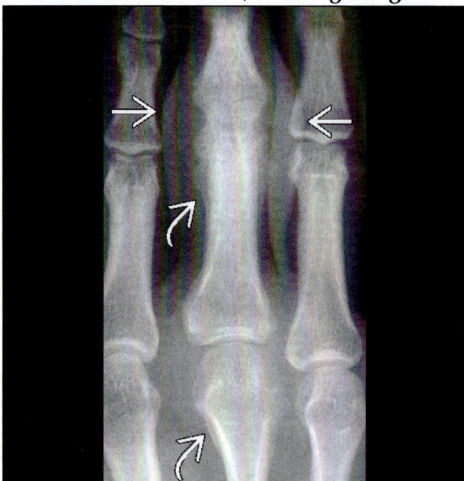

PA radiograph shows tremendous soft tissue swelling of the third digit ➡, along with prominent periostitis of the proximal phalanx and metacarpal ➡. This may be an early indication of psoriatic arthritis. (†MSK Req).

Psoriatic Arthritis, "Sausage Digit"

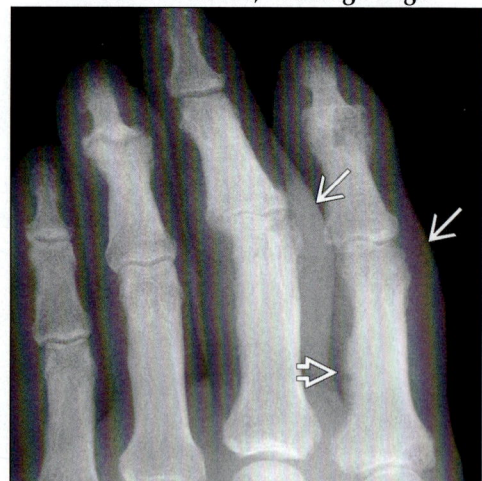

PA radiograph shows second & third "sausage digits", with soft tissue swelling ➡ and periostitis ➡. This patient has erosive changes in the DIP joints; all findings are typical of psoriatic arthritis.

SWELLING & PERIOSTITIS OF DIGIT (DACTYLITIS)

Osteomyelitis

Juvenile Idiopathic Arthritis (JIA)

(Left) PA radiograph shows soft tissue swelling and periosteal reaction ➡. Additionally, there is an oval density with surrounding lysis ➡, which is diagnostic of sequestrum in osteomyelitis. *(Right)* PA radiograph shows soft tissue swelling and periostitis involving the proximal phalanges ➡ of a child. This was the first manifestation of JIA in this patient; erosions and joint disease were not seen until later, as the disease progressed.

Chronic Reactive Arthritis, "Sausage Digit"

HIV-AIDS Related Arthritis

(Left) AP radiograph shows a "sausage digit" of the fourth toe ➡ of a young male who also has symptoms of urethritis and uveitis. The trio of findings make the diagnosis of chronic reactive arthritis. With the radiographic findings alone, psoriatic arthritis or infection should be considered. *(Right)* Lateral radiograph shows soft tissue swelling and periostitis ➡. This constitutes a "sausage digit". There is also mild cartilage loss ➡ in this HIV-positive patient.

Sickle Cell Disease, "Hand-Foot"

Fibroosseous Pseudotumor of Digits

(Left) Anteroposterior radiograph shows periostitis of several of the small bones of the hand ➡. This is an African American child who had her first episode of hand pain; this dactylitis is due to reaction to bone infarcts. *(Right)* PA radiograph shows dense periosteal reaction of the fourth and fifth metacarpals ➡. This is maturing; the patient had a crush injury 3 months earlier. The reactive change is similar to myositis ossificans & is also called florid reactive periostitis.

LESIONS CROSSING A DISC SPACE

DIFFERENTIAL DIAGNOSIS

Common
- Fusion
- Vertebral Body Osteomyelitis
- Pseudoarthrosis

Less Common
- Multiple Myeloma
- Lymphoma
- Metastatic Disease

Rare but Important
- Giant Cell Tumor
- Sarcoma
- Chordoma

ESSENTIAL INFORMATION

Key Differential Diagnosis Issues
- Lesion may extend through disc space or via paraspinal soft tissues
- Neoplasm: Aggressive bone destruction, periostitis, soft tissue mass common
- Hint: Age & history are key factors

Helpful Clues for Common Diagnoses
- Fusion (congenital): Narrow anteroposterior vertebral dimension, narrow disc space, normal endplates; cervical spine
- Fusion (surgical): Marrow & trabecular continuity; endplates not seen
- Vertebral Body Osteomyelitis: Debilitated & immunocompromised patients
  - Pyogenic: Typically single level
  - Fungal: Candida, immunocompromised
  - Granulomatous: Tuberculosis; disc destruction late; may track along anterior longitudinal ligament creating multiple noncontiguous lesions; ± soft tissue calcification
  - Early: Endplate edema, disc enhancement
  - Late: Disc narrowing, endplate destruction, sclerosis ± iliopsoas or epidural abscess
- Pseudoarthrosis: History of surgery, ankylosing spondylitis, DISH, ochronosis
  - Narrow disc space; endplate sclerosis; fragmentation; vacuum phenomenon

Helpful Clues for Less Common Diagnoses
- Multiple Myeloma: Adults; punched-out lytic lesions, expansile lesion(s) or permeative destruction; ± disc destruction
- Lymphoma: Any age, most frequently young adult
  - May cause destruction of intervening disc
- Metastatic Disease: Breast, lung

Helpful Clues for Rare Diagnoses
- Giant Cell Tumor: Young adults; expansile, lesion, well-defined non-sclerotic margins
- Sarcoma
  - Ewing sarcoma: Teens & young adults
  - Osteosarcoma: Teens & young adults, 2nd peak older adults; ranges lytic to sclerotic ± soft tissue ossification
  - Chondrosarcoma: Mesenchymal type; women 3rd & 4th decades; ± mineralization
- Chordoma: Any age, adults most common
  - Sacrum > clivus > remainder of spinal axis

Fusion

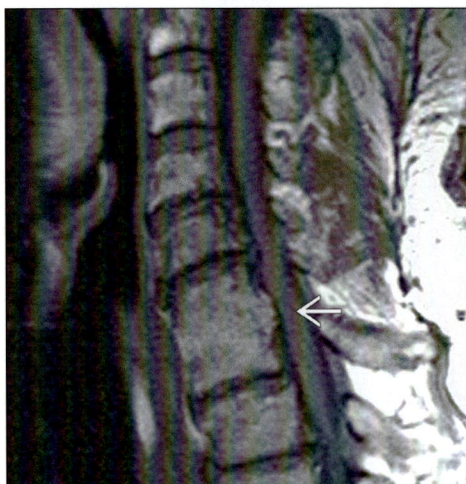

Sagittal T1WI MR shows a solid surgical fusion at C6-7 ➡ with continuous marrow signal between the two vertebral bodies.

Vertebral Body Osteomyelitis

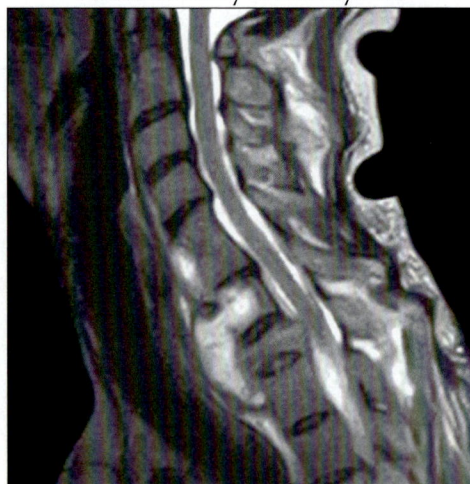

Sagittal T2WI MR shows a destructive process involving C7 & T1 (not seen on this image) with a large prevertebral mass & relative sparing of the intervertebral discs. Typical of an indolent (TB or fungal) infection.

LESIONS CROSSING A DISC SPACE

Pseudoarthrosis

Lymphoma

(Left) Sagittal T1WI MR shows prior solid fusion at L4-5. There is an irregular low signal extending through L5-S1 disc space and through the posterior elements, indicative of pseudoarthrosis ➡. *(Right)* Sagittal T1WI MR shows multiple thoracic vertebra with abnormal low T1 signal within the body and posterior elements, crossing a disc space. There is a large paravertebral ➡ and epidural ➡ mass. The appearance is typical for lymphoma.

Metastatic Disease

Sarcoma

(Left) Coronal T2WI FS MR shows a large mass destroying the right side of T7 & T8 crossing but sparing the disc space, involving the right ribs & costo-vertebral joint. Multiple flow voids ➡ are present within this metastatic renal cell carcinoma. *(Right)* Sagittal T1WI MR shows a lobulated soft tissue mass ➡ involving multiple contiguous vertebral bodies, crossing but sparing the intervening discs, with extension into the neural foramina and spinal canal. Diagnosis: Ewing sarcoma.

Sarcoma

Chordoma

(Left) Sagittal T2WI MR shows an aggressive mass arising from the L5 vertebral body and extending into the posterior elements, spinal canal, paraspinous soft tissues and into the sacrum ➡ in this patient with telangiectatic osteosarcoma. *(Right)* Sagittal STIR MR shows a large destructive mass involving L4 and L5 bodies and intervening disc space ➡ with posterior epidural extension and extension into neural foramen ➡. This patient has a chordoma.

DISCAL MINERALIZATION

DIFFERENTIAL DIAGNOSIS

Common
- Degenerative Spondylosis
- Surgical Spinal Fusion
- Discography (Mimic)
- DISH
- Vertebroplasty Cement (Mimic)
- Congenital Fusion
- Pyrophosphate Arthropathy

Less Common
- Ankylosing Spondylitis (AS)
- Hemochromatosis
- Juvenile Idiopathic Arthritis (JIA)
- Hyperparathyroidism
- Amyloid Deposition
- Tuberculosis

Rare but Important
- Ochronosis (Alkaptonuria)
- Acromegaly
- Paraplegia
- Polio
- Idiopathic, Childhood

ESSENTIAL INFORMATION

Key Differential Diagnosis Issues
- **Hint**: Distinguishing post-operative findings from other causes is essential; with the exception of ochronosis, disc calcification is rarely the defining feature of an entity
- Fusion from long standing immobilization: AS, DISH, JIA, surgical fusion
- **Hint**: Disc space height can be useful feature; may be increased, normal, or decreased
- Common associated nonspecific findings include endplate sclerosis, osteophyte formation, vacuum phenomenon

Helpful Clues for Common Diagnoses
- **Degenerative Spondylosis**
  - Older patient population
  - Thoracolumbar junction most common
  - ± Other degenerative changes
- **Surgical Spinal Fusion**
  - Long standing immobilization leads to disc mineralization & eventual fusion
    - Disc space height may be narrowed as part of underlying degenerative process
  - Interbody fusion

- Early graft is visible; late → solid fusion with bridging bone endplate to endplate or pseudoarthrosis with collapsed graft
  - Cages: Help retain graft within disc space, carbon fiber cages identified by tantalum markers
  - Bone filler/graft substitute: Morselized fragments or plug of material with geometric shape (due to preparation for insertion)
- **Discography (Mimic)**
  - Contrast material within disc space
    - Disc normal (especially if control) or degenerative
  - Patterns of contrast distribution
    - Irregularly distributed through disc: Degeneration
    - Into epidural space: Annular tear
    - Into canal within herniated fragment
- **DISH**
  - Bulky anterior vertebral body ossification involving 4 or more contiguous vertebral levels
  - Disc space normal or narrowed, lacks other changes
  - May see lucency between vertebral corner & anterior ossification
    - Anterior longitudinal ligament tightly adherent at mid portion of anterior vertebral cortex
    - Less tightly attached at vertebral corners
- **Vertebroplasty Cement (Mimic)**
  - Dense material contiguous with cement within collapsed vertebra
  - Indicates fracture or perforation of endplate
- **Congenital Fusion**
  - Usually isolated to one level
  - Vertebra with diminished anterior to posterior dimensions
  - Narrowed but otherwise normal disc space
  - ± Fusion of posterior elements
- **Pyrophosphate Arthropathy**
  - Calcification in outer fibers of annulus
    - Mimics syndesmophytes of ankylosing spondylitis
  - Disc space normal or narrowed
  - ± Ligamentum flava calcification
  - Favors lumbar spine

Helpful Clues for Less Common Diagnoses
- **Ankylosing Spondylitis (AS)**

DISCAL MINERALIZATION

- ○ Preserved disc spaces
- ○ Squaring vertebral bodies
- ○ Syndesmophyte formation (ossification Sharpey fibers), tightly adherent to vertebral corner
- ○ Spinal osteoporosis if long standing
- ○ Associated sacroiliac joint fusion, enthesopathy, large joint arthritis
- • **Hemochromatosis**
  - ○ Mimics pyrophosphate arthropathy
- • **Juvenile Idiopathic Arthritis (JIA)**
  - ○ Predominately cervical spine
  - ○ Preserved disc spaces
  - ○ Associated spinal fusion
- • **Hyperparathyroidism**
  - ○ Mimics pyrophosphate arthropathy
- • **Amyloid Deposition**
  - ○ Favors cervical spine
  - ○ Disc space narrowed, may progress to endplate irregularity, sclerosis, fragmentation
  - ○ Underlying cause of dialysis spondyloarthropathy
- • **Tuberculosis**
  - ○ Initially adjacent endplate destruction with fragmentation
  - ○ Increased density 2° mineralization occurs during healing phase, progresses to ossification
  - ○ Kyphosis
  - ○ May involve multiple contiguous or noncontiguous disc spaces

Helpful Clues for Rare Diagnoses

- • **Ochronosis (Alkaptonuria)**
  - ○ Thick linear mineralization within multiple levels, lumbar spine predominance
  - ○ Osteoporosis, disc space narrowing, subchondral sclerosis, vacuum phenomenon, lack of osteophytes
  - ○ Overall appearance may mimic ankylosing spondylitis, including SI, facet joint fusion, large joint involvement, enthesopathy, ligament mineralization
- • **Acromegaly**
  - ○ Enlarged disc space
  - ○ Increased vertebral body width (AP & medial-lateral)
  - ○ Posterior vertebral scalloping
  - ○ Osteophytes
- • **Paraplegia**
  - ○ Variable changes range from disc space narrowing, endplate sclerosis, osteophytes & vacuum phenomenon to paravertebral ossification mimicking ankylosing spondylitis or psoriasis
- • **Polio**
  - ○ Changes similar to paraplegia, see above
- • **Idiopathic, Childhood**
  - ○ Cervical spine, one or multiple discs
  - ○ Involves nucleus pulposus
  - ○ Systemic symptoms: Fever, elevated WBC, pain, spontaneous resolution without sequelae
  - ○ MR: Inflammatory changes

Degenerative Spondylosis

Lateral radiograph shows mineralization of the annular fibers ➡ with sparing of the nucleus pulposus ➡ in this patient with disc degeneration.

Surgical Spinal Fusion

Lateral radiograph shows 3 level interbody fusion. At C4-5 the graft is partially extruded ➡. At C5-6 solid fusion is seen ➡. A pseudoarthrosis is present at C6-7 ➡ with overgrowth of the endplates.

DISCAL MINERALIZATION

Surgical Spinal Fusion

Surgical Spinal Fusion

(Left) Lateral radiograph shows interbody fusion with cages. The cages are identified by the tantalum markers ➡. The graft material appears as irregular density within the cages ⇉. *(Right)* Sagittal CT myelogram shows interbody cages at L2-3 and L4-5 ⇉. The graft material within the cages is difficult to appreciate. At L3-4 interbody fusion has been performed with a plug of calcium hydroxyapatite graft ➡.

Discography (Mimic)

DISH

(Left) Sagittal bone CT shows contrast material within multiple disc spaces following discography ➡. Contrast extravasation posteriorly at L4-5 ⇉ is the result of a disc herniation. *(Right)* Sagittal bone CT shows extensive anterior longitudinal ligament ossification of DISH ➡ accompanied by extensive ossification of the posterior longitudinal ligament ➡. Discal calcification is present at several levels including C5-6 and C6-7 ➡.

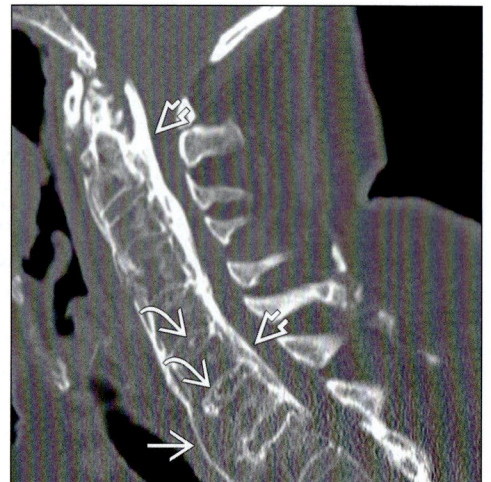

Vertebroplasty Cement (Mimic)

Congenital Fusion

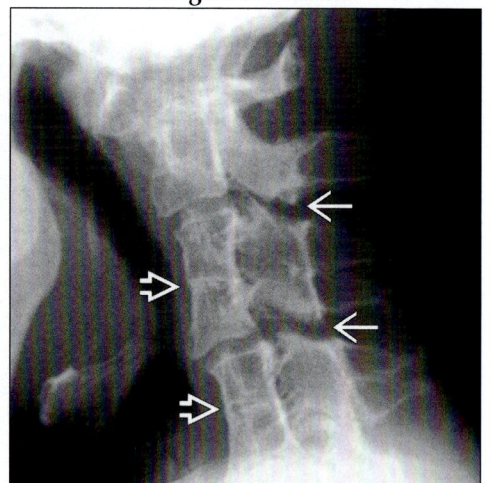

(Left) Lateral radiograph shows cement within the disc space between two vertebra that have been treated with vertebroplasty ➡. The cement is contiguous with the cement in the inferior vertebral body. *(Right)* Lateral radiograph shows congenital fusion of C3 and C4 as well as C5 and C6 ⇉. Widened facet joints at C2-3 and C4-5 ➡ are the result of abnormal motion. The odontoid is absent, and there is widening of the atlantodental distance.

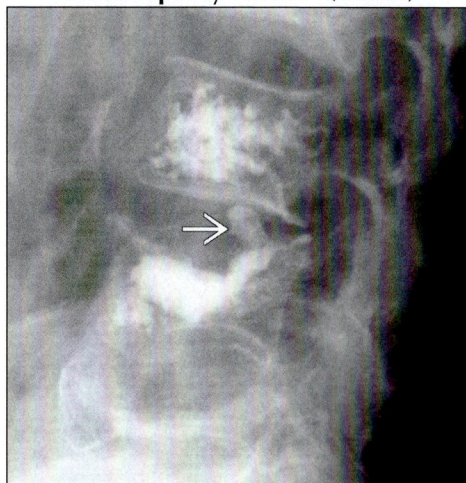

DISCAL MINERALIZATION

Pyrophosphate Arthropathy

Ankylosing Spondylitis (AS)

(Left) Lateral radiograph shows linear calcification ➡ in a degenerated-appearing disc. The disc is narrowed with endplate sclerosis. Vacuum phenomenon is present in the disc above. These findings are nonspecific. However, characteristic findings of CPPD were present elsewhere in the skeleton. *(Right)* Sagittal T1WI MR shows typical squaring of the lumbar vertebral bodies and diffuse disc calcification (T1 hyperintense) from long standing AS.

Juvenile Idiopathic Arthritis (JIA)

Hyperparathyroidism

(Left) Lateral radiograph shows fusion from C2-4 involving the vertebral bodies & posterior elements. Extensive discal mineralization is present within the C3-4 disc space ➡. These findings are commonly seen in juvenile idiopathic arthritis. *(Right)* Sagittal bone CT shows disc space narrowing at many levels. Diffuse annular mineralization mimicking syndesmophyte formation ➡ is present at two levels in this patient with hyperparathyroidism.

Tuberculosis

Ochronosis (Alkaptonuria)

(Left) Sagittal NECT shows destruction of L5 and S1 centered at the intervertebral disc, with anterolisthesis of L5 on S1 in this patient with tuberculous vertebral body osteomyelitis. Extensive paraspinal soft tissue mass is present. In this active stage, the density ➡ is likely from endplate fragmentation. *(Right)* Lateral radiograph shows diffuse osteoporosis, dense linear calcification of most of the discs ➡ with little endplate sclerosis or osteophyte formation in this patient with ochronosis.

OSSIFICATION/CALCIFICATION ANTERIOR TO C1

DIFFERENTIAL DIAGNOSIS

Common
- Calcium Pyrophosphate Deposition Disease

Less Common
- Hydroxyapatite Deposition Disease (HADD)
- Hyperextension (Teardrop) Fracture
- Accessory Ossicle
- Avulsion Fracture Anterior Arch C1
- Stylohyoid Ligament Ossification (Mimic)

Rare but Important
- Progressive Systemic Sclerosis

ESSENTIAL INFORMATION

Helpful Clues for Common Diagnoses
- **Calcium Pyrophosphate Deposition Disease**
  - Rarely symptomatic
  - Flocculent mineralization within midline C1-2 articulation
    - Calcification speckled or linear, irregularly distributed
  - Associated soft tissue mass may be large & may compress spinal canal
  - Varying size cysts in odontoid process & anterior arch C1
  - May see chondrocalcinosis elsewhere including symphysis, knee
    - Not necessary to make diagnosis

Helpful Clues for Less Common Diagnoses
- **Hydroxyapatite Deposition Disease (HADD)**
  - a.k.a., longus colli calcific tendinitis
  - **Hint**: Symptomatic with pain, fever, elevated WBC
  - Amorphous density inferior to C1 arch
  - Soft tissue swelling may be extensive
- **Hyperextension (Teardrop) Fracture**
  - Older, osteopenic patient
  - Pain, history of trauma
  - Soft tissue swelling
  - Fragment from inferior C2 body
    - Vertical dimension > horizontal
- **Accessory Ossicle**
  - Asymptomatic, incidental finding
  - Smooth margins, cortical-medullary architecture
- **Avulsion Fracture Anterior Arch C1**
  - Hyperextension injury
  - Horizontally oriented fx anterior arch C1
  - Avulsion longus colli muscles & atlantoaxial ligament
  - Soft tissue swelling
- **Stylohyoid Ligament Ossification (Mimic)**
  - On lateral view ligament may project anterior to arch C1
  - Eagle-Barrett syndrome: Sore throat, pain during swallowing

Helpful Clues for Rare Diagnoses
- **Progressive Systemic Sclerosis**
  - Cloud-like soft tissue calcification
  - Pain, stiffness, dysphagia, spine or nerve root compression
  - Paraspinal location: Any site cervical, thoracic, lumbar spine

Calcium Pyrophosphate Deposition Disease

Sagittal bone CT shows speckled & linear calcification centered at the C1-2 articulation ➡ with associated calcification of the occipitocervical ligaments ➡ in this patient with CPPD.

Hydroxyapatite Deposition Disease (HADD)

Axial bone CT shows an amorphous calcific density ➡ with mild surrounding soft tissue edema in this patient with hydroxyapatite deposition disease of the longus colli muscle.

OSSIFICATION/CALCIFICATION ANTERIOR TO C1

Hydroxyapatite Deposition Disease (HADD)

Hyperextension (Teardrop) Fracture

(Left) Lateral radiograph shows focal soft tissue swelling in the upper cervical spine ➡ and small calcifications inferior to C1 and anterior to C2 ➡ indicative of longus colli calcification. *(Right)* Sagittal NECT shows hyperextension teardrop fracture at the anterior inferior margin of the C2 body ➡. The fracture fragment is slightly distant to the arch of C1.

Accessory Ossicle

Avulsion Fracture Anterior Arch C1

(Left) Axial NECT shows the typical appearance of an accessory ossicle of C1 ➡ with a well-defined cortex and internal trabecular bone. *(Right)* Lateral radiograph shows longitudinal atlanto-occipital dislocation and C1 fracture. There is prevertebral soft tissue swelling and a transverse fracture of the anterior arch of C1 with a visible fragment inferior to the arch of C1 ➡.

Stylohyoid Ligament Ossification (Mimic)

Progressive Systemic Sclerosis

(Left) Lateral radiograph shows an unusually thick ossification of the stylohyoid ligament ➡. Note its course just anterior to the arch of C1. *(Right)* Lateral radiograph shows cloud-like calcification surrounding the C2 vertebral body and posterior elements ➡. This is a typical appearance of progressive systemic sclerosis, or scleroderma.

PARAVERTEBRAL OSSIFICATION AND CALCIFICATION

DIFFERENTIAL DIAGNOSIS

Common
- Post-Operative Fusion
- Extruded Cement (Mimic)
- Vertebral Body Osteomyelitis, Pyogenic

Less Common
- Psoriatic Arthritis
- Chronic Reactive Arthritis
- Paraplegia
- Charcot, Neuropathic

Rare but Important
- Tumoral Calcinosis
- Osteochondroma
- Progressive Systemic Sclerosis
- Osteoblastoma
- Chondrosarcoma
- Chordoma
- Vertebral Osteomyelitis, Granulomatous
- Osteosarcoma
- Fibrodysplasia Ossificans Progressiva

ESSENTIAL INFORMATION

Key Differential Diagnosis Issues
- Differential excludes syndesmophytes, anterior longitudinal ligament ossification, & associated forms of ossification that are more commonly seen anteriorly & closely adherent to spine
- **Hint**: Determine if associated findings include abnormal disc space or abnormal vertebra or otherwise normal spine

Helpful Clues for Common Diagnoses
- **Post-Operative Fusion**
  - Posterior fusion
    - Initially just small osseous fragments
    - Develops mature ossification with time; may or may not → solid osseous union
    - May extend from transverse process to transverse process or across facet joints
  - Anterior (interbody) fusion
    - Usually confined to disc space
    - Graft material may extrude; initially small mineralized fragments, may progress to mature bone
- **Extruded Cement (Mimic)**
  - Intravascular or within paraspinal muscles
  - Adjacent intravertebral cement, collapsed vertebra

- **Vertebral Body Osteomyelitis, Pyogenic**
  - Disc space destruction
  - Endplate sclerosis & fragmentation
    - Fragmentation may give appearance of soft tissue mineralization/ossification
  - Irregular periosteal new bone formation
  - Paravertebral ossification may be component of healing process
    - Located at disc space
    - Progresses to mature bone
    - May lead to disc ankylosis

Helpful Clues for Less Common Diagnoses
- **Psoriatic Arthritis**
  - Spondyloarthropathy may involve any segment of spine
  - Ranges from immature mineralization to bulky mature bone
    - May fuse with vertebral body & disc
  - More pronounced on the right; formation on the left possibly limited by aortic pulsation
  - Associated appendicular findings
    - Enthesopathy, periosteal new bone
    - Bilateral asymmetric erosive arthritis in hands & feet
    - Sausage digits, phalangeal tuft resorption
- **Chronic Reactive Arthritis**
  - Mimics psoriasis
    - Cervical spine less common
    - Foot involvement more common than upper extremity involvement
- **Paraplegia**
  - Bulky paravertebral ossification mimics psoriasis
  - Other spinal changes
    - Syndesmophyte-like ossification mimicking ankylosing spondylitis
    - Anterior longitudinal ligament ossification mimicking DISH
    - Neuropathic changes
- **Charcot, Neuropathic**
  - Mimics vertebral osteomyelitis
    - Destruction, osseous debris, malalignment more extensive with neuropathic disease

Helpful Clues for Rare Diagnoses
- **Tumoral Calcinosis**
  - Amorphous, cloud-like deposits of calcium
  - Associated with hyperparathyroidism

- Other findings: Bone resorption; subchondral, subperiosteal, subligamentous, subtendinous, cortical tunneling
  ○ Associated with renal osteodystrophy
    - Bone resorption of hyperparathyroidism
    - Ill-defined trabecula of osteomalacia
  ○ Idiopathic form
    - Most common in African-American males, 10-20 years old, familial
- **Osteochondroma**
  ○ Cortical-medullary continuity with vertebra
  ○ Any vertebra surface
    - May cause cord compression
- **Progressive Systemic Sclerosis**
  ○ Amorphous, cloud-like deposits
  ○ Few other spinal changes
  ○ Appendicular changes
    - Osteolysis
    - Soft tissue resorption of distal digits
    - Erosive arthritis in hands & feet
- **Osteoblastoma**
  ○ Any age, most frequent 10-30 years old
  ○ Expansile lytic lesion
    - Wide spectrum of internal calcification or ossification
  ○ Arises in posterior elements
  ○ Most common thoracic, lumbar spine
    - ± Scoliosis, lesion on concavity
- **Chondrosarcoma**
  ○ Osteolytic lesion with mineralization
    - Conventional or mesenchymal type
    - Mineralization stippled, arcs, whorls

- Lobulated growth is characteristic
  ○ Mesenchymal type
    - Women, 3rd & 4th decades
    - May be purely soft tissue
- **Chordoma**
  ○ Any age, adults most common
  ○ Sacral > clivus > remainder of spine
  ○ Osseous destruction ± soft tissue mass
    - Associated mineralization > 50%
- **Vertebral Osteomyelitis, Granulomatous**
  ○ Single or multiple noncontiguous levels of involvement
    - Subligamentous spread
  ○ Disc destruction late
  ○ Endplate sclerosis may be minimal
  ○ Calcification within soft tissue abscesses
    - May be large & remote from disc space
- **Osteosarcoma**
  ○ Teens & young adults
    - 2nd peak older adults
  ○ Spectrum of appearance
    - Primarily lytic ± soft tissue mass; varying degrees of ossification within tumor, may be minimal
    - Diffusely sclerotic ± heavily ossified soft tissue component
- **Fibrodysplasia Ossificans Progressiva**
  ○ Axial changes dominate
  ○ Begins in infancy
  ○ Progresses from proximal to distal
  ○ Changes progress over time
    - Initial soft tissue swelling/nodules
    - Progress to large plaque-like foci of ossification

Extruded Cement (Mimic)

Axial T1WI MR shows extraosseous collection of methacrylate (cement) ➡ following vertebroplasty.

Vertebral Body Osteomyelitis, Pyogenic

Axial NECT shows destruction of the L5-S1 disc space in this patient with pyogenic vertebral body osteomyelitis. Ossific fragments ➡ are seen in the anterior soft tissues within a large paraspinal abscess ➡.

PARAVERTEBRAL OSSIFICATION AND CALCIFICATION

(Left) Anteroposterior radiograph shows a classic presentation of chronic reactive arthritis with abnormal sacroiliac joints and bulky paraspinal ossification ➡. Psoriatic spondyloarthropathy has a similar appearance. (†MSK Req). *(Right)* Lateral radiograph shows significant subluxation and endplate destruction with osseous debris at 2 adjacent levels ➡ in this paraplegic patient. Though infection should be considered, this process was neuropathic (Charcot spine).

Chronic Reactive Arthritis

Paraplegia

(Left) Lateral radiograph shows severe vertebral body destruction, centered on the L2/3 disc space & accompanied by endplate sclerosis, and extensive osseous debris around the vertebrae ➡. This is a typical Charcot (neuropathic) spine *(Right)* Axial bone CT shows a typical appearance of tumoral calcinosis with large calcific mass ➡ associated with posterior elements of lumbar spine.

Charcot, Neuropathic

Tumoral Calcinosis

(Left) Axial NECT shows vertebral body exostosis ➡ without suggestion of degeneration. Note the extension into the canal. This benign neoplasm was highly symptomatic. *(Right)* Lateral radiograph shows cloud-like calcification surrounding the C2 vertebral body and posterior elements ➡. This is a typical appearance of progressive systemic sclerosis, or scleroderma.

Osteochondroma

Progressive Systemic Sclerosis

PARAVERTEBRAL OSSIFICATION AND CALCIFICATION

Osteoblastoma

Chondrosarcoma

(Left) Anteroposterior radiograph shows a densely ossified mass ⮞ arising at the T3 level on the left. The mass proved to be an osteoblastoma arising in the posterior elements. *(Right)* Axial NECT shows a fairly well-defined matrix arising from a lesion in the spinous process ⮞. While osteoblastoma might be strongly considered, this proved to be chondrosarcoma, arising in an exostosis.

Chordoma

Vertebral Osteomyelitis, Granulomatous

(Left) Sagittal NECT shows massive thoracic chordoma with calcific matrix in the paraspinal soft tissues ⮞ and destruction of several adjacent vertebral bodies ⮞. *(Right)* Axial NECT shows thoracic spinal TB in a young child with large epidural and paraspinal abscesses. Peripheral mineralization is present and involves both the intradural and extradural portions of the soft tissue mass ⮞.

Osteosarcoma

Fibrodysplasia Ossificans Progressiva

(Left) Anteroposterior radiograph shows multiple sites of sclerotic dense bone formation ⮞ in this patient with osseous metastases from a primary osteosarcoma. A large paravertebral ossified mass ⮞ accompanies the largest vertebral lesion. *(Right)* Anteroposterior radiograph shows mature ossification within the soft tissues of the back ⮞. A similar ossification was present in the anterior thigh of this patient with fibrodysplasia ossificans progressiva.

LINEAR OSSIFICATION ALONG ANTERIOR SPINE

DIFFERENTIAL DIAGNOSIS

Common
- DISH
- Aortic Calcification
- Ankylosing Spondylitis (AS)
- Inflammatory Bowel Disease Arthritis

Less Common
- Psoriatic Arthritis
- Chronic Reactive Arthritis
- Pyrophosphate Arthropathy
- Renal Osteodystrophy
- Hemochromatosis
- Juvenile Idiopathic Arthritis (Mimic)
- Hyperparathyroidism (HPTH)
- Complications of Retinoids
- Paraplegia

Rare but Important
- Sternoclavicular Hyperostosis (SAPHO)
- Ochronosis (Alkaptonuria)
- Osteomalacia, Hypophosphatemic

ESSENTIAL INFORMATION

Helpful Clues for Common Diagnoses
- **DISH**
  - Flowing anterior longitudinal ligament (ALL) ossification
  - Closely adherent midvertebra, lucency at vertebra corner where loosely adherent
- **Aortic Calcification**
  - Separate from disc
- **Ankylosing Spondylitis (AS)**
  - Spinal fusion & thin syndesmophytes
- **Inflammatory Bowel Disease Arthritis**
  - Spine findings identical to AS

Helpful Clues for Less Common Diagnoses
- **Psoriatic Arthritis**
  - Bulky paravertebral ossification
- **Chronic Reactive Arthritis**
  - Spine findings identical to psoriasis
- **Pyrophosphate Arthropathy**
  - Mineralization anterior annular fibers (MAAF); disc normal or narrowed, favors lumbar spine
- **Renal Osteodystrophy**
  - 2° HPTH; Rugger Jersey spine
- **Hemochromatosis**
  - MAAF; arthritis with subchondral cysts
- **Juvenile Idiopathic Arthritis (Mimic)**
  - Hypoplastic discs mimic syndesmophytes; facet joint fusion
- **Hyperparathyroidism (HPTH)**
  - MAAF, bone resorption, calcific deposits
- **Complications of Retinoids**
  - ALL ossification, spinal osteophytes
- **Paraplegia**
  - MAAF, ALL/paravertebral ossification

Helpful Clues for Rare Diagnoses
- **Sternoclavicular Hyperostosis (SAPHO)**
  - Ossification ALL, cervical spine
- **Ochronosis (Alkaptonuria)**
  - Syndesmophytes, spinal osteoporosis, discal linear mineralization
- **Osteomalacia, Hypophosphatemic**
  - MAAF; ↑ bone density, enthesopathy

DISH

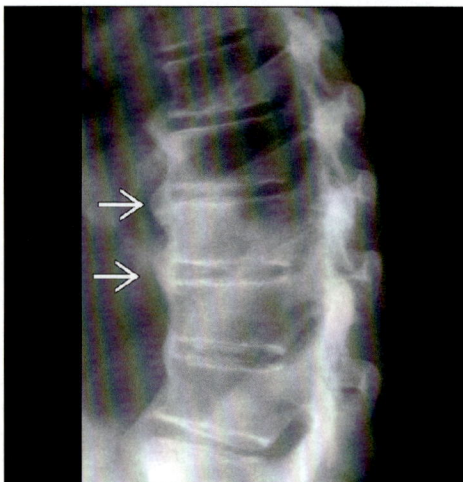

Lateral radiograph shows flowing the anterior longitudinal ligament ossification ➡ characteristic of DISH. Note how the ossification is tightly adherent to the mid-anterior vertebral body cortex.

Aortic Calcification

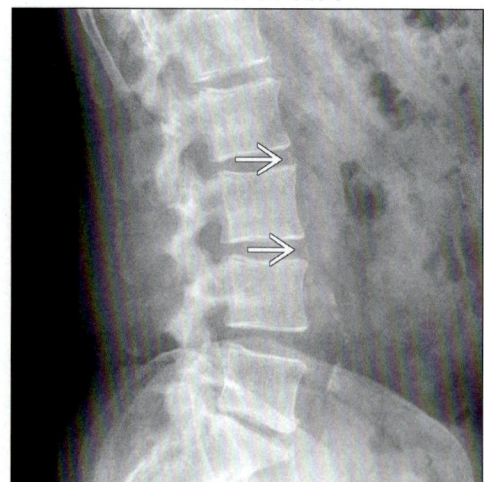

Lateral radiograph shows extensive calcification of the aorta. At two levels the calcification is closely related to the anterior disc space ➡, mimicking mineralization in the annulus fibrosus.

LINEAR OSSIFICATION ALONG ANTERIOR SPINE

Ankylosing Spondylitis (AS)

Inflammatory Bowel Disease Arthritis

(Left) Lateral radiograph shows syndesmophyte formation ➡ throughout the lumbar spine in this patient with ankylosing spondylitis. The syndesmophytes are intimately related to the vertebral body corners. *(Right)* Lateral radiograph shows extensive cervical ankylosis with thin syndesmophytes at multiple levels ➡ in this patient with spondyloarthropathy of inflammatory bowel disease. Posterior fusion is related to prior injury.

Juvenile Idiopathic Arthritis (Mimic)

Hyperparathyroidism (HPTH)

(Left) Sagittal bone CT shows ankylosis of hypoplastic vertebra and facet joints in this patient with juvenile idiopathic arthritis. The discs are also hypoplastic, producing an appearance mimicking syndesmophytes ➡. *(Right)* Sagittal bone CT shows mineralization within the anterior fibers of the annulus fibrosus ➡ mimicking syndesmophytes in this patient with hyperparathyroidism.

Complications of Retinoids

Ochronosis (Alkaptonuria)

(Left) Lateral radiograph shows the productive changes associated with retinoid use ➡ that mimic the anterior longitudinal ligament ossification of DISH. *(Right)* Lateral radiograph shows typical findings of ochronosis with extensive mineralization within the discs and spinal osteoporosis. Less apparent is the thin mineralization in the anterior annular fibers ➡ that mimics syndesmophyte formation.

BULLET SHAPED VERTEBRA/ANTERIOR VERTEBRAL BODY BEAKING

DIFFERENTIAL DIAGNOSIS

Common
- Achondroplasia
- Down Syndrome (Trisomy 21)

Less Common
- Radiation-Induced Growth Deformities
- Hypothyroidism (Congenital)
- Pseudoachondroplasia

Rare but Important
- Morquio Syndrome
- Hurler Syndrome

ESSENTIAL INFORMATION

Key Differential Diagnosis Issues
- Bullet shape: Down, achondroplasia, pseudoachondroplasia, hypothyroidism, Hurler, Morquio
- Anterior beaking: Achondroplasia, radiation-induced, Hurler, Morquio

Helpful Clues for Common Diagnoses
- **Achondroplasia**
  - Rhizomelic dwarf
  - Exaggerated lumbar lordosis, posterior vertebral scalloping, narrow foramen magnum, congenital spinal stenosis, decreased interpediculate distance
  - Squared iliac wings, narrow sciatic notch, horizontal acetabular roof
  - Trident hand, flared anterior ribs
- **Down Syndrome (Trisomy 21)**
  - Congenital heart disease, GI abnormalities
  - Brachycephaly, abnormal facies
  - Short stature, atlanto-axial instability, developmental hip dysplasia

Helpful Clues for Less Common Diagnoses
- **Radiation-Induced Growth Deformities**
  - Regional osteoporosis ± scoliosis
- **Hypothyroidism (Congenital)**
  - Mental retardation, delayed growth, short stature, stippled epiphyses
  - Abnormal skull & face with thick protruding tongue, delayed dentition
- **Pseudoachondroplasia**
  - Rhizomelic dwarf
  - C1-2 subluxation, accentuated lumbar lordosis, early osteoarthritis
  - Short thick tubular bones especially hands & feet, metaphyseal excrescences

Helpful Clues for Rare Diagnoses
- **Morquio Syndrome**
  - Short stature, macrocephaly, coarse facial features, widely spaced teeth
  - Odontoid hypoplasia, increased lumbar lordosis, bell chest, & paddle-shaped ribs
  - Flared iliac wings, inferior tapering iliac bones, steep acetabuli, coxa valga
- **Hurler Syndrome**
  - Mental retardation, short stature
  - Coarse facial features, macrocephaly, & other craniovertebral anomalies including J-shaped sella
  - Small iliac bones with inferior tapering, steep acetabuli, abnormal femoral heads
  - Thickened tubular bones, contractures

Achondroplasia

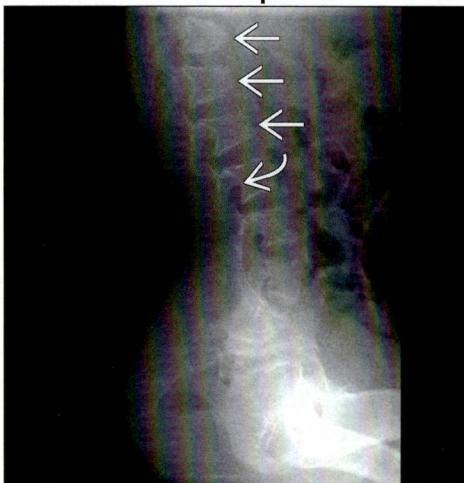

Lateral radiograph shows bullet-shaped vertebrae at the lumbosacral junction ➡ and scalloping of the posterior vertebral cortices ⤹, findings commonly seen in patients with achondroplasia.

Achondroplasia

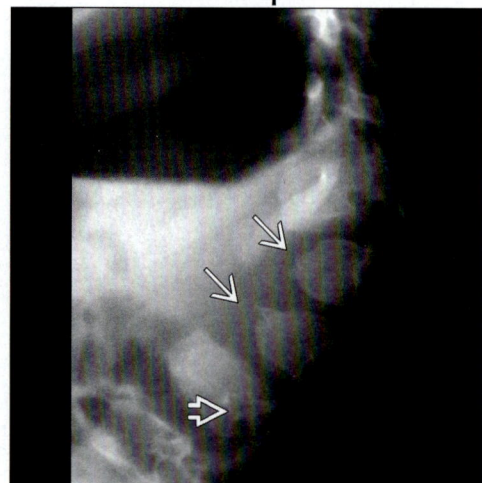

Lateral radiograph shows posterior vertebral scalloping ⮂, hypoplasia of L1 & L2, and anterior beaking ➡ with focal kyphosis in this patient with achondroplasia.

BULLET SHAPED VERTEBRA/ANTERIOR VERTEBRAL BODY BEAKING

Radiation-Induced Growth Deformities

Pseudoachondroplasia

(Left) Lateral radiograph shows a hypoplastic almost bullet-shaped L1 ➡ in a child who was radiated 1 year earlier for Wilms tumor. Radiation of growing bone slows or stops growth due to vascular damage. *(Right)* Lateral radiograph shows very mild platyspondyly, with mild anterior beaking ➡ in a patient with pseudoachondroplasia.

Morquio Syndrome

Morquio Syndrome

(Left) Lateral radiograph shows a thoracolumbar kyphosis, with a hypoplastic oval L1 and central anterior beaking ➡ in this patient with Morquio syndrome. *(Right)* Lateral radiograph shows classic example of Morquio syndrome, including dorsolumbar gibbus with vertebral beaking ➡.

Hurler Syndrome

Hurler Syndrome

(Left) Lateral radiograph shows inferior beaking ➡ of 3 vertebral bodies in this patient with many classic findings of Hurler syndrome. *(Right)* Lateral radiograph shows typical skeletal findings of dysostosis multiplex, including vertebral body beaking ➡ in this patient with Hurler syndrome.

CONGENITAL & ACQUIRED CHILDHOOD PLATYSPONDYLY

DIFFERENTIAL DIAGNOSIS

Common
- Trauma
- Langerhans Cell Histiocytosis
- Leukemia
- Metastatic Disease
- Ewing Sarcoma

Less Common
- Achondroplasia (Homozygous)
- Osteogenesis Imperfecta
- Pseudoachondroplasia
- Mucopolysaccharidoses
- Radiation-Induced
- Spondyloepiphyseal Dysplasia

Rare but Important
- Complications of Bisphosphonates
- Homocystinuria
- Idiopathic Juvenile Osteoporosis
- Cushing Disease
- Thanatophoric Dwarf
- Metatropic Dwarf
- Kniest Dysplasia
- Short Rib Polydactyly
- Hypophosphatasia

ESSENTIAL INFORMATION

Key Differential Diagnosis Issues
- Platyspondyly: Generalized vertebral collapse maintaining relatively parallel endplates
- Differentiating features: Congenital presentation vs. childhood onset; diffuse collapse vs. solitary or multifocal collapse

Helpful Clues for Common Diagnoses
- **Trauma**
  - Solitary or multifocal, history diagnostic
  - Any age
- **Langerhans Cell Histiocytosis**
  - Childhood, thoracic spine mainly
  - Solitary or few vertebra involved
  - May reconstitute during healing
- **Leukemia**
  - Age 2-5 years
  - Variable presentations
    - Generalized osteoporosis, diffuse collapse
    - Focal lesion(s) with permeative destruction, periostitis, soft tissue mass; collapse solitary or multifocal
  - Metaphyseal bands (lucent, dense, or alternating), may involve vertebra
- **Metastatic Disease**
  - Neuroblastoma, retinoblastoma, Wilms
  - ± Soft tissue mass, skeletal imaging nonspecific
- **Ewing Sarcoma**
  - Teens, young adults
  - Solitary lesion
  - Permeative destruction, soft tissue mass

Helpful Clues for Less Common Diagnoses
- **Achondroplasia (Homozygous)**
  - Radiographically & clinically mimics thanatophoric dwarf
  - Both parents have achondroplasia
  - Diffuse collapse
  - Congenital presentation
- **Osteogenesis Imperfecta**
  - Generalized osteoporosis
  - Solitary, multiple, or diffuse vertebra involved
    - Depends on severity of disease
    - Younger patients at presentation have more extensive disease
    - May be congenital
  - Multiple fractures axial & appendicular skeleton
  - Congenital platyspondyly type IIA
  - Micromelia, short ribs
- **Pseudoachondroplasia**
  - Rhizomelic dwarf
  - Normal infancy, manifests age 2-3 years
  - As child develops, mimics spondyloepiphyseal dysplasia
  - Diffuse collapse develops during childhood
- **Mucopolysaccharidoses**
  - Short stature, diffuse skeletal dysplasia
  - Coarse facial features
  - Diffuse collapse
  - Congenital presentation
  - Morquio, Hunter best known
    - Mental retardation with Hunter
- **Radiation-Induced**
  - Regional osteoporosis
  - May affect only one side of vertebra
    - ± Scoliosis
  - May induce osteochondroma formation
- **Spondyloepiphyseal Dysplasia**
  - Truncal dwarfism
  - Diffuse spine deformities
  - Delayed ossification long bone epiphyses

CONGENITAL & ACQUIRED CHILDHOOD PLATYSPONDYLY

○ Coxa vara consistent feature of variable severity
○ Congenita: Congenital presentation
○ Tarda: Develops around puberty
  ▪ Spine changes are not dominant feature

Helpful Clues for Rare Diagnoses
- **Complications of Bisphosphonates**
  ○ Used to treat conditions such osteogenesis imperfecta (OI)
    ▪ See above for discussion of OI
  ○ May cause bone weakening, lead to fractures
  ○ Metaphyseal dense bands including vertebral bodies
- **Homocystinuria**
  ○ Nonspecific osteoporosis
  ○ Scoliosis
  ○ Diffuse collapse develops in childhood
  ○ Body habitus mimics Marfan
  ○ Mental retardation
- **Idiopathic Juvenile Osteoporosis**
  ○ Typically > 2 years
  ○ Axial & appendicular osteoporosis
    ▪ Complicated by fractures
    ▪ Spine involvement solitary, multifocal, diffuse
  ○ May mimic osteogenesis imperfecta tarda
- **Cushing Disease**
  ○ Rare in children
  ○ Produces generalized osteoporosis
    ▪ Solitary or multifocal collapse, especially thoracic & lumbar spine
  ○ May develop osteonecrosis

- **Thanatophoric Dwarf**
  ○ Fatal, rhizomelic dwarf
    ▪ Micromelia, short ribs
  ○ Diffuse collapse
  ○ Congenital presentation
  ○ Telephone receiver femurs (bowing, metaphyseal flaring)
- **Metatropic Dwarf**
  ○ Metatropic: Changing
    ▪ Early life short limb, normal trunk
    ▪ Later life short trunk with severe kyphoscoliosis
  ○ Characteristic short long bones with dramatic metaphyseal flaring
  ○ Diffuse collapse
  ○ Congenital presentation
- **Kniest Dysplasia**
  ○ Short trunk, short limb, large joints
  ○ Diffuse collapse develops in childhood
- **Short Rib Polydactyly**
  ○ Lethal dwarfism
  ○ Short ribs, micromelia, polydactyly
  ○ Diffuse changes
  ○ Congenital presentation
  ○ Includes asphyxiating thoracic dystrophy (Jeune) & Ellis-van Creveld
- **Hypophosphatasia**
  ○ Varying degrees of poor bone mineralization
  ○ Congenital (lethal)
    ▪ Diffuse collapse
  ○ Variable degree & number collapsed vertebra with later presentations

Langerhans Cell Histiocytosis

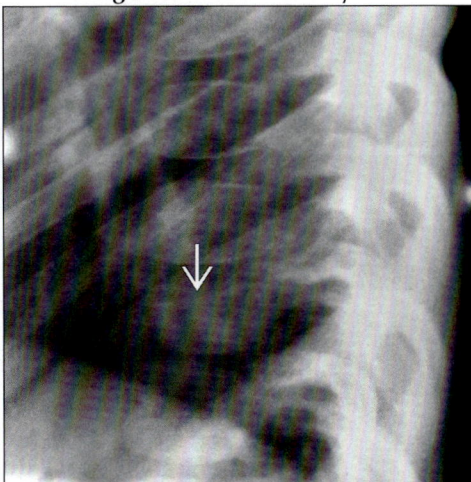

Lateral radiograph shows partial collapse of thoracic vertebral body ➡. The endplates are intact as are the disc spaces and posterior elements. The appearance is common in Langerhans cell histiocytosis.

Langerhans Cell Histiocytosis

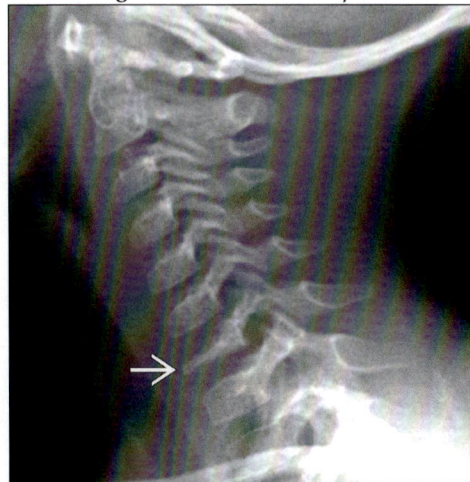

Lateral radiograph shows typical presentation of Langerhans cell histiocytosis with vertebra plana at C7 ➡. Following treatment, this body partially reconstituted its height.

CONGENITAL & ACQUIRED CHILDHOOD PLATYSPONDYLY

Leukemia

Ewing Sarcoma

(Left) Sagittal T1 C+ MR shows the typical appearance of leukemic marrow infiltration with height loss of varying degrees involving all vertebral bodies ➡. Note the contrast-enhancement of all the vertebral bodies in this child. *(Right)* Anteroposterior radiograph shows asymmetric platyspondyly ➡ with destruction of the left pedicle in a 12 year old. This proved to be early destruction in Ewing sarcoma.

Osteogenesis Imperfecta

Pseudoachondroplasia

(Left) Anteroposterior radiograph shows multiple rib, vertebral, and long bone fractures in this fetus with osteogenesis imperfecta, type II. The arms and legs are short due to angulation and deformity resulting from the fractures. *(Right)* Lateral radiograph shows very mild platyspondyly ➡, with mild anterior beaking in this patient with pseudoachondroplasia.

Mucopolysaccharidoses

Radiation-Induced

(Left) Lateral radiograph shows classic example of Morquaio syndrome, with diffuse vertebral body collapse, dorsolumbar gibbus, and vertebral beaking. *(Right)* Anteroposterior radiograph shows relative hypoplasia of the left side of the T12, L1, L2, and L3 vertebral bodies ➡, creating an asymmetric platyspondyly due to radiation of a left Wilms tumor. Note the clips from the left nephrectomy.

CONGENITAL & ACQUIRED CHILDHOOD PLATYSPONDYLY

Spondyloepiphyseal Dysplasia

Complications of Bisphosphonates

(Left) Sagittal T2WI MR shows endplate irregularity and diffuse platyspondyly with rectangular-shaped vertebral bodies. There is a generous bony spinal canal dimension. This is the adult appearance of spondyloepiphyseal dysplasia. *(Right)* AP radiograph shows severe osteopenia, gracile ribs, and diffuse vertebral compressions. Metaphyseal dense bands are present. This patient has osteogenesis imperfecta and was treated with bisphosphonates.

Homocystinuria

Cushing Disease

(Left) Lateral radiograph shows diffuse osteopenia and mild generalized platyspondyly. The findings are nonspecific and, in this case, due to homocystinuria. *(Right)* Anteroposterior radiograph shows minimal platyspondyly of T12 ➡. The 11th ribs have been resected as a surgical approach for adrenalectomy in this patient with Cushing disease.

Thanatophoric Dwarf

Hypophosphatasia

(Left) Lateral radiograph shows short ribs ➡ and classic platyspondyly ➡, with the widened intervertebral disc spaces associated with many dwarfisms, including thanatophoric dwarfism. *(Right)* Lateral radiograph shows a severe deficit in bone formation. Diffuse platyspondyly is present. The cranium is particularly notable for having no ossification, except at the base of skull, a clue to the diagnosis of hypophosphatasia.

FISH (BICONCAVE) OR H-SHAPED VERTEBRA

DIFFERENTIAL DIAGNOSIS

Common
- Senile Osteoporosis (SOP)
- Complications of Steroids
- Paget Disease
- Multiple Myeloma
- Neoplasm
- Renal Osteodystrophy
- Hyperparathyroidism (HPTH)
- Osteomalacia
- Sickle Cell Anemia

Less Common
- Gaucher Disease
- Osteogenesis Imperfecta
- Thalassemia Major

Rare but Important
- Homocystinuria

ESSENTIAL INFORMATION

Key Differential Diagnosis Issues
- H-shape: Osteonecrosis producing central endplate collapse with sharp margins
  - Sickle cell, Gaucher, thalassemia
- Biconcave: Structural weakening, disc impresses upon & remodels vertebra
  - Any entity on list may be biconcave

Helpful Clues for Common Diagnoses
- **Senile Osteoporosis (SOP)**
  - Elderly individuals: Women > men
- **Complications of Steroids**
  - Chronic medical diseases (exogenous) & Cushing disease (endogenous)
- **Paget Disease**
  - Increased vertebral size, coarse trabecula, increased density at vertebral margins
- **Multiple Myeloma**
  - Generalized osteoporosis mimics SOP
- **Neoplasm**
  - Metastatic: Multilevel disease, variable destruction
  - Primary: Ewing, lymphoma; collapse is more common with other neoplasms
- **Renal Osteodystrophy**
  - HPTH, osteomalacia, osteoporosis
- **Hyperparathyroidism (HPTH)**
  - Bone resorption weakens vertebra
- **Osteomalacia**
  - Coarse, ill-defined trabecula
- **Sickle Cell Anemia**
  - Osteoporosis, osteonecrosis, coarse trabecula

Helpful Clues for Less Common Diagnoses
- **Gaucher Disease**
  - Erlenmeyer flask deformity distal femur
- **Osteogenesis Imperfecta**
  - Bones thin & gracile or short & tubular
  - Osteoporosis, bowing, & deformities
- **Thalassemia Major**
  - Osteoporosis, Erlenmeyer flask deformities, "hair on end" skull, rodent facies

Helpful Clues for Rare Diagnoses
- **Homocystinuria**
  - Nonspecific osteoporosis, scoliosis

Senile Osteoporosis (SOP)

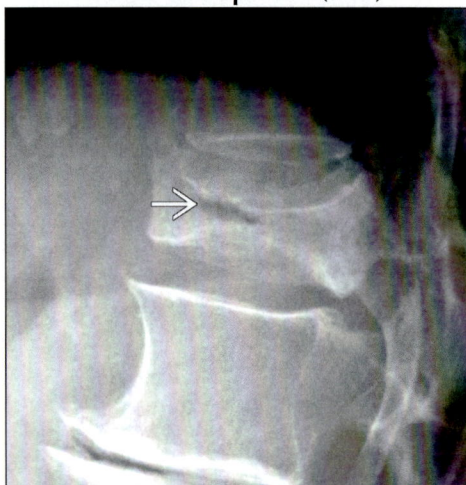

Lateral radiograph shows collapse of T12 vertebral body in this patient with senile osteoporosis. Gas is present within the body ➜, consistent with pseudoarthrosis and intervertebral cleft.

Senile Osteoporosis (SOP)

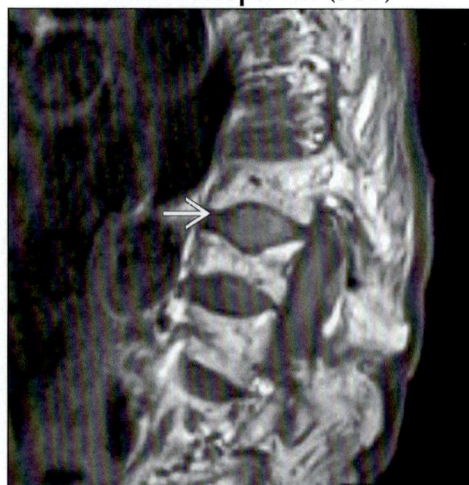

Sagittal T1WI MR shows biconcave T10 vertebra. Ballooning of the T9-10 disc ➜ is due to concave deformities of the adjacent endplates in this patient with senile osteoporosis.

FISH (BICONCAVE) OR H-SHAPED VERTEBRA

Complications of Steroids

Paget Disease

(Left) Sagittal T1WI MR shows multilevel biconcave vertebra ➡ in this patient on long term steroids. Note the edema at T8 ➡, indicative of active compression. *(Right)* Lateral radiograph shows AP dimension enlargement as well as coarsened cortical and trabecular bone in L3, typical of Paget disease ➡. The vertebral height is diminished relative to adjacent vertebra with mild concavity of each endplate.

Multiple Myeloma

Neoplasm

(Left) Lateral radiograph shows diffuse osteoporosis and compression fractures of all the lumbar vertebrae ➡. No focal lesions are seen. Biopsy was required to establish a diagnosis of multiple myeloma. *(Right)* Sagittal STIR MR shows multiple vertebral lesions ➡ with severe compression of L3 ➡. Diagnosis of metastatic disease is facilitated by the multiplicity of lesions.

Sickle Cell Anemia

Sickle Cell Anemia

(Left) Lateral radiograph shows a very abrupt loss of height in the mid portion of the vertebral body ➡. This appearance is known as "H-shaped" vertebral body, as seen in this patient with sickle cell anemia. *(Right)* Coronal NECT shows anteroposterior appearance of "H-shaped" vertebral bodies in this patient with sickle cell anemia. The appearance mimics the changes seen on the lateral view.

SQUARING OF ONE OR MORE VERTEBRA

DIFFERENTIAL DIAGNOSIS

Common
- Anterior Cervical Discectomy & Fusion
- Long-Standing Posterior Fusion
- Paget Disease
- Block Vertebra (Congenital Fusion)
- Ankylosing Spondylitis (AS)

Less Common
- Inflammatory Bowel Disease Arthritis
- Normal Variant
- Juvenile Idiopathic Arthritis
- Psoriatic Arthritis
- Chronic Reactive Arthritis

ESSENTIAL INFORMATION

Key Differential Diagnosis Issues
- Finding is only evident on lateral view
- **Hint**: Vertebral size is a distinguishing feature

Helpful Clues for Common Diagnoses
- **Anterior Cervical Discectomy & Fusion**
  - Osseous-fusion across disc space
  - Normal-sized vertebra
- **Long-Standing Posterior Fusion**
  - Disc may mineralize or completely fuse
  - Normal-sized vertebra
- **Paget Disease**
  - Increased vertebral body size
    - May involve posterior elements
  - Thickened cortices, coarse trabecula
- **Block Vertebra (Congenital Fusion)**
  - Vertebra narrowed anterior to posterior
  - Hypoplastic or fused disc
  - ± Unilateral or bilateral posterior fusion
- **Ankylosing Spondylitis (AS)**
  - Most common at thoracolumbar junction
  - Romanus lesion (early): Corner erosion
  - Shiny corner: 2° new bone at corner
  - Normal size vertebral bodies
  - Associated findings: Anterior & posterior fusion, symmetric sacroiliac (SI) disease, enthesopathy, large joint arthritis

Helpful Clues for Less Common Diagnoses
- **Inflammatory Bowel Disease**
  - Radiographically identical to ankylosing spondylitis, differentiate clinically
- **Normal Variant**: Absence of other features
- **Juvenile Idiopathic Arthritis**
  - Cervical fusion common (anterior & posterior); generalized osteoporosis
  - Other: Erosive arthritis, periostitis, ballooned epiphyses; esp. knee & elbow
- **Psoriatic Arthritis**
  - Vertebral squaring uncommon, mimics AS
  - No spinal fusion, asymmetric SI arthritis
  - Associated findings
    - Enthesopathy, periosteal new bone
    - Bilateral asymmetric erosive arthritis hands & feet, sausage digits, tuft resorption
- **Chronic Reactive Arthritis**
  - Radiographically identical to psoriasis
    - Less cervical spine involvement
    - Foot involvement greater than hand

Anterior Cervical Discectomy & Fusion

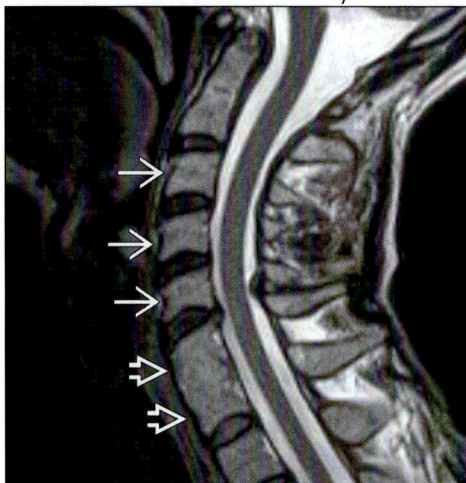

Sagittal T2WI MR shows solid C6-7 anterior fusion. Note the normal concavity along the upper cervical vertebra ➡. The concavity is missing at the fused levels ⇒.

Long-Standing Posterior Fusion

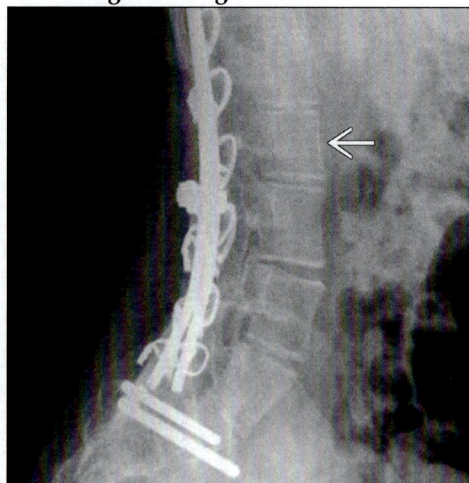

Lateral radiograph shows long-standing posterior spinal fusion. The anterior vertebra body cortices assume a flat contour ➡ rather than the normal mild concavity.

SQUARING OF ONE OR MORE VERTEBRA

Paget Disease

Block Vertebra (Congenital Fusion)

(Left) Lateral radiograph shows the classic "picture frame" appearance of vertebral body Paget disease. With enlargement of the body, the anterior concavity is lost ➡. Note normal concavity in the adjacent body for comparison ➡. *(Right)* Lateral radiograph shows congenital fusion of C3 and C4. Note the relatively flat anterior vertebra contours, especially at C3 ➡.

Ankylosing Spondylitis (AS)

Inflammatory Bowel Disease Arthritis

(Left) Sagittal T2WI MR shows typical squaring of the lumbar vertebral bodies ➡ & diffuse disc calcification (from long-standing ankylosing spondylitis). *(Right)* Lateral radiograph shows squared configuration of anterior vertebral cortices. The squaring is caused by erosions beneath the anterior longitudinal ligament. L2 also shows the characteristic "shiny corner" sign ➡ due to inflammatory reaction seen in patients with seronegative spondyloarthropathy.

Normal Variant

Juvenile Idiopathic Arthritis

(Left) Lateral radiograph shows squaring of several vertebral bodies ➡ with loss of the normal prominent corners and flattening of the anterior cortex. Paget disease of L4 ➡, also with squaring, is an incidental finding in this otherwise normal individual. *(Right)* Sagittal T2WI MR shows long and gracile upper cervical vertebral bodies that are of normal height but thin in anterior posterior direction due to fusion from C2-C6 ➡.

VERTEBRAL BODY SCLEROSIS

DIFFERENTIAL DIAGNOSIS

Common
- Fracture Healing
- Schmorl Node
- Discogenic Sclerosis
- Intraosseous Hemangioma
- Compression Fracture, Acute
- Metastases, Blastic
- Enostosis (Bone Island)
- Vertebral Augmentation (Mimic)
- Paget Disease
- Osteomyelitis, Chronic
- Renal Osteodystrophy

Less Common
- Langerhans Cell Histiocytosis
- Lymphoma
- Fibrous Dysplasia

Rare but Important
- Chordoma
- Myelofibrosis
- Plasma Cell Myeloma
- Osteopetrosis
- Osteosarcoma
- Ewing Sarcoma
- Chondrosarcoma
- Helmut Sclerosis
- Mastocytosis
- Fluorosis
- Axial Osteomalacia
- Melorheostosis
- Tuberous Sclerosis

ESSENTIAL INFORMATION

Key Differential Diagnosis Issues
- Excludes conditions with diffuse polyostotic osteosclerosis unless limited to spine or unusual appearance in spine
- Ivory vertebra (diffusely dense): Lymphoma, Paget, blastic metastases, low grade osteomyelitis

Helpful Clues for Common Diagnoses
- **Fracture Healing**
  - Callus formation, may be seen with any fracture pattern
- **Schmorl Node**
  - Nucleus pulposus herniates through endplate, sclerotic margin; abuts endplate
- **Discogenic Sclerosis**
  - Reactive sclerosis to degenerative disc disease
  - Endplate distribution, or triangular distribution in anterior vertebral body
- **Intraosseous Hemangioma**
  - Corduroy appearance: Thickened vertically oriented struts
  - Seen more often on MR than radiography
- **Compression Fracture, Acute**
  - Superimposed trabecula creates sclerotic appearance
  - Height loss evident, may be along endplate, diffuse or asymmetric
  - Traumatic or insufficiency fracture
- **Metastasis, Blastic**
  - Breast, prostate, lung, colon, stomach, bladder, uterus, rectum, thyroid, kidney, carcinoid
- **Enostosis (Bone Island)**
  - Round or oblong (long axis vertical), brush-like margins, solitary or multiple
- **Vertebral Augmentation (Mimic)**
  - Homogeneously dense cement within collapsed or destroyed vertebra
- **Paget Disease**
  - Picture frame
  - Increased vertebra size, thickened cortices & trabecula
- **Osteomyelitis, Chronic**
  - Disc space destruction ± fragmentation
  - Osteolytic foci may be evident
  - Periosteal new bone formation
  - Paraspinal abscess
- **Renal Osteodystrophy**
  - Rugger jersey spine: Thick sclerosis along endplates
  - Associated changes of hyperparathyroidism & osteomalacia

Helpful Clues for Less Common Diagnoses
- **Langerhans Cell Histiocytosis**
  - Increased density within vertebra plana
  - Protean manifestations: Varying types of osteolytic lesions throughout skeleton
  - Button sequestrum skull
- **Lymphoma**
  - Splenomegaly
  - Hodgkin > non-Hodgkin
- **Fibrous Dysplasia**
  - Spine involvement unusual, more common with polyostotic disease
  - Expansile lesion, ground-glass matrix

VERTEBRAL BODY SCLEROSIS

Helpful Clues for Rare Diagnoses

- **Chordoma**
  - Any age, adults most common
  - Sacrum > clivus > rest of spine
  - Osseous destruction ± soft tissue mass
    - Mineralization > 50%
- **Myelofibrosis**
  - Vertebra, pelvis, ribs, proximal long bones
    - Sclerosis, especially endosteal; loss of corticomedullary distinction
    - Endplate sclerosis = sandwich vertebra
  - Splenomegaly
  - Extra-medullary hematopoiesis
  - Presents in late middle-aged, elderly adults
- **Plasma Cell Myeloma**
  - Typically multiple osteolytic lesions
    - Sclerosis following fx or treatment
  - Plasmacytoma
    - Younger patients than multiple myeloma
    - Rarer than myeloma, rarely sclerotic
    - Solitary, expansile lesion
  - POEMS
    - **P**olyneuropathy, **O**rganomegaly, **E**ndocrinopathy, **M** proteins, **S**kin changes
    - Younger patients than multiple myeloma
- **Osteopetrosis**
  - Diffuse axial & appendicular sclerosis
  - Bone-within-bone appearance
  - Endplate sclerosis = sandwich vertebra
  - Undertubulation of long bones, especially femurs
- **Osteosarcoma**
  - Teens & young adults, 2nd peak older adults
  - Spectrum
    - Primary lytic lesion ± soft tissue mass, variable degrees of mineralization
    - Diffusely sclerotic with extensively ossified soft tissue mass
- **Ewing Sarcoma**
  - Teens & young adults
  - Diffuse vertebral body reactive sclerosis ± soft tissue mass
- **Chondrosarcoma**
  - Expansile lytic lesion with flocculent mineralization (arcs & whorls) ± soft tissue mass, may see lobulated growth pattern
- **Helmut Sclerosis**
  - Women in 40s, pain
  - Isolated hemispherical sclerosis in anterior inferior lumbar vertebra
    - Normal disc space
- **Mastocytosis**
  - Axial ± appendicular involvement
  - Focal or diffuse sclerosis
  - Splenomegaly
- **Fluorosis**
  - Spinal osteophytes, enthesopathy, ligament calcification, periosteal new bone
- **Axial Osteomalacia**
  - Spine involvement only, predominately cervical, coarse trabecula
  - Primarily males
- **Tuberous Sclerosis**
  - Variable size osteosclerotic foci

Schmorl Node

Coronal bone CT shows multiple Schmorl nodes of varying size ➡. There is variable sclerosis at the periphery of the nodes.

Discogenic Sclerosis

Lateral radiograph shows triangular-shaped sclerosis within the anterior vertebral body ➡ with adjacent disc space narrowing, a typical pattern of reactive sclerosis associated with degenerative disc disease.

VERTEBRAL BODY SCLEROSIS

(Left) Sagittal NECT shows the classic honeycomb appearance of hemangioma with thickened trabeculae, intact cortex, and focal low attenuation between trabeculae. **(Right)** Anteroposterior 3D bone CT shows compression fractures at T4 & T5 ➡. At T5 generalized height loss is present, and the vertebra is diffusely sclerotic, an appearance consistent with acute fracture.

Intraosseous Hemangioma

Compression Fracture, Acute

(Left) Sagittal bone CT shows step-off depression of superior endplate ➡ and sclerotic line due to trabecular impaction ➡ following vertebral compression fracture. **(Right)** Sagittal bone CT shows prostate metastases causing uniformly dense L3 vertebral body ➡ and less extensive dense metastases at adjacent levels ➡.

Compression Fracture, Acute

Metastases, Blastic

(Left) Sagittal bone CT shows the characteristic dense sclerosis that is oriented along the long axis of the vertebra with typical irregular "brush-like" margins of a bone island ➡. **(Right)** Lateral radiograph obtained following vertebroplasty shows cement filling a cleft within a compressed vertebral body ➡.

Enostosis (Bone Island)

Vertebral Augmentation (Mimic)

VERTEBRAL BODY SCLEROSIS

Paget Disease

Osteomyelitis, Chronic

(Left) Anteroposterior radiograph shows an "ivory" L1 vertebral body due to Paget disease. The vertebra is enlarged with cortical thickening, findings that are a clue to the underlying etiology. (Right) Sagittal NECT shows marked sclerosis of L3 and L4 bodies with extensive endplate irregularity and bone destruction resulting from chronic osteomyelitis. The endplate destruction is the clue that the abnormality originated at that site as infection.

Renal Osteodystrophy

Renal Osteodystrophy

(Left) Anteroposterior radiograph shows unusually severe sclerosis and thickening of the vertebral endplates ➡. Severe nephrocalcinosis ➡ and small left kidney are a clue to the underlying renal disease that produced this rugger jersey spine. (Right) Lateral radiograph shows unusually severe sclerosis and thickening of the vertebral endplates ➡ in this dramatic case of rugger jersey spine in a patient with renal osteodystrophy.

Langerhans Cell Histiocytosis

Lymphoma

(Left) Lateral radiograph shows vertebra plana with diffuse sclerosis ➡ in this patient with Langerhans cell histiocytosis. (Right) Axial NECT in this patient with lymphoma shows a single sclerotic vertebral body and paraspinal mass ➡. Lymphoma is one of the recognized causes of ivory vertebra.

VERTEBRAL BODY SCLEROSIS

Fibrous Dysplasia

Chordoma

(Left) Coronal bone CT shows characteristic appearance of fibrous dysplasia with extensive "ground-glass" vertebral lesions ➡ & associated lytic lesions. Note expansion of the skull base & clivus ➡.
(Right) Sagittal NECT shows massive thoracic chordoma with a large mediastinal mass & scattered calcifications ➡. The mass destroys the anterior margin of several upper thoracic vertebral bodies. Note the sclerosis within several of the vertebra ➡.

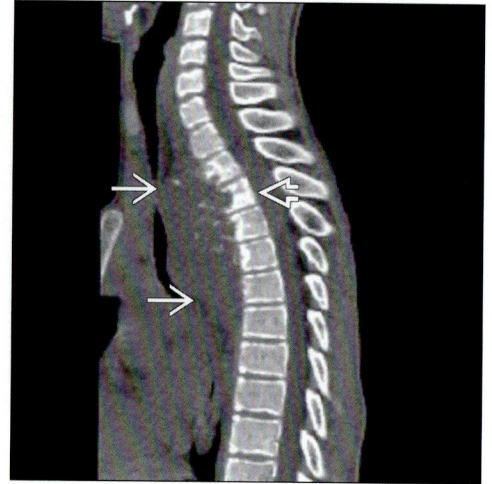

Myelofibrosis

Plasma Cell Myeloma

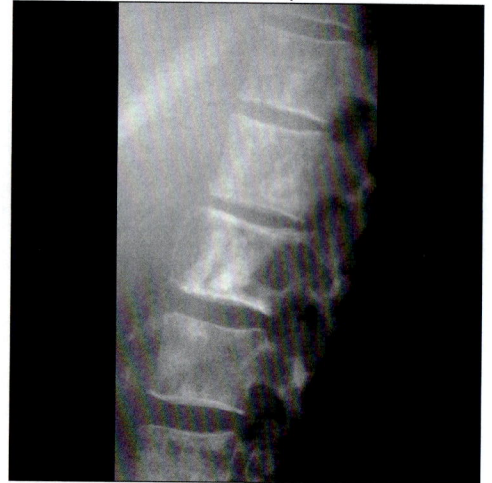

(Left) Anteroposterior radiograph shows diffuse osteosclerosis predominantly involving the medullary space, without thickening of the endosteal cortex. This is typical of myelofibrosis, which results from replacement of the fatty marrow with fibrous tissue.
(Right) Lateral radiograph shows small round lesions too numerous to count, either sclerotic or lytic with sclerotic rings. This pattern is a variant of the purely sclerotic lesions seen in the POEMS form of myeloma.

Osteopetrosis

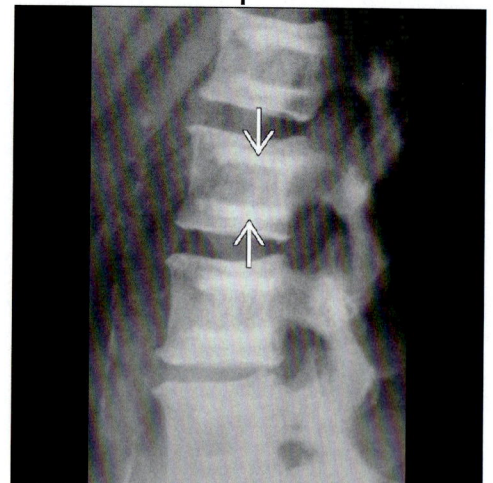

Osteopetrosis

(Left) Axial bone CT shows a typical example of dense vertebral body in a patient with osteopetrosis, demonstrating diffuse bony sclerosis. (Right) Lateral radiograph shows bone-in-bone appearance that can be seen in osteopetrosis ➡. The bones are mildly diffusely sclerotic. The bone-in-bone appearance results from failure of osteoclasts to remodel vertebral bodies during growth.

VERTEBRAL BODY SCLEROSIS

Osteosarcoma

Ewing Sarcoma

(Left) Axial CECT shows metastatic osteosarcoma with an unusual appearance of peripheral sclerosis with central lucency ➡. Some of this appearance may be due to chemotherapy. *(Right)* Lateral radiograph shows a sclerotic lesion occupying the body of S1 ➡. An unmineralized soft tissue mass is present ➡. These findings are typical for Ewing sarcoma, with the sclerosis due to reactive bone formation. The location in the axial skeleton is not unusual.

Chondrosarcoma

Mastocytosis

(Left) Sagittal NECT shows a large expanded mass with flocculent chondroid ("arcs and whorls") matrix involving posterior elements and right posterior vertebral body ➡ in this patient with chondrosarcoma. *(Right)* Lateral radiograph of the thoracic spine shows a classic ivory vertebra ➡ with dense bone replacing the entire body but no change in size. Focal sclerosis such as this is one appearance found in mastocytosis.

Fluorosis

Melorheostosis

(Left) Lateral radiograph shows diffuse sclerosis. There is thickening and indistinctness of the trabeculae. The findings resulted from two years of fluoride treatment. *(Right)* Coronal NECT shows dense sclerosis that involves the right side of the C2 and C3 vertebral bodies. The dermatomal distribution is characteristic of melorheostosis.

SPINAL OSTEOPHYTES

DIFFERENTIAL DIAGNOSIS

Common
- Spondylosis Deformans
- DISH (Mimic)
- Disc Disease

Less Common
- Seronegative Spondyloarthropathy (Mimic)
- Paralysis
- Complications of Retinoids
- Sternoclavicular Hyperostosis/SAPHO

Rare but Important
- Hypoparathyroidism
- Acromegaly
- Ochronosis (Alkaptonuria)
- Fluorosis

ESSENTIAL INFORMATION

Key Differential Diagnosis Issues
- Osteophytes demonstrate cortical & medullary continuity with vertebral body

Helpful Clues for Common Diagnoses
- **Spondylosis Deformans**
  - Independent of disc disease & facet arthritis
- **DISH (Mimic)**
  - Ossification anterior longitudinal ligament
  - Peripheral enthesopathy ± ossification posterior longitudinal ligament
- **Disc Disease**
  - Disc space narrowing, endplate changes
  - Multilevel or diffuse: Degenerative

- Solitary/multifocal: Trauma, infection, neuropathic

Helpful Clues for Less Common Diagnoses
- **Seronegative Spondyloarthropathy (Mimic)**
  - Syndesmophytes in all forms
  - Psoriasis, chronic reactive arthritis
    - Spectrum: Syndesmophytes to bulky paravertebral ossification
    - Enthesopathy, periostitis, bilateral asymmetric erosive arthritis hands & feet, sausage digits, tuft resorption
- **Paralysis**
  - Spectrum: Osteophytes, syndesmophytes, bulky paravertebral ossification
- **Complications of Retinoids**
  - Ligament ossification, especially spinal; enthesopathy
- **Sternoclavicular Hyperostosis/SAPHO**
  - Spectrum: Osteophytes, syndesmophytes, bulky paravertebral ossification

Helpful Clues for Rare Diagnoses
- **Hypoparathyroidism**
  - Normal disc space, enthesopathy
- **Acromegaly**
  - Posterior vertebral scalloping, ↑ disc space height, ossification mimics DISH
- **Ochronosis (Alkaptonuria)**
  - Linear disc mineralization & osteoporosis; osteophytes minimal
- **Fluorosis**
  - Osteosclerosis, enthesopathy, tendon ossification

Spondylosis Deformans

Lateral radiograph shows typical changes of spondylosis deformans with osteophytes of varying sizes ➡, without other changes.

DISH (Mimic)

Lateral radiograph shows anterior "flowing" osteophytes ➡ over multiple levels in this patient with typical changes of DISH.

SPINAL OSTEOPHYTES

Disc Disease

Disc Disease

(Left) Sagittal T2WI MR shows severe disc degeneration with loss of disc height at every cervical level. Large anterior ➡ and smaller posterior osteophytes are present. *(Right)* Axial NECT shows severe multilevel disc degeneration with loss of disc height, bony eburnation, and vacuum phenomenon at L5-S1, L3-4, and L2-3, accompanied by osteophytes ➡.

Seronegative Spondyloarthropathy (Mimic)

Seronegative Spondyloarthropathy (Mimic)

(Left) Anteroposterior radiograph shows bulky, asymmetric paravertebral ossification ➡ in the thoracolumbar spine in this patient with chronic reactive arthritis. *(Right)* Sagittal bone CT shows lower cervical ankylosis in this patient with ankylosing spondylitis ➡. Somewhat prominent syndesmophytes are present in the upper cervical spine ➡. Odontoid fracture is incidentally noted ➡, a result of minor trauma in this patient who has severe osteoporosis.

Complications of Retinoids

Ochronosis (Alkaptonuria)

(Left) Lateral radiograph shows small osteophyte at the anterosuperior margin of L5 ➡ in this patient taking retinoids. Such changes are usually more prominent at the thoracolumbar junction. *(Right)* Lateral radiograph shows classic appearance of ochronosis (alkaptonuria) with disc space narrowing & disc mineralization. Note the small anterior osteophytes ➡.

LESIONS ORIGINATING IN VERTEBRAL BODY

DIFFERENTIAL DIAGNOSIS

Common
- Intraosseous Hemangioma
- Metastases
- Schmorl Node (Mimic)
- Paget Disease
- Multiple Myeloma (MM)
- Limbus Vertebra (Mimic)
- Osteonecrosis
- Vertebral Body Osteomyelitis
- Lymphoma
- Plasmacytoma

Less Common
- Giant Cell Tumor
- Langerhans Cell Histiocytosis
- Fibrous Dysplasia
- Ewing Sarcoma
- Osteochondroma
- Renal Osteodystrophy, Brown Tumor

Rare but Important
- Chondrosarcoma
- Chordoma
- Osteosarcoma
- Echinococcal Disease

ESSENTIAL INFORMATION

Key Differential Diagnosis Issues
- List specifically excludes disc-centered processes such as degenerative disease
- Unless stated, any lesion may extend into posterior elements
- Most lesions have nonspecific appearance: Lytic lesion that may be expansile, geographic non-sclerotic margins ± soft tissue mass

Helpful Clues for Common Diagnoses
- **Intraosseous Hemangioma**
  - Solitary or multiple
  - Rarely extends to posterior elements
  - Common on MR with characteristic rounded hyperintense T1 lesion
  - Immature lesions have nonspecific, often aggressive appearance
  - Corduroy vertebra: Coarse, vertically oriented trabecula seen on CT & X-ray
- **Metastases**
  - Breast, lung, prostate, thyroid, kidney
  - Multiple lytic, blastic, or mixed lesions

- **Schmorl Node (Mimic)**
  - Often multiple, no posterior element involvement
  - Cup-like lesion adjacent to endplate defect, disc continuity into lesion, sclerotic rim; if acute has edema on MR
- **Paget Disease**
  - Typically solitary, may be multiple
  - **Hint**: Enlarged vertebra
    - Thick cortices, coarsened irregular trabecula (picture frame vertebra)
    - May produce ivory vertebra
- **Multiple Myeloma (MM)**
  - Patients typically 40 years or older
  - Multiple vertebra, variable appearance
    - Multiple lytic foci, variable size, non-sclerotic margins
    - Innumerable tiny lesions
    - Solitary lesion: Plasmacytoma
    - Sclerotic lesions: POEMS syndrome
  - Bone scan: Cold lesions or false negative
- **Limbus Vertebra (Mimic)**
  - Well-corticated bone fragment at vertebral corner; anterosuperior most common
  - Matching defect in adjacent vertebra, variable size with sclerotic margin
  - If acute has bright marrow signal on MR, increased uptake on bone scan
  - No posterior element involvement
- **Osteonecrosis**
  - Difficult to see on radiographs
  - MR: Serpiginous low signal rim & internal fat; posterior elements lesions rare, no soft tissue mass
  - May have vertebral collapse
    - H-shaped vertebra
    - Kümmel disease: Gas within cleft
  - Underlying medical condition such as sickle cell, chronic steroid use
- **Vertebral Body Osteomyelitis**
  - Typically destroyed intervertebral disc
  - Coccidiomycosis: Non-contiguous, intraosseous osteolytic foci, disc spared, paraspinal abscesses, rib involvement
  - Tuberculosis: Non-contiguous vertebral lesions with anterior cortical destruction
    - Disc destruction late
    - Paraspinal masses may be extensive
  - No posterior element involvement, lesions not expansile
- **Lymphoma**

LESIONS ORIGINATING IN VERTEBRAL BODY

- Any age, frequently young adult
- Permeative destruction, soft tissue mass even without cortical destruction
- Variant: Ivory vertebra
- **Plasmacytoma**
  - Slightly younger patient than MM
  - Lesion may be quite expansile

Helpful Clues for Less Common Diagnoses
- **Giant Cell Tumor**
  - Adults: 25-40 years old
  - May present with vertebra plana
  - Posterior element involvement unusual
- **Langerhans Cell Histiocytosis**
  - Children: 2-6 years old
  - Thoracic spine most common
  - Posterior element involvement rare
  - Lymphadenopathy, soft tissue mass/edema
  - **Hint**: Vertebra plana common
    - May reconstitute during healing phase
- **Fibrous Dysplasia**
  - Child < 10 years old; lumbar > cervical
  - Vertebral involvement rare in monostotic disease, common in polyostotic disease
  - May have internal septations/striations
  - **Hint**: Ground-glass matrix characteristic
- **Ewing Sarcoma**
  - Teens & young adults
  - Solitary lesion, confined to vertebral body
  - Permeative destruction, large soft tissue mass, often little cortical destruction
  - Variant: Ivory vertebra
- **Osteochondroma**

- **Hint**: Corticomedullary continuity diagnostic
- Usually part of multiple hereditary osteochondromas; evaluate knees to help establish diagnosis
- **Renal Osteodystrophy, Brown Tumor**
  - Other findings of renal osteodystrophy
    - Coarse ill-defined trabecula, bone resorption, soft tissue calcium deposits

Helpful Clues for Rare Diagnoses
- **Chondrosarcoma**
  - Any age; typically adult
  - **Hint**: Lobulated growth pattern, chondroid mineralization (flocculent or arcs & whorls)
- **Chordoma**
  - Any age, adults most common
  - Sacrum > clivus > remainder of spine
  - Mineralization in 50%
- **Osteosarcoma**
  - Teens & young adults, 2nd peak in older adults; solitary or multiple
  - Ranges from purely lytic to densely sclerotic (ivory vertebra) ± soft tissue mass with variable ossification
- **Echinococcal Disease**
  - Spine disease common in endemic areas, usually monostotic
  - Middle-aged & elderly adults, children rare
  - Septated osteolytic lesion ± soft tissue mass with calcification in cyst walls
  - MR & CT: Multicystic lesion with primary cyst & multiple daughter cysts

Intraosseous Hemangioma

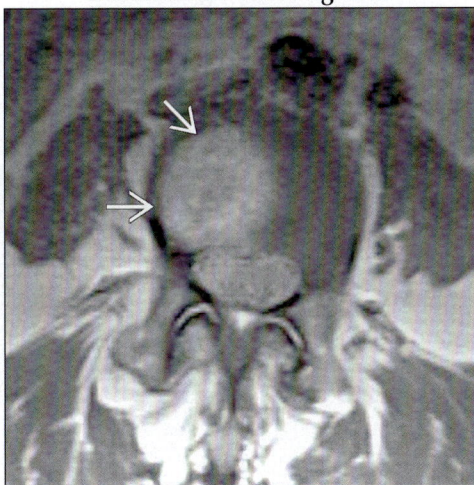

Axial T1WI MR shows a hyperintense L4 vertebral lesion ➡ without epidural expansion. The appearance is characteristic for an intraosseous hemangioma.

Intraosseous Hemangioma

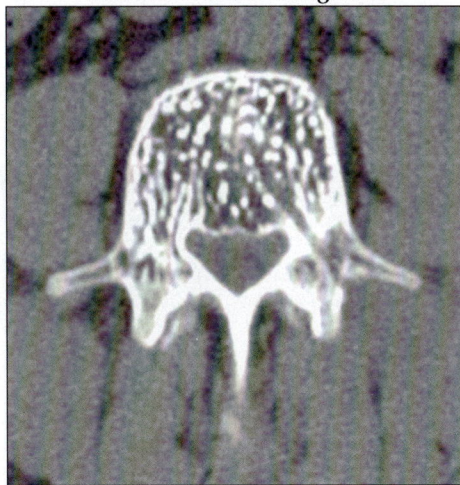

Axial NECT shows the classic honeycomb appearance of a hemangioma with thickened trabeculae, intact cortex, and focal low attenuation between trabeculae.

LESIONS ORIGINATING IN VERTEBRAL BODY

(Left) Sagittal NECT shows multiple blastic metastatic foci involving the thoracic and lumbar vertebral bodies ➡. **(Right)** Sagittal T1WI MR shows multiple focal areas of abnormal low signal due to diffuse metastases. There is confluent involvement of upper thoracic bodies with epidural extension and cord compression ➡, along with a pathologic lower thoracic fracture with no bony retropulsion ➡.

Metastases

Metastases

(Left) Sagittal bone CT shows small lytic-appearing lesions ➡ within several thoracic vertebral bodies. The lesions have sclerotic margins and abut the endplate, which is absent. The appearance is characteristic of Schmorl nodes. **(Right)** Sagittal T1 C+ MR shows a Schmorl node. There is a large, "cup-shaped" depression ➡ within the superior vertebral endplate, with sclerotic margins and no adjacent marrow edema. The disc protrudes directly into the vertebral depression.

Schmorl Node (Mimic)

Schmorl Node (Mimic)

(Left) Anteroposterior radiograph shows an ivory vertebra. Enlargement of the vertebral body ➡, pedicles ➡, and transverse processes ➡ is key to making the diagnosis of Paget disease. **(Right)** Sagittal STIR MR shows a typical appearance of Paget disease. The vertebra is mildly enlarged in anterior-posterior dimension ➡, with slight height loss. Enlargement of the spinous process is also present ➡. Coarsened trabecula are another clue to diagnosis.

Paget Disease

Paget Disease

LESIONS ORIGINATING IN VERTEBRAL BODY

Multiple Myeloma (MM)

Limbus Vertebra (Mimic)

(Left) Sagittal T1WI MR shows typical MR appearance of multiple myeloma, with innumerable ill-defined marrow nodules, subcentimeter in size. Schmorl nodes are also present ➡. *(Right)* Lateral radiograph shows limbus fragments at both L4 and L5 ➡. At both levels, the "divot" in the anterosuperior vertebral body is larger than the limbus fragment because of concurrent Schmorl nodes ➡.

Osteonecrosis

Vertebral Body Osteomyelitis

(Left) Lateral radiograph shows typical H-shaped vertebra of sickle cell disease ➡. The H-shape results from collapse of the central endplate due to osteonecrosis. *(Right)* Sagittal NECT shows multiple focal areas of bone destruction ➡ with preservation of the disc spaces and minimal prevertebral soft tissue involvement in this patient with indolent infection (coccidiomycosis).

Lymphoma

Lymphoma

(Left) Sagittal NECT shows ivory vertebra ➡ without clear destruction, resulting from lymphoma. *(Right)* Axial T1 C+ MR shows marrow replacement throughout the vertebral body, extending into the right neural arch ➡. There is extension of the tumor into the paraspinous soft tissues anterior to the vertebral body and into the epidural space ➡. This pattern of tumor spread is commonly seen in lymphoma.

LESIONS ORIGINATING IN VERTEBRAL BODY

Plasmacytoma

Giant Cell Tumor

(Left) Axial bone CT shows typical appearance of plasmacytoma, with a lytic lesion arising in the vertebral body and mild expansion of the lateral cortical margin ➡ of the vertebra. *(Right)* Lateral radiograph shows lesion with geographic non-sclerotic margins arising in the L1 vertebral body ➡. The lesion was subsequently proven to be a giant cell tumor.

Langerhans Cell Histiocytosis

Langerhans Cell Histiocytosis

(Left) Lateral radiograph shows vertebra plana ➡ at C7 in a child. This is a common presentation of Langerhans cell histiocytosis. Note that the posterior elements are not involved. *(Right)* Coronal T2WI FS MR shows central collapse of C3 ➡, increased signal of C5 ➡, and asymmetric right-sided soft tissue edema ➡. Large soft tissue masses are common during the early phase of Langerhans cell histiocytosis, but they regress with evolution of lesions.

Fibrous Dysplasia

Fibrous Dysplasia

(Left) Anteroposterior radiograph shows a sharply demarcated, slightly expansile lytic lesion of the T2 vertebral body ➡. The lesion has a ground-glass appearance. The findings suggest the diagnosis of fibrous dysplasia. *(Right)* Axial CECT shows lytic lesions ➡ within the vertebra & posterior elements with sharp margins, sclerotic rims, & mild expansion. They contain amorphous ground-glass matrix consistent with fibrous dysplasia.

LESIONS ORIGINATING IN VERTEBRAL BODY

Ewing Sarcoma

Osteochondroma

(Left) Sagittal STIR MR shows a lesion arising in the L1 vertebral body ➡ in a teenager. Posterior soft tissue mass is present. The appearance is consistent with an aggressive process. The patient's age indicates that Ewing sarcoma must be considered. *(Right)* Axial bone CT shows a mature osteochondroma arising from the anterior cortex of the C2 vertebral body ➡. Mineralization is present in the cartilage cap ➡ in this skeletally mature individual.

Chondrosarcoma

Chordoma

(Left) Axial bone CT shows a destructive vertebral body lesion that features stippled chondroid matrix ➡ extending into the prevertebral tissues. The features are characteristic of chondrosarcoma. *(Right)* Axial T1 C+ FS MR shows a large, diffusely enhancing soft tissue mass ➡ arising in the L4 vertebral body. The lesion also crossed the disc space to extend into the L5 vertebra. Such behavior is typical, but not specific, for chordoma.

Osteosarcoma

Echinococcal Disease

(Left) Anteroposterior radiograph shows multiple sites of sclerotic dense bone formation, extending from the bones into the adjacent soft tissue, involving two lumbar spine vertebra ➡ and the left pubic ramus ➡. This patient has developed osseous metastases from osteosarcoma. *(Right)* Coronal T2WI MR shows a complex, predominately left-sided, multicystic mass ➡ involving bone and adjacent soft tissue in this patient with echinococcus infection.

LESIONS ORIGINATING IN POSTERIOR ELEMENTS

DIFFERENTIAL DIAGNOSIS

Common
- Spondylolysis
- Metastases, Bone Marrow
- Acute Trauma

Less Common
- Pedicle Reactive Sclerosis
- Osteoid Osteoma
- Aneurysmal Bone Cyst
- Osteoblastoma
- Hypoplastic/Aplastic Pedicle

Rare but Important
- Brown Tumor

ESSENTIAL INFORMATION

Key Differential Diagnosis Issues
- **Hint**: Most destructive lesions visualize as absent pedicle on AP view
- **Hint**: Sclerotic pedicle should lead one to consider osteoid osteoma, blastic metastasis, or reactive sclerosis

Helpful Clues for Common Diagnoses
- **Spondylolysis**
  - Best seen on lateral or oblique view
  - Anterolisthesis vertebral body if bilateral
  - **Hint**: Retrolisthesis of posterior arch
- **Metastases, Bone Marrow**
  - Typically older patient
  - **Hint**: Usually not solitary lesion
- **Acute Trauma**
  - History definitive, variable mechanism

Helpful Clues for Less Common Diagnoses
- **Pedicle Reactive Sclerosis**
  - 2° abnormal contralateral pedicle: Spondylolysis most common
- **Osteoid Osteoma**
  - Under 30 years; M > F, any spinal level
  - Pain relieved by salicylates
  - Lytic lesion, central nidus, reactive sclerosis (sclerosis less dramatic in spine)
  - Non-rotational scoliosis; lesion on concavity & generally < 1 cm in size
  - MR: Surrounding inflammatory response
- **Aneurysmal Bone Cyst**
  - Any age, typically under 20 years, F > M
  - Any spinal level, favors thoracic, lumbar
  - ± Extension to adjacent bones, across disc
  - Fluid-fluid levels common, not diagnostic
  - MR: Blood products
- **Osteoblastoma**
  - Any age, especially 10-30 years: M > F
  - Expansile lytic lesion
    - Wide spectrum of calcification or ossification ± soft tissue mass
  - Most common thoracic, lumbar spine
    - ± Scoliosis, lesion on concavity
- **Hypoplastic/Aplastic Pedicle**
  - Varying degrees of malformation
  - ± Abnormal lamina
  - Incidental finding when isolated

Helpful Clues for Rare Diagnoses
- **Brown Tumor**
  - Primary or secondary hyperparathyroidism
  - Lytic lesion ± mild expansion

Spondylolysis

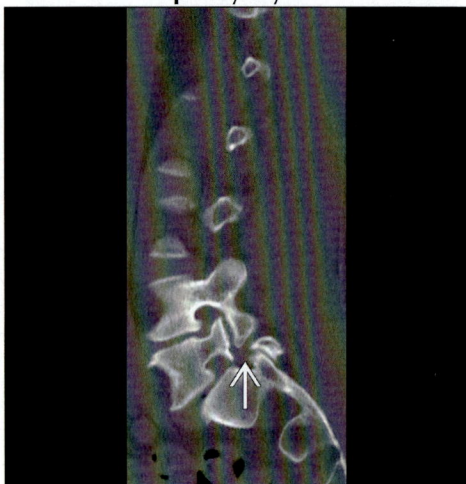

Sagittal bone CT shows defect in pars interarticularis ➡ and grade 2 anterior displacement of L5 vertebral body relative to sacrum.

Metastases, Bone Marrow

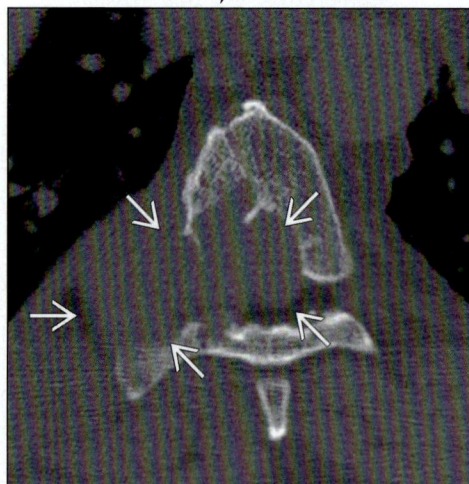

Axial NECT shows hypervascular renal cell metastasis ➡ with a large soft tissue mass. The origin of the lesion is the pedicle.

LESIONS ORIGINATING IN POSTERIOR ELEMENTS

Acute Trauma

Pedicle Reactive Sclerosis

(Left) Lateral radiograph shows typical case of hangman fracture demonstrating fracture between the vertebral body and neural arch ➡. *(Right)* Axial NECT shows left posterior element hypoplasia ⇶ and left pedicle aplasia ➡. There is sclerosis of the compensatory enlarged right pedicle, which contains a central horizontal lucency from an insufficiency fracture ➡.

Osteoid Osteoma

Aneurysmal Bone Cyst

(Left) Axial bone CT shows classic appearance of osteoid osteoma with a sharply demarcated lesion in the neural arch ➡ containing bone matrix. Reactive sclerosis is present around the lesion ⇶. *(Right)* Axial T2WI MR shows a multiloculated mass containing multiple fluid-fluid levels in this aneurysmal bone cyst ➡. Mixed signal intensity reflects the presence of blood products.

Osteoblastoma

Brown Tumor

(Left) Anteroposterior radiograph shows an expansile mass replacing the right L5 pedicle ➡ and indistinct vertebral body cortex resulting from osteoblastoma. *(Right)* Axial bone CT shows an expanded lytic lesion within the posterior elements of this cervical vertebra ➡. The patient had a parathyroid adenoma, and a Brown tumor was proven at biopsy.

307

RIB NOTCHING, INFERIOR

DIFFERENTIAL DIAGNOSIS

Common
- Coarctation Aorta, Thoracic
- Normal Variant
- Post-Operative
- Hyperparathyroidism (Mimic)
- Neurofibromatosis

Less Common
- Decreased Pulmonary Blood Flow
- Congenital Heart Disease, Repaired
- Subclavian Artery Obstruction
- Low Aortic Obstruction
- Thalassemia
- Arteriovenous Malformation

Rare but Important
- Superior Vena Cava Obstruction
- Giant Cell Tumor (Mimic)
- Tuberous Sclerosis (Mimic)

ESSENTIAL INFORMATION

Key Differential Diagnosis Issues
- Rib notching = localized erosion or thinning

Helpful Clues for Common Diagnoses
- **Coarctation Aorta, Thoracic**
  - Commonly involves 4th to 8th ribs
    - Tortuous, dilated intercostal arteries
  - "Figure 3" sign = undulation in distal aortic arch at coarctation site
  - Right unilateral notching if coarctation proximal to left subclavian artery origin
  - Bicuspid aortic valve in 25-50%
- **Normal Variant**
  - Inferior rib often undulating/indistinct
- **Post-Operative**
  - Thoracotomy rib resection/deformity
- **Hyperparathyroidism (Mimic)**
  - Subperiosteal & endosteal bone resorption
  - Bone destruction by Brown tumors
- **Neurofibromatosis**
  - Pressure from intercostal neurofibromas
  - Dysplastic "twisted ribbon" ribs

Helpful Clues for Less Common Diagnoses
- **Decreased Pulmonary Blood Flow**
  - Notching from enlarged transpleural collateral vessels
  - Congenital absence of pulmonary artery, pulmonary stenosis, tetralogy of Fallot, Ebstein anomaly, emphysema
- **Congenital Heart Disease, Repaired**
  - Findings of Blalock-Taussig shunt or cava-pulmonary anastomosis
  - Often unilateral right-sided
- **Subclavian Artery Obstruction**
  - Takayasu arteritis, arteriosclerosis obliterans, Blalock-Taussig procedure, thrombosis
- **Low Aortic Obstruction**
  - Low thoracic or abdominal aorta
  - Notching of lower ribs
- **Thalassemia**
  - Cortical erosion in posteromedial rib
  - Unusual in widened rib
- **Arteriovenous Malformation**
  - Involves intercostal or pulmonary vessels

Coarctation Aorta, Thoracic

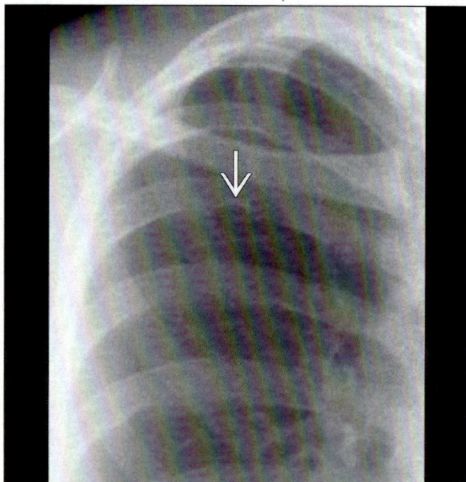

Posteroanterior radiograph shows typical aortic coarctation rib notching ➡ along the inferior surface of the posterior right fifth rib.

Coarctation Aorta, Thoracic

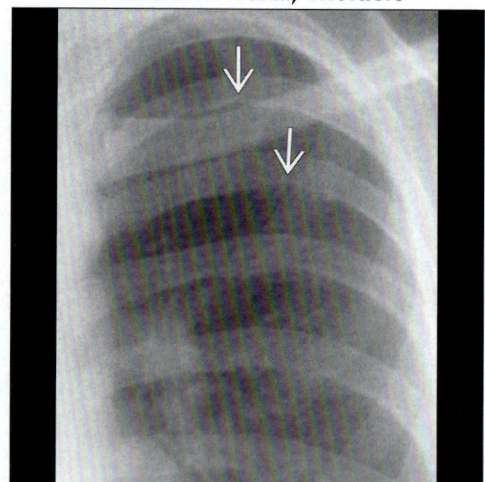

Posteroanterior radiograph shows typical aortic coarctation rib notching ➡ along the inferior surface of the posterior left fourth and fifth ribs.

RIB NOTCHING, INFERIOR

Coarctation Aorta, Thoracic

Coarctation Aorta, Thoracic

(Left) Posteroanterior radiograph shows left-sided inferior rib notching ➡ and post-stenotic dilatation ➡ of the descending aorta due to coarctation. The aortic contour abnormality is referred to as the "figure 3" sign. *(Right)* Posteroanterior radiograph shows a typical case of aortic coarctation with bilateral inferior rib notching ➡.

Post-Operative

Hyperparathyroidism (Mimic)

(Left) Posteroanterior radiograph shows scalloping along the inferior border of the right fourth rib ➡. This was post-operative in origin. Additional signs of surgical intervention includes staples in the middle lobe ➡. *(Right)* Anteroposterior radiograph shows bone resorption along the inferior second rib ➡, mimicking rib notching. This is caused by hyperparathyroidism, seen as a manifestation of renal osteodystrophy. Note signs of rickets in the humerus, with slipped epiphysis.

Neurofibromatosis

Giant Cell Tumor (Mimic)

(Left) Posteroanterior radiograph shows inferior scalloping ➡ of the ribs caused by pressure erosions from intercostal neurofibromas. *(Right)* Axial NECT shows a lytic lesion ➡ originating from and partially destroying the rib. Heterogeneous low density favors either a giant cell tumor containing fluid levels or an aneurysmal bone cyst containing a solid portion.

RIB NOTCHING, SUPERIOR

DIFFERENTIAL DIAGNOSIS

Common
- Normal Variant
- Hyperparathyroidism (Mimic)
- Systemic Lupus Erythematosus
- Rheumatoid Arthritis, Wheelchair
- Progressive Systemic Sclerosis

Less Common
- Coarctation Aorta, Thoracic
- Neurofibromatosis
- Multiple Hereditary Exostosis (Mimic)
- Post-Operative
- Pressure Effect, Thoracic Drainage Tube
- Pressure Effect, Rib Retractor
- Radiation Osteonecrosis

Rare but Important
- Intercostal Muscle Atrophy
- Paraplegia, Complications
- Osteogenesis Imperfecta
- Marfan Syndrome
- Polio
- Restrictive Lung Disease
- Thalassemia
- Progeria

ESSENTIAL INFORMATION

Key Differential Diagnosis Issues
- Rib notching = localized erosion or thinning
- Superior notching is less common than inferior notching and is more likely to be non-neurovascular in origin

Helpful Clues for Common Diagnoses
- **Hyperparathyroidism (Mimic)**
  - Subperiosteal & endosteal bone resorption
    - Unilateral predominance
  - Bone destruction by Brown tumors
- **Systemic Lupus Erythematosus**
  - Third to fifth rib superior border
- **Rheumatoid Arthritis, Wheelchair**
  - Osteoporosis + scapular erosion into ribs

Helpful Clues for Less Common Diagnoses
- **Coarctation Aorta, Thoracic**
  - Usually causes inferior rib notching
  - Superior rib notching seen when intercostal arteries markedly enlarge & erode the superior surface of adjacent rib
- **Neurofibromatosis**
  - Pressure erosions from neurofibromas are usually inferior
  - Dysplastic "twisted ribbon" ribs
  - Vertebral abnormalities
- **Radiation Osteonecrosis**
  - Delayed alteration in bone remodeling

Helpful Clues for Rare Diagnoses
- **Osteogenesis Imperfecta**
  - Dysplastic rib rotation & curvature
- **Marfan Syndrome**
  - Thin ribs with thin cortices
- **Polio**
  - Thin ribs & atrophic intercostal muscles
  - Superior > inferior scalloping → "hourglass" shape
- **Progeria**
  - Thin clavicles & ribs

Hyperparathyroidism (Mimic)

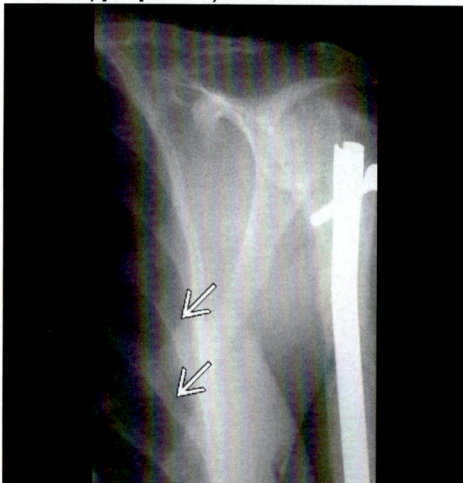

Anteroposterior radiograph shows resorption of the superior rib cortex ➡, which may be mistaken for rib notching.

Systemic Lupus Erythematosus

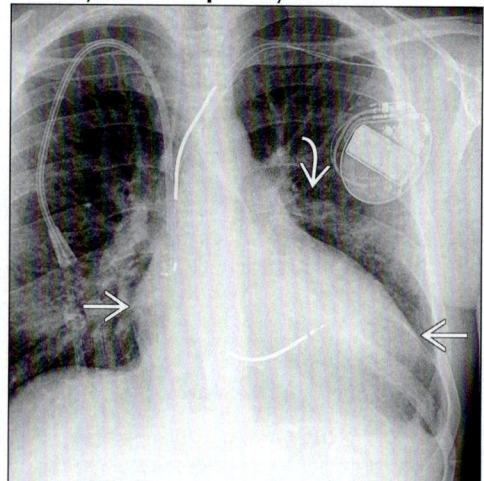

Posteroanterior radiograph shows subtle superior rib notching ➡ and an enlarged heart ➡ due to a pericardial effusion.

RIB NOTCHING, SUPERIOR

Rheumatoid Arthritis, Wheelchair

Neurofibromatosis

(Left) Posteroanterior radiograph shows an ill-defined superior cortex of the posterior mid-thoracic ribs ➡. The combination of osteoporosis & constant rubbing of the scapula against the rib cage results in this pattern of resorption in this rheumatoid arthritis patient who uses a wheelchair. (Right) Anteroposterior radiograph shows a "ribbon rib" on the left ➡, which reflects an osseous dysplasia seen in neurofibromatosis.

Multiple Hereditary Exostosis (Mimic)

Post-Operative

(Left) Posteroanterior radiograph shows deformity and notching of the superior cortex of the ribs ➡ adjacent to a scapular exostosis in this patient with multiple hereditary exostoses. (Right) Posteroanterior radiograph in a patient with a previous left thoracotomy shows a resultant post-operative deformity of the left third rib ➡. The ascending aorta ➡ is enlarged.

Radiation Osteonecrosis

Paraplegia, Complications

(Left) Posteroanterior radiograph shows deformity of the superior rib borders ➡ in a patient with radiation osteonecrosis. Note the elevated hila ➡. The patient had mantle radiation for lymphoma. (Right) Posteroanterior radiograph shows unilateral superior rib notching ➡ in a quadriplegic patient. This erosion is likely due to pressure from the scapula combined with osteopenia and muscle atrophy.

SOLITARY RIB LESION

DIFFERENTIAL DIAGNOSIS

Common
- Fracture Healing Process
- Fibrous Dysplasia (FD)
- Enchondroma
- Multiple Myeloma (MM)
- Metastatic
- Pancoast Tumor
- Osteomyelitis
- Osteochondroma

Less Common
- Langerhans Cell Histiocytosis (LCH)
- Ewing Sarcoma

Rare but Important
- Giant Cell Tumor (GCT)
- Chondrosarcoma
- Askin Tumor
- Osteosarcoma
- Cystic Angiomatosis

ESSENTIAL INFORMATION

Key Differential Diagnosis Issues
- Many entities in the differential may be polyostotic lesions, even if only a single rib lesion is seen in any specific case
  - FD, MM, metastases, LCH, osteochondroma, cystic angiomatosis
  - **Hint:** Look for other skeletal lesions
- Age may be a differentiating factor
  - FD, LCH, Ewing sarcoma, Askin tumor, GCT tend to be seen in younger patients than metastases or MM

Helpful Clues for Common Diagnoses
- **Fracture Healing Process**
  - During callus-producing phase, fracture may appear as a sclerotic metastasis
  - Slightly malaligned healed fracture may appear as a slightly expanded lytic lesion, but without geographic borders
  - Generally will see other fractures in adjacent ribs, making the diagnosis obvious
- **Fibrous Dysplasia (FD)**
  - Most common solitary rib lesion in teenager & young adult
  - Slightly expanded to bubbly; not aggressive
  - Lytic to ground-glass density on radiograph
  - Commonly polyostotic (but < 50%)
- **Enchondroma**
  - Quoted as being most common benign rib lesion in autopsy series
  - Not frequently noted on chest radiograph: Small lesion, chest rather than osseous X-ray technique makes it difficult to see
  - Watch for chondroid matrix (punctate)
  - Generally no geographic margin
- **Multiple Myeloma (MM)**
  - Usually multiple lytic lesions or diffuse infiltration seen only as osteopenia
  - Rarely will find a single rib lesion, with other lesions elsewhere in skeleton
    - If expanded or bubbly, lesion is likely the original plasmacytoma
- **Metastatic**
  - Generally polyostotic
  - Occasional solitary metastasis is found in rib
    - Thyroid or renal cell most common
- **Pancoast Tumor**
  - Tumor in lung apex, may have rib destruction
  - Proximity to nerves & vessels leads to typical clinical symptoms
    - Shoulder & arm pain
    - Horner syndrome
- **Osteomyelitis**
  - Lytic destructive rib lesion
    - Usually wide zone of transition, not geographic
  - Soft tissue mass is most frequently present
  - Elicits pleural effusion
  - Radiographic appearance may be indistinguishable from Ewing sarcoma or Askin tumor
  - MR with contrast usually will differentiate
- **Osteochondroma**
  - Rib osteochondromas less frequent than on long bones
  - Rib osteochondromas often seen as part of multiple hereditary exostosis (MHE)
  - Osteochondroma of rib arises as on long bone
    - Stalk in continuity with rib cortex
    - Marrow extending from rib into osteochondroma
    - Overlying cartilage cap

SOLITARY RIB LESION

- Because rib osteochondromas often project intrathoracically, they may have the appearance of lung nodules
  - Hint: Watch for attaching stalk & osseous character of "nodule"

Helpful Clues for Less Common Diagnoses
- **Langerhans Cell Histiocytosis (LCH)**
  - Frequently involve ribs, skull, flat bones of shoulder & pelvic girdle, long bones
  - Frequently polyostotic
  - Generally occur in a younger age group (children, young teenagers) than the other listed lesions
  - Lytic lesion, ranging from geographic to aggressive
    - Aggressive lesions may have cortical breakthrough and soft tissue mass
  - May advance rapidly & be indistinguishable by imaging from Ewing sarcoma
- **Ewing Sarcoma**
  - Aggressive lytic lesion
    - Cortical breakthrough, large soft tissue mass
    - Rib lesions often elicit a large pleural effusion
  - Proximal & flat bones such as ribs, pelvis, scapula generally involved in older age group; tubular bones in younger children
    - Late teenage and young adults are the prime age group for Ewing of rib
  - May appear polyostotic since osseous metastases are common

Helpful Clues for Rare Diagnoses
- **Giant Cell Tumor (GCT)**
  - Rare rib lesion
  - Lytic lesion, generally geographic but rarely may be aggressive
  - Young to middle-aged adults
  - Characteristic MR features
    - Some low signal regions on T2
    - May occasionally have fluid-fluid levels
- **Chondrosarcoma**
  - May arise in enchondroma or at costochondral junction of rib
  - Lytic, usually containing chondroid matrix
  - Generally low grade & not aggressive in appearance
- **Askin Tumor**
  - Although rare, most common pleural tumor in teenagers & young adults (especially females)
  - Primitive neuroectodermal tumor (PNET) arises in pleura or chest wall
  - Involves rib 23-60% of time
- **Osteosarcoma**
  - Very rare lesion in rib
  - Osteoid matrix, varying aggressiveness
- **Cystic Angiomatosis**
  - One of the vascular tumors that may be polyostotic
  - All may involve a rib; preference is lower extremities
  - Range of aggressiveness; cystic angiomatosis & hemangioma are generally the least aggressive

Fracture Healing Process

Anteroposterior radiograph shows a healed rib fracture ➡. With slight offset, it may appear to be a slightly expanded lytic lesion. Alternatively, during healing, it may appear sclerotic, mimicking metastatic disease.

Fibrous Dysplasia (FD)

Oblique radiograph shows an expanded, bubbly solitary rib lesion ➡. In this young patient, FD is the most likely diagnosis. She had spine and humeral lesions, adding to the probability, as well as a brachial plexopathy.

SOLITARY RIB LESION

Enchondroma

Multiple Myeloma (MM)

(Left) AP radiograph shows a small region of chondroid matrix within the first rib ➡, a typical enchondroma. These lesions are reportedly common in ribs (autopsy series) but infrequently noted on chest X-rays. *(Right)* Coronal STIR MR of the right upper thorax shows high signal in what proved to be a solitary rib lesion ➡. The MR survey showed myeloma lesions in other osseous structures. A single rib involved in MM is unusual; plasmacytoma would be more frequent.

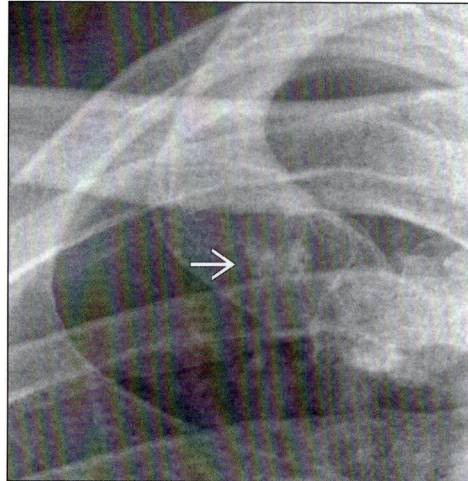

Metastatic

Pancoast Tumor

(Left) PA radiograph shows an expanded solitary rib lesion ➡. While the lesion does not appear highly aggressive, it is important to remember that chest X-ray technique is suboptimal to evaluate osseous structures. This proved to be a solitary kidney metastasis. *(Right)* PA radiograph shows near complete destruction of the first rib ➡ (compare with normal right side), with associated apical lung mass ➡. Pancoast tumors have distinct clinical symptoms.

Osteomyelitis

Osteochondroma

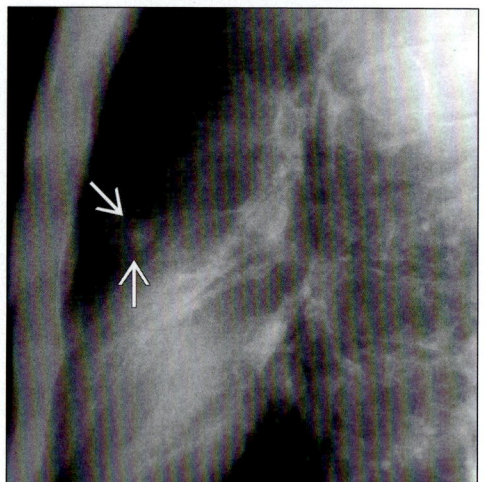

(Left) AP radiograph shows destruction of a solitary rib ➡ with associated large soft tissue mass ➡. While this certainly could represent an aggressive tumor such as Ewing sarcoma, osteomyelitis can have just as aggressive an appearance. *(Right)* Lateral radiograph shows a "lung nodule" which in fact arises from the rib ➡. The lesion contains mature bone and represents an osteochondroma. The chest X-ray technique is suboptimal for evaluating the matrix.

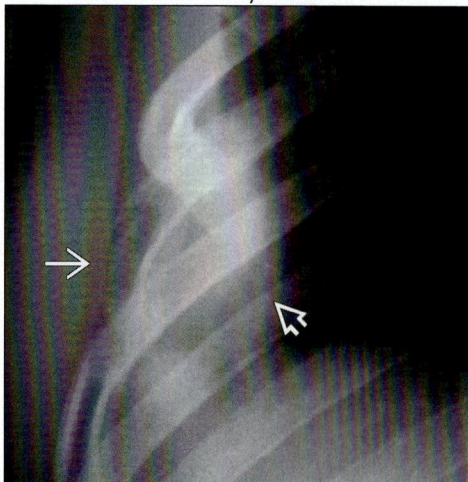

SOLITARY RIB LESION

Langerhans Cell Histiocytosis (LCH)

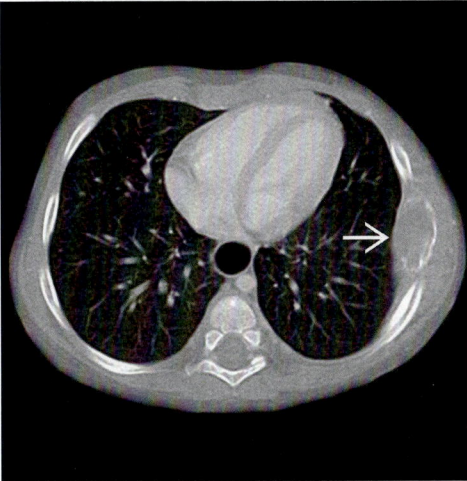

Ewing Sarcoma

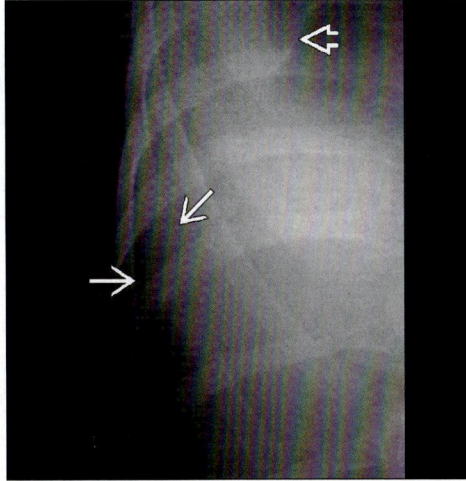

(Left) Axial CECT shows a lytic destructive lesion in the rib of a 2 year old ➡. It was a solitary lesion and proved to be LCH. Note that there is a small associated soft tissue mass. The age of the patient should help suggest the diagnosis. *(Right)* Anteroposterior radiograph shows destruction of a solitary rib ➡ in a 15 year old, along with a large soft tissue mass and pleural effusion ➡. Ewing sarcoma must be strongly considered and proved to be the correct diagnosis.

Giant Cell Tumor (GCT)

Chondrosarcoma

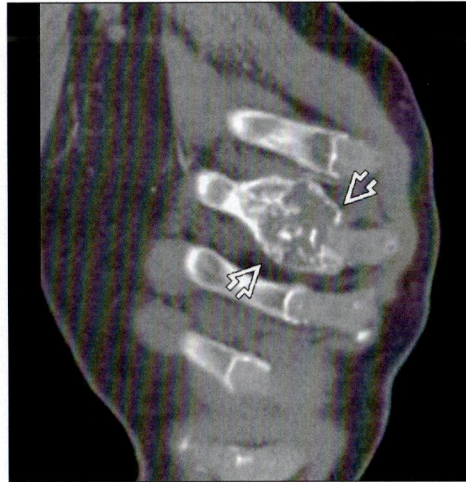

(Left) Axial T2WI MR shows both a solid portion of the rib lesion ➡ and regions containing fluid levels ➡. The appearance is not specific. Aneurysmal bone cyst with a solid component should be considered. Giant cell tumor with fluid levels is the final diagnosis. *(Right)* Sagittal CECT shows an expanded rib end containing a chondroid matrix ➡. The location adjacent to the costochondral cartilage is typical but not exclusive for this tumor.

Askin Tumor

Osteosarcoma

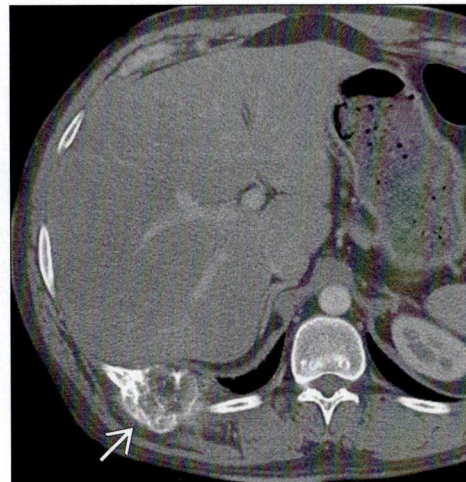

(Left) Axial CECT shows a large pleural-based tumor extending around the hemithorax ➡ in a young adult with associated destruction and reactive change of the adjacent rib ➡. The distribution and age of the patient are typical of Askin tumor; rib involvement is variable. *(Right)* Axial bone CT shows a rare low grade intraosseous osteosarcoma of the rib ➡. Statistically, most rib lesions containing matrix are chondroid in nature, most frequently enchondroma.

SACROILIITIS, BILATERAL SYMMETRIC

DIFFERENTIAL DIAGNOSIS

Common
- Ankylosing Spondylitis (AS)
- Osteoarthritis (Mimic) (OA)
- DISH (Mimic)
- Osteitis Condensans Ilii (Mimic)

Less Common
- Inflammatory Bowel Disease Arthritis (IBD)
- Psoriatic Arthritis, Late (PSA)
- Renal Osteodystrophy (Mimic) (Renal OD)

Rare but Important
- Chronic Reactive Arthritis, Late (CRA)
- Rheumatoid Arthritis (RA)

ESSENTIAL INFORMATION

Key Differential Diagnosis Issues
- Sacroiliac (SI) joint inflammatory disease is most frequently seen in spondyloarthropathies
- Two spondyloarthropathies are particularly noted for bilateral and symmetric involvement
  - **Hint:** Bilateral symmetric sacroiliitis most frequently is due to ankylosing spondylitis, inflammatory bowel disease spondylitis
  - **Hint:** Remember that spondyloarthropathies that are usually bilaterally asymmetric (PSA, CRA) may develop bilaterally symmetric disease at some point
- Purely productive diseases of the SI joints may mimic the sclerosis of sacroiliitis
  - OA, DISH, osteitis condensans ilii
  - Sclerosis is predominantly on iliac side
  - No associated erosive change
  - **Hint:** Watch for location of sclerosis of SI joints to differentiate these mimics from true spondyloarthropathies & from one another

Helpful Clues for Common Diagnoses
- **Ankylosing Spondylitis (AS)**
  - Sacroiliitis begins with erosive change
    - Loss of distinctness of SI joint cortices
    - Erosions lead to widening of joints
    - Usually bilaterally symmetric, but occasionally one side lags behind the other & they appear asymmetric
  - Eventual sclerosis and bilateral fusion

- Eventual profound osteoporosis
- Spine involvement: Tends to be continuous
  - Thin vertical syndesmophytes lead to body fusion
  - Facets fuse as well, leads to bamboo spine
- Peripheral involvement: Large proximal joints (hip, shoulder)
- Male > > female; onset 2nd or 3rd decade
- **Osteoarthritis (Mimic) (OA)**
  - Purely productive; osteophytes tend to bridge anteriorly at superior & inferior ends of synovial portion of SI joint
  - May mimic sclerosis of sacroiliitis, but usually is easily differentiated
  - May appear as a rounded region of sclerosis overlying mid SI joint; may mimic a sclerotic metastatic site
- **DISH (Mimic)**
  - Purely productive, not an articular process
    - Iliolumbar ligaments located superior to SI joints may ossify & bridge
    - Nonarticular superior portion of SI joint may ossify & appear fused
    - Synovial (inferior) portion of SI joint not affected by DISH
  - Ossified superior portions of SI joints appear symmetric & may mimic end-stage sacroiliitis
    - Should be easily differentiated since the true SI joint is not involved
  - Other axial features
    - Ossification sacrotuberous or sacrospinal ligaments
    - Bridging anterior osteophytes along spine, particularly thoracic
- **Osteitis Condensans Ilii (Mimic)**
  - Sclerotic reactive osseous change on iliac side of joint
    - Usually, but not invariably, symmetric
    - Sclerosis may mimic the sclerosis seen in sacroiliitis
  - Sclerosis is generally specific in appearance
    - Involves iliac side of joint, inferiorly
    - Often triangular in shape
  - Not an articular process; joint is normal

Helpful Clues for Less Common Diagnoses
- **Inflammatory Bowel Disease Arthritis (IBD)**
  - Similar in appearance but much less frequent than AS

SACROILIITIS, BILATERAL SYMMETRIC

- ○ Sacroiliitis begins with erosive change
  - ▪ Loss of distinctness of SI joint cortices
  - ▪ Erosions lead to widening of joints
  - ▪ Usually bilaterally symmetric, but occasionally one side lags behind the other & they appear asymmetric
- ○ Eventual sclerosis and bilateral fusion
- ○ Spine involvement: Tends to be continuous
  - ▪ Thin vertical syndesmophytes lead to body fusion
  - ▪ Facets fuse as well, leads to bamboo spine
- ○ Peripheral involvement: Large proximal joints (hip, shoulder)
- ○ Watch for signs of IBD
  - ▪ Staple lines from ileoanal pull-through
  - ▪ Colostomy
  - ▪ Signs of steroid use
  - ▪ Tubular, featureless bowel pattern of colitis
- • **Psoriatic Arthritis, Late (PSA)**
  - ○ Spondyloarthropathy in PSA generally bilateral but asymmetric
    - ▪ May appear symmetric, especially in early or end-stage (bilateral fusion)
  - ○ Differentiating features of end-stage fused sacroiliitis of PSA from AS
    - ▪ Normal bone density
    - ▪ Character of spine involvement (bulky paravertebral osteophytes, skip regions)
    - ▪ Peripheral joint disease favors hands, feet, rather than large proximal joints
    - ▪ Skin disease
- • **Renal Osteodystrophy (Mimic) (Renal OD)**
  - ○ Sacroiliac joints may appear widened & irregular
  - ○ Most frequently bilateral & symmetric
  - ○ Not a true sacroiliitis, but rather a resorptive process
    - ▪ Subchondral resorption on the iliac side
    - ▪ With weight-bearing, resorbed bone collapses, resulting in apparent widening & erosive change
  - ○ Differentiating features: Look for other signs of renal OD or hyperparathyroidism
    - ▪ Abnormal bone density
    - ▪ Other resorptive patterns: Subperiosteal, subligamentous, Brown tumors

Helpful Clues for Rare Diagnoses
- • **Chronic Reactive Arthritis, Late (CRA)**
  - ○ Spondyloarthropathy in CRA generally bilateral but asymmetric
    - ▪ May appear symmetric, especially in early or end-stage (bilateral fusion)
  - ○ Differentiating features of end-stage fused sacroiliitis of CRA from AS
    - ▪ Normal bone density
    - ▪ Character of spine involvement (bulky paravertebral osteophytes, skip regions)
    - ▪ Peripheral joint disease favors ankles & feet, rather than large proximal joints
    - ▪ Clinical symptoms of urethritis & uveitis
- • **Rheumatoid Arthritis (RA)**
  - ○ RA relatively frequently affects SI joints
    - ▪ Erosions, generally bilaterally symmetric
  - ○ Though present, erosions generally not large enough to be observed on imaging

Ankylosing Spondylitis (AS)

AP radiograph shows a "bowl-shaped" pelvis, typical of advanced AS. Both SI joints are completely & symmetrically fused ➡. Note also the prominent enthesopathy ⮞ & the arthritic changes in the hips.

Ankylosing Spondylitis (AS)

AP radiograph shows AS relatively early in the disease process. The SI joints show bilateral and symmetric widening due to erosions, as well as bilateral sclerosis ➡. Osteoporosis has not yet developed.

SACROILIITIS, BILATERAL SYMMETRIC

(Left) AP radiograph shows bilaterally symmetric sacroiliitis which is predominantly erosive ➡ with little productive change at this point. The hips bilaterally show minimal productive change ⟱ in this 18 year old male. **(Right)** AP radiograph shows sclerosis involving both sides of the SI joints, bilaterally symmetric ➡. The iliac side is more prominently involved than the sacral side. There is no erosive change; this is osteoarthritis.

Ankylosing Spondylitis (AS)

Osteoarthritis (Mimic) (OA)

(Left) AP radiograph shows complete & symmetric fusion in the upper non-synovial portions of the SI joints ➡. The synovial portions of the joints are normal ⟱, typical of DISH. Since the synovial portions are not involved, this is not a true sacroiliitis. **(Right)** Axial bone CT shows sclerosis of the iliac side of the SI joints which is bilaterally symmetric ⟱. The sacral side is normal, as are the joints themselves. Since the joints are normal, this form of sclerosis is a mimic rather than a true sacroiliitis.

DISH (Mimic)

Osteitis Condensans Ilii (Mimic)

(Left) AP radiograph shows bilateral & symmetric mixed erosive and productive changes at the SI joints ➡. There is no fusion. The left hip shows productive change ⟱ in this young adult. The appearance is of either AS or IBD; clinical information proved IBD. **(Right)** AP radiograph shows bilateral widening of the SI joints due to erosions, with minimal associated sclerosis ➡. The barium outlines findings of ulcerative colitis ⟱; this patient has IBD spondyloarthropathy.

Inflammatory Bowel Disease Arthritis (IBD)

Inflammatory Bowel Disease Arthritis (IBD)

SACROILIITIS, BILATERAL SYMMETRIC

Inflammatory Bowel Disease Arthritis (IBD)

Psoriatic Arthritis, Late (PSA)

(Left) AP radiograph shows bilateral symmetric mixed erosive & productive sacroiliitis ➡. Staples are seen outlining an ileoanal pull-through in this patient with IBD. Note also the left hip AVN ➡, related to steroid use for the bowel disease. *(Right)* AP radiograph shows bilaterally symmetric nearly fused SI joints ➡ in a patient with psoriatic arthritis. Although we generally think of PSA being asymmetric, in end-stage disease it will be symmetric.

Renal Osteodystrophy (Mimic) (Renal OD)

Renal Osteodystrophy (Mimic) (Renal OD)

(Left) AP radiograph shows widened SI joints, bilaterally symmetric ➡ that could be mistaken for sacroiliitis. These are not true erosions in this patient with renal osteodystrophy but rather regions of subchondral resorption and collapse along the iliac side. *(Right)* AP radiograph shows bilateral severe widening of the SI joints ➡ in a child with renal osteodystrophy. This is resorption with collapse rather than true erosive disease. Note the peritoneal dialysis catheter.

Chronic Reactive Arthritis, Late (CRA)

Chronic Reactive Arthritis, Late (CRA)

(Left) AP radiograph shows end-stage sacroiliitis with complete fusion ➡ which is bilaterally symmetric. The patient had CRA; earlier sacroiliitis is usually bilateral but asymmetric. *(Right)* AP radiograph shows bilateral fusion of the SI joints ➡ in end-stage CRA. The patient also has erosive change in the left hip ➡; the hip is usually involved only late in the process; foot and ankle involvement is generally most prominent.

SACROILIITIS, BILATERAL ASYMMETRIC

DIFFERENTIAL DIAGNOSIS

Common
- Psoriatic Arthritis (PSA)
- Osteoarthritis (OA) (Mimic)

Less Common
- Chronic Reactive Arthritis (CRA)
- Ankylosing Spondylitis (AS)
- Inflammatory Bowel Disease (IBD)
- Renal Osteodystrophy (Renal OD) (Mimic)

Rare but Important
- Juvenile Idiopathic Arthritis (JIA)
- Gout
- Rheumatoid Arthritis (RA)

ESSENTIAL INFORMATION

Key Differential Diagnosis Issues
- Bilateral asymmetric sacroiliac (SI) disease most frequently is seen in PSA & CRA
- Other spondyloarthropathies that are generally bilaterally asymmetric may be asymmetric at some point in the process
  - **Hint**: AS is much more prevalent than either psoriatic or chronic reactive spondyloarthritis, so should be strongly considered with this appearance

Helpful Clues for Common Diagnoses
- **Psoriatic Arthritis (PSA)**
  - Spondyloarthritis is most frequently bilateral & asymmetric
  - Spine involvement: Bulky asymmetric paravertebral osteophytes, skip areas
  - Consider sites & appearance of peripheral arthropathy in making diagnosis
    - Hand > foot; acral > proximal
    - Mixed erosive/productive
    - Sausage digit & periostitis
- **Osteoarthritis (OA) (Mimic)**
  - Not sacroiliitis, but bridging osteophyte is seen
    - Seen as sclerosis, often rounded, more often iliac than sacral side of joint
    - Most prominent at margins of joint

Helpful Clues for Less Common Diagnoses
- **Chronic Reactive Arthritis (CRA)**
  - Identical SI joint & spine findings to PSA
  - MUCH less frequent than PSA sacroiliitis
  - Peripheral involvement: Foot/ankle > hand
- **Ankylosing Spondylitis (AS)**
  - Generally bilateral symmetric sacroiliitis, but early in disease may be asymmetric
  - Osteoporotic; peripheral disease usually has large proximal joints
- **Inflammatory Bowel Disease (IBD)**
  - Generally bilateral symmetric sacroiliitis, but early in disease may be asymmetric
- **Renal Osteodystrophy (Renal OD) (Mimic)**
  - Subchondral resorption & collapse on iliac side may be asymmetric

Helpful Clues for Rare Diagnoses
- **Juvenile Idiopathic Arthritis (JIA), Gout, Rheumatoid Arthritis (RA)**
  - Involvement of SI joint may not be rare, but is rarely seen with imaging

Psoriatic Arthritis (PSA)

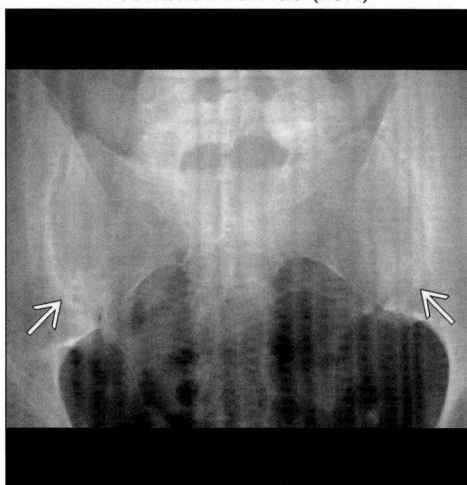

AP radiograph shows bilateral erosive/productive SI joint disease ➡ that is mildly asymmetric, with greater widening on the left than the right. The patient also had psoriatic arthritic changes in the hands.

Osteoarthritis (OA) (Mimic)

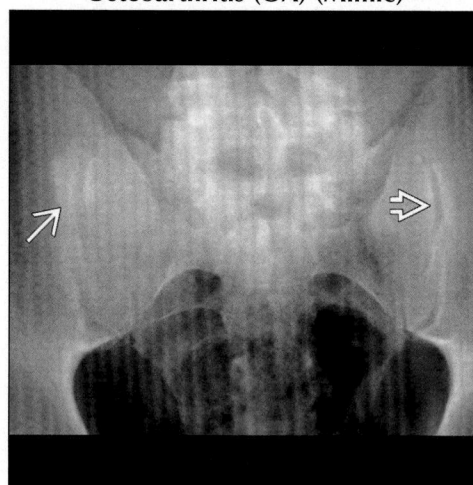

AP radiograph shows a focal site of sclerosis at the superior aspect of the right SI joint ➡, with minimal sclerosis on the left ➡ & normal SI joints otherwise. These represent OA with marginal osteophytes.

SACROILIITIS, BILATERAL ASYMMETRIC

Osteoarthritis (OA) (Mimic)

Chronic Reactive Arthritis (CRA)

(Left) Axial bone CT of the same patient confirms the bridging osteophyte on the right ➡ and sclerosis of OA on the left ➡. These sites of sclerosis tend to form at the margins of the SIJ and could mimic spondyloarthropathy. *(Right)* Anteroposterior radiograph shows bilateral asymmetric SI joint disease in a patient with CRA. The left joint shows far more erosive change as well as sclerosis ➡ compared with mild erosion on the right ➡. Bilateral asymmetry is typical of CRA.

Chronic Reactive Arthritis (CRA)

Ankylosing Spondylitis (AS)

(Left) AP radiograph shows bilateral but significantly asymmetric SI joint disease in a patient with CRA. The left SI joint shows erosions & sclerosis ➡ while the right shows only mild deossification, or very early erosions ➡. *(Right)* AP radiograph shows mild erosive & sclerotic change in the left SI joint ➡ and only minimal deossification on the right ➡. This patient has early manifestations of AS; with early disease, the usually bilaterality of SI joints may not be seen.

Inflammatory Bowel Disease (IBD)

Renal Osteodystrophy (Renal OD) (Mimic)

(Left) AP radiograph in a patient with IBD shows bilateral advanced but asymmetric sacroiliitis, left ➡ less severe than right ➡, which is nearly fused. Even in late disease, symmetry is not always maintained. *(Right)* AP radiograph shows right SI joint widening with iliac sclerosis ➡ typical of the subchondral resorption & collapse seen with renal OD. The left SI joint shows less prominent involvement. Note the vas deferens calcification ➡ in this diabetic.

SACROILIITIS, UNILATERAL

DIFFERENTIAL DIAGNOSIS

Common
- Septic Joint

Less Common
- Psoriatic Arthritis (PSA), Early
- Ankylosing Spondylitis (AS), Early
- Chronic Reactive Arthritis (CRA), Early
- Osteoarthritis (OA) (Mimic)

Rare but Important
- Rheumatoid Arthritis (RA)
- Gout

ESSENTIAL INFORMATION

Key Differential Diagnosis Issues
- **Hint**: True unilateral sacroiliitis must be considered septic joint until proven otherwise
  - Radiographic signs may be subtle
  - Clinical signs may be misleading (buttock, groin, hip pain)
- **Hint**: Consider diagnosis of septic SI joint in at-risk patients
  - HIV-AIDS
  - Diabetic patients

Helpful Clues for Common Diagnoses
- **Septic Joint**
  - Earliest changes
    - Effusion, deossification (lack of distinctness) of subchondral cortex
  - Later changes
    - Erosions, widening of joint
    - If chronic, sclerotic reactive changes
    - Abscess in iliopsoas or gluteal muscles

Helpful Clues for Less Common Diagnoses
- **Psoriatic Arthritis (PSA), Early**
  - PSA sacroiliitis is a bilateral & generally asymmetric process
  - Early in process, changes may be so subtle on one side that the more advanced side appears to mimic unilateral disease
  - Other findings to help differentiate PSA
    - Peripheral mixed erosive/productive disease in hands & feet; skin changes
- **Ankylosing Spondylitis (AS), Early**
  - AS sacroiliitis is a bilateral & generally symmetric process
  - Early in process, changes may be so subtle on one side that the more advanced side appears to mimic unilateral disease
  - Other findings to help differentiate AS
    - Large proximal joint arthritis
- **Chronic Reactive Arthritis (CRA), Early**
  - Like PSA, sacroiliitis is bilateral & asymmetric, but may appear to be unilateral early in the process
- **Osteoarthritis (OA) (Mimic)**
  - Unilateral sclerosis of productive change could mimic a unilateral sacroiliitis

Helpful Clues for Rare Diagnoses
- **Rheumatoid Arthritis (RA)**
  - Bilateral erosive disease & rarely visualized
- **Gout**
  - Rare involvement; rarely visualized

Septic Joint

Axial T2WI MR shows fluid in the right SI joint ➡ without evidence of destruction of the cortices. There is a fluid collection extending into the iliacus ➡. This is a septic joint; the left SI joint is normal.

Septic Joint

Axial T2WI MR in the same patient shows the anterior fluid collection, as well as extension posteriorly ➡. This patient had HIV-AIDS, making him more susceptible to SI joint infection.

SACROILIITIS, UNILATERAL

Septic Joint

Septic Joint

(Left) Oblique axial T1WI MR shows low signal abnormality involving both sides of the left SI joint ➡. Note that the abnormal signal is centered on the synovial portion of the joint. It should not be mistaken for stress fracture. *(Right)* Oblique axial T1 C+ FS MR in the same patient shows high signal, again involving both sides of the left SI joint ➡. There is a small fluid collection adjacent to the joint ➡; there is no diagnosis to consider other than septic joint.

Septic Joint

Septic Joint

(Left) Axial STIR MR shows high signal involving the sacral ala as well as the iliac wing, with fluid in the SI joint ➡. There is a mass extending from the joint anteriorly, deviating the iliacus ➡ which is fluid signal. *(Right)* Coronal T2WI FS MR in the same patient confirms the abnormality centered on the SI joint, with unilateral sacroiliitis ➡ and extension of a soft tissue abscess ➡. This is a septic hip in an HIV-AIDS patient who presented with hip pain.

Psoriatic Arthritis (PSA), Early

Ankylosing Spondylitis (AS), Early

(Left) AP radiograph shows a normal left SI joint ➡ but abnormality on the right side. There is sclerosis on the iliac side ➡, without significant erosive change. This early & apparently unilateral sacroiliitis was seen in a patient with PSA. *(Right)* AP radiograph shows normal width & appearance of the left SI joint in a 14 year old ➡ but widening & erosions on the right ➡. This represents very early and unilateral sacroiliitis in a teenager who proved to have AS.

SYMPHYSIS PUBIS WITH PRODUCTIVE CHANGES/FUSION

DIFFERENTIAL DIAGNOSIS

Common
- Chronic Repetitive Trauma
- Post-Traumatic Instability
- Fracture, Malunion (Mimic)
- Septic Joint
- Osteoarthritis
- DISH
- Pyrophosphate Arthropathy
- Stress Fracture, Adult (Mimic)
- Postpartum
- Post-Operative

Less Common
- Ankylosing Spondylitis
- Juvenile Idiopathic Arthritis (JIA)
- Rheumatoid Arthritis
- Hyperparathyroidism
- Psoriatic Arthritis
- Osteitis Pubis, Late

Rare but Important
- SAPHO
- Complications of Fluoride
- Ochronosis (Alkaptonuria)

ESSENTIAL INFORMATION

Helpful Clues for Common Diagnoses
- **Septic Joint**
  - Irregular bone destruction
  - Sclerosis is sign of healing
- **Osteoarthritis**
  - Osteophytes & joint space narrowing
- **DISH**
  - Bone proliferation at ligamentous insertions
  - Flowing ossification of 4 contiguous vertebral bodies
  - Disc spaces preserved

Helpful Clues for Less Common Diagnoses
- **Ankylosing Spondylitis**
  - Symphysis pubis & sacroiliac joint erosion leading to fusion
  - Proliferative changes predominantly along inferior pubic rami
- **Hyperparathyroidism**
  - Erosion & sclerosis of symphysis pubis in primary hyperparathyroidism; rarely fuses
- **Psoriatic Arthritis**
  - Erosion & sclerosis with asymmetric sacroiliac joint involvement
- **Osteitis Pubis, Late**
  - End stage → spontaneous arthrodesis

Helpful Clues for Rare Diagnoses
- **Complications of Fluoride**
  - Diffuse increased bone density
  - Ligamentous ossification: Paraspinal, sacrotuberous, & iliolumbar in pelvis
  - Bulky spinal osteophytes
- **Ochronosis (Alkaptonuria)**
  - Symphysis pubis fusion
  - Disc spaces narrowed + marginal vertebral body sclerosis
  - Disc calcification progresses to ossification
    - Intervertebral bridging can mimic ankylosing spondylitis

Septic Joint

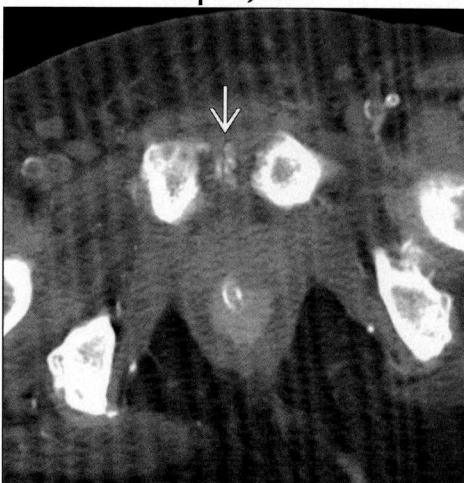

Axial NECT shows significant irregular destruction of the pubic symphysis →. CT was performed for biopsy guidance, which cultured Staphylococcus.

DISH

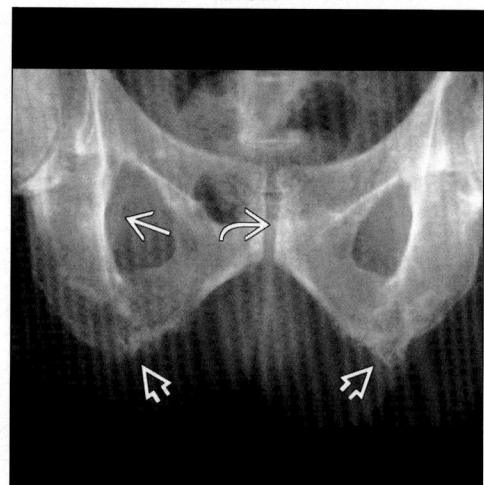

Anteroposterior radiograph shows sacrotuberous ligament calcification → as well as enthesopathy of the ischial tuberosities ⇉ and sclerosis of pubic symphysis →.

SYMPHYSIS PUBIS WITH PRODUCTIVE CHANGES/FUSION

Stress Fracture, Adult (Mimic)

Ankylosing Spondylitis

(Left) Axial T1WI MR shows changes typical of nondisplaced insufficiency fractures in the pelvis. Edema and fracture lines are seen not only in the left pubic ramus ➡ but also in the right pubic ramus ➡. *(Right)* Anteroposterior radiograph shows solid bony fusion of the symphysis pubis ➡ and symmetric fusion of the sacroiliac joints ➡. Characteristic enthesopathic changes are present along the ischial tuberosities ➡.

Rheumatoid Arthritis

Hyperparathyroidism

(Left) Anteroposterior radiograph shows mild erosion of the symphysis pubis ➡. Note the typical appearance of the hips ➡ in rheumatoid arthritis. There are small erosions and concentric joint space narrowing without any suggestion of productive change. *(Right)* Anteroposterior radiograph shows that the sacroiliac joints ➡ and symphysis pubis ➡ are fused, consistent with the patient's history of secondary hyperparathyroidism.

Osteitis Pubis, Late

Ochronosis (Alkaptonuria)

(Left) Anteroposterior radiograph shows irregular sclerosis and fusion of the symphysis pubis ➡. This reflects chronic changes from osteitis pubis. *(Right)* Anteroposterior radiograph shows fusion of the symphysis pubis ➡. Changes in the spine including disc calcification and marked disc space narrowing ➡, along with large marginal osteophytes, are typical for ochronosis.

SYMPHYSIS PUBIS, WIDENING

DIFFERENTIAL DIAGNOSIS

Common
- Osteitis Pubis
- Pregnancy
- Trauma, Pelvic Injury
- Stress Fracture, Malunion
- Chronic Repetitive Trauma
- Septic Joint

Less Common
- Metastasis, Osteolytic
- Radiation Osteonecrosis
- Hyperparathyroidism (Mimic)
- Ankylosing Spondylitis, Early
- Rheumatoid Arthritis, Early
- Achondroplasia
- Chronic Reactive Arthritis

Rare but Important
- Langerhans Cell Histiocytosis
- Pycnodysostosis
- Marfan Syndrome
- Ehlers-Danlos
- Chondrodysplasia Punctata
- Hypophosphatasia
- Prune Belly Syndrome (Eagle-Barrett)
- Cleidocranial Dysplasia
- Imperforate Anus
- Bladder Extrophy
- Urethral Duplication
- Hypospadias
- Epispadius
- Spondyloepiphyseal Dysplasia
- Dyggve-Melchior-Clausen Syndrome

ESSENTIAL INFORMATION

Key Differential Diagnosis Issues
- Normal symphysis pubis width varies with age & gender
  - 10 mm wide in early childhood
  - 6 mm wide in early adulthood
  - 3 mm wide in middle to late adulthood
  - Females have greater symphysis mobility than males

Helpful Clues for Common Diagnoses
- **Osteitis Pubis**
  - Mild widening → osteolysis & erosions → sclerosis
  - ± Periosteal reaction
  - Symphysis may fuse late in course

- **Pregnancy**
  - Symphysis pubis mobility increases to 8-12 mm during last trimester of pregnancy
  - Air in symphysis pubis is normal < 24 hours postpartum
- **Trauma, Pelvic Injury**
  - Injury patterns include diastasis, straddle fracture, intraarticular fracture, overlapping dislocation, and fracture-dislocations
  - Diastasis is most common injury
  - Widening > 10 mm in adult males or > 15 mm in females, suggests instability
  - Widening > 25 mm suggests associated sacroiliac joint injury
- **Stress Fracture, Malunion**
  - Insufficiency fractures of pubic bone are more common than overuse stress fractures
  - Typically these fractures are not immobilized & thus prone to malunion
- **Chronic Repetitive Trauma**
  - Repetitive microtrauma leads to fatigue fracture or ligamentous injury
  - Widening, erosions, & sclerosis
- **Septic Joint**
  - Moth-eaten destruction of bone
  - Pyogenic infection has rapid destruction
  - Tuberculosis has more indolent course
  - Intravenous drug abuse increases risk of infection with unusual organisms

Helpful Clues for Less Common Diagnoses
- **Metastasis, Osteolytic**
  - Metastases are the most likely of any tumor to involve both pubic bones
- **Radiation Osteonecrosis**
  - Located in distribution of radiation port
  - Damage is related to radiation dose
- **Hyperparathyroidism (Mimic)**
  - Subchondral bone resorption causing symmetric symphyseal widening
  - Osteopenia
  - Focal bone lesions in pelvis
- **Ankylosing Spondylitis, Early**
  - Symphysis pubis less commonly involved than sacroiliac joints
  - Erosive changes early, fusion late
  - Proliferative new bone at muscle attachments
- **Rheumatoid Arthritis, Early**
  - Marginal erosions & osteopenia

SYMPHYSIS PUBIS, WIDENING

- **Achondroplasia**
  - Champagne glass pelvis
  - Square iliac wings
  - Narrow sciatic notch
- **Chronic Reactive Arthritis**
  - Erosions produce widening

Helpful Clues for Rare Diagnoses

- **Langerhans Cell Histiocytosis**
  - Well-defined border of lytic lesions
- **Pycnodysostosis**
  - Narrow ilia
  - Wide cranial sutures
  - Generalized osteosclerosis
  - Distal phalangeal aplasia or resorption
- **Marfan Syndrome**
  - Protrusio acetabuli
  - Kyphoscoliosis + spondylolisthesis
  - Sacral abnormalities
- **Ehlers-Danlos**
  - Pubic symphysis distraction during birth
  - Heterotopic bone around hips
  - Lumbar platyspondyly
- **Chondrodysplasia Punctata**
  - Punctate calcifications of epiphyses & spine
  - Vertebral coronal clefts
  - Shortened limbs
- **Hypophosphatasia**
  - Skeletal ossification delay
  - Thoracolumbar vertebral wedging
- **Prune Belly Syndrome (Eagle-Barrett)**
  - Absent abdominal musculature
  - Flared iliac wings

- Hip dysplasia
- Urogenital abnormalities
- **Cleidocranial Dysplasia**
  - Absent or delayed pubic bone ossification
  - Hypoplastic iliac wings
  - Coxa vara or valga
  - Other midline structure dysplasia: Cranium, mandible, teeth, clavicles, neural arches
- **Imperforate Anus**
  - Widened symphysis
- **Bladder Extrophy**
  - Pubic bones completely separated
    - Absent symphysis
  - Laterally flared innominate bones
    - Posterolateral facing acetabula
  - Midline anterior soft tissues unfused
  - Bladder mucosa exposed
- **Urethral Duplication**
  - Widened or completely separated pubis
- **Hypospadias**
  - Widened or completely separated pubis
- **Spondyloepiphyseal Dysplasia**
  - Small iliac wings
  - Hypoplastic acetabular roof
  - Epiphyseal ossification delay
- **Dyggve-Melchior-Clausen Syndrome**
  - Small iliac wings with lacy calcification of iliac crests
  - Wide public ramus & ischiopubic synchondrosis
  - Wide sacroiliac joints
  - Flat acetabular roof

Osteitis Pubis

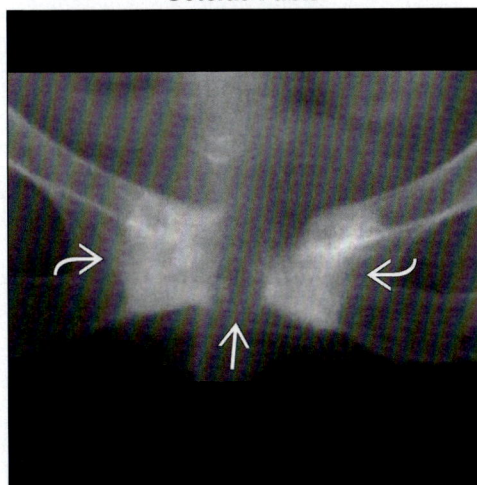

Anteroposterior radiograph shows a wide symphysis pubis ➡ with ill-defined borders. Note the marked sclerosis ➡ involving each side of the pubic bone.

Trauma, Pelvic Injury

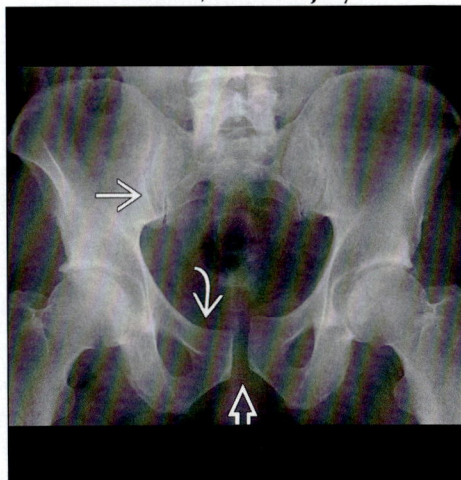

Anteroposterior radiograph shows a wide symphysis pubis ➡, inferior displacement of the right hemipelvis ➡, and widening of the right sacroiliac joint ➡.

SYMPHYSIS PUBIS, WIDENING

Trauma, Pelvic Injury

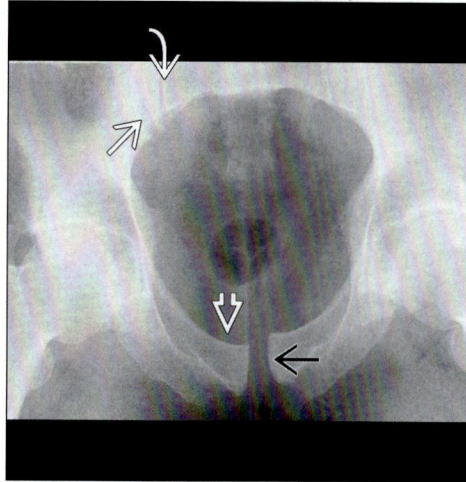

Stress Fracture, Malunion

(Left) Radiograph outlet view shows anterior to posterior displacement through the pelvic ring. The right hemipelvis is minimally displaced anteriorly ⇥, and the pubic symphysis is widened ⇥. The outlet view nicely demonstrates the anterior sacroiliac joint widening ⇥ and the normal posterior aspect of the joint ⇥. *(Right)* Anteroposterior radiograph shows widening of the symphysis pubis ⇥ due to malunion of a left pubic bone stress (insufficiency) fracture ⇥.

Septic Joint

Septic Joint

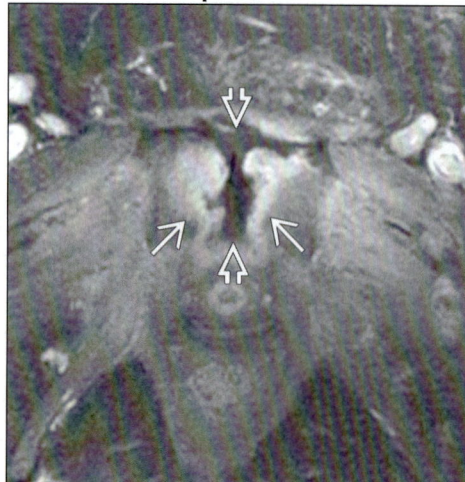

(Left) Axial T1 C+ FS MR shows enhancement within the osseous structures on both sides of the pubic symphysis ⇥, representing osteomyelitis. There is also a collection of fluid within the widened symphysis ⇥, representing a septic joint. *(Right)* Axial NECT shows gross destruction of the symphysis pubis ⇥ giving it a widened appearance, with osseous destruction of both the superior and inferior pubic rami. CT was used for needle aspiration guidance.

Metastasis, Osteolytic

Ankylosing Spondylitis, Early

(Left) Axial STIR MR shows metastatic prostate carcinoma foci in the right pubic ramus ⇥ and left hip ⇥. These were osteolytic on radiographs and caused a widened appearance of the symphysis pubis due to adjacent bone destruction. *(Right)* Anteroposterior radiograph shows loss of cortical definition and mature enthesopathy involving the ischial tuberosities ⇥. Erosive changes are mildly widening the symphysis pubis ⇥.

SYMPHYSIS PUBIS, WIDENING

Langerhans Cell Histiocytosis

Hypophosphatasia

(Left) Anteroposterior radiograph shows irregular destruction of the left pubic bone ➡, giving the symphysis a widened appearance. Bone destruction extends into the left superior pubic ramus ➡. This child also had lytic skull lesions. (Right) Anteroposterior radiograph demonstrates significantly softened bones, showing severe osteoporosis, symphysis pubis diastasis ➡, protrusio of the hips ➡, and bowing of the long bones ➡ with fractures.

Cleidocranial Dysplasia

Imperforate Anus

(Left) Anteroposterior radiograph shows a midline defect at the pubic symphysis ➡. The presence of additional midline defects suggests cleidocranial dysplasia (or dysostosis). (Right) Anteroposterior high-pressure colostogram was performed to evaluate imperforate anus and rectal fistula prior to definitive repair. It shows filling of the distal rectal segment ➡ from the mucous fistula of the colostomy. A mildly widened symphysis pubis ➡ is a common finding.

Imperforate Anus

Spondyloepiphyseal Dysplasia

(Left) Anteroposterior radiograph obtained in an infant with imperforate anus diagnosed at birth shows a widened symphysis pubis ➡ and mildly dysmorphic sacrum ➡. (Right) Anteroposterior radiograph shows a widened symphysis pubis ➡. The epiphyses are irregular and flattened ➡. The spine was more obviously abnormal, with diffuse mild flattening of the vertebral bodies. The combination of findings suggests spondyloepiphyseal dysplasia.

SUPRA-ACETABULAR ILIAC DESTRUCTION

DIFFERENTIAL DIAGNOSIS

Common
- Subchondral Cyst
- Metastases, Bone Marrow
- Arthroplasty Loosening & Dislocation
- Arthroplasty Component Wear/Particle Disease
- Multiple Myeloma
- Plasmacytoma
- Osteomyelitis, Adult
- Radiation Osteonecrosis
- Paget Disease
- Ewing Sarcoma

Less Common
- Aneurysmal Bone Cyst
- Osteosarcoma
- Chondroblastoma
- Hyperparathyroidism
- Fibrous Dysplasia
- Fibrosarcoma
- Lymphoma
- Angiosarcoma, Osseous
- Hemophilia, Pseudotumor
- Chondromyxoid Fibroma
- Giant Cell Tumor

Rare but Important
- Syphilis, Secondary or Tertiary
- Hemangiopericytoma, Osseous
- Gaucher Disease

ESSENTIAL INFORMATION

Helpful Clues for Common Diagnoses
- **Subchondral Cyst**
  - Well-defined lytic lesion, often with sclerotic border
  - Most common cause is osteoarthritis
    - Associated findings of joint space narrowing & osteophytes
  - Numerous less common causes include gout, PVNS, synovial osteochondromatosis, inflammatory arthropathy, & seronegative spondyloarthropathy
- **Metastases, Bone Marrow**
  - Well-defined lytic to ill-defined, permeative lesions
  - Breast, lung, & renal carcinoma metastases common
  - Multiple lesions are usually evident

- **Arthroplasty Loosening & Dislocation**
  - Lucency greater than 2 mm at the cement-bone or prosthesis-bone interface of acetabular component of total hip replacement
  - Evaluate multiple projections to assess for component malposition or dislocation
- **Arthroplasty Component Wear/Particle Disease**
  - Polyethylene wear evident by progressive eccentric location of femoral component within the acetabular component
  - Periprosthetic lucency, as described above
- **Multiple Myeloma**
  - Multiple sharply demarcated lytic lesions
  - Intramedullary with endosteal scalloping
  - Lacks periosteal new bone formation
  - ± Soft tissue mass
  - Spine > ribs > femur > pelvis
- **Plasmacytoma**
  - Solitary focus of myeloma
  - Larger & more expansile lesion than multiple myeloma
- **Osteomyelitis, Adult**
  - Permeative bone destruction
  - Periosteal new bone
  - Soft tissue abscess
  - Late surrounding sclerosis + sequestrum
  - More rapid bone destruction than tumor, except for Langerhans cell histiocytosis
- **Radiation Osteonecrosis**
  - Ill-defined bone destruction ± fracture
  - Lacks a soft tissue mass
  - Latent period of at least one year before bone changes are seen in pelvis
- **Paget Disease**
  - Well-defined lytic lesions in active stage
  - Enlarged bone with coarse trabeculae
  - Thickened iliopectineal line
  - Acetabular protrusio
  - Polyostotic in 70%
  - Pelvis > spine > skull
- **Ewing Sarcoma**
  - Osteolysis, cortical destruction, periosteal reaction, & soft tissue mass
    - Can mimic osteomyelitis
  - Aggressive periosteal new bone
    - Laminated, onion skin, sunburst, or "hair on end"
  - Lower skeletal involvement in 2/3 of cases
    - Femur > ilium > tibia

SUPRA-ACETABULAR ILIAC DESTRUCTION

Helpful Clues for Less Common Diagnoses

- **Aneurysmal Bone Cyst**
  - Well-defined osteolysis with bone expansion
  - Internal fluid-fluid levels
  - ± Surrounding bone sclerosis
- **Osteosarcoma**
  - Mixed osteolytic & osteosclerotic lesion depending on subtype
  - Aggressive periosteal reaction
  - Cortical violation with soft tissue mass
  - Osteoid matrix present
- **Chondroblastoma**
  - Located around acetabulum in pelvis
    - Epiphyseal equivalent
  - Well-defined round to oval lytic lesion with thin sclerotic rim
  - Periosteal reaction in adjacent metaphysis or diaphysis
- **Hyperparathyroidism**
  - Brown tumors in primary or secondary hyperparathyroidism
  - Well-defined lytic lesion ± bone expansion
  - May undergo necrosis, producing a cyst
- **Fibrous Dysplasia**
  - Hazy radiolucent, or ground-glass, lesions ± mild bone expansion
  - Usually polyostotic when pelvis is involved
  - Protrusio acetabula present
- **Lymphoma**
  - Cancellous bone erosion early
  - Cortex destroyed late

- **Hemophilia, Pseudotumor**
  - Intraosseous and subperiosteal bleeds produce pressure erosion of bone
  - Soft tissue mass may extend into the iliopsoas and gluteal muscles
- **Giant Cell Tumor**
  - Lytic metaphyseal lesion without sclerotic border
    - Bones around the acetabulum are metaphyseal and epiphyseal equivalents

Helpful Clues for Rare Diagnoses

- **Syphilis, Secondary or Tertiary**
  - Secondary syphilis → irregular bone lysis
    - Skull involvement is characteristic
  - Tertiary syphilis → neuropathic changes
  - Periostitis is common
- **Hemangiopericytoma, Osseous**
  - Lobulated lytic foci with honeycomb appearance
  - Mild bone expansion
  - Aggressive features include soft tissue mass, cortical destruction, ill-defined borders
  - 10% of cases in innominate bone
- **Gaucher Disease**
  - Younger patients with generalized osteopenia
  - Marrow infiltration causing cortical scalloping can mimic metastasis, myeloma, or pseudotumor of hemophilia
  - Additional findings of abdominal organomegaly, "H-shaped" vertebral bodies, & femoral head avascular necrosis

Subchondral Cyst

Anteroposterior radiograph shows a large subchondral cyst ➡ present within the superior aspect of the acetabulum. Note the joint space narrowing ➡.

Metastases, Bone Marrow

Anteroposterior radiograph shows a fairly non-aggressive acetabular lesion ➡ that distorts the normal trabecular pattern. This was a solitary breast metastasis.

SUPRA-ACETABULAR ILIAC DESTRUCTION

Arthroplasty Component Wear/Particle Disease

Multiple Myeloma

(Left) Coronal bone CT shows acetabular lysis →. Note that the distance between the femoral head and acetabular rim is less on the superolateral side → than the inferomedial side →, indicating wear of the polyethylene liner. (Right) Coronal T1WI MR shows the multifocal presentation of myeloma as hypointense deposits → adjacent to the normal bone marrow. This has the appearance of multiple "punched out" lytic lesions on radiographs, typical of myeloma.

Plasmacytoma

Osteomyelitis, Adult

(Left) Anteroposterior radiograph shows a well-defined, lytic bubbly lesion → that occupies the superior pubic ramus and extends well into the acetabulum. The lesion is mildly expansile. This is a typical appearance of plasmacytoma. (Right) Coronal T1WI MR demonstrates the extent of the right hip infection →, which destroys both acetabular and femoral bone. Antibiotic beads → and surrounding soft tissue edema → are also evident.

Paget Disease

Aneurysmal Bone Cyst

(Left) Anteroposterior radiograph shows bone overgrowth and trabecular thickening of the pelvis and femurs. The bones have a mixed sclerotic and lytic → appearance. Protrusio at the hips → and femoral deformity reflect bone softening. (Right) Coronal T2WI MR shows an expansile lesion → involving the superomedial acetabulum. Multiple loculations contain fluid intensity material, and fluid-fluid levels were seen on axial images.

SUPRA-ACETABULAR ILIAC DESTRUCTION

Anatomy Based: Pelvis

Osteosarcoma

Hyperparathyroidism

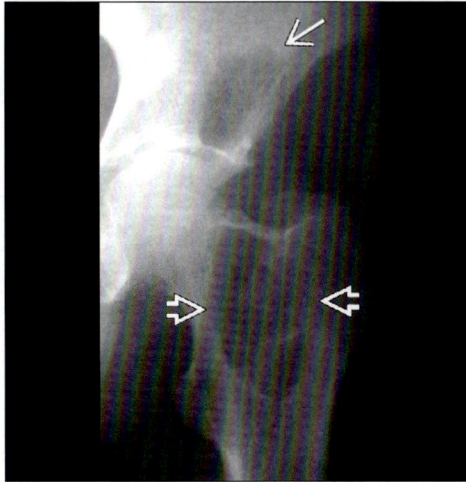

(Left) Anteroposterior radiograph shows a mixed osteosclerotic and osteolytic lesion ➡ in the supra-acetabular region. There is an associated large soft tissue mass ➡ that contains osteoid matrix. *(Right)* Anteroposterior radiograph shows a supra-acetabular lytic lesion with indistinct borders ➡ and a similar femoral ➡ lesion. The combination of multiple lytic lesions with cortical and trabecular indistinctness is typical of Brown tumors.

Fibrous Dysplasia

Fibrosarcoma

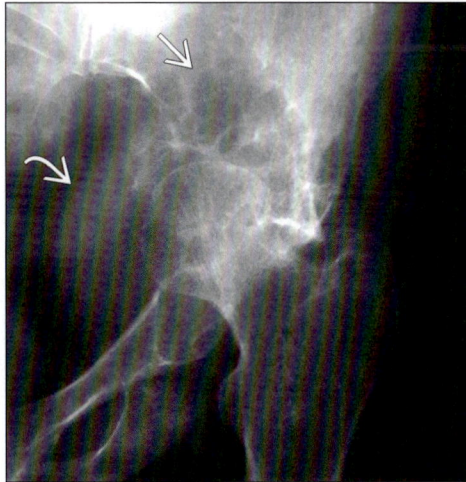

(Left) Anteroposterior radiograph shows a large, lobulated lesion ➡ with a sclerotic border in the supra-acetabular region. This lesion has a faint ground-glass appearance. A similar lesion in the proximal femur ➡ produces a shepherd's crook deformity. *(Right)* Anteroposterior radiograph shows severe and rapid progression of bone destruction ➡, with an obvious soft tissue mass ➡ as well as pathologic fracture. This case is classic for fibrosarcoma.

Lymphoma

Giant Cell Tumor

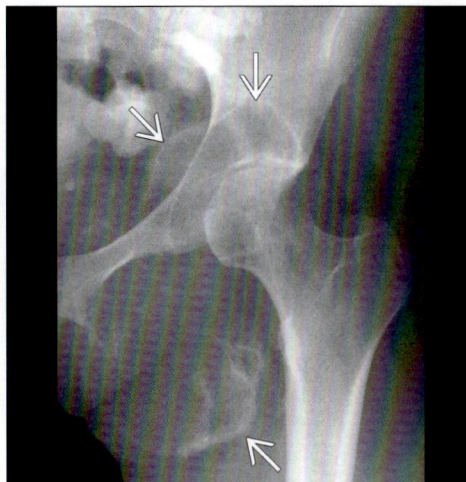

(Left) AP radiograph shows a highly permeative, infiltrating lesion involving the superior acetabulum ➡ and extending into both the superior pubic ramus ➡ and ischium ➡. This is a highly aggressive lesion. (†MSK Req). *(Right)* Anteroposterior radiograph shows an extremely expansile lesion ➡ involving the left acetabulum, inferior pubic ramus, and ischium. There is a narrow zone of transition. Despite the degree of expansion it does not appear aggressive.

333

PROTRUSIO ACETABULI

DIFFERENTIAL DIAGNOSIS

Common
- Arthritis
  - Osteoarthritis
  - Rheumatoid Arthritis, Hip
  - Ankylosing Spondylitis
  - Juvenile Idiopathic Arthritis (JIA)
  - Crystalline Arthropathy
- Trauma
- Paget Disease

Less Common
- Renal Osteodystrophy
- Septic Joint
- Osseous Neoplasm

Rare but Important
- Sickle Cell Anemia
- Otto Disease
- Hyperparathyroidism
- Osteomalacia
- Rickets
- Idiopathic Chondrolysis
- Hypophosphatasia
- Collagen Vascular Disorders
- Osteogenesis Imperfecta
- Fibrous Dysplasia

ESSENTIAL INFORMATION

Key Differential Diagnosis Issues
- Acetabular protrusion = intrapelvic bulging of acetabular wall, ± joint space loss
  - Diagnosis of dramatic contour abnormalities (acetabular wall/femoral head protruding into pelvis) are not difficult
  - Diagnosis of subtle or early changes may be challenging
  - **Hint**: Acetabular line projecting medial to ilioischial line is most reliable sign
    - Adults: Male > 3 mm; female > 6 mm
    - Children: Male > 1 mm; female > 3 mm
  - **Hint**: Other methods are less accurate in evaluating subtle protrusio including center edge angle of Wiberg > 45 °, teardrop "crossing"

Helpful Clues for Common Diagnoses
- **Arthritis**
  - **Osteoarthritis**
    - Most common cause of protrusio

- Protrusio is more frequent in RA, but OA is so much more common than RA that, in absolute numbers, protrusio is more common in OA
    - Axial or medial femoral head migration, joint space narrowing
    - Normal mineralization; osteophytes
    - May be asymmetric, unilateral
  - **Rheumatoid Arthritis, Hip**
    - Osteopenia, erosions of femoral head & acetabulum
    - Axial femoral head migration; bilateral & symmetrical joint space loss
  - **Ankylosing Spondylitis**
    - Axial femoral head migration with uniform, symmetric joint space loss; femoral neck ring osteophytes
    - **Hint**: Look at adjacent sacroiliac joints for erosion or fusion
  - **Juvenile Idiopathic Arthritis (JIA)**
    - Due to erosions & mechanical remodeling from compressive forces
    - Periarticular osteopenia
  - **Crystalline Arthropathy**
    - Pyrophosphate arthropathy: Axial femoral head migration, osteophytes
    - **Hint**: Look for rapid fragmentation & destruction of both femoral head & acetabulum with resultant protrusio
- **Trauma**
  - Protrusio may result from
    - Acute trauma: Periacetabular fracture, particularly quadrilateral plate
    - Late complications: Malalignment at time of healing; secondary osteoarthritis
    - Post-operative complications: Hardware failure due to loosening, infection, etc.
  - Underlying osteoporosis increases risk of protrusio development
- **Paget Disease**
  - Patchy lytic, sclerotic pattern with relative overgrowth of involved bone
  - Osteoarthritis changes with medial/axial joint space loss & axial femoral head migration
  - Protrusio may result from inherently weakened acetabular bone or associated osteoarthritis
  - **Hint**: Look for trabecular thickening, particularly along iliopectineal line

Helpful Clues for Less Common Diagnoses
- **Renal Osteodystrophy**
  - Osteomalacia combined with hyperparathyroidism in chronic renal failure
  - Osteopenia with extensive bone resorption
  - Soft tissue calcification, osteosclerosis, periostitis, Brown tumors
- **Septic Joint**
  - Results in cartilage destruction; ± osteomyelitis with acetabular remodeling or destruction
  - Unilateral, rapid onset destruction; requires aspiration for diagnosis
- **Osseous Neoplasm**
  - Metastases & myeloma most common
  - Replacement/destruction of quadrilateral plate leads to protrusio
  - Protrusio may be late complication of pelvic radiation therapy & osteonecrosis

Helpful Clues for Rare Diagnoses
- **Sickle Cell Anemia**
  - Marrow hyperplasia may contribute to bone weakness & remodeling from compressive forces across hip
- **Otto Disease**
  - Primary protrusio acetabuli
  - Due to abnormal triradiate cartilage development
  - Familial; female > male
  - Bilateral, symmetric, normal joint space in early stages progressing to osteoarthritis
- **Hyperparathyroidism**
  - May be 1° due to adenoma, etc., or 2° due to renal failure
  - Bone resorption is hallmark of disease
  - Diffuse osteopenia, Brown tumors, soft tissue calcification
- **Osteomalacia**
  - Vitamin D production failure = osteomalacia
  - Rickets: Osteomalacia in child
  - Osteopenia with coarsened & indistinct trabeculae, Looser zones, acetabular remodeling
- **Idiopathic Chondrolysis**
  - Monoarticular; acute onset occurring in adolescent females; no history of trauma
  - Rapid cartilage loss/joint space narrowing with subchondral erosion, osteoporosis
  - Mimics inflammatory arthritis, septic arthritis; requires aspiration to exclude infection
- **Hypophosphatasia**
  - Defective bone mineralization similar to osteomalacia
  - Protrusio due to abnormal bone; ± associated pyrophosphate arthropathy
- **Collagen Vascular Disorders**
  - Marfan syndrome, Ehlers-Danlos
- **Osteogenesis Imperfecta**
  - Defective collagen matrix synthesis & mineralization
- **Fibrous Dysplasia**
  - Lytic expansile lesion(s) with ground-glass matrix; abnormally weak bone allows deformity with weight-bearing

Osteoarthritis

Anteroposterior radiograph shows acetabular medial wall ⊳ projecting > 3 mm medial to ilioischial line ➡ in this male with mild secondary OA due to trauma. Note heterotopic ossification near acetabular rim ➘.

Osteoarthritis

Anteroposterior radiograph shows protrusio ⊳ due to osteoarthritis with medial femoral head migration & joint space loss ➡. Acetabular & femoral osteophytes ➘ are seen with subchondral sclerosis ➡.

335

PROTRUSIO ACETABULI

(Left) *Anteroposterior radiograph shows rheumatoid arthritis with bilateral, symmetric joint narrowing* ➡ *& axial femoral head migration with small erosions but no osteophytes. Note diffuse osteopenia & mild protrusio* ➡. *(Right) Anteroposterior radiograph shows bilateral hip joint space narrowing & erosion* ➡ *with protrusio acetabuli on the right* ➡. *The bilateral sacroiliac fusion* ➢ *confirms ankylosing spondylitis.*

Rheumatoid Arthritis, Hip

Ankylosing Spondylitis

(Left) *Anteroposterior radiograph shows classic JIA in a 22 yo female with severe bilateral femoral head erosion* ➡ *as well as erosive acetabular remodeling, protrusio* ➡, *& diffuse osteopenia. (Right) Axial NECT shows left hip protrusio from a comminuted acetabular fracture* ➢. *The right hip demonstrates a mild protrusio* ➡ *from osteoarthritis, characterized by joint space narrowing, subchondral cysts* ➡, *& osteophytic ridging* ➡.

Juvenile Idiopathic Arthritis (JIA)

Trauma

(Left) *Anteroposterior radiograph shows secondary osteoarthritis* ➡ *& protrusio* ➢ *from comminuted acetabular fracture treated with multiple plates & screws that are loose, with screws* ➡ *projecting into the pelvic soft tissues. (Right) Anteroposterior radiograph shows Paget disease with marked thickening of cortical & trabecular bone* ➡ *as well as disuse osteoporosis. Despite the apparent thickening, the bone is weak & protrusio* ➡ *results.*

Trauma

Paget Disease

PROTRUSIO ACETABULI

Renal Osteodystrophy

Septic Joint

(Left) Posteroanterior radiograph shows residua from renal osteodystrophy with bone resorption of 2° hyperparathyroidism & osteomalacia resulting in a shepherd crook deformity ⇨ & protrusio ⇨. *(Right)* Coronal reformation NECT shows extensive femoral head ⇨ & acetabular destruction ⇨ with a large joint effusion ⇨ & protrusio ⇨ in this patient with septic arthritis/osteomyelitis.

Osseous Neoplasm

Otto Disease

(Left) Anteroposterior radiograph shows protrusio ⇨ due to metastasis from lung adenocarcinoma. Note the permeative lytic acetabular lesion ⇨ while the femoral head is normal. *(Right)* Anteroposterior radiograph shows bilateral protrusio ⇨ of Otto disease in this young woman whose mother had similar signs & symptoms at age 41. Secondary osteoarthritis often develops over time, but the primary failure is in triradiate cartilage development.

Hypophosphatasia

Fibrous Dysplasia

(Left) Anteroposterior radiograph shows severe osteopenia, protrusio ⇨, & disordered bone formation. There is widening of the zone of provisional ossification at the femoral head metaphysis. *(Right)* Anteroposterior radiograph shows diffuse expansile lytic lesions ⇨ throughout pelvis & femora with ground-glass matrix typical of fibrous dysplasia with marked deformity of femoral necks & bilateral protrusio ⇨.

COXA MAGNA DEFORMITY

DIFFERENTIAL DIAGNOSIS

Common
- Developmental Dysplasia Hip (DDH)

Less Common
- Slipped Capital Femoral Epiphysis (SCFE)
- Legg-Calvé-Perthes (LCP)

Rare but Important
- Septic Hip
- Hip/Femur Trauma

ESSENTIAL INFORMATION

Key Differential Diagnosis Issues
- Coxa magna: Short broad femoral head sitting on a short broad femoral neck
  - Results in limb length discrepancy
  - Relatively proximal displacement of greater & lesser trochanters
- Coxa magna is secondary to an insult to femoral head or epiphysis

Helpful Clues for Common Diagnoses
- **Developmental Dysplasia Hip (DDH)**
  - Lack of coverage of femoral head during development due to deficient acetabulum
  - Without coverage, head cannot develop spherical shape
    - Head becomes short, broad
    - With head & neck shortening, limb becomes short, with proximal displacement of both trochanters
  - Congenital abnormality
    - Severe DDH develops coxa magna
  - Subtle DDH does not show coxa magna, but seen as ↓ center-edge angle of Wiberg
  - **Hint**: Shallow acetabulum distinguishes coxa magna of DDH from other etiologies of coxa magna

Helpful Clues for Less Common Diagnoses
- **Slipped Capital Femoral Epiphysis (SCFE)**
  - Femoral capital epiphysis slips medially & posteriorly
    - As head slips, appears short & broad, on a short & broad neck
  - Most frequently occurs 8-14 years of age
  - **Hint**: Position of femoral head on neck & a normal acetabulum distinguish coxa magna of SCFE from other etiologies
- **Legg-Calvé-Perthes (LCP)**
  - Avascular necrosis femoral head in a child, generally 4-8 years of age
  - Flattening of head leads to coxa magna deformity
  - **Hint**: Head remains centered on femoral neck & acetabulum is normal, distinguishing this etiology of coxa magna from others

Helpful Clues for Rare Diagnoses
- **Septic Hip**
  - Chronic hip infection during childhood
    - Hyperemia results in overgrowth of femoral head & neck
- **Hip/Femur Trauma**
  - Resorption/impaction of neck or malalignment mimics coxa magna
  - Salter fracture with early fusion

Developmental Dysplasia Hip (DDH)

AP radiograph shows right DDH. Note short broad head ⇥ & neck, compared with normal left side. Coxa magna is due to DDH, with shallow acetabulum seen ⇥, resulting in decrease in femoral head coverage.

Slipped Capital Femoral Epiphysis (SCFE)

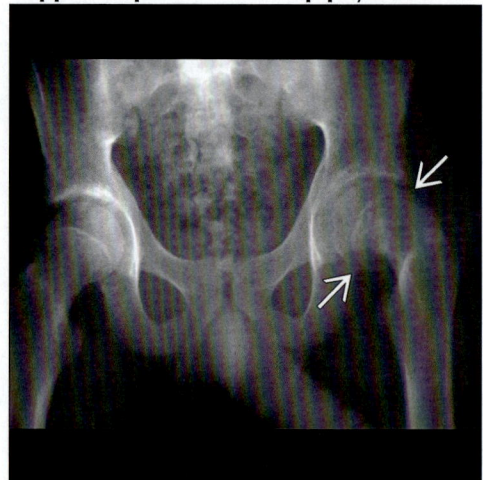

AP radiograph shows SCFE, with medial & posterior femoral head slip ⇥. This results in the appearance of a short broad femoral head; the neck also appears broad. Note the lateral femoral neck is not covered by head.

COXA MAGNA DEFORMITY

Legg-Calvé-Perthes (LCP)

Legg-Calvé-Perthes (LCP)

(Left) AP radiograph shows flattened & dense femoral capital epiphysis typical of LCP. This is already chronic disease, & morphologic change of short broad head & neck is seen in its early form. (†MSK Req). (Right) AP radiograph in same patient 12 years later shows typical coxa magna deformity. Head is not medially displaced to suggest SCFE, & acetabulum is normal, ruling out DDH. Even without prior X-ray, this should be diagnosed as coxa magna due to LCP.

Legg-Calvé-Perthes (LCP)

Septic Hip

(Left) Coronal T2WI FS MR shows old LCP, with the short broad femoral head ➡ on a shortened femoral neck, resulting in a coxa magna deformity. This has resulted in a significant labral tear ➡ & early arthritic change. (Right) Anteroposterior radiograph shows an enlarged, short femoral capital femoral epiphysis ➡, with broadening & slight shortening of the femoral neck. This 12 year old had a septic hip treated 9 months earlier. The growth deformity results from hyperemia.

Hip/Femur Trauma

Hip/Femur Trauma

(Left) AP radiograph shows an old subcapital fracture treated with pins. The fracture has impacted, with resorption of much of the neck ➡ & backing out of the pins ➡. This results in the appearance of a short femoral head on a short broad neck, similar to a coxa magna deformity. (Right) AP radiograph shows enlarged femoral head with early fusion ➡ & subsequent limb shortening in a teenager. This coxa magna deformity resulted from Salter II fracture.

HIP LABRAL TEARS, ETIOLOGY

DIFFERENTIAL DIAGNOSIS

Common
- Degenerative
  - Osteoarthritis (OA)
- Femoral Acetabular Impingement, CAM-Type
  - Lateral Femoral Neck "Bump"
  - Elliptical Femoral Head Morphology
- Femoral Acetabular Impingement, Pincer-Type
  - Retroverted Acetabulum
- Hip Dysplasia (DDH)
  - Acetabular Dysplasia
  - Coxa Valga

Less Common
- Femoral Acetabular Impingement, CAM-Type
  - Slipped Femoral Capital Epiphysis (SCFE)
  - Legg-Perthes, Coxa Magna
  - Femoral Neck Fracture, Malunited
- Femoral Acetabular Impingement, Pincer-Type
  - Hip Protrusio, Secondary
  - Otto Disease
  - Ossification of Acetabular Rim
  - Overcorrection Osteotomy for DDH

Rare but Important
- Hip Dysplasia
  - Reduced Femoral Anteversion

ESSENTIAL INFORMATION

Key Differential Diagnosis Issues
- Labral tears likely are common in OA, but are rarely specifically imaged
- Cartilage damage is as important as labral damage, but more difficult to accurately diagnose
- Femoral acetabular impingement (FAI) is an important etiology of labral tears
  - Hint: Important to diagnose morphologic abnormalities early in order to avoid early damage and development of osteoarthritis at a young age
- Impingement has been separated into "cam" and "pincer" types, based on different hip morphologies & etiologies
  - Hint: There is often overlap between "cam" and "pincer" types, with contributions of both in an individual

- DDH results in several abnormalities that can result in impingement & subsequent labral tears
  - Hint: DDH morphologic abnormalities can be very subtle, and must be carefully sought out
- May make diagnosis on routine MR, but MR arthrograph increases specificity & confidence
  - Consider traction on hip during arthrography to better visualize cartilage
- Note that different morphologic abnormalities resulting in CAM or pincer FAI or DDH may be more or less common; hence, examples of FAI and DDH are found in "common", "less common", and "rare" lists

Helpful Clues for Common Diagnoses
- **Osteoarthritis (OA)**
  - OA is most common abnormality of hip
  - Cartilage damage in weight-bearing region
  - Advanced disease usually results in superolateral subluxation of femoral head
    - Shear stress may result in labral tear
  - Though labral & cartilage damage are common, advanced imaging generally not utilized for OA
    - Salvage or arthroplasty situation rather than surgical reconstruction
- **Lateral Femoral Neck "Bump"**
  - Etiology of the bump unknown
  - ↓ Cutback at femoral head/neck junction
  - Conflict between bump & labrum when hip in flexion, internal rotation, adduction: "Cam" mechanism of FAI
  - Cartilage damage earlier than labrum
  - Labral injury is often detachment
- **Elliptical Femoral Head Morphology**
  - Functions the same as the lateral femoral neck bump
    - ↓ Cutback at femoral head/neck junction
    - "Cam" mechanism of FAI
- **Retroverted Acetabulum**
  - Acetabulum is generally anteverted
  - Usually only the cranial portion is retroverted in FAI
    - Seen as crossover sign of anterior rim overlapping posterior rim on X-ray
    - Directly visualized on axial MR or CT
  - → Focal acetabular rim overcoverage
    - "Pincer" mechanism of FAI
    - Labral tear > detachment

HIP LABRAL TEARS, ETIOLOGY

- **Acetabular Dysplasia**
  - Acetabular coverage of head may be deficient either laterally or anteriorly
    - Abnormal lateral coverage if center-edge angle of Wiberg < 25°
    - Abnormal anterior coverage seen on false profile view; vertical-center angle < 25°
  - DDH also frequently has cranial acetabular retroversion
  - Labrum frequently hypertrophied
    - Shear stress on hypertrophied labrum makes it at high risk for tear
  - Watch for morphologic changes from childhood acetabular surgery
    - Gives hint of diagnosis
    - May have overcoverage anteriorly
- **Coxa Valga**
  - Form of DDH with decreased femoral neck/shaft angle
  - Associated with pulvinar hypertrophy & labral tear

Helpful Clues for Less Common Diagnoses
- **Slipped Femoral Capital Epiphysis (SCFE)**
  - SCFE: Head slips medially & posteriorly
  - → Coxa magna deformity with decreased α angle & femoral head/neck offset
  - Acts as a "cam" type of FAI, with same association of labral & cartilage injury
- **Legg-Perthes, Coxa Magna**
  - Short broad femoral head & neck resulting from childhood AVN → "cam" type of FAI
- **Femoral Neck Fracture, Malunited**

- Impaction of femoral neck fx may shorten neck & ↓ femoral head/neck cutback
- May result in "cam" type of FAI
- **Hip Protrusio, Secondary**
  - Many secondary causes of hip protrusio
    - Rheumatoid arthritis, Paget disease, or renal osteodystrophy
    - Acetabular fx that heals in protrusio
  - → Relative over-coverage by acetabular rim
    - "Pincer" type of FAI
- **Otto Disease**
  - Hereditary type of OA, resulting from abnormal fusion of triradiate cartilage
  - Primary protrusio of hip → relative overcoverage of head by acetabular rim
    - "Pincer" type of FAI
- **Ossification of Acetabular Rim**
  - Anterosuperior acetabular rim may become overgrown & hyperossified
  - → Relative overcoverage of femoral head
    - "Pincer" type of FAI
- **Overcorrection Osteotomy for DDH**
  - Periacetabular osteotomy to improve femoral head coverage in DDH may result in overcoverage, especially anteriorly
    - Iatrogenic acetabular retroversion
    - "Pincer" type of FAI

Helpful Clues for Rare Diagnoses
- **Reduced Femoral Anteversion**
  - Femoral head/neck is generally anteverted
  - If retroverted, increased shear stress on posterior labrum, increasing risk for tear

Osteoarthritis (OA)

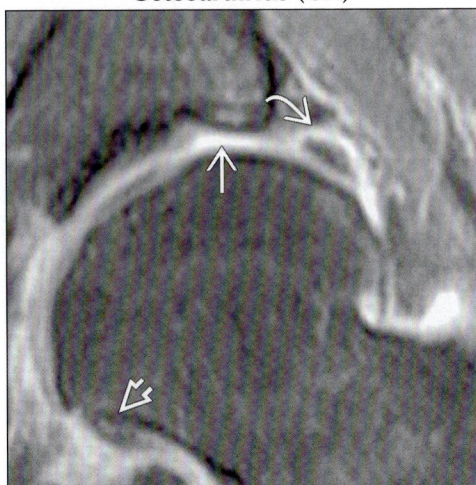

Coronal T1WI FS MR arthrogram shows osteoarthritis with osteophytes, cartilage loss, and a detached labrum. OA is the most common etiology of cartilage & labral damage but is rarely imaged with MR.

Lateral Femoral Neck "Bump"

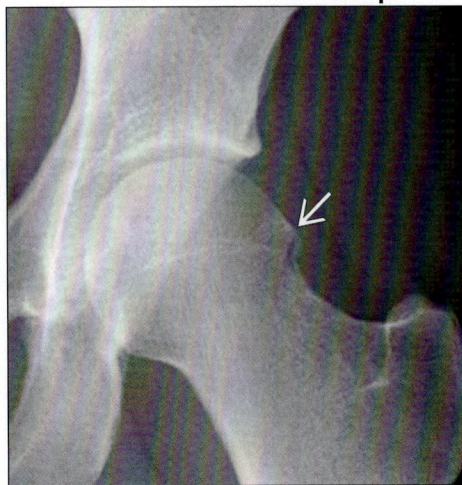

AP radiograph shows a lateral femoral neck "bump" causing cam type impingement; note the lack of normal cutback at the femoral head/neck junction. This is the most common type of femoral acetabular impingement.

HIP LABRAL TEARS, ETIOLOGY

(Left) AP radiograph shows an elliptical morphology of the femoral head, with small lateral femoral neck bump ➡. There is no femoral head/neck cutback. This appearance has been likened to a pistol, also called pistol grip deformity. **(Right)** Coronal T1WI FS MR arthrogram in the same patient shows the elliptical head morphology, along with a complex labral tear ➡. This was a young adult with early onset of hip pain related to femoral acetabular impingement.

Elliptical Femoral Head Morphology

Elliptical Femoral Head Morphology

(Left) AP radiograph shows acetabular retroversion. The anterior acetabular rim ➡ crosses over the posterior rim ➡ superiorly (crossover sign). This results in focal relative overcoverage by the anterosuperior acetabular rim which contributes to the pincer type of femoral acetabular impingement. **(Right)** Axial T1WI FS MR arthrogram on the same patient shows the retroversion of the anterior acetabular rim ➡ relative to the posterior ➡, confirming the retroverted acetabulum.

Retroverted Acetabulum

Retroverted Acetabulum

(Left) Sagittal T1WI FS MR arthrogram on the same patient shows the large labral tear ➡ associated with the acetabular retroversion & subsequent femoral acetabular impingement. **(Right)** Anteroposterior radiograph shows a normal right hip but shallow acetabulum on the left. The center-edge angle of Wiberg on the left is less than 25°, indicating acetabular dysplasia. With this abnormality, the labrum becomes hypertrophied and is at significant risk for tear.

Retroverted Acetabulum

Acetabular Dysplasia

HIP LABRAL TEARS, ETIOLOGY

Acetabular Dysplasia

Acetabular Dysplasia

(Left) Coronal T1WI FS MR arthrogram of the same patient shows the shallow acetabulum ⇨ that does not cover the femoral head. The labrum is hypertrophied, and there is an extensive tear ⇨, which continued over a significant distance. (Right) Axial T1WI FS MR arthrogram of the same patient shows a hypertrophied ligamentum teres ⇨. This and a hypertrophied pulvinar occupy medial joint space in patients with DDH.

Coxa Valga

Slipped Femoral Capital Epiphysis (SCFE)

(Left) Anteroposterior radiograph shows abnormal straightening of the femoral neck, termed coxa valga. There is no acetabular dysplasia, but coxa valga is a form of DDH. It may result in femoral acetabular impingement and labral/cartilage damage. (Right) AP radiograph shows an old SCFE, pinned during childhood. The medial slip of the femoral head results in lack of normal femoral head/neck cutback ⇨, or a form of femoral neck bump. This results in cam-type FAI.

Legg-Perthes, Coxa Magna

Femoral Neck Fracture, Malunited

(Left) Coronal T2WI FS MR shows a coxa magna deformity ⇨ with normal acetabular coverage and no evidence of SCFE. This deformed head & neck is due to Legg-Perthes, and puts the labrum at risk for a cam-type of impingement and tear ⇨. (Right) AP radiograph shows subcapital fracture which was pinned but impacted, developing a varus deformity. This results in lack of femoral head/neck cutback & lateral bump ⇨. This alignment may result in cam-type FAI.

HIP LABRAL TEARS, ETIOLOGY

Hip Protrusio, Secondary

Otto Disease

(Left) AP radiograph shows protrusio of the right hip ➡ (due to old acetabular fracture) compared to a normal left hip. This results in relative overcoverage of the right femoral head & neck ➡, resulting in a pincer-type of FAI. Labral tear was found at surgery. (Right) AP radiograph shows protrusio acetabulae ➡, which was bilateral & hereditary. This is Otto disease, which results in pincer type impingement and early OA, including labral and cartilage damage.

Ossification of Acetabular Rim

Ossification of Acetabular Rim

(Left) Anteroposterior radiograph shows abnormal excessive ossification of the acetabular rim ➡ that can cause a pincer-type of FAI. Note there is also a lateral femoral bump ➡, contributing to a cam impingement. These often coexist. (Right) Coronal T1WI FS MR arthrogram shows the overgrown acetabular rim to be fragmented ➡. The femoral neck bump is seen as well ➡. Both contributed to the labral tear and cartilage damage found at surgery.

Ossification of Acetabular Rim

Ossification of Acetabular Rim

(Left) AP radiograph shows excess ossification of the acetabular rim ➡, along with a lateral femoral neck bump ➡. This patient is highly symptomatic; one must alert the surgeon to the combined pincer & cam mechanisms. (Right) Coronal T1WI FS MR arthrogram on the same patient shows the overgrown ossification of the acetabular rim ➡ and confirms the femoral bump ➡. The combined impingement mechanisms resulted in severe labral and cartilage damage ➡.

Overcorrection Osteotomy for DDH

Overcorrection Osteotomy for DDH

(Left) AP radiograph shows left hip DDH, with coxa magna deformity. The patient had a Salter opening wedge osteotomy of the acetabulum to increase coverage of the left femoral head ➔. This results in acetabular retroversion (note the crossover sign) & pincer-type FAI. *(Right)* AP radiograph during arthrogram shows subtle DDH, with an abnormally small center-edge angle of Wiberg. Additionally, there is evidence of prior surgery to deepen the acetabulum ➔.

Overcorrection Osteotomy for DDH

Overcorrection Osteotomy for DDH

(Left) Coronal T1WI FS MR arthrogram on the same patient shows DDH with shallow acetabulum, as expected. As is frequently seen in DDH, the labrum is hypertrophied and has an extensive tear ➔. *(Right)* Sagittal T1WI FS MR arthrogram from the same study shows that the acetabulum has been overcorrected. While it did not sufficiently cover the femoral head laterally, it has too much anterior coverage, creating retroversion ➔. Note the associated tear ➔.

Reduced Femoral Anteversion

Reduced Femoral Anteversion

(Left) Axial bone CT shows retroversion of the femoral neck ➔. Normally the femoral head and neck are anteverted. This unusual form of dysplasia results in abnormal force on the posterior labrum. *(Right)* Sagittal T1WI FS MR arthrogram on the same patient shows a large posterior labral tear ➔, associated with the retroversion of the femoral neck.

ENLARGEMENT OF INTERCONDYLAR NOTCH DISTAL FEMUR

DIFFERENTIAL DIAGNOSIS

Common
- Post-Operative (Notchplasty)
- Hemophilia: MSK Complications
- Inflammatory Arthritis

Less Common
- Pigmented Villonodular Synovitis (PVNS)
- Septic Joint

Rare but Important
- Gout
- Synovial Osteochondromatosis
- Hemangioma, Synovial
- Inherited Skeletal Disorders

ESSENTIAL INFORMATION

Key Differential Diagnosis Issues
- Intercondylar notch widening, remodeling due to abnormal bone growth, hyperemia, surgical intervention

Helpful Clues for Common Diagnoses
- **Post-Operative (Notchplasty)**
  - Notch osteoplasty of lateral wall & roof to limit impingement in ACL reconstruction
- **Hemophilia: MSK Complication**
  - Chronic hyperemia → femoral epiphyseal overgrowth & notch widening, accentuated by flexion of knee
  - Osteopenia, intraosseous cysts, radiodense joint effusion
- **Inflammatory Arthritis**
  - Juvenile idiopathic arthritis

- Hyperemia, epiphysis overgrowth, notch widening, minimal erosion or cysts initially
- Late disease mimics hemophilia
  - Rheumatoid arthritis
    - Profound osteopenia, erosions, bilateral

Helpful Clues for Less Common Diagnoses
- **Pigmented Villonodular Synovitis (PVNS)**
  - Nodular soft tissue masses, ± ↓ SI on all sequences due to hemosiderin
- **Septic Joint**
  - More common with indolent non-pyogenic infection (e.g., mycobacterium, fungal)
  - Monoarticular, poorly defined erosions, effusion, juxtaarticular osteopenia, gradual joint space loss

Helpful Clues for Rare Diagnoses
- **Gout**
  - Sharp erosions, effusion, tophi
- **Synovial Osteochondromatosis**
  - Multiple intraarticular bodies ± ossification
  - Rare pressure erosions may mimic notch widening
- **Hemangioma, Synovial**
  - Phleboliths, serpentine vascular tangle of vessels, may be diffuse or localized
- **Inherited Skeletal Disorders**
  - Mucopolysaccharidoses
  - Dysplasia epiphysealis hemimelica
  - Engelmann disease (Engelmann-Camurati)
  - Klippel-Trenaunay-Weber syndrome
  - Kasabach-Merritt syndrome

Post-Operative (Notchplasty)

AP radiograph shows an ACL reconstruction with interference screws ⇨ in place to secure the bone-patellar tendon-bone graft. A notchplasty ⇨ widens the notch to reduce impingement on the graft.

Post-Operative (Notchplasty)

Coronal PD FSE MR shows the lateral wall portion of a notchplasty ⇨ performed to limit osseous impingement of the reconstructed ACL ⇨.

ENLARGEMENT OF INTERCONDYLAR NOTCH DISTAL FEMUR

Hemophilia: MSK Complications

Inflammatory Arthritis

(Left) AP radiograph shows femoral condylar overgrowth with widened notch ➡. Significant erosions ➡ & subchondral cysts ⮞, as seen in this young male with hemophilia, may mimic juvenile idiopathic arthritis. **(Right)** AP radiograph shows severe juvenile idiopathic arthritis with profound osteopenia, femoral epiphyseal overgrowth ⮞, notch widening ➡, early growth plate closure, and marked joint space loss with accompanying erosions ➡.

Pigmented Villonodular Synovitis (PVNS)

Gout

(Left) Axial PD FSE FS MR shows multiple ↓ SI masses ⮞ of pigmented villonodular synovitis, mechanically eroding the femoral condyles and widening the intercondylar notch ➡. **(Right)** Coronal bone CT reformation shows erosive notch widening ➡ from gouty tophi ⮞ in this 88 year old man with longstanding tophaceous gout.

Synovial Osteochondromatosis

Hemangioma, Synovial

(Left) Axial bone CT shows both intraarticular ➡ and conglomerate extraarticular ⮞ synovial osteochondromatosis, with widening of the intracondylar notch ➡ due to pressure erosion. **(Right)** Lateral radiograph shows severe erosive change in the tibia ➡ secondary to an intraarticular synovial hemangioma. The bowed Blumensaat line ⮞ indicates that there is also focal erosion of the intercondylar notch.

347

PATELLAR LYTIC LESIONS

DIFFERENTIAL DIAGNOSIS

Common
- Subchondral Cyst, Osteoarthritis
- Subchondral Cyst, Pyrophosphate Arthropathy
- Gout
- Hyperparathyroidism, Brown Tumor (HPTH)

Less Common
- Amyloid Deposition
- Chondroblastoma (CB)
- Giant Cell Tumor (GCT)
- Paget Disease
- Pigmented Villonodular Synovitis (PVNS)
- Unicameral Bone Cyst (UBC)
- Aneurysmal Bone Cyst (ABC)
- Metastases, Bone Marrow
- Dorsal Defect of Patella (Mimic)
- Osteomyelitis

Rare but Important
- Langerhans Cell Histiocytosis (LCH)
- Vascular Tumors
- Lymphoma
- Osteoblastoma
- Osteosarcoma

ESSENTIAL INFORMATION

Key Differential Diagnosis Issues
- Patellar tumor distribution published by Kransdorf
  - Benign: 38% chondroblastoma, 19% GCT, others: UBC, hemangioma, exostosis, osteoblastoma
  - Malignant: Lymphoma > hemangioendothelioma
- Patellar tumor distribution published by Mercuri
  - Benign: 33% GCT, 16% chondroblastoma, others: Enchondroma, ABC, osteoid osteoma, osteoblastoma, hemangioma
  - Malignant: Osteosarcoma > lymphoma > hemangioendothelioma
- Some arthritides result in prominent subchondral cyst formation; may mimic lytic lesion
  - In correct age group, may be more likely diagnosis than neoplasm

Helpful Clues for Common Diagnoses
- **Subchondral Cyst, Osteoarthritis**
  - Cysts may be large, mimicking lytic lesion
    - Generally in tibia rather than femur or patella
    - Watch for osteophytes & other cysts
- **Subchondral Cyst, Pyrophosphate Arthropathy**
  - Pyrophosphate arthropathy develops particularly large cysts
    - Generally in tibia rather than femur or patella
    - Watch for chondrocalcinosis, prominence of patellofemoral disease
- **Gout**
  - Lytic, often well-defined lesion
  - Often associated disease such as end-stage renal disease (ESRD)
    - With ESRD, lytic lesions may be due to gout, amyloid deposition, or Brown tumor
  - MR inhomogeneous low T2 signal; enhances with contrast
- **Hyperparathyroidism, Brown Tumor (HPTH)**
  - Radiographic appearance depends on stage
    - Active stage: Lytic, often well-defined
    - Healing stage: Various degrees of ossification in lesion; may be entirely hyperossified
  - MR inhomogeneous low T2 signal; may enhance with contrast
  - Often has associated ESRD findings
    - Abnormal bone density, disordered trabeculae
    - Quadriceps tendon rupture

Helpful Clues for Less Common Diagnoses
- **Amyloid Deposition**
  - Often secondary (ESRD, myeloma, rheumatoid arthritis)
  - Lytic, well-defined lesion
  - MR inhomogeneous low T2 signal; enhances with contrast
  - Watch for thickening of tendons, soft tissue deposits with same MR characteristics
- **Chondroblastoma (CB)**
  - Lytic, well-marginated lesion
  - MR: Lobulated high T2 signal, typical of cartilage
  - Typically seen in skeletally immature or young adult patient
- **Giant Cell Tumor (GCT)**

PATELLAR LYTIC LESIONS

○ Lytic lesion; may not have sclerotic margin
○ MR: Inhomogeneous high T2 signal (patchy low signal within); enhances with contrast
- **Pigmented Villonodular Synovitis (PVNS)**
  ○ Common in knee
  ○ Nodular or diffuse low signal material within synovium
  ○ May develop erosions or large subchondral cysts
    ▪ More frequent in femur or tibia than patella
- **Unicameral Bone Cyst (UBC)**
  ○ Lytic, well-marginated lesion
  ○ Fluid signal on MR
  ○ Generally in skeletally immature patients; rare in adults
- **Aneurysmal Bone Cyst (ABC)**
  ○ Lytic, well-marginated lesion
  ○ MR: Fluid-fluid levels in most cases
- **Metastases, Bone Marrow**
  ○ Rare patellar involvement
- **Dorsal Defect of Patella (Mimic)**
  ○ Lytic, round lesion in upper outer quadrant of patella
  ○ Located on articular surface
  ○ Overlying cartilage is intact
- **Osteomyelitis**
  ○ Lytic, often serpiginous lesion
  ○ Direct inoculation likely; watch for foreign body or tracking ulcer/air
  ○ Effusion
  ○ Reactive edema in Hoffa fat pad
  ○ MR: Enhancing rim with contrast

Helpful Clues for Rare Diagnoses
- **Langerhans Cell Histiocytosis (LCH)**
  ○ Lytic lesion
  ○ May be well-defined or more aggressive
  ○ Nonspecific on MR
  ○ May be polyostotic
  ○ Either indolent or extremely rapid growth
  ○ Generally seen in child or young teenager
- **Vascular Tumors**
  ○ Range from benign to malignant
  ○ Benign: Hemangioma
    ▪ Coarsened trabeculae, well-defined lesion
  ○ Indeterminate: Hemangioendothelioma, hemangiopericytoma
    ▪ May appear non-aggressive or aggressive
  ○ Malignant: Angiosarcoma
  ○ Vascular tumors often are located within fatty stroma; demonstrated on MR
  ○ Often polyostotic
    ▪ Lower extremity favored
- **Lymphoma**
  ○ Malignant tumors involving patella rare
  ○ Of these, lymphoma is one of the two more frequent lesions
- **Osteoblastoma**
  ○ Rare benign bone-forming tumor
  ○ Extremely rare location
  ○ ± Osteoid formation
- **Osteosarcoma**
  ○ Common tumor but extremely rare location; aggressive lesion
  ○ May be lytic, but generally has immature osteoid matrix

Subchondral Cyst, Osteoarthritis

Lateral radiograph shows a subchondral cyst ⇒ along with prominent osteophyte formation & cartilage loss. The combination is typical of osteoarthritis. Cysts are more common in the femur/tibia than patella in OA.

Subchondral Cyst, Pyrophosphate Arthropathy

Lateral radiograph shows an ill-defined subchondral cyst ⇒ within the patella, along with erosive changes. The AP view showed chondrocalcinosis. Cysts may be large in pyrophosphate arthropathy, especially in the tibia.

PATELLAR LYTIC LESIONS

Gout

Gout

(Left) Lateral radiograph shows a large lytic lesion within the patella ➡, with no signs of arthritic change. This is a 20 year old with end-stage renal disease; the lesion proved to be gout at biopsy. *(Right)* Lateral radiograph shows a lytic lesion ➡ without other distinct changes of arthritis in the knee. However, the patient had more classic evidence of gout involving the hands. This lesion improved with treatment for gout.

Hyperparathyroidism, Brown Tumor (HPTH)

Hyperparathyroidism, Brown Tumor (HPTH)

(Left) Lateral radiograph shows a lytic lesion in the patella ➡ as well as the distal femur ➡ in this patient with end-stage renal disease. *(Right)* Axial T2WI MR in the same patient shows both the patellar ➡ and femoral ➡ lesions to be inhomogeneously low signal. In this renal patient, this could represent Brown tumors, gout, or amyloid deposits. With treatment of the underlying disease, these lesions hyperossified, proving that they were Brown tumors.

Amyloid Deposition

Giant Cell Tumor (GCT)

(Left) Lateral radiograph shows lytic lesions in the patella ➡ and proximal femur ➡ in a patient with end-stage renal disease. Biopsy proved amyloid, but there is nothing on imaging to distinguish it from gout or Brown tumors. *(Right)* Lateral radiograph shows a lytic lesion within the patella ➡. It is nonspecific in appearance, well-marginated, and without matrix. Since there is no effusion, either chondroblastoma or GCT should be suspected.

PATELLAR LYTIC LESIONS

Giant Cell Tumor (GCT)

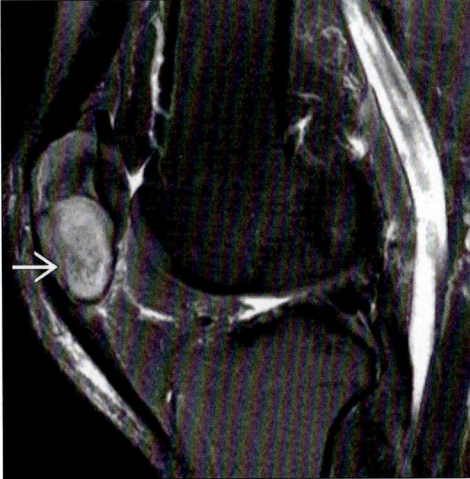

Unicameral Bone Cyst (UBC)

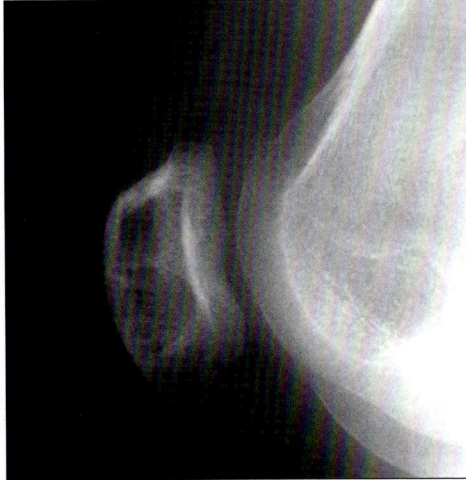

(Left) Sagittal T2WI FS MR of the patient shown in the previous image demonstrates the lesion to be inhomogeneously high signal, containing patchy areas of low signal ➡. This is a typical T2 appearance for giant cell tumor. *(Right)* Lateral radiograph shows a lytic lesion with pseudotrabeculations. The patient is middle-aged, so it is surprising that this lesion proved to be a unicameral bone cyst at biopsy. GCT or cartilage tumor would be more likely in this age group.

Dorsal Defect of Patella (Mimic)

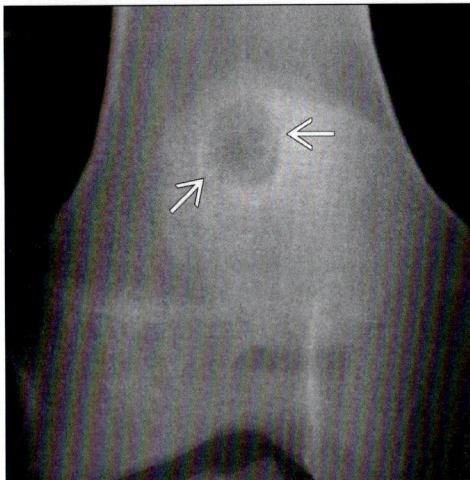

Dorsal Defect of Patella (Mimic)

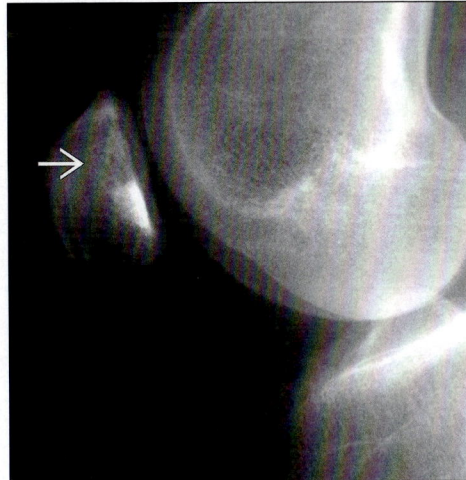

(Left) Anteroposterior radiograph shows a round lytic "lesion" occupying the upper outer quadrant of the patella ➡. *(Right)* Lateral radiograph of the same patient confirms the lytic lesion is within the patella ➡. The location is typical of dorsal defect of the patella, which is a normal variant. If MR were performed, it would show normal cartilage overlying this lesion.

Osteomyelitis

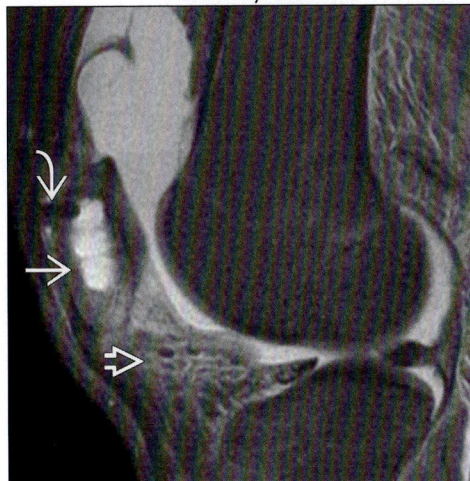

Langerhans Cell Histiocytosis (LCH)

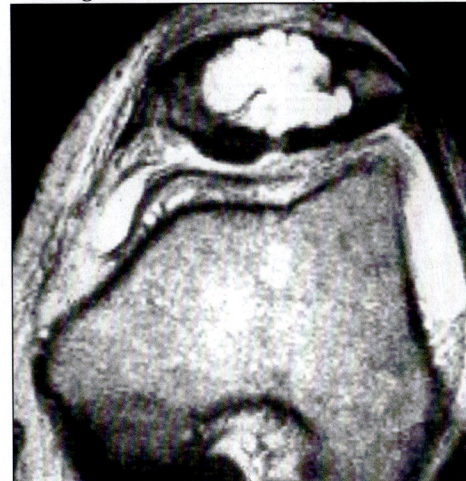

(Left) Sagittal T2WI FSE MR shows a fluid signal lesion within the patella ➡ with adjacent blooming low signal metal artifact ➡; this suggests penetrating foreign body. There is edema in Hoffa fat pad ➡, substantiating the diagnosis of osteomyelitis, proven Staphylococcus. *(Right)* Axial T2WI FS MR shows pathologic fracture through a large lesion in the patella. The appearance is nonspecific, and biopsy showed a rare lesion for the patella: LCH.

TIBIAL BOWING

DIFFERENTIAL DIAGNOSIS

Common
- Physiologic
- Fracture Malunion
- Paget Disease
- Hyperparathyroidism/Renal OD
- Rickets
- Blount Disease

Less Common
- Fibrous Dysplasia (FD)
- Neurofibromatosis

Rare but Important
- Congenital Pseudoarthrosis
- Osteogenesis Imperfecta
- Adamantinoma
- Osteofibrous Dysplasia
- Tertiary Syphilis
- Hypophosphatasia
- Ollier Disease
- Maffucci Syndrome
- Metaphyseal Chondrodysplasia
- Turner Syndrome (Mimic)

ESSENTIAL INFORMATION

Key Differential Diagnosis Issues
- Tibial bowing is generally anterior
  - Normal slight anterior bowing is accentuated when bearing weight on abnormal bone
- Lateral bowing most frequently due to
  - Physiologic causes
  - Abnormalities of the medial physis
    - Fracture malunion
    - Blount disease
    - Turner syndrome
    - Rickets
    - Hypophosphatasia
- Neurofibromatosis may lead to tibial bowing in any direction

Helpful Clues for Common Diagnoses
- **Physiologic**
  - Tibial bowing (varus, bowlegged) common in infants
  - Mild bowing may persist into adulthood
- **Fracture Malunion**
  - Salter III or IV at the proximal tibia with cessation of medial growth & continued lateral growth → proximal varus bowing

- Diaphyseal fractures may malunite
  - Anterior or posterior bowing may be compensated by hinge joints (knee/ankle)
  - Medial or lateral bowing > 5° cannot be compensated
- **Paget Disease**
  - Tibia is common location
  - Unlike other long bones, lesion may originate at diaphysis of tibia
  - Anterior cortical origin is common; with overgrowth, develops anterior bowing
  - Watch for abrupt sclerotic line at margin with normal bone ("blade of grass")
- **Hyperparathyroidism/Renal OD**
  - Resorption of bone results in weakening
  - Incomplete insufficiency fractures result in bowing, especially of tibia & femur
- **Rickets**
  - Poor mineralization of bone → weakening
  - Insufficiency fractures attempt to heal by laying down osteoid, which in turn is not properly mineralized
    - → Looser zone (wide, non-healing fx line)
  - Bowing at fracture sites, anterior or lateral
- **Blount Disease**
  - Abnormal vertical orientation of physis at medial tibia → abnormal tilt & growth abnormality of medial tibial condyle
    - → Varus bowing at proximal tibia
  - Frequently bilateral

Helpful Clues for Less Common Diagnoses
- **Fibrous Dysplasia (FD)**
  - Common process which results in mild expansion & thinning of endosteum
  - Most frequently arises in central diaphysis, but in tibia, may be based in cortex
    - Cortical fibrous dysplasia frequently results in bowing, usually anteriorly
- **Neurofibromatosis**
  - Dysplasia of bone
    - Several sites may be affected, but of the tubular bones, tibia is most frequent
  - Dysplastic bone is fragile & develops incomplete fractures, usually transverse
  - Continued weight bearing → deformities
    - Healed incomplete fracture may result in bowing, in any direction
    - Completed fracture may develop pseudarthrosis, with attenuated ends at fracture site and no callus formation

TIBIAL BOWING

○ 50% of tibial pseudoarthroses associated with neurofibromatosis

Helpful Clues for Rare Diagnoses
- **Congenital Pseudoarthrosis**
  ○ Anterior or anterolateral tibiofibular bowing at birth
  ○ Progresses to fracture within 2 years
  ○ Fracture develops fibrous union or pseudarthrosis
    ▪ Smoothly tapered bone at fracture site
  ○ Cannot be differentiated from pseudarthrosis of neurofibromatosis without clinical information
- **Osteogenesis Imperfecta**
  ○ Congenita: Short, broad tubular bones
    ▪ Bowing results from multiple intrauterine fractures
  ○ Tarda form: Either thin, gracile tubular bones or normal tubulation
    ▪ Osteoporosis & multiple incomplete fractures with weight bearing → bowing
- **Adamantinoma**
  ○ Rare lesion that occurs nearly exclusively in the tibia (usually anterior tibial cortex)
  ○ Over time, may develop bowing, most frequently anteriorly
  ○ Lytic lesion ranges from nonaggressive to moderately aggressive
  ○ Differential is cortical fibrous dysplasia & osteofibrous dysplasia; imaging does not differentiate the 3 entities
- **Osteofibrous Dysplasia**
  ○ Rare anterior tibial lesion that may cause bowing (lytic or with osteoid matrix)
- **Tertiary Syphilis**
  ○ Mixed lytic & sclerotic; expanded with anterior bowing
  ○ Termed "saber shin"; may not be easily distinguished from chronic osteomyelitis or Paget disease
- **Hypophosphatasia**
  ○ Similar appearance to rickets: Osteoporotic with bowed bones & widened physes
- **Ollier Disease**
  ○ Metaphyseal dysplasia results in growth abnormality; bowing is uncommon
- **Maffucci Syndrome**
  ○ Same as Ollier disease, plus soft tissue hemangiomas
- **Metaphyseal Chondrodysplasia**
  ○ Heterogeneous group of dysplasias involving metaphyses
    ▪ Enlarged, widened, cupped metaphysis appears similar to rickets
  ○ Schmid type particularly shows genu varum & tibial bowing
- **Turner Syndrome (Mimic)**
  ○ Hypoplasia medial tibial metaphysis; may have compensatory overgrowth of medial femoral condyle
  ○ Results in mild varus deformity; mimics Blount disease, but medial physis is not vertical (as in Blount)

Fracture Malunion

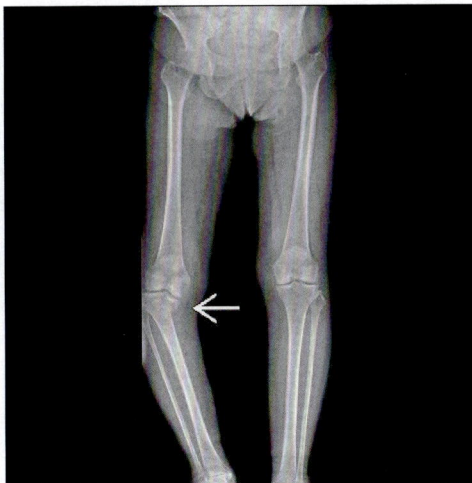

Anteroposterior radiograph shows clinical bowing of the right tibia resulting from medial tibial condylar fracture with depression and malunion ➡. If untreated, this will progress to early osteoarthritis.

Paget Disease

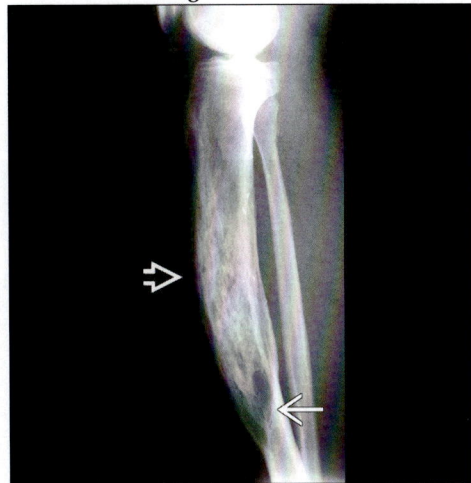

Lateral radiograph shows anterior bowing of the diaphysis ➡, with associated cortical thickening & mixed lytic/sclerotic density. Note the sharp border with normal bone ➡, typical of Paget disease.

TIBIAL BOWING

Hyperparathyroidism/Renal OD

Rickets

(Left) Lateral radiograph shows anterior bowing of the femur ➔ & posterior bowing of the tibia ⇒ in a patient with renal osteodystrophy, now being treated. Note the ossified Brown tumors. *(Right)* Lateral radiograph shows osteoporosis with thickened trabeculae. There is a fracture with wide lucency, termed a Looser zone ➔; anterior tibial bowing is occurring at this site of particularly fragile bone. Findings are classic for rickets.

Blount Disease

Fibrous Dysplasia (FD)

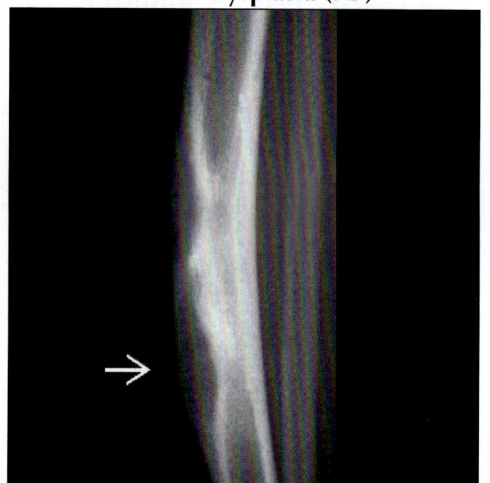

(Left) Anteroposterior radiograph shows underdevelopment of medial tibial metaphysis resulting from vertical orientation of physis ➔. Final result is a severe varus deformity of the knee due to acute bowing of the proximal tibia. *(Right)* Anteroposterior radiograph shows a cortically based lytic lesion occupying the mid-tibia. Though fibrous dysplasia is generally a central process, it may be cortically based in the tibia and often results in tibial bowing ➔.

Neurofibromatosis

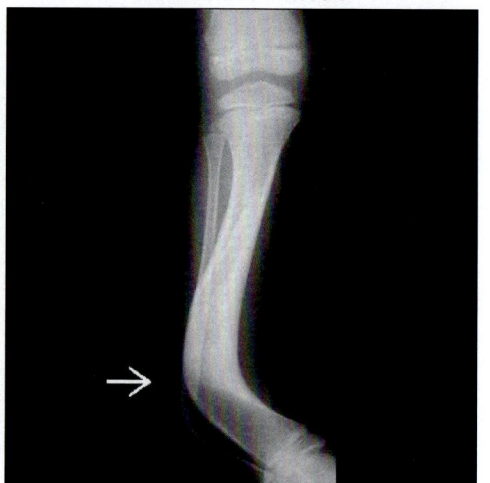

Neurofibromatosis

(Left) Anteroposterior radiograph shows dysplastic bone of the tibia, with incomplete transverse fractures that are resistant to normal healing ➔. With continued weight bearing, the tibia bows laterally. *(Right)* Anteroposterior radiograph shows severe lateral bowing ➔ in bone that otherwise appears normal. The tibia is the most frequently involved long bone in the dysplastic process seen with neurofibromatosis.

TIBIAL BOWING

Congenital Pseudoarthrosis

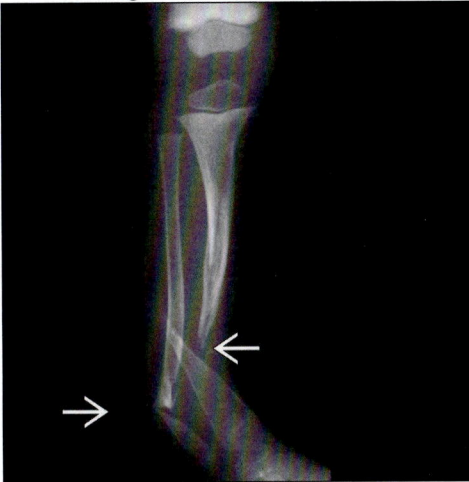

Osteogenesis Imperfecta

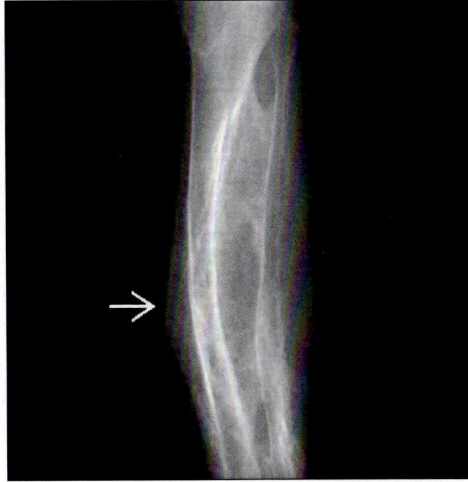

(Left) Anteroposterior radiograph shows complete fracture through the mid-tibia and fibula at the junction of the mid and distal 1/3 of the diaphyses ➡. The fracture margins are smoothly tapered, without callus. This appearance is classic for congenital pseudoarthrosis. *(Right)* Anteroposterior radiograph shows a gracile tibia & fibula with medial bowing ➡ and hypertrophic callus bridging them in a patient with typical osteogenesis imperfecta tarda.

Adamantinoma

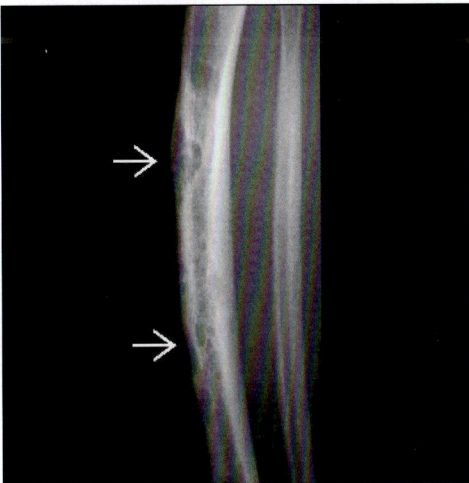

Osteofibrous Dysplasia

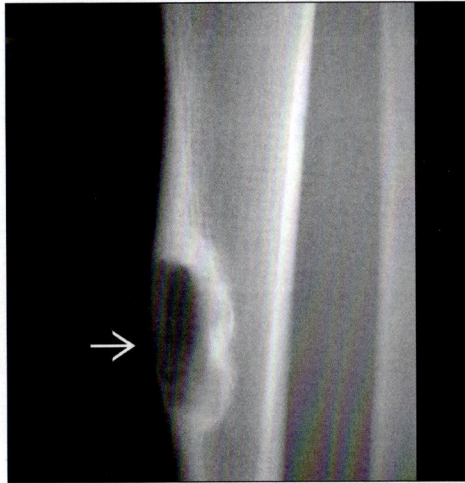

(Left) Lateral radiograph shows a cortically based lytic lesion of the anterior tibia in a child ➡ with associated anterior tibial bowing. This lesion is most suggestive of either adamantinoma or cortical FD; former was proven. (†MSK Req). *(Right)* Lateral radiograph shows a cortically based lytic lesion in the anterior tibia ➡ with mild associated anterior bowing. This proved to be osteofibrous dysplasia, though adamantinoma or FD might be considered. (†MSK Req).

Tertiary Syphilis

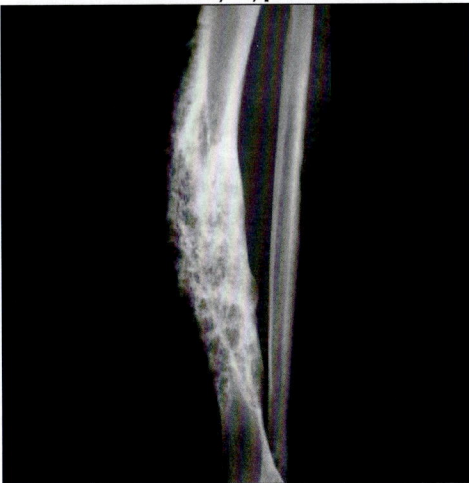

Turner Syndrome (Mimic)

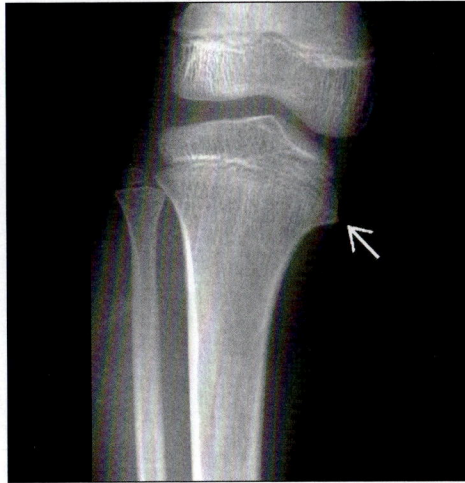

(Left) Lateral radiograph shows enlargement and anterior bowing of the diaphysis of the tibia, with mixed lytic & sclerotic density. This is a typical "saber shin" deformity of tertiary syphilis. *(Right)* Anteroposterior radiograph shows mild hypoplasia of the medial tibial metaphysis ➡ resulting in slight tibial bowing. This, along with the associated small excrescence, is seen in Turner syndrome.

FLUID COLLECTIONS ABOUT THE KNEE

DIFFERENTIAL DIAGNOSIS

Common
- Popliteal Cyst
- Popliteal Cyst, Ruptured
- Meniscal Cyst
- Synovitis, Knee
- Hematoma
- Patellar (Anterior) Bursitis
- Mucoid Degeneration, Cruciate Ligament
- Medial Bursitis, Pes Anserine
- Medial Bursitis, Collateral Ligament
- Gastrocnemius Strain
- Popliteus Myotendinous Injury
- Intercondylar Notch Cyst
- Ganglion, Knee
- Iliotibial Bursitis
- Soft Tissue Abscess

Less Common
- Bursitis Surrounding Osteochondroma
- Infectious Bursitis
- Semimembranosus Bursitis
- Proximal Tibio-Fibular Joint Synovial Processes
- Popliteal Artery Aneurysm

Rare but Important
- Synovial Osteochondromatosis within a Bursa
- Pigmented Villonodular Synovitis within a Bursa

ESSENTIAL INFORMATION

Key Differential Diagnosis Issues
- Bursae: Suprapatellar, prepatellar, superficial infrapatellar, deep infrapatellar, anserine, MCL, semimembranosus-MCL, iliotibial, LCL-biceps
  - Isolated suprapatellar bursa (by non-perforated plica) may mimic a cyst
- **Hint**: Analysis of location often leads to correct diagnosis

Helpful Clues for Common Diagnoses
- **Popliteal Cyst**
  - Located in semimembranosus/gastrocnemius bursa
  - Connects to knee joint, but thin connecting neck may be difficult to visualize
- **Popliteal Cyst, Ruptured**
  - At site of rupture, may dissect through adjacent tissues, giving an infiltrative appearance
  - Follow "lesion" to origin where it will appear more cystic
- **Meniscal Cyst**
  - Associated with meniscal tear
    - Lateral meniscal cyst: Most frequently anterolateral
    - Medial meniscal cyst: May arise from any portion of meniscus & may dissect away from site of tear
- **Synovitis, Knee**
  - Low signal enhancing material lining synovium; effusion
- **Hematoma**
  - MR signal characteristics of blood products, depending on age of injury
  - Frequently found within the prepatellar bursa
- **Patellar (Anterior) Bursitis**
  - Fluid interposed between subcutaneous tissues and patella or inferior patellar tendon
- **Mucoid Degeneration, Cruciate Ligament**
  - May involve anterior cruciate (ACL), posterior cruciate (PCL), or both
  - High signal separating fibers from one another, with fibers continuing through; ligament may appear enlarged overall
- **Medial Bursitis, Pes Anserine**
  - Bursa surrounding fibers of pes (sartorius, gracilis, semitendinosus)
  - Approach to insertion: Wraps from posteromedial above knee to anteromedial location below knee joint
- **Medial Bursitis, Collateral Ligament**
  - Bursa is normally present between deep and superficial fibers
- **Gastrocnemius Strain**
  - Strain most frequently located in proximal calf rather than at knee
  - May occur at gastrocnemius origin
    - High signal in fibers at femoral origin
    - ± Edema in adjacent bone
- **Popliteus Myotendinous Injury**
  - Popliteus injury most frequent at myotendinous junction, posterior to knee
  - May present with large fluid collection surrounding fibers
- **Intercondylar Notch Cyst**

- Cyst may split ACL or PCL or arise between them
- Fluid collection with adjacent normal-appearing cruciate fibers
- **Ganglion, Knee**
  - Intraarticular ganglia: Usually arise from cruciate ligament; sometimes in Hoffa fat pad
  - Insertional cysts (tibial insertions of cruciates & menisci) common
- **Iliotibial Bursitis**
  - Bursitis arising secondary to friction of iliotibial band against lateral femoral epicondylar prominence
  - Fluid collection adjacent to lateral femoral condyle, associated with iliotibial (IT) band
  - ± Adjacent marrow edema & IT band thickening
- **Soft Tissue Abscess**
  - Fluid-filled mass; enhancing rim on MR
  - Watch for adjacent periosteal reaction &/or osteomyelitis

Helpful Clues for Less Common Diagnoses
- **Bursitis Surrounding Osteochondroma**
  - Osteochondromas are particularly common around knee
  - With mechanical trauma, may develop an overlying bursa
  - Watch for stalk of exostosis projecting into fluid collection
- **Infectious Bursitis**
  - Bursitis with irregular margins

- Adjacent edema
- Thick enhancing rim on MR
- **Semimembranosus Bursitis**
  - U-shaped fluid collection surrounding the anterior, medial, & posterior portions of semimembranosus tendon near its tibial insertion
- **Proximal Tibio-Fibular Joint Synovial Processes**
  - 15% of proximal tibiofibular joints connect with knee joint
  - Synovial joint; at risk for synovial process
  - Posterolateral location is diagnostic
- **Popliteal Artery Aneurysm**
  - Round mass in path of popliteal artery
  - Lamellated appearance due to
    - Mural thrombus
    - Differing rates of blood flow

Helpful Clues for Rare Diagnoses
- **Synovial Osteochondromatosis within a Bursa**
  - Remember that bursae may develop synovial processes, just as joints
  - Multiple round bodies, all of similar size
    - Generally visible as calcified/ossified bodies on X-ray; occasionally lucent
- **Pigmented Villonodular Synovitis within a Bursa**
  - Rarely arises within a bursa
  - MR characteristics typical for PVNS
    - Inhomogeneous low T2 signal
    - "Blooms" on gradient echo due to hemosiderin

Popliteal Cyst

Axial T2WI FS MR shows a large popliteal cyst, located in the expected position of the semimembranosus gastrocnemius bursa. These may dissect far proximally or distally, may become bilobed, or may contain debris.

Popliteal Cyst, Ruptured

Axial PD FSE FS MR shows high signal located between the gastrocnemius & semimembranosus muscles ➔. There is not a mass-like configuration. A popliteal cyst can appear infiltrative at the point of rupture.

FLUID COLLECTIONS ABOUT THE KNEE

Meniscal Cyst

Meniscal Cyst

(Left) Sagittal T2 GRE MR shows a large multilobulated cyst ⇨ located anteriorly to, and arising from, a degenerated anterior horn lateral meniscus ⇨. The patient is a gymnast; such injuries are common in this population. (Right) Coronal T2WI MR shows a large multilobulated cyst arising from a meniscal tear of the medial meniscus. The cyst is distorting the pes anserinus tendons ⇨. Medial meniscus cysts frequently dissect far from the original meniscal tear.*

Synovitis, Knee

Hematoma

(Left) Sagittal T1 C+ FS MR shows a huge popliteal cyst containing mildly enhancing synovitis ⇨. The erosive and edematous changes in the bone help confirm the underlying diagnosis of rheumatoid arthritis. (Right) Sagittal PD FSE MR shows an intermediate signal intensity fluid collection within the prepatellar bursa ⇨, typical of hematoma. There is associated elevation of the tibial apophysis ⇨ and metaphyseal fracture ⇨ in this Salter II injury.

Patellar (Anterior) Bursitis

Mucoid Degeneration, Cruciate Ligament

(Left) Axial PD FSE FS MR shows fluid within the pre-patellar bursa ⇨ resulting from direct trauma; note also the contusion in the vastus medialis ⇨ in this patient who "caught" a medicine ball with his knee. (Right) Sagittal T2WI FS MR shows a cystic structure within the posterior cruciate ligament ⇨, displacing fibers that are otherwise intact. This is the typical appearance of mucoid degeneration of a cruciate ligament.

FLUID COLLECTIONS ABOUT THE KNEE

Mucoid Degeneration, Cruciate Ligament

Medial Bursitis, Pes Anserine

(Left) Axial PD FSE FS MR shows fluid signal within the anterior cruciate ligament that displaces fibers that are otherwise intact ➡. This is a typical appearance of mucoid degeneration. The normal posterior cruciate ligament is seen as well ➡. *(Right)* Sagittal T2WI FS MR located far medially shows fluid surrounding the tendons of the pes anserinus ➡ as they approach their insertion site.

Medial Bursitis, Pes Anserine

Medial Bursitis, Collateral Ligament

(Left) Axial PD FSE MR shows fluid surrounding the pes anserinus tendons ➡ (sartorius, gracilis, semitendinosus) as they approach their insertion on the anteromedial portion of the tibial metaphysis. *(Right)* Coronal PD FSE FS MR shows a variant case of medial bursitis involving an adventitial bursa overlying the medial femoral condyle. There is a calcific density ➡ surrounded by inflammation that is clearly within the medial collateral bursa rather than the pes anserine bursa.

Gastrocnemius Strain

Popliteus Myotendinous Injury

(Left) Sagittal PD FSE FS MR shows a low grade partial thickness strain at the medial gastrocnemius origin, with increased signal and thickening at the muscle origin ➡ & adjacent edema ➡. *(Right)* Coronal T2WI MR located far posterior in the knee shows increased fluid at the musculotendinous junction of the popliteus ➡ (popliteus tendon seen proximally ➡ and muscle seen distally ➡), typical of injury.

FLUID COLLECTIONS ABOUT THE KNEE

(Left) Sagittal T2WI FS MR shows increased fluid surrounding the musculotendinous junction of the popliteus ➡ in a patient with posterolateral corner injury. Edema in the fabella ➡ indicates fabellofibular ligament injury. Edema in the anterior tibia ➡ suggests hyperextension injury. *(Right)* Sagittal T2WI MR shows normal fibers of the ACL ➡ that are split by an intercondylar notch cyst. The fibers do not appear degenerated. These cysts may be symptomatic.

Popliteus Myotendinous Injury

Intercondylar Notch Cyst

(Left) Axial T2WI FS MR shows a small teardrop-shaped ganglion ➡ arising anterior to the distal fibers of the anterior cruciate ligament ➡. The ligament appeared intact in this case, but such ganglia are often related to prior partial cruciate ligament tear. *(Right)* Axial PD FSE FS MR shows fluid ➡ interposed between a normal iliotibial band ➡ and prominence of the lateral femoral condyle ➡. This is the typical site of friction, resulting in iliotibial band syndrome.

Ganglion, Knee

Iliotibial Bursitis

(Left) Sagittal T2WI MR shows a high signal complex mass posterior to the knee ➡. There is adjacent osseous destruction ➡. Contrast imaging proved this to be an abscess which has progressed to osteomyelitis. *(Right)* Coronal T2WI FS MR shows a bursa ➡ surrounding an osteochondroma ➡ of the proximal tibia. Trauma to an osteochondroma may result in development of such a bursa, which may clinically mimic degeneration to chondrosarcoma.

Soft Tissue Abscess

Bursitis Surrounding Osteochondroma

FLUID COLLECTIONS ABOUT THE KNEE

Infectious Bursitis

Semimembranosus Bursitis

(Left) Sagittal T1 C+ FS MR shows irregular thick enhancing rim about a fluid collection ➡ within the pre-patellar bursa. There is surrounding edema; this represents infectious bursitis. (Right) Axial T2WI MR shows fluid ➡ surrounding the semimembranosus tendon ➡, indicating semimembranosus bursitis. The configuration of the fluid is typically U-shaped in this entity.

Proximal Tibio-Fibular Joint Synovial Processes

Popliteal Artery Aneurysm

(Left) Coronal T2WI MR shows multiple loose bodies ➡. The bodies are within the proximal tibiofibular joint (note the fibula ➡). It is important to remember that this is a synovial joint, which may develop any articular process. (Right) Axial T1WI FS MR shows a lamellated mass ➡ in the popliteal fossa of the knee. This mass is in the expected location of the popliteal artery. Signal characteristics are due to mural thrombus and blood flow of varying speed and turbulence.

Synovial Osteochondromatosis within a Bursa

Pigmented Villonodular Synovitis within a Bursa

(Left) Axial PD FSE FS MR shows innumerable small bodies located within a large fluid collection ➡ which surrounds the popliteal musculotendinous junction. This is synovial chondromatosis, extending from the knee through the popliteal hiatus. (Right) Coronal T1 C+ FS MR shows a mass containing low signal elements ➡ which proved to be PVNS within the pes anserinus bursa. Remember that bursae may develop many of the same processes as synovial joints.

POPLITEAL MASS, EXTRAARTICULAR

DIFFERENTIAL DIAGNOSIS

Common
- Popliteal Cyst
- Popliteal Cyst, Ruptured
- Popliteal Cyst, Synovitis
- Pigmented Villonodular Synovitis (PVNS) (Mimic)
- Osteosarcoma, Conventional
- Osteosarcoma, Parosteal
- Synovial Sarcoma
- Benign Peripheral Nerve Sheath Tumor (BPNST)
- Lymph Node (Mimic)
- Soft Tissue Abscess

Less Common
- Gastrocnemius Muscle Variant
- Hemangioma, Soft Tissue
- Popliteal Artery Aneurysm
- Malignant Peripheral Nerve Sheath Tumor (MPNST)
- Semimembranosus Bursa

Rare but Important
- Synovial Osteochondromatosis, Extraarticular

ESSENTIAL INFORMATION

Key Differential Diagnosis Issues
- **Hint**: Carefully identify nerves, vessels, & normal musculature to help identify etiology of popliteal mass

Helpful Clues for Common Diagnoses
- **Popliteal Cyst**
  - Simple fluid collection within semimembranosus/gastrocnemius bursa
  - Connects with joint, though thin connecting neck may not be visible
  - When large, may dissect far proximally or distally
- **Popliteal Cyst, Ruptured**
  - Routine popliteal cyst that ruptures
  - At ruptured site, fluid is not contained
    - Dissects through tissues
    - Identify by tracking it back to semimembranosus/gastrocnemius bursa
- **Popliteal Cyst, Synovitis**
  - Popliteal cyst in classic location of semimembranosus/gastrocnemius bursa

- Cyst may appear complex, containing nodular densities, especially along lining
- Watch for osseous erosions
- Watch for similar appearance of synovitis in suprapatellar bursa
- **Pigmented Villonodular Synovitis (PVNS) (Mimic)**
  - PVNS occasionally appears as a focal mass
  - If mass is located posteriorly in joint, it may mimic extraarticular popliteal mass
    - Watch for overlying capsule to define intraarticular position
  - Usually inhomogeneously low signal on T2 MR; enhances
    - "Blooms" on gradient echo imaging due to hemosiderin deposition
- **Osteosarcoma, Conventional**
  - Most common malignant osseous tumor in 1st two decades
  - Distal femoral metaphysis is one of most common locations
    - If cortical breakthrough is posterior, soft tissue mass may present as a popliteal mass
  - Watch for permeative osseous destruction & amorphous osteoid formation
- **Osteosarcoma, Parosteal**
  - Surface osteosarcoma occurring in 2nd & 3rd decades
  - Most common location is distal femoral metaphysis
  - Fairly mature osteoid extends from cortical bone
    - More mature centrally than peripherally
    - Commonly involves intramedullary bone as well
- **Synovial Sarcoma**
  - Relatively common sarcoma in young adults
  - Most frequent in lower extremity, especially around knee
    - Almost never intraarticular
  - May contain dystrophic calcification
- **Benign Peripheral Nerve Sheath Tumor (BPNST)**
  - Popliteal mass when sciatic, tibial, or peroneal nerves involved
  - Target sign (central low signal on T2 imaging) is frequent but nonspecific
  - Watch for elongated shape with associated nerve

POPLITEAL MASS, EXTRAARTICULAR

- **Lymph Node (Mimic)**
  - Generally multiple nodes
  - May have fatty tissue in hilum
- **Soft Tissue Abscess**
  - Enhancing rim about fluid collection
  - Watch for adjacent osteomyelitis & reactive bone formation

Helpful Clues for Less Common Diagnoses

- **Gastrocnemius Muscle Variant**
  - Aberrant origin of a portion of gastrocnemius
    - Usually lateral head arising from medial femoral condyle
  - Forms a sling around popliteal vessels
  - Rarely presents as a mass; not symmetric to opposite limb on palpation
  - More frequently presents with claudication
  - Most frequently is an incidental finding
- **Hemangioma, Soft Tissue**
  - May occur in popliteal fossa
  - When located as intramuscular mass (in gastrocnemius), symptoms are of calf spasm
  - Watch for tortuous vessels within fatty stroma
- **Popliteal Artery Aneurysm**
  - Aneurysm presents as round mass, in path of popliteal artery
  - Lamellated appearance due to
    - Walled-off thrombus
    - Different rates of blood flow through aneurysm

- **Malignant Peripheral Nerve Sheath Tumor (MPNST)**
  - Associated with sciatic, tibial, or peroneal nerves in popliteal fossa
  - May have target sign on T2 imaging (as does BPNST)
  - Often seen in association with neurofibromatosis
    - Watch for dominant mass & multiple smaller masses associated with nerve tissue
- **Semimembranosus Bursa**
  - U-shaped fluid collection surrounding semimembranosus tendon near its tibial insertion
  - Does not extend up between semimembranosus and gastrocnemius, so should not be mistaken for popliteal cyst

Helpful Clues for Rare Diagnoses

- **Synovial Osteochondromatosis, Extraarticular**
  - Multiple round bodies
  - Generally calcified or ossified; may be confirmed on radiograph
    - Occasionally no matrix within bodies, so seen only on MR
  - Knee is common location
  - Generally contained within joint space
  - Rarely becomes more aggressive, extending from joint into surrounding soft tissues
    - Invades muscle, fascial planes, bursae

Popliteal Cyst

Axial T2WI MR shows a typical popliteal cyst ▷ located within the semimembranosus-gastrocnemius bursa, with a neck extending towards the joint space ▶. Large cysts may dissect far proximally or distally.

Popliteal Cyst, Ruptured

Axial PD FS MR shows uncontained mass-like fluid ▶ dissecting within the semimembranosus/gastrocnemius bursa within the popliteal fossa. A ruptured popliteal cyst appears infiltrative at the point of rupture.

POPLITEAL MASS, EXTRAARTICULAR

Popliteal Cyst, Synovitis

Pigmented Villonodular Synovitis (PVNS) (Mimic)

(Left) Axial T2WI FS MR shows a complex popliteal cyst arising between the displaced semimembranosus ➡ & gastrocnemius ➡ tendons. There is synovitis within the cyst and joint; the patient has rheumatoid arthritis. *(Right)* Sagittal PD FSE MR shows a mass posterior to the cruciate ligaments ➡. Low signal persisted in T2 & GRE imaging, & this proved to be PVNS, which may appear mass-like. It is a mimic, however, as it is actually intraarticular.

Osteosarcoma, Conventional

Osteosarcoma, Parosteal

(Left) Lateral radiograph shows a large popliteal fossa soft tissue mass ➡ in a teenaged patient, along with lytic permeative destruction within the metaphysis ➡. This appearance is typical of a lytic osteosarcoma. *(Right)* Sagittal T2WI MR shows a large popliteal mass that contains inhomogeneous areas of low signal ➡. The mass extends from the posterior surface of the femur, & there is invasion of the adjacent femoral metaphysis. This is typical parosteal OS.

Synovial Sarcoma

Benign Peripheral Nerve Sheath Tumor (BPNST)

(Left) Sagittal T2WI MR shows a large inhomogeneous mass within the popliteal fossa ➡. The extraarticular location in the lower extremity, in a young adult, should make one strongly consider the diagnosis of synovial sarcoma. *(Right)* Sagittal T1WI MR shows a large inhomogeneous mass within the popliteal fossa ➡ with a "tail" of nerve extending from it ➡. The location and associated nerve makes the diagnosis of PNST; this proved to be a schwannoma.

POPLITEAL MASS, EXTRAARTICULAR

Soft Tissue Abscess

Hemangioma, Soft Tissue

(Left) Sagittal T1 C+ MR shows a thick enhancing rim surrounding an abscess ⇨ in the popliteal fossa. There is adjacent osseous destruction ➡. This patient had been camping in the western U.S. desert and acquired a Yersinia pestis infection. *(Right)* Axial T2WI MR shows tortuous vessels within an intramuscular hemangioma ➡. This presented as a popliteal mass. It also resulted in calf muscle spasm.

Popliteal Artery Aneurysm

Malignant Peripheral Nerve Sheath Tumor (MPNST)

(Left) Axial T2WI FS MR shows a mass at the expected location of the popliteal artery ➡. The lamellated appearance is due to mural thrombus in this aneurysm, as well as differing rates of blood flow. *(Right)* Axial T2WI MR shows a large inhomogeneous popliteal fossa mass ➡ as well as adjacent smaller masses within the neurovascular bundle ➡. This patient has neurofibromatosis; the dominant mass is an MPNST.

Semimembranosus Bursa

Synovial Osteochondromatosis, Extraarticular

(Left) Axial T2WI MR shows a typical U-shaped fluid collection ➡ that surrounds the semimembranosus tendon just prior to its insertion on the posterior tibia. This is in an extraarticular position. *(Right)* Sagittal T1 C+ FS MR shows large extraarticular popliteal masses that contain calcified bodies ➡. Similar masses are seen intraarticularly ➡. This patient has synovial osteochondromatosis, which may rarely extend into an extraarticular location.

ALTERATIONS IN MENISCAL SIZE

DIFFERENTIAL DIAGNOSIS

Common
- Enlarged, Medial (MM) or Lateral (LM)
  - Discoid Meniscus
  - Lateral Meniscal Bucket-Handle Tear with Flipped Fragment (Mimic)
- Diminutive Meniscus
  - Post-Operative Meniscus Change
  - Meniscal Bucket-Handle Tear
  - Meniscal Degeneration
  - Meniscal Extrusion (Mimic)

Less Common
- Enlarged Meniscus
  - Chondrocalcinosis
  - Meniscal Ossicle
  - Intrameniscal Cyst
  - Meniscal Flounce (Mimic)
  - Ligament Merging with LM (Mimic)
- Diminutive Meniscus
  - Small Anterior Root, MM (Mimic)

Rare but Important
- Intraarticular Air (Mimic)

ESSENTIAL INFORMATION

Key Differential Diagnosis Issues
- Menisci have typical normal size & morphology
  - Posterior horn is largest portion of medial meniscus (long triangle)
  - Anterior horn shorter than posterior, but body is shortest (small equilateral triangle)
  - Lateral meniscus is symmetric in size through all portions
- Either enlargement or diminution of meniscus indicates pathology, with few exceptions

Helpful Clues for Common Diagnoses
- Discoid Meniscus
  - Enlarged meniscus from peripheral to central free edge
    - In axial plane, assumes more of a discoid than C-shaped outline
    - May be partial, making the diagnosis more difficult
    - Lateral more frequently involved than medial
    - Occasionally involves both MM & LM
    - Morphology of posterior horn tends to be abnormal, with popliteal hiatus and popliteus tendon more prominent
    - Diagnosis most often suggested when sagittal plane shows body of meniscus over more than 3 images (bow-tie)
    - Confirmed on coronal or axial imaging
  - Generally diagnosed at a younger age than routine traumatic meniscal injury
  - Enlarged meniscus is at ↑ risk for tear
  - **Hint:** If a portion of the meniscus appears too wide from peripheral to central, consider discoid meniscus
- **Lateral Meniscal Bucket-Handle Tear with Flipped Fragment (Mimic)**
  - Vertical tear continuing over a significant longitudinal extent that detaches at either anterior or posterior end
  - Detached end of meniscus, often with a large amount of meniscal tissue, may flip over the opposite end of meniscus
    - Flipped meniscal fragment generally is superimposed on native anterior horn, making it appear to be double in size (↑ height from superior to inferior)
    - Flipped fragment may be obliquely superimposed (↑ in size both height & width)
    - Flip from torn posterior horn, superimposed over native anterior horn is more frequent than anterior horn fragment over posterior horn
    - This pattern of tear with flipped fragment is more frequent in lateral meniscus than true bucket handle
    - True bucket-handle tear is more frequent in MM than is flipped fragment
  - **Hint:** If one portion of meniscus appears ↓ & another portion appears ↑ (height or width), consider flipped fragment
- **Post-Operative Meniscus Change**
  - Results in smaller meniscus in the portion that was trimmed
  - Free edge often blunt; may have adjacent cartilage defect
  - May continue to show abnormal signal within meniscus, extending to free edge
  - **Hint:** If considering diagnosis of post-operative change for an abnormally small meniscus, watch for linear fibrotic changes in Hoffa fat pad from arthroscope

ALTERATIONS IN MENISCAL SIZE

- **Meniscal Bucket-Handle Tear**
  - Vertical longitudinal tear that remains intact at anterior & posterior horns, with fragment flipped centrally into intercondylar notch
  - Results in diminutive meniscus throughout nearly its entire extent
  - Bucket-handle tear seen in medial meniscus more frequently than lateral
  - **Hint**: If entire meniscus appears small, do not assume it is post-operative; look for meniscal tissue in intercondylar notch
- **Meniscal Degeneration**
  - Degeneration may result in tears at free edge of meniscus which detach
  - Involved portion of meniscus appears to have a blunt edge, without necessarily having increased signal of a tear
  - **Hint**: With this pattern, search for free intraarticular meniscal fragments
- **Meniscal Extrusion (Mimic)**
  - With severe degenerative change, & especially with radial tears, a portion of meniscus may be extruded beyond joint line; meniscus appears small

Helpful Clues for Less Common Diagnoses
- **Chondrocalcinosis**
  - Extensive meniscal chondrocalcinosis may result in enlargement of meniscus
    - Enlargement usually in height, rarely enlarged from periphery to free edge
  - Chondrocalcinosis generally appears low signal on all sequences, but infrequently may be high signal
    - High signal may be solid or speckled
    - High signal may be mistaken for degenerative tear
  - **Hint**: When meniscus appears enlarged in height, particularly with central high signal, consider chondrocalcinosis
    - May confirm on radiograph
- **Meniscal Ossicle**
  - Intraarticular osseous structure, usually MM posterior horn, causes ↑ in meniscal size
  - Follows MR bone signal; confirm on X-ray
- **Intrameniscal Cyst**
  - Cystic signal within meniscus → size ↑
- **Meniscal Flounce (Mimic)**
  - Positionally dependent wavy appearance of "extra" meniscal tissue
- **Ligament Merging with LM (Mimic)**
  - Meniscofemoral or transverse ligaments merging with posterior or anterior horns, respectively, may mimic focal ↑ in size
- **Small Anterior Root, MM (Mimic)**
  - Anterior horn medial meniscus may be small & have variable attachments (anterior to joint line, transverse ligament)

Helpful Clues for Rare Diagnoses
- **Intraarticular Air (Mimic)**
  - Intraarticular air appears as low signal that blooms on GRE imaging; adjacent meniscus may appear enlarged

Discoid Meniscus

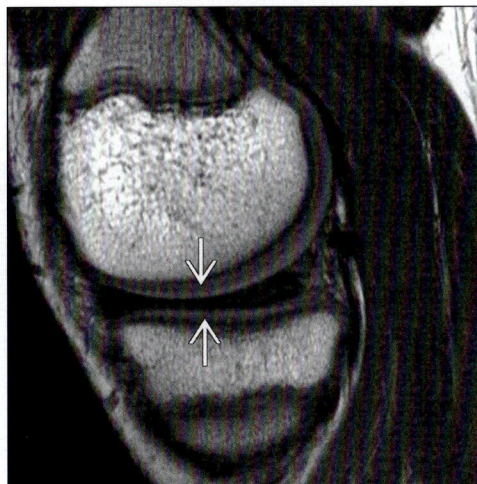

Sagittal PD FSE MR located just medial to the intercondylar notch shows a continuous "bowtie" meniscus, with body still in evidence ➡. This indicates an abnormally large body, termed discoid meniscus.

Discoid Meniscus

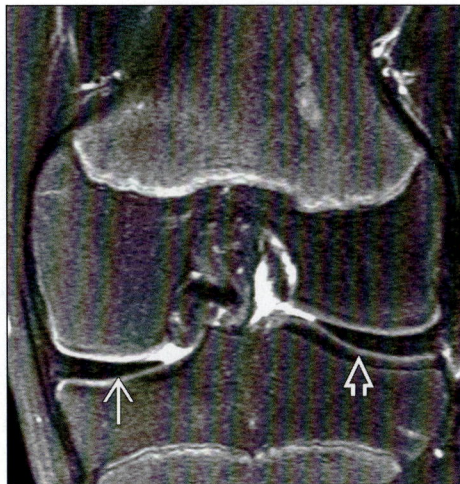

Coronal T2WI FS MR shows enlargement of both the body of medial meniscus ➡ and body of lateral meniscus ➡. This was confirmed on sagittal imaging. Lateral discoid is more frequently seen than medial.

ALTERATIONS IN MENISCAL SIZE

(Left) Sagittal T2WI MR shows an apparently enlarged anterior horn ➡ but small torn posterior horn ➡ of the lateral meniscus. This is a longitudinal vertical tear of the posterior horn and body, flipped over the anterior horn, mimicking enlargement. *(Right)* Sagittal PD FSE MR shows an unusual flipped body fragment which doubles the size of both the anterior & posterior horns. The flipped fragments ➡ are superimposed on the native meniscus ➡.

Lateral Meniscal Bucket-Handle Tear with Flipped Fragment (Mimic)

Lateral Meniscal Bucket-Handle Tear with Flipped Fragment (Mimic)

(Left) Sagittal T2WI MR shows a blunt & irregular posterior horn ➡ with adjacent cartilage damage ➡. Though a degenerative tear may result in meniscal blunting, this appearance is more frequently seen following arthroscopic repair. *(Right)* Coronal T2WI FS MR shows a small, blunt body of medial meniscus ➡. While it is possible for this to be a degenerative tear, one must look for the displaced fragment ➡, generally in the intercondylar notch. This is a bucket-handle tear.

Post-Operative Meniscus Change

Meniscal Bucket-Handle Tear

(Left) Sagittal PD FSE FS MR shows an enlarged anterior horn containing speckled high signal ➡. The signal might be mistaken for meniscal degeneration, but the enlargement should make one consider other etiologies. *(Right)* Lateral radiograph of the same patient shows chondrocalcinosis ➡. Though meniscal chondrocalcinosis is generally dark or not seen on MR, it rarely will exhibit high signal and cause enlargement of the meniscus.

Chondrocalcinosis

Chondrocalcinosis

ALTERATIONS IN MENISCAL SIZE

Meniscal Ossicle

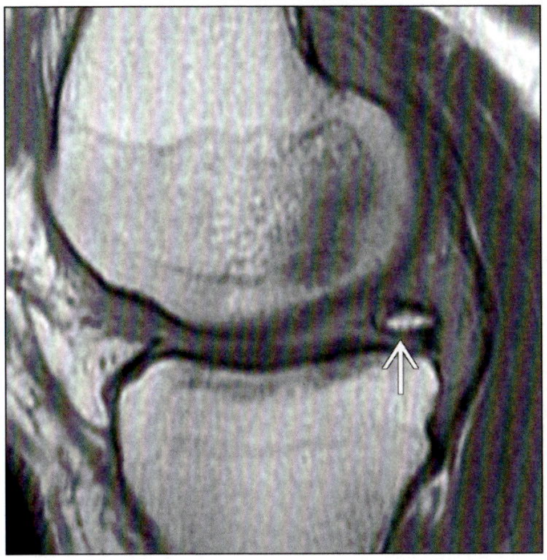

Meniscal Ossicle

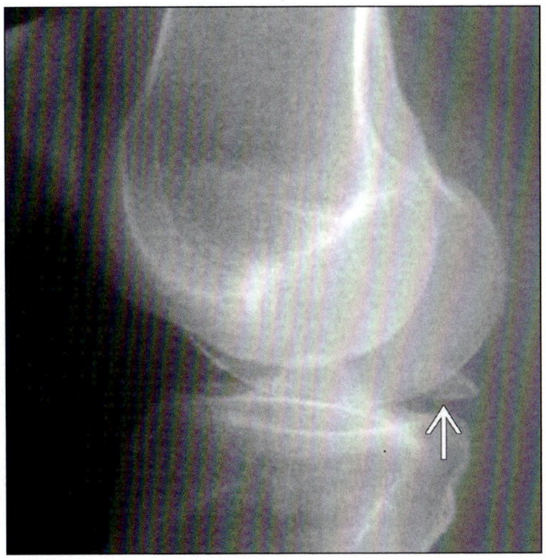

(Left) Sagittal PD FSE MR shows a body with signal identical to bone occupying the posterior horn medial meniscus →, causing mild enlargement of that structure. The signal followed that of bone on all sequences and is typical of meniscal ossicle. (Right) Lateral radiograph of the same knee confirms the ossicle →. Its location in the posterior horn of the medial meniscus is typical; it generally results in meniscal enlargement & degeneration.

Intrameniscal Cyst

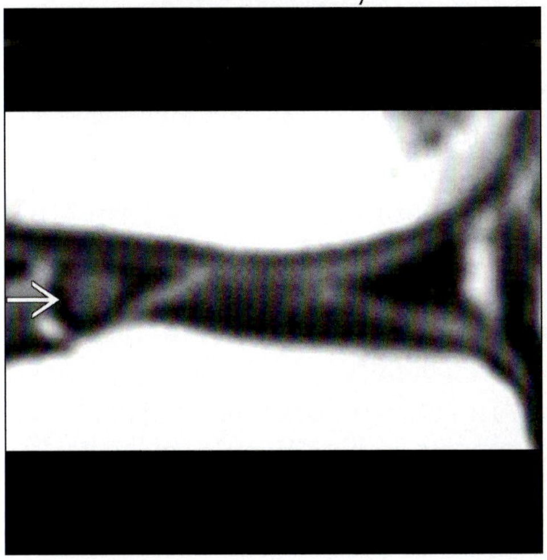

Meniscal Flounce (Mimic)

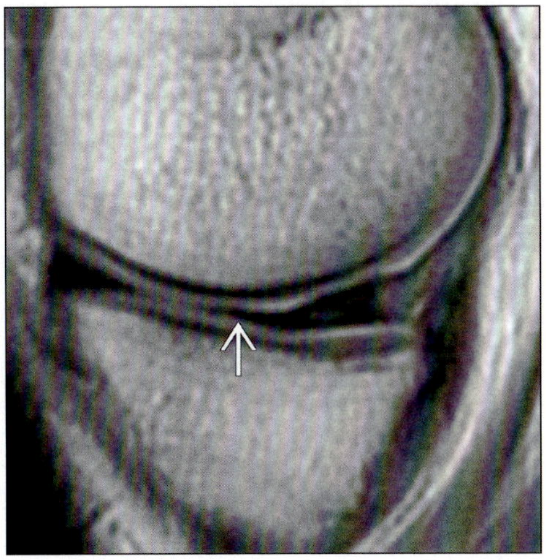

(Left) Sagittal PD FSE MR shows an enlarged anterior horn of the lateral meniscus. The enlargement results from a distended intrameniscal cyst →. (Right) Sagittal PD FSE MR shows a meniscal flounce →, a single meniscal fold along the free edge that is a normal variant. It is not associated with a meniscal tear. The appearance is typical and does not represent true meniscal enlargement.

Ligament Merging with LM (Mimic)

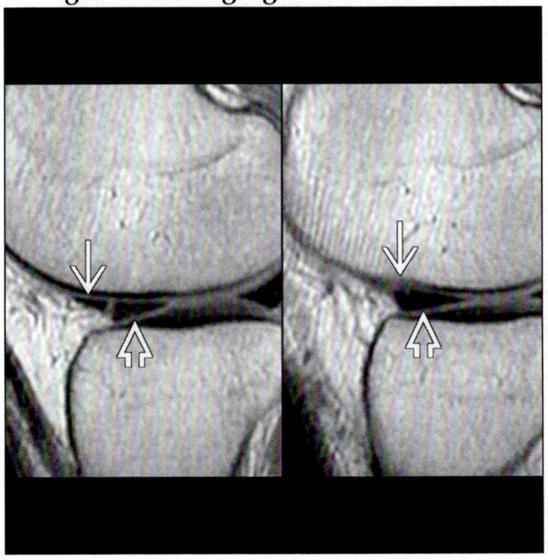

Intraarticular Air (Mimic)

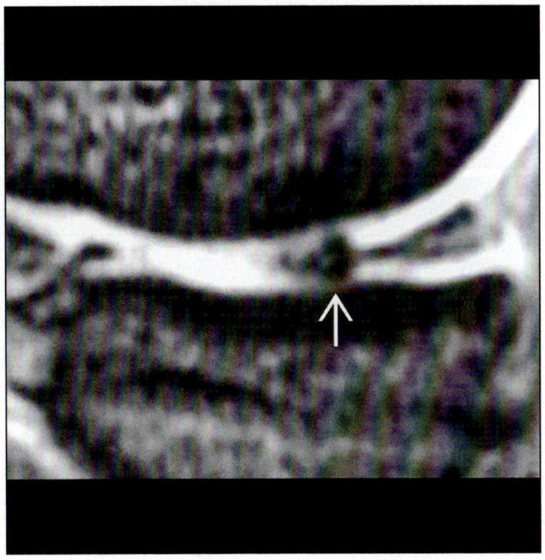

(Left) Sagittal PD FSE MR of two adjacent images through the lateral compartment shows a large transverse ligament → merging with the anterior horn →. Once fully merged, it gives the appearance of an enlarged anterior horn. (Right) Sagittal T2* GRE MR shows an apparently irregularly enlarged posterior horn medial meniscus →. This is a gradient echo image, which allows "blooming" of either metal or air. In this case, the radiograph showed a focus of intraarticular air.

GENU VALGUM (KNOCK KNEES)

DIFFERENTIAL DIAGNOSIS

Common
- Idiopathic
- Arthritis
- Physeal Fractures
- Renal Osteodystrophy (Renal OD)
- Rickets
- Osteomyelitis

Less Common
- Fibrous Dysplasia
- Osteochondromatosis
- Fluorosis
- Homocystinuria
- Spondyloepiphyseal Dysplasia
- Multiple Epiphyseal Dysplasia
- Osteogenesis Imperfecta
- Trevor Fairbank (Dysplasia Epiphysealis Hemimelica)
- Hypophosphatasia
- Ollier Disease
- Nail Patella Disease (Fong)
- Mucopolysaccharidoses

Rare but Important
- Vitamin C Deficiency
- Pseudoachondroplasia
- Chondroectodermal Dysplasia (Ellis-van Creveld)
- Spondyloepimetaphyseal Dysplasia
- Chondrodysplasia Punctata
- Cleidocranial Dysplasia
- Pyle Dysplasia
- Radiation-Induced Growth Deformities

ESSENTIAL INFORMATION

Key Differential Diagnosis Issues
- Genu valgum: 2 measurements
  - Angle described by line bisecting distal femur & line bisecting proximal tibia (normal angle 6° ± 2°; valgus > 8°)
  - Mechanical axis: Line drawn from center of femoral head to center of tibial plafond
    - Should fall through middle of knee
- Consider joint-related abnormalities
  - Arthritis, differentially affecting lateral compartment cartilage (RA > OA)
  - Morphologic abnormalities of epiphyses, resulting in relatively larger medial femoral condyle or flat lateral femoral condyle
    - Spondyloepiphyseal dysplasia, multiple epiphyseal dysplasia, Trevor Fairbank, etc.
- Consider abnormalities differentially affecting lateral physis
  - Early bony bridging laterally following Salter fracture or osteomyelitis
  - Differential radiation to lateral portion of knee prior to skeletal maturation
- Consider osseous abnormalities resulting in dysmorphic change in metaphysis/diaphyses → bowing of femur or tibia
  - Not a true genu valgus deformity, but mimics one clinically
  - Renal OD, rickets, hypophosphatasia, fibrous dysplasia, osteochondromatosis, osteogenesis imperfecta, Ollier disease, etc.

Arthritis

AP radiograph shows osteopenia, uniform cartilage loss, and a valgus deformity. Note the medial-lateral translation of the tibia, indicating ligamentous instability. The findings are typical of rheumatoid arthritis.

Renal Osteodystrophy (Renal OD)

AP radiograph shows a femoral bowing deformity ➡, which in turn mimics genu valgum clinically. There is patchy increased density in the bones, as well as ossified brown tumors ➡ in this treated renal OD.

GENU VALGUM (KNOCK KNEES)

Rickets

Osteomyelitis

(Left) AP radiograph shows bilateral genu valgus. There is widening of the provisional zone of calcification ➡ with impaction and fraying of the metaphyses, contributing to the deformity in this patient with nutritional rickets. *(Right)* Coronal T2WI MR shows a focus of osteomyelitis within the metaphysis of the lateral femoral condyle ➡, crossing the physis. With healing, a bony bar will form, inhibiting growth. Continued medial growth will result in genu valgum. (†MSK Req).

Fibrous Dysplasia

Osteochondromatosis

(Left) AP radiograph shows a focus of polyostotic fibrous dysplasia in the femur ➡ that, with weight bearing, has resulted in a focal medial bowing. This bowing clinically mimics a valgus deformity of the knee. *(Right)* AP radiograph shows sessile osteochondromas ➡ lining the femoral metaphyses. These, along with hip exostoses, result in mechanical abnormalities promoting early osteoarthritis ➡ centered in the lateral compartment and a resulting valgus deformity.

Spondyloepiphyseal Dysplasia

Trevor Fairbank (Dysplasia Epiphysealis Hemimelica)

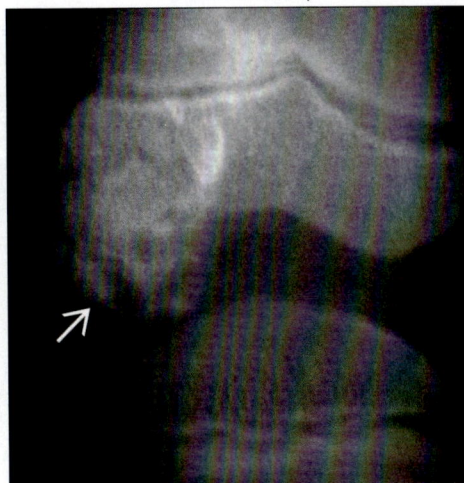

(Left) AP radiograph shows enlarged, flattened, slightly dysmorphic epiphyses in a patient with a mild form of spondyloepiphyseal dysplasia. The morphologic abnormalities can result in abnormal alignment (genu valgum) and early osteoarthritis. *(Right)* AP radiograph shows lobulated cartilage attached to the medial femoral condyle ➡, an example of Trevor Fairbank disease. With weight bearing, this forces the knee into a genu valgum position. (†MSK Req).

GENU VARUM (BOW LEG DEFORMITY)

DIFFERENTIAL DIAGNOSIS

Common
- Physiologic Bowing
- Arthritis
- Physeal Fractures
- Blount Disease
- Renal Osteodystrophy (Renal OD)

Less Common
- Osteogenesis Imperfecta (OI)
- Osteomyelitis
- Charcot, Neuropathic
- Osteochondromatosis
- Achondroplasia
- Spondyloepiphyseal Dysplasia
- Multiple Epiphyseal Dysplasia

Rare but Important
- Turner Syndrome (Mimic)
- Mucopolysaccharidoses
- Ollier Disease
- Lead Poisoning
- Hypochondroplasia
- Fluorosis
- Hypophosphatemic Rickets (X-Linked)
- Metaphyseal Chondrodysplasia
- Radiation-Induced Growth Deformities

ESSENTIAL INFORMATION

Key Differential Diagnosis Issues
- Genu varum = < 4° valgus, or mechanical axis falling lateral to mid-knee
- General categories resulting in genu varum
  - Joint-related abnormalities (arthritis, morphologic abnormalities of epiphyses)
  - Abnormalities differentially affecting medial physis (trauma, osteomyelitis, Blount disease, radiation, Turner)
  - Abnormalities resulting in bowing of femur/tibia, mimicking genu varum (renal OD, OI, osteochondromatosis, Ollier, etc.)

Helpful Clues for Common Diagnoses
- **Physiologic Bowing**
  - Seen in infants; occasionally persists
- **Arthritis**
  - Osteoarthritis (OA) most frequently affects medial compartment, resulting in varus
- **Physeal Fractures**
  - Salter fx (usually III or IV) of medial femoral or tibial condyle → early bony bridging medially → genu varum
- **Blount Disease**
  - Vertical & irregular medial tibial growth plate → undergrowth of medial tibial condyle (beaking) → varus

Helpful Clues for Less Common Diagnoses
- **Osteogenesis Imperfecta (OI)**
  - Congenita form has short, bowed femora & tibia, giving exaggerated bowed leg
- **Spondyloepiphyseal Dysplasia**
  - Any epiphyseal dysplasia may have larger lateral femoral condyle, resulting in varus

Helpful Clues for Rare Diagnoses
- **Turner Syndrome (Mimic)**
  - Underdevelopment & flattening medial tibial metaphysis; may mimic Blount dz

Arthritis

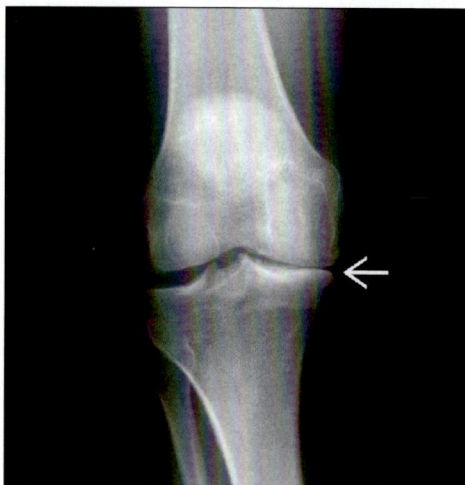

AP radiograph shows differential narrowing of the medial compartment ➡, resulting in genu varum. Normal bone density, sclerosis of the subchondral bone, & mild osteophyte formation are all typical of OA.

Physeal Fractures

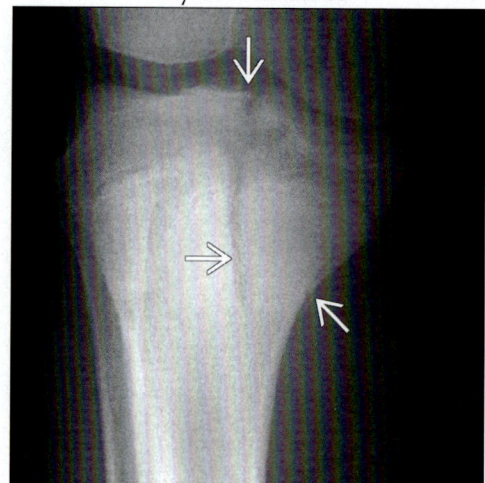

AP radiograph shows a Salter IV fracture crossing the medial tibial epiphysis, physis, & metaphysis ➡. There is mild depression of the fragment. Healing occurred in this position, resulting in a varus deformity.

GENU VARUM (BOW LEG DEFORMITY)

Blount Disease

Osteogenesis Imperfecta (OI)

(Left) Coronal PD FSE FS MR shows typical case of Blount disease or tibial vara, with a vertically oriented irregular medial tibial growth plate ➡. This results in a beak-like appearance of the proximal tibial metaphysis ➡. *(Right)* Anteroposterior radiograph shows OI congenita, with short, broad, & bowed tubular bones of the lower extremity ➡. The bowing of the tibia & femur typically is in a lateral direction, resulting in a clinical appearance of genu varum.

Osteomyelitis

Charcot, Neuropathic

(Left) AP radiograph shows abnormalities at femoral & tibial epiphyses, with early bony bridging at the medial tibial physis ➡. With continued growth laterally, a genu varum deformity develops. The underlying cause in this case was meningococcemia. *(Right)* AP radiograph shows destruction of the joint, predominantly medially ➡, resulting in genu varum. Note the bony debris dissecting down fascial tissue planes ➡ in this patient with tabes-related Charcot joint.

Achondroplasia

Turner Syndrome (Mimic)

(Left) AP radiograph shows short tubular bones of the lower extremity, with broad dysmorphic metaphyses. The abnormal growth at the metaphyses often results in genu varum in patients with achondroplasia. *(Right)* AP radiograph shows relative underdevelopment and flattening of the medial tibial metaphysis ➡ in Turner syndrome. There is some compensatory overgrowth of the medial femoral condyle ➡, but varus deformity may occur. This may mimic Blount disease.

373

ACHILLES TENDON THICKENING/ENLARGEMENT

DIFFERENTIAL DIAGNOSIS

Common
- Tendinosis/Tear
- Retrocalcaneal Bursitis
- Haglund Syndrome

Less Common
- Post-surgical Thickening
- Arthritis

Rare but Important
- Xanthoma (Fibroxanthoma)
- Accessory Soleus (Mimic)
- Neoplasm

ESSENTIAL INFORMATION

Helpful Clues for Common Diagnoses
- **Tendinosis/Tear**
  - Tendon thickening ± increased SI
  - Most common 2-6 cm proximal to insertion
  - Results in rounding of normal crescentic tendon in axial plane
  - Intrasubstance, partial & complete tears = ↑ SI on T2
  - ± Peritendinous edema & retrocalcaneal bursitis
- **Retrocalcaneal Bursitis**
  - Inflammation/swelling of bursa between calcaneus & tendon
  - Typically ↑ SI (T2) due to bursal effusion ± synovial hypertrophy

  - Seen with degenerative tendinopathy, inflammatory or seronegative arthritis
- **Haglund Syndrome**
  - Enlarged posterosuperior calcaneal process, retrocalcaneal bursitis, Achilles tendinosis
  - Aggravated by tight shoes = "pump bump"

Helpful Clues for Less Common Diagnoses
- **Post-surgical Thickening**
  - Marked thickening with extensive intrasubstance increased SI typical in repaired tendon
  - Failed repair marked by extensive fiber disruption
- **Arthritis**
  - Inflammatory arthritis: Osteopenia, retrocalcaneal bursitis, erosions
  - Seronegative spondyloarthropathies: ± Osteopenia, mixed erosive-productive arthritis, periostitis
  - Gout: Tophaceous calcific deposition

Helpful Clues for Rare Diagnoses
- **Xanthoma (Fibroxanthoma)**
  - Thickened tendon with speckled intermediate SI due to lipid deposition in hyperlipoproteinemia
- **Accessory Soleus (Mimic)**
  - Located anteromedial to Achilles tendon, obscuring Kager fat pad; intermediate SI = muscle
- **Neoplasm**
  - Rare reports of pigmented villonodular synovitis, lymphoma, chondrosarcoma, fibroma

Tendinosis/Tear

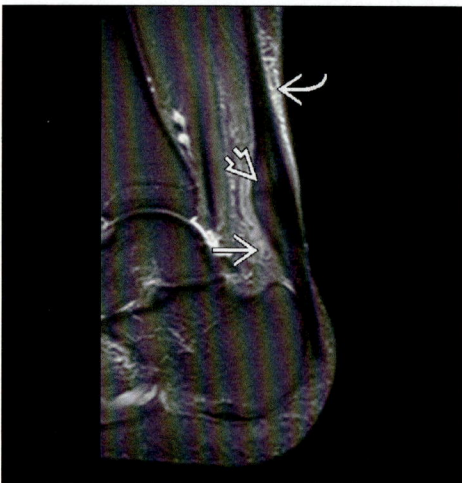

Sagittal PD FSE FS MR shows intermediate SI tendon thickening ⇒ 4-5 cm proximal to tendon insertion, representing Achilles tendinosis. Note adjacent soft tissue edema ⇒ & Kager fat pad edema ⇒.

Tendinosis/Tear

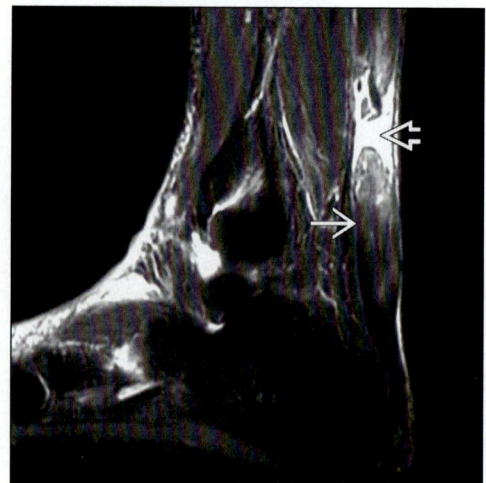

Sagittal PD FSE FS MR shows complete Achilles tendon tear ⇒ at the musculotendinous junction with fiber retraction leaving a 2.5 cm gap. The more distal tendon is markedly thickened ⇒.

ACHILLES TENDON THICKENING/ENLARGEMENT

Retrocalcaneal Bursitis

Haglund Syndrome

(Left) Sagittal PD FSE FS MR shows retrocalcaneal bursitis with intermediate & ↑ SI due to synovial hypertrophy ⇒ & effusion ➡, respectively. Note the adjacent heterogeneity & thickening of tendinosis ➡. *(Right)* Sagittal T2WI FS MR shows a prominent posterosuperior calcaneal "bump" with mild marrow edema ➡ & retrocalcaneal bursitis ➡. There is a partial tear of the thickened Achilles tendon ➡. The combination is typical of Haglund syndrome.

Post-surgical Thickening

Arthritis

(Left) Sagittal T1WI MR shows an intact Achilles tendon debridement & repair with diffuse intermediate thickening ➡ & post-surgical change in the adjacent soft tissues ➡ including small foci of micrometallic debris ➡. *(Right)* Sagittal bone CT reformation shows Achilles tendon thickening ➡ with periostitis ➡ & enthesitis ➡ in this middle-aged man with chronic reactive arthritis.

Xanthoma (Fibroxanthoma)

Accessory Soleus (Mimic)

(Left) Sagittal T1WI MR shows a diffuse Achilles tendon mass ➡ with slightly heterogeneous ↓ SI on all sequences, typical of a xanthofibroma. This patient has hypercholesterolemia. *(Right)* Sagittal T1WI MR shows an accessory soleus muscle ➡ extending to the medial posterior calcaneal tubercle. This normal variant may present as a "thickened Achilles tendon" but in fact is a separate structure. Note the normal SI of muscle throughout.

CALCANEAL EROSIONS, POSTERIOR TUBERCLE

DIFFERENTIAL DIAGNOSIS

Common
- Rheumatoid Arthritis (RA)
- Chronic Reactive Arthritis (CRA)
- Psoriatic Arthritis (PSA)

Less Common
- Ankylosing Spondylitis (AS)
- Inflammatory Bowel Disease Arthritis (IBD)
- Haglund Syndrome
- Achilles Tendinitis
- Plantar Fasciitis
- Osteomyelitis

Rare but Important
- Gout
- Repair of Achilles Tendon (Mimic)
- Juvenile Idiopathic Arthritis (JIA)

ESSENTIAL INFORMATION

Key Differential Diagnosis Issues
- Classic calcaneal erosive disease is CRA
  - CRA much less prevalent relative to other inflammatory arthritides that may occasionally affect the calcaneus
  - **Hint**: Remember that RA eroding the calcaneus may actually be more common than CRA
- **Hint**: Watch for osteoporosis
  - Present in RA, AS, & JIA
  - Present focally with local inflammatory change (Achilles bursitis & early inflammatory arthritis)
- **Hint**: Location of other erosions is an important parameter

Helpful Clues for Common Diagnoses
- **Rheumatoid Arthritis (RA)**
  - Most common inflammatory arthritis
  - Purely erosive process; osteoporotic
  - Foot disease more prevalent than is commonly thought
    - MTP (especially 5th)
    - Ankle, including posterior calcaneus
  - **Hint**: Purely erosive change in osteoporotic posterior calcaneus results from RA more frequently than CRA
- **Chronic Reactive Arthritis (CRA)**
  - Combined syndrome of uveitis, urethritis (cervicitis), & inflammatory arthritis

- Inflammatory arthritis may be axial &/or peripheral
  - Axial: Spondyloarthropathy, generally with bilaterally asymmetric sacroiliitis
  - Peripheral: Foot/ankle most frequently involved
- Arthritis is mixed erosive & productive; either may predominate
  - Digits may show sausage swelling & periostitis
- **Hint**: Calcaneal involvement is thought to be the hallmark of CRA
  - CRA is relatively rare process, but calcaneal involvement is frequent if one has the disease
- **Psoriatic Arthritis (PSA)**
  - Relatively common inflammatory arthritis
  - Arthritis may occur prior to development of skin lesions
  - May be axial &/or peripheral
    - Axial: Spondyloarthropathy, generally with bilaterally asymmetric sacroiliitis
    - Peripheral: Hand most frequently involved, though foot/ankle may be as well
  - Arthritis is mixed erosive & productive, with either predominating
    - Digits may show sausage swelling & periostitis
  - **Hint**: PSA may involve calcaneus, but not as frequently as CRA

Helpful Clues for Less Common Diagnoses
- **Ankylosing Spondylitis (AS)**
  - Most common of the spondyloarthritides (bilaterally symmetric sacroiliitis)
  - Does not often involve foot/ankle
    - Generally involves large proximal joints (hip, shoulder)
  - Advanced disease (generally not treated) may involve peripheral joints, including ankle & calcaneus
  - Mixed erosive/productive
  - Osteoporosis
- **Inflammatory Bowel Disease Arthritis (IBD)**
  - Similar appearance to AS, with symmetric & bilateral sacroiliitis
  - Generally involves proximal large joints (hip, shoulder)
  - Rarely involves peripheral joints & calcaneus

CALCANEAL EROSIONS, POSTERIOR TUBERCLE

- **Haglund Syndrome**
  - "Pump bump"
  - Prominent posterior calcaneal osseous & bursal projection
  - Thickening of Achilles tendon at insertion
  - Achilles bursitis
  - True erosive change of posterior calcaneus is rare, but deossification may occur, related to bursal inflammation
- **Achilles Tendinitis**
  - Most often occurs at the musculotendinous junction, well above posterior calcaneal tubercle
  - Occasionally may occur more distally
    - Thickening & signal abnormality within tendon
    - Elicits pre-Achilles bursitis
    - Does not cause true erosion, but adjacent inflammation may result in posterior calcaneal cortical deossification
- **Plantar Fasciitis**
  - Thickening, increased signal intensity of plantar fascia
  - Usually at plantar aponeurosis insertion on plantar aspect posterior calcaneal tubercle
  - Generally there is an associated plantar spur
  - May have edema within adjacent bone
  - Inflammatory changes may result in deossification of bone, though generally not true erosion
- **Osteomyelitis**
  - Calcaneal metaphysis & apophysis are typical locations for infection in child
    - Hematogenous spread
    - Direct inoculation
  - Direct inoculation in adults, particularly diabetics with heel ulceration
  - Destructive change, but usually not at typical location for true erosive disease

Helpful Clues for Rare Diagnoses
- **Gout**
  - Tibiotalar involvement may extend as juxtaarticular involvement of posterior calcaneus
  - Scalloped erosive change on posterior tubercle with associated soft tissue mass
    - Mass may be dense (tophus) or even subtly calcified
- **Repair of Achilles Tendon (Mimic)**
  - Tunnel or direct attachment of reconstruction into posterior tubercle
    - One technique is to loop flexor hallucis tendon through tunnel & attach to residual Achilles fibers
  - Site of tunnel or attachment may cause a defect in posterior calcaneus mimicking an erosion
- **Juvenile Idiopathic Arthritis (JIA)**
  - Ankle involvement in JIA is generally tibiotalar destructive change, similar to that of hemophilic arthropathy
  - Rare true erosive change in posterior calcaneal tubercle

Rheumatoid Arthritis (RA)

Lateral radiograph shows extensive erosive disease at the posterior tubercle ➤. The bones are osteopenic for age & gender, and there is no productive change. Prominent MTP erosions help make the diagnosis of RA.

Rheumatoid Arthritis (RA)

Lateral radiograph shows focal osteopenia and a dot-dash cortical pattern ➤ typical of early erosive change. This patient has convincing RA at other sites; later erosive change in the calcaneus is not uncommon.

CALCANEAL EROSIONS, POSTERIOR TUBERCLE

Chronic Reactive Arthritis (CRA)

Chronic Reactive Arthritis (CRA)

(Left) Lateral radiograph shows normal bone density, very large erosions ➡, and mild productive change adjacent to the erosions. The patient was a young male with urethritis; this is CRA. *(Right)* Lateral radiograph shows mild erosive change at the posterior calcaneus ➡ with surrounding more prominent fluffy productive change ➡. This pattern of periostitis in the calcaneus is typical of CRA, though less frequently could be seen with psoriatic arthritis.

Psoriatic Arthritis (PSA)

Ankylosing Spondylitis (AS)

(Left) Lateral radiograph shows an erosion ➡ with mild periostitis ➡ as well as a heel spur. Though this could represent the changes of CRA, in this case the diagnosis is PSA; the patient had skin changes as well as arthritis involving the hand. *(Right)* Lateral radiograph shows posterior calcaneal deossification & early erosion ➡ along with severe erosions in the Chopart joints ➡ & subtalar fusion. This patient had long-standing AS, not treated with medication.

Inflammatory Bowel Disease Arthritis (IBD)

Haglund Syndrome

(Left) Lateral radiograph shows inflammatory change at the posterior calcaneus ➡ and an early erosion ➡. The more inferior osseous density is ossification of the calcaneal apophysis. This is IBD arthritis in a 10 year old child who had 3 months of diarrhea. *(Right)* Sagittal T1WI MR shows an osseous bump ➡ at the posterior tubercle with thickened overlying Achilles ➡, typical of Haglund syndrome. There is fluid distending the pre-Achilles bursa and adjacent deossification ➡.

CALCANEAL EROSIONS, POSTERIOR TUBERCLE

Achilles Tendinitis

Plantar Fasciitis

(Left) Sagittal PD FSE FS MR shows high signal of Achilles tendinitis ➡ with adjacent distended pre-Achilles bursa ⇨. There is mild calcaneal edema at the insertion ➡ that may be seen as deossification on radiograph. *(Right)* Sagittal STIR MR shows thickening & high signal in the plantar fascia ➡ with surrounding soft tissue edema ➡. There is edema within the calcaneus ⇨ that may eventually develop into a plantar spur; at this point, it may appear as deossification on X-ray.

Osteomyelitis

Osteomyelitis

(Left) Lateral radiograph shows erosive and destructive change in the metaphysis of the calcaneus as well as the apophysis ➡. This is typical of, and proved to be, osteomyelitis. *(Right)* Lateral radiograph shows severe erosive destructive change at the posterior calcaneus, along with air in the soft tissues ➡. This is advanced osteomyelitis in a diabetic patient.

Gout

Repair of Achilles Tendon (Mimic)

(Left) Lateral radiograph shows a dense soft tissue mass ➡ with erosions of the posterior talus ➡ and calcaneus ⇨. This proved to be gout in a young woman with end-stage renal disease. *(Right)* Sagittal T1WI MR shows the looped flexor hallucis tendon interposition ➡ for an Achilles tendon repair (which has failed). There is an associated surgical defect in the superior aspect of the posterior calcaneus ⇨ that might be mistaken for an erosion.

RETROCALCANEAL BURSITIS

DIFFERENTIAL DIAGNOSIS

Common
- Achilles Tendon Tear & Tendinopathy
- Haglund Deformity
- Inflammatory Arthritis

Less Common
- Gout
- Seronegative Spondyloarthropathy
- Calcaneal Fractures
- Osteomyelitis

Rare but Important
- Sever Disease (Calcaneal Apophysitis)

ESSENTIAL INFORMATION

Key Differential Diagnosis Issues
- Inflammation of deep Achilles bursa interposed between Achilles tendon & posterior calcaneal tubercle
- May have ↑ SI from bursal effusion &/or synovial hypertrophy (intermediate SI)
- May be unilateral or bilateral depending on etiology

Helpful Clues for Common Diagnoses
- **Achilles Tendon Tear & Tendinopathy**
  - Tendon thickening with intrasubstance signal; ± bursal thickening, effusion
- **Haglund Deformity**
  - Also known as "pump bump"; related to wearing tight shoes with closed back
  - Prominent posterosuperior calcaneal tubercle (squaring or enthesophyte)

- **Inflammatory Arthritis**
  - Rheumatoid & juvenile idiopathic arthritis
  - Diffuse osteopenia, erosion of posterosuperior calcaneus from synovial inflammation; joint space loss & erosions in hindfoot joints

Helpful Clues for Less Common Diagnoses
- **Gout**
  - Discrete, marginated erosions; ± soft tissue tophi
- **Seronegative Spondyloarthropathy**
  - Psoriatic, chronic reactive, ankylosing spondylitis & inflammatory bowel disease arthritis
  - Posterosuperior calcaneus erosions, soft tissue thickening, periosteal reaction ("whiskering") near tendon insertions
- **Calcaneal Fractures**
  - Consider this diagnosis when evaluating bone & soft tissue edema on MR; fractures may be less evident on MR than radiography/CT
- **Osteomyelitis**
  - Soft tissue swelling, cortical loss, marrow edema, ± abscess

Helpful Clues for Rare Diagnoses
- **Sever Disease (Calcaneal Apophysitis)**
  - Calcaneal apophysitis: Inflammation of apophysis in active boys 10-13 years
  - Sclerotic calcaneal apophysis with associated pain; marrow edema with intact cortical surfaces

Achilles Tendon Tear & Tendinopathy

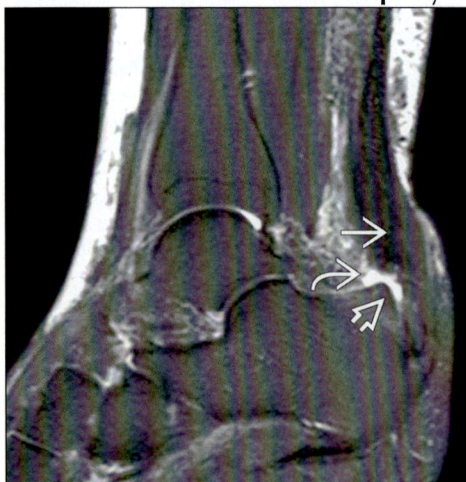

Sagittal T2WI FS MR shows Achilles tendon thickening ➡ with associated retrocalcaneal bursitis ➡. Note the prominent posterior calcaneal tubercle ➡, resulting in "pump bump".

Haglund Deformity

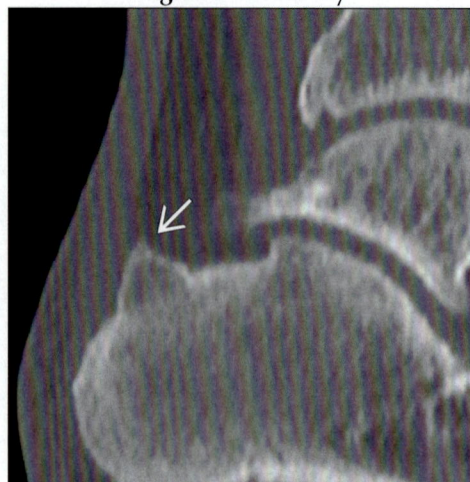

Sagittal bone CT reformation shows marked prominence of the posterosuperior calcaneal tubercle ➡, typical of Haglund deformity.

RETROCALCANEAL BURSITIS

Inflammatory Arthritis

Seronegative Spondyloarthropathy

(Left) Lateral radiograph shows diffuse osteopenia & multiple small posterior calcaneal erosions ⮕ in this patient with rheumatoid arthritis. Note the marked tibiotalar joint space narrowing ⮕ & absence of reparative bone. *(Right)* Lateral radiograph shows posterior calcaneal erosions ⮕ with soft tissue swelling of the retrocalcaneal bursa ⮕ in this patient with psoriatic arthritis. Note the large tibiotalar joint effusion ⮕.

Seronegative Spondyloarthropathy

Calcaneal Fractures

(Left) Sagittal bone CT reformation shows retrocalcaneal bursitis ⮕ with a mixed erosive-productive arthropathy in this 40 year old man with chronic reactive arthritis. Note the "whiskering" ⮕ of reparative bone. *(Right)* Sagittal STIR MR shows the retrocalcaneal bursal effusion ⮕ accompanying a calcaneal fracture ⮕ that runs perpendicular to the main trabecular struts with surrounding marrow edema.

Osteomyelitis

Sever Disease (Calcaneal Apophysitis)

(Left) Sagittal T1 C+ MR shows intense calcaneal marrow edema ⮕ with a small fluid collection ⮕ in apophysis as well as soft tissue swelling & bursitis ⮕ in this biopsy proven osteomyelitis. *(Right)* Sagittal T2WI FS MR shows inflammation with calcaneal apophyseal & metaphyseal edema ⮕ with retrocalcaneal bursitis ⮕ as well as subcutaneous edema ⮕ but no discrete fluid collection. The apophysis is sclerotic on radiograph (not shown).

SOFT TISSUE MASS IN THE FOOT

DIFFERENTIAL DIAGNOSIS

Common
- Bursitis
- Tendon, Injury
- Plantar Fasciitis
- Ganglion Cyst
- Plantar Fibroma
- Morton Neuroma
- Gouty Tophus
- Lipoma, Soft Tissue

Less Common
- Charcot, Neuropathic
- Hemangioma, Soft Tissue
- Soft Tissue Abscess
- Giant Cell Tumor Tendon Sheath
- Pigmented Villonodular Synovitis (PVNS)
- Glomus Tumor

Rare but Important
- Rheumatoid Nodule
- Xanthoma (Fibroxanthoma)
- Aneurysm
- Accessory Muscle
- Soft Tissue Neoplasms
- Granuloma Annulare
- Tumoral (Idiopathic) Calcinosis
- Macrodystrophia Lipomatosa
- Skin & Subcutaneous Lesions

ESSENTIAL INFORMATION

Key Differential Diagnosis Issues
- While radiographs demonstrate the osseous changes, MR is the imaging tool of choice for soft tissue evaluation

Helpful Clues for Common Diagnoses
- **Bursitis**
  - Inflammation of space interposed between muscle, tendon, skin, & adjacent bone
  - Retrocalcaneal: Between calcaneus & Achilles
  - Intermetatarsal: Between 2 metatarsal heads, dorsal to intermetatarsal ligament
  - Adventitious: Plantar fat pad near metatarsal head (1st & 5th, most commonly); often with accompanying fibrosis
- **Tendon, Injury**
  - Tendinopathy/partial intrasubstance tear: Intermediate to ↑ SI in tendon

- Complete tendon tear with minimal diastasis: ↑ SI in tear defect
  - Tenosynovitis: Distended ↑ SI in sheath, ± tendon abnormality
- **Plantar Fasciitis**
  - Thickening fascia (usually medial band); ± plantar fat pad edema, calcaneal marrow edema
  - May lead to rupture
- **Ganglion Cyst**
  - Thin-walled discrete fluid collection, ± multiseptate, often near joint line
- **Plantar Fibroma**
  - Single or multiple nodular thickenings arising from plantar fascia
  - Intermediate to ↓ SI on all sequences, ± enhancement
- **Morton Neuroma**
  - Nodule plantar to intermetatarsal ligament; intermediate T1 SI, ↓ T2 SI, ± enhancement
  - May be associated with intermetatarsal bursitis
- **Gouty Tophus**
  - Soft tissue nodular calcification, ↓ SI (T1 & T2); osseous erosions, predilection for Lisfranc, MTP joints
- **Lipoma, Soft Tissue**
  - SI similar to subcutaneous fat; may have associated calcification, ossification, hemorrhage, or fibrosis

Helpful Clues for Less Common Diagnoses
- **Charcot, Neuropathic**
  - Mimics soft tissue mass due to marked joint distension, dissolution, destruction, disorganization, dislocation
- **Hemangioma, Soft Tissue**
  - ↓ SI (T1) mass with interdigitating fat; striated or septated ↑ SI (T2); ± phleboliths
- **Soft Tissue Abscess**
  - Look for sinus tract, foreign body implant
  - Fluid collection with thickened, irregular walls; ± surrounding soft tissue edema
- **Giant Cell Tumor Tendon Sheath**
  - Intermediate to ↓ SI (T1 & T2) mass associated with tendon, + enhancement; ± calcification
- **Pigmented Villonodular Synovitis (PVNS)**
  - Intermediate to ↓ SI (T1 & T2) mass; ↓ SI on GRE due to hemosiderin; ± calcification; + enhancement; erodes adjacent bones

SOFT TISSUE MASS IN THE FOOT

- **Glomus Tumor**
  - Well-defined, ↑ SI (T2/STIR), intense enhancement
  - Tumor of neuromyoarterial glomus of nail bed

Helpful Clues for Rare Diagnoses

- **Rheumatoid Nodule**
  - Subcutaneous nodule with homogeneous ↓ SI, peripheral enhancement; adjacent joint erosions
- **Xanthoma (Fibroxanthoma)**
  - Seen in hypercholesterolemia; ↓ SI (T1 & T2) masses within tendons, speckled in appearance
- **Aneurysm**
  - Look for vessel of origin, may be saccular or fusiform; flow voids
- **Accessory Muscle**
  - Soleus, flexor digitorum accessorius longus, peroneocalcaneus internus, tibiocalcaneus internus
- **Soft Tissue Neoplasms**
  - Benign: Lipoma, hemangioma, nerve sheath tumor, soft tissue chondroma, desmoid type fibromatosis
  - Malignant: Fibrosarcoma, dermatofibrosarcoma protuberans, clear cell sarcoma, malignant fibrous histiocytoma, synovial sarcoma, leiomyosarcoma, Kaposi sarcoma, chondrosarcoma, rhabdomyosarcoma
- **Granuloma Annulare**

  - Ill-defined, intermediate to ↓ SI nodule with enhancement
- **Tumoral (Idiopathic) Calcinosis**
  - Lobular calcification in muscles & soft tissues; heterogeneous ↓ SI due to calcification intermixed with edema, fibrosis
  - More common in African Americans
- **Macrodystrophia Lipomatosa**
  - Macrodactyly associated with neural fibrolipoma; osseous/soft tissue overgrowth
  - Look for nerve enlargement
- **Skin & Subcutaneous Lesions**
  - Plantar warts, epidermal inclusion cyst

Other Essential Information

- Differential considerations may be further subdivided by anatomic location
  - Forefoot
    - Morton neuroma, intermetatarsal bursitis, adventitious bursitis, rheumatoid nodule, gout, glomus tumor
  - Plantar fascia
    - Fasciitis, fascial rupture, plantar fibromatosis, soft tissue abscess, foreign body
  - Retrocalcaneal palpable mass
    - Retrocalcaneal bursitis, Achilles tendinopathy, xanthoma, accessory muscle

Bursitis

Sagittal STIR MR shows retrocalcaneal bursitis (↑ SI fluid) ➡ *accompanying Achilles tendinosis/partial intrasubstance tear with striated intermediate SI* ➡ *in the tendon.*

Bursitis

Coronal PD FSE FS MR shows a slightly nodular fluid collection ➡ *interposed between 3rd & 4th metatarsal heads dorsal to the intermetatarsal ligament, typical of intermetatarsal bursitis.*

SOFT TISSUE MASS IN THE FOOT

Bursitis

Bursitis

(Left) Coronal T1WI MR shows a focal uniform ↓ SI mass ⇨ under the 5th metatarsal head that is palpable & relatively painless. The adjacent metatarsal is normal. *(Right)* Coronal PD FSE FS MR shows the same soft tissue mass with slightly heterogeneous ↑ SI in the patient with an adventitious bursa ⇨ & fibrosis ⇨. This benign subcutaneous bursitis is biopsy proven.

Tendon, Injury

Tendon, Injury

(Left) Sagittal PD FSE FS MR shows an ankle mass ⇨ anterior to the talus. Thickening & intermediate SI ⇨ represent an anterior tibialis tendinosis/partial tear with a small amount of tenosynovitis ⇨. *(Right)* Sagittal PD FSE FS MR shows a normal flexor hallucis longus tendon ⇨ with a distended tendon sheath ⇨ in this patient with osteoarthritis & tenosynovitis. Note the degenerative subchondral cyst ⇨.

Plantar Fasciitis

Plantar Fasciitis

(Left) Sagittal STIR MR shows plantar fat pad ⇨ & muscle edema ⇨ with complete plantar plate rupture ⇨ 15 mm distal to calcaneal origin ⇨ of fascia. *(Right)* Coronal T2WI FS MR shows medial plantar fascial band thickening ⇨ just distal to the calcaneal origin with mild adjacent plantar fat pad edema ⇨.

SOFT TISSUE MASS IN THE FOOT

Ganglion Cyst

Plantar Fibroma

(Left) Coronal PD FSE FS MR shows a thin-walled multiseptate ganglion ➡ that arises lateral to the 1st metatarsal head & tracks to the dorsal subcutaneous soft tissues. *(Right)* Sagittal PD FSE FS MR shows a small intermediate signal nodule ➡ arising in the planter fascia, typical of a plantar fibroma. In addition, there is a small but ill-defined soft tissue ganglion ➡ arising from the arthritic 1st tarsometatarsal joint ➡.

Morton Neuroma

Morton Neuroma

(Left) Coronal T1WI MR shows a slightly dumbbell-shaped nodule ➡ arising between the 3rd & 4th metatarsal heads plantar to the intermetatarsal ligament and extending into the plantar soft tissue. *(Right)* Coronal T1 C+ FS MR shows heterogeneous enhancement ➡ of the same lesion, typical of a Morton neuroma, which is a perineural fibrosis of a plantar digital nerve, resulting in entrapment of the nerve itself.

Gouty Tophus

Lipoma, Soft Tissue

(Left) Sagittal T1WI MR shows a large soft tissue mass ➡, low signal intensity, which remained largely low SI on T2 weighted imaging. The lesion is destructive but involves the 1st MTP joint. It proved to be gout. *(Right)* Coronal T1WI MR shows a dumbbell shaped ↑ SI mass ➡ similar to the adjacent subcutaneous fat. This encapsulated lipoma results in a widened intermetatarsal space.

SOFT TISSUE MASS IN THE FOOT

(Left) Sagittal T1WI MR shows the typical destruction of a Charcot joint with talonavicular dislocation ➡. There is joint effusion ➡ filled with ossific debris ➡ in this patient with diabetes. The large distended and disrupted joints may present as a soft tissue mass. **(Right)** Coronal T2WI FS MR shows a mass composed of ↑ SI tubular structures ➡ with interdigitating fat (↓ SI on fat suppression sequence) ➡, displacing the flexor digitorum tendons ➡ & infiltrating the muscle belly.

Charcot, Neuropathic

Hemangioma, Soft Tissue

(Left) Sagittal T1WI FS MR shows a plantar mass in a young girl with a history of a toothpick puncture wound 2 months earlier with incomplete removal. There is subsequent abscess ➡ formation around the retained foreign body ➡. **(Right)** Sagittal PD FSE FS MR shows a focal subcutaneous fluid collection ➡ & sinus tract ➡ to a deeper fluid collection with a thickened, irregular wall ➡ in this patient with diabetes.

Soft Tissue Abscess

Soft Tissue Abscess

(Left) Sagittal PD FSE FS MR shows an intermediate SI mass ➡ within the anterior tibialis tendon sheath ➡ displacing the tendon. This giant cell tumor of tendon sheath enhanced uniformly (not shown). **(Right)** Sagittal T2WI MR shows a large, predominantly low signal intensity mass within the ankle joint ➡, which produces an anterior foot mass. Since it is intraarticular, the low signal should be suggestive of either PVNS or gout; the former was proven.

Giant Cell Tumor Tendon Sheath

Pigmented Villonodular Synovitis (PVNS)

SOFT TISSUE MASS IN THE FOOT

Glomus Tumor

Xanthoma (Fibroxanthoma)

(Left) Coronal T1WI FS MR shows an intensely enhancing nodule ➡ in the tip of the nailbed. There was subtle erosion of the distal phalanx on initial radiograph (not shown). (Right) Axial T1WI MR shows xanthofibromatosis of Achilles tendon ➡ with slightly heterogeneous low signal. There are similar findings in the posterior tibial tendon ➡ in this patient with hypercholesterolemia.

Accessory Muscle

Soft Tissue Neoplasms

(Left) Axial PD FSE MR shows a palpable, painless mass ➡ (isointense to muscle) that originates from the tibia anterior to soleus & inserts on the superior calcaneus, typical of an accessory soleus. (Right) Sagittal T2WI MR shows the multiple lobulate, ↑ SI lesion ➡ destroying the tarsals & invading the adjacent soft tissues. This aggressive lesion is a chondrosarcoma.

Macrodystrophia Lipomatosa

Skin & Subcutaneous Lesions

(Left) Anteroposterior radiograph shows a normal hind & midfoot, as well as normal 4th & 5th rays ➡. However, there is giantism of both the soft tissues & bones of 1st three digits ➡, typical of macrodystrophia lipomatosa. (Right) Sagittal T1WI MR shows an elliptical epidermal mass ➡ that is ↓ SI & corresponds to a slightly flattened nodule with a small central petechiae, typical of a plantar wart.

TALAR BEAK

DIFFERENTIAL DIAGNOSIS

Common
- Talar Ridge
- Hypertrophied Talar Ridge
- Osteophyte

Less Common
- Tarsal Coalition

ESSENTIAL INFORMATION

Key Differential Diagnosis Issues
- Osseous excrescence located along the dorsal surface of the talus
- Location & size of bony outgrowth is most important for diagnosis
- a.k.a., talar spur, talar lip, or talar crest
- Best demonstrated on lateral radiographs & sagittal MR or CT

Helpful Clues for Common Diagnoses
- **Talar Ridge**
  - Located 7-14 mm from trochlear surface
  - Several millimeters high
  - Straight to convex configuration
    - Sloped along proximal border
    - More acute angle along distal border
  - Normal ridge of bone at junction of
    - Ankle joint capsule
    - Talonavicular ligament
    - Anterior talofibular ligament
  - Largest along lateral border
  - Normal, flat portion of talus between talar ridge & talar head articular surface

- **Hypertrophied Talar Ridge**
  - Same location as talar ridge
  - Subjectively enlarged talar ridge, but no specific size to delineate normal from hypertrophied
  - Key finding: Bony ridge is located proximal to the talar head articular surface with an intervening normal segment
  - Seen in athletic patients or patients with diffuse enthesopathy

- **Osteophyte**
  - Located along cartilage margins
    - Proximally at ankle with associated anterior tibial osteophytes
    - Distally at talonavicular joint with associated joint space narrowing
  - Degenerative or post-traumatic finding

Helpful Clues for Less Common Diagnoses
- **Tarsal Coalition**
  - Anteriorly directed, triangular outgrowth extending from the talar ridge to, or near, the level of the talar head articular surface
  - May be extreme hypertrophy of talar ridge
  - Look for osseous or fibrous union of the talus & calcaneus or calcaneus & navicular
  - Secondary signs of coalition include the "C-sign" & non-visualization of the subtalar joint middle facet

SELECTED REFERENCES

1. Resnick D: Talar ridges, osteophytes, and beaks: a radiologic commentary. Radiology. 151(2):329-32, 1984

Talar Ridge

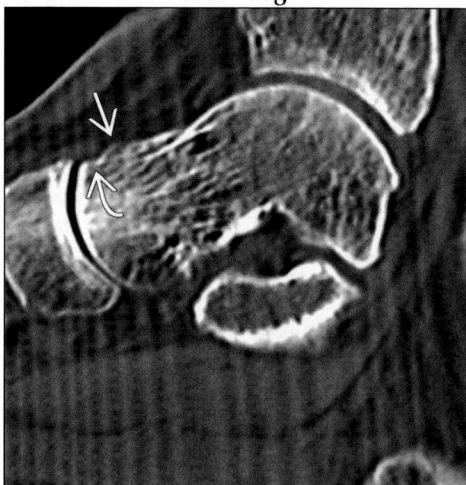

Sagittal NECT shows a normal talar ridge ➡ along the dorsum of the talus. Note the short, flat segment ➡ between the ridge and articular surface.

Talar Ridge

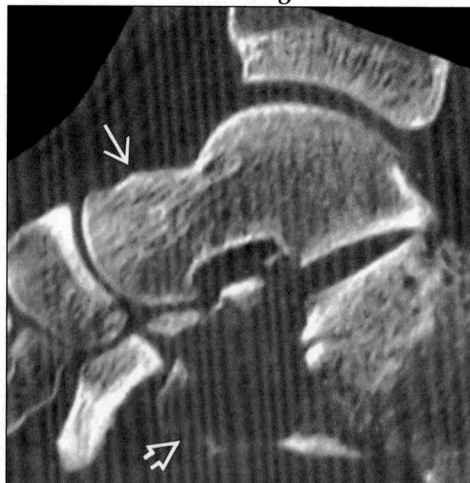

Sagittal NECT shows a normal talar ridge ➡ located proximal to the talar head articular surface. This patient also had an unrelated but extensively comminuted calcaneus fracture ➡.

TALAR BEAK

Hypertrophied Talar Ridge

Hypertrophied Talar Ridge

(Left) Sagittal T1WI FS MR shows hypertrophy ➡ of the normal talar ridge. This is likely caused, at least in part, by traction from a thickened talonavicular ligament ➡ in this athletic patient. (Right) Sagittal NECT shows a hypertrophied talar ridge ➡. The location of the excrescence proximal to the talar head articular surface, with a short intervening normal segment ➡ is typical. This patient had a CT to characterize the comminuted distal tibial fracture ➡.

Osteophyte

Osteophyte

(Left) Lateral radiograph shows a talar osteophyte ➡ that extends all the way to the articular surface. Note also the talonavicular joint space narrowing ➡ and mild osteophyte formation ➡ on the navicular side of the joint. (Right) Sagittal NECT shows a proximally located dorsal talar osteophyte ➡ along the articular margin of the anterior ankle joint. This is secondary to degenerative changes, as seen by an associated small anterior tibial osteophyte ➡.

Tarsal Coalition

Tarsal Coalition

(Left) Lateral radiograph shows a large talar beak ➡ due to talocalcaneal coalition. Notice that the talar dome is rounded, as is the medial aspect of the tibial plafond, producing the "C-sign" ➡. The normal lucency of the subtalar joint middle facet ➡ is obscured. (Right) Sagittal NECT shows a small talar beak ➡ in a patient with talocalcaneal coalition. Solid bone bridges the subtalar joint middle facet ➡ and partially fuses the subtalar joint posterior facet ➡.

TARSAL CYSTIC/LYTIC LESIONS

DIFFERENTIAL DIAGNOSIS

Common
- Subchondral Cyst
  - Osteoarthritis
  - Gout
  - Rheumatoid Arthritis
  - Juvenile Idiopathic Arthritis (JIA)
  - Pyrophosphate Arthropathy
  - Amyloid Deposition
  - Pigmented Villonodular Synovitis (PVNS)
- Intraosseous Ganglion
- Intraosseous Lipoma
- Osteomyelitis
- Charcot, Neuropathic
- Osteonecrosis

Less Common
- Osteochondral Lesion of the Talus
- Hemophilia, Pseudotumor
- Unicameral Bone Cyst (UBC)
- Aneurysmal Bone Cyst
- Giant Cell Tumor
- Enchondroma
- Ewing Sarcoma
- Hyperparathyroidism/Renal Osteodystrophy, Brown Tumor
- Chondroblastoma
- Chondrosarcoma
- Soft Tissue Tumor, Locally Invasive
- Silicone-Induced Synovitis

Rare but Important
- Metastases, Bone Marrow
- Multiple Myeloma
- Paget Disease
- Osteosarcoma, Telangiectatic
- Angiosarcoma, Osseous
- Hemangioendothelioma, Osseous
- Sarcoidosis

ESSENTIAL INFORMATION

Helpful Clues for Common Diagnoses
- **Subchondral Cyst**
  - a.k.a., synovial cyst, geode, pseudocyst
  - Rounded radiolucent lesion near bone surface
  - Signal intensity on MR varies with cyst content: Fluid, gas, fibrous, adipose, myxoid, or proteinaceous material
  - **Osteoarthritis**
    - Joint space narrowing
    - Surrounding sclerotic bone
    - Preferential involvement of pressure portion of joint
  - **Gout**
    - Oval erosions with overhanging edges
    - Preserved joint spaces
    - Normal mineralization
    - Soft tissue tophi
  - **Rheumatoid Arthritis**
    - Inflammatory erosions located in juxtaarticular regions
    - Lack sclerotic border
    - Joint space narrowing with osteoporosis
    - Lytic lesions may also be due to secondary osteoarthritis
  - **Pyrophosphate Arthropathy**
    - Large, widespread lesions
    - Surrounding sclerotic bone
    - Joint space narrowing with bone collapse
  - **Amyloid Deposition**
    - Intraosseous amyloid collections have variable appearance on MR
    - May show communication with articular surface
    - History of hemodialysis is common
  - **Pigmented Villonodular Synovitis (PVNS)**
    - Blooming signal of soft tissue masses on gradient echo MR sequences
- **Intraosseous Ganglion**
  - Single lesion with sclerotic border
  - ± Soft tissue mass
- **Intraosseous Lipoma**
  - Typical location in mid-calcaneus
  - Fat content can be confirmed with CT
  - ± Central calcification or fluid
- **Osteomyelitis**
  - Osteopenia
  - Ill-defined bone erosion
  - Soft tissue abscess
  - Sinus tract
  - ± Sequestrum
- **Charcot, Neuropathic**
  - Bone collapse & fragmentation
  - Joint disorganization & debris
  - Can be difficult to differentiate from osteomyelitis
- **Osteonecrosis**
  - Single or multiple lesions
  - Weight-bearing area of joint
  - Bone collapse & fragmentation

TARSAL CYSTIC/LYTIC LESIONS

Helpful Clues for Less Common Diagnoses

- **Hemophilia, Pseudotumor**
  - Subchondral bone erosion, joint space narrowing, osteopenia, & soft tissue masses from hemorrhage
  - Calcaneus: 1 of 3 most common sites of hemophiliac pseudotumor
- **Giant Cell Tumor**
  - Eccentric, expansile lytic lesion in epiphysis
  - Lacks sclerotic border
  - ± Soft tissue mass
- **Ewing Sarcoma**
  - Lytic or sclerotic lesion with cortical breakthrough
  - Classic onion-skin periosteal reaction is rare in foot
- **Chondroblastoma**
  - Epiphyseal or apophyseal lytic lesion with sclerotic border & chondroid matrix
- **Chondrosarcoma**
  - Lytic lesion with chondroid matrix
  - Endosteal scalloping or cortical breakthrough
  - ± Soft tissue mass
- **Soft Tissue Tumor, Locally Invasive**
  - Soft tissue mass not centered in bone
  - Signs of extrinsic mass effect, such as scalloping, in addition to invasion
  - Bone invasion favors synovial sarcoma, clear cell sarcoma, or epithelioid sarcoma
- **Silicone-Induced Synovitis**
  - Well-defined periprosthetic lytic lesions
  - Onset months to years after placement of silicone joint prosthesis
  - Normal surrounding bone mineralization helps exclude osteomyelitis

Helpful Clues for Rare Diagnoses

- **Metastases, Bone Marrow**
  - History of colon, genitourinary, or lung malignancy in adults
  - History of neuroblastoma, rhabdomyosarcoma, or clear cell renal carcinoma in children
- **Multiple Myeloma**
  - Lytic lesions with well-defined margins
  - Faint sclerotic rim is rare
- **Paget Disease**
  - Osteolytic lesion with blade of grass or flame shape
  - Disease progression includes coarsened trabeculae, cortical thickening, bone enlargement, & sclerosis
- **Osteosarcoma, Telangiectatic**
  - Fluid-fluid levels
  - ± Aggressive periosteal reaction
- **Angiosarcoma, Osseous**
  - Clustered, multicentric lytic lesions
  - Ill-defined borders
- **Hemangioendothelioma, Osseous**
  - Similar but less aggressive appearance than angiosarcoma
  - May have faint sclerotic borders
- **Sarcoidosis**
  - Punched-out round to oval lytic lesions
  - Honeycomb or lattice trabeculae

Gout

Anteroposterior radiograph shows marked lytic erosion ➡ of the tarsals and metatarsals. Overhanging edges ➡ and calcified soft tissue tophi ➡ are typical of gout.

Gout

Coronal NECT shows a focal lytic lesion in the talus ➡ with a subtle overhanging edge ➡. An additional lesion in the fibula ➡ supports the diagnosis of gout.

TARSAL CYSTIC/LYTIC LESIONS

Rheumatoid Arthritis

Juvenile Idiopathic Arthritis (JIA)

(Left) Axial T1WI MR shows periarticular erosions ➡ involving the metatarsal heads. The bones were osteopenic on radiographs. This is typical for rheumatoid arthritis. *(Right)* Lateral radiograph shows severe joint space narrowing at the tibiotalar joint and a moderate joint effusion ➡. A few small ossifications in the effusion are likely intraarticular osteochondral bodies. Subchondral cystic changes ➡ involve both the talus and tibia.

Pigmented Villonodular Synovitis (PVNS)

Pigmented Villonodular Synovitis (PVNS)

(Left) Anteroposterior radiograph shows 2 lytic lesions ➡ in the 1st metatarsal head. The smooth borders of the lesions suggest extrinsic erosion of the bone. This was due to pigmented villonodular synovitis of the 1st metatarsophalangeal joint. *(Right)* Sagittal T1WI MR shows multiple isointense lesions ➡ eroding the calcaneus and cuboid bones. There is an intraarticular soft tissue mass ➡ extending from the region of the anterior and middle facet of the subtalar joint.

Intraosseous Lipoma

Osteomyelitis

(Left) Lateral radiograph shows an oval, sharply demarcated, radiolucent lesion ➡ in the middle portion of the calcaneus. The lesion has a central focus of calcification ➡. Fat content of the lesion was confirmed with computed tomography. *(Right)* Anteroposterior radiograph shows osteopenia and a focal, ill-defined erosion involving the tibial side of the 3rd metatarsal ➡. An infectious etiology is also suggested by the prior amputation of the 3rd digit ➡.

TARSAL CYSTIC/LYTIC LESIONS

Osteomyelitis

Osteomyelitis

(Left) Coronal T2WI FS MR shows a fluid collection ➜ located between the 3rd and 4th digits at the level of the MTP joints. This collection communicates with the joint via a small sinus tract ➜. Bone enhancement favors septic arthritis and osteomyelitis. *(Right)* Sagittal T1WI MR shows irregular destruction of the talus ➜ and intraarticular soft tissue ➜, which extends posteriorly in the joint space. These findings were due to an indolent fungal infection.

Osteomyelitis

Charcot, Neuropathic

(Left) Sagittal T2WI MR shows a typical case of osteomyelitis. There is a focal erosion ➜ and abnormal signal ➜ involving the calcaneus and calcaneal apophysis, with extension into the adjacent soft tissues. Biopsy confirmed infection. *(Right)* Anteroposterior radiograph shows a neuropathic deformity of the midfoot with collapse, fragmentation, dislocations, and cystic changes ➜. There are amputations ➜ through the 1st metatarsal and 3rd toe.

Osteochondral Lesion of the Talus

Hemophilia, Pseudotumor

(Left) Sagittal T1WI FS MR arthrogram shows an osteochondral lesion ➜ involving the medial talar dome. Intraarticularly administered contrast ➜ extends into the osteochondral lesion, suggesting instability. *(Right)* Lateral radiograph shows lytic expanded lesions ➜ in the calcaneus. The clinical history is key. This represents a pseudotumor, resulting from repeated intraosseous bleeds in a young man with hemophilia.

TARSAL CYSTIC/LYTIC LESIONS

Unicameral Bone Cyst (UBC)

Unicameral Bone Cyst (UBC)

(Left) Lateral radiograph shows a lytic lesion ➡ in the calcaneal neck. The calcaneus is one of the most common locations of UBC in adults. A paucity of trabeculae in this region, as an anatomic variant, can mimic a bone cyst. *(Right)* Sagittal T1 C+ FS MR shows an ovoid lesion ➡ in the mid calcaneus. The lesion followed fluid signal intensity on all MR imaging sequences. UBC typically shows mild peripheral enhancement ➡ without central enhancement.

Aneurysmal Bone Cyst

Aneurysmal Bone Cyst

(Left) Anteroposterior radiograph shows a typical aneurysmal bone cyst ➡ involving the base of the first metatarsal. Note the thin, intact cortex surrounding the expanded portion of the lesion. *(Right)* Sagittal T1WI MR shows an eccentrically located lesion ➡ in the base of the 1st metatarsal. Note the intact surrounding cortex ➡. These findings in this location suggest ABC, unicameral bone cyst, and possibly giant cell tumor as a potential diagnoses.

Chondroblastoma

Chondrosarcoma

(Left) Coronal oblique CECT shows a lytic lesion with geographic borders ➡ involving the right talus. The lesion has a faintly sclerotic border and internal chondroid matrix ➡, suggestive of a chondroblastoma. *(Right)* Lateral radiograph shows multiple lytic lesions ➡, which cause frank destruction of most of the tarsal bones and metatarsal bases. These aggressive lesions have an associated soft tissue mass ➡.

TARSAL CYSTIC/LYTIC LESIONS

Silicone-Induced Synovitis

Metastases, Bone Marrow

(Left) Anteroposterior radiograph shows lucency in the distal first metatarsal ➔ and great toe proximal phalanx ➔. This patient with rheumatoid arthritis had a 1st MTP joint replacement and a silicone prosthesis. Prosthesis failure has led to a granulomatous reaction eroding bone. (Right) Sagittal T1WI MR shows a low signal mass ➔ destroying the medial cuneiform bone. Cortical disruption and a subtle soft tissue mass are present. This was due to lytic metastatic breast carcinoma.

Metastases, Bone Marrow

Multiple Myeloma

(Left) Coronal NECT shows a large, aggressive-appearing lytic lesion ➔ involving multiple bones of the hindfoot. Metastases below the elbow or knee are unusual; however, the diagnosis in this case was metastatic adenocarcinoma. (Right) Axial T1WI MR shows a focal low signal lesion ➔ involving the 3rd metatarsal. This lesion was lytic on radiographs. A pathologic fracture is faintly visible as a nondisplaced low signal line ➔. Myeloma was proven on biopsy.

Paget Disease

Angiosarcoma, Osseous

(Left) Sagittal T1WI MR shows an abnormal talus ➔. On radiographs the appearance was of mixed sclerosis and lucency. The MR best demonstrates the cortical and trabecular thickening with mild bone enlargement, typical of Paget disease. (Right) Sagittal T1WI MR shows an extensive case of polyostotic osseous angiosarcoma. Multiple focal, aggressive destructive lesions ➔ involve, to some extent, nearly every bone of the right foot and ankle.

PART II
Image Based

POLYOSTOTIC LESIONS, ADULT

DIFFERENTIAL DIAGNOSIS

Common
- Enostosis (Bone Island)
- Metastases, Bone Marrow
- Multiple Myeloma
- Paget Disease
- Fibrous Dysplasia, Polyostotic
- Bone Infarcts
- Brown Tumor: HPTH/Renal OD
- Enchondromas
- Osteochondroma, Multiple Hereditary Exostosis
- Ewing Sarcoma, Metastatic
- Leukemia
- Lymphoma, Multifocal

Less Common
- Osteomyelitis
- Angiosarcoma, Osseous
- Hemangiopericytoma, Osseous
- Hemangioendothelioma, Osseous
- Cystic Angiomatosis
- Tuberculosis
- Bacillary Angiomatosis
- Sarcoidosis
- Ollier Disease
- Osteoma
- Maffucci Syndrome
- Osteosarcoma, Metastatic

Rare but Important
- Mastocytosis
- Giant Cell Tumor, Skull or Phalanges

ESSENTIAL INFORMATION

Key Differential Diagnosis Issues
- Long list, with wide spectrum of lesions ranging from benign, "leave me alone" (don't further image) to aggressive nonspecific lesions
- List can be modified into shorter, more helpful lists (see "alternative differential approaches")
- Even with this lengthy list, knowing that a lesion is polyostotic helps to limit differential considerations & is extremely useful
  - MR survey, PET/CT, or bone scans are useful in identifying polyostotic nature of disease & thus limiting differential

Helpful Clues for Common Diagnoses
- **Enostosis (Bone Island)**
  - Bone islands may be multiple without having a pattern that suggests osteopoikilosis
  - Bone islands are densely & uniformly sclerotic, differentiating them from some less densely sclerotic metastases
  - Metastases tend to be axial or shoulder girdle/proximal humerus & pelvis/proximal femora; bone islands less location-specific
  - If questions remain, MR or PET/CT may indicate inactivity of bone islands vs. activity of sclerotic metastases
    - **Caveat:** This is not always reliable with the latter
- **Multiple Myeloma**
  - Vast majority are lytic, punched out lesions or else diffusely osteopenic
  - Those presenting with osteopenia + gammopathy are best evaluated by MR survey
  - There may be a dominant lesion (plasmacytoma), with multiple smaller lytic lesions
  - Distribution is heavily axial (including skull), shoulder girdle/humerus, & pelvis/proximal femora
- **Fibrous Dysplasia, Polyostotic**
  - New lesions do not generally develop in adults
  - May see residual lesions which developed during childhood
  - **Hint:** Watch for residual deformities (Shepherd's Crook, bowing, protrusio of hips) & expanded bone
- **Brown Tumor: HPTH/Renal OD**
  - Location not specific; may be axial or appendicular; often noted in digits
  - Watch for abnormal bone density which is always present
  - Watch for bone resorption patterns (subperiosteal, subligamentous, subchondral, tuft)
  - Watch for indications of dialysis (such as central catheter, peritoneal catheter, shunt)
  - Watch for clips in neck region of parathyroids
- **Ewing Sarcoma, Metastatic**

POLYOSTOTIC LESIONS, ADULT

- Young adults, with primary more likely in proximal flat bone than long bone
  - Primary lesion will be larger, more aggressive in appearance
  - Ewing sarcoma is more likely to metastasize to bone than other bone sarcomas; equal likelihood of metastases to bone & lung
  - Osteosarcoma less frequent in adult population, metastasizes to lung & local lymph nodes more frequently than bone
- **Leukemia**
  - Focal lesions rare on X-ray; **hint:** Osteoporosis inappropriate for age/gender
  - Diagnosis & tumor burden determined by MR which shows infiltrative pattern
  - Given normal radiographs, MR differential is myeloma & multifocal lymphoma
- **Lymphoma, Multifocal**
  - Lymphoma usually is monostotic in adults, but often polyostotic in children
  - **Hint:** Serpiginous pattern on MR suggests the diagnosis; otherwise infiltrative

Helpful Clues for Less Common Diagnoses
- **Vascular Tumors**
  - No imaging discrimination between angiosarcoma, hemangiopericytoma, hemangioendothelioma
  - **Hint:** Vascular tumors favor lower extremity locations; polyostotic lytic lesions predominantly involving lower extremities should raise this consideration
- **Cystic Angiomatosis**

- Multiple lesions with either prominent trabeculae or cystic appearance
- Expand slowly but significantly over time

Alternative Differential Approaches
- Consider subdividing the list into 2 which are easier to handle
  - Polyostotic lesions which are easily identified by imaging (when their appearance is classic)
    - Paget disease
    - Fibrous dysplasia
    - Bone infarcts
    - Enchondromas
    - Osteochondromas, multiple hereditary exostoses
    - Sarcoidosis
    - Ollier disease
    - Osteoma
    - Maffucci syndrome
  - Polyostotic lesions which have a moderately to severely aggressive appearance but are otherwise nonspecific
    - Metastases, bone marrow (including primary bone sarcomas)
    - Multiple myeloma
    - Brown tumor: Hyperparathyroidism/renal osteodystrophy
    - Leukemia
    - Lymphoma, multifocal
    - Vascular tumors
    - Osteomyelitis (including TB)

Enostosis (Bone Island)

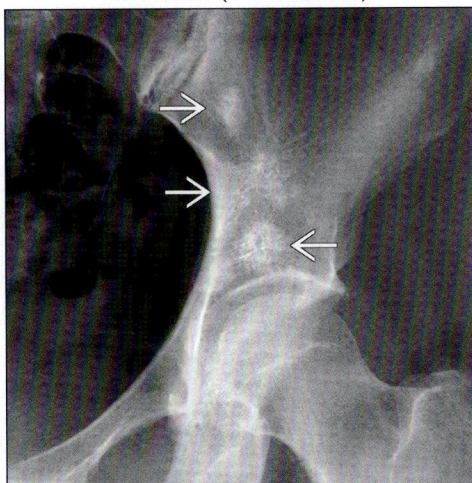

AP radiograph shows multiple sclerotic lesions restricted to the left iliac wing ➡. These were stable over a 4 year period and represent multiple bone islands. At initial presentation, one might consider sclerotic metastases.

Metastases, Bone Marrow

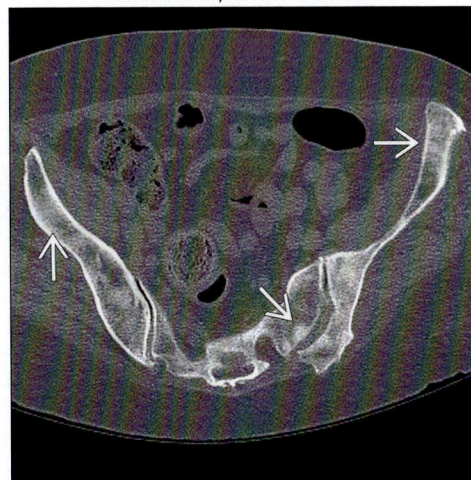

Axial CECT shows multiple sclerotic bone lesions ➡ scattered throughout the pelvis. They were extensively seen in the entire axial skeleton; the primary was non-small cell lung adenocarcinoma.

POLYOSTOTIC LESIONS, ADULT

Multiple Myeloma

Multiple Myeloma

(Left) Lateral radiograph shows multiple "punched out lytic lesions, of different sizes. There is no sclerotic border. This appearance is typical of multiple myeloma, & the skull is a favorite location. *(Right)* Coronal STIR MR in a patient with normal radiographs & gammopathy shows a lesion in the clavicle ⮕ and another, larger, lesion in the sternum ⮕. Myeloma may appear as osteopenia without focal lesions on radiograph; MR survey helps determine tumor burden.

Paget Disease

Paget Disease

(Left) Lateral radiograph shows a mixed lytic/sclerotic lesion in a thoracic vertebra ⮕. The alert radiologist will recognize slight enlargement of the body and suggest Paget disease. *(Right)* Posteroanterior bone scan of the same patient, distal to the thoracic lesion shows an additional L5 lesion as well as uptake extending along the ilioischial line of the right hemipelvis ⮕ and involvement of the right hip. This distribution is classic, and confirms the diagnosis.

Fibrous Dysplasia, Polyostotic

Bone Infarcts

(Left) Oblique radiograph shows multiple lesions, both lytic ⮕ & ground-glass ⮕ in the left hemipelvis. there is no aggressive feature, and fibrous dysplasia is the only reasonable diagnosis to consider. *(Right)* Axial T1WI MR shows multiple serpiginous bone infarcts, paralleling the bone outline ⮕. When this is the presentation (rather than a subtle density change without serpiginous outline), the diagnosis is secure.

POLYOSTOTIC LESIONS, ADULT

Brown Tumor: HPTH/Renal OD

Enchondromas

(Left) AP radiograph shows a supraacetabular lesion with indistinct borders ➡ & a femoral neck lesion with distinct borders ➡. The bone density is abnormal & trabeculae indistinct, suggesting metabolic disease. *(Right)* Lateral radiograph shows multiple lytic lesions, some containing chondroid matrix ➡. Each is a typical enchondroma. The patient had no other lesions to suggest Ollier disease; she had multiple enchondromas but not multiple enchondromatosis.

Osteochondroma, Multiple Hereditary Exostosis

Osteochondroma, Multiple Hereditary Exostosis

(Left) Axial NECT shows an exophytic osteochondroma ➡. It might be easy to overlook the additional small sessile osteochondromas at the iliac spines ➡. *(Right)* Axial NECT more distally in the same patient shows a portion of the exophytic osteochondroma ➡ as well as multiple small sessile osteochondromas draped along the iliac wings ➡. It is important not to overlook these; multiple hereditary exostosis carries a different prognosis than solitary exostosis.

Ewing Sarcoma, Metastatic

Ewing Sarcoma, Metastatic

(Left) Anteroposterior radiograph shows a highly aggressive permeative lytic lesion of the scapula ➡ with cortical breakthrough & soft tissue mass. This lesion in a flat bone of a 21 year old is typical of Ewing sarcoma. *(Right)* Bone scan obtained in the same patient is part of the workup, looking for osseous metastases. Unfortunately, there were several, scattered throughout the skeleton. Chest CT at the same setting showed no lung metastases.

POLYOSTOTIC LESIONS, ADULT

(Left) Axial T1 C+ FS MR shows enhancement of all the imaged osseous structures, indicating diffuse marrow infiltration. Radiographs were normal, as can be the case with infiltrative disease. Biopsy proved leukemia. **(Right)** Coronal STIR MR shows multiple lesions in both femora in this 60 year old. Additionally, lesions were seen throughout the axial skeleton. This proved to be multifocal lymphoma, an unusual presentation of lymphoma in the adult.

Leukemia

Lymphoma, Multifocal

(Left) Sagittal T2WI FS MR shows a septic joint with superinfection of both the humerus and radius ➡ in a patient with rheumatoid arthritis. Polyostotic osteomyelitis in adults tends to be in contiguous bones, unlike the child. **(Right)** Sagittal T1WI MR shows multiple lesions involving the ankle and foot ➡. Vascular tumor should be considered with polyostotic lesions, particularly of the lower extremities. This proved to be angiosarcoma.

Osteomyelitis

Angiosarcoma, Osseous

(Left) Lateral radiograph shows lytic lesions of the talus and calcaneus ➡. These moderately aggressive lesions are typical of vascular tumors, but otherwise nonspecific. Biopsy showed hemangioendothelioma. **(Right)** AP radiograph shows significant expansion of the pubic rami ➡, which has occurred over at least 2 decades. The patient had other lower extremity cystic-appearing lesions. The slow growth is typical of this benign vascular multicentric lesion.

Hemangioendothelioma, Osseous

Cystic Angiomatosis

POLYOSTOTIC LESIONS, ADULT

Tuberculosis

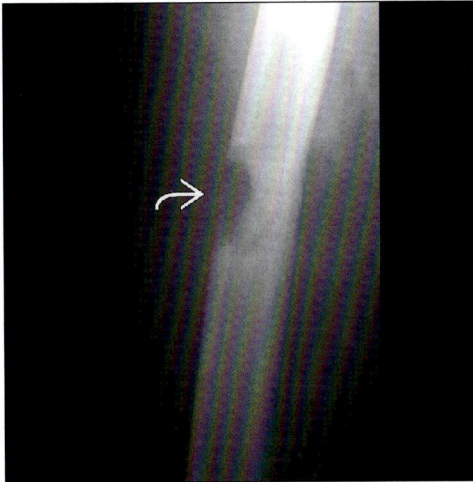

Tuberculosis

(Left) Oblique radiograph shows a moderately aggressive lesion ➘ with cortical breakthrough. This is a nonspecific appearance. *(Right)* Anteroposterior radiograph coned from a chest image of the same patient shows a lytic lesion of the rib ➘. The patient had complete white-out of the left lung, with mediastinal shift to the right. The combination of chest findings plus multiple lytic osseous lesions is typical for TB.

Sarcoidosis

Sarcoidosis

(Left) Coronal T1WI MR shows multiple tiny lesions scattered throughout the humeral head/neck ➘. These showed high signal on fluid sensitive sequences. There were also lesions of similar size in the muscles. These are sarcoid granulomas. *(Right)* Oblique radiograph shows typical lacy lytic lesions of the phalanges ➘, which are seen in osseous sarcoidosis.

Ollier Disease

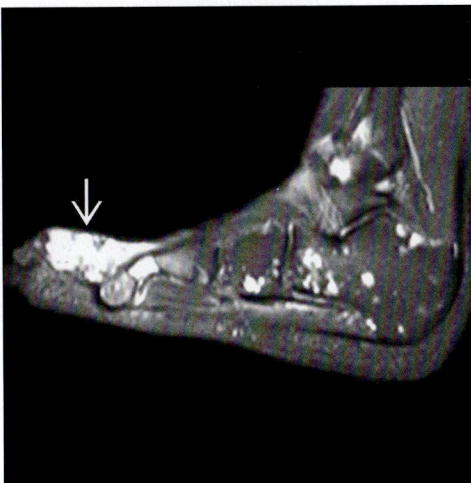

Maffucci Syndrome

(Left) Sagittal T2WI FS MR shows multiple lobulated high signal cartilaginous lesions. There is one lesion which is expanded significantly ➘. Radiographs showed chondroid matrix; this is Ollier disease. *(Right)* Posteroanterior radiograph shows multiple lytic lesions with chondroid matrix. Additionally, there is a soft tissue mass containing phleboliths ➘; the combination yields a diagnosis of Maffucci syndrome. (†MSK Req).

DIFFERENTIAL DIAGNOSIS

Common
- Fibroxanthoma (Non-Ossifying Fibroma)
- Fibrous Dysplasia, Polyostotic
- Langerhans Cell Histiocytosis (LCH)
- Osteomyelitis, Pediatric
- Osteochondroma, Multiple Hereditary Exostosis
- Leukemia
- Ewing Sarcoma, Metastatic
- Metastases, Bone Marrow

Less Common
- Lymphoma, Multifocal
- Osteosarcoma, Metastatic
- Hyperparathyroidism/Renal Osteodystrophy, Brown Tumor
- Melorheostosis

Rare but Important
- Ollier Disease
- Maffucci Syndrome
- Chronic Recurrent Multifocal Osteomyelitis
- Sarcoidosis
- Trevor Fairbank

ESSENTIAL INFORMATION

Key Differential Diagnosis Issues
- Polyostotic nature of a lesion can narrow the differential substantially & is a highly valuable characteristic
  - Information regarding multiple sites can be gained by bone scan, PET/CT, or clinical exam
- Lesions listed above range from benign (leave me alone) lesions, through "Aunt Minnie" lesions, through highly aggressive lesions
  - It is most reasonable to have an alternative approach to sort these out

Helpful Clues for Common Diagnoses
- **Fibroxanthoma (Non-Ossifying Fibroma)**
  - Benign fibrous cortical defects (same histologically as NOF, but smaller) are often multiple in children
  - Non-ossifying fibroma is not commonly multiple, except in patients with neurofibromatosis
  - Both have same natural history of healing
  - Both are cortically-based and metadiaphyseal
- **Fibrous Dysplasia, Polyostotic**
  - Lesion may have different appearance in different locations
    - Skull: Sclerotic
    - Pelvis: Bubbly, lytic
    - Long bones: Generally central, metadiaphyseal, mildly expanded, with variable homogeneous ground-glass density
- **Langerhans Cell Histiocytosis (LCH)**
  - Lesions may be lytic, geographic, & nonaggressive
  - Lesions may also be extremely aggressive in appearance: Permeative, cortical breakthrough, soft tissue mass, periosteal reaction, with rapid growth
  - **Hint**: Skull lesions may have beveled edge appearance due to differential involvement of inner & outer tables
- **Osteomyelitis, Pediatric**
  - Hematogenous spread usually results in metaphyseal sites
  - Osteomyelitis can appear extremely aggressive, with permeative change & cortical breakthrough with soft tissue mass: May not be distinguishable from aggressive tumor
  - Sickle cell patients at risk for multifocal osseous infection; higher predilection for Salmonella
- **Osteochondroma, Multiple Hereditary Exostosis**
  - Not a difficult diagnosis if exophytic (cauliflower) lesions are present
  - May have only sessile exostoses at the metaphyses which can give the appearance of a dysplasia; diagnosis often missed
- **Leukemia**
  - Diffuse marrow infiltration may result in appearance of osteopenia, easily overlooked
  - Metaphyseal lucent bands may highlight the degree of osteopenia
  - MR shows the extent of the abnormalities
- **Ewing Sarcoma, Metastatic**
  - Primary lesion usually highly aggressive: Lytic, permeative, cortical breakthrough, large soft tissue mass

POLYOSTOTIC LESIONS, CHILD

○ May have extensive reactive bone formation, giving the appearance of osteoid, with potential confusion with osteosarcoma
  ▪ Reactive bone formation restricted to bone, does not extend into soft tissue mass (as it does in osteosarcoma)
○ Most common sarcoma to have osseous metastases; lung & osseous metastases present with equal frequency

Helpful Clues for Less Common Diagnoses
• **Lymphoma, Multifocal**
  ○ 50% of childhood bone lymphoma is polyostotic (much less frequent in adults)
  ○ Lesions highly aggressive: Permeative, cortical breakthrough with soft tissue mass
  ○ Generally lytic, but may have reactive sclerosis within osseous lesion
  ○ In same differential as Ewing sarcoma with metastases, multifocal osteomyelitis, LCH, & metastases

Alternative Differential Approaches
• "Aunt Minnie" lesions can generally be identified immediately
  ○ Fibroxanthoma (non-ossifying fibroma)/benign fibrous cortical defect
  ○ Osteochondroma (multiple hereditary exostoses): Remember they can be sessile & resemble a metaphyseal dysplasia
  ○ Melorheostosis
  ○ Sarcoidosis (when lacy appearance is obvious)
  ○ Trevor Fairbank

• Polyostotic lesions which are usually monomelic
  ○ Fibrous dysplasia (generally unilateral)
  ○ Melorheostosis
  ○ Ollier disease
  ○ Trevor Fairbank
  ○ Maffucci syndrome
• Polyostotic lesions with an intermediately aggressive appearance
  ○ Fibrous dysplasia: Generally central, poorly marginated, but geographic
  ○ Langerhans cell histiocytosis: Appearance ranges from nonaggressive geographic to extremely aggressive permeative
  ○ Hyperparathyroidism/renal osteodystrophy, Brown tumor: Generally the lesion is geographic, but surrounding bone abnormal in density & trabecular pattern
• Polyostotic lesions with an aggressive appearance: These can be indistinguishable from one another by imaging!
  ○ Langerhans cell histiocytosis: Range in appearance from nonaggressive to highly aggressive
  ○ Osteomyelitis
  ○ Leukemia
  ○ Ewing sarcoma, metastatic
  ○ Metastases, bone marrow
  ○ Lymphoma, multifocal
  ○ Osteosarcoma, metastatic
  ○ Chronic recurrent multifocal osteomyelitis

Fibroxanthoma (Non-Ossifying Fibroma)

Anteroposterior radiograph shows a small lytic cortical lesion ➡ (benign fibrous cortical defect) and a sclerotic healing non-ossifying fibroma ➡. The two lesions have the same histology, & the natural history is to heal.

Fibroxanthoma (Non-Ossifying Fibroma)

Oblique radiograph (same patient) shows a lytic cortically based lesion; this is another non-ossifying fibroma, but one which is still active in this child. These images show the 3 expected appearances of this lesion.

POLYOSTOTIC LESIONS, CHILD

Fibrous Dysplasia, Polyostotic

Fibrous Dysplasia, Polyostotic

(Left) Anteroposterior radiograph shows mixed lytic and sclerotic lesion involving the metadiaphysis of the femur, tibia, & fibula. The lesions are central & nonaggressive, typical of fibrous dysplasia. *(Right)* Anteroposterior radiograph shows the mildly expanded and sclerotic, otherwise featureless "ground-glass" appearance of fibrous dysplasia in the tibial diaphysis ➔, with lytic talar lesion ➔ in this teenager with polyostotic fibrous dysplasia.

Langerhans Cell Histiocytosis (LCH)

Langerhans Cell Histiocytosis (LCH)

(Left) Anteroposterior radiograph shows a geographic lytic lesion of the femoral neck ➔. This is compatible with a diagnosis of Langerhans cell histiocytosis (LCH). *(Right)* Lateral radiograph (same child) shows multiple skull lesions. These lesions have a more aggressive appearance, and in fact grew quite rapidly. The polyostotic and relatively geographic appearance overall makes the diagnosis of LCH highly probable, proven in this case.

Osteomyelitis, Pediatric

Osteomyelitis, Pediatric

(Left) Anteroposterior radiograph shows lytic lesions within the metaphysis ➔ which have an aggressive appearance. *(Right)* Lateral radiograph of the contralateral heel in the same patient as previous image, at the same setting, shows lytic lesions within both the metaphysis and apophysis ➔. The metaphyseal location makes hematogenous spread of osteomyelitis the most likely diagnosis, proven here.

POLYOSTOTIC LESIONS, CHILD

Osteochondroma, Multiple Hereditary Exostosis

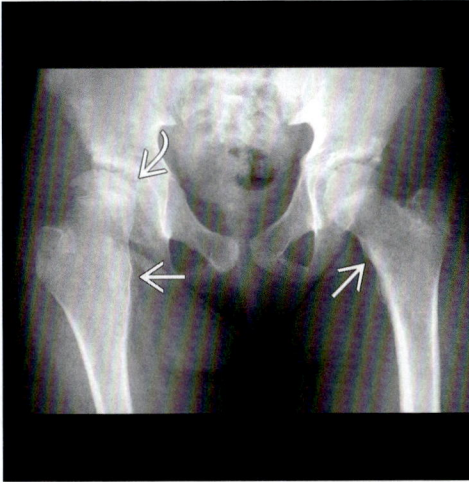

Leukemia

(Left) Anteroposterior radiograph shows sessile osteochondromas along the medial femoral metaphyses ➡ in this teenager. Note the subluxation of the right femoral head ➡; this was proven to be an intraarticular exostosis. *(Right)* AP radiograph shows diffuse osteopenia & metaphyseal lucent lines ➡ in this child. He also had mild compression fractures in the spine. Leukemia may present as diffuse osteopenia rather than focal lesions, as in this case.

Ewing Sarcoma, Metastatic

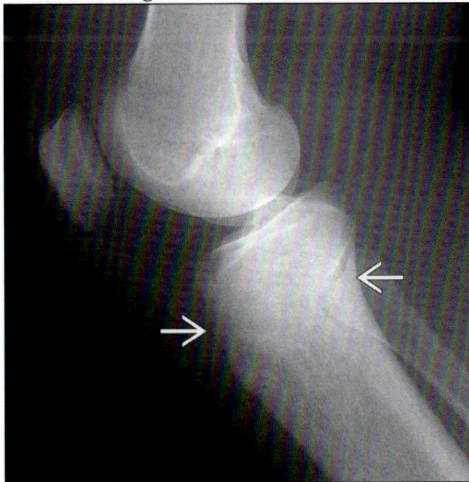

Ewing Sarcoma, Metastatic

(Left) Lateral radiograph shows faint permeative change and sclerosis within the proximal tibia ➡ in a teenager. The lesion is so subtle as to be easily missed; this makes it aggressive. With the reactive sclerosis, Ewing sarcoma is highly probable. *(Right)* Anteroposterior bone scan of the same patient as previous image, shows the tibial lesion, with extended uptake ➡. However, there is also a lesion within the contralateral fibula ➡; the diagnosis is Ewing sarcoma with osseous metastasis.

Metastases, Bone Marrow

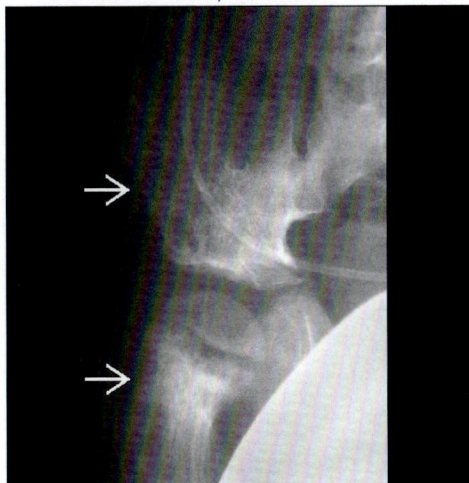

Lymphoma, Multifocal

(Left) AP radiograph shows multiple lesions in a child ➡. These are metaphyseal, suggesting hematogenous spread. The major differential is multifocal osteomyelitis & metastases; the primary was medulloblastoma (note the VP shunt). *(Right)* Axial STIR MR shows polyostotic lesions involving the iliac wings & sacrum in this child. A serpiginous pattern is seen ➡, which is typical. 50% of children developing lymphoma of bone present with polyostotic lesions.

POLYOSTOTIC LESIONS, CHILD

(Left) *Anteroposterior radiograph shows multiple osseous sites of amorphous bone formation ➔ within the spine and pelvis in a teenager whose left hip was disarticulated 1 year earlier for osteosarcoma (note the recurrence in the acetabulum ➔).* ***(Right)*** *Posteroanterior radiograph shows severe renal osteodystrophy in a teenager with end stage renal disease. Besides the subperiosteal and tuft resorption, there are multiple lytic lesions, Brown tumors ➔.*

Osteosarcoma, Metastatic

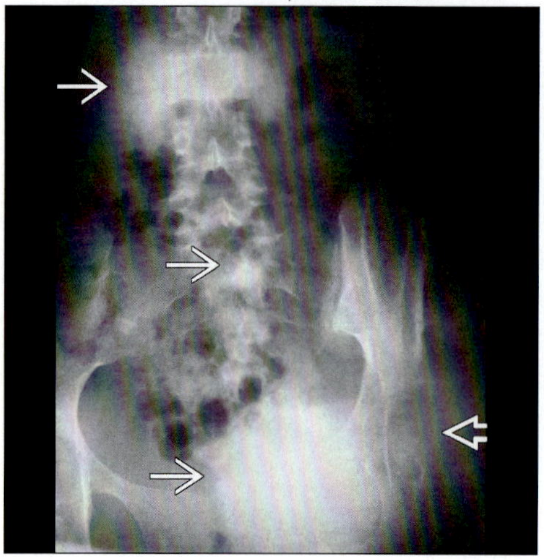

Hyperparathyroidism/Renal Osteodystrophy, Brown Tumor

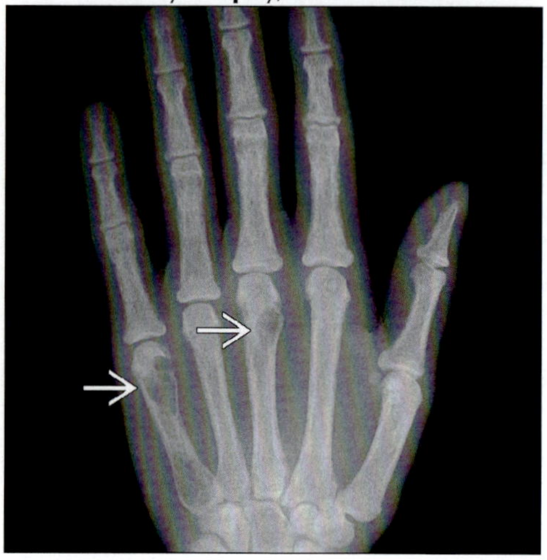

(Left) *Anteroposterior radiograph shows dense sclerotic endosteal bone extending down the femur ➔ with what has been termed a "dripping candle wax" appearance. This is typical melorheostosis, a sclerosing dysplasia.* ***(Right)*** *Oblique radiograph (same patient as previous image) shows linear as well as punctate regions of sclerosis ➔, in a sclerotomal pattern. The lesions are restricted to one extremity (monomelic).*

Melorheostosis

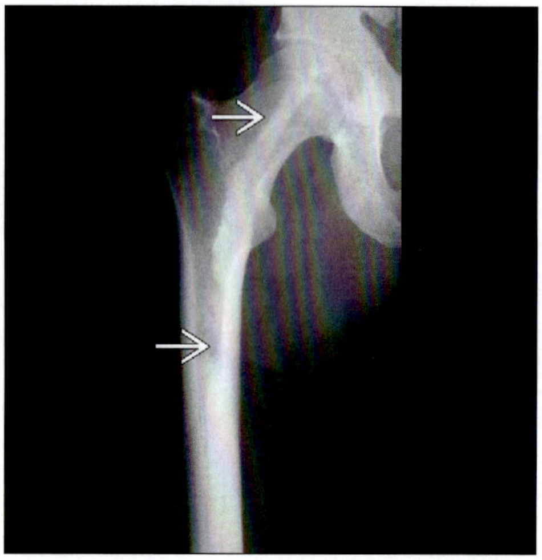

Melorheostosis

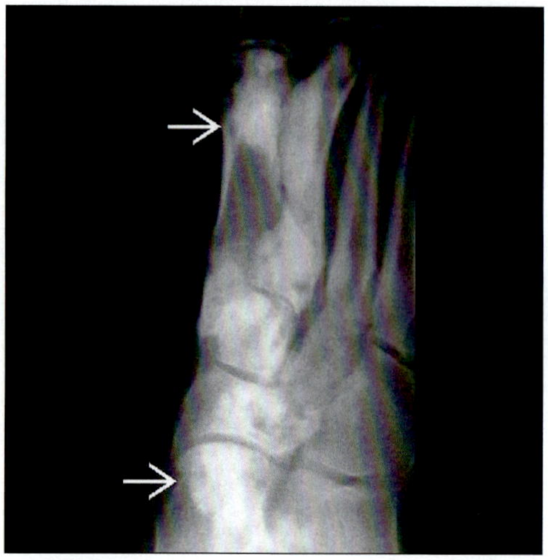

(Left) *Oblique radiograph shows multiple lytic lesions in the hand ➔, some with prominent expansion. These do not have distinct cartilage matrix, but nonetheless are typical for multiple enchondromatosis.* ***(Right)*** *AP radiograph shows a lytic lesion occupying the metaphysis, with faintly seen linear striations ➔. No distinct matrix is seen. Remember that the lesions in Ollier disease often do not have the same appearance as solitary enchondromas.*

Ollier Disease

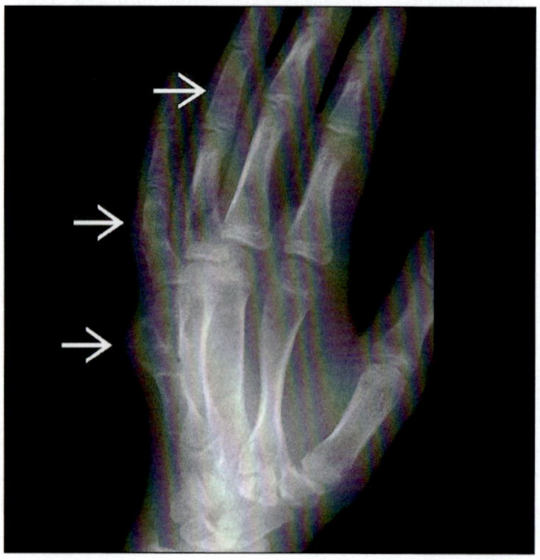

Ollier Disease

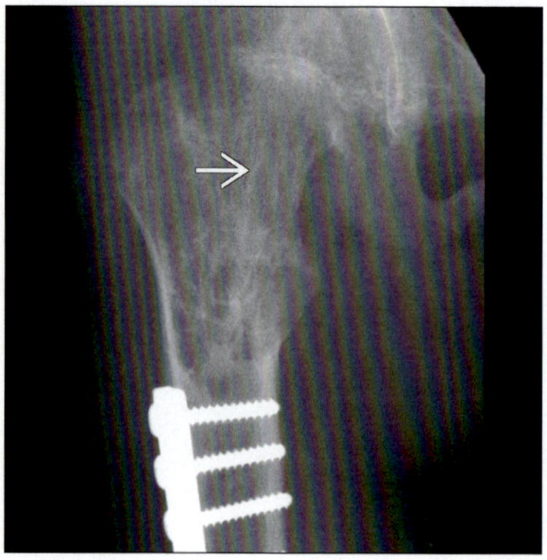

POLYOSTOTIC LESIONS, CHILD

Maffucci Syndrome

Maffucci Syndrome

(Left) Lateral radiograph shows the linear striations within a lytic metaphyseal lesion ➡; note the proximal fibula is abnormal as well. The findings are typical of multiple enchondromatosis. *(Right)* Anteroposterior radiograph (same patient as previous image) shows a lytic lesion in the proximal humerus, as well as phleboliths in the adjacent soft tissues ➡; these change the diagnosis to Maffucci syndrome. Note: Patient is undergoing limb lengthening. (†MSK Req).

Chronic Recurrent Multifocal Osteomyelitis

Sarcoidosis

(Left) Coronal T2WI FS MR shows signal abnormalities in the sacrum ➡, iliac wing ➡, and ischium ➡. There is no soft tissue mass. The patient had chronic pain for 1 year but normal radiograph & no constitutional symptoms. *(Right)* Posteroanterior radiograph shows the lacy lytic lesion ➡ typical of sarcoidosis of the hands and feet. This teen-age patient had lesions in her foot as well, and massive pulmonary fibrosis.

Trevor Fairbank

Trevor Fairbank

(Left) Anteroposterior radiograph shows abnormal bone formation in the ankle ➡. Other radiographs demonstrate this to be intraarticular and attached to the talus. This represents an intraarticular exostosis, or Trevor disease. *(Right)* Anteroposterior radiograph of the hip in the same patient as previous image, shows abnormal ossification arising from the acetabulum ➡. It is not uncommon for Trevor disease to be polyarticular; it is monomelic.

SOLITARY GEOGRAPHIC LYTIC LESIONS

DIFFERENTIAL DIAGNOSIS

Common
- Subchondral Cyst
- Enchondroma
- Metastases, Bone Marrow
- Fibroxanthoma (Non-Ossifying Fibroma)
- Plasmacytoma
- Unicameral Bone Cyst (UBC)
- Giant Cell Tumor (GCT)
- Aneurysmal Bone Cyst (ABC)
- Fibrous Dysplasia
- Chondrosarcoma
- Langerhans Cell Histiocytosis
- Chondroblastoma
- Osteomyelitis

Less Common
- Arthroplasty Component Wear/Particle Disease
- Amyloid Deposition
- Intraosseous Lipoma
- Paget Disease
- Pyrophosphate Arthropathy
- Renal Osteodystrophy
- Osteosarcoma, Telangiectatic
- Osteosarcoma, Conventional

Rare but Important
- Adamantinoma
- Chondromyxoid Fibroma
- Tertiary Syphilis
- Sarcoidosis
- Hemophilia: Pseudotumor
- Osteofibrous Dysplasia
- Benign Peripheral Nerve Sheath Tumor
- Gout
- Pigmented Villonodular Synovitis (PVNS)

ESSENTIAL INFORMATION

Key Differential Diagnosis Issues
- Lucent lesion with narrow zone of transition
  - May be due to intraosseous lesion or erosion of lesion into bone

Helpful Clues for Common Diagnoses
- **Subchondral Cyst**
  - Location around synovial joints
  - Associated findings of subchondral sclerosis, marginal osteophytes, joint space narrowing
- **Enchondroma**
  - Need not have matrix
  - Most common lesion of the phalanx
  - Well-defined and may be mildly expansile
- **Metastases, Bone Marrow**
  - Lack of multiplicity & aggressive features does not exclude metastatic disease
- **Fibroxanthoma (Non-Ossifying Fibroma)**
  - Cortically based, lobulated lesion with narrow zone of transition
  - No aggressive features
- **Plasmacytoma**
  - Solitary myeloma lesion
  - Lytic & bubbly, often with cortical breakthrough
  - Usually lacks a large soft tissue mass
- **Unicameral Bone Cyst (UBC)**
  - Associated fallen fragment sign
- **Giant Cell Tumor (GCT)**
  - Metaphyseal lesion extending to subchondral region of bone
  - Lacks sclerotic margin
- **Aneurysmal Bone Cyst (ABC)**
  - Expansile eccentric lesion, intact cortex
- **Fibrous Dysplasia**
  - Classic well-demarcated lesion with "ground-glass" attenuation
  - Pelvic lesions particularly may be lytic
- **Chondrosarcoma**
  - Cortical thinning or thickening; low grade lesion may appear non-aggressive; no matrix necessary
- **Langerhans Cell Histiocytosis**
  - Elicits periosteal reaction near the lesion
- **Chondroblastoma**
  - Epiphyseal lesion with sclerotic border
  - Often with associated periosteal reaction along the metaphysis
- **Osteomyelitis**
  - Well-defined foci of osteomyelitis are typically due to tuberculosis or fungi
    - Less host reaction & bone destruction than Staphylococcus osteomyelitis

Helpful Clues for Less Common Diagnoses
- **Arthroplasty Component Wear/Particle Disease**
  - Location in bone adjacent to joint replacement
  - Associated findings of polyethylene wear: Narrowing or asymmetry of the liner
- **Amyloid Deposition**
  - Erosion of amyloid deposits into bone

SOLITARY GEOGRAPHIC LYTIC LESIONS

- Patients with end stage renal disease & multiple myeloma
- **Intraosseous Lipoma**
  - Location in long bone metaphysis and calcaneus most common
  - Presence of fat and central calcification differentiates from normal variant or solitary bone cyst
- **Paget Disease**
  - Osteoporosis circumscripta of skull
    - Typical location in frontal & occipital regions
  - Associated findings of widened diploic space & traversed suture lines
- **Pyrophosphate Arthropathy**
  - May result in very large subchondral cysts
  - Associated finding of chondrocalcinosis
- **Renal Osteodystrophy**
  - Lytic lesions in patients with end stage renal disease include Brown tumors, amyloid and gout
  - Subchondral location of these lesions can simulate an erosion or subchondral cyst
- **Osteosarcoma, Telangiectatic**
  - Can have less permeative appearance than conventional osteosarcoma
  - Associated finding of fluid-fluid levels
- **Osteosarcoma, Conventional**
  - Highly aggressive appearance typical
    - Geographic appearance is uncommon except in low grade intraosseous variety

Helpful Clues for Rare Diagnoses
- **Adamantinoma**

- Anterior tibial metadiaphysis
- Multilobulated, expansile lesion
- Associated cortical breakthrough and soft tissue mass
- **Chondromyxoid Fibroma**
  - Multilobulated expansile lesion without cortical breakthrough
- **Hemophilia: Pseudotumor**
  - Pseudotumor can have significant destruction without a permeative pattern
- **Osteofibrous Dysplasia**
  - Similar to adamantinoma & chondromyxoid fibroma; tibial cortex
- **Benign Peripheral Nerve Sheath Tumor**
  - Well-differentiated nerve sheath tissue mass
  - May erode into the adjacent bone
  - Rare intraosseous tumors occur predominantly in the mandible
- **Gout**
  - Masses of crystal deposition typically cause juxtaarticular erosions of bone
  - Depending on the imaging plane on radiographs, erosions can mimic intraosseous lesions
    - Alternatively sodium urate crystals can form masses within subchondral bone
  - Large erosions can cause significant bone destruction, simulating tumor
- **Pigmented Villonodular Synovitis (PVNS)**
  - Intraarticular, nodular masses with blooming signal on gradient echo MR
  - Masses erode adjacent bone, similar to gout

Subchondral Cyst

Anteroposterior radiograph shows cartilage loss in the weight-bearing area of the hip, femoral neck marginal osteophytes and a large subchondral cyst ➡ in the acetabulum, due to osteoarthritis.

Enchondroma

AP radiograph shows a lytic lesion in metaphysis ➡. An enchondroma need not contain radiographically visible chondroid matrix. Without matrix, differential includes SBC, GCT, & ABC. (†MSK Req).

SOLITARY GEOGRAPHIC LYTIC LESIONS

(Left) AP radiograph shows an expanded lytic lesion ➔ in the region of the acetabulum, which normally has a lucent triangle. A solitary lytic lesion in a woman should always lead to consideration of metastatic breast cancer. *(Right)* AP radiograph shows a geographic lytic lesion ➔ in the metadiaphysis of a skeletally immature patient. Lateral view (not shown) shows it is cortically based, non-aggressive and has a narrow zone of transition.

Metastases, Bone Marrow

Fibroxanthoma (Non-Ossifying Fibroma)

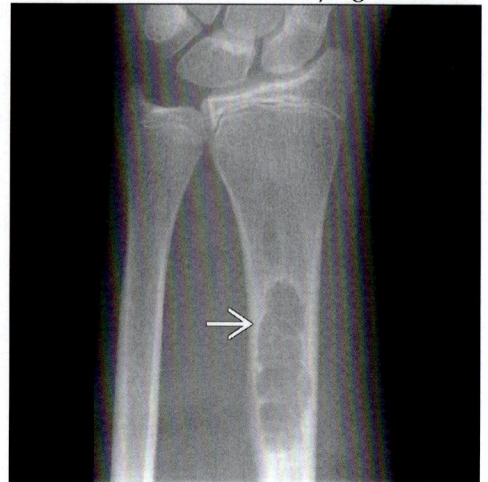

(Left) Anteroposterior radiograph shows a bubbly lesion ➔ occupying the superior pubic ramus and extending well into the acetabulum. In a patient over 50 years of age, metastatic disease or myeloma should be considered first. *(Right)* Anteroposterior radiograph shows a lytic lesion ➔ with sclerotic borders and thinned cortices. This case also shows the fallen fragment sign ➔, due to a fracture fragment within the fluid of the lesion. (†MSK Req).

Plasmacytoma

Unicameral Bone Cyst (UBC)

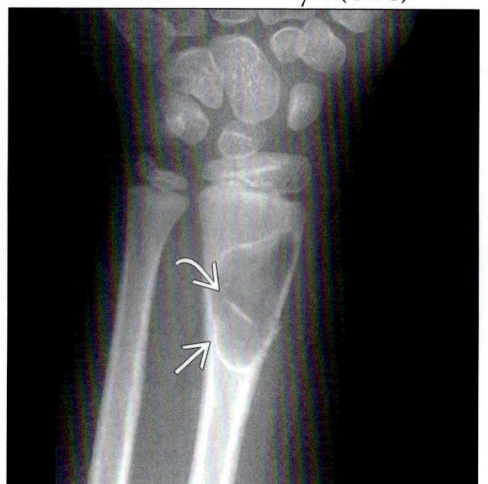

(Left) AP radiograph shows an eccentric metaphyseal lytic lesion ➔ extending to the end of bone. The lesion is geographic, with a narrow zone of transition but no sclerotic margin. This appearance and location is classic for giant cell tumor. *(Right)* Anteroposterior radiograph shows an eccentric, expanded lytic lesion ➔ with intact cortex in a teenager. An MR demonstrated fluid levels typical for an aneurysmal bone cyst.

Giant Cell Tumor (GCT)

Aneurysmal Bone Cyst (ABC)

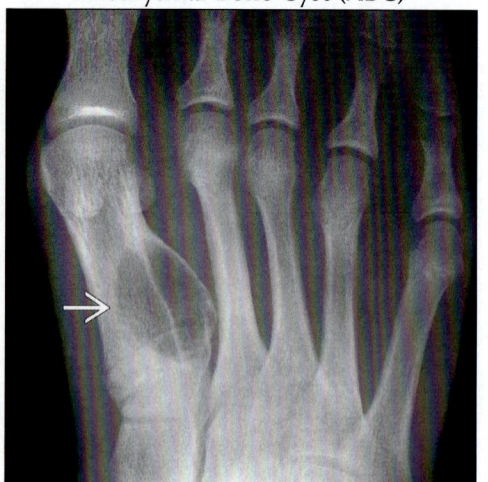

SOLITARY GEOGRAPHIC LYTIC LESIONS

Fibrous Dysplasia

Chondrosarcoma

(Left) Anteroposterior radiograph shows a bubbly expansile lesion ➡, without aggressive features. Bubbly lytic non-aggressive pelvis lesions are typical of fibrous dysplasia. *(Right)* AP radiograph shows a completely lytic lesion in the pelvis ➡, with a pathologic fracture through the superior acetabulum. It is important to remember that chondrosarcoma need not show radiographic evidence of chondroid matrix.

Langerhans Cell Histiocytosis

Chondroblastoma

(Left) AP radiograph shows a lytic geographic lesion ➡ in the proximal humeral metaphysis with periosteal reaction ➡. In this location and young age group, Langerhans cell histiocytosis, infection, and metastatic neuroblastoma should be considered. *(Right)* AP radiograph shows a lytic epiphyseal lesion ➡ without significant chondroid matrix. There is dense periosteal reaction in metaphysis ➡. These findings are classic for chondroblastoma. (†MSK Req).

Osteomyelitis

Arthroplasty Component Wear/Particle Disease

(Left) AP radiograph shows a well-defined lesion ➡ with soft tissue swelling ➡, and no periosteal reaction. This suggests a slower process than is usually seen with bacterial osteomyelitis. Blastomycosis was the infecting agent. *(Right)* Coronal bone CT shows acetabular lysis ➡ from particle disease. Note the offset of the femoral head in the cup on the superolateral side ➡ compared with the inferomedial side ➡, indicating polyethylene wear.

SOLITARY GEOGRAPHIC LYTIC LESIONS

(Left) Sagittal T2WI MR shows a humeral head erosion ➡. Rotator cuff tendons are thick & uniformly low in signal ➡. Biopsy confirmed amyloid deposition in this patient with end stage renal disease. (†MSK Req). (Right) Lateral radiograph shows a lucent lesion ➡, containing a central calcific density ⮊. Lytic calcaneal lesions in this location usually represent normal variant, bone cyst, or lipoma; a central calcific density confirmed lipoma.

Amyloid Deposition

Intraosseous Lipoma

(Left) Lateral radiograph shows a geographic lytic region in the occiput ➡. The skull shows a diffusely widened diploic space ⮊. Osteoporosis circumscripta is an early destructive phase of Paget disease of the skull. (Right) Anteroposterior radiograph shows osteophyte formation, cartilage narrowing, and a large lytic lesion in the medial tibial plateau ➡. Chondrocalcinosis ➡ leads one to consider the diagnosis of pyrophosphate arthropathy.

Paget Disease

Pyrophosphate Arthropathy

(Left) Lateral radiograph shows diffuse mottled density in the bones due to bone infarcts ⮊ and a lytic lesion of the anterior distal femoral metaphysis ➡ due to a Brown tumor in this patient with end stage renal disease. (Right) Oblique radiograph shows a lytic lesion with fairly geographic borders ➡ extending to the end of the bone. Cortical breakthrough and soft tissue mass were subtle findings. Telangiectatic osteosarcoma is not as permeative as classic osteosarcoma.

Renal Osteodystrophy

Osteosarcoma, Telangiectatic

SOLITARY GEOGRAPHIC LYTIC LESIONS

Adamantinoma

Chondromyxoid Fibroma

(Left) Anteroposterior radiograph shows an expansile lytic lesion ➔ with sclerotic margins. Cortical destruction and a soft tissue mass were visible with CT, suggesting the diagnosis of adamantinoma. *(Right)* Anteroposterior radiograph shows an eccentric, expansile, lytic lesion ➔ in the tibial metadiaphysis, without cortical breakthrough. The large size is unusual for a chondromyxoid fibroma. (†MSK Req).

Hemophilia: Pseudotumor

Osteofibrous Dysplasia

(Left) Anteroposterior radiograph shows a highly expanded lytic lesion ➔ of the right iliac wing. This is typical of pseudotumor; despite the extensive destructive change, there is no permeative pattern. *(Right)* Lateral radiograph shows a geographic lytic lesion ➔ in the proximal tibial diaphysis with cortical breakthrough ➔ anteriorly. The differential diagnosis includes chondromyxoid fibroma, osteofibrous dysplasia, and adamantinoma.

Benign Peripheral Nerve Sheath Tumor

Gout

(Left) Anteroposterior radiograph shows a lytic lesion in the capitellum ➔. Peripheral nerve sheath tumors may excavate the cortex of adjacent bone, but frank bone invasion such as was proven in this case is distinctly uncommon. *(Right)* Lateral radiograph shows a large erosion or lytic lesion within the patella ➔. Biopsy proved gout in this patient with end stage renal disease.

SCLEROTIC BONE LESION, SOLITARY

DIFFERENTIAL DIAGNOSIS

Common
- Enostosis (Bone Island)
- Stress or Insufficiency Fracture
- Fibroxanthoma (Non-Ossifying Fibroma)
- Bone Infarct
- Enchondroma
- Osteoma
- Osteoid Osteoma
- Osteosarcoma, Conventional
- Intraosseous Lipoma
- Metastases, Bone Marrow

Less Common
- Paget Disease
- Cement & Bone Fillers
- Ewing Sarcoma
- Osteosarcoma, Parosteal
- Osteosarcoma, Periosteal
- Lymphoma, Hodgkin Disease
- Fibrous Dysplasia, Skull Base
- Liposclerosing Myxofibrous Tumor
- Osteitis Condensans of Clavicle

Rare but Important
- Sarcoidosis
- Mastocytosis

ESSENTIAL INFORMATION

Key Differential Diagnosis Issues
- Differential for solitary sclerotic bone lesion is wide
  ○ Ranges from malignant to "leave me alone" lesions
  ○ Important to differentiate; may depend on clinical factors or, finally, biopsy
- Location may be an important differentiating factor
  ○ Some of the lesions are site specific
  ○ Most are site-preferred
- It is crucial to differentiate type of sclerosis if possible
  ○ If matrix, osteoid vs. chondroid
  ○ Dystrophic or reactive sclerosis

Helpful Clues for Common Diagnoses
- **Enostosis (Bone Island)**
  ○ Sub-centimeter to giant (10 cm); most frequently metaphyseal
  ○ Homogeneously sclerotic, featureless, with edges "fading" into normal bone
  ○ Low signal on all MR sequences, non-enhancing
- **Stress or Insufficiency Fracture**
  ○ Best clue is linear pattern of sclerosis; fracture line may be obscured by healing callus
  ○ Fracture line seen well on T1 MR; may be obscured on fluid sensitive sequences
- **Fibroxanthoma (Non-Ossifying Fibroma)**
  ○ Cortically based, metadiaphyseal; location is best clue
  ○ Natural history is for the lytic lesion to heal; it often appears mildly sclerotic prior to development of normal trabecular pattern
- **Bone Infarct**
  ○ Metaphyseal, metadiaphyseal, or subchondral
  ○ When dystrophic calcification is present, may be focal or serpiginous; serpiginous pattern is fairly specific
- **Enchondroma**
  ○ Metaphyseal, metadiaphyseal
  ○ Best clue: Usually contains chondroid matrix: Punctate densities, C's & J's
- **Osteoma**
  ○ Homogeneously densely sclerotic, featureless, like bone island
  ○ Best clue: Usually calvarial or within paranasal sinuses
  ○ May see on long bones in patients with polyposis syndrome; appearance may be similar to melorheostosis
- **Osteoid Osteoma**
  ○ May have central sclerotic nidus within lytic lesion
  ○ In long bone, nidus is cortically-based
    ▪ Surrounding sclerosis in diaphyseal lesion may obscure nidus
    ▪ May be difficult to differentiate from healing stress fracture by radiograph
    ▪ CT or MR differentiates the two
- **Osteosarcoma, Conventional**
  ○ Eccentric, metaphyseal
  ○ Best clue: Subtle, amorphous osteoid matrix is formed in bone & soft tissue mass; immature & appears aggressive
  ○ Other aggressive features: Periosteal reaction, permeative bone destruction, soft tissue mass

SCLEROTIC BONE LESION, SOLITARY

Helpful Clues for Less Common Diagnoses

- **Paget Disease**
  - Rarely appears purely sclerotic; lytic active component generally present
  - Watch for active edge of lesion (blade-of-grass)
  - Usually originates at one end of long bone, advancing away from subchondral bone
- **Cement & Bone Fillers**
  - Generally seen within a geographic (curetted) lesion
  - Cement: Homogeneous sclerosis: Featureless
  - Bone graft: Either structural (large piece of bone) or multiple small pieces, often squared
- **Ewing Sarcoma**
  - Lesion itself is lytic & highly permeative, with aggressive periosteal reaction & soft tissue mass
  - May elicit tremendous reactive bone formation
    - Reactive bone may simulate tumor osteoid, but it is contained entirely within the bone
    - No bone formation within soft tissue mass; differentiates from osteosarcoma
- **Osteosarcoma, Parosteal**
  - Location is constant: Metadiaphyseal, distal femur > proximal tibia > proximal femur > proximal humerus
  - Surface lesion, but usually involves some marrow
  - Tumor osteoid is more mature bone than conventional osteosarcoma
  - Zoning of tumor bone formation: More mature centrally, less mature peripherally
- **Osteosarcoma, Periosteal**
  - Surface lesion, no marrow involvement
  - Metadiaphyseal
  - Tumor osteoid is more mature than conventional osteosarcoma, but less than parosteal
  - Often scallops underlying cortex
- **Fibrous Dysplasia, Skull Base**
  - Dense homogeneous bone: May be slightly ground-glass & less densely sclerotic than osteoma
  - Density is different from the mild ground glass appearance in long bones or lytic bubbly fibrous dysplasia of pelvis
  - Involved bone is usually enlarged, as in all cases of fibrous dysplasia
- **Liposclerosing Myxofibrous Tumor**
  - Location specific: Neck of femur
  - Geographic; variably sclerotic or mixed lytic/sclerotic
- **Osteitis Condensans of Clavicle**
  - Proximal clavicular sclerosis, without soft tissue mass or manubrial abnormality

Helpful Clues for Rare Diagnoses

- **Sarcoidosis**
  - Rarely may present as focal sclerotic bone: Dense, inhomogeneous
- **Mastocytosis**
  - Focal sclerotic presentation rare

Enostosis (Bone Island)

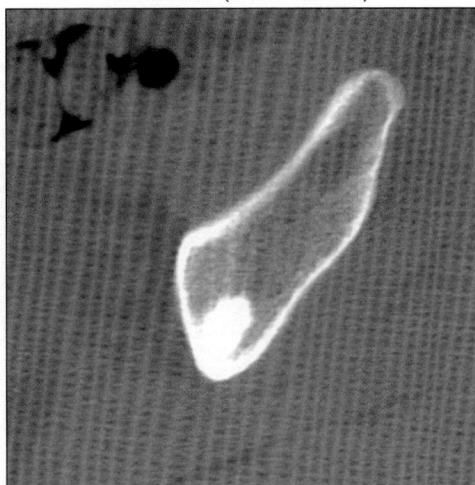

Axial NECT shows a solitary densely sclerotic lesion. Note that the edge of the lesion is not completely geographic, but rather somewhat spiculated, fading out into the adjacent normal bone. This is typical.

Stress or Insufficiency Fracture

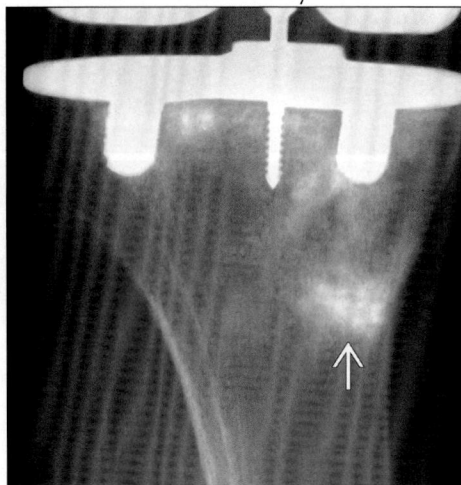

Anteroposterior radiograph shows a patient who is osteopenic & has a knee arthroplasty, putting her at risk for insufficiency fracture. Note the subtle linear pattern of the sclerotic lesion ➡, confirming fracture.

SCLEROTIC BONE LESION, SOLITARY

Fibroxanthoma (Non-Ossifying Fibroma)

Bone Infarct

(Left) Anteroposterior radiograph shows a cortically based elongated metaphyseal lesion which is mildly sclerotic ➡. This is a fibroxanthoma, undergoing the natural course of healing with sclerosis. These lesions are common. *(Right)* Lateral radiograph shows an irregularly-shaped densely sclerotic metaphyseal lesion ➡. It has a somewhat serpiginous pattern, which is characteristic although not a required feature of bone infarct.

Enchondroma

Osteoma

(Left) Anteroposterior radiograph shows a metaphyseal lesion containing punctate sclerotic densities ➡. There is no sclerotic margin, though the lesion has a geographic appearance. This chondroid lesion is a classic enchondroma. *(Right)* Axial NECT shows a densely sclerotic, rather featureless lesion of the cranium ➡, typical of osteoma. These hamartomas are usually located in a paranasal sinus or the calvarium.

Osteoid Osteoma

Osteoid Osteoma

(Left) Coronal bone CT shows a densely sclerotic nidus located centrally within a lytic lesion ➡. Lesion was intensely hot on bone scan, & was extremely painful. The appearance & clinical presentation is typical of osteoid osteoma. *(Right)* Lateral radiograph shows a densely sclerotic cortically based lesion ➡. Osteoid osteoma of the tubular bones may elicit so much reactive bone formation that it obscures the lytic nidus. This nidus is seen by MR or CT. (†MSK Req).

SCLEROTIC BONE LESION, SOLITARY

Osteosarcoma, Conventional

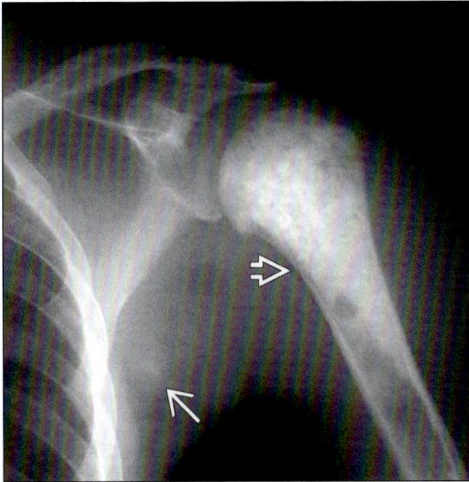

Osteosarcoma, Conventional

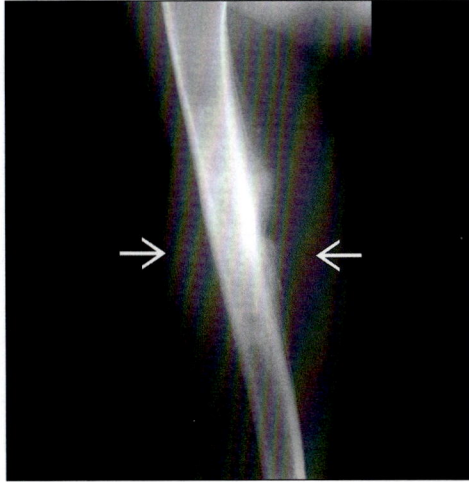

(Left) Anteroposterior radiograph shows dense osteoid formation within a permeative lesion of the humerus ➡. There is a wide zone of transition & soft tissue mass, as well as an ossified lymph node metastasis ➡. *(Right)* Anteroposterior radiograph shows amorphous osteoid formation within the bone, with cortical breakthrough and osteoid formation within a large soft tissue mass ➡. The presence of immature osteoid confirms the diagnosis of osteosarcoma.

Intraosseous Lipoma

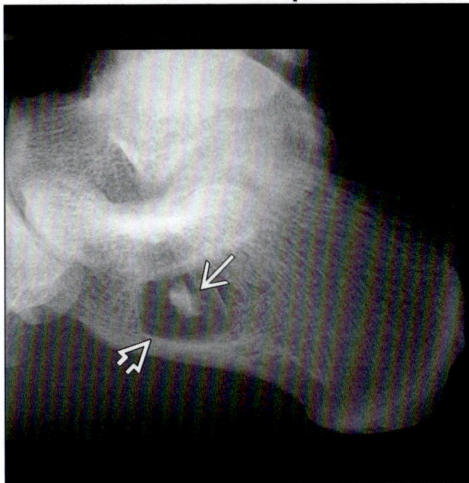

Metastases, Bone Marrow

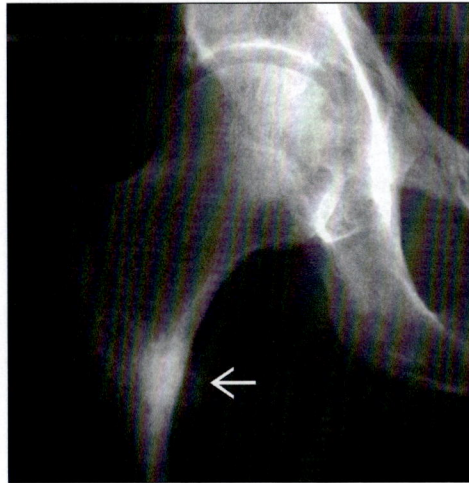

(Left) Lateral radiograph shows a geographic lytic lesion in the central calcaneus ➡ containing a central sclerotic nidus ➡. Location & appearance are pathognomonic for intraosseous lipoma. (†MSK Req). *(Right)* AP radiograph shows an amorphous sclerotic lesion occupying the lesser trochanter ➡. Although lesion fades off into normal bone, as is seen in a bone island, the destructive change at medial border helps secure dx of metastatic prostate carcinoma.

Paget Disease

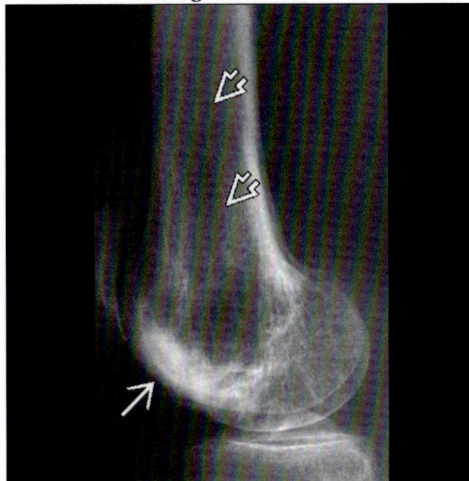

Paget Disease

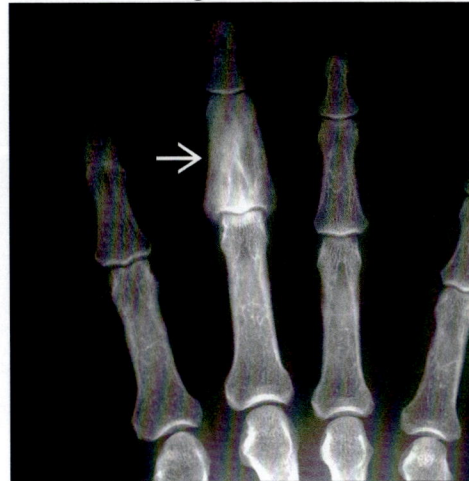

(Left) Lateral radiograph shows a densely sclerotic focus in the subchondral bone ➡. However, there is an additional clue; there is an adjacent lytic region, demarcated by a sharp "blade of grass" ➡, making the diagnosis of Paget disease. *(Right)* AP radiograph shows an isolated densely sclerotic phalanx ➡. The bone is expanded, with thickened trabeculae. There is no destructive change. Findings are typical of Paget disease, despite the somewhat unusual location.

SCLEROTIC BONE LESION, SOLITARY

Cement & Bone Fillers

Cement & Bone Fillers

(Left) AP radiograph shows cement ➡ placed following curettage for giant cell tumor (GCT). The cement has a smooth, homogeneous appearance, & should not be mistaken for a matrix-producing tumor. Note local recurrence of the lytic GCT ➡. *(Right)* AP radiograph shows bone chips ➡ placed following curettage of a GCT. Some of the chips are squared, suggesting they are not matrix, but iatrogenic. There is a tumor recurrence ➡.

Ewing Sarcoma

Ewing Sarcoma

(Left) AP radiograph shows dense sclerosis of the epiphysis ➡ in a child. Axial imaging demonstrated a soft tissue mass and permeative lytic lesion in the metaphysis, typical of Ewing sarcoma. Remember that this disease can elicit tremendous osseous reaction. *(Right)* Axial NECT shows a sclerotic lesion occupying a portion of S1 in a child ➡. This could represent either osteoid formation in osteosarcoma, or reactive bone in Ewing sarcoma; the latter was proven.

Osteosarcoma, Parosteal

Osteosarcoma, Periosteal

(Left) Lateral radiograph shows a sclerotic surface lesion arising at the posterior distal metaphysis ➡. Axial imaging confirmed the surface origin and zoning pattern diagnostic of parosteal osteosarcoma. *(Right)* Anteroposterior radiograph shows fairly mature osteoid matrix arising from the surface of the tibial metadiaphysis ➡. Axial imaging is important to confirm the pattern of bone formation and lack of marrow involvement.

SCLEROTIC BONE LESION, SOLITARY

Lymphoma, Hodgkin Disease

Fibrous Dysplasia, Skull Base

(Left) *Lateral radiograph shows a sclerotic lesion in the vertebral body* ➔*, demonstrated to be Hodgkin disease. This process is most frequently sclerotic; primary lymphoma of bone may be lytic or mixed.* *(Right)* *Axial bone CT shows dense "ground-glass" sclerosis of the maxilla and skull base* ➔*. The bones are expanded. The lesion is not as sclerotic as with an osteoma. This is a typical appearance of fibrous dysplasia in this location.*

Liposclerosing Myxofibrous Tumor

Osteitis Condensans of Clavicle

(Left) *Anteroposterior radiograph shows a well-marginated sclerotic lesion located in the femoral neck* ➔*. This case of LSMFT is predominantly sclerotic; others are mixed lytic-sclerotic. Location is a prime factor in considering the diagnosis.* *(Right)* *Axial NECT shows sclerosis of the distal clavicle* ➔*, compared with the normal left side* ➔*. The adjoining manubrium was normal, eliminating infection as a possibility. The lesion was stable over 1 year.*

Sarcoidosis

Mastocytosis

(Left) *Anteroposterior radiograph shows a homogeneous dense sclerotic lesion within the femoral head (trocar present for biopsy). Rarely, osseous sarcoid may present as a sclerotic lesion.* *(Right)* *Anteroposterior radiograph shows a densely sclerotic, enlarged diaphysis of the clavicle* ➔*. The patient had GI and skin symptoms which led to the diagnosis of mastocytosis, biopsy proven.*

SCLEROTIC BONE LESIONS, MULTIPLE

DIFFERENTIAL DIAGNOSIS

Common
- Metastatic, Breast
- Metastatic, Prostate
- Metastatic, Lung
- Multiple Healing Rib Fractures (Mimic)
- Paget Disease
- Enostosis (Bone Island)
- Bone Infarct
- Brown Tumors, Healing
- Fibrous Dysplasia, Skull
- Metastatic, Osteosarcoma
- Metastatic, Medulloblastoma
- Fibroxanthoma (NOF), Healing
- Melorheostosis
- Osteopoikilosis

Less Common
- Osteoma
- Renal Osteodystrophy, Neostosis
- Hyperparathyroidism (Mimic)
- Hyperparathyroidism, Treated
- Metastatic, Lymphoma
- Metastatic, Carcinoid

Rare but Important
- Sarcoidosis
- Mastocytosis
- POEMS
- Tuberous Sclerosis

ESSENTIAL INFORMATION

Key Differential Diagnosis Issues
- Diagnosis ranges from malignant (metastases) to benign, to "leave me alone" lesions (bone islands)
- Clues which may help differentiate
  - Patient age
  - Clinical information, esp. known primary tumors or metabolic bone disease
  - Specific location of lesions
- If necessary, MR or PET CT may differentiate active lesions (such as metastases) from inactive lesions (such as bone islands)

Helpful Clues for Common Diagnoses
- **Sclerotic Metastases**
  - Most common: Breast, prostate
  - Less common: Lung, Hodgkin disease, lymphoma, carcinoid, medulloblastoma, osteosarcoma, transitional cell, GI tumors

- Lung metastases are more frequently lytic, but sclerotic mets are seen in non-small cell lung cancer
  - **Hint**: Expect to see common diseases with uncommon appearances
  - Location of metastases: Axial, shoulder girdle, pelvis, proximal humeri & femora
  - Compared with bone islands, at least some lesions should enhance on MR or appear active on PET CT
- **Multiple Healing Rib Fractures (Mimic)**
  - Healing may be bulky & round, obscure the fracture line, & mimic sclerotic lesions
  - **Hint**: Generally multiple & in a linear pattern in adjacent ribs
- **Paget Disease**
  - Usually the pattern is mixed lytic & sclerotic, but mature Paget disease may result in homogeneous sclerosis
  - **Hint**: Location in long bones (end of bone, extending to subchondral surface, with abrupt cut-off adjacent to normal bone)
  - **Hint**: Enlargement of bone
  - Skull pattern of round "cotton wool" sclerotic foci is classic; foci appear "fuzzier" at margin than sclerotic metastases
- **Enostosis (Bone Island)**
  - May have several foci, scattered without a pattern to suggest osteopoikilosis
  - Characteristics are same as solitary bone island, dense sclerosis, fading at edges
  - Inactive lesion on MR or PET CT
- **Bone Infarct**
  - Different patterns; some easy to diagnose
    - Most difficult: Patchy but homogeneous sclerosis, most often in femoral or humeral head: Early AVN, particularly in sickle cell patients
    - Diffuse increased density: Often overlooked, but not confused with sclerotic bone lesions; most often in sickle cell patients
    - Serpiginous dystrophic calcification, usually metaphyseal: Rarely may be confused with enchondroma, but not other sclerotic bone lesions
- **Fibrous Dysplasia, Skull**
  - Fibrous dysplasia usually has different manifestations in different parts of body
  - Skull: Sclerotic foci (base of skull most frequent, but may involve cranium)

○ Sclerotic foci in the skull may be homogeneously dense, or may be slightly less dense than an osteoma, tending towards a "ground-glass" opacity
○ **Hint**: Enlarged bone, polyostotic in 50%
• **Fibroxanthoma (NOF), Healing**
○ May occasionally be multiple, especially in patients with neurofibromatosis
○ Natural history is to heal in (sclerosis → normal trabeculation)
○ **Hint**: Location is cortical & metaphyseal
• **Melorheostosis**
○ **Hint**: Watch for pattern of involvement
  ▪ Linear, endosteal or periosteal, monomelic
• **Osteopoikilosis**
○ Metaphyseal, round

Helpful Clues for Less Common Diagnoses
• **Osteoma**
○ Multiple in polyposis syndromes
• **Renal Osteodystrophy, Neostosis**
○ Renal osteodystrophy (ROD) may show focal sclerosis of bone, at various stages of disease, with various etiologies
  ▪ ROD, active: Generally osteopenic, but osteoblast activation may result in superimposed generalized sclerosis; foci may be seen (Rugger jersey spine)
  ▪ ROD, treated: New bone formation
○ **Hint**: Watch for other manifestations
  ▪ Resorptive processes: Subperiosteal, subligamentous, subchondral
  ▪ Soft tissue calcification

▪ Bowed bones, protrusio hips
▪ Evidence of dialysis (central line, peritoneal catheter, shunt)
• **Hyperparathyroidism (Mimic)**
○ a.k.a. HPTH, active: Generally osteopenic, in skull may develop a trabecular resorptive pattern which leaves punctate sclerotic foci ("salt & pepper" skull)
• **Hyperparathyroidism, Treated**
○ HPTH & ROD, healing: New bone is formed which may appear patchy, often along with periosteal new bone
○ HPTH & ROD, healing: New bone fills in Brown tumors, often appearing hyperossified (distinct, round sclerotic foci); these may remain sclerotic or eventually develop normal trabeculae

Helpful Clues for Rare Diagnoses
• **Sarcoidosis**
○ Rare osseous manifestation: Sclerotic foci
○ **Hint**: Skin involvement highly likely; pulmonary involvement less likely
• **Mastocytosis**
○ Rarely may develop sclerotic bone foci
○ **Hint**: Clinical manifestations of skin rash, episodic vomiting & diarrhea
• **POEMS**
○ Homogeneous sclerotic or sclerotic rim
○ Clinical: Peripheral neuropathy, organomegaly, endocrinopathy, skin manifestations

Metastatic, Breast

Anteroposterior radiograph shows multiple sclerotic (as well as lytic) lesions in this young woman with pathologic fx. The presence of axillary clips helps secure the diagnosis of metastatic breast cancer. (†MSK Req).

Metastatic, Prostate

Coronal bone CT shows multiple sclerotic lesions scattered through the axial skeleton & pelvis ➡. There are clips in the pelvis from inguinal node dissection; this is sclerotic metastatic prostate cancer.

SCLEROTIC BONE LESIONS, MULTIPLE

Metastatic, Lung

Multiple Healing Rib Fractures (Mimic)

(Left) Sagittal MIP shows diffuse small sclerotic metastases scattered throughout the vertebrae and sternum ➡. The primary lung cancer (non-small cell) is seen on the same image ➡. *(Right)* PA radiograph shows multiple sclerotic "lesions" of the ribs ➡. These sclerotic foci are aligned in a linear fashion, making it clear that they are healing rib fractures rather than metastases in this patient who happens also to have a primary cancer.

Paget Disease

Paget Disease

(Left) Anteroposterior radiograph shows sclerosis and enlargement of both the clavicle ➡ and axillary border of the scapula ➡. Both of these lesions are mature sclerotic foci of Paget disease. *(Right)* Lateral radiograph shows multiple rounded, rather fuzzy-appearing sclerotic lesions, along with generalized thickening of the cranium. This is the "cotton wool" appearance typically seen in late Paget disease of the skull.

Bone Infarct

Brown Tumors, Healing

(Left) Anteroposterior radiograph shows multiple sclerotic foci ➡, representing the relative sclerosis of bone infarcts in a patient with sickle cell anemia. The contralateral hip showed collapse, indicating a higher grade of AVN. *(Right)* Anteroposterior radiograph shows multiple sclerotic lesions throughout the pelvis of a young man. The patient is on dialysis for end stage renal disease, and these are healed Brown tumors.

SCLEROTIC BONE LESIONS, MULTIPLE

Fibrous Dysplasia, Skull

Metastatic, Osteosarcoma

(Left) Axial bone CT shows right maxillary & pterygoid replacement by ground-glass sclerosis ➡, typical of fibrous dysplasia of the skull. Note the bones are enlarged. 50% of skull lesions in fibrous dysplasia are polyostotic. *(**Right**)* Anteroposterior radiograph shows amorphous bone formation in two vertebral bodies, left iliac wing, & left pubis, all sites of metastasis from osteosarcoma. Note the disarticulated left hip, treatment for the primary 1 year earlier.

Metastatic, Medulloblastoma

Fibroxanthoma (NOF), Healing

*(**Left**)* Lateral radiograph shows sclerotic ulnar lesion with prominent sunburst type of periosteal reaction ➡. This child had medulloblastoma; osseous metastases may be lytic, sclerotic, or mixed. *(**Right**)* Anteroposterior radiograph shows multiple cortically based nonossifying fibromas, in the sclerotic phase of healing ➡. This is the natural history of these lesions, and they generally eventually acquire normal trabeculation. The patient had neurofibromatosis.

Melorheostosis

Osteopoikilosis

*(**Left**)* Anteroposterior radiograph shows linear as well as rounded sclerotic densities which were confined to the left extremity. This is melorheostosis, one of the sclerosing dysplasias. *(**Right**)* Axial NECT shows multiple small rounded sclerotic densities. If MR were performed, they would be low signal on all sequences. When bone islands are clustered in the metaphyses like this, it is termed osteopoikilosis.

SCLEROTIC BONE LESIONS, MULTIPLE

Osteoma

Osteoma

(Left) Anteroposterior radiograph shows multiple osteomas arising from the cortex of the femur ⇗. The patient had similar lesions on the contralateral femur. *(Right)* Oblique radiograph shows osteoma of the mandible ⇘ in the same patient as previous image. Multiple osteomas may be seen in patients with polyposis, termed Gardner syndrome.

Renal Osteodystrophy, Neostosis

Hyperparathyroidism (Mimic)

(Left) Anteroposterior radiograph shows generalized bone sclerosis, plus sclerotic osseous excrescences ➡. This is neostosis, which may occur with effective treatment of end stage renal disease. *(Right)* Lateral radiograph of the skull shows the "salt & pepper" pattern of trabecular resorption in hyperparathyroidism. The appearance is of multiple round sclerotic lesions, but it is due to resorption around residual bone.

Hyperparathyroidism, Treated

Metastatic, Lymphoma

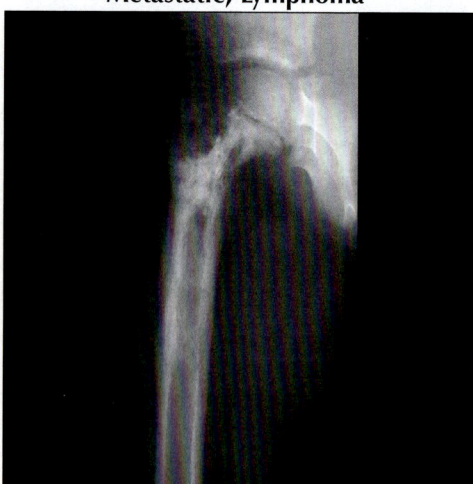

(Left) Lateral radiograph shows several smudgy areas of sclerosis ➡ within bones which show generalized increased density. This patient had a parathyroidectomy for intractable hyperparathyroidism, and the sclerosis shows healing of bone. *(Right)* AP radiograph shows a sclerotic aggressive lesion in the metadiaphysis of a child. This is a case of polyostotic lymphoma; 50% of childhood bone lymphoma presents with multiple lesions.

SCLEROTIC BONE LESIONS, MULTIPLE

Metastatic, Carcinoid

Sarcoidosis

(Left) Axial bone CT shows two of the multiple densely sclerotic lesions in this patient with known carcinoid. The lesions are typical of the osseous metastases in this disease. *(Right)* Anteroposterior radiograph shows two sites of osseous sclerosis ➡, without other features, in a patient with sarcoidosis. Sarcoid occasionally presents with sclerotic bone lesions, as in this case, but more frequently the lesions are lytic.

Mastocytosis

Mastocytosis

(Left) Lateral radiograph shows an ivory vertebral body, without enlargement or other distinguishing features. There was another sclerotic focus in the lumbar spine. Mastocytosis may present with sclerotic osseous lesions. *(Right)* Anteroposterior radiograph shows multiple sclerotic lesions, some rather confluent to give the appearance of generalized sclerosis in this patient with mastocytosis. (†MSK Req).

POEMS

POEMS

(Left) Anteroposterior radiograph shows one large and several subcentimeter round sclerotic skull lesions ➡. Metastatic disease should certainly be considered, but this proved to be POEMS, or sclerotic myeloma. *(Right)* Anteroposterior radiograph shows a mixture of multiple sclerotic lesions, and others which are lytic with a sclerotic rim. This is one manifestation of POEMS, the rare sclerosing myeloma. (†MSK Req).

SCLEROTIC LESION WITH CENTRAL LUCENCY

DIFFERENTIAL DIAGNOSIS

Common
- Osteoid Osteoma
- Fibroxanthoma (Non-Ossifying Fibroma)
- Stress Fracture, Adult
- Paget Disease
- Bone Infarct

Less Common
- Chronic Osteomyelitis
- Enchondroma
- Loose Bodies (Mimic)

Rare but Important
- Osteoblastoma
- Langerhans Cell Histiocytosis
- POEMS
- Tertiary Syphilis

ESSENTIAL INFORMATION

Helpful Clues for Common Diagnoses
- **Osteoid Osteoma**
  - Highly vascular nidus of osteoid tissue (lucency) surrounded by reactive bone (sclerosis)
    - Intracortical, intramedullary or subperiosteal
    - Less reactive bone when intraarticular (femoral neck) than when located in diaphyseal cortex
    - Nidus can calcify
  - > 50% in tibia and femur
  - 90% of cases age < 25 years
- **Fibroxanthoma (Non-Ossifying Fibroma)**
  - Eccentric, parallel to long axis of bone
  - Ovoid or lobulated lesion
    - Greater than 2 cm
    - Sclerotic medullary margin
  - Metaphyses of lower extremities most common
  - Spontaneous healing of lesions
    - Sclerosis varies based on stage of healing
    - Tends to progress peripheral to central
    - Healed lesions may persist as regions of sclerosis or develop normal trabeculation
- **Stress Fracture, Adult**
  - Appearance dependent on location and duration of injury
  - Localized cortical thickening of tubular bones
    - Periosteal reaction along shaft

- Fracture line not always evident
  - Typical location in tibia and metatarsals
  - Pain worsened by activity
- **Paget Disease**
  - Cortical thickening with bone enlargement is typical
  - Mixed sclerotic and lytic lesions
    - Reparative phase
    - More common than purely sclerotic phase
  - Sclerotic phase causes uniform areas of increased density
    - "Cotton wool" skull
    - "Ivory" vertebral body
- **Bone Infarct**
  - Dense bone in the medullary space
  - Serpiginous or "smoke up the chimney" outline with lucent center
  - Proximal or distal long bones
    - Metaphyseal most common
    - Can extend to subchondral plate
  - Associated with steroids, alcohol use + numerous other disease states

Helpful Clues for Less Common Diagnoses
- **Chronic Osteomyelitis**
  - Mixed osteosclerotic and osteolytic lesions with periosteal reaction
  - Solitary lesion with sequestrum is classic
  - Can have multiple lesions
  - Metaphyseal or diaphyseal location
  - Cortical thickening, periosteal new bone
- **Enchondroma**
  - Lytic lesion with chondroid matrix
    - Located in medullary cavity
    - Single or multiple lesions
    - Expansile without cortical breech or periosteal reaction, excluding pathologic fracture
    - Epiphyses spared when skeletally immature
  - Pattern of matrix can outline central lucency
  - Can mimic a bone infarct when heavily calcified
  - 50% in tubular bones of hand
    - Proximal phalanges
    - Mid to distal metacarpals
  - Transformation to chondrosarcoma is rare
- **Loose Bodies (Mimic)**
  - Osteochondral fragments
  - Vary in number and size

SCLEROTIC LESION WITH CENTRAL LUCENCY

- Synovial osteochondromatosis = numerous loose bodies due to synovial metaplasia
  - Distribution limited to extent of joint space
    - Can be mobile or fixed to synovium
  - Ossified ± central lucency
    - Solidly ossified loose bodies projected over other bones on radiographs can artifactually simulate sclerotic lesion with lucent center
  - May have accelerated arthritis due to associated prior injury or impingement

Helpful Clues for Rare Diagnoses

- **Osteoblastoma**
  - Large osteoid osteoma, > 1.5 to 2 cm
  - > 50% involve vertebral body posterior elements
  - Can have central lucency or calcification
  - Majority show cortical expansion and reactive sclerosis
  - Unlikely to spontaneously regress as osteoid osteomas may
- **Langerhans Cell Histiocytosis**
  - Abnormal proliferation of Langerhans cell histiocytes in reticuloendothelial system
  - Single or multiple lesions, rapid growth
  - Predilection for skull, mandible, ribs, femur, pelvis, spine
  - Lesion is generally lytic
  - Healing lesion may develop peripheral sclerosis, giving the appearance of a sclerotic lesion with central lucency

- Healing lesions can appear similar to fibrous dysplasia
- **POEMS**
  - **P**olyneuropathy, **O**rganomegaly, **E**ndocrinopathy, **M** protein, **S**kin changes
  - Solitary or multiple lesions
  - At ligamentous attachment sites, lesions appear as fluffy, spiculated hyperostosis
  - Multiple lesions in a similar location to standard lytic myeloma show sclerosis ± central lucency
- **Tertiary Syphilis**
  - Osteitis and osteomyelitis from Treponema pallidum spirochetes
  - Skull involvement = lucency or sclerosis of outer table, relatively preserved inner table
    - Worm-eaten appearance on CT
  - Gummatous destruction of bone with periosteal reaction and sclerosis is seen late in disease

Alternative Differential Approaches

- Sclerotic lesion with central lucency which is solitary
  - Osteoid osteoma, stress fracture, chronic osteomyelitis, enchondroma, osteoblastoma, secondary syphilis
- Sclerotic lesions with central lucency which may be either solitary or multiple
  - Fibroxanthoma (non-ossifying fibroma), Paget disease, bone infarct, loose body, Langerhans cell histiocytosis, POEMS
- Sclerotic lesions with central lucency which are generally multiple: POEMS, Paget disease

Osteoid Osteoma

Lateral radiograph demonstrates a markedly thickened, sclerotic anterior tibial cortex ➡. Within this oblong region of sclerosis, there is a focal lucency ➡. This lucency represents the osteoid osteoma nidus.

Fibroxanthoma (Non-Ossifying Fibroma)

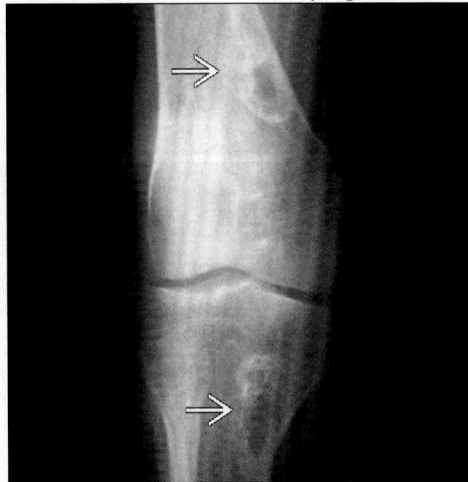

Oblique radiograph shows two metaphyseal, cortically based lesions which are sclerotic with a central lucency ➡. These are partially healed nonossifying fibromas, sclerosing from the periphery.

SCLEROTIC LESION WITH CENTRAL LUCENCY

Stress Fracture, Adult

Stress Fracture, Adult

(Left) Axial bone CT shows periosteal bone formation with focus of lucency ➡. This lucency continued longitudinally down the femur, consistent with a stress fracture. Note: Osteoid osteoma, stress fracture & osteomyelitis can be indistinguishable on a single axial CT image. *(Right)* Coronal bone CT (same patient as previous) shows central longitudinal lucency of the stress fracture ➡, surrounded by thick cortex. This reconstruction helps define the stress fracture.

Stress Fracture, Adult

Paget Disease

(Left) Anteroposterior radiograph shows a linear lucency ➡ surrounded by sclerosis. One does not usually visualize a stress fracture this distinctly, but this runner refused to rest his leg. *(Right)* Lateral radiograph shows a sclerotic vertebral body with central lucency ➡. This is the mixed phase of Paget disease, not as advanced as the classic "picture frame"; a bone scan indicated the patient had two other lesions as well.

Bone Infarct

Chronic Osteomyelitis

(Left) Axial NECT of both proximal tibias show serpiginous dystrophic calcification, with central lucency, typical of bone infarcts ➡. *(Right)* Axial NECT is suboptimal, since it was obtained using soft tissue technique. However, it shows a focal lucency ➡ with sequestrum in the thickened, sclerotic tibial cortex ➡ in this patient with chronic osteomyelitis. Also note inflammatory stranding in the adjacent subcutaneous fat.

SCLEROTIC LESION WITH CENTRAL LUCENCY

Enchondroma

Enchondroma

(Left) Lateral radiograph shows a ring-like sclerotic lesion, with apparent central lucency ➡. The sclerosis is chondroid matrix; occasionally the matrix is arranged such that there is central non-calcified cartilage. *(Right)* Sagittal PD FSE FS MR (same patient as previous image) shows the low signal ring of calcified chondroid matrix ➡, being surrounded by lobular cartilage in this classic enchondroma, incidentally noted on MR.

Loose Bodies (Mimic)

Osteoblastoma

(Left) Anteroposterior radiograph of the left hip shows a sclerotic lesion with central lucency ➡ projected over the femoral head. On cross sectional imaging, the density was shown to represent a loose body. *(Right)* Axial NECT shows mild expansion of the sacrum by a peripherally sclerotic lesion ➡ with central lucency ➡ and osteoid matrix. The presence of osteoid matrix favors osteoblastoma over aneurysmal bone cyst or chordoma.

Langerhans Cell Histiocytosis

POEMS

(Left) Anteroposterior radiograph shows a sclerotic lesion in the ischium with central lucency ➡. Langerhans cell histiocytosis normally is lytic, but this patient was treated with low dose radiation, and the sclerosis indicates healing. *(Right)* Anteroposterior radiograph shows multiple lytic lesions with sclerotic rims ➡, along with purely sclerotic lesions. This is a variant appearance of POEMS, or sclerosing myeloma. (†MSK Req).

SEQUESTRATION

DIFFERENTIAL DIAGNOSIS

Common
- Chronic Osteomyelitis
- Osteoid Osteoma (Mimic)
- Langerhans Cell Histiocytosis
- Lymphoma

Less Common
- Fibrosarcoma
- Malignant Fibrous Histiocytoma, Bone
- Metastases, Bone Marrow
- Removed Hardware
- Bisphosphonate-Related Osteonecrosis
- Intraosseous Hemangioma (Mimic)
- Charcot, Neuropathic

Rare but Important
- Pseudohypoparathyroidism
- Chordoma
- Tertiary Syphilis
- Vascular Channel

ESSENTIAL INFORMATION

Key Differential Diagnosis Issues
- Classically, sequestrum refers to devascularized bone surrounded by purulent material
- Lytic lesions with radiodense foci can have similar appearance to true sequestra on radiographs & CT
  - Calcific densities due to residual bone fragments
  - Calcification from chondroid matrix
  - Dystrophic calcification
  - Ossification

Helpful Clues for Common Diagnoses
- **Chronic Osteomyelitis**
  - True sequestrum of necrotic bone surrounded by viable infectious material
    - Seen in subacute to chronic osteomyelitis
  - Poorly defined lytic lesion with cortical destruction
  - Enhancement of surrounding tissue
  - Periosteal reaction common
  - Sinus tracts develop to extrude the sequestrum
- **Osteoid Osteoma (Mimic)**
  - Typically a well-defined lytic lesion with surrounding sclerosis
  - Can have calcification of the central nidus

- Prominent smooth surrounding sclerosis is typical unless lesion is intraarticular
- **Langerhans Cell Histiocytosis**
  - Geographic lesions
  - Lack sclerotic border
  - May contain button sequestrum (especially skull)
  - Polyostotic in about 25% of cases
    - Polyostotic lesions may be less aggressive
- **Lymphoma**
  - Permeative destruction of bone with sequestrum in 11%
  - Disproportionally large soft tissue mass
    - Intact bone cortex; may be thickened
  - Metaphysis or diaphysis of long, tubular bones, with pelvis second most common

Helpful Clues for Less Common Diagnoses
- **Fibrosarcoma**
  - Relatively uncommon diagnosis that commonly has a sequestrum related to residual bone fragment
  - Eccentric, metaphyseal location typical
  - Expands marrow space with endosteal scalloping
  - Can appear similar to osteomyelitis
- **Malignant Fibrous Histiocytoma, Bone**
  - Metaphysis of long bones
  - Similar radiographic appearance to fibrosarcoma
    - Sequestrum less common in this entity than seen in fibrosarcoma
    - Residual calcification of infarct may mimic sequestrum
  - Can simulate osteomyelitis
- **Metastases, Bone Marrow**
  - Nidus of residual bone in lytic lesion
  - Metastatic lesions are typically multiple and varying in size
  - Can be seen with any primary malignancy producing lytic metastases
    - Breast carcinoma most commonly have button sequestra
  - Cortical destruction and soft tissue mass are associated findings
- **Removed Hardware**
  - Lucent region from prior instrumentation
  - Central dystrophic calcification along tract
    - Alternatively, infection along tract
  - Typical pattern of pin, screw or rod holes with evidence of prior trauma or surgical intervention

SEQUESTRATION

- **Bisphosphonate-Related Osteonecrosis**
  - Poorly circumscribed, mixed sclerotic and lytic lesion in mandible or maxilla
  - Lacks periosteal reaction or soft tissue mass (differentiate from osteomyelitis, metastases)
- **Intraosseous Hemangioma (Mimic)**
  - Well-circumscribed lytic lesion without periosteal reaction/cortical breakthrough
  - Coarse vertical trabeculae can simulate punctate bone sequestra on axial imaging
  - Common location in vertebral body
    - Uncommonly extend into pedicles, as metastases frequently do
- **Charcot, Neuropathic**
  - "Six D's"
    - Normal bone **density**
    - Joint **distention**
    - **Destruction** of joint or cartilage
    - **Deformity**
    - **Debris** (may mimic sequestrum)
    - **Dislocation**
  - Location suggests etiology
    - Shoulder = syringomyelia
    - Spine = cord injury, diabetes, syphilis
    - Hip = alcohol, syphilis
    - Knee = insensitivity to pain, steroid injection, syphilis
    - Foot & ankle = diabetes

Helpful Clues for Rare Diagnoses
- **Pseudohypoparathyroidism**
  - Multiple lytic lesions with button sequestra, especially in skull
  - Short fourth & fifth metacarpals/tarsals
  - Calcification in basal ganglia & dentate nuclei
  - Pseudo-pseudohypoparathyroidism has same radiographic appearance
- **Chordoma**
  - Midline axial skeletal lesions from notochord remnants
  - May be very large at presentation, especially in sacrum
  - Bone destruction with soft tissue extension
  - Intratumoral calcification = residual bone fragments
- **Tertiary Syphilis**
  - Neuropathic joint disease
  - Late neurosyphilis = tabes dorsalis
    - Predilection for hip, knee & ankle
- **Vascular Channel**
  - Intraosseous vascular loop surrounds an island of normal bone
  - Tubular nature is evident on axial imaging

Alternative Differential Approaches
- Button Sequestrum in Skull
  - Langerhans cell histiocytosis
  - Metastases
  - Hemangioma
  - Meningioma
  - Epidermoid or dermoid cyst
  - Osteomyelitis
  - Radiation necrosis
  - Osteonecrosis of craniotomy sites
  - Burr hole
  - Pseudohypoparathyroidism

Chronic Osteomyelitis

Anteroposterior radiograph shows an oval lytic lesion ➡ with central density ➡ representing a sequestrum, plus prominent periosteal reaction ➡ and marrow osseous reactive bone, typical of osteomyelitis.

Osteoid Osteoma (Mimic)

Axial bone CT shows a sharply demarcated lesion in the neural arch ➡ containing bone matrix and surrounding reactive sclerosis. Lesions with central ossification or calcification ➡ can mimic a sequestrum.

SEQUESTRATION

Langerhans Cell Histiocytosis

Lymphoma

(Left) Anteroposterior radiograph shows multiple calvarial lesions ➡ with beveled edges. It is not pathognomonic for Langerhans cell histiocytosis but is typical and is a useful finding when present. Sequestra ➡ are common. *(Right)* Lateral radiograph shows a permeative lesion involving the diaphysis of the femur with cortical thickening posteriorly ➡ and scalloped endosteum anteriorly ➡. A sequestrum ➡ favors primary bone lymphoma.

Fibrosarcoma

Malignant Fibrous Histiocytoma, Bone

(Left) Anteroposterior radiograph shows a highly destructive lytic lesion ➡ involving both sides of the pubic symphysis. There is no matrix, but internal residual bone fragments ➡ mimic sequestra. *(Right)* Lateral radiograph shows a lytic lesion ➡ arising in the central diaphysis. There is a wide zone of transition, cortical breakthrough, host reaction, and a small sequestrum ➡. These findings are not specific beyond appearing aggressive.

Metastases, Bone Marrow

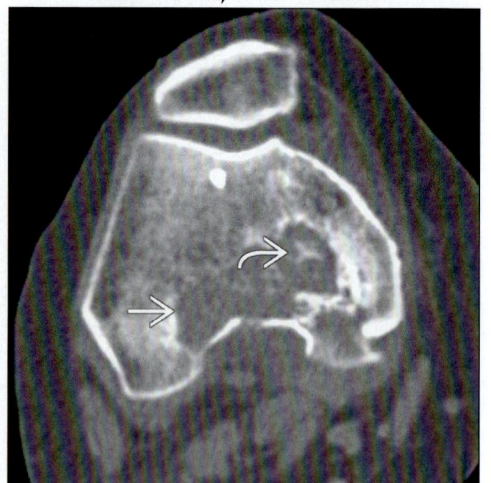

Metastases, Bone Marrow

(Left) Axial NECT shows a predominately lytic mass involving the vertebral body ➡ and left facet & lamina of C3. This has the typical "soap bubble" appearance of metastatic thyroid carcinoma. Residual internal bone trabeculae ➡ mimic sequestra. *(Right)* Axial bone CT shows a lytic lung carcinoma metastasis ➡ in the distal femur. Small foci of calcification in the lesion ➡ represent residual bone fragments rather than matrix, and appear as sequestra.

SEQUESTRATION

Removed Hardware

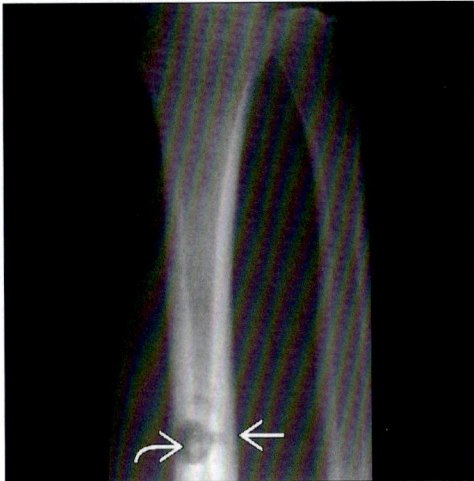

Bisphosphonate-Related Osteonecrosis

(Left) Anteroposterior radiograph shows an old thin pin tract ➡, which has widened into a round lytic lesion with central sclerosis ➡. The central sclerosis is a sequestrum in this pin tract infection. *(Right)* Axial NECT shows a mixed sclerotic and lytic ➡ mandibular lesion, at the site of a recent tooth extraction. Note the cortical loss ➡ and sequestrum ➡ in the defect, typical for mandibular osteonecrosis in a patient taking long-term IV bisphosphonates.

Intraosseous Hemangioma (Mimic)

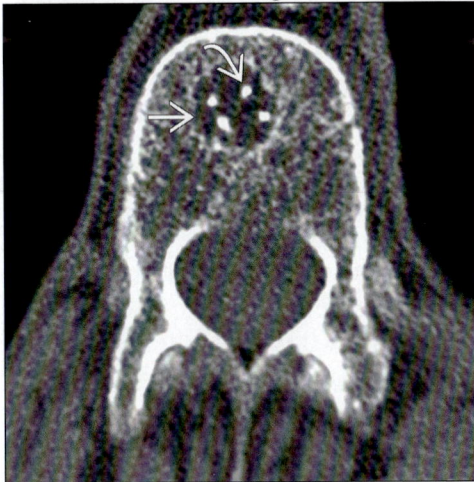

Charcot, Neuropathic

(Left) Axial bone CT shows typical hemangioma characteristics of a well-circumscribed lytic lesion ➡ with sparse, even, thickened trabeculae ➡ mimicking sequestra. *(Right)* Axial bone CT shows chronic L5 vertebral body fracture ➡ with exuberant osteophytes and bone debris. Destruction and debris is also centered around the facet joints ➡. Bone destruction and debris ➡ mimics chronic osteomyelitis with sequestra.

Pseudohypoparathyroidism

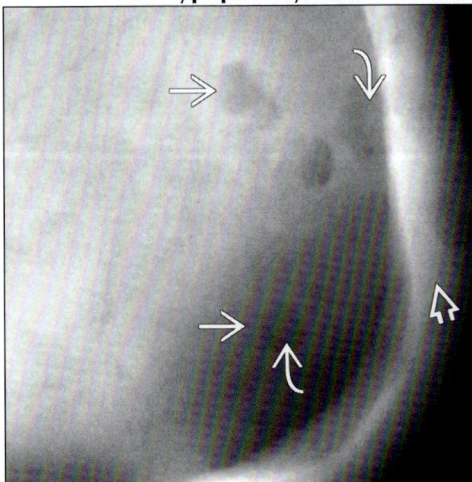

Chordoma

(Left) Lateral radiograph shows multiple calvarial lytic lesions ➡, suggestive of multiple myeloma. However, many of these lytic lesions contain radiodense "button" sequestra ➡ and the skull is thickened ➡, which is not expected in myeloma and suggests the true diagnosis. *(Right)* Axial CECT demonstrates complete destruction of the clivus ➡. There is no significant calcified matrix with the bulk of the lesion but small bony "sequestra" (retained fragments) are present ➡.

39

TARGET LESIONS OF BONE

DIFFERENTIAL DIAGNOSIS

Common
- Osteoid Osteoma
- Intraosseous Lipoma
- Pinhole Sequestra
- Chronic Osteomyelitis
- Fracture Healing Process
- Cement & Bone Fillers, Normal
- Cement & Bone Fillers, Complications

Less Common
- Metastases, Bone Marrow
- Liposclerosing Myxofibrous Tumor
- Bone Infarct
- Enchondroma
- Chondroblastoma
- Chondrosarcoma
- Arthroplasty Loosening & Dislocation (Mimic)
- Chordoma
- Pseudohypoparathyroidism

Rare but Important
- Dermoid Cyst, Skull
- Aneurysmal Bone Cyst

ESSENTIAL INFORMATION

Key Differential Diagnosis Issues
- Lytic lesion of bone with central radiodensity from any cause (calcification, ossification, bone fragment)
- Location & associated findings most helpful for differentiation

Helpful Clues for Common Diagnoses
- **Osteoid Osteoma**
  - Classic: Lucent central nidus within bone cortex may itself have central calcification
  - Surrounding reactive bone sclerosis
- **Intraosseous Lipoma**
  - Well-defined lytic lesion containing fat
  - Typical location in the calcaneus
  - Presence of central calcification differentiates from normal area of bone with paucity of trabeculae
- **Pinhole Sequestra**
  - After removal of pins, screws and rods, central area can calcify
  - Infection along a hardware tract may produce a bone sequestrum centrally within the pin track

- **Chronic Osteomyelitis**
  - Sequestrum of devitalized bone surrounded by infectious material produces target appearance
  - Poorly defined lytic lesion with marked enhancement of surrounding tissues
  - Associated findings of periosteal reaction, sinus tract, skin ulceration
  - Appearance is not pathognomonic for infection, as malignancy can have an identical appearance
- **Fracture Healing Process**
  - Irregular endosteal bone healing or irregular external bone callus may surround bone fragments
- **Cement & Bone Fillers, Normal**
  - Can have a normal halo of lucency at cement-bone interface
  - Lucency will remain stable relative to immediate postoperative images
- **Cement & Bone Fillers, Complications**
  - Tumor recurrence along border of curettage & cement packing
  - Lucency at cement-bone interface progresses from postoperative appearance

Helpful Clues for Less Common Diagnoses
- **Metastases, Bone Marrow**
  - Breast metastases are most likely to have central bone fragments
  - Osteosarcoma metastases produce osteoid
  - Metastases in various stages of both healing and progression may have alternating regions of lucency & sclerosis
  - Associated findings of soft tissue mass, cortical destruction, additional lesions of varying size
- **Liposclerosing Myxofibrous Tumor**
  - Classic location in proximal metadiaphysis of femur
  - Lytic lesion containing fat & calcification, confirm with CT
  - Sclerotic border, no aggressive features
- **Bone Infarct**
  - Dense medullary bone in metaphyses of long bones
  - Tends to have serpiginous borders, rather than smooth target appearance
  - No cortical destruction, soft tissue mass, or cortical breakthrough unless malignant transformation
- **Enchondroma**

TARGET LESIONS OF BONE

- ○ Central chondroid matrix in medullary lytic lesion (cortical lesions less common)
- ○ Typical location in hands
- ○ Associated findings of bone expansion or pathologic fracture when occurring in small tubular bones
- **Chondroblastoma**
  - ○ Focal lytic lesion with internal chondroid matrix occurring at end of bone in skeletally immature patient
  - ○ Associated findings of thin sclerotic border, geographic bone destruction & periosteal reaction in metaphysis, distant from epiphyseal lesion
- **Chondrosarcoma**
  - ○ Ill-defined, destructive lytic lesion with chondroid matrix
  - ○ Associated findings of endosteal scalloping or cortical breakthrough, ring & arc calcification; non-mineralized cartilaginous tumor hypodense to muscle
- **Arthroplasty Loosening & Dislocation (Mimic)**
  - ○ Component failure with migration of portions of prosthesis within joint
  - ○ Lucency from particle disease rarely has central calcification or bone fragments
- **Chordoma**
  - ○ Midline lytic lesion containing residual osseous fragments
    - Sacral chordomas more likely to have target appearance than vertebral lesions
- **Pseudohypoparathyroidism**

- ○ Uncommon entity but common central calcification of the multiple lytic lesions
- ○ Associated findings of short metacarpals & metatarsals and basal ganglia & dentate nuclei calcification

Helpful Clues for Rare Diagnoses
- **Dermoid Cyst, Skull**
  - ○ Well-defined lytic lesion containing mature skin & fat
  - ○ Predilection for sutures & diploic region
  - ○ No enhancement
- **Aneurysmal Bone Cyst**
  - ○ Expansile lytic lesion, central regions of dystrophic calcification may rarely be seen
  - ○ Associated findings of fluid-fluid levels, sclerotic border, septations & intact cortex, unless pathologic fracture

Alternative Differential Approaches
- Reverse target lesions of bone
  - ○ Sclerotic bone lesion with lucent center
    - Osteoid osteoma
    - Fibroxanthoma (non-ossifying fibroma)
    - Stress fracture
    - Paget disease
    - Bone infarct
    - Chronic osteomyelitis
    - Enchondroma
    - Loose bodies
    - Osteoblastoma
    - Langerhans cell histiocytosis
    - POEMS
    - Tertiary syphilis

Osteoid Osteoma

Axial NECT shows a classic osteoid osteoma in the femoral neck. It demonstrates the lytic lesion within the anterior cortex of the femoral neck, with a sclerotic nidus sitting within the lesion ➡. (†MSK Req).

Intraosseous Lipoma

Lateral radiograph shows a lytic calcaneal lesion ➡ with a central sclerotic nidus ➡. Although this region often is relatively lucent because of normal trabecular pattern, this is a true geographic lesion. (†MSK Req).

TARGET LESIONS OF BONE

Pinhole Sequestra

Chronic Osteomyelitis

(Left) Anteroposterior radiograph demonstrates an old, thin, pin tract ➡, which has widened into a round lytic lesion with central sclerosis ⇨. The central sclerosis is a sequestrum in this pin tract infection. *(Right)* Lateral radiograph shows a region of irregular lucency ⇨ surrounding a more sclerotic piece of bone ➡. This is a focus of osteomyelitis with a sequestrum seen centrally. (†MSK Req).

Cement & Bone Fillers, Complications

Metastases, Bone Marrow

(Left) Anteroposterior radiograph shows bone chips ➡ which have been placed following curettage of a giant cell tumor. Residual or recurrent tumor is seen at the periphery ➡ causing an eccentric target sign. *(Right)* Axial CECT shows metastatic osteosarcoma ➡ to the sacrum and ilium. The sacral lesion has a target appearance due to the formation of osteoid matrix.

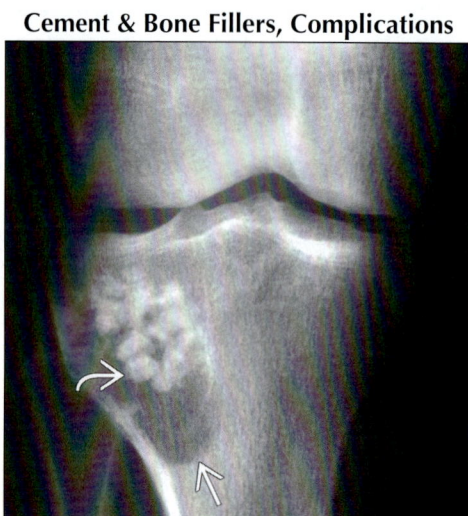

Liposclerosing Myxofibrous Tumor

Bone Infarct

(Left) Axial NECT shows a lesion in the intercondylar region of the femoral neck with geographic borders and central sclerotic matrix ⇨. Additionally, fat is present within the lesion ➡. These have rare malignant transformation. *(Right)* Axial NECT shows a bone infarct ➡ in the right tibia with a target appearance. A bone infarct in the left tibia shows cortical breakthrough ⇨, due to degeneration into a malignant fibrous histiocytoma.

TARGET LESIONS OF BONE

Enchondroma

Chondroblastoma

(Left) AP radiograph shows a small, expansile, lytic lesion with a small central density ➡ that resembles a target. This case is unusual; enchondromas are more commonly located in the medullary space than in the cortex. *(Right)* AP radiograph shows a lytic lesion in the epiphysis ➡ containing small foci of calcific matrix ➡. There is prominent dense periosteal reaction in the metaphyseal region ➡, giving an overall appearance of chondroblastoma. (†MSK Req).

Chondrosarcoma

Arthroplasty Loosening & Dislocation (Mimic)

(Left) Anteroposterior radiograph shows a pathologic fracture ➡ through a large lytic lesion ➡ containing dense central matrix ➡. This expansile lesion has thinned the cortex suggesting it was originally slow growing but cortical breakthrough indicates more recent increased activity. *(Right)* Anteroposterior radiograph shows a rounded density located superior to the patella ➡, representing dissociation of the metal backing from the patellar button.

Chordoma

Pseudohypoparathyroidism

(Left) Axial CECT shows a large lytic lesion ➡ destroying the majority of the sacrum and extending into the adjacent soft tissues ➡. Amorphous intratumoral calcification ➡ has a target appearance and is due to bone destruction. *(Right)* Lateral radiograph shows multiple lytic lesions of the skull ➡, some of which contain central sclerosis ➡ giving a target appearance. When seen in the skull, this central calcification is termed button sequestra.

MATRIX-CONTAINING BONE LESIONS

DIFFERENTIAL DIAGNOSIS

Common
- Enchondroma
- Bone Infarct
- Osteochondroma
- Fibrous Dysplasia
- Osteosarcoma, Conventional
- Osteoid Osteoma
- Chondrosarcoma, Conventional
- Fibroxanthoma (Non-Ossifying Fibroma), Healing
- Fracture Callus Formation, Early
- Osteosarcoma, Parosteal
- Intraosseous Lipoma
- Malignant Fibrous Histiocytoma, Bone
- Periosteal Chondroma
- Osteosarcoma, Periosteal
- Liposclerosing Myxofibrous Tumor (LSMFT)

Less Common
- Radiation-Induced Sarcoma
- Paget Degeneration to Osteosarcoma
- Osteoblastoma
- Chondroblastoma
- Chondromyxoid Fibroma
- Ollier Disease
- Maffucci Syndrome

ESSENTIAL INFORMATION

Key Differential Diagnosis Issues
- For the purpose of this topic, differential diagnosis excludes hamartomatous bone formation (enostosis, osteoma)
- **Hint**: Differentiate by the type and degree of aggressiveness of matrix
  - Bone-producing (osteoid)
    - Aggressive: Amorphous, immature bone; barely visible density, less dense than normal bone
    - Less aggressive: More dense osteoid, forming recognizable bone, sometimes with trabeculae (more mature)
    - Less aggressive tumor bone formation may have a zoning pattern: More mature bone centrally, less mature peripherally
  - Cartilage-producing (chondroid)
    - Punctate matrix, often denser than bone
    - Described as "C's & arcs", ring-like

- If a portion of lesion shows less organization of matrix, termed "snowstorm", it is more aggressive
  - Mixed osteoid and chondroid elements
    - No discernible separate elements; gives smooth opaque ground-glass appearance
    - No trabeculae seen
  - Dystrophic calcification (matrix mimic)
    - Often globular, but may be serpiginous; generally denser than bone
- **Hint**: Use the degree of aggressiveness of the underlying lesion as a differentiating factor between benign and malignant lesions

Helpful Clues for Common Diagnoses
- **Enchondroma**
  - Conventional
    - Ranges from dense punctate matrix to fine, subtle matrix or entirely lytic
    - Small bones of hand/foot or metaphysis/metadiaphysis tubular bones
    - Appears geographic because of matrix, but no sclerotic margin or true demarcating structure
  - **Ollier Disease**
    - May be typical enchondroma, or may have striated appearance in metaphyses
    - Generally monomelic; short extremity
  - **Maffucci Syndrome**
    - Same as Ollier, + soft tissue hemangioma
- **Bone Infarct**
  - May be lytic, but often develops dystrophic calcification
  - Classic pattern of serpiginous dense Ca++
  - May assume other forms difficult to differentiate from enchondroma
- **Osteochondroma**
  - Must have normal bone marrow and cortex extending into excrescence
  - May have chondroid matrix in the more peripheral portions
- **Fibrous Dysplasia**
  - May have calcification of small spicules of osteoid and chondroid
    - Leads to the ground-glass appearance of smooth increased density without trabeculation
  - Density of ground-glass component varies
    - Depends on amount of calcified osteoid and chondroid
    - Therefore not surprising to see different densities, even in same patient

MATRIX-CONTAINING BONE LESIONS

- **Osteosarcoma, Conventional**
  - Aggressive tumor osteoid, amorphous & immature; may be quite subtle
  - Secondary: Most frequently degeneration of Paget or radiated bone; Tumor osteoid is immature, aggressive, and amorphous
- **Osteosarcoma, Parosteal**
  - Mature osteoid, often containing trabeculae
  - Zoning of lesion with more mature bone centrally than peripherally
- **Osteosarcoma, Periosteal**
  - Intermediate grade of maturation of osteoid; may be spiculated
- **Chondrosarcoma, Conventional**
  - When matrix is present, it is chondroid
  - High grade lesion: Chondroid matrix in obvious soft tissue mass
  - May not be able to differentiate low grade central chondrosarcoma & enchondroma
- **Malignant Fibrous Histiocytoma, Bone**
  - Degeneration of bone infarct may → MFH
  - Dystrophic calcification of infarct is seen, often with lytic destructive change arising in a portion of it
- **Fracture Callus Formation, Early**
  - Early callus is amorphous osteoid
    - Same appearance as tumor osteoid radiographically & histologically
  - Generally can see fracture and avoid confusion; osteopenic bone or pathologic fractures are potentially difficult

Alternative Differential Approaches

- Divide into types of matrix and degrees of aggressiveness of matrix
  - Osteoid, aggressive
    - Conventional osteosarcoma
    - Fracture callus, early
    - Radiation or Paget-induced osteosarcoma
  - Osteoid, less aggressive
    - Parosteal osteosarcoma
    - Osteoid osteoma
    - Osteoblastoma
    - Fibroxanthoma, healing
    - Periosteal osteosarcoma
  - Chondroid
    - Enchondroma, including Ollier and Maffucci
    - Osteochondroma
    - Chondrosarcoma
    - Periosteal chondroma
    - Chondroblastoma
    - Chondromyxoid fibroma
  - Ground-glass (mixed osteoid/chondroid)
    - Fibrous dysplasia
    - Liposclerosing myxofibrous tumor
  - Dystrophic calcification
    - Bone infarct
    - Intraosseous lipoma
    - Malignant fibrous histiocytoma, arising in infarct

Enchondroma

Lateral radiograph shows the punctate matrix ➡ which is typical of chondroid. There is minor endosteal scalloping ➡. Note that the lesion has no sclerotic margin. The appearance is typical of enchondroma.

Enchondroma

AP radiograph shows minimal punctate chondroid matrix ➡ in a typical enchondroma which was discovered incidentally on MR. Note the lesion is not geographic and has no defined margin; this is expected.

MATRIX-CONTAINING BONE LESIONS

(Left) Lateral radiograph shows the serpiginous pattern of dystrophic calcification in two sites of bone infarct ➡. This is a typical, though not required pattern for an infarct. (Right) Lateral radiograph shows a small site of punctate density ➡ in the tibia which could represent either chondroid matrix in an enchondroma or dystrophic calcification in a bone infarct. The more serpiginous pattern of infarct in the femur ⇨ makes the diagnosis of bone-infarcts.

Bone Infarct

Bone Infarct

(Left) Lateral radiograph shows punctate regions of chondroid matrix ➡ within the cartilaginous cap of an osteochondroma, with normal bone in the stalk ⇥. Matrix may be seen in osteochondroma without implying chondrosarcoma. (Right) Lateral radiograph shows chondroid matrix within the peripheral portion ➡ of this exostosis, but clearly normal bone extends from the posterior tibial metaphysis into the stalk of the exostosis itself ⇨. (†MSK Req).

Osteochondroma

Osteochondroma

(Left) Anteroposterior radiograph shows the rather featureless increased density which has been termed "ground-glass" ⇨, typical of fibrous dysplasia in tubular bones. Note the absence of normal trabeculae. (Right) Axial NECT shows the smooth increased density of ground-glass matrix ⇨ at a site of fibrous dysplasia in a different patient. There is a lytic focus in an adjacent lesion ➡. Fibrous dysplasia often shows features of both.

Fibrous Dysplasia

Fibrous Dysplasia

MATRIX-CONTAINING BONE LESIONS

Osteosarcoma, Conventional

Osteosarcoma, Conventional

(Left) Lateral radiograph shows the amorphous, featureless density of immature osteoid ➡ within the bone as well as soft tissue mass in this patient with osteosarcoma. The less the matrix appears to be distinctly bone, the more aggressive it is. *(Right)* AP radiograph shows regions of very dense tumor bone formation ➡, mixed with areas that are less dense ➡ in this advanced tumor. Despite areas of density, the matrix is all amorphous and typical of osteosarcoma.

Osteoid Osteoma

Chondrosarcoma, Conventional

(Left) Axial NECT shows a round lytic lesion containing a focus of calcification ➡, buried within densely sclerotic cortex ➡. There is an adjacent nutrient vessel ➡. The radiograph only showed the dense reactive sclerosis. (†MSK Req). *(Right)* Anteroposterior radiograph shows the "snowstorm" appearance of punctate chondroid matrix ➡ of a chondrosarcoma, arising from an underlying osteochondroma ➡ which has better organized chondroid matrix.

Fibroxanthoma (Non-Ossifying Fibroma), Healing

Fracture Callus Formation, Early

(Left) Oblique radiograph shows two NOF lesions, both undergoing the natural process of healing ➡. The new bone formation contains trabeculae and does not have the amorphous appearance of tumor bone. *(Right)* Anteroposterior radiograph shows typical fibrous dysplasia ➡. The mid-humeral lesion which is more expanded, with matrix, and pathologic fracture ➡ is concerning for sarcomatous transformation; biopsy showed healing fracture callus.

MATRIX-CONTAINING BONE LESIONS

Osteosarcoma, Parosteal

Intraosseous Lipoma

(Left) AP radiograph shows a large osteoid-producing lesion appearing to wrap around tibial metaphysis ➡. Note: Matrix is not amorphous, but well-defined ⇨, typical of the less aggressive parosteal variety. *(Right)* Lateral radiograph shows a well-defined lytic lesion in the mid calcaneus ⇨ containing dense calcification ➡. The location and appearance are typical for intraosseous lipoma. The calcification is not required for the diagnosis. (†MSK Req).

Malignant Fibrous Histiocytoma, Bone

Periosteal Chondroma

(Left) Anteroposterior radiograph shows a lytic aggressive lesion ⇨ associated with a serpiginous calcific density typical of bone infarct ➡. MFH may arise secondary to bone infarct; watch for a change in character of the lesion. *(Right)* Anteroposterior radiograph shows matrix of indeterminate type arising from the surface of bone ➡. This is a periosteal (juxtacortical) chondroma; the matrix may appear osseous or chondroid; it is a surface lesion.

Osteosarcoma, Periosteal

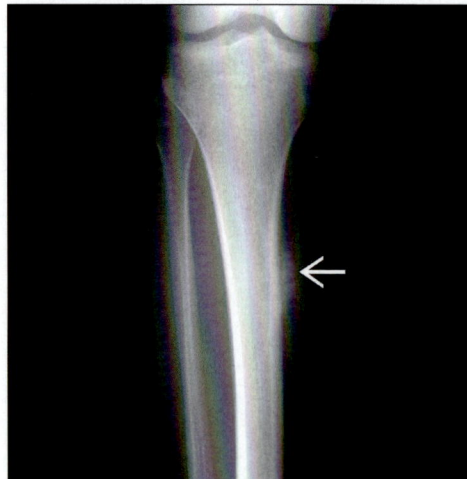

Liposclerosing Myxofibrous Tumor (LSMFT)

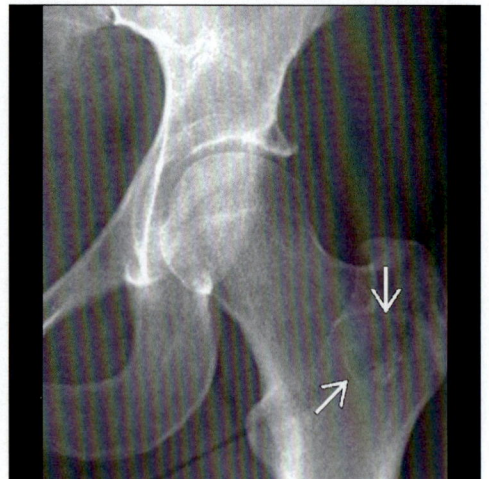

(Left) AP radiograph shows a fairly mature appearing osteoid matrix within a lesion arising from the surface of bone ➡, which proved to be periosteal osteosarcoma. The matrix in this lesion occasionally appears a bit more aggressive than this. *(Right)* AP radiograph shows an intertrochanteric lesion which is geographic and contains both fat and a ground glass matrix ➡. LSMFT usually contains a mixture of lipomatous, fibrous, myxomatous, and osteoid matrix.

MATRIX-CONTAINING BONE LESIONS

Radiation-Induced Sarcoma

Paget Degeneration to Osteosarcoma

(Left) Y view radiograph shows a large soft tissue mass arising from a permeative lesion of the body of scapula. The bone and soft tissue mass contains an amorphous osteoid ➡. This is a radiation-induced osteosarcoma. *(Right)* Lateral radiograph shows destructive change and expansion of the sacrum, with osteoid matrix replacing the entire bone ➡. Individuals with longstanding and diffuse Paget disease are at risk for degeneration to sarcoma.

Osteoblastoma

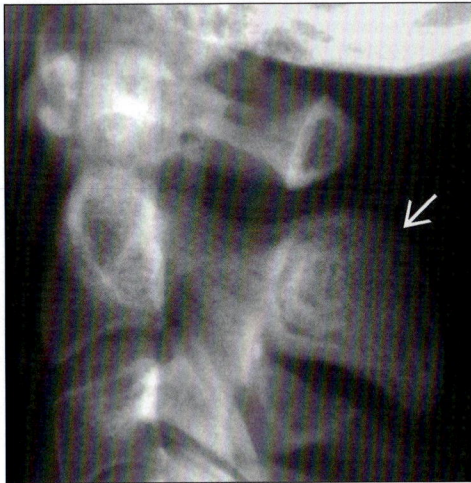

Chondroblastoma

(Left) Lateral radiograph shows an expanded lesion of C2 spinous process which contains fairly mature appearing osteoid matrix ➡. Osteoblastoma need not contain matrix, but this appearance and location are classic. (†MSK Req). *(Right)* Axial NECT shows a mostly lytic, eccentric lesion of the epiphysis which contains a small amount of chondroid matrix ➡. This was a skeletally immature patient, and the appearance is classic for chondroblastoma.

Chondromyxoid Fibroma

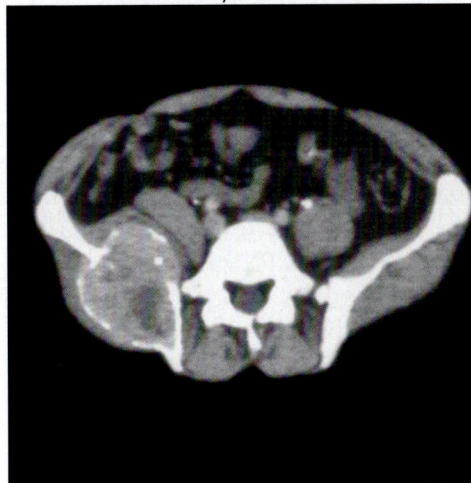

Ollier Disease

(Left) Axial CECT shows an unusual appearance for chondromyxoid fibroma. It is in an unusual location, has central necrosis, and a small amount of chondroid matrix. CMF most frequently arises in the proximal tibia. *(Right)* Lateral radiograph shows an abnormally short ulna, dislocated proximal radius, and ulnar metaphyseal lesion containing chondroid matrix ➡. This is a case of Ollier disease; the metaphyseal lesions more frequently appear striated.

BENIGN OSSEOUS LESIONS THAT CAN APPEAR AGGRESSIVE

DIFFERENTIAL DIAGNOSIS

Common
- Osteomyelitis, Adult
- Osteomyelitis, Pediatric
- Langerhans Cell Histiocytosis (LCH)
- Arthroplasty Wear/Particle Disease
- Hyperparathyroidism, Brown Tumor
- Insufficiency Fracture (Mimic)
- Stress Fracture, Metatarsal (Mimic)
- Radiation Osteonecrosis
- Giant Cell Tumor
- Aneurysmal Bone Cyst
- Disuse Osteoporosis
- Paget Disease
- Enchondroma, Phalanx
- Fibrous Dysplasia
- Garden IV Subcapital Fracture (Mimic)

Less Common
- Fibroxanthoma (Non-Ossifying Fibroma)
- Hemangioma, Spine
- Osteoblastoma
- Chronic Recurrent Multifocal Osteomyelitis
- Charcot, Neuropathic

Rare but Important
- Pseudotumor of Hemophilia
- Hemangiopericytoma, Osseous
- Hemangioendothelioma, Osseous
- Rapidly Destructive Osteoarthritis of Hip
- Massive Osteolysis of Gorham

ESSENTIAL INFORMATION

Key Differential Diagnosis Issues
- Many of these entities do not behave at all in an aggressive fashion, so the imaging can be more confounding than helpful
- Hint: Always consider both osteomyelitis and Langerhans cell histiocytosis when in the "small, round, blue cell" differential
  - i.e., when considering Ewing sarcoma, leukemia, lymphoma
- Certain traumatic entities may appear aggressive; these are usually site-specific: Sacral alar insufficiency, subcapital hip insufficiency, and metatarsal stress fractures

Helpful Clues for Common Diagnoses
- **Osteomyelitis, Adult or Pediatric**
  - Active osteomyelitis, especially bacterial, may show significant bone destruction
    - Lytic, permeative pattern
    - Periosteal reaction, marrow and soft tissue edema
    - Hint: Soft tissue fat planes tend to be obliterated with infection, but displaced with tumor
    - Marrow and soft tissue abscess differentiate osteomyelitis from tumor
    - Reminder: Tumor necrosis may mimic abscess; be critical in assessment
  - Chronic recurrent multifocal osteomyelitis may have completely normal radiograph; biopsy required to differentiate from round cell tumor
- **Langerhans Cell Histiocytosis (LCH)**
  - Often geographic, but may also appear lytic & permeative
  - May have soft tissue mass; imaging may be indistinguishable from malignant tumor such as Ewing sarcoma or lymphoma
  - Hint: Beveled edge in skull lesions (differential destruction of inner & outer tables) suggests LCH
  - Hint: LCH may show much more rapid destruction than sarcoma; this may be a differentiating factor
- **Arthroplasty Wear/Particle Disease**
  - Lysis from particle disease usually geographic but may appear aggressive
  - Age: High risk for metastases or myeloma, which also must be considered
  - Hint: Watch for sources of particles (component wear, bead shedding, bone or cement debris) to suggest associated particle disease
- **Hyperparathyroidism, Brown Tumor**
  - Lytic lesion virtually always associated with other signs of HPTH
    - Abnormal bone density (osteopenic or mixed), generalized pattern
    - Osseous resorption patterns: Subperiosteal, subchondral
- **Stress or Insufficiency Fracture**
  - Hint: These tend to be site-specific; search for fracture line when "lesion" involves sacral ala, pubic ramus, subcapital femoral neck, metatarsals
  - Hint: Fracture line often obscured, particularly by edema in fluid-sensitive sequences; search carefully for fracture line, which may be on only a single image

BENIGN OSSEOUS LESIONS THAT CAN APPEAR AGGRESSIVE

○ Metatarsal fractures
  ▪ Particularly prone to having surrounding soft tissue (as well as marrow) edema; appears aggressive on fluid sequences or post-contrast MR
  ▪ **Hint:** Always look at radiograph before suggesting tumor in a metatarsal
○ Sacral insufficiency fractures
  ▪ Pattern of bilateral vertical abnormality is most suggestive
  ▪ Edema can obscure fracture line & even vertical pattern; may be confusing if unilateral
  ▪ Radiographs generally not helpful since fracture line rarely seen; trabeculae appear smudged
○ Pubic ramus insufficiency fractures
  ▪ Often do not heal well, particularly in elderly osteoporotic patient
  ▪ Constant motion at fracture site results in appearance of a lytic destructive lesion, particularly on MR
  ▪ Radiograph usually shows fracture, but itself may be confusing due to mechanical destruction of bone
○ Garden IV subcapital fracture
  ▪ Rotation of fragments and varus alignment results in an apparent lytic lesion at fracture site
  ▪ **Hint:** Be aware and expect this appearance; should not require a work-up for underlying tumor; MR is confounded by the hematoma and granulation tissue of fracture healing

• **Radiation Osteonecrosis**
  ○ Mixed lytic and sclerotic pattern may appear aggressive
  ○ Abnormal bone at risk for fx, osteomyelitis
  ○ **Hint:** Watch for radiation port-like distribution of osseous abnormalities
  ○ Since there is a primary tumor, differential includes metastatic disease; MR may be required to evaluate for soft tissue mass
  ○ Differential also includes radiation-induced sarcoma; watch for tumor osteoid or more aggressive regions
• **Giant Cell Tumor**
  ○ Benign GCT may appear and behave aggressively, with cortical destruction & soft tissue mass
  ○ Usually there is a suggestion of moderately slow growth (expanded bone prior to cortical breakthrough)
  ○ Subchondral location suggests diagnosis
• **Aneurysmal Bone Cyst**
  ○ ABC may be so significantly expanded that surrounding cortex is no longer visible
  ○ Fluid levels within lesion are suggestive, but not pathognomonic
  ○ Remember that ABC may be solid, which may confound the issue
  ○ **Hint:** If there is anything of concern about suspected ABC lesion (focally wide zone of transition, nodularity within regions of fluid), consider telangiectatic osteosarcoma
    ▪ Alert pathologist to carefully examine all submitted tissue; lesion is easily missed

Osteomyelitis, Adult

Lateral radiograph shows no distinct osseous lesion, but obliteration of fat planes posteriorly ➡. Osteomyelitis can be so highly permeative that no distinct lesion may be seen. It therefore appears aggressive. (†MSK Req).

Osteomyelitis, Adult

Axial T2WI MR shows high signal within the bone ➡, with surrounding soft tissue mass ➡. Osteomyelitis frequently results in adjacent abscesses in the soft tissues; contrast differentiates abscess from tumor.

BENIGN OSSEOUS LESIONS THAT CAN APPEAR AGGRESSIVE

Osteomyelitis, Pediatric

Osteomyelitis, Pediatric

(Left) Oblique radiograph shows dramatic permeative lytic destruction of the radius ➡ in this child. Periosteal reaction & soft tissue mass is present. Differential includes aggressive tumor such as Ewing sarcoma. *(Right)* Sagittal T1 C+ MR in the same case, shows diffuse enhancement of the radius ➡. There is an abscess ➡, but also so much reactive change in the soft tissues that it might be mistaken for soft tissue tumor mass with necrosis. Biopsy proved Staphylococcal infection.

Langerhans Cell Histiocytosis (LCH)

Langerhans Cell Histiocytosis (LCH)

(Left) Lateral radiograph shows an aggressive permeative lytic lesion of the mid diaphysis with prominent periosteal reaction ➡. LCH may present either as a geographic lesion, or with an aggressive appearance as seen here. *(Right)* Axial PD FSE MR shows destructive change of the acetabulum ➡, along with a large soft tissue mass ➡. LCH may be surprisingly rapidly destructive, mimicking a malignant tumor.

Arthroplasty Wear/Particle Disease

Hyperparathyroidism, Brown Tumor

(Left) Anteroposterior radiograph shows a large, lytic, somewhat permeative lesion occupying the acetabulum ➡. The offset of the femoral head in the cup indicates polyethylene wear, resulting in massive osteolysis. *(Right)* AP radiograph shows a poorly delineated lytic lesion in the humeral diaphysis ➡. While this appears moderately aggressive, the correct diagnosis of Brown tumor is secured by the abnormal bone density & resorption of the distal clavicle ➡.

BENIGN OSSEOUS LESIONS THAT CAN APPEAR AGGRESSIVE

Insufficiency Fracture (Mimic)

Stress Fracture, Metatarsal (Mimic)

(Left) Axial STIR MR shows diffuse high signal in both sacral ala ➡. The actual fracture lines of insufficiency fractures may be obscured by fluid sensitive sequences, and are usually not seen on radiographs. *(Right)* Coronal T1 C+ FS MR shows high signal within the marrow ➡, with an apparent circumferential "mass" ➡, mimicking tumor. Stress fracture elicits edema within marrow as well as in the adjacent soft tissues. Misdiagnosis of tumor occurs surprisingly often.

Radiation Osteonecrosis

Giant Cell Tumor

(Left) AP radiograph shows moderately aggressive mixed lytic and sclerotic bone in a square "port-like" configuration. The rest of the skeleton was normal. The patient had axillary node radiation for breast cancer. Radiation osteonecrosis can be difficult to differentiate from metastases. *(Right)* Lateral radiograph shows a giant cell tumor which is so expanded that the cortex is no longer seen ➡. Despite the appearance, this proved to be a benign giant cell tumor.

Aneurysmal Bone Cyst

Disuse Osteoporosis

(Left) Lateral radiograph shows a lytic lesion occupying the distal femur, with a fairly wide zone of transition ➡. The lesion has expanded into a large soft tissue mass ➡, with an extremely thin cortical rim. This proved to be aneurysmal bone cyst. *(Right)* AP radiograph shows such severe osteoporosis that it has a moth-eaten appearance ➡, distal to a fracture nonunion ➡. This osteoporosis can be rather focal, related to fracture hyperemia & disuse.

BENIGN OSSEOUS LESIONS THAT CAN APPEAR AGGRESSIVE

Paget Disease

Enchondroma, Phalanx

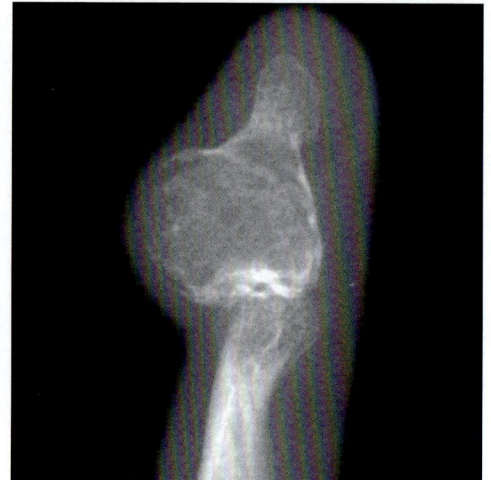

(Left) Lateral radiograph shows osteoporosis circumscripta ➡, the lytic phase of Paget disease in the skull. The early lytic phase, or even the mixed lytic/sclerotic disordered bone phase may appear aggressive. *(Right)* Lateral radiograph shows significant expansion, with severe cortical thinning and chondroid matrix. Enchondroma may appear more aggressive in the phalanges than in more proximal locations, yet behave in a benign manner.

Fibrous Dysplasia

Garden IV Subcapital Fracture (Mimic)

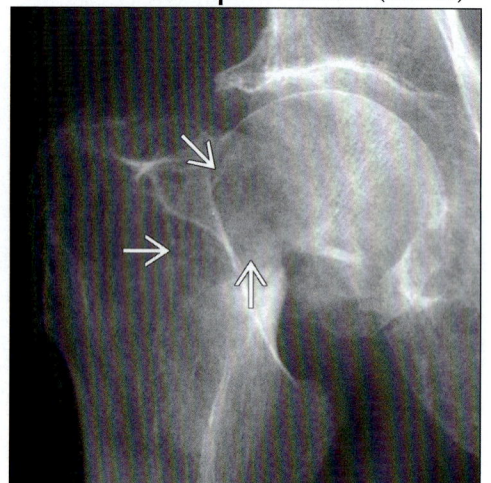

(Left) AP radiograph shows extensive fibrous dysplasia, but focal expansion, cortical break, & central matrix ➡. Concern is for degeneration to sarcoma (extremely rare) vs. the proven diagnosis, pathologic fracture. *(Right)* Anteroposterior radiograph shows a displaced subcapital fracture. The angulation and rotation, combined with osteoporosis, results in the appearance of a lytic lesion in the femoral neck ➡, mimicking underlying pathology.

Fibroxanthoma (Non-Ossifying Fibroma)

Hemangioma, Spine

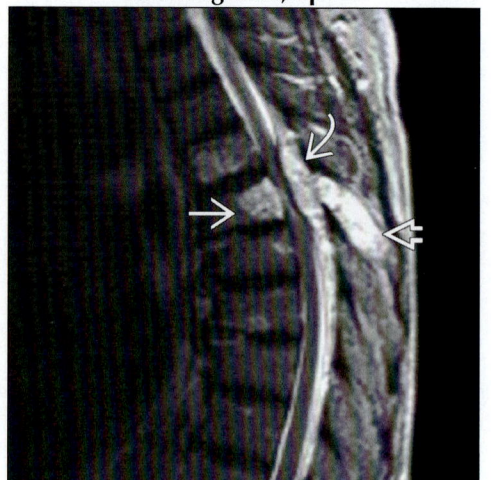

(Left) AP radiograph shows a lytic expanded somewhat aggressive lesion in the fibula ➡. It is important to remember that NOF, when it arises in small bones like the fibula, may appear central and more aggressive than usual. *(Right)* Sagittal T2WI MR shows hemangioma within a vertebral body ➡, extending to the posterior elements ➡, & expanding into a large epidural mass ➡. Occasionally this degree of aggressiveness is seen in hemangioma.

BENIGN OSSEOUS LESIONS THAT CAN APPEAR AGGRESSIVE

Osteoblastoma

Chronic Recurrent Multifocal Osteomyelitis

(Left) Lateral radiograph shows a mixed lytic and sclerotic lesion in the vertebral body, with destruction of the posterior cortex ➡. Rarely an osteoblastoma will show this degree of aggressiveness. (Right) Coronal T2WI FS MR shows high signal in the sacral ala ➡ & iliac wing ➡. The radiograph was normal; this is worrisome for highly permeative lesions. The differential for multifocal osteomyelitis includes Ewing, leukemia, & lymphoma.

Charcot, Neuropathic

Pseudotumor of Hemophilia

(Left) AP radiograph shows dislocation & destruction of the humeral head. There is osseous debris within a distended joint ➡. A shoulder Charcot joint can be so destructive that, with the debris, it is mistaken for chondrosarcoma. (Right) Anteroposterior radiograph shows expansile lytic lesion of the iliac wing, with fracture through the acetabulum by the femoral head. This appears destructive; however, the margination is sclerotic, typical of pseudotumor.

Hemangiopericytoma, Osseous

Hemangioendothelioma, Osseous

(Left) Lateral radiograph shows a moderately aggressive osseous lesion ➡. There were additional osseous lesions raising the concern for a vascular tumor. Hemangiopericytoma has a spectrum ranging from benign to malignant. (Right) PA radiograph shows a highly destructive lesion of the 2nd metacarpal. The appearance is nonspecific. Biopsy proved hemangioendothelioma, which has an appearance & behavior ranging from benign to malignant.

Image Based: Radiograph/CT, Osseous

55

METASTASES TO BONE

DIFFERENTIAL DIAGNOSIS

Common
- Breast Carcinoma
- Lung Carcinoma
- Prostate Carcinoma
- Renal Cell Carcinoma (Hypernephroma)
- Thyroid Carcinoma

Less Common
- Lymphoma
- Leukemia
- Osteosarcoma
- Neuroblastoma
- Ewing Sarcoma
- Malignant Melanoma
- Gastrointestinal Carcinoma
- Medulloblastoma
- Carcinoid
- Wilms Tumor
- Testicular Carcinoma

Rare but Important
- Retinoblastoma
- Adrenal Carcinoma
- Squamous Cell Carcinoma
- Cervical Carcinoma
- Uterine Carcinoma
- Hepatoma
- Transitional Cell Carcinoma
- Fibrosarcoma

ESSENTIAL INFORMATION

Key Differential Diagnosis Issues
- Demographics
  - Metastases are far more common than primary bone tumors (25:1)
  - 80% of skeletal metastases are due to lung, breast, prostate, and kidney carcinomas
  - 50% of all patients with cancer will eventually develop skeletal metastases
- Skeletal distribution
  - Predilection for regions containing red marrow: Skull, spine, ribs, pelvis, humeri, femora
- Typical appearance
  - Single or multiple lesions of varying sizes
  - Joint spaces & intervertebral disks preserved
  - Periosteal reaction rare
  - Density of lesions can change with response or lack of response to therapy
    - Sclerotic healing
    - Sclerotic or lytic progression
    - Radiation osteonecrosis

Helpful Clues for Common Diagnoses
- **Breast Carcinoma**
  - Lytic or sclerotic lesions
  - May contain button sequestra, especially in skull
  - Normal skull thickness differentiates extensive metastases from Paget disease
- **Lung Carcinoma**
  - Typically lytic lesions, but can be sclerotic (esp. small cell lung carcinoma)
  - Majority of lytic metastases to the hands & feet are from lung primary
- **Prostate Carcinoma**
  - Sclerotic lesions typical but can be lytic
    - Homogeneously dense vertebral body, "ivory vertebra"
    - Lack of bone enlargement differentiates from Paget disease
  - Can produce long, solitary expansile rib lesions
  - Diffuse skeletal involvement results in "super scan" pattern on bone scan
- **Renal Cell Carcinoma (Hypernephroma)**
  - Expansile, poorly demarcated osteolytic lesions
    - "Soap bubble" appearance
  - Tremendously vascular metastases make biopsy dangerous; consider embolization first
  - Can contain fat, producing false negative drop out on opposed phase MR imaging
    - Image kidneys if multiple bone lesions are identified on MR and are shown to contain microscopic fat
- **Thyroid Carcinoma**
  - Expansile, poorly demarcated osteolytic lesions
  - Often solitary and highly vascular
  - Similar imaging appearance to renal cell carcinoma metastases

Helpful Clues for Less Common Diagnoses
- **Lymphoma**
  - Oval, lytic lesions
  - Can be faintly sclerotic
  - Extensive permeative lesions in Burkitt lymphoma
  - Sclerotic lesions with Hodgkin lymphoma and histiocytic lymphoma

- Ivory vertebral body with Hodgkin lymphoma
- **Leukemia**
  - Moth eaten bone destruction
  - Sub-epiphyseal rarefaction
  - Transverse radiolucent metaphyseal bands
  - "Sunburst" appearance in skull
- **Osteosarcoma**
  - Metastases ossify, including soft tissue deposits
- **Neuroblastoma**
  - Similar to leukemia
- **Ewing Sarcoma**
  - Ill-defined, lytic lesions
  - May become confluent
- **Malignant Melanoma**
  - Lytic or faintly sclerotic lesions
- **Gastrointestinal Carcinoma**
  - Lytic or sclerotic lesions
    - Sclerotic more common with gastric carcinoma and carcinoid
- **Medulloblastoma**
  - Mixed lytic and sclerotic lesions
  - Most common in children
  - Cerebrospinal metastases before bone

Helpful Clues for Rare Diagnoses

- **Squamous Cell Carcinoma**
  - Nodal involvement usually seen before lytic bone lesion
- **Cervical & Uterine Carcinoma**
  - Lytic lesions from hematogenous spread or direct extension to bone
- **Hepatoma**

- Lytic lesions, can be large & solitary
- **Transitional Cell Carcinoma**
  - Sclerotic lesions
- **Fibrosarcoma**
  - Lytic lesions originating from soft tissue or bone primary

Alternative Differential Approaches

- Lytic metastases to bone
  - Non small cell lung carcinoma
  - Renal cell carcinoma
  - Breast carcinoma
  - Thyroid carcinoma
  - Gastrointestinal carcinoma
  - Neuroblastoma
- Blastic metastases to bone
  - Prostate carcinoma
  - Breast carcinoma
  - Transitional cell carcinoma
  - Gastrointestinal carcinoma
  - Small cell lung carcinoma
  - Medulloblastoma
  - Any carcinoma
- Metastases in children
  - Neuroblastoma
  - Leukemia
  - Lymphoma
  - Medulloblastoma
  - Ewing sarcoma
  - Wilms tumor

Breast Carcinoma

AP radiograph shows mixed sclerotic & lytic metastases ➡ in the ribs & shoulder, with pathologic fracture ➡. Axillary clips suggest lymph node dissection & thus metastatic breast carcinoma. (†MSK Req).

Lung Carcinoma

Axial CECT shows multiple sclerotic lesions ➡ in the pelvis. Additional imaging identified a primary non-small cell lung carcinoma. Metastatic lung carcinoma metastases are typically lytic but can be sclerotic.

METASTASES TO BONE

(Left) Anteroposterior radiograph demonstrates a small cortically-based lesion ➡. Few cortically-based lesions are seen in older patients, & metastases must be suspected. Lung & breast are the most frequent primaries causing cortically-based lesions. (†MSK Req). **(Right)** Axial bone CT shows multiple prostate carcinoma metastases ➡. Even though sclerotic metastases can appear more dense than cortical bone, these lesions have an increased risk for fx.

(Left) Lateral radiograph shows diffuse sclerosis involving all the ribs, vertebral bodies, and posterior elements. The bones are normal in size. This remarkably homogeneous osseous replacement is metastatic prostate disease. **(Right)** Anteroposterior radiograph demonstrates a severely destructive, lytic, and expanded lesion ➡. This was a solitary lesion. It is important to consider metastatic kidney or thyroid disease in older patients.

(Left) Anteroposterior radiograph shows an avulsed lesser trochanter ➡, with lucency extending into the subtrochanteric region ➡. A lesser trochanteric avulsion in an adult is pathologic until proven otherwise. **(Right)** Axial bone CT demonstrates vague sclerosis in a lesion ➡ identified on PET/CT. Since the bone marrow is the "organ" involved in this patient's primary disease, return of the disease, even in a different bone, is more accurately termed a recurrence.

Lung Carcinoma

Prostate Carcinoma

Prostate Carcinoma

Renal Cell Carcinoma (Hypernephroma)

Thyroid Carcinoma

Lymphoma

METASTASES TO BONE

Osteosarcoma

Neuroblastoma

(Left) Axial CECT shows a metastasis with osteoid matrix ➡. The central lucency may be due to response to chemotherapy. Osteosarcoma metastases are typically ossified. *(Right)* Anteroposterior radiograph shows vertebral plana of L1 ➡ with preservation of posterior elements, but complete flattening of the body. In addition, there is a paraspinous mass ➡, as well calcifications in the mass superior to the right kidney ➡ representing the primary tumor.

Malignant Melanoma

Medulloblastoma

(Left) Axial CECT shows a sclerotic lesion with vague central lucency ➡. There were additional metastases to the liver, peritoneum, spleen and thoracic spine. Bone metastases from melanoma are typically lytic or faintly sclerotic. *(Right)* Lateral radiograph shows medulloblastoma metastasis with prominent periosteal reaction in the ulna ➡. These metastases may have either a lytic, sclerotic, or mixed appearance.

Hepatoma

Fibrosarcoma

(Left) Axial bone CT shows a large destructive mass ➡ obliterating the proximal humerus. A thin rim of residual bone is present anteriorly ➡. Hepatocellular metastases to bone are typically lytic. Most patients have nonosseous metastatic sites identified before skeletal metastases develop. *(Right)* Axial bone CT shows vague medullary sclerosis and endosteal scalloping ➡. The patient had a paravertebral soft tissue mass as well as other osseous lesions, any of which could be the primary.

GENERALIZED INCREASED BONE DENSITY, ADULT

DIFFERENTIAL DIAGNOSIS

Common
- Metastases, Bone Marrow
- Renal Osteodystrophy, Healed
- Sickle Cell Anemia: MSK Complications
- Paget Disease
- Myelofibrosis

Less Common
- Radiation Osteonecrosis (Mimic)
- Gaucher Disease
- Complications of Fluoride

Rare but Important
- Hypertrophic Osteoarthropathy (Mimic)
- Hypoparathyroidism
- Mastocytosis
- Osteopetrosis
- Pycnodysostosis
- Engelmann Disease (Engelmann-Camurati) (Mimic)
- Erdheim-Chester
- POEMS

ESSENTIAL INFORMATION

Key Differential Diagnosis Issues
- Increased density may be related to altered osteogenesis or overlying periosteal new bone

Helpful Clues for Common Diagnoses
- **Metastases, Bone Marrow**
  - Breast & prostate most common metastases to progress to diffuse involvement
  - Bone scintigraphic superscan with intense diffuse bone uptake & minimal renal activity
- **Renal Osteodystrophy, Healed**
  - Increased density results from excessive osteoid, subperiosteal new bone, &/or healing resorption
  - "Rugger jersey" spine results from endplate sclerosis
- **Sickle Cell Anemia: MSK Complications**
  - Bone infarctions with dystrophic calcification; periostitis in children
  - Normally contoured bones with no cortical destruction
- **Paget Disease**

- Begins focally but can become diffuse over time
  - Mixed lytic-sclerotic pattern depending on phase; sclerotic in late phase
  - Thickened, coarsened, disorganized trabeculae & bone overgrowth
  - "Picture frame" vertebra due to peripheral sclerosis with central lucency
- **Myelofibrosis**
  - Axial osteosclerosis with uniform density, cortical thickening, endosteal sclerosis
  - Hepatosplenomegaly, extramedullary hematopoiesis
  - May have secondary gout

Helpful Clues for Less Common Diagnoses
- **Radiation Osteonecrosis (Mimic)**
  - Due to osteonecrosis, dystrophic calcification &/or insufficiency fractures with hypertrophic callus formation
  - Look for sharp transition of abnormal to normal bone defining the radiation port
- **Gaucher Disease**
  - Marrow packing results in bone expansion with thinned cortices; Erlenmeyer flask deformities (undertubulation)
  - Density due to mixed lytic/sclerotic pattern with endosteal bone formation resulting in bone-within-bone appearance
  - Osteonecrosis with dystrophic calcification may contribute to density
- **Complications of Fluoride**
  - Ranges from trabecular coarsening to uniform sclerosis; ± periosteal reaction
  - Involves axial > appendicular skeleton
  - Ligament calcification, particularly in sacrospinous ligaments

Helpful Clues for Rare Diagnoses
- **Hypertrophic Osteoarthropathy (Mimic)**
  - Skin thickening, paw-like hands & feet
  - 1° - Pachydermoperiostosis: Inherited
    - Shaggy periostitis; involves all segments tubular bones
  - 2° - Secondary hypertrophic osteoarthropathy: Related most frequently to pulmonary or congenital heart disease
    - Painful, smooth periostitis; involves tubular bones except epiphyses
- **Hypoparathyroidism**
  - Characterized by hypocalcemia & neuromuscular signs & symptoms

GENERALIZED INCREASED BONE DENSITY, ADULT

- ○ Osteosclerosis may be focal or generalized; increased density along iliac crests, vertebral margins, metaphyseal bands
- ○ Calcification of ligaments (esp. paraspinous), tendons, soft tissues
- **Mastocytosis**
  - ○ Diffuse or focal; ± osteolysis
  - ○ Tends to be homogeneous in axial skeleton
  - ○ ± Osteonecrosis
- **Osteopetrosis**
  - ○ Diffuse osteosclerosis with undertubulation & cortical thickening; bone within bone appearance
- **Pycnodysostosis**
  - ○ Diffuse osteosclerosis with short stature, short broad hands
- **Engelmann Disease (Engelmann-Camurati) (Mimic)**
  - ○ Bilateral symmetric cortical thickening & medullary cavity narrowing
  - ○ Spindle-shaped long bones with expanded diaphyses, periosteal & endosteal sclerosis; epiphyses spared
  - ○ Involves (with decreasing frequency) tibia, femur, humerus, ulna, radius, hands, feet, clavicle, ribs, pelvis
- **Erdheim-Chester**
  - ○ Diffuse or patchy density results from trabecular coarsening, medullary sclerosis
  - ○ Metadiaphyseal cortical thickening with epiphyses spared
  - ○ Appendicular common, axial rare
- **POEMS**
  - ○ Syndrome: **P**olyneuropathy, **O**rganomegaly, **E**ndrocrinopathy, **M** proteins, **S**kin changes
  - ○ Affects axial skeleton (spine & pelvis)
  - ○ Diffuse sclerosis seen in about 3% of patients with plasma cell myeloma

Alternative Differential Approaches

- **Hint**: Assess the extent & distribution of osteosclerosis when considering diagnosis
- Diffuse vs. regional sclerosis
  - ○ Diffuse: Metastases, renal osteodystrophy, sickle cell anemia, myelofibrosis, fluorosis, hypoparathyroidism, osteopetrosis, pycnodysostosis, Erdheim-Chester, Engelmann-Camurati
  - ○ Regional: Metastases, sickle cell anemia, Paget, radiation osteonecrosis, Gaucher, hypertrophic osteoarthropathy, mastocytosis, plasma cell myeloma
- Axial versus appendicular sclerosis
  - ○ Involves axial & appendicular skeleton
    - Metastases, renal osteodystrophy, sickle cell disease, Gaucher, hypoparathyroidism, osteopetrosis, pycnodysostosis
  - ○ Predominates in axial skeleton
    - Paget disease, myelofibrosis, fluorosis, mastocytosis, POEMS
  - ○ Predominates in appendicular skeleton
    - Hypertrophic osteoarthropathy, Engelmann-Camurati, Erdheim-Chester

Metastases, Bone Marrow

Lateral radiograph shows diffuse sclerosis of prostatic metastases throughout the lumbar spine (anterior & posterior elements) as well as visualized ribs ➡.

Renal Osteodystrophy, Healed

Anteroposterior radiograph shows diffuse increased bone density with periosteal new bone ➡ & indistinct trabeculae related to new mineralization of previously excessive unmineralized osteoid of osteomalacia.

GENERALIZED INCREASED BONE DENSITY, ADULT

(Left) *Lateral radiograph shows diffuse patchy sclerosis in the metadiaphyses* ➡ *of this patient with sickle cell anemia, representing dystrophic calcification in healing bone infarctions.* **(Right)** *AP radiograph shows mixed lytic-sclerotic pattern of thickened disorganized trabeculae & osteoporosis in a patient with diffuse Paget disease. Bone overgrowth & remodeling results in protrusio* ➡ *& bowing deformity* ➡ *of proximal femurs.*

Sickle Cell Anemia: MSK Complications

Paget Disease

(Left) *Anteroposterior radiograph shows diffuse patchy osteosclerosis. Normal fatty marrow has been replaced by fibrous tissue, typical of myelofibrosis. The patient also had splenomegaly (not shown).* **(Right)** *Anteroposterior radiograph shows osteosclerosis of sacrum & visualized pelvis* ➡ *as well as lower lumbar spine. Note vascular clips* ➡ *from lymph node dissection. Patient was treated 15 years prior for endometrial carcinoma.*

Myelofibrosis

Radiation Osteonecrosis (Mimic)

(Left) *Anteroposterior radiograph shows diffuse patchy increased bone density* ➡. *Note the right hip resurfacing hemiarthroplasty* ➡, *placed because of avascular necrosis in this patient with longstanding Gaucher disease.* **(Right)** *Lateral radiograph shows diffuse trabecular thickening & coarsening, involving anterior* ➡ *& posterior* ➡ *spinal elements. Patient is being treated with fluoride for osteoporosis.*

Gaucher Disease

Complications of Fluoride

GENERALIZED INCREASED BONE DENSITY, ADULT

Hypertrophic Osteoarthropathy (Mimic)

Hypoparathyroidism

(Left) AP radiograph shows heavy periosteal new bone ➡ in the tibia & fibula, mimicking diffuse increased density. The hand and all other imaged long bones demonstrate similar periosteal reaction. Patient has 1° hypertrophic osteoarthropathy (pachydermoperiostosis). *(Right)* Lateral radiograph shows diffuse increased bone density with marked bowing deformity of femur ➡ & patchy sclerosis of femoral neck ⋗, related to chronic hypoparathyroidism.

Mastocytosis

Osteopetrosis

(Left) Anteroposterior radiograph shows diffuse mixed lytic & sclerotic density. Although mastocytosis generally produces either focal sclerosis or diffuse osteoporosis, this patient has a mixture of both. *(Right)* Anteroposterior radiograph shows diffuse increased density throughout the axial and appendicular skeleton. The appearance is of "marble bone", or osteopetrosis.

Erdheim-Chester

POEMS

(Left) Anteroposterior radiograph shows generalized increased density in the marrow of both the femur and tibia ➡, sparing the cortices and epiphyses ⋗. The findings were bilateral and the axial skeleton was normal. Appearance is typical of Erdheim-Chester disease. *(Right)* AP radiograph shows the unusual sclerosing pattern ⋗ of myeloma in this patient with POEMS syndrome. The sclerosis may be focal, or more diffuse as in this case.

GENERALIZED INCREASED BONE DENSITY, CHILD

DIFFERENTIAL DIAGNOSIS

Common
- Physiologic Periosteal Reaction of Newborn (Mimic)
- Renal Osteodystrophy (Healing)
- Child Abuse (Mimic)

Less Common
- Sickle Cell Anemia: MSK Complications
- Complications of Prostaglandins (Mimic)
- Congenital Cyanotic Heart Disease
- Complications of Vitamin A
- Complications of Vitamin D
- Scurvy (Mimic)
- Neuroblastoma (Mimic)
- Leukemia (Mimic)
- Osteomyelitis

Rare but Important
- Caffey Disease (Infantile Cortical Hyperostosis) (Mimic)
- Idiopathic Hypercalcemia of Infancy
- Erythroblastosis Fetalis
- Osteopetrosis
- Pycnodysostosis
- Polyostotic Fibrous Dysplasia
- Hypoparathyroidism
- Complications of Fluoride
- Engelmann-Camurati Disease
- Osteosclerotic Dysplasias
- Hyperphosphatasia (Juvenile Paget)
- Melorheostosis
- Tuberous Sclerosis
- Van Buchem Disease
- Ribbing Disease

ESSENTIAL INFORMATION

Key Differential Diagnosis Issues
- Generalized density due to intrinsic alteration of bone vs. dense circumferential overlay of periosteal new bone
- Hint: Consider age at presentation
- Hint: May involve diaphysis, metaphysis &/or epiphysis

Helpful Clues for Common Diagnoses
- Physiologic Periosteal Reaction of Newborn (Mimic)
  - Seen in 35% of infants age 1-4 months
  - Thin, uniform symmetric periosteal new bone; in humerus, femur, tibia

- Renal Osteodystrophy (Healing)
  - Patchy sclerosis as unmineralized osteoid (osteomalacia) calcifies and bone resorption (hyperparathyroidism) heals
  - Coarsened trabeculae, periosteal new bone, widened metaphyses
- Child Abuse (Mimic)
  - Average age: 1-4 years
  - Fractures of varying ages, metaphyseal corner fractures, periosteal new bone

Helpful Clues for Less Common Diagnoses
- Sickle Cell Anemia: MSK Complications
  - Bone pain begins after age 2-3
  - Multiple bone infarctions may create "bone within bone" appearance
  - Long bone periostitis and generalized patchy increased density
- Complications of Prostaglandins (Mimic)
  - IV prostaglandins used in ductus-dependent congenital heart disease
  - Soft tissue swelling, periosteal elevation and extensive periosteal new bone
- Congenital Cyanotic Heart Disease
  - Represents 2° hypertrophic osteoarthropathy
  - Thick, widespread periostitis in diaphysis, metaphysis, and epiphysis
- Complications of Vitamin A
  - Excessive intake; occurs after age 1 year
  - Cortical thickening, soft tissue nodules
  - Involves ulna, metatarsal, clavicle, tibia, other tubular bones, ribs
- Complications of Vitamin D
  - Excessive intake; given for rickets
  - Dense metaphyseal bands; variable cortical thickening & thinning
- Scurvy (Mimic)
  - Occurs later than 8 months
  - Typically osteopenic but coarsened trabeculae, subperiosteal hemorrhage and periosteal new bone may dominate
- Neuroblastoma (Mimic)
  - Typically aggressive osteolytic process but may have periostitis & periosteal new bone
- Leukemia (Mimic)
  - Similar to neuroblastoma, particularly metadiaphyseal
- Osteomyelitis
  - Congenital syphilis-transplacental

GENERALIZED INCREASED BONE DENSITY, CHILD

- Symmetric diaphyseal periosteal reaction; widened, serrated metaphysis; epiphyses spared
  - Rubella-1st trimester maternal infection
    - Irregular, alternating sclerotic and lytic areas create "celery stick" pattern

Helpful Clues for Rare Diagnoses
- **Caffey Disease (Mimic)**
  - Seen first 5 months
  - Involves mandible, clavicles, scapulae, ribs, tubular bones; ± asymmetric
  - Spindle-shaped bones due to diaphyseal involvement; lamellated periosteal reaction when healing
- **Idiopathic Hypercalcemia of Infancy**
  - Seen after first 5 months; looks similar to hypervitaminosis D
- **Erythroblastosis Fetalis**
  - Diffuse diaphyseal sclerosis and transverse metaphyseal bands
- **Osteopetrosis**
  - Osteosclerosis with mottled metaphyses; "bone within bone" appearance
- **Pycnodysostosis**
  - Like osteopetrosis but with short stature, short broad hands, acroosteolysis
- **Polyostotic Fibrous Dysplasia**
  - Triad: Polyostotic fibrous dysplasia, cutaneous pigmentation, precocious puberty; female > male
  - Mildly expanded, ground-glass matrix; generally not diffuse dense sclerosis
- **Hypoparathyroidism**

- Axial skeleton osteosclerosis with sclerotic metaphyseal bands
- **Complications of Fluoride**
  - Excessive intake; axial skeletal changes predominate
  - Coarsened trabeculae; ± diffuse periosteal new bone; extensive ligament calcification
- **Engelmann-Camurati Disease**
  - Presents 4-12 years with waddling gait, muscle weakness
  - Spindle-shaped with diaphyseal cortical thickening; metaepiphyses spared
- **Osteosclerotic Dysplasias**
  - Frontometaphyseal: Prominent cranial involvement, flared iliac wings
  - Craniometaphyseal: Prominent cranial involvement, normal pelvis
  - Pyle: Minimal cranial involvement, marked metaphyseal flaring
- **Hyperphosphatasia (Juvenile Paget)**
  - Sclerosis with narrowed medullary space
  - Short, large skull, bowed long bone
- **Melorheostosis**
  - Cortical and/or endosteal hyperostosis; usually limited to one extremity
- **Tuberous Sclerosis**
  - Sclerotic bone blends with normal bone; involves hands, feet, long bones & spines
- **Van Buchem Disease**
  - a.k.a., Hyperostosis corticalis generalisata
  - Normal stature, diffuse osteosclerosis, enlarged mandible, ribs, clavicles
- **Ribbing Disease**
  - Hyperostosis, predilection for femur/tibia

Physiologic Periosteal Reaction of Newborn (Mimic)

Anteroposterior radiograph shows subtle diffuse increased density of the upper extremity long bones which is bilaterally symmetric and results from subtle diaphyseal periostitis ➔.

Renal Osteodystrophy (Healing)

Posteroanterior radiograph shows growth plate widening ➔ as a result of unmineralized osteoid of osteomalacia. The trabeculae are coarsened, and there is generalized increased density.

GENERALIZED INCREASED BONE DENSITY, CHILD

*(**Left**) Lateral radiograph shows new bone formation resulting from subperiosteal hemorrhage in this child with nonaccidental trauma. Note the metaphyseal corner fracture, typical of this trauma. (**Right**) Anteroposterior radiograph shows sclerosis in the proximal tibial metaphysis due to infarction and dystrophic calcification. Multiple long bone infarctions in sickle cell anemia can result in apparent diffuse increased bone density.*

Child Abuse (Mimic)

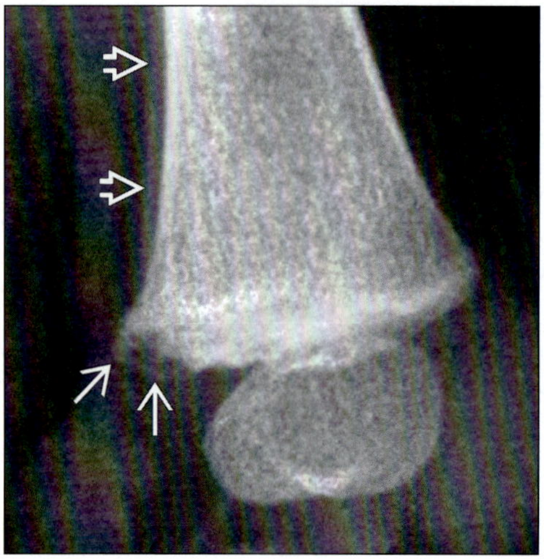

Sickle Cell Anemia: MSK Complications

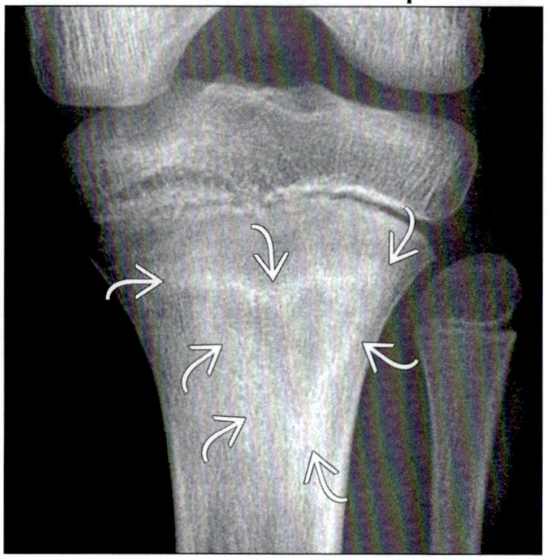

*(**Left**) Anteroposterior radiograph shows uniform, thick, periosteal new bone formation in the humerus in this patient who received prostaglandins for several days to maintain a patent ductus arteriosus. (**Right**) Anteroposterior radiograph shows cortical hyperostosis of the ulna which does not involve the metaphysis or epiphysis. If the hypervitaminosis continues, it may result in deformity of the metaphyses and epiphyses.*

Complications of Prostaglandins (Mimic)

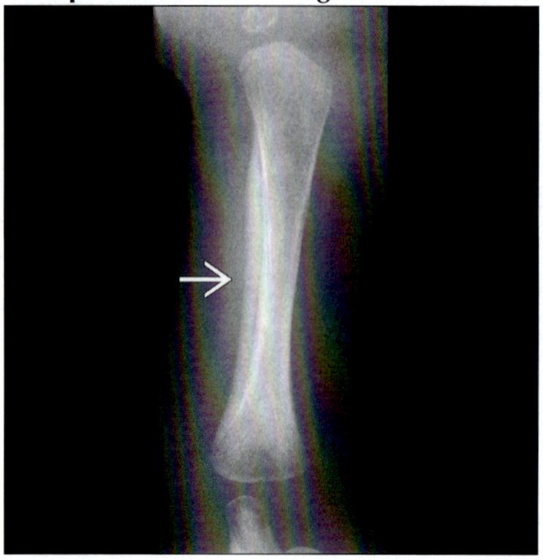

Complications of Vitamin A

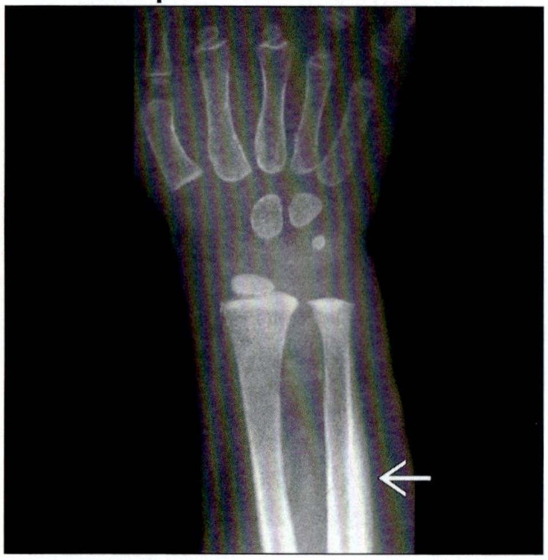

*(**Left**) Anteroposterior radiograph shows diffuse increased density of diaphyses due to subperiosteal hemorrhage and periosteal new bone. Note dense metaphyseal bands (white line of Frankel) and metaphyseal (Pelken) fracture. (**Right**) Lateral radiograph shows diffuse soft tissue swelling and moth-eaten appearing humerus with extensive cloaking periostitis resulting in increased density. Findings represent metastatic neuroblastoma.*

Scurvy (Mimic)

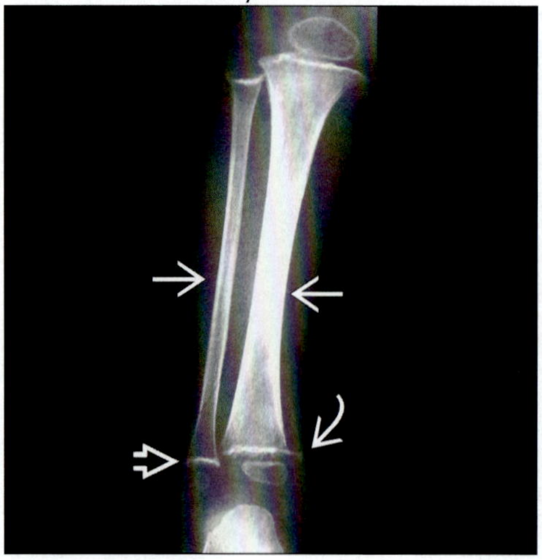

Neuroblastoma (Mimic)

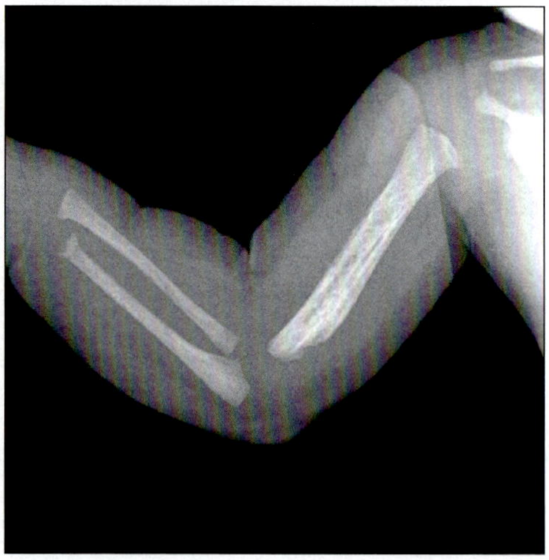

GENERALIZED INCREASED BONE DENSITY, CHILD

Osteomyelitis

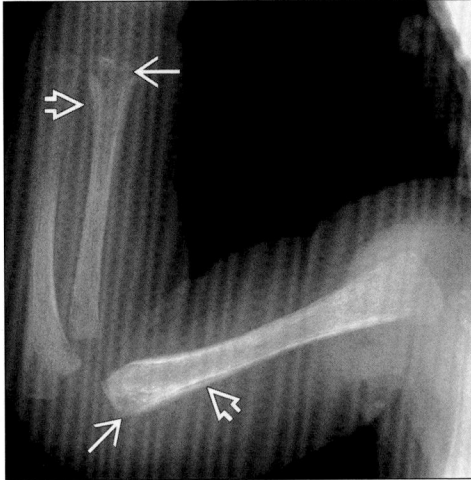

Caffey Disease (Infantile Cortical Hyperostosis) (Mimic)

(Left) Anteroposterior radiograph shows widened provisional calcification zone of syphilitic osteochondritis. There are lucent metaphyseal bands ➡ with subtle diaphyseal periostitis ➡ along the long bones, typical of congenital syphilis. *(Right)* Anteroposterior radiograph shows Caffey disease at age one month with the typical marked thick, wavy periosteal new bone ➡, typical of cortical hyperostosis. This patient's mandible was also involved (not shown).

Osteopetrosis

Pycnodysostosis

(Left) Anteroposterior radiograph shows uniform increased density in osteopetrosis. There is mild undertubulation ➡, with relative widening of the distal femoral metadiaphyses. *(Right)* Anteroposterior radiograph in a child with pycnodysostosis also shows uniformly dense bone, similar to osteopetrosis. This short-limbed dwarf also has micrognathia and shortened fingers (not shown) typical of pycnodysostosis.

Polyostotic Fibrous Dysplasia

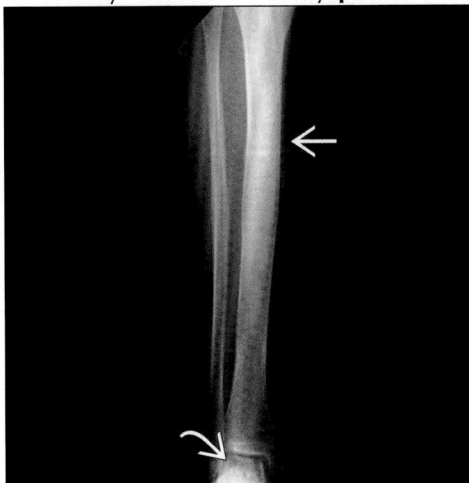

Engelmann-Camurati Disease

(Left) Anteroposterior radiograph shows a long, mildly expansile tibial diaphyseal lesion ➡ with ground-glass matrix, typical of fibrous dysplasia. Additional lesions are present in distal tibia and talus ➡ in this female with precocious puberty. *(Right)* Anteroposterior radiograph shows bilateral diaphyseal cortical thickening ➡ with normal metaphyses and epiphyses. Process becomes smoother and thicker, involving entire diaphysis, as patient matures.

SCLEROSING DYSPLASIAS

DIFFERENTIAL DIAGNOSIS

Common
- Enostosis (Bone Island)
- Melorheostosis (Leri-Weill)
- Sclerotic Metastasis (Mimic)
- Osteitis Condensans Ilii (Mimic)
- Osteitis Pubis (Mimic)
- Osteitis Condensans of Clavicle (Mimic)
- Osteoma (Mimic)
- Osteopoikilosis
- Hyperossified Brown Tumors (Mimic)
- POEMS (Mimic)

Less Common
- Osteopetrosis (Albers-Schonberg)
- Osteopathia Striata (Voorhoeve)
- Engelmann-Camurati Disease (Progressive Diaphyseal Dysplasia)
- Ribbing Disease (Hereditary Multiple Diaphyseal Sclerosis)
- Sarcoid (Mimic)

Rare but Important
- Pycnodysostosis (Maroteaux-Lamy)
- Erdheim-Chester Disease (Mimic)
- Intramedullary Osteosclerosis
- Osteosclerosis (Worth Disease)
- Pyle Dysplasia
- Hyperostosis Corticalis Generalisata (Van Buchem)
- Kenny-Caffey Syndrome (Mimic)
- Mastocytosis (Mimic)

ESSENTIAL INFORMATION

Key Differential Diagnosis Issues
- Sclerosing dysplasias are a spectrum of disease, ranging from the innocuous bone island through the severely disabling osteopetrosis
  - Most are identified by their radiographic distribution, which can be quite specific
  - Sclerosing dysplasias can be mixed (particularly melorheostosis + bone islands/osteopoikilosis/osteopathia striata)
  - Histology usually does not differentiate the sclerosing dysplasias from one another; dense hamartomatous bone is nonspecific
- Aside from the two most common (bone island & melorheostosis), sclerosing dysplasias are uncommon or rare diseases

- Mimics of bone island or generalized sclerosis are relatively common
- Distribution of osseous abnormality, clinical history, or other radiographic clues are most useful for differentiation

Helpful Clues for Common Diagnoses
- **Enostosis (Bone Island)**
  - Focal dense sclerosis, generally rounded, in medullary space
  - Edges "fade" into normal bone, making the lesion appear somewhat spiculated
  - MR low signal on all sequences, non-enhancing
- **Melorheostosis (Leri-Weill)**
  - Irregular cortical hyperostosis; may involve either periosteal or endosteal cortical thickening, or both
  - Usually monostotic or monomelic (single limb)
  - May follow sclerotome distribution (medial or lateral distribution in limb)
  - "Flowing" elongated pattern likened to dripping candle wax
- **Sclerotic Metastasis (Mimic)**
  - Solitary: May be radiographically indistinguishable from bone island; enhance with MR
  - Generalized: Rarely breast or prostate metastases will have a symmetric generalized distribution making them difficult to distinguish from osteopetrosis in the pelvis or spine
- **Osteitis Condensans Ilii (Mimic)**
  - Location-specific, often bilaterally symmetric
  - High signal on fluid-sensitive MR sequences; enhancing
- **Osteitis Pubis (Mimic)**
  - Same as Osteitis Condensans Ilii
- **Osteitis Condensans of Clavicle (Mimic)**
  - Same as Osteitis Condensans Ilii
- **Osteoma (Mimic)**
  - Hamartoma which may be radiographically indistinguishable from bone island
  - Location within paranasal sinus or calvarium is usually diagnostic
  - Familial polyposis: Cortical surface osteomas in long bones
- **Osteopoikilosis**
  - Metaphyseal or epiphyseal

SCLEROSING DYSPLASIAS

○ Low signal on all sequences, non-enhancing
- **Hyperossified Brown Tumors (Mimic)**
  ○ Patients treated for hyperparathyroidism/renal osteodystrophy may hyperossify their brown tumors during the healing process
  ○ If small, gives appearance of osteopoikilosis
  ○ If large, gives appearance of bone islands or sclerotic metastases
  ○ Search for other radiographic hints of hyperparathyroidism (resorptive patterns, abnormal bone density)

Helpful Clues for Less Common Diagnoses
- **Osteopetrosis (Albers-Schonberg)**
  ○ Diffuse & dense sclerosis of all bones, axial & appendicular
  ○ Range of severity; severe "marble bone" is most easily diagnosed
  ○ Impaired osteoclasts do not allow normal bone remodeling during skeletal growth
    - Undertubulation (dense, widened metadiaphyses)
    - "Bone-in-bone" appearance: Particularly vertebrae & iliac wing
- **Osteopathia Striata (Voorhoeve)**
  ○ Striated densities, metaphyseal
- **Engelmann-Camurati Disease (Progressive Diaphyseal Dysplasia)**
  ○ Fusiform thickening of cortical bone, bilaterally symmetric in long bones; hyperostosis of calvarium

○ Affects diaphyses; over long term may extend to metaphyses
○ Normal axial skeleton
○ Autosomal dominant, male > female, begins in 1st decade
- **Ribbing Disease (Hereditary Multiple Diaphyseal Sclerosis)**
  ○ Asymmetric intramedullary diaphyseal sclerosis
  ○ Long bones; no axial or calvarial involvement
  ○ Autosomal recessive; onset after puberty

Helpful Clues for Rare Diagnoses
- **Pycnodysostosis (Maroteaux-Lamy)**
  ○ Severe sclerosis involving entire skeleton
  ○ Distinguished from osteopetrosis by 3 findings
    - Acroosteolysis (resorption of phalangeal tufts)
    - Diminutive (obtuse) angle of mandible
    - Wormian bones
- **Erdheim Chester (Mimic)**
  ○ Intramedullary sclerosis, without cortical thickening; bilaterally symmetric
  ○ Restricted to metadiaphyses of long bones; no axial involvement
  ○ Lipidosis, not dysplasia
- **Intramedullary Osteosclerosis**
  ○ Intramedullary sclerosis without cortical thickening; may not be bilateral
  ○ Mid-tibia is most common location
  ○ Not hereditary; this is most reliable differentiating factor from Ribbing disease

Enostosis (Bone Island)

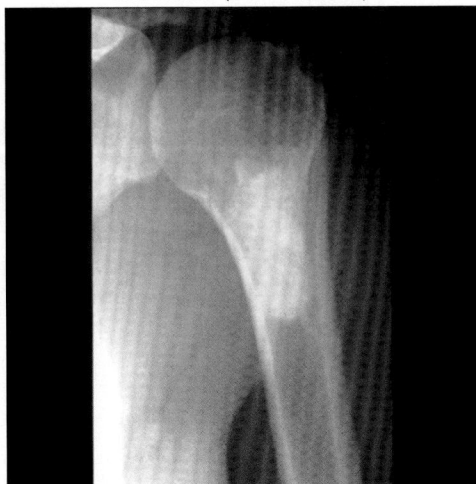

Anteroposterior radiograph shows a giant bone island, incidentally noted during another examination. It is asymptomatic. Note that the margins "fade" off into normal bone; sometimes they can appear spiculated.

Enostosis (Bone Island)

Coronal T1WI MR is identical to any other sequence, showing uniform low signal, fading into normal marrow; this mirrors exactly the radiographic picture of bone island. There is no enhancement if contrast is given.

SCLEROSING DYSPLASIAS

(Left) Anteroposterior radiograph shows the elongated, rather flowing (termed "dripping candle wax") endosteal sclerosis ➡ in this patient with melorheostosis. In this process, the dense bone may form either on the periosteal or endosteal cortex, or both. **(Right)** Oblique radiograph shows sclerosis in the sclerodermal pattern ➡ (medial side) in the same patient as previous image. The dysplasia is polyostotic but monomelic, typical for melorheostosis.

Melorheostosis (Leri-Weill)

Melorheostosis (Leri-Weill)

(Left) Lateral radiograph in a patient with melorheostosis shows many of the lesions are round, typical of bone island ➡. This dysplasia often displays not only the elongated "dripping wax" but also rounded or striated patterns. **(Right)** Sagittal PD FSE FS MR shows a lobulated dense bone lesion exclusively involving the cortex of the ulna ➡, low signal on all sequences. The location & dense sclerosis is typical.

Melorheostosis (Leri-Weill)

Melorheostosis (Leri-Weill)

(Left) Anteroposterior radiograph shows sclerosis within the lesser trochanter ➡. The cortical destruction of the lesser trochanter should differentiate this prostate metastasis lesion from bone island. **(Right)** Axial bone CT shows sclerosis along the iliac margin of the SI joint ➡ typical of osteitis condensans illi. It often appears triangular on a radiograph. It is usually symmetric, but may be unilateral, and is easily distinguished from a sclerosing dysplasia.

Sclerotic Metastasis (Mimic)

Osteitis Condensans Ilii (Mimic)

SCLEROSING DYSPLASIAS

Osteitis Pubis (Mimic)

Osteitis Condensans of Clavicle (Mimic)

(Left) Coronal T2WI FS MR shows high signal within the pubic rami ➡ in a typical MR appearance of osteitis pubis. Though the radiographic appearance is of sclerosis, the MR is distinctly different from the uniformly low signal of a sclerosing dysplasia. *(Right)* Axial NECT shows sclerosis of the medial clavicle ➡. The lesion was intensely hot on bone scan, & mostly low signal on T2 MR. It remained stable over a 1-year follow-up period.

Osteoma (Mimic)

Osteoma (Mimic)

(Left) AP radiograph shows dense sclerosis within the frontal sinus ➡. The appearance is of a bone island, but the location within a paranasal sinus is typical of osteoma. Histology does not differentiate the two. *(Right)* AP radiograph shows lobulated cortically based sclerotic lesions ➡. Although these may not be distinguishable from melorheostosis (and is histologically identical), in a patient with intestinal polyposis, they are considered osteomas.

Osteopoikilosis

Hyperossified Brown Tumors (Mimic)

(Left) Coronal T1WI MR shows multiple round low signal lesions in a metaphyseal distribution ➡. They remained low signal on fluid sequences, as well as post-contrast, confirming the diagnosis of osteopoikilosis. *(Right)* Posteroanterior radiograph shows multiple round sclerotic lesions ➡ suggesting osteopoikilosis. This patient had a parathyroid adenoma removed; these are Brown tumors, hyperossified in the healing phase.

SCLEROSING DYSPLASIAS

Hyperossified Brown Tumors (Mimic)

POEMS (Mimic)

(Left) Posteroanterior radiograph shows dense sclerosis in the tuft ➡. Prior image showed a lytic lesion; the patient had a parathyroid adenoma resected and the Brown tumor healed with dense ossification. *(Right)* Anteroposterior radiograph shows diffuse sclerosis of the pelvic osseous structures. This is a case of sclerosing myeloma. Most cases show more discrete round sclerotic lesions, but occasionally they are diffuse, mimicking osteopetrosis.

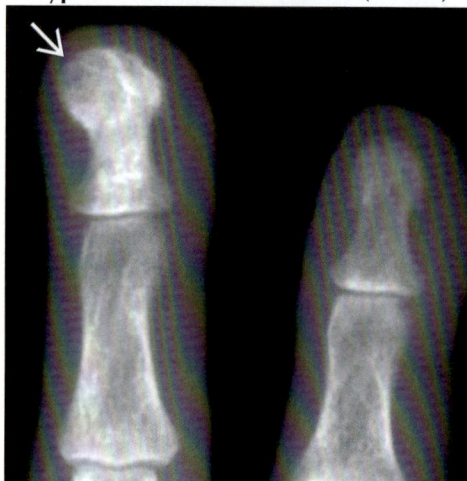

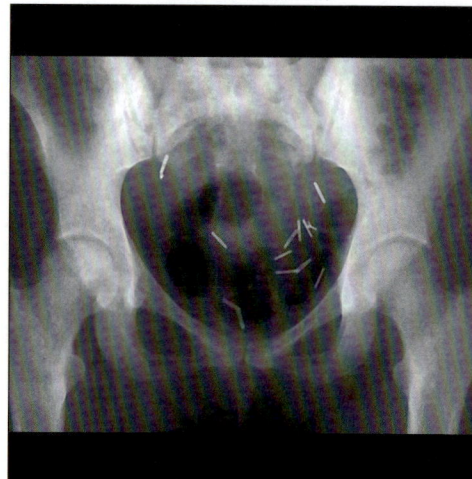

Osteopetrosis (Albers-Schonberg)

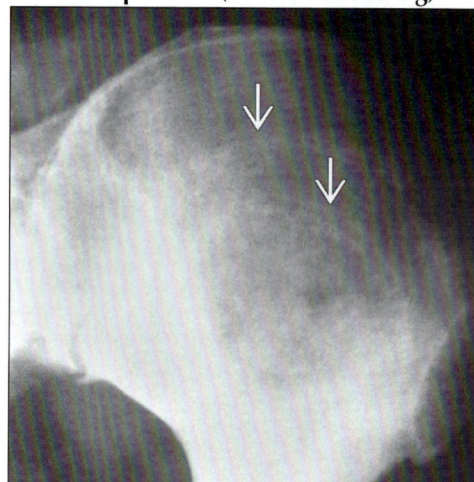

Osteopetrosis (Albers-Schonberg)

(Left) Anteroposterior radiograph shows dense sclerosis of the entire skeleton. There is undertubulation in the proximal & distal femora ➡ due to inadequate osteoclast resorption during the remodeling process of growth. *(Right)* Anteroposterior radiograph shows the bone-in-bone appearance ➡, seen secondary to failure of osteoclastic activity during growth of the bone.

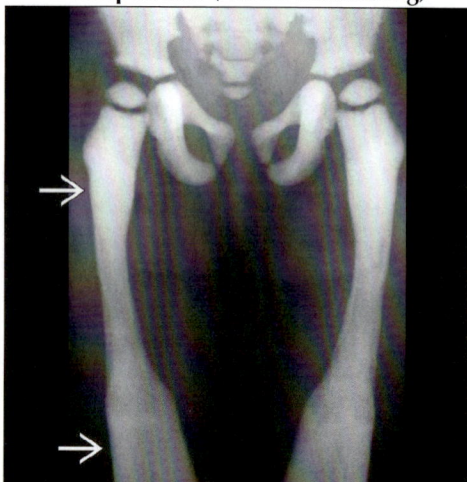

Engelmann-Camurati Disease (Progressive Diaphyseal Dysplasia)

Engelmann-Camurati Disease (Progressive Diaphyseal Dysplasia)

(Left) AP radiograph shows dense sclerosis of the cortical bone, both endosteal & periosteal. It is limited to the diaphysis (note normal metaphyses) & is symmetric, typical of Engelmann-Camurati disease. *(Right)* Anteroposterior radiograph shows the early manifestation of diaphyseal cortical thickening and sclerosis in a young patient with Engelmann-Camurati disease.

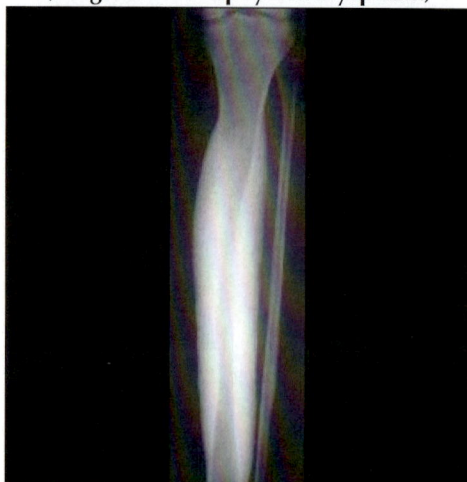

SCLEROSING DYSPLASIAS

Sarcoid (Mimic)

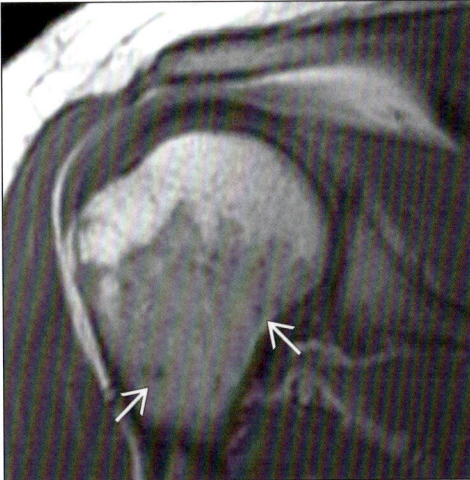

Sarcoid (Mimic)

(Left) Coronal T1WI MR shows multiple, round, low signal metaphyseal lesions ➡, which might mimic osteopoikilosis. However, fluid sensitive sequences show high signal in this case of sarcoid granulomas. *(Right)* Anteroposterior radiograph shows dense sclerosis occupying the femoral head (biopsy trocar in place), which could suggest either giant bone island or solitary sclerotic metastasis. Biopsy showed sarcoid.

Pycnodysostosis (Maroteaux-Lamy)

Pycnodysostosis (Maroteaux-Lamy)

(Left) Anteroposterior radiograph shows diffuse dense sclerosis, with mild undertubulation, suggesting osteopetrosis. However, the patient also had a decreased angle of the mandible, more typical of pycnodysostosis. *(Right)* Posteroanterior radiograph in the same patient as previous image, shows severe acroosteolysis ➡, along with dense sclerosis of all the bones. This feature differentiates pycnodysostosis from osteopetrosis.

Erdheim-Chester Disease (Mimic)

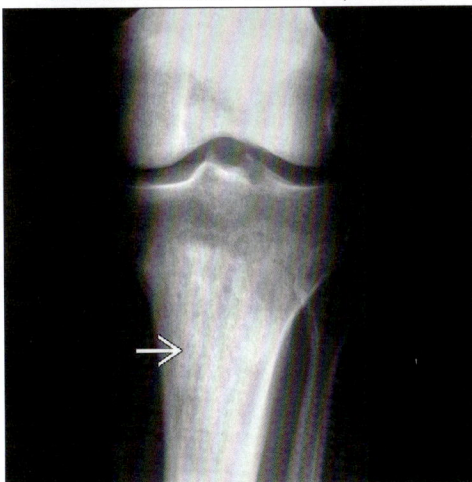

Intramedullary Osteosclerosis

(Left) Anteroposterior radiograph shows dense sclerosis of the medullary canal of the diaphysis ➡, sparing the epiphysis. The process is limited to the medullary space; the cortex is of normal width & density. *(Right)* Lateral radiograph shows diffuse sclerosis within the medullary canal of the mid tibial diaphysis ➡. This finding was bilateral in this patient which is a common but not required feature of intramedullary osteosclerosis.

HYPERTROPHIC CALLUS FORMATION

DIFFERENTIAL DIAGNOSIS

Common
- Motion (Poor Immobilization)
- Fracture, Nonunion
- Fracture, Delayed Union
- Bone Graft (Mimic)
- Infection

Less Common
- Complications of Steroids
- Cushing Disease
- Brain and Spinal Cord injury
- Fracture with Thermal Injury, Burns

Rare but Important
- Osteogenesis Imperfecta

ESSENTIAL INFORMATION

Key Differential Diagnosis Issues
- **Hint:** External callus with hardware fixation concerning for complication
  - Infection or delayed union

Helpful Clues for Common Diagnoses
- **Motion (Poor Immobilization)**
  - Hardware failure or delayed treatment
- **Fracture, Nonunion**
  - Rounded, sclerotic fracture edges
- **Fracture, Delayed Union**
  - Represent continuum of healing
  - Time frame varies by location, type of fixation, patient age, condition of tissues
- **Bone Graft (Mimic)**
  - Seen on post-operative images

  - Over time decreased density, more ill-defined: Resorbs or incorporates
- **Infection**
  - Open fracture or open reduction (ORIF)
  - **Hint:** Worsening pain

Helpful Clues for Less Common Diagnoses
- **Complications of Steroids**
  - Insufficiency or rib fxs: Prominent callus
  - Atrophic callus more typical
  - Generalized osteoporosis
  - Spine compression fxs, AVN
- **Cushing Disease**
  - Endogenous steroid production
  - Finding same as with steroid use
- **Brain and Spinal Cord injury**
  - Disuse osteoporosis with poorly controlled motion of body → fx & hypertrophic callus
- **Fracture with Thermal Injury, Burns**
  - Overlying soft tissues abnormal or grafted

Helpful Clues for Rare Diagnoses
- **Osteogenesis Imperfecta**
  - Femur most common
  - Generalized osteoporosis
  - Limb, vertebral deformities
  - Other fractures, varied ages

Other Essential Information
- Degree of callus formation dependent on age, site of fracture, type of immobilization
  - Minimal external callus with hardware
- Diaphyseal callus > metaphyseal callus
- Callus thick cortex > thin cortex
- Minimal external callus with carpal, tarsal bones, bone protuberances (i.e., malleoli)

Motion (Poor Immobilization)

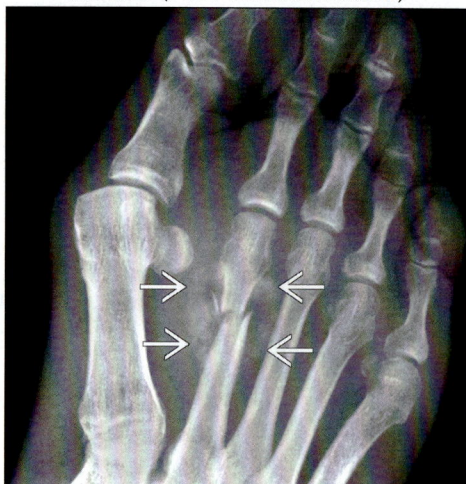

Anteroposterior radiograph shows second metatarsal fracture. The callus ➡ lacks organization and is larger than expected, consistent with hypertrophic callus due to lack of immobilization.

Motion (Poor Immobilization)

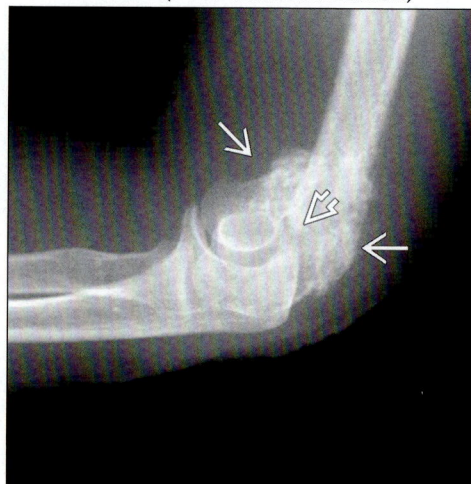

Lateral radiograph shows a transverse supracondylar humerus fracture ⇒. The extensive callus ➡ does bridge the fracture, but is disorganized and results from motion due to lack of immobilization.

HYPERTROPHIC CALLUS FORMATION

Motion (Poor Immobilization)

Fracture, Nonunion

(Left) Anteroposterior radiograph shows a nonunited fibular fracture ➡. The callus is mature and more extensive than expected; this is a result of continued motion. Secondary stress fractures are present ⇉ in the tibia. *(Right)* Lateral radiograph shows plate fixation. The plate has lifted from the bone (not shown). The fracture line is still visible. External hypertrophic callus extends from the fracture margins without evidence of union ➡.

Fracture, Nonunion

Bone Graft (Mimic)

(Left) Anteroposterior radiograph shows ulnar diaphyseal fracture with plate fixation. The plate is fractured ⇉ allowing motion. This leads to development of a nonunion with extensive callus formation a without solid osseous union ➡. *(Right)* Anteroposterior radiograph shows dense granular material surrounding the distal tibial diaphysis ⇉. This bone substitute/filler is placed to fill the gap created by distraction through the fracture.

Infection

Osteogenesis Imperfecta

(Left) Anteroposterior radiograph shows sequelae from hardware for tibiotalar fusion ➡. Extensive external callus is present around the distal tibia ⇉ and is the result of infection during healing. *(Right)* Anteroposterior radiograph shows thin, osteoporotic, bowed tibia & fibula. Extensive callus surrounds & bridges between the bones. This finding may be seen in patients with osteogenesis imperfecta tarda.

BONE WITHIN BONE APPEARANCE

DIFFERENTIAL DIAGNOSIS

Common
- Neonatal Spine, Normal
- Osteopetrosis
- Renal Osteodystrophy, Healing
- Immobilization
- Paget Disease

Less Common
- Osteomyelitis, with Involucrum
- Hypervitaminosis D
- Leukemia
- Subperiosteal Hemorrhage
- Bone Infarct
- Acromegaly
- Reflex Sympathetic Dystrophy
- Linea Aspera Hypertrophy (Mimic)
- Cement & Bone Fillers (Mimic)
- Sickle Cell Anemia: MSK Complications
- Gaucher Disease

Rare but Important
- Tuberculosis
- Heavy Metal Poisoning
- Erdheim Chester
- Oxalosis
- Thorotrast Exposure

ESSENTIAL INFORMATION

Key Differential Diagnosis Issues
- Alternating bands of sclerosis producing similar outline of bone in marrow space
- During stress or severe illness, osteoblasts form a thin line under the zone of proliferative cartilage
  - Line ossifies when chondroblastic and osteoblastic activity resumes
- "Bone within bone" appearance is not classic for any particular diagnosis without history

Helpful Clues for Common Diagnoses
- **Neonatal Spine, Normal**
  - Approximately half of 1-2 month old infants have this finding
  - Spontaneously resolves
  - Ovoid vertebral shape with dense superior and inferior endplates is normal
- **Osteopetrosis**
  - Primary bone dysplasia causing failure of osteoclast activity

  - Systemic, symmetric increase in bone density
  - Normal serum calcium, alkaline phosphatase and phosphorus levels
- **Renal Osteodystrophy, Healing**
  - Skeletal response to any chronic renal disease
  - Primary hyperparathyroidism causes sclerosis only in healing stage
  - Rugger jersey spine more common appearance than "bone in bone"
    - Striped appearance of spine
    - Dense endplates with lucent vertebral body centers
- **Immobilization**
  - Induces osteopenia
  - Produces growth arrest and recovery lines
- **Paget Disease**
  - Spine and iliac wings commonly affected
  - Cortical thickening producing bone enlargement is the classic finding
  - Mixed sclerotic and lytic phase is more common than purely sclerotic phase
  - Polyostotic form results in deformed, sclerotic skeleton in end stage

Helpful Clues for Less Common Diagnoses
- **Osteomyelitis, with Involucrum**
  - Infarction of bone with fibroosseous wall
  - Focal disease
  - Long bones
- **Hypervitaminosis D**
  - Disrupts enchondral bone formation
  - Excessive calcification of cartilage cells
  - Dense metaphyseal bands, generalized sclerosis in children
- **Leukemia**
  - Growth arrest and resumption
  - Radiolucent metaphyseal bands
    - Bone involvement in 50% of cases
    - Can be presenting radiologic appearance
- **Subperiosteal Hemorrhage**
  - Blood tracking along periosteum calcifies → outline of underlying bone
  - Due to trauma, scurvy
  - Scurvy has radiolucent band beneath widened zone of provisional calcification
    - "Trümmerfeld zone"
- **Bone Infarct**
  - Irregularly calcified lesions in medullary cavity

BONE WITHIN BONE APPEARANCE

- ○ Serpiginous or streaky region of infarction can follow outline of bone cortex
- ○ Most often in ends of long tubular bones
- ○ Associated with other entities
  - ▪ Sickle cell anemia, pancreatitis, collagen vascular disease, occlusive vascular disease, Gaucher disease, Caisson disease
- ○ Enchondromas can rarely have a similar appearance
- • **Acromegaly**
  - ○ Additional differentiating radiographic findings
    - ▪ Tubular bone widening in skeletally mature patient
    - ▪ Enlarged sella on CT, MR, radiographs
    - ▪ Phalangeal and heel pad thickening
    - ▪ Excessively pneumatized sinuses
    - ▪ Increased vertebral body and disk height
    - ▪ Spadelike phalangeal tufts
    - ▪ Bony proliferation at entheses
- • **Reflex Sympathetic Dystrophy**
  - ○ Subcortical osteoporosis
  - ○ Predilection for this appearance in wrist and foot
- • **Linea Aspera Hypertrophy (Mimic)**
  - ○ Dense parallel lines along middle third of femur visible on AP radiograph
  - ○ Longitudinal ridges along posterior femur
    - ▪ Hypertrophy of medial and lateral ridge from muscle attachments
- • **Cement & Bone Fillers (Mimic)**
  - ○ Associated with post-operative changes, usually removal of pin or rod from long axis of bone, with residual cement

- ▪ Periphery of the rod tract, without cement, can calcify
- ○ Allographic bone (fibula) is typically split and placed superficial to native bone

Helpful Clues for Rare Diagnoses
- • **Tuberculosis**
  - ○ Localized bone-in-bone changes
  - ○ Appearance can be related to fusion of bones or periostitis with bone expansion
  - ○ Slow clinical course compared with bacterial osteomyelitis
- • **Heavy Metal Poisoning**
  - ○ Lead and bismuth most commonly
    - ▪ Faulty resorption of calcified cartilage
  - ○ Phosphorus blocks resorption of bone trabeculae
- • **Erdheim Chester**
  - ○ Symmetric patchy or diffuse osteosclerosis
  - ○ a.k.a. lipid granulomatosis
  - ○ Metadiaphyseal and diaphyseal cortical thickening
    - ▪ Epiphyses relatively spared
- • **Oxalosis**
  - ○ Deposition of calcium oxalate crystals → excessive cartilage calcification
  - ○ Sclerotic metaphyseal bands
  - ○ Pagetic and "woolly" sclerosis
- • **Thorotrast Exposure**
  - ○ Reticuloendothelial cells phagocytize radioactive thorium dioxide producing radiation osteitis
  - ○ Dense opacification of liver, spleen and lymph nodes

Neonatal Spine, Normal

Lateral radiograph of the spine demonstrates oval-shaped vertebral bodies with peripheral lucency and a central bone-in-bone appearance ➡. This is a normal variant that spontaneously resolves.

Osteopetrosis

Lateral radiograph shows diffuse sclerosis and bone-in-bone appearance ➡, due to osteoclast remodeling failure, leaving cortical bone within the enlarged mature bone.

BONE WITHIN BONE APPEARANCE

Osteopetrosis

Renal Osteodystrophy, Healing

(Left) Anteroposterior radiograph shows the typical bone-in-bone appearance which can be seen in osteopetrosis ➡. The bones are mildly diffusely sclerotic. *(Right)* Lateral radiograph shows the bone-in-bone appearance ➡ which can be seen in vertebral bodies in children with renal osteodystrophy. Note the generalized osteopenia and the peritoneal dialysis catheter ➡.

Immobilization

Paget Disease

(Left) Anteroposterior radiograph shows severe disuse osteoporosis in a patient with Paget disease, which has caused overgrowth of the femur. With disuse, the femur has acquired a bone-in-bone appearance ➡. *(Right)* Anteroposterior radiograph shows classic Paget disease with thickened, enlarged bone ➡ extending from the subarticular region to end in a blade of grass configuration proximally. The central cavity ➡ has a bone-in-bone appearance.

Paget Disease

Osteomyelitis, with Involucrum

(Left) Lateral radiograph of the tibia shows sclerotic ➡ and lytic regions consistent with the mixed phase of Paget disease. The distal blade of grass or flame-shaped pattern ➡ outlines the proximal sclerosis producing an outline of the overlying bone. *(Right)* Anteroposterior radiograph shows sequestrum ➡ with surrounding involucrum ➡, giving a bone-in-bone appearance in a patient with osteomyelitis in the pre-antibiotics era.

BONE WITHIN BONE APPEARANCE

Bone Infarct

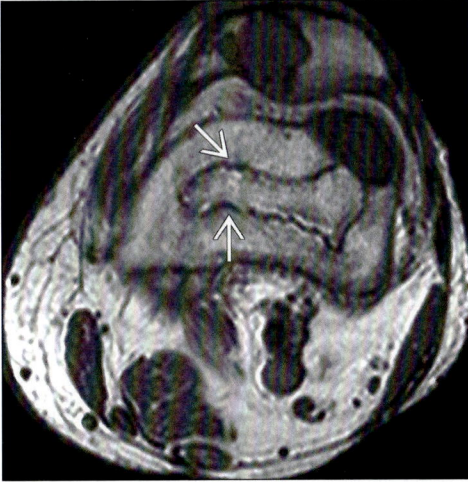

Linea Aspera Hypertrophy (Mimic)

(Left) Axial T1WI MR shows a classic bone infarct ➡, with serpiginous low signal. The infarct pattern matches the outline of the bone, and gives a bone-in-bone appearance. The low signal lesions in the patella and condyle are Brown tumors. *(Right)* Anteroposterior radiograph of the middle third of the femoral diaphysis shows two parallel sclerotic lines ➡, representing the medial and lateral lips of the linea aspera, located along the posterior aspect of the femur.

Cement & Bone Fillers (Mimic)

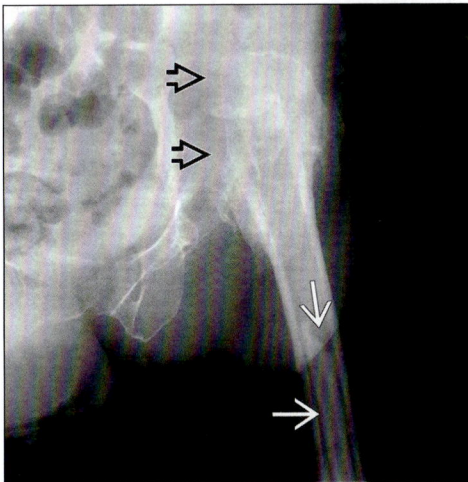

Cement & Bone Fillers (Mimic)

(Left) Oblique radiograph shows Girdlestone anatomy ▷ of the hip after removal of a total hip prosthesis. A longitudinal sclerotic density ➡ with a lucent center in the femoral medullary space is due to a cement fragment left when the femoral prosthesis stem was removed. This mimics a bone-in-bone appearance. *(Right)* Coronal bone CT in the same patient as previous image, better demonstrates the Girdlestone configuration of the hip ➡ and cement fragment ➡.

Gaucher Disease

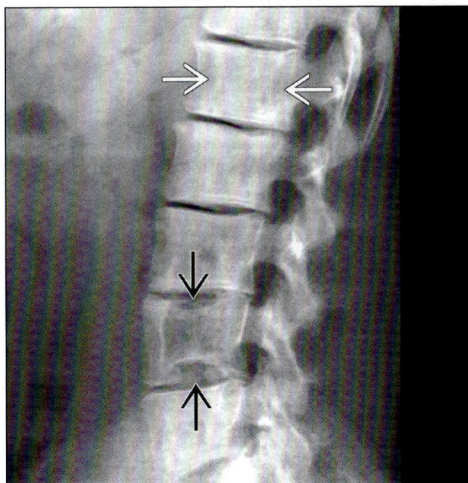

Erdheim Chester

(Left) Lateral radiograph shows rectangular regions of increased density in central portion of each vertebral body ➡ from bone infarcts, which have a faint bone-in-bone appearance. Central endplate depression ➡ of L4 mimics sickle cell disease. *(Right)* Anteroposterior radiograph shows medullary sclerosis, with trabecular thickening ➡, producing a faint bone-in-bone appearance. This was bilaterally symmetric and did not involve the cortices.

OSTEOPENIA

DIFFERENTIAL DIAGNOSIS

Common
- Osteoporosis
- Radiographic Technique (Mimic)

Less Common
- Osteomalacia/Rickets
- Renal Osteodystrophy
- Multiple Myeloma
- Neoplasm

ESSENTIAL INFORMATION

Key Differential Diagnosis Issues
- Terms **osteoporosis** and **osteopenia** in context of bone mineral density (DEXA scans) are different from their use in context of this chapter
  - In the context of this chapter
    - **Osteopenia**: Radiographic finding indicative of decreased bone density
    - **Osteoporosis**: Decrease in amount of normally formed bone
  - Relative to DEXA
    - Osteopenia and osteoporosis are degrees of decreased bone mineral density relative to a control population
    - Multitude of causes including all those in this differential

Helpful Clues for Common Diagnoses
- **Osteoporosis**
  - Multiple causes of decreased bone volume including steroids, chronic medical disease
  - Separate differential diagnosis for osteoporosis available: See "Osteoporosis"
- **Radiographic Technique (Mimic)**
  - Correlate with other radiographic examinations, clinical history

Helpful Clues for Less Common Diagnoses
- **Osteomalacia/Rickets**
  - Abnormal bone formation due to the inability to mineralize osteoid
  - Coarse, ill-defined trabeculae
  - Looser zones, pseudofractures
  - Cortical tunneling
  - Pediatric: Metaphyseal cupping & fraying
  - Osteopenia also seen with related diseases such as hypophosphatasia
- **Renal Osteodystrophy**
  - Combination of osteomalacia and HPTH
  - Osteomalacia: See above
  - Hyperparathyroidism (HPTH)
    - Bone resorption: Subperiosteal, subchondral, subligamentous, subtendinous, cortical tunneling
- **Multiple Myeloma**
  - Osteopenia 2° to diffuse tumor infiltration and osteoporosis induced by tumor itself
  - Generalized osteopenia may be only abnormality
  - Otherwise, may see lytic lesions typical of multiple myeloma or plasmacytoma
- **Neoplasm**
  - Osteopenia 2° to tumor infiltration (leukemia most frequent)
  - May have associated lytic or blastic lesions

Osteoporosis

Anteroposterior radiograph shows gracile limbs of normal length with severe osteopenia and subacute fracture ➡. This patient suffers from a severe case of osteogenesis imperfecta tarda.

Osteoporosis

Lateral radiograph shows osteopenia and fusion of several lower cervical vertebral bodies ➡ as a result of ankylosing spondylitis (AS). Osteoporosis is typically seen in late AS due to fusion and immobility.

OSTEOPENIA

Osteomalacia/Rickets

Renal Osteodystrophy

(Left) Anteroposterior radiograph shows severe generalized bone loss as well as metaphyseal cupping and fraying ➡ in this child with rickets. *(Right)* Anteroposterior radiograph shows osteopenia and dysmorphic femoral necks ➡ and trochanters which are the result of renal osteodystrophy. The osteopenia in end stage renal osteodystrophy is secondary to a combination of hyperparathyroidism and osteomalacia (rickets).

Multiple Myeloma

Multiple Myeloma

(Left) Anteroposterior radiograph of the pelvis shows diffuse osteopenia which is atypical for the patient's age and consistent with his multiple myeloma. *(Right)* Lateral radiograph of the spine shows diffuse osteopenia. Note the mild superior endplate compression fractures ➡. This appearance proved to be the result of multiple myeloma. Myeloma may present with diffuse infiltration and osteopenia, without focal lesions.

Neoplasm

Neoplasm

(Left) Anteroposterior radiograph of the pelvis shows diffuse osteopenia and metaphyseal lucent lines ➡ in a child. *(Right)* Lateral radiograph of the spine from the same patient as previous image, shows diffuse and severe osteopenia. A mild compression deformity of the L1 vertebra ➡ is also seen which was out of proportion to a mild injury. The findings represent a diffuse infiltrative process which proved to be leukemia.

OSTEOPOROSIS, GENERALIZED

DIFFERENTIAL DIAGNOSIS

Common
- Senile Osteoporosis
- Postmenopausal
- Steroids
- Alcohol
- Smoking
- Non-Weightbearing
- Diabetes Mellitus
- Chronic Liver Disease
- Renal Osteodystrophy
- Malnutrition & Anorexia
- Multiple Myeloma
- Rheumatoid Arthritis

Less Common
- Sickle Cell Anemia
- Juvenile Idiopathic Arthritis
- Ankylosing Spondylitis
- Hyperparathyroidism
- Hyperthyroidism
- Cushing Disease
- Pregnancy
- Thalassemia
- Calcium Deficiency
- Amyloid Deposition
- Estrogen Deficiency (Non-Menopausal)
- Gaucher Disease
- Hemochromatosis (Primary)
- Ochronosis (Alkaptonuria)

Rare but Important
- Heparin
- Hypogonadism
- Homocystinuria
- Osteogenesis Imperfecta
- Mastocytosis
- Scurvy
- Acromegaly
- Idiopathic Juvenile Osteoporosis
- Fabry Disease (Vertebral Bodies)

ESSENTIAL INFORMATION

Key Differential Diagnosis Issues
- Osteoporosis
  - Decreased amount of normal bone
  - Insufficiency fractures common to all
- Osteopenia: Radiographic finding indicative of decreased bone density; nonspecific
  - Osteoporosis is one cause of osteopenia

- AVN & infarcts are common associations with steroids, alcohol, sickle cell anemia, Gaucher disease as etiologies

Helpful Clues for Common Diagnoses
- **Senile Osteoporosis**
  - No distinguishing radiographic features
  - Same for postmenopausal, alcohol, smoking, non-weightbearing, chronic liver disease
- **Steroids**
  - AVN, infarcts, hypertrophic callus
- **Renal Osteodystrophy**
  - Combination HPTH & osteomalacia
  - Osteomalacia: Coarse ill-defined trabeculae, Looser's zones, pseudofractures, cortical tunneling, metaphyseal cupping & flaring (rickets)
- **Malnutrition & Anorexia**
  - Generalized soft tissue wasting
- **Multiple Myeloma**
  - Focal lesions most common in skull, spine
  - Multiple punched out lytic lesions
  - Expansile lytic lesions uncommon
  - May present as osteoporosis without focal lesions
- **Rheumatoid Arthritis**
  - Bilateral symmetric arthritis, hands & feet; also hips, knees, SI joints, elbow
  - Uniform joint space narrowing, marginal erosions, peri-articular osteoporosis

Helpful Clues for Less Common Diagnoses
- **Sickle Cell Anemia**
  - Osteoporosis most severe in the spine
  - Multiple bone infarcts & AVN common
  - H-shaped vertebra, coarse trabecula
  - Widening diploic space sparing skull base
  - Osteomyelitis, septic arthritis, dactylitis
- **Juvenile Idiopathic Arthritis**
  - Range monoarticular to bilateral symmetric polyarticular arthritis
  - Small joints of hands, feet; also wrist, shoulder, knee, ankle, cervical spine
  - Uniform joint space narrowing, marginal erosions, peri-articular osteoporosis
- **Ankylosing Spondylitis**
  - Hip, shoulder arthritis
  - Fusion spine & SI joints
  - Enthesopathy
- **Hyperparathyroidism**

OSTEOPOROSIS, GENERALIZED

- Bone resorption: Subperiosteal, subchondral, subligamentous, subtendinous, cortical tunneling
- Chondrocalcinosis, soft tissue calcium deposition, Brown tumors
- **Hyperthyroidism**
  - Cortical tunneling
  - Accelerated skeletal maturation
- **Cushing Disease**
  - Hypertrophic callus
  - Limited appendicular involvement
- **Thalassemia**
  - Marrow hyperplasia: Widened diploic space, hair on end appearance, rodent facies, diaphyseal widening, deformity mimicking Erlenmeyer flask
  - H-shaped vertebra, coarse trabecula
  - Extramedullary hematopoiesis
- **Calcium Deficiency**
  - Mimics osteomalacia
- **Amyloid Deposition**
  - Soft tissue masses; bilateral symmetric arthritis with subchondral cysts, erosions, joint spaces normal to widened
- **Estrogen Deficiency (Non-Menopausal)**
  - No specific radiographic changes
- **Gaucher Disease**
  - Erlenmeyer flask deformity & AVN characteristic, H-shaped vertebra
- **Hemochromatosis (Primary)**
  - Arthropathy of MCP joints, wrists, elbows, shoulder with chondrocalcinosis; uniform joint space narrowing, osteophytes, large subchondral cysts

- **Ochronosis (Alkaptonuria)**
  - Disc changes: Extensive mineralization, narrowing, vacuum, endplate sclerosis

Helpful Clues for Rare Diagnoses
- **Heparin**
  - No specific radiographic changes
- **Hypogonadism**
  - No specific changes
- **Homocystinuria**
  - Scoliosis, abnormal vertebral shape
- **Osteogenesis Imperfecta**
  - Wormian bones, kyphoscoliosis, fractures
  - Bowing & deformities due to "soft bones"
  - Bones thin & gracile or short & tubular
- **Mastocytosis**
  - May see ill-defined focal lytic lesions
  - Characteristic cutaneous manifestations
  - Extensive marrow infiltration on MR
- **Scurvy**
  - Metaphyseal lucent & dense lines, beaking
  - Wimberger sign, periostitis
- **Acromegaly**
  - Enlarged bones: Mandible, skull, face
  - Thickened cortices, increased medullary canal, spade-like (phalangeal) tufts
  - Enthesopathy, cortical tunneling
  - Widened joints, thickened heel pad
  - Enlarged disc space & costochondral junctions
- **Idiopathic Juvenile Osteoporosis**
  - Diagnosis of exclusion
- **Fabry Disease (Vertebral Bodies)**
  - Characteristic skin lesion

Senile Osteoporosis

Lateral radiograph shows multiple compression fractures ➡ in this elderly woman with senile osteoporosis. Patient has already been treated with vertebroplasty ➡.

Postmenopausal

Sagittal NECT shows marked postmenopausal osteoporosis involving all vertebral bodies and posterior elements. At this time, vertebral body shape and height continue to be maintained.

OSTEOPOROSIS, GENERALIZED

(Left) Anteroposterior radiograph from a renal transplant patient on steroids shows diffuse osteopenia and AVN within the lunate ➡ and proximal pole of the scaphoid ➡. *(Right)* AP radiograph shows a patient with Paget disease who has been bedridden for a year. The bones are severely osteoporotic from non-weightbearing, superimposed on the sclerotic Pagetic changes. Osteoporosis results in deformities, including protrusio ➡.

Steroids

Non-Weightbearing

(Left) Lateral radiograph shows vascular calcification ➡ in this young diabetic patient. There is diffuse osteopenia, typically seen in this disease, which has resulted in calcaneal insufficiency avulsion fracture ➡. *(Right)* Anteroposterior radiograph shows diffuse osteoporosis, coarsening of trabeculae, resorption of the distal clavicle ➡, and a large Brown tumor ➡. Findings are typical of renal osteodystrophy.

Diabetes Mellitus

Renal Osteodystrophy

(Left) Lateral radiograph shows insufficiency fracture ➡ through an osteoporotic calcaneus in this young woman with anorexia. *(Right)* Lateral radiograph of the lumbar spine shows diffuse osteoporosis and multiple compression fractures ➡ which are not normal for a patient of this age and sex (50 year old man). There were no focal lytic lesions. Myeloma may present with diffuse marrow infiltration.

Malnutrition & Anorexia

Multiple Myeloma

OSTEOPOROSIS, GENERALIZED

Rheumatoid Arthritis

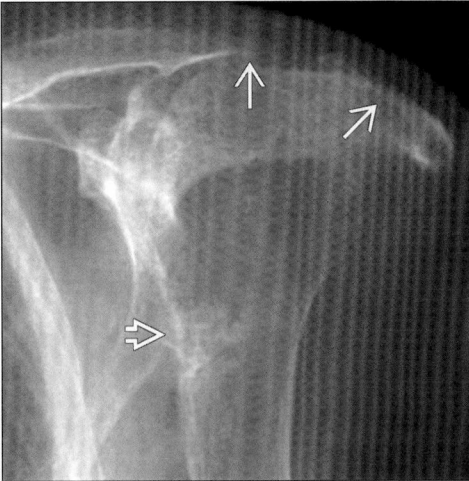

Sickle Cell Anemia

(Left) Anteroposterior radiograph shows advanced rheumatoid arthritis with severe osteopenia, erosion of the distal clavicle and acromion ➡, insufficiency fracture of the proximal humerus ➡, and changes of long-standing rotator cuff tear. *(Right)* Lateral radiograph shows diffuse osteoporosis in a patient with sickle cell anemia. There are H-shaped vertebra ➡ seen throughout the thoracic spine, typical of the AVN and collapse pattern seen in these patients.

Juvenile Idiopathic Arthritis

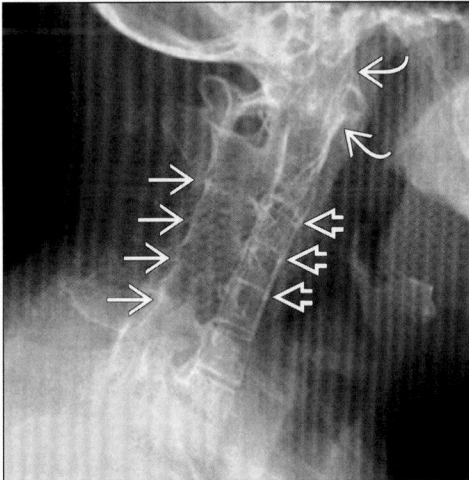

Ankylosing Spondylitis

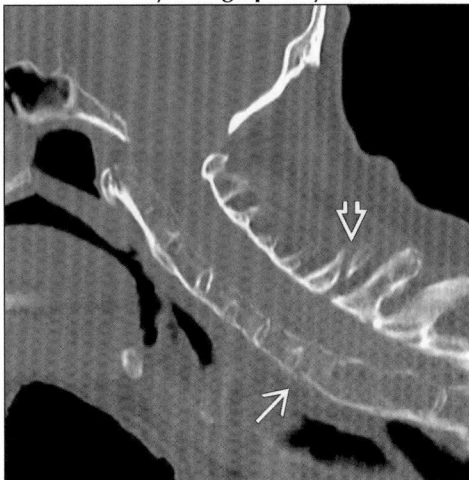

(Left) Lateral radiograph reveals extensive osteoporosis which is a common finding in JIA. Extensive fusion of the facet joints ➡ and disc spaces ➡ is present and has extended cephalad to involve the occipito-cervical junction ➡. *(Right)* Lateral radiograph shows diffuse osteopenia of the lumbar spine atypical for a 29 year old man. Squaring of the vertebral body corners is present ➡, consistent with early changes of ankylosing spondylitis.

Ankylosing Spondylitis

Hyperparathyroidism

(Left) Sagittal bone CT shows complete ankylosis of the cervical spine and diffuse osteopenia in this patient with ankylosing spondylitis. Fracture through the C7 vertebra ➡ and posterior elements ➡ (termed pseudarthrosis) is seen following minor motor vehicle crash. *(Right)* AP radiograph shows severe osteopenia of the humerus, typical of all the osseous structures in this patient with hyperparathyroidism. There is a Brown tumor located within the cortex ➡.

OSTEOPOROSIS, GENERALIZED

Hyperparathyroidism

Cushing Disease

(Left) Anteroposterior radiograph shows diffuse osteopenia and an expansile lytic lesion of the right ilium ➔ in this patient with hyperparathyroidism and a brown tumor of the iliac wing. *(Right)* Anteroposterior radiograph shows diffuse osteopenia in this patient with Cushing disease. Sclerosis in the femoral head from AVN ➔ is present, an uncommon finding with endogenous steroid excess.

Thalassemia

Amyloid Deposition

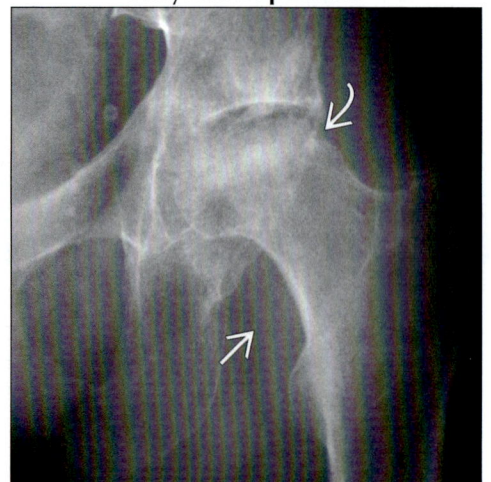

(Left) Anteroposterior radiograph shows typical findings of thalassemia with "squaring" of the bones, especially the metacarpals ➔, due to marrow packing with accompanying thinning of the endosteal cortex. (†MSK Req). *(Right)* Anteroposterior radiograph shows diffuse osteoporosis, as well as a distended hip joint ➔. Erosions are seen at the femoral head, with collapse ➔. This is a patient with myeloma and focal amyloid deposition within the hip joint.

Gaucher Disease

Ochronosis (Alkaptonuria)

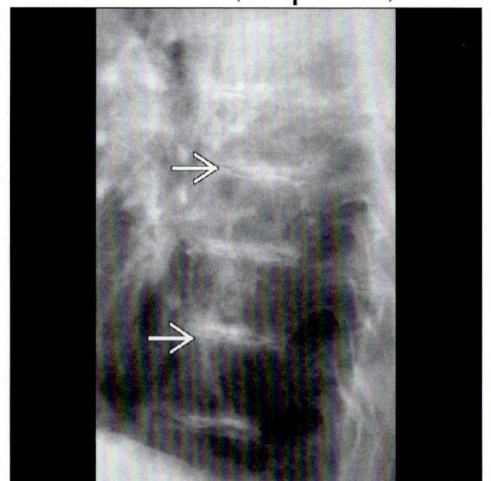

(Left) Anteroposterior radiograph shows diffuse osteopenia and an Erlenmeyer flask deformity of the distal femur. These findings are characteristic of Gaucher disease, related to marrow packing. *(Right)* Lateral radiograph shows calcification within the disks ➔ as well as diffuse osteoporosis in a patient with ochronosis.

OSTEOPOROSIS, GENERALIZED

Homocystinuria

Osteogenesis Imperfecta

(Left) Lateral radiograph shows severe osteoporosis and early compression fractures in a teenager with homocystinuria. Other images, not shown, include hands showing arachnodactyly. (Right) Anteroposterior radiograph shows severe osteopenia, gracile bones with "growth" lines ➡ *in the metaphyses in this skeletally immature individual with osteogenesis imperfecta tarda.*

Osteogenesis Imperfecta

Mastocytosis

(Left) AP radiograph shows short broad, multiply fractured femora ➡ *and tibiae* ➡. *The bones are severely osteopenic, which helps distinguish this case of osteogenesis imperfecta congenita from a dwarf syndrome. (Right) AP radiograph shows severe osteopenia and a midshaft femoral fracture. While these findings are suggestive of osteogenesis imperfecta, the history of GI complaints was consistent with the biopsy diagnosis of mastocytosis. (†MSK Req).*

Scurvy

Idiopathic Juvenile Osteoporosis

(Left) AP radiograph shows classic signs of scurvy. The bones are diffusely osteopenic. Associated findings include Wimberger sign (sclerotic ring around epiphysis) ➡ *and the white line of Frankel (dense metaphyseal line)* ➡. *(Right) AP radiograph shows a basicervical femoral neck fracture* ➡ *in this skeletally immature patient with no history of trauma. The patient was eventually diagnosed with idiopathic juvenile osteoporosis, a diagnosis of exclusion.*

DIFFERENTIAL DIAGNOSIS

Common
- Disuse/Immobilization
- Loss or Absence of Overlying Soft Tissues (Mimic)
- Complex Regional Pain Syndrome (CRPS)
- Inflammatory Arthritis
  - Rheumatoid Arthritis
  - Juvenile Idiopathic Arthritis
  - Ankylosing Spondylitis
  - Inflammatory Bowel Disease Arthritis
- Septic Joint

Less Common
- Regional Migratory Osteoporosis
- Transient Osteoporosis of the Hip
- Hemophilia

Rare but Important
- Hypothyroidism

ESSENTIAL INFORMATION

Key Differential Diagnosis Issues
- Need to correlate with clinical information
- Important to determine if monoarticular or polyarticular
- Beware: Must exclude septic arthritis if monoarticular; consider a clinical emergency
- Varied radiographic appearance of osteoporosis
  - Uniform
  - Mottled or spotty
  - Band-like lucency either subchondral or metaphyseal
  - Cortical tunneling & scalloping
  - Subperiosteal and endosteal resorption (unusual, mainly CRPS)
- **Hint**: Mottled or band-like appearance implies rapid onset; consider disuse, CRPS
- **Hint**: Cortical tunneling suggests inflammatory arthritis, CRPS
- Peri-articular osteoporosis may be subjective if other changes not apparent
- **Hint**: Distribution may suggest etiology
  - Segmental (i.e., spine, foot, hand): Consider disuse or CRPS
  - Peri-articular: Consider inflammatory
  - Focal (limited portion of a bone usually part of epiphysis) or digit: Consider partial regional migratory osteoporosis, CRPS
  - Single joint: Consider infection

- Large joints lower extremity: Consider transient osteoporosis/regional migratory osteoporosis

Helpful Clues for Common Diagnoses
- **Disuse/Immobilization**
  - Clinically evident cause
  - Segmental (foot, hand)
  - Larger joint (elbow, knee) involvement not common, only with distal joint involvement
  - Occurs after 6-8 weeks immobilization
  - Increased fracture risk
  - Rapid bone turnover
- **Loss or Absence of Overlying Soft Tissues (Mimic)**
  - Segmental distribution
  - Uniform appearance
  - Mastectomy most common cause
  - Surgical resection overlying soft tissues
    - Forequarter amputation or hip disarticulation
  - Atrophy
    - Stroke
    - Neuromuscular disorders
    - Associated osteoporosis from disuse
  - Rotation may mimic, especially on CXR, pelvis
  - Grid cutoff may mimic
- **Complex Regional Pain Syndrome (CRPS)**
  - a.k.a. reflex sympathetic dystrophy, RSD, Sudeck atrophy
  - Segmental distribution most common
  - Involvement of multiple digits less common
  - Lower extremity more common
  - Early clinical phase: Severe burning pain, soft tissue swelling, hypersensitivity, sweating, vasomotor alterations
  - Late clinical phase: Muscle atrophy, joint contracture, skin changes
  - Joint space preservation
  - Radiographic changes 3-6 months after clinical symptoms
  - Bone scan or MR changes earlier
- **Inflammatory Arthritis**
  - General comments
    - Peri-articular
    - Secondary to hyperemia
    - Uniform appearance
    - Pain, limited range of motion
  - **Rheumatoid Arthritis**

REGIONAL OSTEOPOROSIS

- Bilateral symmetric
- Small joint of hands, feet; also wrist, elbow, knee, shoulder, ankle
- Periarticular osteopenia may be earliest manifestation of arthritis
- Uniform joint space narrowing
- Marginal erosions
  - **Juvenile Idiopathic Arthritis**
    - JIA: Childhood onset
    - Ranges from monoarticular to symmetric polyarticular disease
    - Small joints of hands, feet; also wrist, elbow, knee, shoulder, ankle
    - Marginal erosions
    - Periosteal new bone
    - Uniform joint space narrowing
  - **Ankylosing Spondylitis**
    - AS: Peri-articular osteoporosis less frequent than other arthridites
    - Hip, shoulder more common than smaller joints
    - Evaluate SI joints & spine to aid diagnosis
    - Segmental osteoporosis in the spine with long-standing disease
  - **Inflammatory Bowel Disease Arthritis**
    - Skeletal manifestations identical to AS
    - Clinical history of bowel disease
- **Septic Joint**
  - Monoarticular
  - Uniform joint space narrowing
  - Marginal erosions; cortical indistinctness
  - Low grade fever, elevated WBC
  - Aspirate to confirm diagnosis

Helpful Clues for Less Common Diagnoses
- **Regional Migratory Osteoporosis**
  - Peri-articular osteoporosis
  - Joint space preservation
  - Partial transient osteoporosis involves only portion of joint or 1-2 contiguous digits
  - Lower extremity joints predominate
  - Diagnosis requires multiple joint involvement, staggered clinical onset
  - Pain, swelling, no history of trauma
  - Clinical onset precedes radiographic changes by 6-8 weeks
  - MR bone marrow edema pattern earlier
- **Transient Osteoporosis of the Hip**
  - Osteoporosis femoral head > acetabulum
  - Joint space preservation
  - Pain, swelling, decreased range of motion
  - Clinical onset precedes radiographic changes by 6-8 weeks
  - Early MR bone marrow edema pattern
- **Hemophilia**
  - Peri-articular osteoporosis
  - Knee, elbow, ankle, hip, shoulder common
  - Ballooned epiphyses, dense effusion

Helpful Clues for Rare Diagnoses
- **Hypothyroidism**
  - Osteoporosis uncommon; clinical manifestations varied

Other Essential Information
- Causes of immobilization include paralysis, stroke, polio, fracture fixation, weightlessness (astronauts)

Disuse/Immobilization

AP radiograph shows severe osteoporosis ➡ distal to a nonunion of the tibia-fibula ➡. The moth-eaten pattern of osteoporosis develops due to disuse/immobilization, and can appear highly aggressive.

Disuse/Immobilization

Axial bone CT shows a pattern of spotty osteoporosis scattered within the distal femur and patella including small lucencies in the subchondral bone ➡, cortical thinning ➡ and medullary lucencies ➡, due to disuse.

REGIONAL OSTEOPOROSIS

Disuse/Immobilization

Loss or Absence of Overlying Soft Tissues (Mimic)

(Left) Anteroposterior radiograph shows decreased density of the right hemipelvis and proximal femur. This decreased density is due to atrophy of the overlying soft tissues and diminished bone density due to disuse in this patient with polio. *(Right)* Posteroanterior radiograph shows that the left hemithorax is less dense than the right due to surgical resection of the soft tissues and osseous structures of the shoulder girdle for sarcoma.

Complex Regional Pain Syndrome (CRPS)

Complex Regional Pain Syndrome (CRPS)

(Left) Oblique radiograph shows linear subchondral lucency within base of the middle and lateral cuneiforms ➡. Subchondral lucency at the metatarsal bases has a spotted appearance ➡ in this patient with CRPS. *(Right)* Posteroanterior radiograph shows severe osteopenia in a speckled or spotty distribution centered around the carpus ➡. This patient developed CRPS following an episode of luxatio erecta of the shoulder.

Rheumatoid Arthritis

Rheumatoid Arthritis

(Left) Posteroanterior radiograph shows peri-articular osteoporosis involving the carpus and MCP joints ➡. Many other RA features are noted, including soft tissue nodules, joint space loss, and marginal erosions. *(Right)* Anteroposterior radiograph shows decreased bone density for a 41 year old male. There is diffuse joint space loss, cortical indistinctness and several focal marginal erosions ➡, all typical of rheumatoid arthritis.

REGIONAL OSTEOPOROSIS

Juvenile Idiopathic Arthritis

Ankylosing Spondylitis

(Left) Lateral radiograph shows decreased bone density in this patient with JIA. Thinning of the cortices, especially the radial head and capitellum is apparent ➡. The patient also had advanced maturation of these epiphyses relative to the opposite elbow. (†MSK Req). (Right) Lateral radiograph shows osteopenia of the lower cervical spine ➡ with fusion of several lower cervical vertebral bodies. Findings suggest the diagnosis of ankylosing spondylitis.

Ankylosing Spondylitis

Septic Joint

(Left) Anteroposterior radiograph shows aggressive osteoporosis with a pattern of lucent metaphyseal bands ➡. This pattern is more commonly seen in disuse osteoporosis, but is present with early inflammation in this patient with AS. (Right) Anteroposterior radiograph shows peri-articular osteopenia of the IP joint of the great toe. Associated bone destruction ➡ and periostitis lead to the diagnosis of septic arthritis with osteomyelitis.

Regional Migratory Osteoporosis

Transient Osteoporosis of the Hip

(Left) Lateral radiograph shows diffuse osteopenia with thinning of the anterior cortex of the distal femur, proximal tibia ➡, and generalized decreased patellar density in a young man. His hip developed the same process 6 months later. (Right) AP radiograph shows diffuse osteopenia of the left hip. Note loss of the normal cortical line of the femoral head ➡ and the central portion of the acetabulum ➡. Septic hip must be considered, but this proved to be transient osteoporosis.

CORTICAL TUNNELING

DIFFERENTIAL DIAGNOSIS

Common
- Disuse Osteoporosis
- Immobilization
- Rheumatoid Arthritis
- Hyperparathyroidism (HPTH)
- Renal Osteodystrophy
- Osteomalacia/Rickets

Less Common
- Complex Regional Pain Syndrome (CRPS)
- Thyrotoxicosis
- Acromegaly

Rare but Important
- Hypophosphatasia

ESSENTIAL INFORMATION

Key Differential Diagnosis Issues
- **Hint:** Usually not an isolated finding; this is an aggressive pattern of bone resorption & other associated processes are likely present
- Appearance of cortical tunneling is due to widening of haversian canals
- Indicative of high bone turnover, but with several different etiologies
  - ↑ Osteoclastic activity: Hyperparathyroidism
  - Hyperemia: CRPS
  - ↓ Stress on bone: Disuse/immobilization osteoporosis
  - Unmineralized osteoid: Osteomalacia/rickets

Helpful Clues for Common Diagnoses
- **Disuse Osteoporosis and Immobilization**
  - Lower extremity common
  - Regional pattern of osteoporosis
- **Rheumatoid Arthritis**
  - Hands, feet predominate early in disease
  - Peri-articular osteopenia, marginal erosions
  - Uniform joint space narrowing
  - Includes juvenile onset disease
- **Hyperparathyroidism (HPTH)**
  - Hands commonly show findings well
  - Generalized osteoporosis
  - Subperiosteal, subchondral, subligamentous, subtendon resorption
- **Renal Osteodystrophy**
  - Combination osteomalacia & HPTH
- **Osteomalacia/Rickets**
  - Diffuse skeletal involvement
  - Ill-defined, coarse trabeculae
  - Looser zones, pseudofractures
  - Rickets: Metaphyseal cupping, fraying

Helpful Clues for Less Common Diagnoses
- **Complex Regional Pain Syndrome (CRPS)**
  - Lower extremity common
  - Regional pattern of osteoporosis
  - May have trophic soft tissue changes
- **Thyrotoxicosis**
  - Phalanges of hands, feet
  - Generalized osteoporosis
- **Acromegaly**
  - Generalized osteoporosis
  - Spade-like phalangeal tufts
  - Cortical thickening, enthesopathy

Disuse Osteoporosis

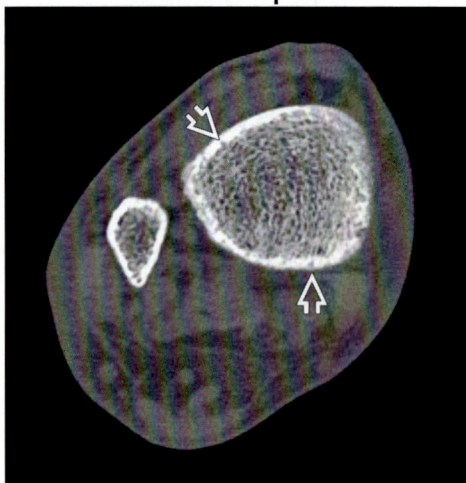

Axial NECT nicely demonstrates the findings of disuse osteoporosis including worm-like lucencies within the cortex consistent with resorption of bone from the margins of the Haversian canals ➡.

Rheumatoid Arthritis

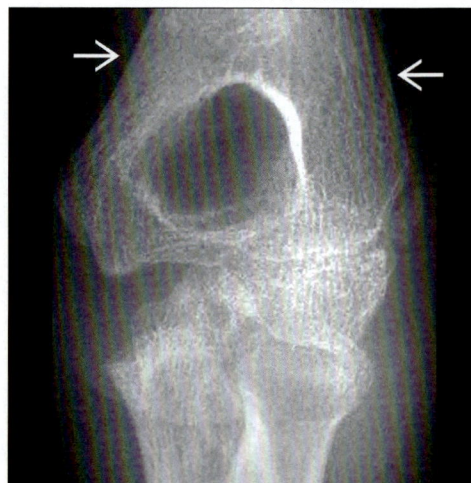

Anteroposterior radiograph shows typical changes of juvenile idiopathic arthritis, many of which are due to hyperemia. The hyperemia leads to rapid bone turnover, in turn causing intracortical tunneling ➡.

CORTICAL TUNNELING

Hyperparathyroidism (HPTH)

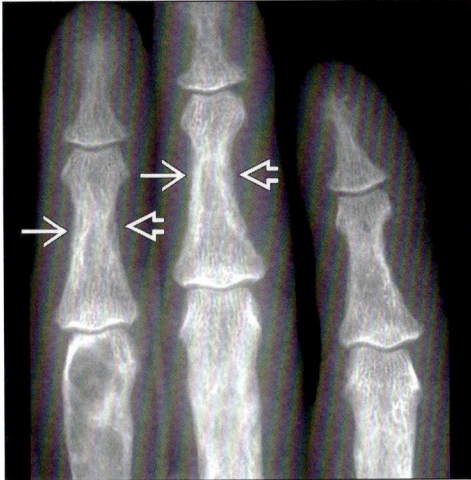

Renal Osteodystrophy

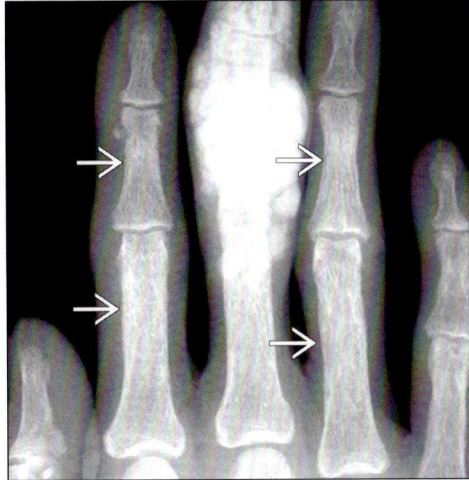

(Left) Posteroanterior radiograph shows cortical tunneling appearing as longitudinal lucencies ➡ with adjacent subperiosteal resorption ➡, characteristic findings of hyperparathyroidism. *(Right)* Posteroanterior radiograph shows metastatic calcium deposition and cortical striations within the phalanges ➡ in this patient with renal osteodystrophy.

Osteomalacia/Rickets

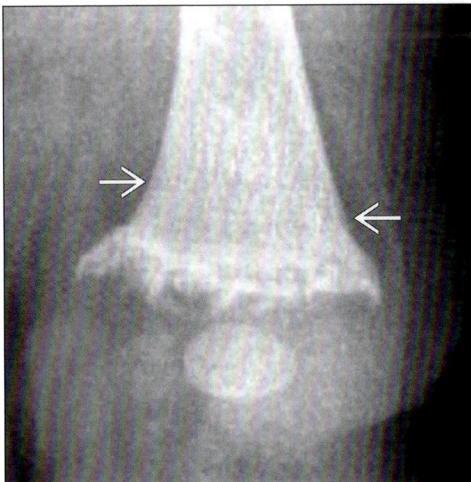

Osteomalacia/Rickets

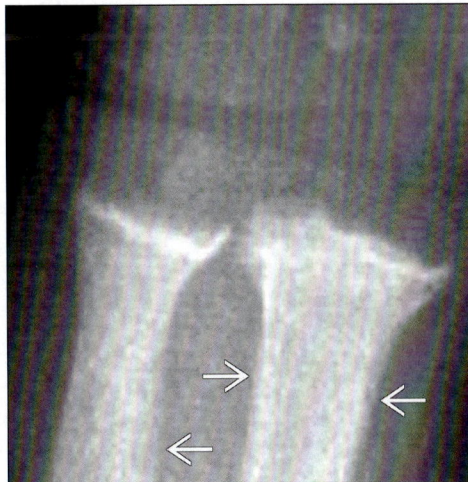

(Left) Anteroposterior radiograph shows intracortical lucencies ➡ in this child with rickets. These findings are due to nonmineralized osteoid lining Haversian canals. *(Right)* Posteroanterior radiograph shows lack of distinction between medullary and cortical bone of the distal radius and ulna ➡ as a result of cortical tunneling in this patent with rickets.

Complex Regional Pain Syndrome (CRPS)

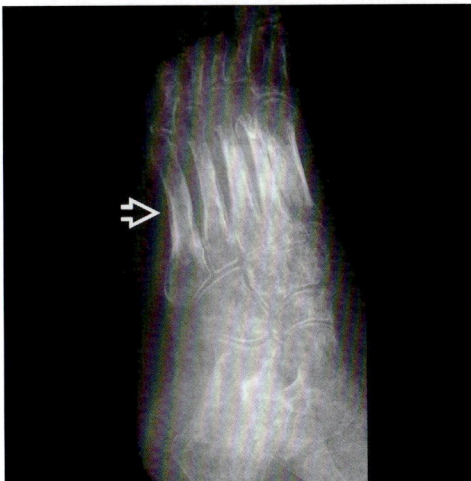

Hypophosphatasia

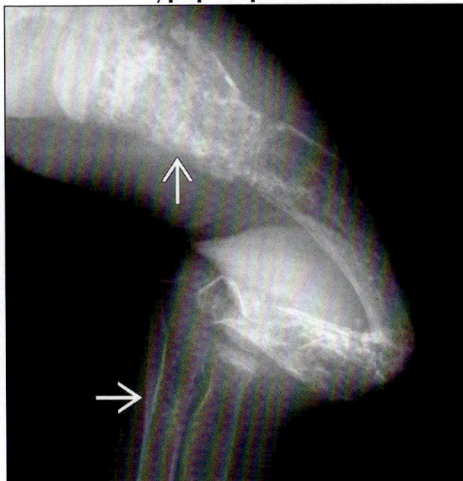

(Left) Oblique radiograph shows cortical tunneling ➡ along with a moth-eaten pattern in a patient with complex regional pain syndrome, related to nonunion of a tibial fracture. *(Right)* Anteroposterior radiograph shows severe cortical tunneling ➡, along with extreme osteoporosis and metaphyseal widening in this patient with hypophosphatasia.

PSEUDOARTHROSIS

DIFFERENTIAL DIAGNOSIS

Common
- Fracture, Nonunion
- Failed Graft

Less Common
- Ankylosing Spondylitis, Post-Trauma
- DISH, Post-Trauma
- Fibrous Dysplasia

Rare but Important
- Neurofibromatosis
- Congenital Pseudoarthrosis
- Ochronosis (Alkaptonuria)
- Osteogenesis Imperfecta

ESSENTIAL INFORMATION

Key Differential Diagnosis Issues
- **Hint**: Similar spinal risk of pseudoarthrosis with ankylosing spondylitis, DISH, ochronosis

Helpful Clues for Common Diagnoses
- **Post-Operative (Nonunion & Failed Graft)**
  - **Hint**: Motion, especially in spine
  - **Hint**: Look for hardware failure
  - Tibia common due to poor blood supply
  - Nonbridging callus, may be hypertrophic
  - Smooth sclerotic margins

Helpful Clues for Less Common Diagnoses
- **Ankylosing Spondylitis, Post-Trauma**
  - Following disruption of fused spine
  - Syndesmophytes, facet joint ankylosis
  - Interspinous, supraspinous ligament ossification
  - Sacroiliac joint fusion
  - Enthesopathy, hip & shoulder arthritis
- **DISH, Post-Trauma**
  - Following disruption of fused spine
  - Ligament ossification
    - ALL, iliolumbar, sacrotuberous, sacrospinous, stylohyoid, OPLL
  - Enthesopathy
  - Sacroiliac joint changes
    - Fusion upper 1/3, bridging osteophytes
- **Fibrous Dysplasia**
  - Mildly expansile, ground-glass matrix
  - Well-defined ± sclerotic margins
  - Monostotic or polyostotic

Helpful Clues for Rare Diagnoses
- **Neurofibromatosis**
  - Tibia, clavicle, radius, ulna
  - Fracture by age 2
  - May be only manifestation of neurofibromatosis
  - Congenital pseudoarthrosis similar
- **Ochronosis (Alkaptonuria)**
  - Following disruption of fused spine
  - Vertebral osteoporosis, extensive discal mineralization
  - OA-like changes SI joints, hips, knees
  - Absence of osteophytes
- **Osteogenesis Imperfecta**
  - Generalized osteoporosis
  - Bowing & other deformities of "soft" bones
  - Multiple fractures of varying ages

Fracture, Nonunion

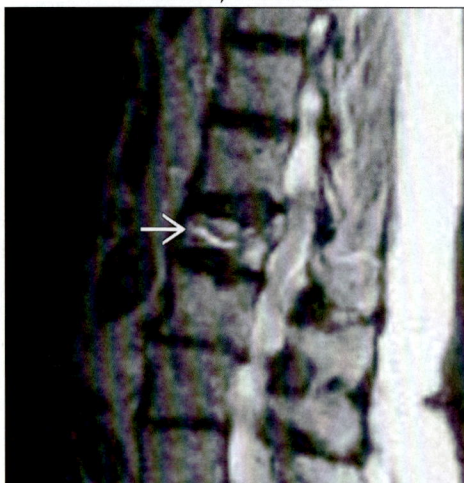

Lateral T2WI FSE MR shows a fluid-filled cleft ➡ within a midthoracic vertebra in this patient with osteoporosis and a compression fracture following minor trauma.

Fracture, Nonunion

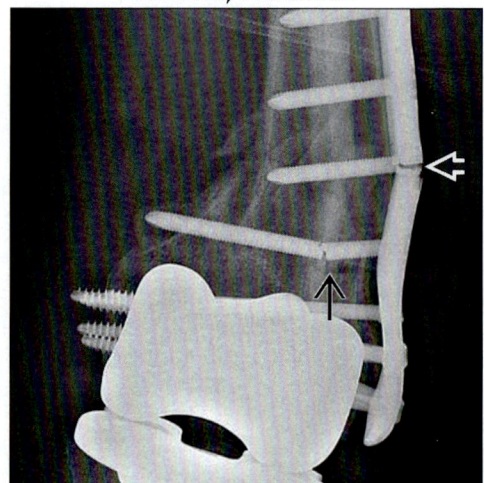

AP radiograph shows screw ➡ & plate ➡ fractures in a patient who has developed pseudarthrosis. The original construct was too rigid to permit the micromotion required to promote osteoblastic activity.

PSEUDOARTHROSIS

Failed Graft

Ankylosing Spondylitis, Post-Trauma

(Left) Sagittal NECT reveals a C5 corpectomy and a strut graft from C4 to C6 ➡. The margins of the graft-C6 interface are smooth and sclerotic ➡ consistent pseudoarthrosis. *(Right)* Sagittal STIR MR shows a pronounced oblique fracture involving the lower thoracic spine with a fluid-filled pseudoarthrosis ➡ in this patient with ankylosing spondylitis.

DISH, Post-Trauma

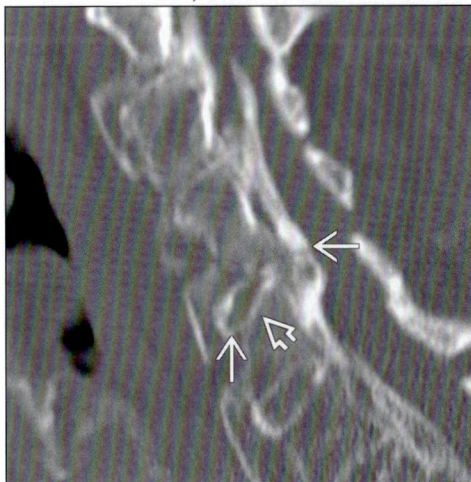

Neurofibromatosis

(Left) Sagittal bone CT demonstrates OPLL and DISH ➡. Fracture is present resulting in deformity of the inferior vertebra ➡. The fracture margins are smooth and sclerotic consistent with pseudoarthrosis. *(Right)* Anteroposterior radiograph shows two sites of osseous dysplasia ➡ in this child with the cystic type of pseudoarthrosis associated with neurofibromatosis.

Congenital Pseudoarthrosis

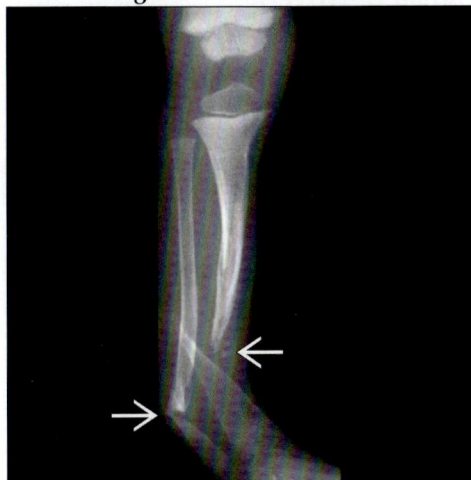

Osteogenesis Imperfecta

(Left) Anteroposterior radiograph shows complete fracture through the tibia and fibula with smoothly tapered fracture margins ➡. The appearance is classic for congenital pseudoarthrosis. *(Right)* Anteroposterior radiograph shows intramedullary rodding of both femora. The right femoral rod is fractured with pseudoarthrosis of the mid femoral diaphysis ➡ in this patient with osteogenesis imperfecta.

DIFFERENTIAL DIAGNOSIS

Common
- Degenerative
- DISH
- Baastrup Disease
- Subacromial Spur
- Plantar Fasciitis
- Haglund Syndrome
- Tendon/Ligament Microtrauma with Calcification (Mimic)
- Ankylosing Spondylitis
- Avulsion Fractures, Pelvic (Mimic)
- Inflammatory Bowel Disease Arthritis (IBD)
- Psoriatic Arthritis

Less Common
- Chronic Reactive Arthritis
- Rheumatoid Arthritis

Rare but Important
- Fluorosis
- Hypoparathyroidism
- Hypophosphatasia
- Hypophosphatemia (Vitamin D Resistant Rickets)

ESSENTIAL INFORMATION

Key Differential Diagnosis Issues
- Enthesis: Insertion of tendon or ligament onto bone
- Enthesopathy: Bone proliferation within enthesis
- Enthesitis: Inflammation at enthesis
  - May lead to erosion, bone formation
- **Hint**: Calcaneus common site RA, seronegative spondyloarthropathies
  - Retrocalcaneal bursitis/erosions in all
  - Achilles enthesophyte in all
    - Least common: Chronic reactive arthritis
  - Plantar surface reflects overall characteristics of arthritis
    - RA: Well-defined erosion, sharp enthesophytes
    - Seronegative: Ill-defined erosion, whiskering new bone formation, sclerosis
  - Subligamentous bone resorption plantar fascia in hyperparathyroidism may mimic
- **Hint**: Lower extremity common
  - Especially pelvis, proximal femur
  - Nonspecific
- Upper extremity

- Olecranon most common site
- Nonspecific

Helpful Clues for Common Diagnoses
- **Degenerative**
  - No specific distribution
  - Well-defined
  - No erosions or soft tissue swelling
- **DISH**
  - Especially pelvis, calcaneus, patella, olecranon
    - Well-defined
    - May be "bulky"
  - Ligament ossification
    - Anterior longitudinal (ALL), iliolumbar, sacrotuberous, sacrospinous, stylohyoid
  - Sacroiliac joint
    - Fusion upper 1/3, osteophytes
- **Baastrup Disease**
  - Supraspinous ligament
  - Spinous processes abnormal
    - Hypertrophied
    - Marginal sclerosis and cysts
    - Bursa between hypertrophied processes
- **Subacromial Spur**
  - Result of impingement
  - Associated bone proliferation on greater tuberosity
- **Plantar Fasciitis**
  - Well-defined plantar enthesophyte
  - Enthesophyte not causative
  - Thickened plantar fascia
  - Fascial, perifascial edema
  - Bone marrow edema at insertion
- **Haglund Syndrome**
  - Achilles enthesophyte
  - Achilles tendinosis
  - Retrocalcaneal bursitis (no erosion)
  - Prominent bump on superior surface posterior process of calcaneus
- **Tendon/Ligament Microtrauma with Calcification (Mimic)**
  - Atypical sites
  - Consider when absence of other findings
- **Ankylosing Spondylitis & IBD**
  - Pelvis, proximal femur, calcaneus, patella
    - Associated erosion, sclerosis at enthesis
  - Spinal fusion
    - Syndesmophytes
    - Interspinous, supraspinous ligament ossification
  - Sacroiliac joint fusion (synovial portion)

○ Hips, shoulder arthritis
• **Avulsion Fractures, Pelvic (Mimic)**
  ○ Result of healing process
  ○ Especially ASIS, ischial tuberosity
• **Psoriatic Arthritis**
  ○ Pelvis, proximal femur, calcaneus, patella
  ○ Calcaneal involvement
    ▪ Ill-defined plantar enthesophyte, erosion
    ▪ Achilles enthesophyte
    ▪ Retrocalcaneal bursitis, erosion
  ○ Erosive and proliferative arthritis
    ▪ Hands, feet most common
    ▪ Bilateral, asymmetric distribution
    ▪ Uniform joint space narrowing
    ▪ Spectrum: Marginal erosions to arthritis mutilans
    ▪ New bone formation at erosion margins
    ▪ Joint fusion
    ▪ Paravertebral ossification
    ▪ Periostitis
    ▪ Phalangeal tuft bone resorption

Helpful Clues for Less Common Diagnoses
• **Chronic Reactive Arthritis**
  ○ Calcaneus involvement characteristic
    ▪ Plantar enthesophyte common: Ill-defined appearance, ± erosion
    ▪ Achilles enthesophyte uncommon
    ▪ Retrocalcaneal bursitis, erosion
  ○ Enthesopathy at other sites less common than other spondyloarthropathies
  ○ Erosive and proliferative arthritis
    ▪ Lower extremity, spine dominate
    ▪ Otherwise similar to psoriasis

• **Rheumatoid Arthritis**
  ○ Calcaneus only site of enthesopathy
    ▪ Plantar enthesophyte well-defined
    ▪ Achilles enthesophyte
    ▪ Retrocalcaneal bursitis, erosion
  ○ Erosive arthritis
    ▪ Hands, feet predominate in early disease
    ▪ Bilateral symmetric disease
    ▪ Peri-articular osteopenia
    ▪ Marginal erosions
    ▪ Uniform joint space narrowing

Helpful Clues for Rare Diagnoses
• **Fluorosis**
  ○ Enthesopathy most common in pelvis, ribs
  ○ ALL, iliolumbar, sacrotuberous ligament ossification, OPLL
  ○ Spine, pelvis changes dominate
    ▪ Diffuse sclerosis
    ▪ Osteophytes
  ○ Appendicular periostitis
• **Hypoparathyroidism**
  ○ Nonspecific enthesopathy distribution
  ○ ALL ossification
  ○ Diffuse sclerosis
  ○ Spinal osteophytes
  ○ Calvarial thickening, subcutaneous calcifications, hypoplastic teeth
• **Hypophosphatasia & Vitamin D Resistant Rickets**
  ○ Nonspecific enthesopathy distribution
  ○ Ill-defined, coarse trabeculae
  ○ Looser's zones, pseudofractures

Degenerative

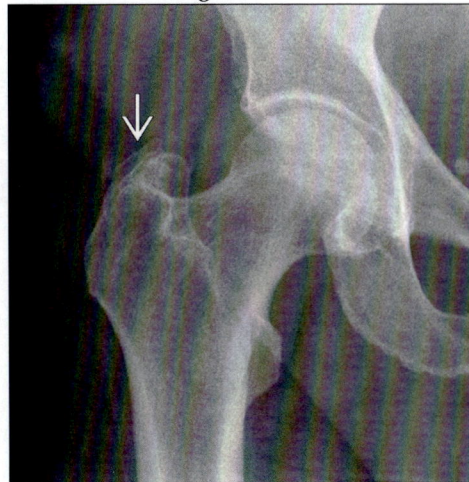

Lateral radiograph shows degenerative enthesophytes at the attachment of the plantar fascia ⇒ and the insertion of the Achilles tendon ⇒.

Degenerative

Anteroposterior radiograph shows new bone formation along the superior aspect of the greater trochanter in this elderly individual with degenerative enthesopathy ⇒.

ENTHESOPATHY

DISH

Subacromial Spur

(Left) Anteroposterior radiograph shows a classic case of DISH with pelvic enthesopathy including enthesopathy along the ischial tuberosity ➡. *(Right)* Anteroposterior radiograph shows a large subacromial spur ➡ which arises from the acromial attachment of the coracoacromial ligament as a result of impingement.

Plantar Fasciitis

Haglund Syndrome

(Left) Sagittal T1WI MR shows plantar fasciitis with a thickened ligament. An associated marrow-containing enthesophyte ➡ is present. *(Right)* Sagittal T1WI MR shows typical changes of Haglund syndrome including prominent "bump" ➡ and marked thickening of the Achilles tendon ➡. A small focus of ossification is present near the Achilles tendon insertion ➡.

Tendon/Ligament Microtrauma with Calcification (Mimic)

Ankylosing Spondylitis

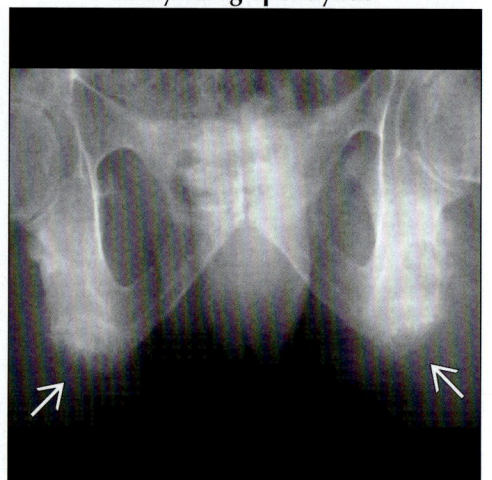

(Left) Axial NECT shows linear calcification within the gluteus maximus tendon near its insertion ➡ as well as irregularity at the tendon insertion onto the posterior femoral cortex ➡, likely from prior trauma. *(Right)* Anteroposterior radiograph shows classic signs of ankylosing spondylitis with enthesopathy at the ischial tuberosities ➡.

ENTHESOPATHY

Avulsion Fractures, Pelvic (Mimic)

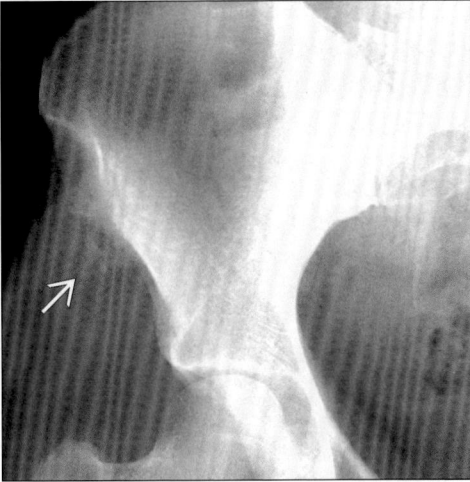

Psoriatic Arthritis

(Left) Anteroposterior radiograph shows typical case of an avulsion of the anterior superior iliac spine. At four weeks follow-up new bone formation is seen at the site ➡. *(Right)* Anteroposterior radiograph shows extensive ill-defined enthesopathy at the malleoli ➡. The productive changes seen here are typical of either psoriatic arthritis or chronic reactive arthritis.

Psoriatic Arthritis

Chronic Reactive Arthritis

(Left) Anteroposterior radiograph shows prominent enthesopathy seen at the anterior superior iliac spine ➡ in this patient with psoriatic arthritis. *(Right)* Lateral radiograph shows dense reactive change with ill-defined enthesopathy at the attachment of the plantar fascia ➡ in this patient with chronic reactive arthritis.

Chronic Reactive Arthritis

Hypophosphatemia (Vitamin D Resistant Rickets)

(Left) Anteroposterior radiograph shows loss of normal cortical definition on the ischial tuberosity, an early indicator of enthesopathy ➡. This finding is commonly seen in any of the spondyloarthropathies. *(Right)* Anteroposterior radiograph of a patient with vitamin D resistant rickets who must take massive doses of vitamin D, resulting in prominent enthesopathy at the ischial tuberosity ➡ and anterior superior iliac spine ➡.

TENDON & LIGAMENTOUS OSSIFICATION

DIFFERENTIAL DIAGNOSIS

Common
- DISH
- Post-Traumatic
- Ossification Posterior Longitudinal Ligament (OPLL)
- Ankylosing Spondylitis
- Idiopathic Achilles Tendon Ossification

Less Common
- Fluorosis
- Stylohyoid Ligament Ossification & Eagle-Barrett Syndrome

Rare but Important
- Hypophosphatasia
- Hypoparathyroidism

ESSENTIAL INFORMATION

Key Differential Diagnosis Issues
- **Hint**: Similar spinal manifestations in DISH, OPLL, fluorosis, hypoparathyroidism

Helpful Clues for Common Diagnoses
- **DISH**
  - Anterior longitudinal ligament (ALL)
  - Iliolumbar, sacrotuberous, sacrospinous, stylohyoid ligaments
  - Enthesopathy
  - Sacroiliac joint changes
    - Fusion upper 1/3, osteophytes
  - 50% have OPLL
- **Post-Traumatic**
  - Random sites

- **Ossification Posterior Longitudinal Ligament (OPLL)**
  - All levels, especially cervical
  - 20% have DISH
- **Ankylosing Spondylitis**
  - Interspinous, supraspinous ligaments
    - Dagger sign
  - Syndesmophytes
  - Enthesopathy
  - Sacroiliac joint fusion (synovial portion)
  - Hip, shoulder arthritis
- **Idiopathic Achilles Tendon Ossification**
  - Isolated finding

Helpful Clues for Less Common Diagnoses
- **Fluorosis**
  - ALL, iliolumbar, sacrotuberous lig., OPLL
  - Spine, pelvis changes dominate
    - Diffuse sclerosis, osteophytes
  - Appendicular periostitis, enthesopathy
- **Stylohyoid Ligament Ossification & Eagle-Barrett Syndrome**
  - Syndrome: Throat, swallowing pain

Helpful Clues for Rare Diagnoses
- **Hypophosphatasia**
  - Diffuse skeletal involvement
  - Ill-defined coarse trabeculae
  - Looser's zones, pseudofractures
- **Hypoparathyroidism**
  - ALL
  - Diffuse sclerosis, spinal osteophytes
  - Calvarial thickening, subcutaneous calcifications, hypoplastic teeth

DISH

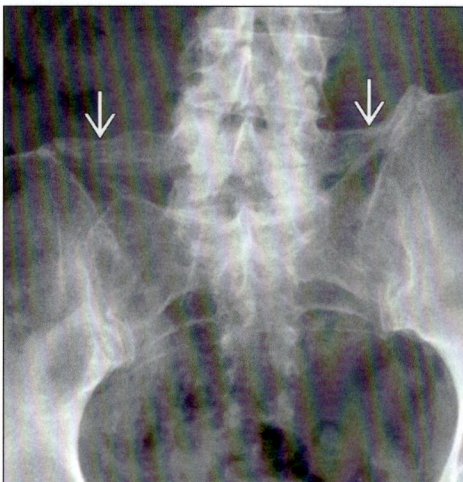

Anteroposterior radiograph shows extensive ossification within the iliolumbar ligament bilaterally ➡. Ossification of this ligament may be seen with many conditions, most commonly DISH.

DISH

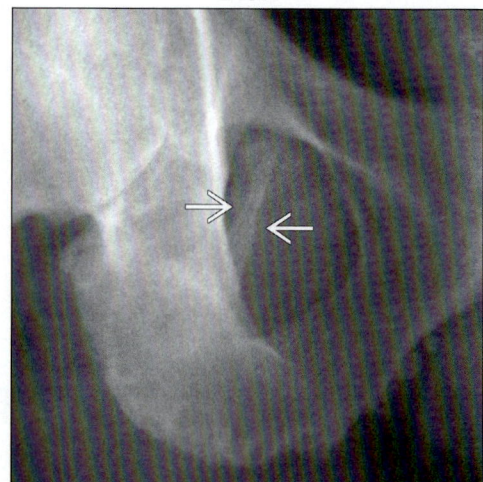

Anteroposterior radiograph shows linear calcification superimposed on the obturator foramen ➡, representing sacrotuberous ligament ossification, commonly seen in DISH.

TENDON & LIGAMENTOUS OSSIFICATION

Post-Traumatic

Ossification Posterior Longitudinal Ligament (OPLL)

(Left) Coronal bone CT shows irregular linearly oriented ossification ➡ which follows the course of the ligamentum teres. An unusual finding, this mineralization is either the result of intrinsic degeneration or prior injury to the ligament. (Right) Lateral radiograph shows thick ossification of the posterior longitudinal ligament extending along the anterior spinal canal ➡. The finding is typical of OPLL.

Ankylosing Spondylitis

Idiopathic Achilles Tendon Ossification

(Left) Anteroposterior radiograph shows extensive enthesopathy, or ossification of the tendon insertions at the ischial tuberosities ➡. Note the fused SI joints in this patient with ankylosing spondylitis. (Right) Lateral radiograph shows ossification of the distal Achilles tendon, slightly proximal to the tendinous insertion ➡. It is slightly rounded and smoothly marginated, contrasting with the more angular plantar fascial enthesophyte ➡.

Fluorosis

Stylohyoid Ligament Ossification & Eagle-Barrett Syndrome

(Left) Anteroposterior radiograph shows calcification of the sacrospinous ligaments ➡ which is a common finding in patients with fluorosis. (Right) Sagittal oblique NECT shows extensive ossification of the stylohyoid ligament ➡. The finding is bilateral and symmetric in this patient with Eagle-Barrett syndrome.

BONE AGE, ADVANCED

DIFFERENTIAL DIAGNOSIS

Common
- Familial Tall Stature
- Idiopathic Precocious Puberty
- Excessive Sex Hormone
- Juvenile Idiopathic Arthritis (JIA)
- Hemophilia
- Physeal Fractures
- Radiation-Induced Growth Deformities

Less Common
- Hyperthyroidism
- Hypothalamic Mass
- Pituitary Gigantism
- Adrenocortical Tumor
- Adrenal Hyperplasia
- Exogenous Obesity
- Ectopic Gonadotropin Tumor
- Polyostotic Fibrous Dysplasia, McCune-Albright

Rare but Important
- Chronic Septic Arthritis, Non-Bacterial
- Encephalitis
- Primary Hyperaldosteronism
- Beckwith-Wiedemann Syndrome

ESSENTIAL INFORMATION

Key Differential Diagnosis Issues
- Skeletal maturation more than two standard deviations above the mean
- Determining etiology highly dependent on lab findings and clinical presentation
- Marked advancement in bone age is more likely to indicate elevated sex hormones

Helpful Clues for Common Diagnoses
- **Excessive Sex Hormone**
  - Induces early growth plate maturation
- **Juvenile Idiopathic Arthritis (JIA)**
  - Chronic hyperemia causes growth centers to ossify early, enlarge, & fuse prematurely
- **Hemophilia**
- Similar JIA, + dense effusion
- **Radiation-Induced Growth Deformities**
  - Vascular obliteration → premature fusion
  - Associated with bone hypoplasia, slipped capital femoral epiphysis, scoliosis
  - Watch for "port-like" distribution
  - Associated radiation-induced sarcoma

Helpful Clues for Less Common Diagnoses
- **Hypothalamic Mass**
  - Early onset of normal maturation process
  - Hypothalamic hamartoma or mass effect from suprasellar tumors
- **Adrenocortical Tumor or Hyperplasia**
  - Hypersecretion of androgens and cortisol
- **Ectopic Gonadotropin Tumor**
  - Hepatoblastoma/teratoma/chorioepithelioma
- **Polyostotic Fibrous Dysplasia**
  - Ground-glass bone lesions + cafe au lait spots + precocious puberty

Other Essential Information
- MR brain to exclude hypothalamic lesion
- Pelvic ultrasound (females) for evidence of gonadotropin/estrogen stimulation

Juvenile Idiopathic Arthritis (JIA)

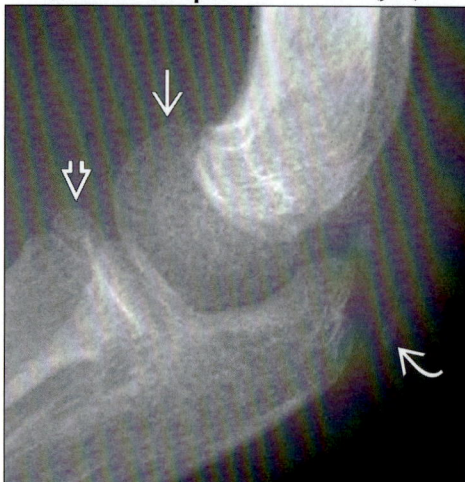

Lateral radiograph of the affected left elbow shows advanced skeletal maturation in the capitellum ➡, radial head ➡, & olecranon ➡. This early skeletal maturation is due to chronic hyperemia. (†MSK Req).

Juvenile Idiopathic Arthritis (JIA)

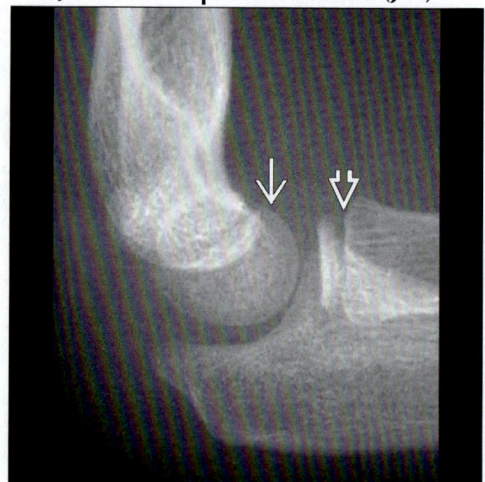

Lateral radiograph of the unaffected right elbow, in the same patient as previous image, for comparison. The capitellum ➡ and radial head ➡ are normal. (†MSK Req).

BONE AGE, ADVANCED

Hemophilia

Hemophilia

(Left) Lateral radiograph of a teenager's knee shows a huge effusion ➡ and overgrowth of the epiphyses ➡ with the femoral condyles particularly enlarged in a male patient with hemophilia. *(Right)* Anteroposterior radiograph of the same knee as previous image, shows epiphyseal overgrowth ➡ and intercondylar notch widening ➡, which can be seen with hemophilia or juvenile idiopathic arthritis. Bone age was advanced.

Physeal Fractures

Radiation-Induced Growth Deformities

(Left) Coronal bone CT shows a remote fracture of the distal tibia ➡ and development of bridging of bone across the physeal plate ➡. This will result in a short limb from premature growth plate closure. *(Right)* 3D bone CT shows focal convex left scoliosis ➡ in a patient treated with radiation therapy for neuroblastoma. The affected thoracolumbar vertebrae are short on the right from early physeal fusion, yielding a flattened curvature without congenital segmentation anomalies.

Radiation-Induced Growth Deformities

Polyostotic Fibrous Dysplasia, McCune-Albright

(Left) Anteroposterior radiograph shows a short humerus (relative to thorax) in a patient radiated at a young age for Ewing sarcoma. Note the aggressive osteoid-producing tumor ➡, an associated radiation-induced osteosarcoma. *(Right)* Anteroposterior radiograph shows numerous lesions ➡ of mixed density and with a narrow zone of transition. The right femoral lesion extends to the epiphyseal plate resulting in a shepherd's crook deformity.

BONE AGE, DELAYED

DIFFERENTIAL DIAGNOSIS

Common
- Constitutional Delay of Puberty (Normal Variant)
- Chronic Disease
  - Chronic Liver Disease
  - Renal Osteodystrophy
  - Congenital Heart Disease
  - Rickets
  - Juvenile Idiopathic Arthritis
  - Thalassemia
  - Cerebral Palsy
- Excessive Exercise
- Malnutrition
  - Anorexia
  - Malabsorption Conditions
- Complications of Steroids
- Fetal Alcohol Syndrome

Less Common
- Lead Poisoning
- Down Syndrome (Trisomy 21)
- Cushing Disease
- Hypopituitarism
- Pseudohypoparathyroidism
- Craniopharyngioma

Rare but Important
- HIV-AIDS: MSK Complications
- Growth Hormone Deficiency
- Hypogonadism
- Hypothyroidism
- Warfarin Embryopathy

ESSENTIAL INFORMATION

Key Differential Diagnosis Issues
- Skeletal maturation more than two standard deviations below the mean
  - Formally evaluated with serial PA radiographs of left hand
  - Standards of Greulich and Pyle classically used for comparison

Helpful Clues for Common Diagnoses
- Majority of common diagnoses cause delayed bone age due to delay of puberty
  - Are identifiable by clinical history

Helpful Clues for Less Common Diagnoses
- **Lead Poisoning**
  - Widened metaphyses, dense metaphyseal lines
- **Down Syndrome (Trisomy 21)**
  - Additional findings = flared iliac wing, flat acetabular roof, clinodactyly, microcephaly, atlantoaxial instability

Helpful Clues for Rare Diagnoses
- **Hypogonadism**
  - Results in long limbs with disproportionally short trunk

Alternative Differential Approaches
- Stippled epiphyses: Hypothyroidism, Warfarin embryopathy, chondrodysplasia punctata, multiple epiphyseal dysplasia, trisomy 21, trisomy 18, prenatal infection, Morquio syndrome

Chronic Disease

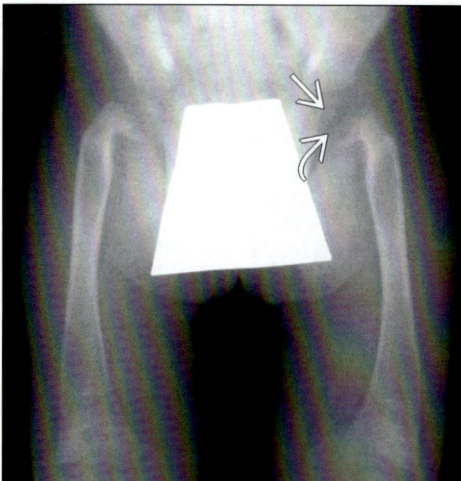

AP radiograph shows delayed skeletal maturation in this 5 year old. Note the tiny femoral head ossification centers ➡. The widened metaphyses ➡ indicate rickets in this patient with long-term renal disease.

Renal Osteodystrophy

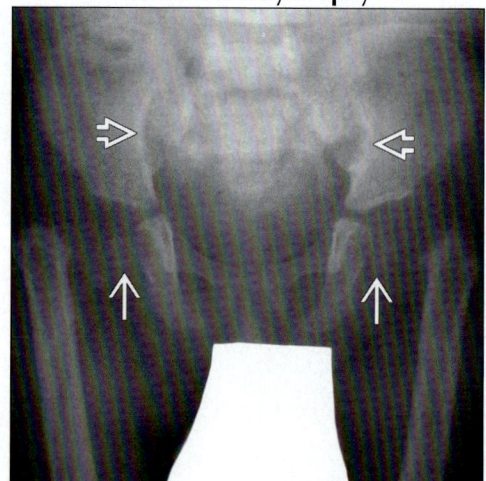

AP radiograph shows subchondral resorption at the SIJ ➡ & slipped capital femoral epiphyses from rickets ➡ in this 10 year old with renal osteodystrophy. The skeletal maturation is severely delayed.

BONE AGE, DELAYED

Rickets

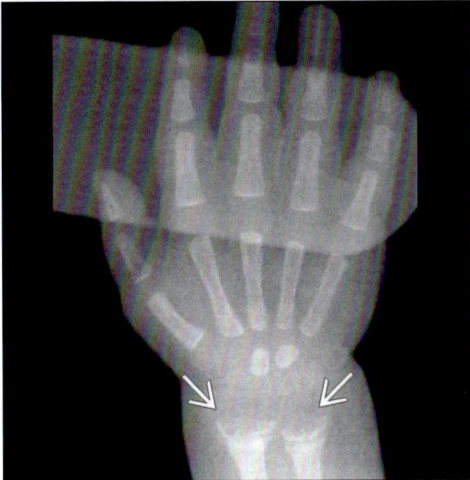

Juvenile Idiopathic Arthritis

(Left) Posteroanterior radiograph shows the widened zone of provisional calcification with frayed, cupped metaphysis at the distal radius and ulna ➡, typical of rickets. Note that despite the chronologic age of 1 year, the skeletal maturation is severely delayed. (Right) Posteroanterior radiograph shows an open physis ➡ in a 22 year old patient with JIA, indicating delayed bone age. Note also the fused carpals and significant metacarpal erosive disease.

Excessive Exercise

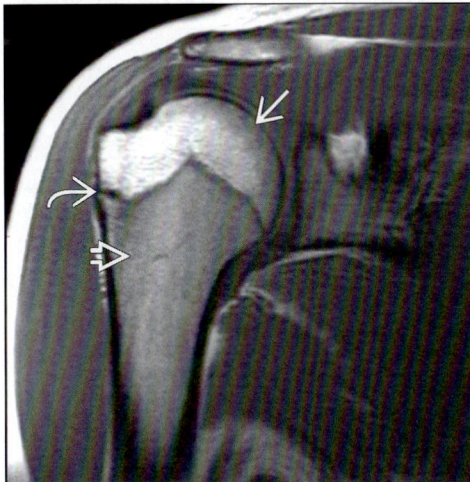

Excessive Exercise

(Left) Coronal T1WI MR shows open physis ➡, as well as immature bone marrow distribution with a crescent of red marrow in the epiphysis ➡ and solid red marrow in the metadiaphysis ➡. She is a 19 year old competitive gymnast who practices 5 hours daily. (Right) PA radiograph of the wrist in the same patient as previous image, shows open physes at the distal radius & ulna ➡. This patient is at least 2 standard deviations younger than her chronologic age.

Thalassemia

Lead Poisoning

(Left) Anteroposterior radiograph shows the squared bones, indicating severe marrow packing in a patient with thalassemia. This five year old patient also shows delayed bone age, related to the chronicity of the disease. (Right) Anteroposterior radiograph shows the dense metaphyseal lines ➡, resulting from deposition of lead during growth. Chronic lead poisoning can lead to a delay in skeletal maturation.

SOFT TISSUE OSSIFICATION

DIFFERENTIAL DIAGNOSIS

Common
- Heterotopic Ossification
  - Myositis Ossificans (Late)
- Loose Bodies

Less Common
- Fracture Fragment (Mimic)
- DISH
- Leiomyoma, Deep
- Cement & Bone Fillers (Mimic)
- Hematoma
- Synovial Osteochondromatosis
- OPLL
- Osteosarcoma, Parosteal
- Extraskeletal Osteosarcoma
- Osteosarcoma, Metastasis

Rare but Important
- Liposarcoma, Soft Tissue
- Lipoma, Soft Tissue
- Post-Operative Scar
- Rhabdomyosarcoma, Embryonal
- Fibrodysplasia Ossificans Progressiva
- Giant Cell Tumor, Soft Tissue Implants

ESSENTIAL INFORMATION

Key Differential Diagnosis Issues
- Calcification is not the same as ossification
  - Ossification has mature features, such as trabeculae and cortex

Helpful Clues for Common Diagnoses
- **Heterotopic Ossification**
  - Numerous causes of soft tissue ossification
    - Blunt trauma, tendon tear, burns, paralysis, tumor, neurologic infection (poliomyelitis, tetanus, Guillain-Barré)
  - Calcifies at approximately one month post insult, then ossifies later
  - Ossification is most mature peripherally, with center less mature
  - Common sites of injury may suggest this diagnosis when changes are early
    - Thigh after trauma and hip after joint replacement or paralysis
- **Myositis Ossificans (Late)**
  - Implies muscle ossification
    - Term is sometimes used interchangeably with heterotopic ossification

- Timing & zoning identical to heterotopic ossification
- **Loose Bodies**
  - Ossified round to oval masses located in & around joints
    - May migrate away from joint within tendon sheath
  - Location & typical appearance can be confirmed with CT, MR

Helpful Clues for Less Common Diagnoses
- **Fracture Fragment (Mimic)**
  - Borders of bone fragment angular when acute, rounded when chronic
  - Donor site usually has identifiable deformity
  - Cartilage fragments may or may not ossify
- **DISH**
  - Enthesopathic changes in spine and pelvis predominate
    - Flowing ossification anterior to vertebral bodies
  - Ligamentous ossification, with iliolumbar most common
- **Leiomyoma, Deep**
  - Smooth muscle benign neoplasm with dense popcorn ossification
  - Very commonly seen on pelvic imaging due to uterine fibroids
- **Cement & Bone Fillers (Mimic)**
  - Bone graft may extrude into soft tissues
  - Cement extravasation may mimic bone
- **Hematoma**
  - Peripheral ossification if chronic
    - Most commonly involving intracranial epidural hematomas
  - Subperiosteal hemorrhage ossifies with more mature bone in the periphery
- **Synovial Osteochondromatosis**
  - Intraarticular ossified masses may appear to be in soft tissue, depending on imaging plane
  - Extraarticular extension into surrounding soft tissues may occur
  - Bursal synovial osteochondromatosis projects outside joint on radiographs
- **OPLL**
  - Multilevel ossification of posterior longitudinal ligament in spine
    - Mid cervical spine level most commonly involved
  - Look for changes of myelopathy on MR

SOFT TISSUE OSSIFICATION

- **Osteosarcoma, Parosteal**
  - Dense ossified mass most commonly posterior to distal femur
    - Contiguous with underlying femoral cortex
  - Seen in older patients compared with conventional osteosarcoma
  - Low grade lesion
- **Extraskeletal Osteosarcoma**
  - Older patients than conventional osteosarcoma
  - Slow growing mass may be large at presentation
  - Difficult to differentiate from other soft tissue sarcomas
    - 50% demonstrate mineralization
    - Separate from adjacent bone
  - Lower extremities & pelvis most commonly involved
  - Metastases common at diagnosis
- **Osteosarcoma, Metastasis**
  - Metastases ossify in a similar fashion to the primary tumor
  - Lung and nodal soft tissue masses most common
  - Other "bone forming metastases" (including breast, colon and urinary tract carcinomas), tend to calcify, rather than ossify

Helpful Clues for Rare Diagnoses
- **Liposarcoma & Lipoma, Soft Tissue**
  - Fat-containing soft tissue mass

- Malignant liposarcoma contains nodular soft tissue elements or thick septations
  - Ossification is uncommon but can occur in both benign and malignant tumors
- **Post-Operative Scar**
  - Ossification follows course of operative incision
  - Most common in anterior abdominal wall, above umbilicus
  - Male predominance
- **Rhabdomyosarcoma, Embryonal**
  - Embryonal subtype more common in children
  - Soft tissue mass with metaplastic foci of ossification
    - Mass may invade adjacent bone
- **Fibrodysplasia Ossificans Progressiva**
  - Abnormal ossification of the soft tissues
    - Accelerated by minor trauma
  - Ossification fatally limits respiratory movement
  - Associated finding of short great toe with valgus orientation
- **Giant Cell Tumor, Soft Tissue Implants**
  - Foci of benign giant cell tumor implanted into soft tissue
    - Iatrogenic from surgery or biopsy
    - Post-traumatic from pathologic fracture through primary lesion
  - Characteristic peripheral ossification in 1-2% of soft tissue implants
    - Ossification histologically identifiable in high proportion of soft tissue implants

Heterotopic Ossification

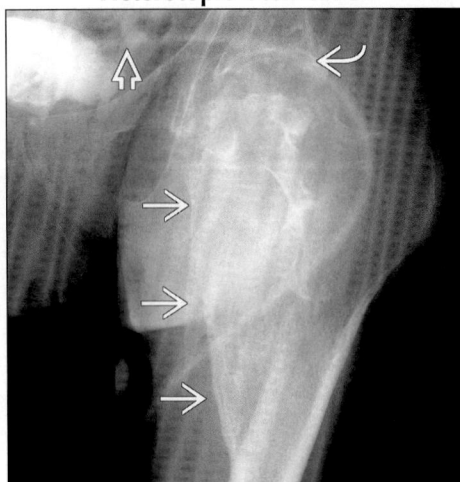

Anteroposterior radiograph shows mature ossification ⇒ involving the medial thighs in this horseback rider. Note the peripheral cortex and central trabeculae, suggesting it is likely at least several months old.

Heterotopic Ossification

Anteroposterior radiograph shows a solid sheet of mature ossification ⇒ around the hip. The hip joint space is narrowed ⇉ and there is a suprapubic catheter ⇒ in place, suggesting paralysis.

SOFT TISSUE OSSIFICATION

Heterotopic Ossification

Myositis Ossificans (Late)

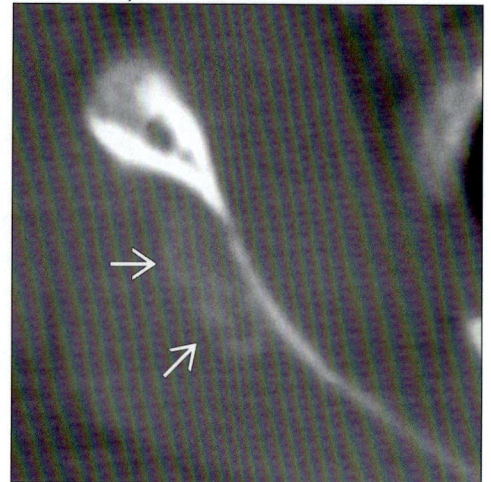

(Left) Anteroposterior radiograph shows a grade III acromioclavicular dislocation, with elevation of the clavicle ➡ relative to the acromion. Ossification ➡ between the clavicle and coracoid indicates disruption of the coracoclavicular ligaments. (Right) Axial bone CT shows osseous matrix ➡ at the surface of the scapula. Ossification zoning, with mature peripheral ossification, is typical of myositis. Osteosarcoma typically has more mature matrix centrally.

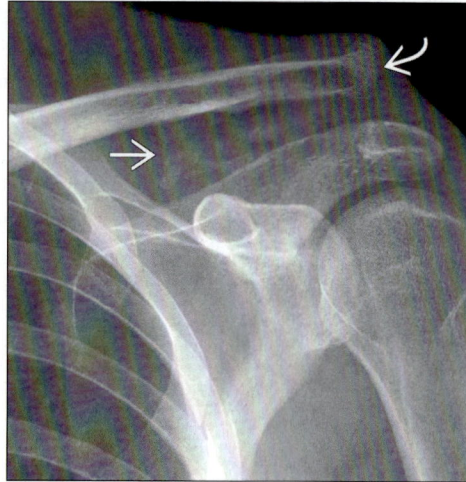

Fracture Fragment (Mimic)

DISH

(Left) Axial NECT shows an osseous body ➡ in the soft tissues, which separated from the posterior acetabular rim ➡, indicating a recent episode of posterior subluxation or dislocation of the hip. (Right) Anteroposterior radiograph shows ossification of the iliolumbar ligament bilaterally ➡. This may be seen with DISH, sacroiliac joint osteoarthritis, trauma, fluorosis and X-linked hypophosphatemia.

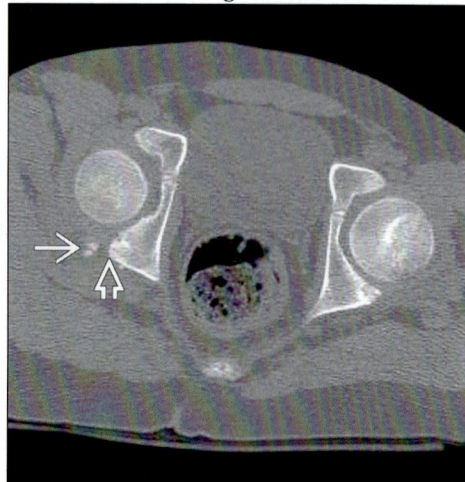

Cement & Bone Fillers (Mimic)

Synovial Osteochondromatosis

(Left) Anteroposterior radiograph shows dense material ➡ in the soft tissues surrounding a tibia fracture. This material is hydroxyapatite, a bone substitute that is osteoconductive, acting as a scaffold for the ingrowth of new bone. (Right) Lateral radiograph shows an elevated anterior fat pad ➡, with the joint containing several large, similarly sized ossified rounded bodies ➡.

SOFT TISSUE OSSIFICATION

Osteosarcoma, Parosteal

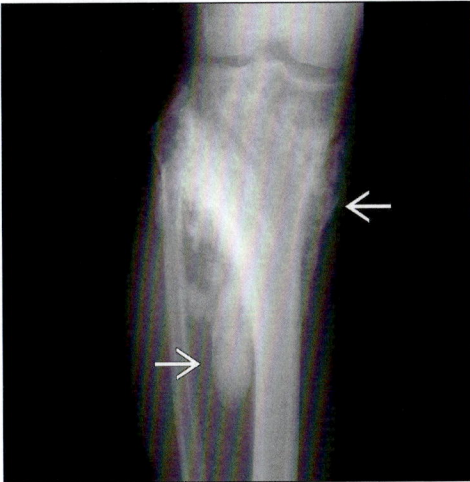

Extraskeletal Osteosarcoma

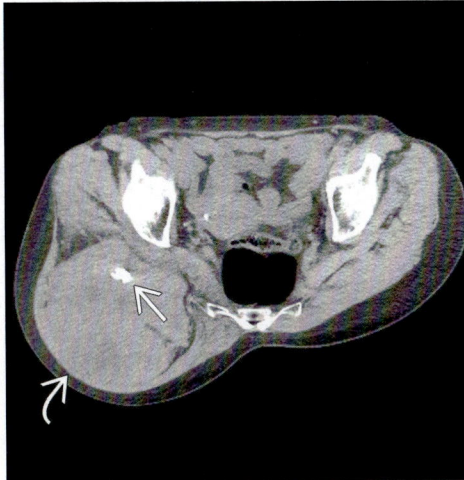

(Left) Anteroposterior radiograph shows well-differentiated ossification ➡ wrapping around and appearing "pasted" on the metaphyseal region of the tibia. The tumor bone is quite mature. *(Right)* Axial NECT shows a large mass ➡ between the right gluteus maximus and medius muscles. The mass contains areas of dense calcification or ossification ➡. Extraskeletal osteosarcoma is seen in older patients than conventional osteosarcoma.

Osteosarcoma, Metastasis

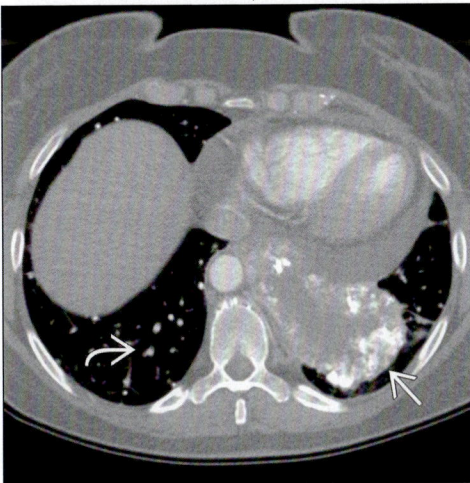

Osteosarcoma, Metastasis

(Left) Axial CECT shows ossification of a retrocardiac mass ➡ in this patient with known metastatic osteosarcoma. Innumerable bilateral pulmonary nodules ➡ are also present, some of which are clearly ossified similar to the primary tumor. *(Right)* Axial CECT shows ossification of an enlarged lymph node ➡ from metastatic osteosarcoma. This showed increased radiotracer uptake on bone scan.

Liposarcoma, Soft Tissue

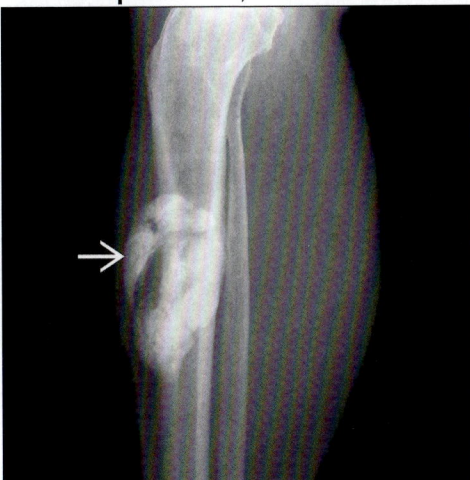

Fibrodysplasia Ossificans Progressiva

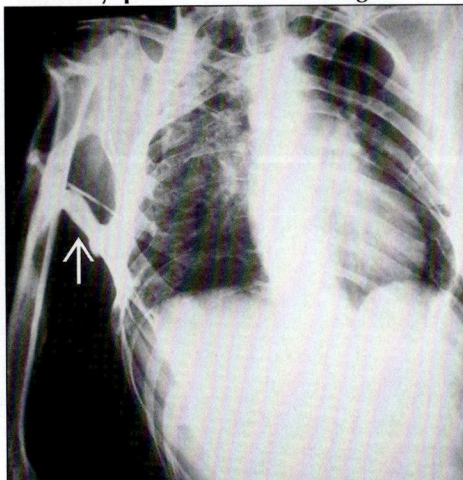

(Left) Lateral radiograph shows a fatty mass containing prominent dystrophic calcification appearing ossified ➡. MR showed fat, calcification and soft tissue regions of the mass making it suspicious for malignancy, proven liposarcoma. *(Right)* AP radiograph shows mature bone bridging between ribs, as well as between the humerus and rib cage ➡. The end result is complete loss of motion of the rib cage, increasing risk of pneumonia and early death.

NODULAR CALCIFICATION

DIFFERENTIAL DIAGNOSIS

Common
- Phlebolith
- Pyrophosphate Arthropathy
- Tendinitis, Calcific
- Bursitis, Calcific
- Injection Granuloma
- Myositis Ossificans (Early)
- Progressive Systemic Sclerosis
- Loose Body (Mimic)

Less Common
- Gout
- Avulsion Fractures (Early)
- Dermatomyositis
- Hyperparathyroidism/Renal Osteodystrophy
- Mixed Connective Tissue Disease
- Hypervitaminosis D
- Hematoma
- Synovial Osteochondromatosis
- Rheumatoid Nodule
- Soft Tissue Tumors Containing Nodular Calcification
  - Hemangioma, Soft Tissue
    - Maffucci Syndrome
  - Uterine Fibroid
  - Synovial Sarcoma
  - Hemangiopericytoma

Rare but Important
- Metastatic Calcification
- Systemic Lupus Erythematosus
- Calcific Myonecrosis
- Tumoral (Idiopathic) Calcinosis
- Trevor Fairbank (Dysplasia Epiphysealis Hemimelica)
- Thermal Injury, Burns
- Sarcoidosis
- Chondrodysplasia Punctata (Mimic)
- Pseudohypoparathyroidism
- Parasites
- Melorheostosis

ESSENTIAL INFORMATION

Key Differential Diagnosis Issues
- Overlap in radiographic appearance of calcified collections
  - Calcification = structureless density
  - Ossification = organized density with cortex and/or trabeculae
- Maintain a high suspicion for malignancy when calcification is present with a mass

Helpful Clues for Common Diagnoses
- **Phlebolith**
  - Small round calcification in vessel
  - Characteristic central lucency
  - Common in lower extremities & pelvis
- **Pyrophosphate Arthropathy**
  - Calcium pyrophosphate dihydrate (CPPD) crystal deposition
  - Chondrocalcinosis in knee menisci, wrist TFCC & hip labrum can be nodular
- **Tendinitis, Calcific**
  - Hydroxyapatite Deposition Disease (HADD) in tendons
  - Additional deposition in capsule, ligaments & bursae
- **Bursitis, Calcific**
  - HADD involving the bursa
  - Shoulder & hip most common
- **Injection Granuloma**
  - Classic gluteal location; central lucency
- **Myositis Ossificans (Early)**
  - Amorphous calcification one month post trauma, before ossification
  - Radiolucent zone between bone and myositis, unlike malignancy
  - Correlate with history of regional trauma, although patients may not recall trauma
- **Progressive Systemic Sclerosis**
  - Lobulated calcifications + tuft resorption
- **Loose Body (Mimic)**
  - Intraarticular; features of ossification

Helpful Clues for Less Common Diagnoses
- **Gout**
  - Calcified tophi → pressure erosions & intraosseous collections
  - First MTP joint, Achilles tendon insertion & olecranon bursa common
- **Avulsion Fractures (Early)**
  - Cartilaginous fragments may calcify
  - Small osseous fragments can mimic calcification
- **Dermatomyositis**
  - Inter- & intramuscular calcification
- **Hyperparathyroidism/Renal Osteodystrophy**
  - Subperiosteal resorption, vascular calcification & evidence of renal failure
  - Wrist, knee, hip, shoulder & elbow
- **Mixed Connective Tissue Disease**

NODULAR CALCIFICATION

- ○ Dermatomyositis & scleroderma findings
- **Hypervitaminosis D**
  - ○ Large, calcified, periarticular masses
  - ○ Associated ligamentous & intervertebral disc calcification
- **Hematoma**
  - ○ Even with history of trauma, need follow-up to exclude malignancy unless there is complete lack of enhancement on MR
- **Synovial Osteochondromatosis**
  - ○ Multiple intraarticular densities
- **Rheumatoid Nodule**
  - ○ Soft tissue masses with periarticular erosions, osteopenia, joint space narrowing
- **Soft Tissue Tumors Containing Nodular Calcification**
  - ○ Hemangioma, Soft Tissue
    - Mass with fat, vessels & phleboliths
    - Maffucci syndrome = enchondromatosis + hemangiomas
  - ○ **Uterine Fibroid**
    - Popcorn calcifications in midline pelvis
  - ○ Synovial sarcoma
    - Up to 50% contain dystrophic calcification, usually peripheral
    - Vast majority are extraarticular
  - ○ Hemangiopericytoma
    - Cannot differentiate from a benign hemangioma by imaging alone

Helpful Clues for Rare Diagnoses
- **Metastatic Calcification**
  - ○ Large deposits around large joints

- ○ Disturbance of calcium or phosphorus metabolism (can resolve with treatment)
- **Systemic Lupus Erythematosus**
  - ○ Rare calcifications, most common in lower extremity
  - ○ Joint subluxation without erosion
- **Calcific Myonecrosis**
  - ○ Amorphus or plaque-like calcification in muscle compartment, usually lower extremity
- **Tumoral (Idiopathic) Calcinosis**
  - ○ Diagnosis of exclusion, with same appearance as metastatic calcification
- **Trevor Fairbank (Dysplasia Epiphysealis Hemimelica)**
  - ○ Lobulated intraarticular osteochondroma mimics calcification
  - ○ May simulate loose bodies
- **Thermal Injury, Burns**
  - ○ Stippled calcification in area of burn or along contracture bands
- **Sarcoidosis**
  - ○ Large calcified periarticular masses are rare
- **Chondrodysplasia Punctata (Mimic)**
  - ○ Dwarfism with congenital stippled epiphyses
- **Pseudohypoparathyroidism**
  - ○ Calcifications + short metatarsals & metacarpals
- **Parasites**
  - ○ Variable by type
- **Melorheostosis**
  - ○ Classic undulating cortical hyperostosis + rare soft tissue calcification

Phlebolith

Anteroposterior radiograph shows several nodular calcifications ➡ of varying sizes in the low pelvis. These are typical for phleboliths. A lucent center ➡ is classic but not always present.

Pyrophosphate Arthropathy

Anteroposterior radiograph shows nodular calcification ➡ in the medial meniscus due to chondrocalcinosis. More typical linear hyaline ➡ & triangular meniscal chondrocalcinosis ➡ involves the lateral compartment.

NODULAR CALCIFICATION

(Left) *Anteroposterior radiograph shows nodular calcification* ➡ *in the expected region of the distal supraspinatus tendon, consistent with calcific tendonitis.* **(Right)** *Anteroposterior radiograph shows a nodular calcific deposit* ➡ *located superior to the greater tuberosity. While the deposit looks solid in this radiograph, the distribution became linear on internal rotation, confirming location in the bursa, rather than tendon, as is illustrated in the prior case.*

Tendinitis, Calcific

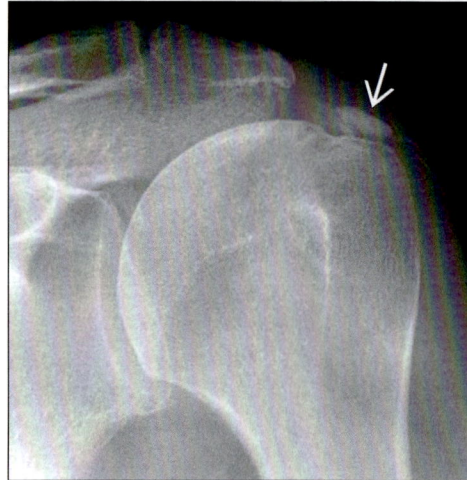

Bursitis, Calcific

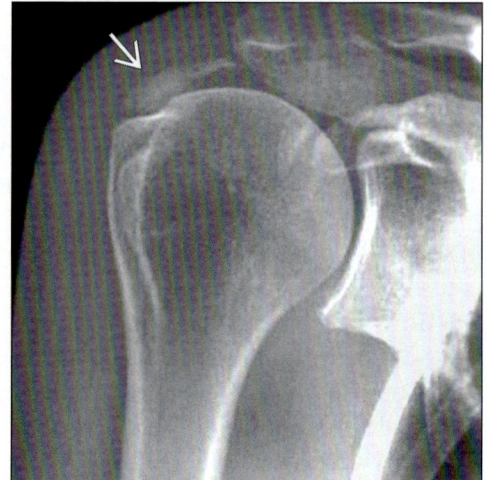

(Left) *Anteroposterior radiograph shows several peripherally calcified lesions* ➡ *in the right gluteal region from prior injections. The central lucency is commonly seen but can also be present in phleboliths.* **(Right)** *Lateral radiograph shows early myositis in the antecubital fossa & forearm. Note that the early bone formation is amorphous* ➡*, appearing nodular & calcified at this time. This appearance suggests an injury 4-8 weeks earlier, possibly an elbow dislocation.*

Injection Granuloma

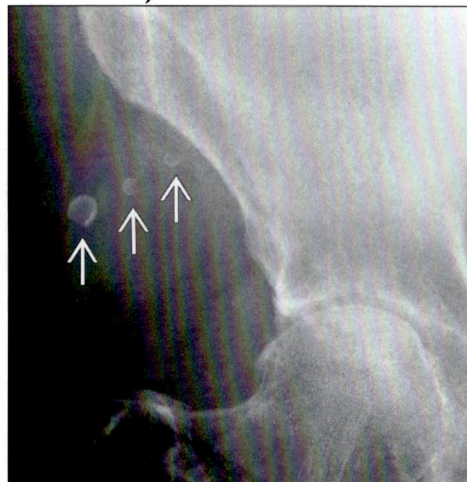

Myositis Ossificans (Early)

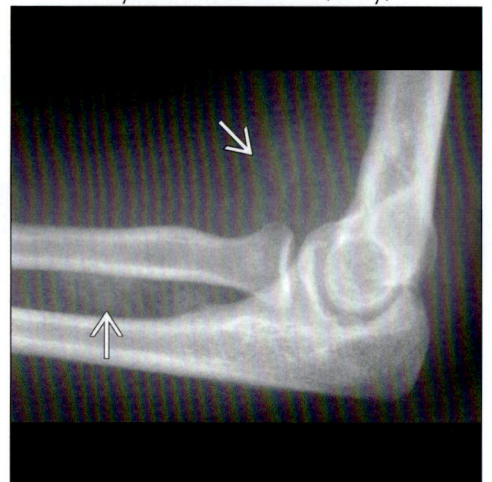

(Left) *Lateral radiograph shows an extraarticular globular calcification* ➡ *along the volar aspect of the index finger with a typical appearance for scleroderma.* **(Right)** *Anteroposterior radiograph shows multiple nodular bodies* ➡ *in the axillary recess and along the biceps tendon sheath. These loose bodies are technically ossified but can appear calcified, depending on their maturity.*

Progressive Systemic Sclerosis

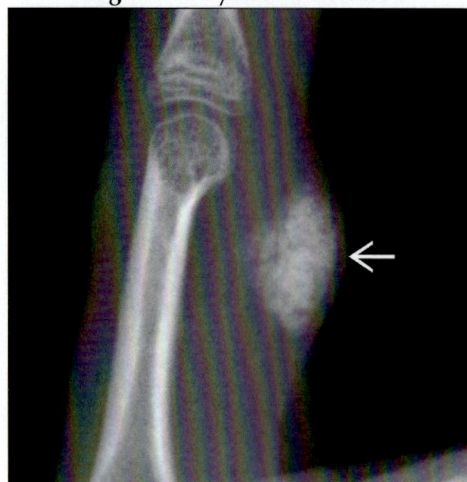

Loose Body (Mimic)

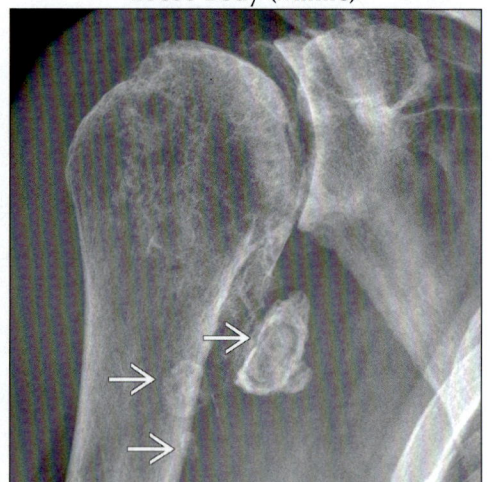

NODULAR CALCIFICATION

Gout

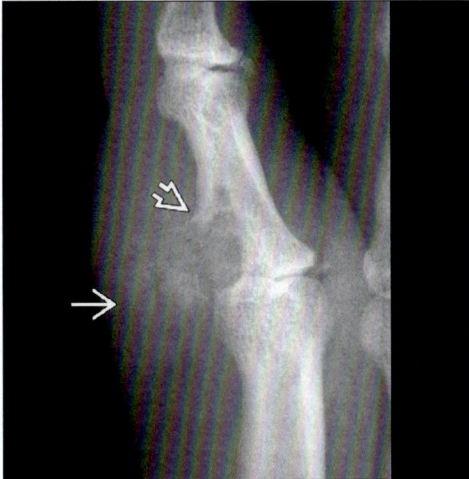

Avulsion Fractures (Early)

(Left) *Oblique radiograph shows an impressive soft tissue tophus ➡️, containing density typical of sodium urate deposition. There is a large erosion at the PIP which has resulted in a classic overhanging edge ➡️. (Right) Lateral radiograph shows an avulsion fracture ➡️ from the base of the middle phalanx. This is a volar plate fracture, most commonly seen following dorsal dislocation. The size of the fracture fragment varies from a sliver of bone to a sizable fragment.*

Dermatomyositis

Hyperparathyroidism/Renal Osteodystrophy

(Left) *Axial NECT shows extensive myofascial calcification with focal areas of more confluent nodular calcification ➡️. (Right) Posteroanterior radiograph shows severe osteopenia, prominent vascular calcification and globular soft tissue calcification ➡️ suggesting hyperparathyroidism. The patient proved to have a parathyroid adenoma.*

Synovial Osteochondromatosis

Rheumatoid Nodule

(Left) *Axial bone CT shows numerous, rounded, calcified bodies within the knee joint ➡️, as well as extension of the collection into the posterior soft tissues ➡️ of the knee. (Right) Posteroanterior radiograph shows a focal nodular density ➡️ which causes scalloping of the underlying bone ➡️. While this could represent a giant cell tumor of the tendon sheath, narrowing of the second MCP joint and a marginal erosion ➡️ suggests rheumatoid arthritis.*

NODULAR CALCIFICATION

Hemangioma, Soft Tissue

Hemangioma, Soft Tissue

(Left) Lateral radiograph shows multiple round calcifications ➡ associated with a soft tissue mass in the thigh. These are phleboliths within a hemangioma. *(Right)* Axial NECT in the same patient as the prior case illustrates the round, calcified phleboliths ➡ within the fatty stroma ➡ that is typical for hemangiomas.

Maffucci Syndrome

Uterine Fibroid

(Left) Posteroanterior radiograph shows multiple enchondromas ➡ within the phalanges and metacarpals and a soft tissue hemangioma containing multiple round phleboliths ➡. Enchondromatosis + soft tissue hemangiomas = Maffucci syndrome. (†MSK Req). *(Right)* Anteroposterior radiograph shows a large mass in the pelvis containing nodular calcification ➡. This type of calcification is typical for uterine fibroids, although this is an unusually large example.

Synovial Sarcoma

Hemangiopericytoma

(Left) Lateral radiograph shows a mass ➡ posteromedial to the knee in a young adult containing peripheral, dystrophic, nodular calcification ➡. One should always consider this dx if there is a mass in the lower extremity of a young adult. (†MSK Req). *(Right)* Axial NECT shows an anterior compartment mass containing phleboliths ➡, which enhance intensely. Vascular tumors range from benign to malignant and it is not easy to differentiate them by imaging features.

NODULAR CALCIFICATION

Metastatic Calcification

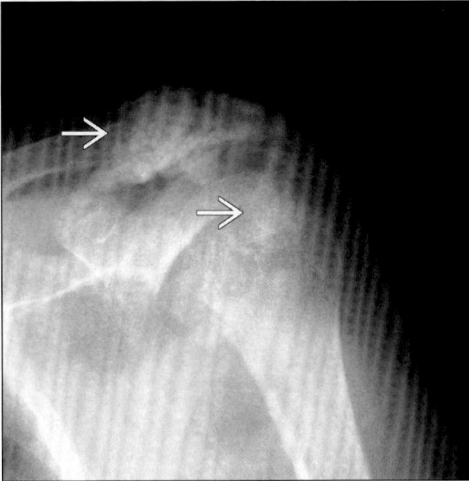

Systemic Lupus Erythematosus

(Left) Anteroposterior radiograph shows extensive amorphous calcification ➡, consistent with metastatic calcium deposition, around the shoulder in a dialysis patient. Amorphous calcium deposition is commonly bilateral and asymptomatic. *(Right)* Frog lateral radiograph shows dense globular soft tissue calcifications ➡ around the hip. SLE patients occasionally develop dystrophic soft tissue calcification, predominantly in the lower extremities. (†MSK Req).

Calcific Myonecrosis

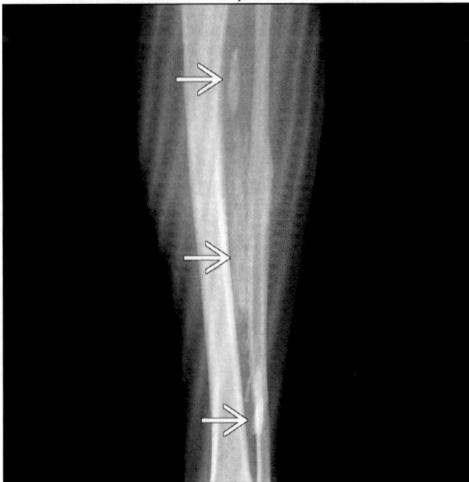

Tumoral (Idiopathic) Calcinosis

(Left) Anteroposterior radiograph shows nodular to sheet-like calcification ➡ involving the anterior compartment of the lower leg. This is a common location for the sequelae of compartment syndrome. *(Right)* Anteroposterior radiograph shows a dense, cloud-like collection of nodular calcifications ➡ surrounding an otherwise normal shoulder. Renal failure and collagen vascular diseases may cause a similar appearance.

Trevor Fairbank (Dysplasia Epiphysealis Hemimelica)

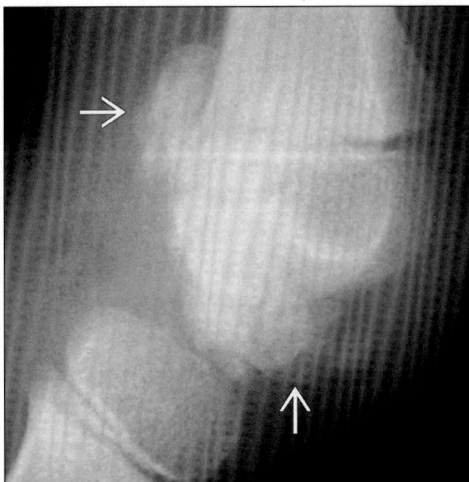

Pseudohypoparathyroidism

(Left) Lateral radiograph shows lobulated ossification ➡ which is intraarticular and apparently arises from the medial femoral condyle. It is a calcification mimic and represents Trevor Fairbank, essentially an intraarticular osteochondroma. *(Right)* Anteroposterior radiograph shows subtle soft tissue calcification ➡, as well as short first metatarsal ➡. This is the combination of findings that makes the diagnosis of pseudo-hypoparathyroidism.

LINEAR AND CURVILINEAR CALCIFICATION

DIFFERENTIAL DIAGNOSIS

Common
- Arteriosclerosis
- Chondrocalcinosis
- Aneurysm
- Hemangioma, Soft Tissue
- Hyperparathyroidism/Renal Osteodystrophy
- DISH

Less Common
- Dermatomyositis
- Progressive Systemic Sclerosis
- Synovial Sarcoma
- Hypercalcemia
- Calcified Chronic DVT
- Thermal Injury, Burns

Rare but Important
- OPLL
- Systemic Lupus Erythematosus
- Pseudohypoparathyroidism
- Cysticercosis
- Echinococcal Cyst
- Filariasis
- Leprosy
- Dracunculiasis
- Complications of Fluoride
- Armillifer Armillatus Infection

ESSENTIAL INFORMATION

Key Differential Diagnosis Issues
- Extremely common finding
- Key factors: Location & pattern of calcification

Helpful Clues for Common Diagnoses
- **Arteriosclerosis**
  - Follows expected course of blood vessels
  - Three types: Atherosclerosis, Mönckeberg arteriosclerosis, arteriolar sclerosis
  - Atherosclerosis consists of intimal plaques that narrow the vessel lumen
    - Coarse, irregular, patchy calcifications
    - Morbidity and mortality with involvement of aorta, coronary and cerebral arteries
    - Plaques can cause ulceration, thrombosis and embolic complications
  - Mönckeberg (medial) arteriosclerosis refers to calcification of the middle vessel wall (media)
    - Most commonly seen type of arteriosclerosis on extremity radiographs
    - Pipe stem appearance with contiguous, granular calcification
    - Medium-sized vessels involved
    - Common in diabetics
    - No narrowing of vessel lumen
  - Arteriolar sclerosis involves small arteries and arterioles
    - Causes wall thickening and luminal narrowing
    - Predominantly affects kidneys
- **Chondrocalcinosis**
  - Nonspecific cartilage calcification
    - Involves hyaline or fibrocartilage
    - Linear to globular configuration depending on location
  - Common in knee menisci, wrist triangular fibrocartilage complex, symphysis pubis
  - Can involve joint capsule, synovium, ligaments, and tendons
  - Associated with numerous entities
    - Calcium pyrophosphate deposition disease (CPPD), gout, hemochromatosis, hyperparathyroidism, ochronosis, oxalosis, acromegaly, Wilson disease, degenerative/idiopathic causes
- **Aneurysm**
  - Arteriosclerosis outlines a larger than expected caliber for vessel on radiographs
  - Attention to aorta on chest, thoracic, and lumbar studies
  - Attention to popliteal artery on lateral knee radiographs
- **Hemangioma, Soft Tissue**
  - Soft tissue mass consisting of abnormal blood vessels
    - 7% of all benign soft tissue masses
  - Usually intramuscular
  - Curvilinear calcification of blood vessels
  - Linear dystrophic calcification in thrombus
  - Partially/completely calcified phleboliths
- **Hyperparathyroidism/Renal Osteodystrophy**
  - Cartilage calcification in wrist, knee, hip, or shoulder in 20-40%
  - Also, Rugger jersey spine, distal clavicular osteolysis, subperiosteal bone resorption, Brown tumors, or salt-and-pepper skull

LINEAR AND CURVILINEAR CALCIFICATION

Helpful Clues for Less Common Diagnoses

- **Dermatomyositis**
  - Irregular calcification with wide variety of appearances
  - Involves striated muscle, fascia, and skin
  - Can be extensive, involving the trunk and extremities
  - Associations: Muscle atrophy and/or osteoporosis
  - Other findings include interstitial lung disease, esophageal dysmotility
  - Sometimes seen with occult neoplasm in patients > 50 years old
- **Progressive Systemic Sclerosis**
  - Synonym: Scleroderma
  - Elongated globular calcifications most common
    - Curvilinear appearance early
  - Associated findings
    - DIP and PIP erosions
    - Soft tissue atrophy
    - Acroosteolysis
- **Hypercalcemia**
  - Extensive clinical differential diagnosis
    - 90% due to hyperparathyroidism or malignancy
    - Differentiate with associated lab abnormalities
  - Cartilage calcification caused by hyperparathyroidism is most common
- **Calcified Chronic DVT**
  - Irregular calcifications along venous distribution

- Calcifications can outline venous valves
- **Thermal Injury, Burns**
  - Fine, stippled linear calcification
  - Localized to area of injury or can extend along contracture bands

Helpful Clues for Rare Diagnoses

- **Cysticercosis**
  - "Rice grain" linear to oval calcifications
    - Noncalcified central area
  - Oriented parallel to muscle fibers
  - Intracranial calcifications seen on CT
- **Echinococcal Cyst**
  - Hydatid cysts in organs, muscle, or subcutaneous tissue peripherally calcify
- **Filariasis**
  - Dead coiled or linear worms calcify
  - Very fine calcifications best seen in web spaces of hands and feet
- **Leprosy**
  - Linear calcification of affected nerves
- **Dracunculiasis**
  - Small crescentic calcifications
- **Complications of Fluoride**
  - Iliolumbar, sacrotuberous, and paraspinal ligamentous calcification most common
- **Armillifer Armillatus Infection**
  - Snake parasite larvae calcifies in soft tissues
    - Liver, mesentery, intestinal wall, lung, pleura, scrotum
  - West Africa infection rate 23% (visible on radiographs in up to 7%)
  - 4-8 mm coiled, horseshoe, crescentic, or linear calcifications

Arteriosclerosis

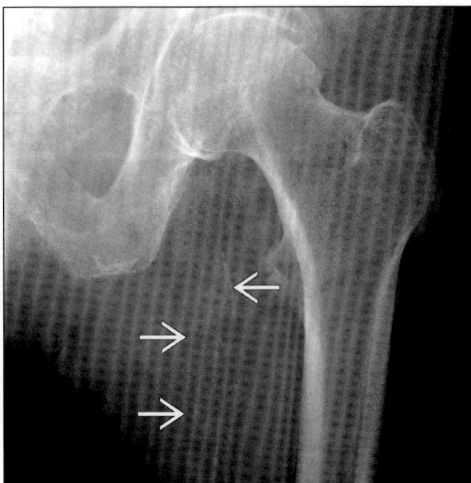

Anteroposterior radiograph shows Mönckeberg (medial) arteriosclerosis, one of the three types of arteriosclerosis, which has fine, granular calcification with a pipestem appearance ➡.

Arteriosclerosis

Axial CECT demonstrates coarse, irregular calcifications ➡ of the abdominal aorta that narrow the vessel lumen, typical for atherosclerosis, the most common form of arteriosclerosis.

LINEAR AND CURVILINEAR CALCIFICATION

(Left) Anteroposterior radiograph of the knee shows a typical case of chondrocalcinosis with calcification of the fibrocartilage (meniscus) ➡ and articular hyaline cartilage ➡. *(Right)* Anteroposterior radiograph of first MTP joint shows chondrocalcinosis not only in the articular cartilage ➡, but also in the joint capsule/ligaments ➡ and bursa ➡.

Chondrocalcinosis

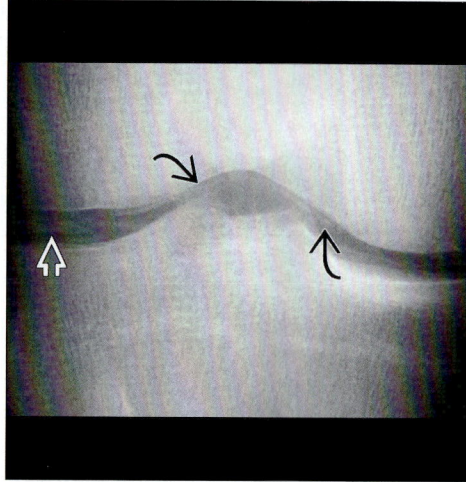

Chondrocalcinosis

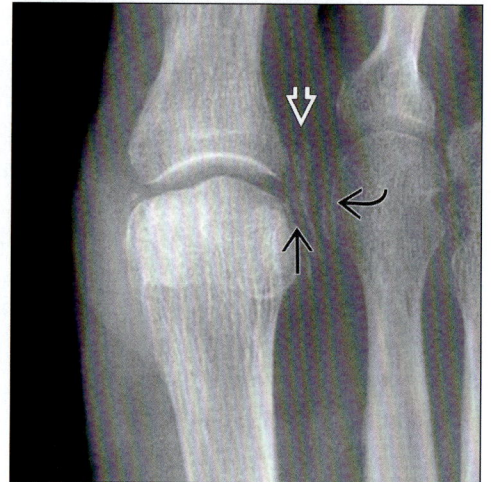

(Left) Axial NECT demonstrates a partially calcified aortic aneurysm ➡ measuring up to 6.3 cm. The rupture rate of aneurysms increases with maximal diameter. *(Right)* Lateral radiograph shows a hemangioma containing several calcified phleboliths ➡ with varying shape depending on projection and associated pathologic fracture ➡ from pressure erosion. (†MSK Req).

Aneurysm

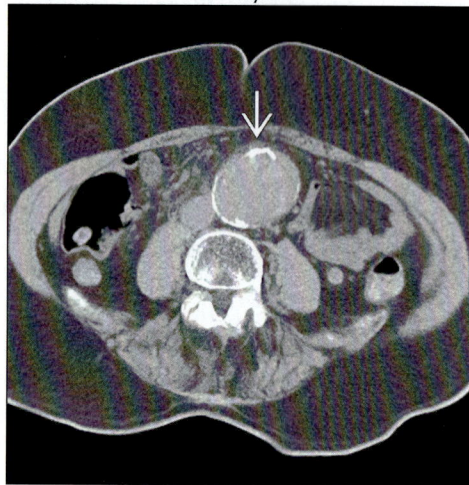

Hemangioma, Soft Tissue

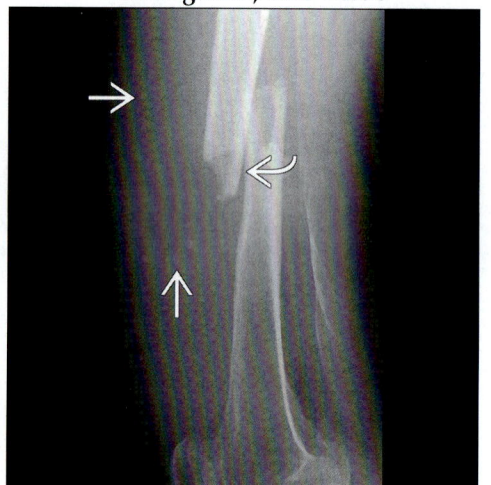

(Left) Anteroposterior radiograph shows diffuse, intermediate density soft tissue calcification ➡. This is a prominent feature in hyperparathyroidism. *(Right)* Axial NECT of the symphysis pubis shows chondrocalcinosis ➡ due to renal osteodystrophy from this patient's end stage renal disease.

Hyperparathyroidism/Renal Osteodystrophy

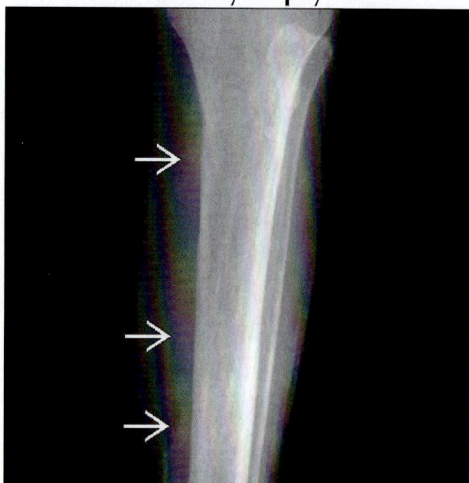

Hyperparathyroidism/Renal Osteodystrophy

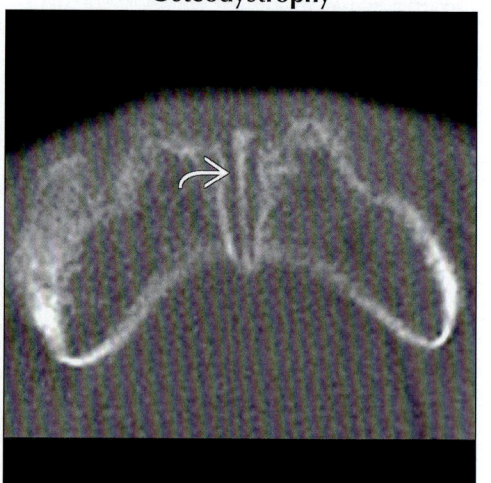

LINEAR AND CURVILINEAR CALCIFICATION

DISH

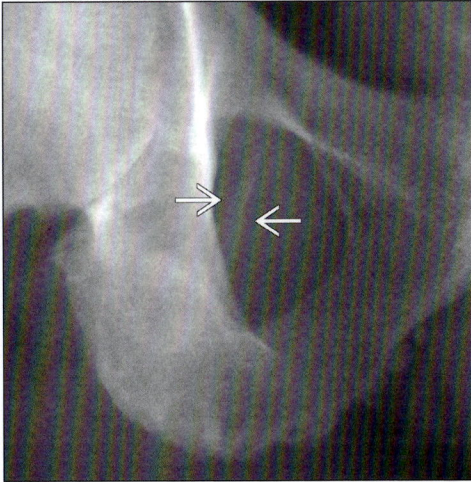

DISH

DISH

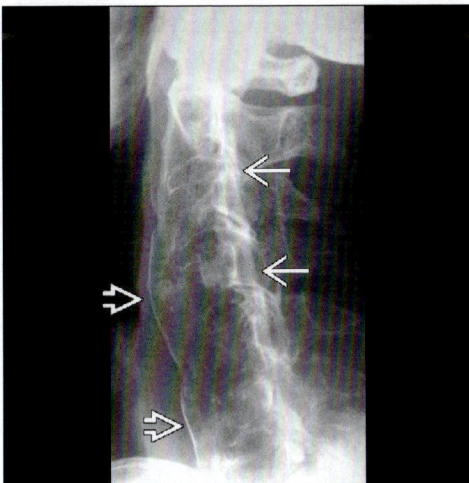

Dermatomyositis

Dermatomyositis

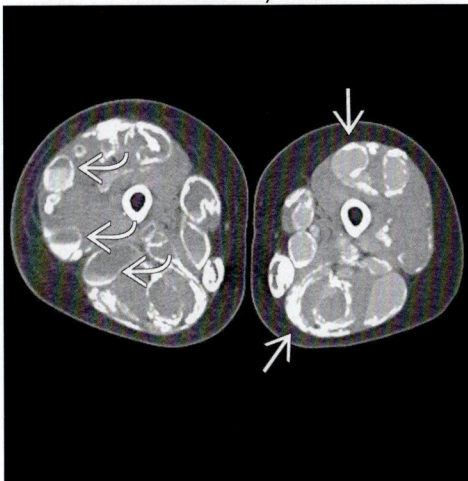

Progressive Systemic Sclerosis

(Left) Anteroposterior radiograph shows sacrotuberous ligament calcification ➡ which is seen in DISH; sacrospinous ligament calcification may be seen as well. *(Right)* Anteroposterior radiograph shows iliolumbar ligamentous calcification ➡ frequently seen in DISH. Note the fusion of the non-articular portions of the sacroiliac joints as well ➡.

(Left) Lateral radiograph shows ossification of the posterior longitudinal ligament ➡. Though this is seen more frequently on OPLL, it may be seen in DISH as well. Note the flowing anterior osteophytes which have effectively fused the spine ➡. (†MSK Req). *(Right)* Lateral radiograph of the right thigh shows extensive, sheet-like calcification of the muscles and fascial planes ➡ in this patient with dermatomyositis.

(Left) Axial NECT of both thighs shows extensive, sheet-like calcification of the muscles and fascial planes ➡ and also demonstrates scattered fluid-fluid levels ➡. *(Right)* Lateral radiograph shows linear sheet-like calcification in the subcutaneous tissues. Although this pattern of calcification most often evokes the diagnosis of dermatomyositis, it can be seen in scleroderma (PSS) as well.

LINEAR AND CURVILINEAR CALCIFICATION

(Left) Lateral radiograph shows curvilinear calcification in an extraarticular location posterior to the knee ➡. Though any soft tissue tumor may contain dystrophic calcification, it occurs most frequently in synovial sarcoma. (†MSK Req).
(Right) AP radiograph shows chondrocalcinosis in the pubic symphysis & labrum of the hip ➡, as well as juxtaarticular calcifications ➡ in a patient with paraneoplastic syndrome & hypercalcemia.

Synovial Sarcoma

Hypercalcemia

(Left) Lateral radiograph of the leg demonstrates a serpiginous, calcified mass in the calf ➡ corresponding to a previously documented area of venous thrombus. Varicose veins ➡ and phleboliths ➡ are also present. *(Right)* Anteroposterior radiograph demonstrates a pin tract ➡ through the distal femoral diaphysis, related to suspension of the burned extremity, and resultant myositis ossificans ➡.

Calcified Chronic DVT

Thermal Injury, Burns

(Left) Lateral radiograph shows linear ossification of the posterior longitudinal ligament ➡, typical of the disease termed OPLL. Although it is quite obvious in this case, the ossification may be thinner and much more subtle. (†MSK Req).
(Right) Axial bone CT confirms the ossification seen in the previous image to be of the posterior longitudinal ligament ➡, and demonstrates the degree of stenosis suffered by this patient.

OPLL

OPLL

LINEAR AND CURVILINEAR CALCIFICATION

Systemic Lupus Erythematosus

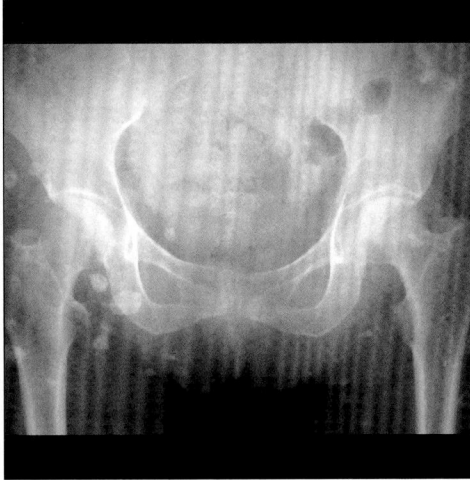

Pseudohypoparathyroidism

(Left) Anteroposterior radiograph shows both globular and linear calcification in the soft tissues in a patient with SLE. It is unusual, but not unheard of, for such calcifications to be seen in this disease. *(Right)* Anteroposterior radiograph shows soft tissue calcification ➡ as well as a short first metatarsal ➡. This combination is considered the radiographic hallmark of pseudo- or pseudohypoparathyroidism.

Cysticercosis

Echinococcal Cyst

(Left) Anteroposterior radiograph shows rice-shaped calcified bodies ➡ within the soft tissues. The size and shape of these bodies is typical of the parasite Cysticercosis. *(Right)* Axial NECT demonstrates a dominant cyst ➡ with an adjacent daughter cyst ➡ in the spleen, due to infection with the Echinococcus tapeworm resulting in hydatid disease (echinococcosis).

Leprosy

Complications of Fluoride

(Left) Posteroanterior radiograph of the hand shows tremendous acroosteolysis, which has destroyed most of the phalanges. Additionally, there is linear calcification in the location of a digital nerve ➡. (†MSK Req). *(Right)* Anteroposterior radiograph shows calcification of the sacrospinous ligaments ➡ in a patient with fluorosis. Note the character and location of the calcifications are both slightly different than that of pelvic arterial calcification.

SOFT TISSUE NEOPLASM CONTAINING CALCIFICATION

DIFFERENTIAL DIAGNOSIS

Common
- Myositis Ossificans (Mimic)
- Synovial Sarcoma
- Periosteal Chondroma (Mimic)
- Hemangioma, Soft Tissue
- Soft Tissue Chondroma
- Intraarticular Chondroma

Less Common
- Malignant Fibrous Histiocytoma (MFH)
- Liposarcoma, Soft Tissue
- Nerve Sheath Tumors
- Osteosarcoma, Periosteal or Surface (Mimic)
- Mesenchymal Chondrosarcoma
- Dystrophic Calcification within any Soft Tissue Tumor
- Parosteal Lipoma

Rare but Important
- Extraskeletal Osteosarcoma
- Extraskeletal Myxoid Chondrosarcoma

ESSENTIAL INFORMATION

Key Differential Diagnosis Issues
- **Hint**: Whenever possible, determine the nature of the calcification
  - If calcification can be identified as either osteoid, chondroid, or dystrophic, go to the alternative differential approach (below), segmented by type
  - Calcified osteoid: Amorphous, less dense than bone
  - Calcified chondroid: Denser than bone, rings and arcs or punctate
  - Dystrophic calcification: Often globular, very dense
- **Hint**: Be very careful to avoid confusing early myositis ossificans with tumor!
  - To differentiate, use zoning pattern and timing of bone formation
  - Biopsy of myositis in its early amorphous phase mimics osteosarcoma histologically

Helpful Clues for Common Diagnoses
- **Myositis Ossificans (Mimic)**
  - Related to trauma which may not be recalled by patient (or may be denied)
  - Appearance varies significantly with time
    - 0-4 weeks: Doughy mass, but no calcification

- 4-10 weeks: Earliest formation of osteoid; appears subtle, not dense, amorphous
- 10 weeks-6 months: Progressive maturation; with maturation, develops the zoning typical of myositis (immature at center, mature bone peripherally)
- 6+ months: May begin to resolve and decrease in size
  - Time of greatest risk for confusion: 4-10 weeks post trauma, when the osteoid formation is amorphous and appears similar to aggressive tumor bone formation
  - MR shows the halo of more mature bone, even at 4-10 weeks post trauma; helps to differentiate from tumor
    - Be aware that there may be periosteal reaction adjacent to myositis, with marrow and soft tissue edema; this may mimic a greater level of aggressiveness
- **Synovial Sarcoma**
  - Relatively common soft tissue sarcoma (though less frequently seen than malignant fibrous histiocytoma or liposarcoma)
  - Most frequent soft tissue sarcoma to contain dystrophic calcification
    - 50% of synovial sarcomas contain dystrophic calcification
    - Pattern of calcification is linear or globular, central or peripheral; therefore, not predictable
  - Preferential location: Extraarticular, lower extremity
  - Prime age group is young to middle aged adult; generally younger than patients with MFH or liposarcoma
  - Hint: Soft tissue mass in the lower extremity containing dystrophic calcification in a young to middle aged adult is most likely synovial sarcoma
- **Periosteal Chondroma (Mimic)**
  - Considered a mimic since it is an osseous surface lesion rather than soft tissue mass
  - Chondroid matrix adjacent to osseous cortex; often causes underlying scalloping (but not invasion) of bone
- **Hemangioma, Soft Tissue**
  - Phleboliths (central lucency within round calcifications) in tangle of vessels; lipomatous stroma
- **Soft Tissue Chondroma**

SOFT TISSUE NEOPLASM CONTAINING CALCIFICATION

○ Generally dense rings and arcs pattern of chondroid in a painless soft tissue mass

• **Intraarticular Chondroma**
  ○ Usually site-specific; arises in Hoffa fat pad
  ○ Rounded calcific densities

Helpful Clues for Less Common Diagnoses

• **Soft Tissue Neoplasms**
  ○ Any soft tissue tumor may develop dystrophic calcification
  ○ Character of the dystrophic calcification is not specific or helpful in differentiation
  ○ Most common is synovial sarcoma (50%)
  ○ Others in which it is (uncommonly) seen
    ▪ Malignant Fibrous Histiocytoma: No other specific features, except relative frequency of MFH in older patients
    ▪ Liposarcoma: Appearance of lipomatous tissue varies significantly with grade of lesion; low grade shows fatty tissue, often with thickened septa or nodularity; high grade may have so much cellularity that no lipomatous tissue remains
    ▪ Nerve Sheath Tumors: Lesion in distribution of nerve, often shows nerve entering or exiting lesion; shape may be oval, elongated, or teardrop; target sign (central low signal on T2 imaging) often seen, either with benign or malignant peripheral nerve sheath tumors
• **Parosteal Lipoma**
  ○ Lipoma closely associated with cortex of long bone
  ○ Lipoma is simple in appearance

○ May have associated bone formation, often arising from the underlying cortex
○ Bone may extend horizontally from the osseous cortex, giving the appearance of a bizarre periosteal reaction

Helpful Clues for Rare Diagnoses

• **Extraskeletal Osteosarcoma**
  ○ Older adult age group
  ○ Lower extremity predominates

Alternative Differential Approaches

• Differentiate into groups according to type of calcification
  ○ Osteoid
    ▪ Myositis ossificans (mimic of soft tissue neoplasm)
    ▪ Osteosarcoma, periosteal or surface (mimic of soft tissue neoplasm)
    ▪ Extraskeletal osteosarcoma
  ○ Chondroid
    ▪ Periosteal chondroma
    ▪ Soft tissue chondroma
    ▪ Intraarticular chondroma
    ▪ Mesenchymal chondrosarcoma
    ▪ Extraskeletal myxoid chondrosarcoma
  ○ Dystrophic calcification
    ▪ Synovial sarcoma
    ▪ Hemangioma
    ▪ Malignant fibrous histiocytoma
    ▪ Liposarcoma, soft tissue
    ▪ Nerve sheath tumors
    ▪ Dystrophic calcification within any soft tissue tumor
    ▪ Parosteal lipoma

Myositis Ossificans (Mimic)

Anteroposterior radiograph shows amorphous osteoid formation in the soft tissues ➡ with dense periosteal reaction elicited in the adjacent femoral shaft ➡. This is myositis, but mimics a surface osteosarcoma.

Synovial Sarcoma

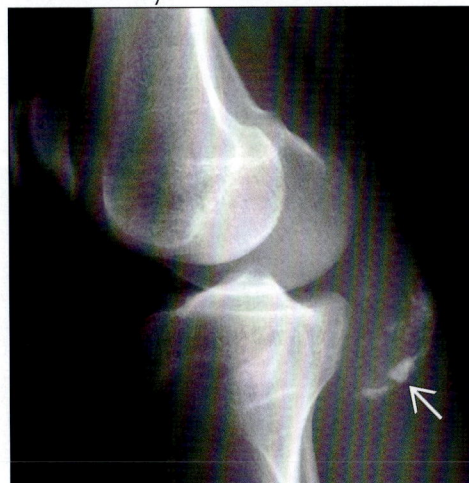

Oblique radiograph shows dense dystrophic calcification surrounding and within a round soft tissue mass ➡. Synovial sarcoma is the most frequent soft tissue sarcoma to contain calcium. (†MSK Req).

SOFT TISSUE NEOPLASM CONTAINING CALCIFICATION

(Left) Anteroposterior radiograph shows an apparent soft tissue lesion containing tumor matrix ➡, causing extrinsic scalloping of the underlying humerus ⧫➡. While it mimics a soft tissue neoplasm, it is actually a surface lesion of bone. *(Right)* Anteroposterior radiograph shows a soft tissue mass containing round calcific densities which have a distinct lucent center ➡. These are typical phleboliths, seen in hemangioma.

Periosteal Chondroma (Mimic)

Hemangioma, Soft Tissue

(Left) Lateral radiograph shows dense chondroid matrix, with well-formed rings and arcs ⧫➡. The mass was painless, but resected because it bothered the patient. It is typical of a soft tissue chondroma. *(Right)* Lateral radiograph shows punctate chondroid matrix located entirely within the Hoffa fat pad ➡. The mass has caused a small focal erosion in the anterior tibia ➡. The appearance is typical for intraarticular chondroma.

Soft Tissue Chondroma

Intraarticular Chondroma

(Left) Axial NECT shows a large subcutaneous lesion ➡ which contains dense dystrophic calcification. This is an unusual lesion, since MFH more frequently is a deep lesion, and only rarely contains dystrophic calcification. *(Right)* AP radiograph shows dense soft tissue calcification within a large soft tissue mass. Fat density is faintly seen proximally and distally within the mass ➡. This is unusual dystrophic calcification occupying the majority of a low grade liposarcoma.

Malignant Fibrous Histiocytoma (MFH)

Liposarcoma, Soft Tissue

SOFT TISSUE NEOPLASM CONTAINING CALCIFICATION

Nerve Sheath Tumors

Osteosarcoma, Periosteal or Surface (Mimic)

(Left) Axial NECT shows eccentrically located dystrophic calcification within a mass ➡; the sciatic nerve is not identified as a separate structure. A peripheral nerve sheath tumor must be strongly suspected. *(Right)* Anteroposterior radiograph shows a tumor osteoid located adjacent to the humeral diaphysis ➡. This proved to be a high grade surface osteosarcoma, slightly different from a periosteal osteosarcoma.

Mesenchymal Chondrosarcoma

Dystrophic Calcification within any Soft Tissue Tumor

(Left) Axial CECT shows a large soft tissue mass ➡ containing a chondroid matrix and extensive necrosis. The mass is retroperitoneal, and does not arise from the iliac wing. This is a rare form of chondrosarcoma. *(Right)* Lateral radiograph shows dystrophic calcification ➡ within a large soft tissue mass which also contains fat ➡. Biopsy showed pleomorphic spindle cell sarcoma. Any soft tissue mass may contain dystrophic calcification.

Parosteal Lipoma

Extraskeletal Osteosarcoma

(Left) Axial NECT shows dystrophic calcification ➡ within a large lipoma ➡. This is a rare type of lipoma, termed parosteal lipoma, which may elicit prominent reactive bone formation. *(Right)* Axial NECT shows osteoid matrix ➡ within a large soft tissue mass ➡ in the buttocks of an elderly patient. There is tumor necrosis. Extraskeletal osteosarcoma is rare, and tends to be seen in an older patient age group than conventional osteosarcoma.

BONE MARROW EDEMA SYNDROMES (PROXIMAL FEMUR)

DIFFERENTIAL DIAGNOSIS

Common
- Arthritis
- Insufficiency Fracture
- Osteonecrosis, Hip
- Stress Reaction
- Stress Fracture
- Metastases, Bone Marrow

Less Common
- Transient Bone Marrow Edema
- Septic Joint
- Osteomyelitis
- Rapidly Destructive Osteoarthritis of Hip

Rare but Important
- Peritumoral Reactive Marrow Edema
- Leukemia
- Lymphoma

ESSENTIAL INFORMATION

Key Differential Diagnosis Issues
- Bone marrow edema is a nonspecific MR appearance
- Presents as low signal on T1; high signal on T2 & fluid sensitive sequences
- **Hint**: Survey surrounding structures including acetabulum, soft tissues, etc. when considering differential diagnosis
- **Hint**: Correlate appearance with patient age & relevant history
- **Hint**: Radiograph appearance will assist with diagnosis

Helpful Clues for Common Diagnoses
- **Arthritis**
  - Marrow edema often results from reactive marrow related to adjacent cartilage damage
  - Most common: Osteoarthritis
  - Other arthropathies: Inflammatory arthritis, crystalline arthritis (gout & CPPD), spondyloarthropathies
  - Both femoral head and acetabulum show abnormalities including joint space narrowing, subchondral edema & eburnation, subchondral cyst formation & osteophytic ridging
- **Insufficiency Fracture**
  - Typically originates in the lateral femoral neck & propagates medially
  - Failure of the tensile trabeculae
  - Tends to occur in older and/or physically inactive patients
  - Radiograph key to evaluate bone density
- **Osteonecrosis, Hip**
  - Stages of osteonecrosis
    - Ill-defined subchondral and femoral head edema, may be mistaken for transient bone marrow edema
    - Progresses to well-defined, slightly heterogeneous lesions
    - May develop subchondral fracture and subsequently collapse
    - Develops secondary osteoarthritis
  - Tends to exclude joint space and acetabulum until late stages
  - **Hint**: Look at both hips; often bilateral even when symptoms initially present unilaterally
- **Stress Reaction**
  - Ill-defined endosteal edema parallels the medial femoral cortex/calcar region
  - No definable fracture
  - Represents microtrabecular fracture along compressive trabeculae
  - Result of abnormal stress on normal bone; seen in distance runners, military recruits
- **Stress Fracture**
  - Marrow edema along medial femoral neck and/or proximal femur may mask cortical break
  - Cortical break often best seen on T1 MR
  - Typically located along the medial femoral neck and proximal femur (compressive trabeculae)
  - Occurs as a result of abnormal stress on normal bone; seen in distance runners, military recruits
- **Metastases, Bone Marrow**
  - Consider age, history of primary neoplasm
  - Lesion may be infiltrative without or with cortical breakthrough and soft tissue mass
  - **Hint**: Lesions in lesser trochanter should be considered metastatic disease until proven otherwise
  - **Hint**: Look for additional osseous lesions

Helpful Clues for Less Common Diagnoses
- **Transient Bone Marrow Edema**
  - Acute onset hip pain, most common in middle-age men
  - Joint space normal; no arthritis present

BONE MARROW EDEMA SYNDROMES (PROXIMAL FEMUR)

- Small joint effusion often present
  - Mimics septic arthritis or acute gout or pseudogout
  - Hip aspiration needed to exclude infection or crystals
  - Radiograph demonstrates focal osteopenia of femoral head
- **Septic Joint**
  - Joint effusion always present
    - Hip aspiration needed to evaluate for infection or crystals
  - Radiographs initially normal
    - Develops regional osteopenia over time
  - Cortex may lose crispness or distinctness
  - Underlying arthritis may co-exist
    - Look for joint space narrowing, regional osteopenia, erosions or osteophytes
- **Osteomyelitis**
  - May occur as extension of septic joint, hematogenous or direct implantation (e.g., trauma, hardware, etc.)
  - Progressive regional osteopenia of proximal femur and acetabulum; progressive joint space loss
  - **Hint**: Look for soft tissues changes such as cellulitis, abscess or sinus tract
- **Rapidly Destructive Osteoarthritis of Hip**
  - Rapid dissolution of hip joint over weeks to months
    - Femoral head flattening and lateral subluxation
    - Joint space loss, subchondral cysts, sclerosis of both sides of joint
    - Osteophytes uncommon

- Resembles a neuropathic or infected joint
  - Hip aspiration needed to exclude these diagnoses

Helpful Clues for Rare Diagnoses
- **Peritumoral Reactive Marrow Edema**
  - Reactive (non-neoplastic) marrow edema in the area surrounding a primary or secondary tumor
  - Generally associated with malignant tumors (e.g., osteosarcoma, chondrosarcoma, giant cell tumor)
  - May also be seen with benign tumors such as osteoid osteoma
  - Edema tends to overestimate actual tumor extent; gadolinium may help distinguish tumor from edema
- **Leukemia**
  - Most common childhood malignancy; also seen in adults
  - Nonspecific increased marrow signal on fluid-sensitive sequences; replaces normal marrow fat on T1
  - Radiographs are key and reveal regional or diffuse osteopenia; band-like metaphyseal lucent zone
    - Diffuse osteopenia, metaphyseal radiolucent bands; osteolysis; periostitis
- **Lymphoma**
  - May be so infiltrative as to appear only as osteopenia on radiograph
  - Nonspecific marrow signal on MR, as in leukemia

Arthritis

Coronal T2WI FS MR shows cartilage thinning ➡ & subchondral edema ➡ of acetabulum & femoral head, so called "kissing" lesions. Ring osteophytes ➡ encircle the femoral neck in this patient with osteoarthritis.

Insufficiency Fracture

Coronal STIR MR shows intense edema of femoral head/neck ➡ with focal flattening of the articular surface & low signal of subchondral fracture ➡. Surrounding soft tissue edema is also noted ➡.

BONE MARROW EDEMA SYNDROMES (PROXIMAL FEMUR)

Osteonecrosis, Hip

Stress Reaction

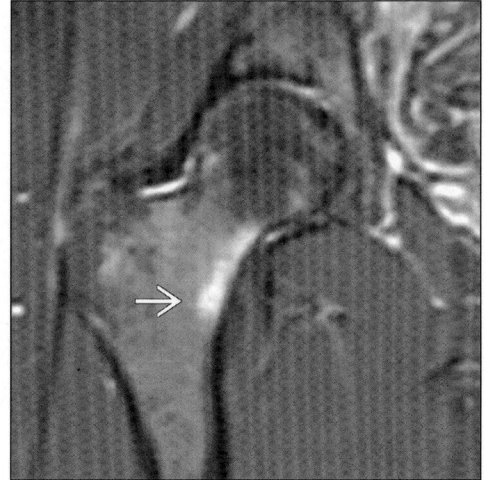

(Left) Coronal STIR MR shows crescentic subchondral high signal ➡ in the right hip with no associated arthritis. Subtle signal abnormality suggesting AVN is also present in the anterior left femoral head ➡. (Right) Coronal T2WI FS MR shows high signal along the medial femoral neck ➡ without a discrete fracture line. The location & orientation of this signal indicates stress reaction, rather than stress fracture.

Stress Fracture

Metastases, Bone Marrow

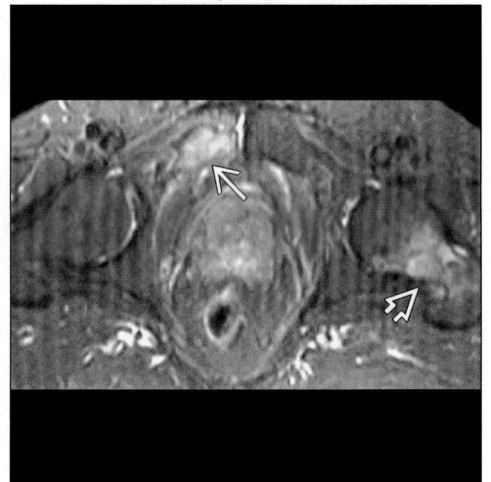

(Left) Coronal T2WI FS MR shows focal linear low signal ➡ in the medial femoral neck with extensive surrounding edema ➡, typical of an acute basicervical stress fracture. (Right) Axial STIR MR shows marrow infiltration ➡ in the left femoral neck with diffuse signal but no obvious cortical destruction. A second lesion ➡ in the right symphysis shows cortical break in this patient with prostate metastases.

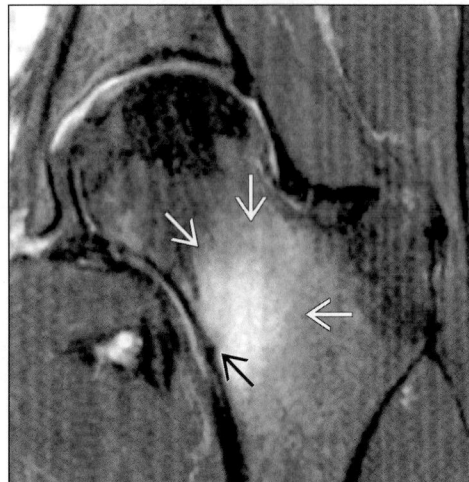

Transient Bone Marrow Edema

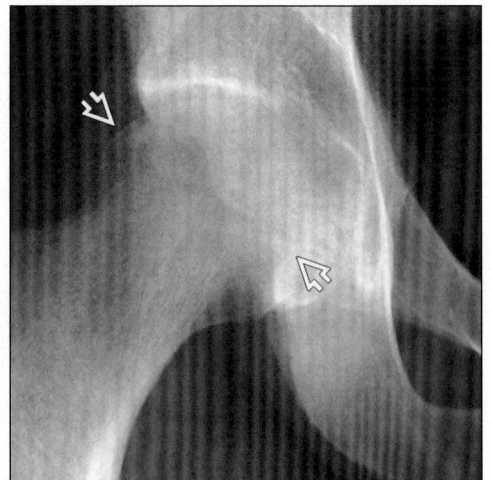

Transient Bone Marrow Edema

(Left) Coronal STIR MR shows intense edema in right femoral head & neck ➡ with acute onset hip pain 6 weeks prior. There is no cartilage loss or arthritis. The acetabulum is normal. Small joint effusion ➡ is typical of transient edema. (Right) Anteroposterior radiograph in the same patient as previous image, reveals focal osteopenia ➡ of the femoral head & neck with a normal adjacent acetabulum. Hip aspirate was normal.

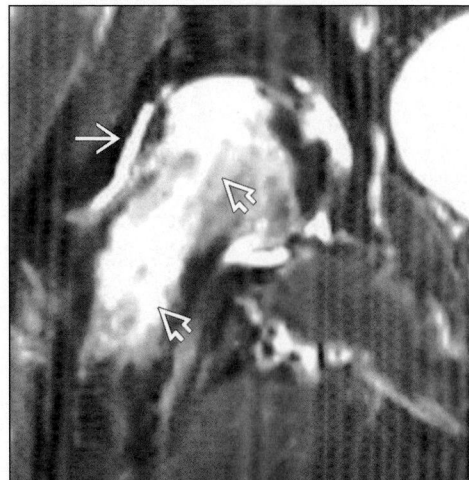

BONE MARROW EDEMA SYNDROMES (PROXIMAL FEMUR)

Septic Joint

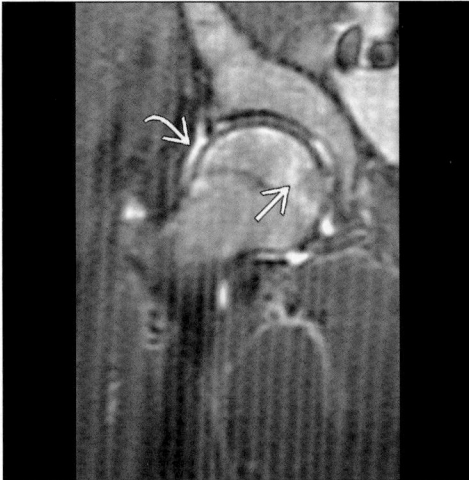

Osteomyelitis

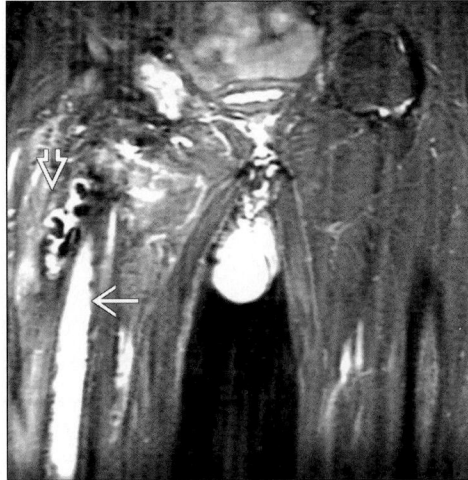

(Left) Coronal STIR MR shows moderate right hip joint effusion ➡ with arthritis. There is mild femoral head reactive marrow edema ➡. Hip aspirate yielded Staphylococcus aureus. *(Right)* Coronal T2WI MR shows Girdlestone arthroplasty following infection of THA. Prosthesis is removed & replaced by multiple antibiotic-impregnated beads ➡. Intense edema of proximal femoral shaft ➡ confirms ongoing osteomyelitis.

Rapidly Destructive Osteoarthritis of Hip

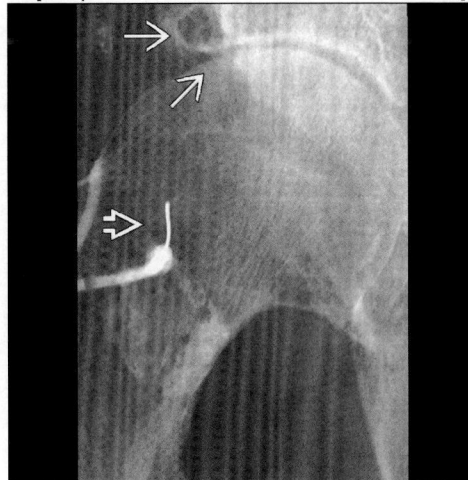

Rapidly Destructive Osteoarthritis of Hip

(Left) Coronal STIR MR shows edema in the collapsed & distorted right femoral head ➡ as well as the adjacent acetabulum ➡. Note the right iliacus fluid ➡ which is an extension of a large debris-filled iliopsoas bursal effusion. *(Right)* Anteroposterior radiograph obtained 1 month earlier, during an arthrogram ➡, shows moderate osteoarthritis with joint space narrowing, subchondral eburnation & cyst formation ➡. Note the spherical femoral head.

Peritumoral Reactive Marrow Edema

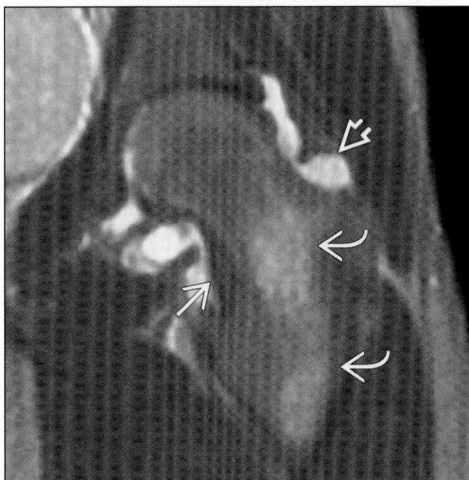

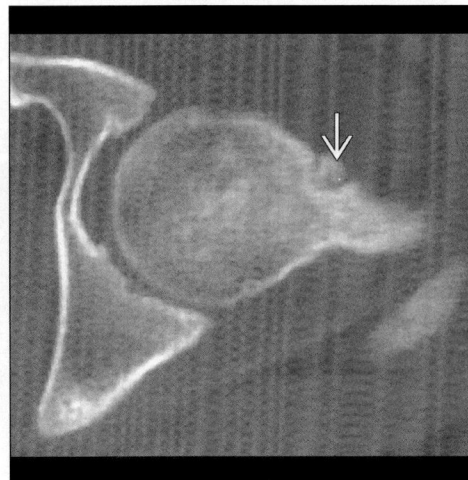

Peritumoral Reactive Marrow Edema

(Left) Coronal T2WI MR shows a moderate joint effusion ➡ in this 17 yo. Diffuse marrow edema ➡ involves neck & subtrochanteric femur. Calcar buttressing is present ➡. This is confusing, until CT is seen (next image). *(Right)* Axial NECT in the same patient, reveals an osteoid osteoma. This lytic lesion with central radiodense nidus ➡ incites an intense reactive marrow edema on MR which may obscure underlying tumor. (†MSK Req).

SUBCHONDRAL EDEMATOUS-LIKE SIGNAL

DIFFERENTIAL DIAGNOSIS

Common
- Trauma
  - Bone Bruise
  - Osteochondral Fracture
  - Reactive Marrow Edema
- Arthritis
  - Osteoarthritis
  - Inflammatory Arthritis
  - Crystalline Arthropathy
- Insufficiency Fracture
- Osteonecrosis

Less Common
- Transient Bone Marrow Edema Syndrome
- Septic Joint
- Osteomyelitis
- Peritumoral Edema

ESSENTIAL INFORMATION

Key Differential Diagnosis Issues
- Signal intensity: Hypointense T1WI; hyperintense T2WI, STIR just deep to osteochondral interface

Helpful Clues for Common Diagnoses
- **Bone Bruise**
  - Compression or impaction injury
  - **Hint**: Look for associated soft tissue injury
- **Osteochondral Fracture**
  - Injury crossing chondral plate into adjacent subchondral bone
  - Osteochondral fragment may stay in place, become flattened, or become completely loose & displaced
- **Reactive Marrow Edema**
  - Bone & adjacent cartilage normal but adjacent tissues are not (e.g., meniscal tear)
- **Arthritis**
  - Osteoarthritis: Cartilage loss; osteophytes
  - Inflammatory: Marrow edema ± cartilage defects; effusions; erosions
  - Crystalline: Crystals penetrating cartilage/subchondral bone with resultant edema; ± erosions or osteophytes
- **Insufficiency Fracture**
  - Intense edema out of proportion to arthritis; may obscure fracture line
- **Osteonecrosis**
  - Subchondral edema may progress to hemorrhage & fluid in fracture/collapse stage; late subchondral edema from cartilage loss & secondary OA

Helpful Clues for Less Common Diagnoses
- **Transient Bone Marrow Edema Syndrome**
  - Diagnosis of exclusion; acute onset pain, typically in middle aged men
- **Septic Joint vs. Osteomyelitis**
  - Septic joint: Effusion, synovial thickening
  - Osteomyelitis: Edema on one side of joint, marginal erosions, periostitis
- **Peritumoral Edema**
  - Osteoid osteoma, giant cell tumor, malignant tumors such as osteosarcoma & chondrosarcoma

Bone Bruise

Axial STIR MR shows subchondral edema in the lateral femoral condyle ➡ & posterolateral tibial plateau ➡. There is a large joint effusion ➡ & ACL tear (not shown). This bruise pattern is common with ACL injury.

Osteochondral Fracture

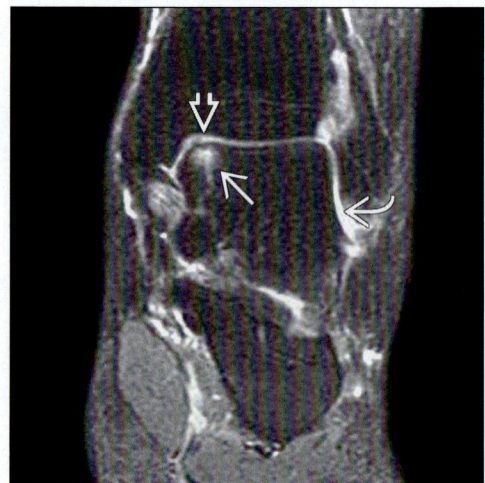

Coronal STIR MR shows a small hyperintense area in the talar subchondral bone ➡ with adjacent hyaline cartilage injury ➡. An ATFL tear (not shown) is accompanied by a small joint effusion ➡ in this injury.

SUBCHONDRAL EDEMATOUS-LIKE SIGNAL

Reactive Marrow Edema

Arthritis

(Left) Coronal PD FSE FS MR shows subtle reactive marrow edema ➡ in patient with medical meniscal tear (not shown). Note the intact cartilage. There was no cartilage damage at surgery. *(Right)* Axial T1 C+ FS MR shows edema in the lateral patella & extensive prepatellar soft tissue swelling ➡. There is a joint effusion with synovial enhancement ➡. A small non-displaced fracture has occurred through a gouty erosion ➡.

Insufficiency Fracture

Septic Joint

(Left) Sagittal PD FSE MR shows hypointense posterior lateral femoral condylar signal ➡ paralleling the articular surface with slight flattening of the articular surface due to an insufficiency fracture. *(Right)* Coronal PD FSE FS MR shows high signal within multiple carpal bones ➡ & multiple joint effusions with synovial thickening ➡. This proved to be Staphylococcus septic arthritis.

Osteomyelitis

Peritumoral Edema

(Left) Coronal T2WI FS MR shows high signal at multiple subchondral sites within the pelvis (sacral ala ➡ & iliac wing ➡) in a child with normal radiograph. Biopsy proved chronic multifocal osteomyelitis. *(Right)* Sagittal T2WI FS MR shows a mildly expansile hyperintense patellar lesion ➡ with a thin rim and no cortical breakthrough. The bone adjacent to this giant cell tumor demonstrates non-neoplastic peritumoral edema ➡.

ABNORMAL EPIPHYSEAL MARROW SIGNAL

DIFFERENTIAL DIAGNOSIS

Common
- Reactive Marrow Edema
- Bone Bruise
- Fracture
- Osteonecrosis
- Transient Bone Marrow Edema
- Legg-Calvé-Perthes
- Osteomyelitis
- Septic Joint
- Arthritis
  - Osteoarthritis
  - Inflammatory Arthritis
  - Juvenile Idiopathic Arthritis (JIA)

Less Common
- Anemia
- Neoplasm
  - Metastases, Bone Marrow
  - Primary Bone Neoplasm
- Stem Cell Stimulation

Rare but Important
- Myelofibrosis
- Gaucher Disease

ESSENTIAL INFORMATION

Key Differential Diagnosis Issues
- Epiphyses convert to fatty (yellow) marrow before 1 year of age
- Abnormal epiphyseal marrow defined as change in normal fatty signal
  - Normal: T1WI - hyperintense; T2WI - intermediate; fat-suppression - hypointense
- Differential diagnoses include epiphysis, apophyses or epiphyseal equivalent (carpals, tarsals)
- Other differentials may be tailored to location, such as proximal femur

Helpful Clues for Common Diagnoses
- **Reactive Marrow Edema**
  - Marrow edema typically related to adjacent abnormality (e.g., tendon or meniscal tear)
  - No history of direct trauma; no cartilage damage, infection or neoplasm
- **Bone Bruise**
  - Marrow contusion related to microtrabecular fracture

- History of acute or subacute trauma
- **Hint**: Look for adjacent soft tissue injury
- **Fracture**
  - Intense diffuse edema may obscure fracture line
  - Traumatic - **Hint**: Look for adjacent soft tissue injury
  - Insufficiency - **Hint**: Look for articular surface flattening
- **Osteonecrosis**
  - Serpentine margin between normal & avascular bone
  - "Double line" sign: Outer margin low signal while inner margin high signal
- **Transient Bone Marrow Edema**
  - Diagnosis of exclusion; may require hip aspiration to exclude septic arthritis
  - History is key: No trauma, minimal arthritis, acute onset
- **Legg-Calvé-Perthes**
  - Edema which may progress to femoral head low signal & flattening
  - Small femoral ossification center; thickened articular cartilage
  - Boys > girls; age 4-8 at risk as foveal arteries regress
- **Osteomyelitis**
  - May be difficult to distinguish from septic joint in early stages
  - Marrow edema on one side of joint, marginal erosions, periostitis; ± bone or soft tissue abscess
  - Brodie abscess: Abscesses may be epiphyseal or in carpals/tarsals in infants; meta-epiphyseal in children
- **Septic Joint**
  - Effusion, synovial thickening, ± adjacent marrow edema
- **Arthritis**
  - Osteoarthritis: Cartilage loss, osteophytes, subchondral edema &/or cysts
  - Inflammatory: Marrow edema, effusion, ± erosions, ± cartilage loss
  - Juvenile idiopathic: Soft tissue swelling, periostitis, erosions are late finding

Helpful Clues for Less Common Diagnoses
- **Anemia**
  - Marrow undergoes reconversion from fatty to hematopoietic marrow in an orderly fashion

ABNORMAL EPIPHYSEAL MARROW SIGNAL

○ Epiphyses are last to reconvert; thus epiphyseal involvement is indicative of chronic long standing anemia
○ Sickle cell anemia & thalassemia at risk for osteonecrosis

- **Neoplasm**
  ○ May be primary or secondary (metastatic)
  ○ Epiphyseal involvement is less common than metadiaphyseal
  ○ Marrow replacement may be patchy or diffuse
  ○ ± Cortical breakthrough with associated soft tissue mass
  ○ **Hint**: Age is a useful determinate
    ▪ Child: Leukemia, metastases, chondroblastoma
    ▪ Young adult: Giant cell tumor, leukemia, lymphoma
    ▪ Older adult: Metastases, lymphoma, leukemia, clear cell chondrosarcoma
- **Stem Cell Stimulation**
  ○ Medication related: Erythropoietin, Neupogen
  ○ Facilitates stem cell repopulation; often used in conjunction with chemotherapy
  ○ Marrow reconversion is patchy & can mimic metastatic disease
  ○ In- & out-of-phase imaging may help distinguish normal hematopoiesis from metastatic infiltration

Helpful Clues for Rare Diagnoses
- **Myelofibrosis**
  ○ Fibrosis most common in areas of normal adult hematopoiesis (spine, pelvis, ribs)
  ○ Associated anemia results in reconversion of fatty marrow including epiphyses
  ○ Epiphyses subsequently become fibrotic with trabecular thickening & sclerosis
- **Gaucher Disease**
  ○ Marrow packing disorder results in anemia, undertubulation, osteonecrosis, osteopenia
  ○ Associated anemia results in reconversion of fatty marrow including epiphyses
  ○ Undertubulation: Erlenmeyer flask deformity, cortical thinning
  ○ Osteonecrosis of epiphyses, metaphyses & diaphyses as well as axial skeleton
  ○ Osteopenic: At risk for fractures
  ○ Most common in Ashkenazi Jews

Alternative Differential Approaches
- **Adult Versus Child**
  ○ Adult
    ▪ Trauma, osteonecrosis, transient bone marrow edema syndrome, osteomyelitis, arthritis, metastases, multiple myeloma, lymphoma, giant cell tumor, stem cell stimulation, myelofibrosis, Gaucher disease
  ○ Child
    ▪ Trauma, Legg-Calvé-Perthes, osteomyelitis, juvenile idiopathic arthritis, leukemia, lymphoma, chondroblastoma, stem cell stimulation, Gaucher disease

Reactive Marrow Edema

Coronal STIR MR shows a radial medial meniscus tear at the posterior meniscal root ➡ with adjacent epiphyseal reactive marrow edema ➡. The ligaments & cartilage were normal at arthroscopy.

Fracture

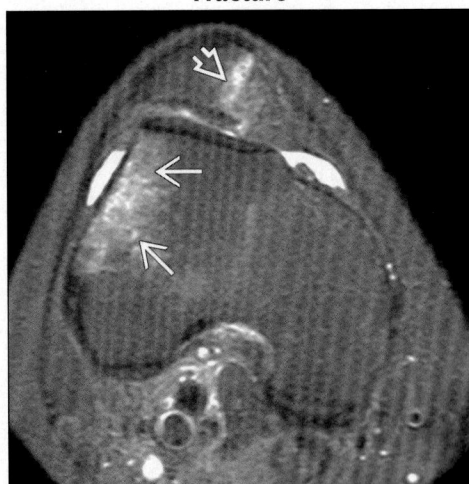

Axial PD FSE FS MR shows an impaction fracture of the medial patellar facet ➡ with a bone bruise of the distal lateral femoral condyle ➡ in this patient with transient lateral patellar dislocation.

ABNORMAL EPIPHYSEAL MARROW SIGNAL

Osteonecrosis

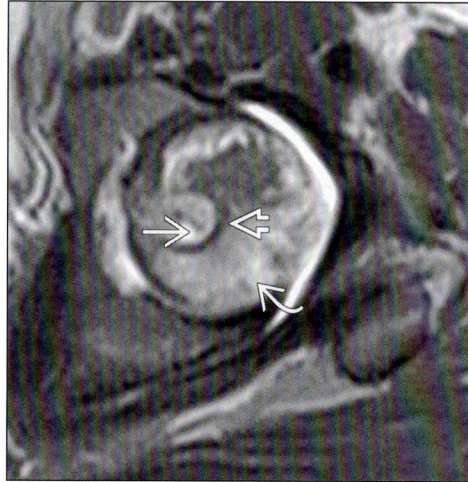

Transient Bone Marrow Edema

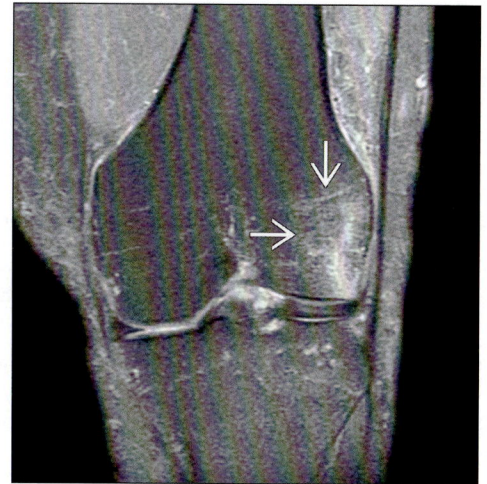

(Left) Axial T2WI FS MR shows a serpentine "double line" sign of avascular necrosis with outer low ➡ & inner high ➡ signal intensity marking the avascular region. Note adjacent reactive marrow edema ➡. *(Right)* Coronal T2WI FS MR shows diffuse marrow edema ➡ in the lateral femoral condyle. Prior history of similar process in the medial femoral condyle which resolved about 3 months prior to this presentation represents the migratory form of this process.

Legg-Calvé-Perthes

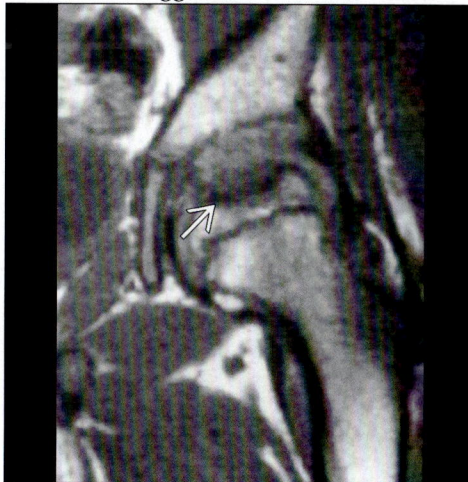

Osteomyelitis

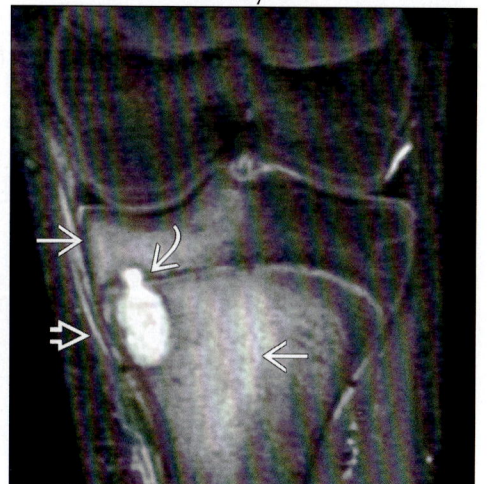

(Left) Coronal T1WI MR shows capital femoral epiphysis flattening with a well-demarcated hypointense ➡ ischemic area in Legg-Calvé-Perthes. Mild coxa magna deformity is present. *(Right)* Coronal STIR MR shows diffuse edema of epiphysis & metaphysis ➡ with a discrete rim-enhancing lesion ➡ spanning the physis, representing a subacute osteomyelitis/Brodie abscess. There is mild periosteal edema ➡.

Osteoarthritis

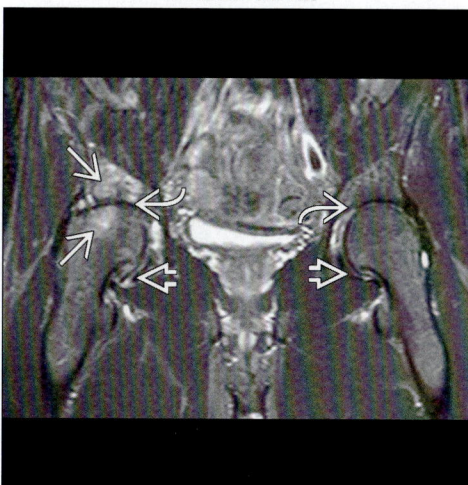

Juvenile Idiopathic Arthritis (JIA)

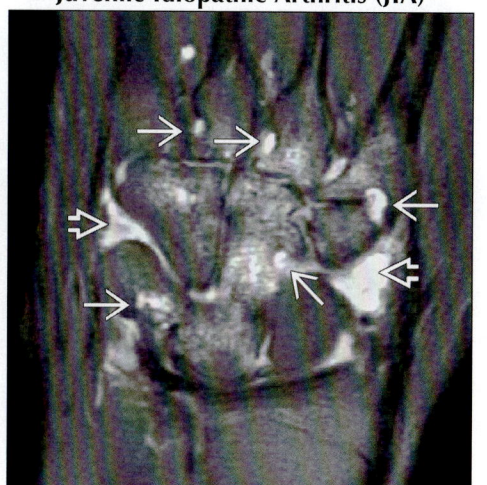

(Left) Coronal STIR MR shows typical endstage osteoarthritis (R > L) with joint space loss, femoral head flattening, acetabular remodeling, & subchondral (epiphyseal) marrow edema ➡. Involvement of both sides of the joint ➡ & osteophytic ridging ➡ assist in diagnosis. *(Right)* Coronal T2WI MR shows dramatic diffuse marrow edema throughout the carpals (epiphyseal equivalent) with extensive synovitis ➡ & multiple erosions ➡ (a late finding in JIA).

ABNORMAL EPIPHYSEAL MARROW SIGNAL

Anemia

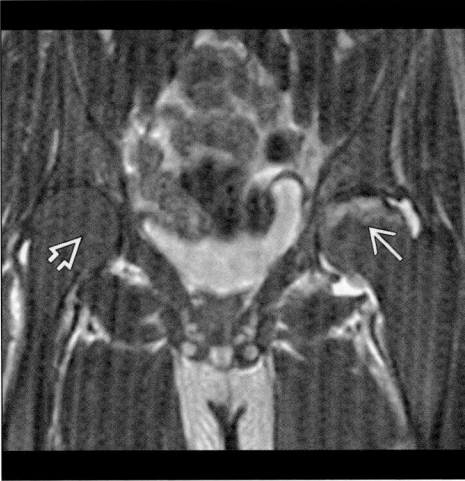

Metastases, Bone Marrow

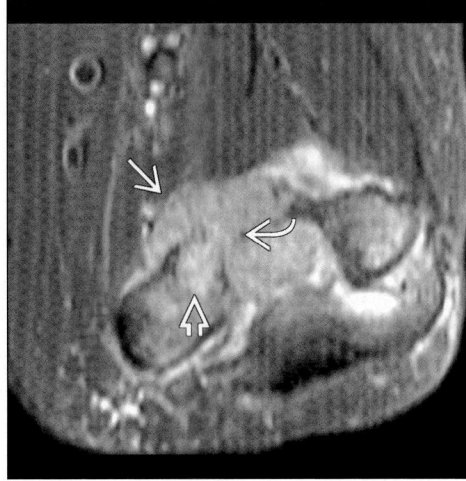

(Left) Coronal T2WI MR shows absence of normal fatty marrow signal. This sickle cell patient's marrow is fully hematopoietic including the normal fatty epiphyses ➡. Note left femoral head avascular necrosis with edema, flattening & collapse ➡. *(Right)* Axial T1 C+ FS MR shows a renal cell metastatic lesion in the trochlear epiphyseal region with marrow replacement ➡ & cortical breakthrough ➡ with a soft tissue mass ➡ in the joint. Moderate enhancement is present.

Primary Bone Neoplasm

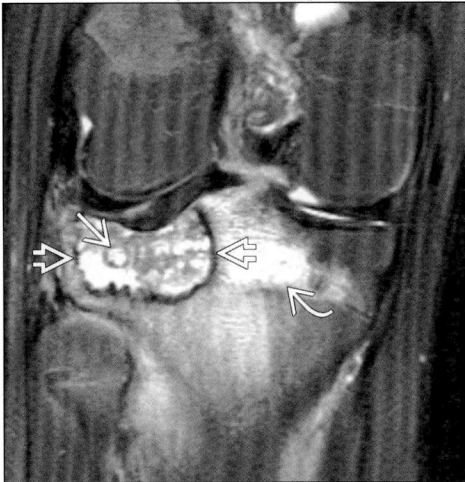

Primary Bone Neoplasm

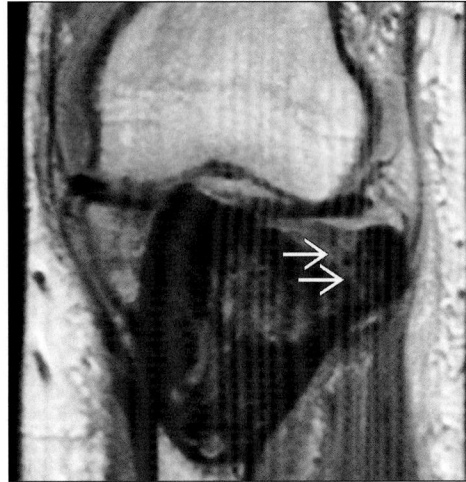

(Left) Coronal T1 C+ FS MR shows a well-circumscribed enhancing tibial epiphyseal lesion ➡ with intense peritumoral edema ➡. The cartilage lobules ➡ as well as the location are typical in this chondroblastoma. *(Right)* Coronal PD FSE MR shows a large low signal meta-epiphyseal lesion extending to the subchondral bone. The low signal is due to intralesional calcification in this giant cell tumor. Note the pathological fracture in the lateral tibial plateau ➡.

Myelofibrosis

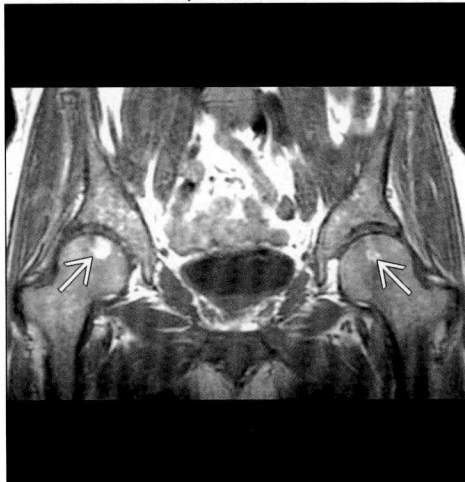

Gaucher Disease

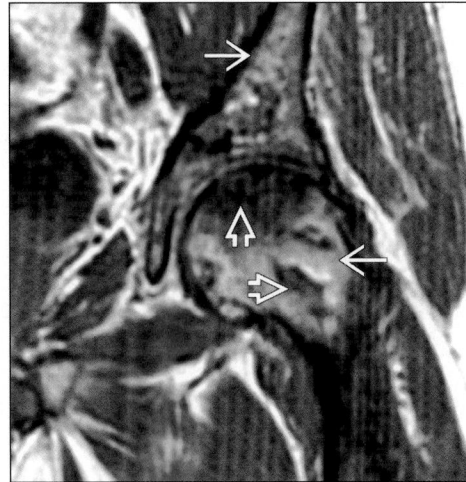

(Left) Coronal T1WI MR shows bland intermediate marrow replacement including the epiphyses, which are normally high signal on T1WI. This is fibrotic marrow typical of myelofibrosis. Note the small islands of retained normal fat ➡. *(Right)* Coronal T1WI MR shows slightly speckled, intermediate signal of diffuse Gaucher infiltration ➡. This is complicated by osteonecrosis ➡ of the femoral head, neck & acetabulum.

INCREASED MARROW FAT

DIFFERENTIAL DIAGNOSIS

Common
- Osteoporosis
- Normal Aging
- Focal Fatty Deposition
- Discogenic Endplate Changes

Less Common
- Intraosseous Hemangioma
- Intraosseous Lipoma
- Steroid-Induced Increased Fat
- Radiation-Induced Increased Fat
- Osteonecrosis

Rare but Important
- Bone Marrow Failure
- Anorexia
- Liposclerosing Myxofibrous Tumor
- Hypopituitarism
- Weightlessness

ESSENTIAL INFORMATION

Key Differential Diagnosis Issues
- Increased marrow fat may be focal or diffuse
  - Represents either a true increase in fat or a marked decrease in hematopoietic marrow elements
- Normal adult marrow
  - Hematopoietic (red) marrow content: 40% fat, 40% water, 20% protein
    - Intermediate signal intensity (SI) on T1, T2 & fluid-sensitive sequences
  - Fatty (yellow) marrow content: 80% fat, 15% water, 5% protein
    - High SI on T1
    - Lower SI on T2 & fluid-sensitive sequences
- Normal red vs. yellow marrow distribution
  - Predominantly red marrow at birth
  - Epiphyses/apophyses convert to yellow marrow in 1st year of life
  - Red to yellow marrow proceeds distal to proximal; appendicular to axial skeleton
- **Hint**: Radiographs may be useful in differential diagnosis

Helpful Clues for Common Diagnoses
- **Osteoporosis**
  - Pronounced osteopenia may be confirmed by radiograph

  - Primary trabecular struts thicken as secondary trabeculae are resorbed
  - May be diffuse or focal
- **Normal Aging**
  - Diffuse increased yellow marrow in aging population
  - Retains hematopoietic elements in proximal femurs, flat bones of pelvis & spine longer than in the extremities
  - Minimal osteopenia by radiograph
- **Focal Fatty Deposition**
  - Typically visible in those of advancing age
  - Tend to be rounded and discrete lesions in the vertebral bodies but can involve entire vertebral body
  - Trabeculae are normal within and around the lesion
  - T2 signal may be low, intermediate, or high SI
- **Discogenic Endplate Changes**
  - Degenerative changes in vertebral endplate resulting from red marrow being replaced by fatty yellow marrow
  - Also known as Modic type 2 changes
  - Modic degenerative endplate types
    - Type 1: Low SI T1 and high SI T2
    - Type 2: High SI T1 and isointense SI T2
    - Type 3: Low SI T1 and T2

Helpful Clues for Less Common Diagnoses
- **Intraosseous Hemangioma**
  - Most common in vertebra and skull
  - High SI T1 due to fat in interstices of tumor
  - High SI T2 due to vascular components and interstitial edema
  - May or may not enhance
  - Radiographs show intralesional vertical striations due to thickened trabeculae
- **Intraosseous Lipoma**
  - Most common in proximal femur and calcaneus
  - Appears predominantly high SI while adipocytes viable but becomes cystic with dystrophic calcification as it evolves due to ischemia and necrosis
  - Radiographs show well-circumscribed, mildly expansile lucent lesion with variable dystrophic calcification
- **Steroid-Induced Increased Fat**
  - Corticosteroids shown to actually enlarge the adipocytes

INCREASED MARROW FAT

- At increased risk for AVN, insufficiency fractures
- **Hint**: Look for fat deposition in surrounding soft tissues
- **Radiation-Induced Increased Fat**
  - Complete loss of hematopoietic elements accounts for apparent increase in marrow fat
  - **Hint**: Distinct transition between irradiated and nonirradiated marrow
  - **Hint**: Look for radiation changes in surrounding soft tissues
- **Osteonecrosis**
  - High SI T1 seen in early infarction as adipocytes are the last to die following acute ischemic event
  - High SI T1 in chronic stages may represents mummified fat cells or fatty replacement of fibrosis
  - **Hint**: Look for serpentine margin bordering necrotic area
  - **Hint**: Double line sign represents interface between necrotic and reparative marrow

Helpful Clues for Rare Diagnoses

- **Bone Marrow Failure**
  - Includes acquired (aplastic anemia and myelodysplastic syndromes) and inherited (Fanconi anemia, etc.)
  - Profound depletion of hematopoietic elements
  - Appearance similar to radiation changes but without discrete transition between normal and depleted marrow

- **Anorexia**
  - Radiographs show marked osteopenia
  - **Hint**: Look for marked soft tissue and muscle wasting
- **Liposclerosing Myxofibrous Tumor**
  - Benign fibroosseous tumor with mixed content which may include lipoma, myxoma, fibrous dysplasia, fat necrosis and ossification in varying amounts
- **Hypopituitarism**
  - Findings similar to bone marrow failure
- **Weightlessness**
  - Long periods of weightlessness result in diffuse (disuse) osteoporosis

Alternative Differential Approaches

- Diffuse increased marrow fat
  - Osteoporosis
  - Normal aging
  - Steroid-induced increased fat
  - Bone marrow failure
  - Anorexia
  - Hypopituitarism
  - Weightlessness
- Focal increased marrow fat
  - Focal fatty marrow
  - Discogenic fatty deposition
  - Intraosseous hemangioma
  - Radiation-induced increased fat
  - Intraosseous lipoma
  - Osteonecrosis

Osteoporosis

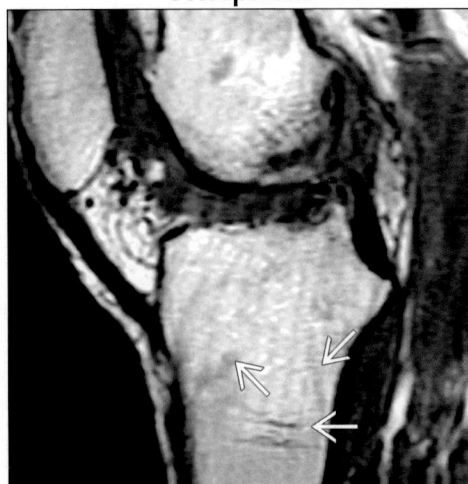

Sagittal PD FSE MR shows loss of secondary trabeculae, reinforced primary trabeculae (bone struts) ➡ and increased marrow fat, typical of osteoporosis in this 86 year old woman.

Normal Aging

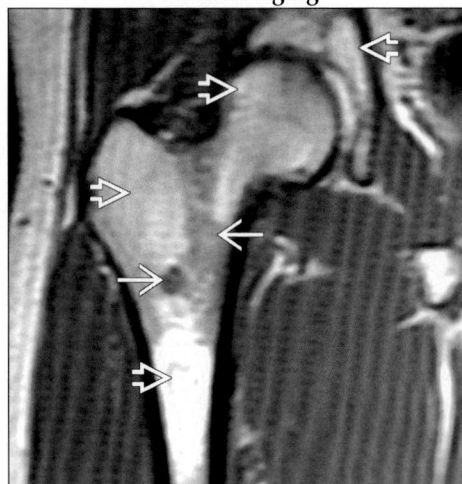

Coronal T1WI MR shows fatty marrow distribution in a normal 70 year old man with patchy intermediate signal red marrow ➡ in intertrochanteric and subtrochanteric bone; yellow marrow ➡ in all other osseous regions.

INCREASED MARROW FAT

Focal Fatty Deposition

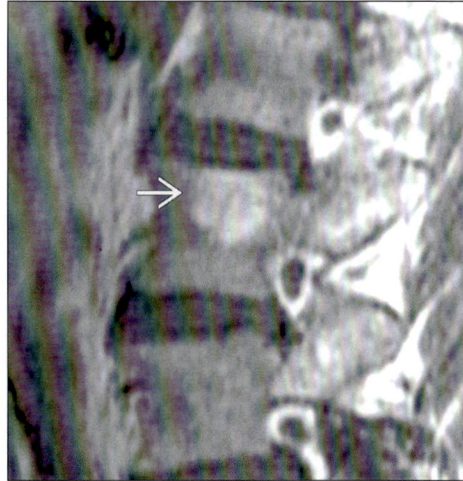

Discogenic Endplate Changes

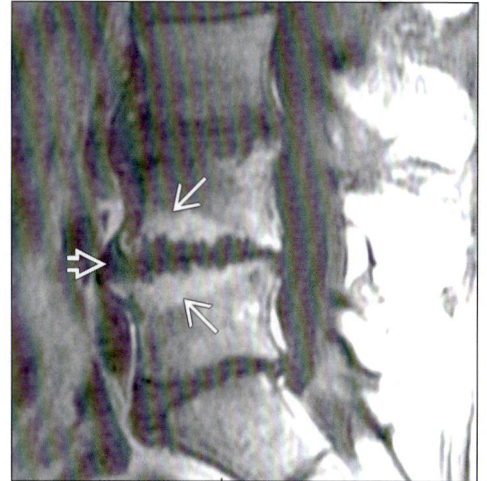

(Left) Sagittal T1WI MR shows focal rounded high signal area ➡ in left paracentral L3 vertebra with a normal trabecular pattern within and around the area, typical of focal fatty deposit. This was also bright on T2WI (not shown). *(Right)* Sagittal T1WI MR shows the significant disc height loss and endplate irregularity of degenerative disc disease ➡. The high signal of fatty marrow in the adjacent endplates ➡ is seen in endstage discogenic changes.

Intraosseous Hemangioma

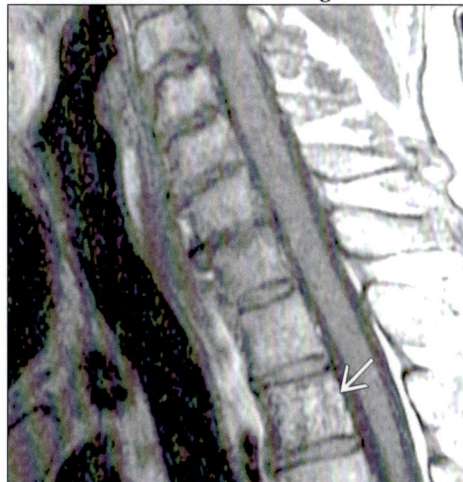

Intraosseous Hemangioma

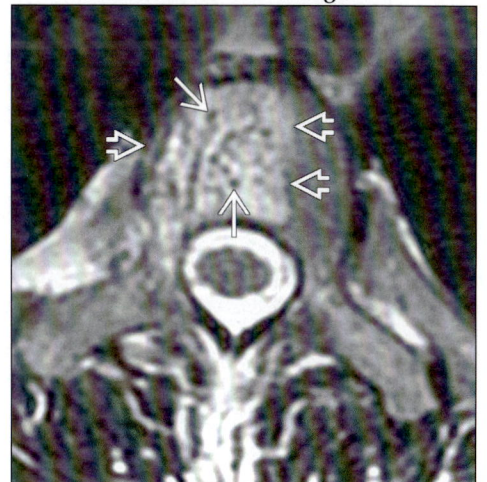

(Left) Sagittal T1WI MR shows mixed high signal ➡ of fatty infiltration admixed with low signal, representing the trabecular thickening often seen in osseous hemangioma. This lesion was high signal in T2WI (not shown). *(Right)* Axial T2WI MR shows the extent of this focal high signal lesion ➡ in this thoracic intraosseous hemangioma in the same patient. Note the punctate appearance of the low signal thickened trabecular struts ➡ seen in cross-section.

Intraosseous Lipoma

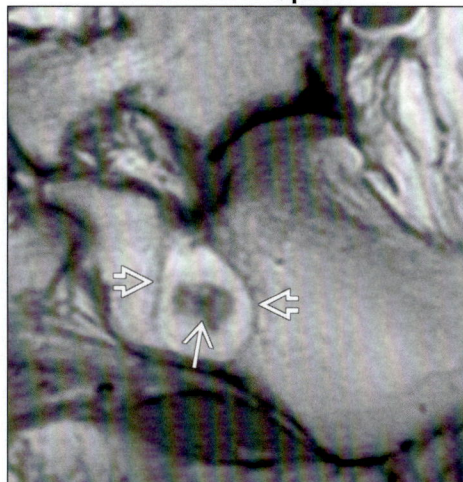

Steroid-Induced Increased Fat

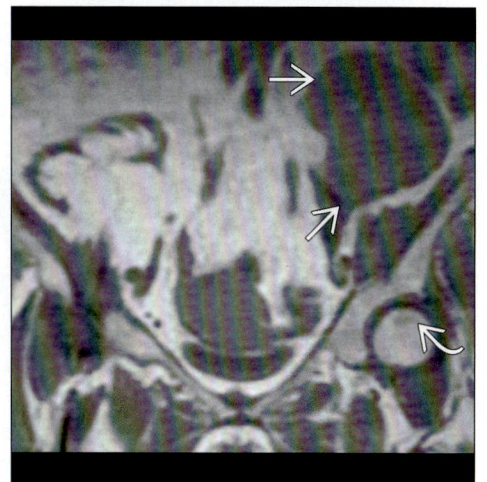

(Left) Sagittal T1WI MR shows a well-defined fat signal intensity lesion ➡ with central low signal ➡ intensity due to mineralization. This is typical of intraosseous lipoma. The calcaneus and proximal femur are common locations for this lesion. *(Right)* Coronal T1WI MR shows diffuse increased marrow fat in left hip of a patient treated with corticosteroids for renal transplantation ➡. Note the crescent-shaped signal in femoral head ➡, suggesting early AVN.

INCREASED MARROW FAT

Radiation-Induced Increased Fat

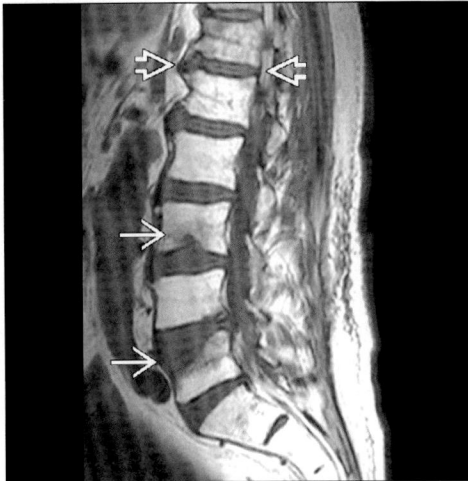

Osteonecrosis

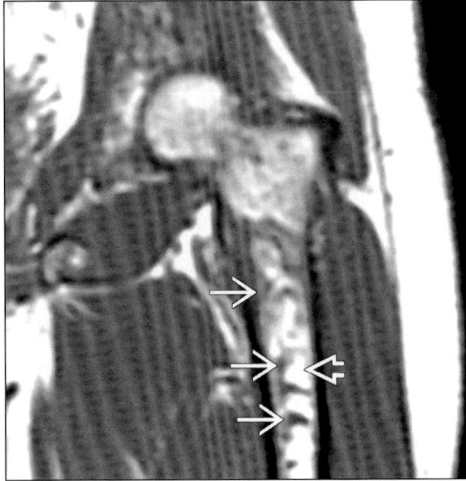

(Left) Sagittal T1WI MR shows diffuse increased signal in the lumbar spine and sacrum with sharp demarcation between irradiated and non-irradiated bone at the T12-L1 level ➡. Note two associated insufficiency fractures ➡. *(Right)* Coronal T1WI MR shows increased fatty marrow ➡ in the femoral shaft, surrounded by a thin, serpentine rim of calcium (low signal, ➡). This is chronic bone infarction in Gaucher disease.

Bone Marrow Failure

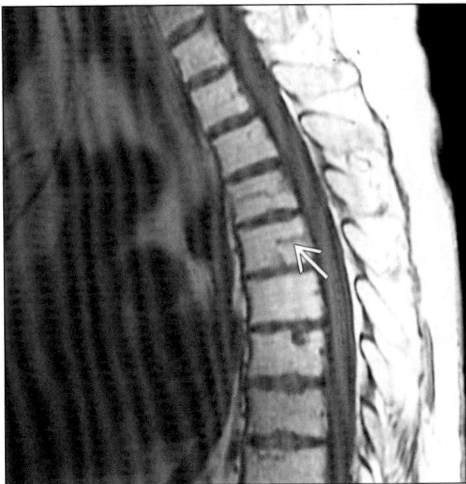

Anorexia

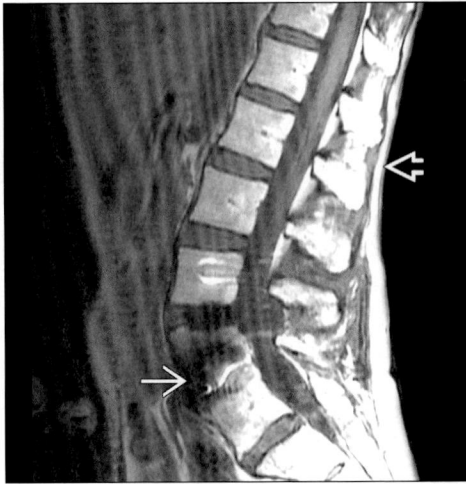

(Left) Sagittal T1WI MR shows a paucity of cellular elements in this 68 year old with aplastic anemia. This results in an apparent increase in marrow fat. Note the prominent basivertebral plexus ➡. *(Right)* Sagittal T1WI MR reveals diffuse increased fatty marrow in a patient status post L4-5 anterior fusion ➡. There is a paucity of subcutaneous fat ➡ in this anorexic female who is 4'10" & weighs 78 pounds.

Liposclerosing Myxofibrous Tumor

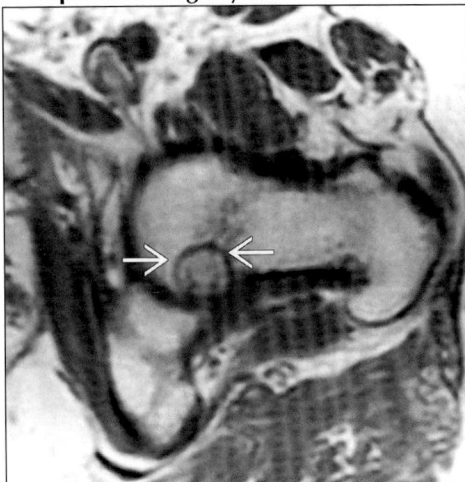

Liposclerosing Myxofibrous Tumor

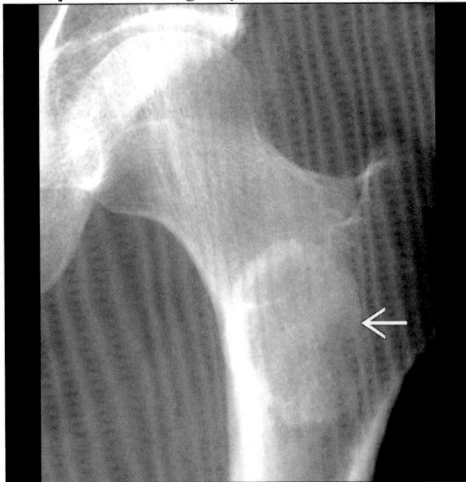

(Left) Axial T1WI MR shows well-circumscribed, non-aggressive, lesion ➡ in posterior subcapital femur with thin sclerotic margin and slight heterogeneity but no cortical breakthrough, confirmed to be an LSMFT by biopsy. *(Right)* Anteroposterior radiograph AP radiograph, in a different patient, shows the more typical location (intertrochanteric) and appearance (geographic with sclerotic margin and subtle internal mineralization ➡) of a LSMFT.

DIFFERENTIAL DIAGNOSIS

Common
- Anemia
- Complications of Smoking
- Sports Anemia
- Sickle Cell Anemia: MSK Complications
- Thalassemia

Less Common
- Hematopoietic Stimulation
- Polycythemia Vera
- Leukemia
- Myelofibrosis

Rare but Important
- Anti-Viral Drug Effect
- Spherocytosis

ESSENTIAL INFORMATION

Key Differential Diagnosis Issues
- Marrow hyperplasia results from an increase in one or more marrow cell lines including RBC, WBC, platelets or their precursors
- Hematopoietic (red or cellular) versus fatty (yellow) marrow
- Marrow appearance should be age appropriate
  - Predominantly red marrow at birth
  - Epiphyses/apophyses convert to yellow marrow in 1st year
  - Red to yellow marrow conversion proceeds from distal to proximal; appendicular to axial skeleton
- **Hint**: In diffuse hyperplasia, look for "flip-flop" sign-vertebral body marrow darker than adjacent discs on T1WI

Helpful Clues for Common Diagnoses
- **Anemia**
  - Three main classes: Acute loss, excessive destruction, decreased production
  - Marrow capable of response will do so in predictable pattern
    - Fatty marrow "re-converted" to red marrow in reverse order
    - Reconversion proceeds from axial to appendicular skeleton; proximal to distal long bones
    - Epiphyses/apophyses recruit late in process

- Osteopenia often a key radiographic feature
- Selected types of anemia are discussed below
- **Complications of Smoking**
  - Seen in smokers; mild to moderate obesity; female > male
  - Etiology unknown; mild leukocytosis noted
  - Patchy reconversion marrow in distal femoral metaphysis
- **Sports Anemia**
  - Seen in marathon runners & other high-performance athletes
  - Group known to have chronic low grade anemia of uncertain etiology
  - Patchy metaphyseal hematopoiesis in distal femur/proximal tibia with epiphyseal sparing
- **Sickle Cell Anemia: MSK Complications**
  - Inherited anemia
  - Radiographs: Osteopenia, widening of medullary spaces, trabecular & cortical thinning
  - MR: Widespread marrow reconversion or failure of initial red to yellow marrow conversion
  - Bone infarction more common than in thalassemia
- **Thalassemia**
  - Inherited anemia
  - MR: Marked increased hematopoietic marrow may include epiphyses
  - Radiographs: Osteopenia, widened medullary space, cortical thinning, coarsened trabeculae, Erlenmeyer flask deformity
  - Bone scan: Generalized decreased uptake

Helpful Clues for Less Common Diagnoses
- **Hematopoietic Stimulation**
  - Marrow stem cell stimulation (e.g., erythrocyte or granulocyte colony-stimulating factor)
  - Used in chemotherapy, anemia of chronic disease, renal disease
  - Typically stimulates somewhat patchy reconversion of marrow which may simulate metastatic disease
    - **Hint**: In- & out-of-phase imaging may help distinguish normal versus neoplastic marrow

MARROW HYPERPLASIA

- Reconversion proceeds axial to appendicular, proximal to distal, ± epiphyseal involvement
- **Polycythemia Vera**
  - Erythrocytosis, leukocytosis, thrombocytosis affects older adults
  - Marrow reconversion in proximal long bones typically spares epiphyses/apophyses until late stage
  - Femoral osteonecrosis due to vascular thrombosis
  - May evolve to myelofibrosis over time
  - Hyperuricemia may present as gouty arthritis
- **Leukemia**
  - Neoplastic proliferation of one or more marrow cell lines
  - Children
    - Acute lymphocytic leukemia (ALL) most common
    - Osteopenia with metaphyseal sclerotic bands, osteolytic lesions, periostitis
    - Marrow hyperplasia from disease & associated anemia; may be focal or diffuse
  - Adults
    - Acute myelocytic leukemia (AML) most common
    - Acute: Bone pain, rheumatoid-like arthritis may be present, diffuse marrow infiltration
    - Chronic lymphocytic leukemia (CLL) most common
    - Chronic: Osteopenia, may progress to myelofibrosis, diffuse marrow infiltration
- **Myelofibrosis**
  - Chronic myeloproliferative disease
  - Cellularity varies ranging from hypercellularity to marked hypocellularity as fibrosis worsens
  - Marrow infiltration typically follows reconversion pattern: Axial to appendicular, proximal to distal, epiphyses spared until late
  - Progresses to osteosclerosis
  - Massive splenomegaly is key finding

Helpful Clues for Rare Diagnoses
- **Anti-Viral Drug Effect**
  - Anti retroviral medications in HIV population
  - Significant drug-related osteopenia
  - HIV-associated avascular necrosis
  - Anemia results in marrow reconversion
  - Look for myositis in combination with significant marrow reconversion
- **Spherocytosis**
  - Inherited hemolytic anemia with onset in early adolescence
  - Marrow fails to convert from red to yellow marrow
  - Osteopenia, cortical thinning, extramedullary hematopoiesis

Anemia

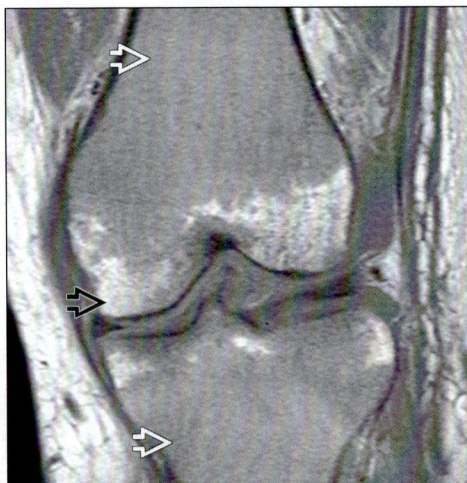

Coronal T1WI MR shows extensive hematopoiesis in the knee metadiaphyses with partial replacement of the normal epiphyseal fatty marrow as well. Patient has known hemolytic anemia.

Complications of Smoking

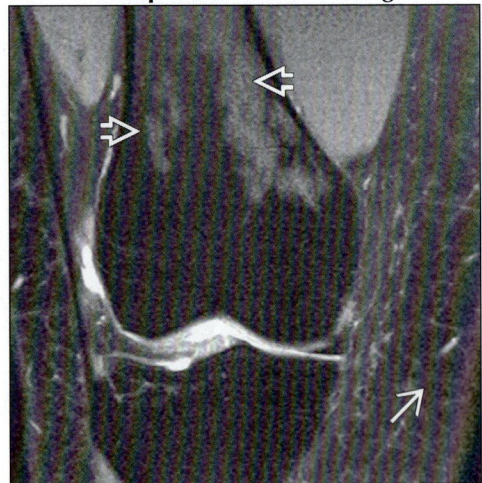

Coronal STIR MR shows islands of reconverted red marrow in the distal femoral metaphysis. Note the body habitus in this 36 year old female smoker.

141

MARROW HYPERPLASIA

(Left) *Sagittal PD FSE FS MR shows patchy, somewhat striated intermediate signal ➡ in the distal femoral metaphysis representing reconversion marrow in this 27 year old marathon runner.* **(Right)** *Sagittal STIR MR shows a stress fracture ➡ of the plantar calcaneus. The marrow shows diffuse intermediate marrow signal ➡. This is related to significant marrow hyperplasia in this 25 year old anorexic female who runs to "control her weight".*

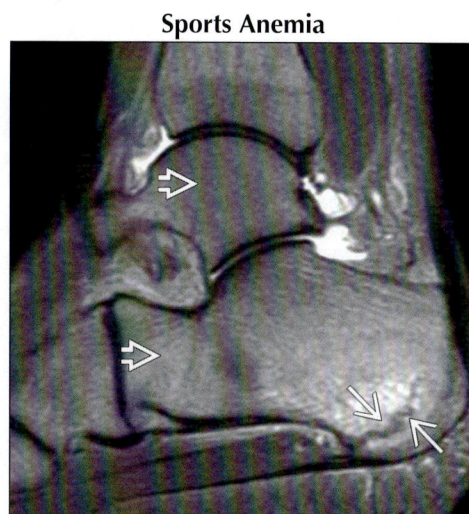

Sports Anemia

Sports Anemia

(Left) *Coronal STIR MR shows fatty marrow replacement in the pelvis & proximal femur ➡. High signal ➡ results from an apophyseal bone infarction in this sickle cell patient. Epiphyseal fatty marrow ➡ is still present.* **(Right)** *Sagittal T1WI MR shows homogeneous vertebral body signal lower than adjacent discs, related to patient's sickle cell anemia & hemosiderin from multiple transfusions. Vertebral body signal should be higher than discs on T1 sequence.*

Sickle Cell Anemia: MSK Complications

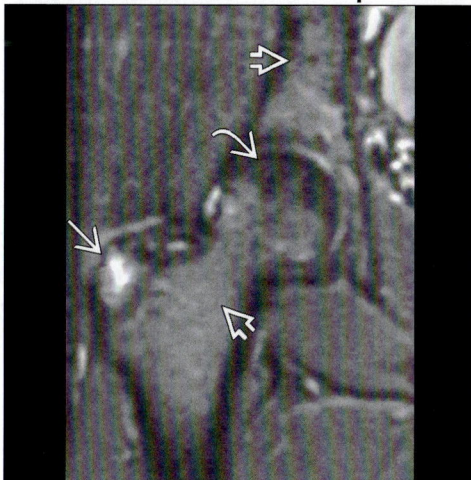

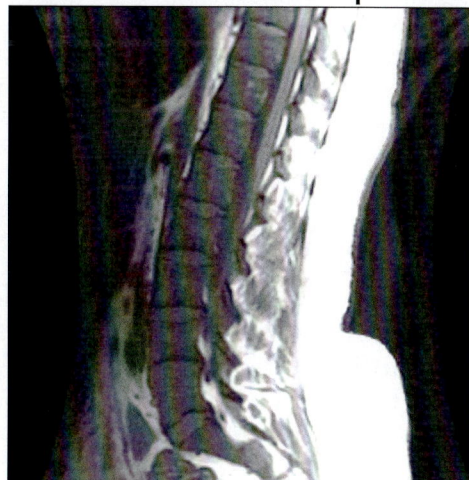

Sickle Cell Anemia: MSK Complications

(Left) *AP radiograph shows the radiographic pattern of marrow hyperplasia in this 11 year old thalassemic. Cortical thinning, "squaring" of small hand bones & profound osteopenia ➡ are due to a marrow space packed with cells. (†MSK Req).* **(Right)** *Lateral radiograph shows medullary (diploic) space widening & trabecular thickening resulting in "hair on end" appearance.*

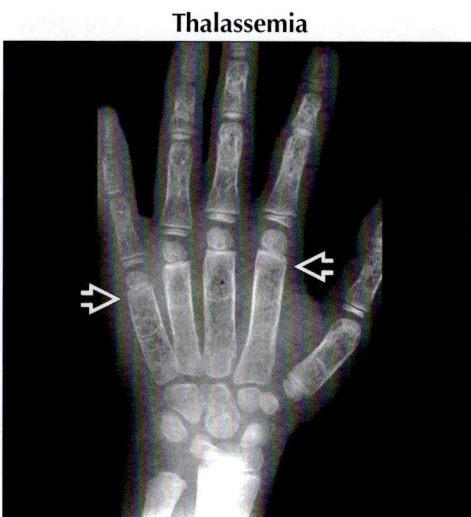

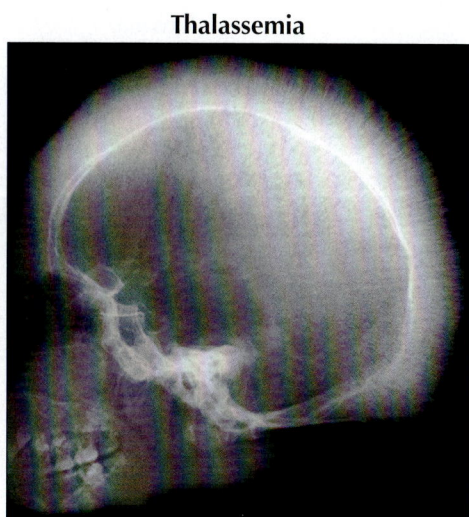

Thalassemia

Thalassemia

MARROW HYPERPLASIA

Hematopoietic Stimulation

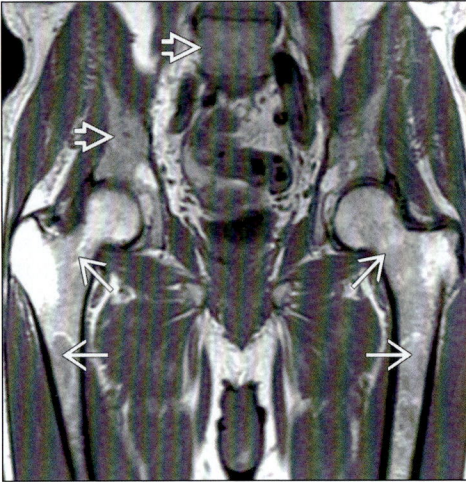

Polycythemia Vera

(Left) Coronal T1WI MR shows reconversion of yellow to red marrow throughout the proximal femurs ➡ & pelvis/spine ⧩ in response to erythropoietin therapy for chemotherapy-related anemia. (Right) Coronal T1WI MR shows diffuse, intermediate-signal marrow replacement ➡ of the femoral metadiaphyses with epiphyseal sparing ⧩. This signal is a combination of marrow hyperplasia & developing fibrosis in this 66 year old.

Leukemia

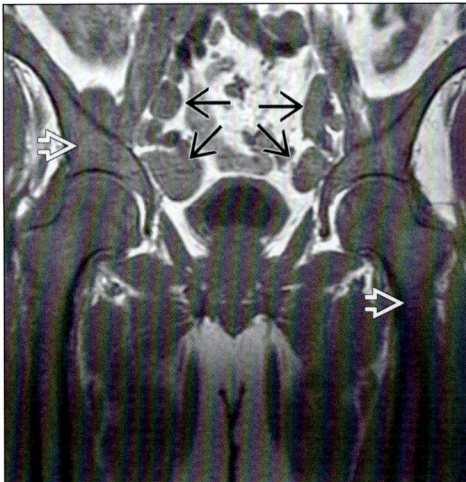

Leukemia

(Left) Coronal T1WI MR shows profound marrow hyperplasia with bland intermediate signal marrow ⧩ in all visualized bones. Note the marked lymphadenopathy ➡ in this case of chronic lymphocytic leukemia in this 75 year old. (Right) Coronal T1WI MR shows diffuse leukemic infiltration with hypointense metadiaphyses ➡ & patchy epiphyseal involvement ⧩. Note the similarity to the first image in this series, hemolytic anemia. Clinical history is key in diagnosis.

Myelofibrosis

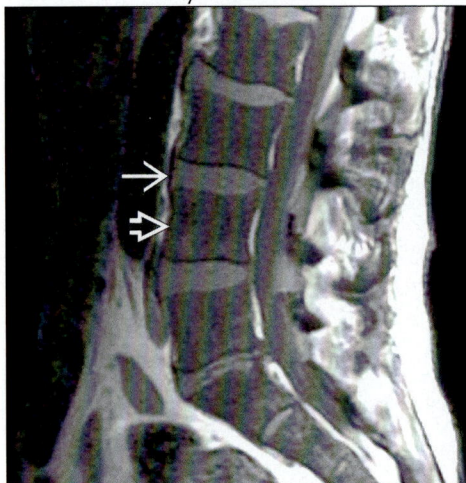

Anti-Viral Drug Effect

(Left) Sagittal T1WI MR shows typical diffuse dark T1 marrow of myelofibrosis. This results from a mix of hypercellularity & developing fibrosis. Note vertebral bodies are darker ⧩ than discs ➡, the so-called "flip-flop" sign. (Right) Sagittal T1WI MR shows profound diffuse marrow hyperplasia with only a few remnants of normal marrow fat at the endplates ➡ & basivertebral plexus ⧩. This is multifactorial due to AIDS & long term anti-viral therapy in this 52 year old.

BONE LESIONS WITH FLUID/FLUID LEVELS

DIFFERENTIAL DIAGNOSIS

Common
- Aneurysmal Bone Cyst (ABC)
- Osteosarcoma, Telangiectatic

Less Common
- Giant Cell Tumor (GCT)
- Unicameral Bone Cyst
- Chondroblastoma

Rare but Important
- Hyperparathyroidism, Brown Tumor
- Teratoma, Sacrococcygeal
- Osteoblastoma

ESSENTIAL INFORMATION

Key Differential Diagnosis Issues
- Fluid-fluid levels can be present in benign and malignant entities
- **Hint**: A high proportion of fluid-fluid levels have been suggested to favor a benign process, but this finding should never be relied upon for diagnosis

Helpful Clues for Common Diagnoses
- **Aneurysmal Bone Cyst (ABC)**
  ○ Expansile, lytic lesion with septations & and fluid-fluid levels, usually in long bone
  ○ Majority of patients < 20 years old
- **Osteosarcoma, Telangiectatic**
  ○ Aggressive features such as periosteal reaction, cortical breakthrough and soft tissue mass may not always be present

  ○ Less permeative appearance than conventional osteosarcoma
  ○ Can be entirely lytic and mimic ABC
  ○ Watch for any hint of aggressiveness

Helpful Clues for Less Common Diagnoses
- **Giant Cell Tumor (GCT)**
  ○ Expansile subchondral lesion in skeletally mature patient lacking a sclerotic border
  ○ May coexist with aneurysmal bone cyst
- **Unicameral Bone Cyst**
  ○ Centrally located, well-defined, lytic lesion
  ○ Fluid-filled cavity; "fallen fragment" sign
  ○ Mild or no bone expansion
- **Chondroblastoma**
  ○ Lytic epiphyseal lesion with sclerotic margin in skeletally immature patient

Helpful Clues for Rare Diagnoses
- **Hyperparathyroidism, Brown Tumor**
  ○ Lytic, expansile lesion without matrix
  ○ Classic term "osteitis fibrosis cystica" better describes cystic appearance of this reactive giant cell lesion from hyperparathyroidism
- **Teratoma, Sacrococcygeal**
  ○ Mixed solid and cystic lesion with enhancement of solid areas
  ○ Large sacral mass with components of all 3 germ cell layers
    ▪ Fluid, soft tissue, fat, bone, teeth, hair
- **Osteoblastoma**
  ○ Circumscribed, lytic lesion with reactive sclerosis and variable calcification/matrix
  ○ Fluid-fluid levels are rare unless due to secondary aneurysmal bone cyst

Aneurysmal Bone Cyst (ABC)

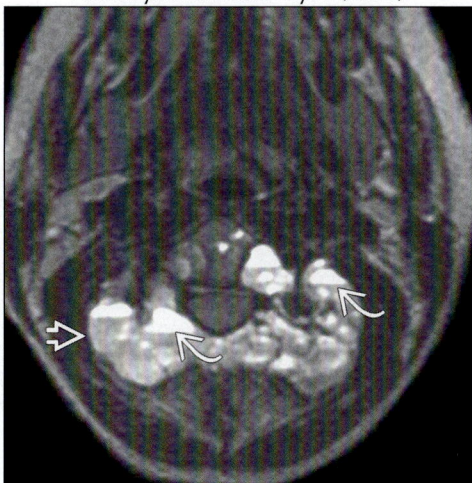

Axial T2WI MR shows an expansile mass involving posterior elements of C3 ➡, which has mixed signal, with low signal areas as well as many cystic-appearing, high signal regions w/fluid-fluid levels ➡. (†MSK Req).

Osteosarcoma, Telangiectatic

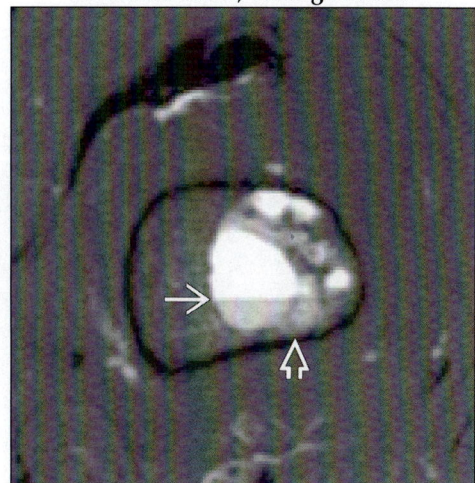

Axial T2WI MR shows a mixed intensity lesion ➡ in the distal femur. Fluid-fluid levels ➡ without a soft tissue mass suggested aneurysmal bone cyst but pathology revealed telangiectatic osteosarcoma.

BONE LESIONS WITH FLUID/FLUID LEVELS

Osteosarcoma, Telangiectatic

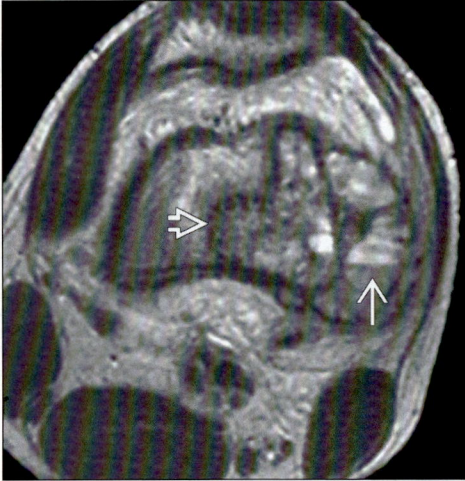

Giant Cell Tumor (GCT)

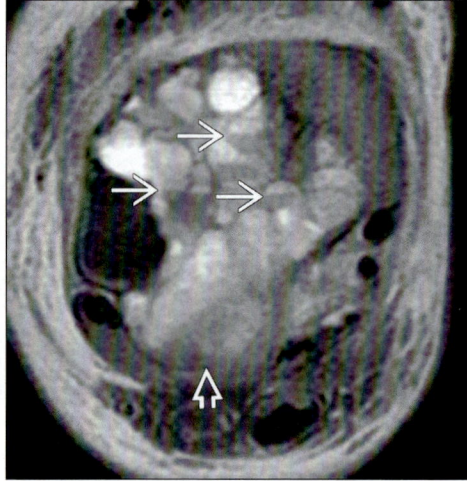

(Left) Axial T2WI MR shows a distal femoral lesion with aggressive features including cortical breakthrough & soft tissue mass ⮕. It has high signal areas which appear lobulated and a few fluid levels ⮕. Regions without fluid levels & the cortical breakthrough alert one that this is not ABC. (†MSK Req). *(Right)* Axial T2WI FS MR shows a multiloculated, expansile mass ⮕ in distal tibia extending into posterior soft tissues. Scattered fluid-fluid levels ⮕ are present in this GCT.

Unicameral Bone Cyst

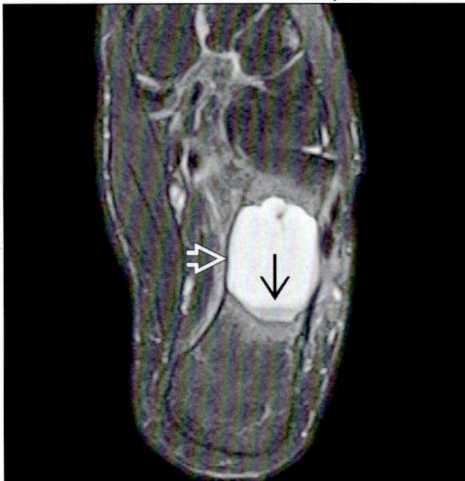

Chondroblastoma

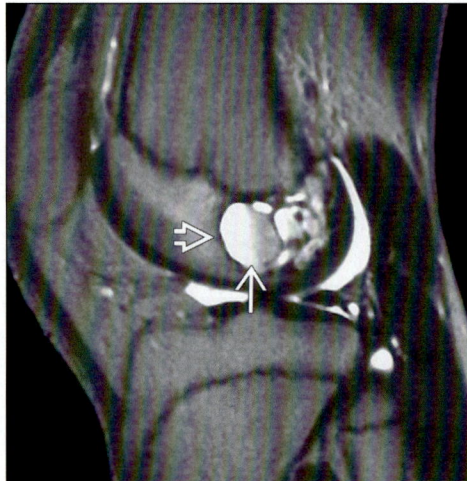

(Left) Axial T2WI FS MR shows a cystic lesion in the calcaneus ⮕. A fluid-fluid level ⮕ is frequently seen in bone cysts. A post-contrast image demonstrated an enhancing rim around the low signal central fluid collection. *(Right)* Sagittal T2WI FS MR shows a skeletally immature patient with an epiphyseal lesion ⮕ having a rather lobulated cartilaginous appearance as well as fluid-fluid levels ⮕. The latter are uncommon in chondroblastoma. (†MSK Req).

Hyperparathyroidism, Brown Tumor

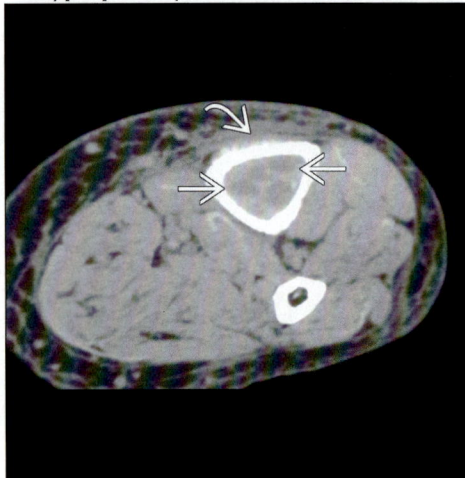

Teratoma, Sacrococcygeal

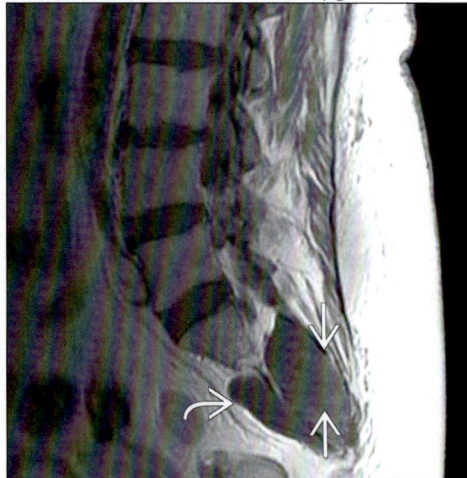

(Left) Axial NECT shows multiple fluid-fluid levels in this Brown tumor ⮕. Note the subperiosteal resorption at the tibial cortex ⮕. This aggressive resorption was secondary to a parathyroid adenoma. *(Right)* Sagittal T1WI MR shows a mixed intensity sacral mass ⮕ involving the bone and extending into the anterior and posterior soft tissues. A fluid-fluid level is evident along the dependent portion of this sacral teratoma ⮕.

LESION WITH BRIGHT T1 SIGNAL

DIFFERENTIAL DIAGNOSIS

Common
- Lipoma, Soft Tissue
- Atypical Lipomatous Tumor
- Hematoma, Subacute
- Hemangioma, Soft Tissue

Less Common
- Liposarcoma, Soft Tissue
- Liposarcoma, Myxoid
- Fat Necrosis
- Hemangiopericytoma
- Intervertebral Disc Calcification
- Chondrocalcinosis
- Lipomatosis

Rare but Important
- Lipoma Arborescens, Knee
- Lipomatosis, Nerve
- Hibernoma

ESSENTIAL INFORMATION

Key Differential Diagnosis Issues
- Bright T1 signal = higher signal intensity than skeletal muscle on T1WI
- Relatively short list of entities that have high T1 signal on MR
  - Fat
  - Blood
  - Protein
  - Crystal
- Bright T1 signal does not differentiate benign from malignant soft tissue lesions

Helpful Clues for Common Diagnoses
- **Lipoma, Soft Tissue**
  - High T1 signal mass similar to subcutaneous fat
  - With or without identifiable capsule
    - Capsule may enhance
  - May contain fine septations
    - < 2 mm in thickness
  - May have mildly increased signal on T2WI
  - Homogeneous fat suppression
  - No nodules or soft tissue elements
  - Located in any area of the body that contains fat
    - Intramuscular lipomas may have traversing or indenting muscle fibers
    - Follow course of fibers to differentiate from thick septations of liposarcoma

- **Atypical Lipomatous Tumor**
  - Appearance of fatty mass can be similar to lipoma or liposarcoma
    - May have thickened septae or nodularity
  - Needs biopsy or excision to exclude malignancy
    - More cellular than typical lipoma upon pathologic examination
- **Hematoma, Subacute**
  - Subacute musculoskeletal hemorrhage has high T1 signal
    - Acute & chronic blood has low T1 signal
  - Must prove lack of underlying malignancy before dismissing as simple hematoma
    - Resolution or significant decrease in size on follow-up
    - Lack of enhancement with subtraction post-processing helpful
- **Hemangioma, Soft Tissue**
  - Vascular mass, classically containing fat and phleboliths
    - Small lesions are less likely to contain fat than larger lesions
  - May be associated with erosion or cortical thickening of underlying bone
  - Maffucci syndrome when present with multiple enchondromas

Helpful Clues for Less Common Diagnoses
- **Liposarcoma, Soft Tissue**
  - Complex fatty mass
    - Septae > 2 mm in thickness
    - Internal enhancement
    - Nodular soft tissue elements
  - Size greater than 5 cm increases suspicion of malignancy
  - Deep location as an indicator of malignancy has been challenged
- **Liposarcoma, Myxoid**
  - Myxoid soft tissue mass with predominantly low T1 signal
  - Look for at least a small region of lacy or amorphous fat, producing high T1 signal
    - Some lesions will have no identifiable fat on MR
- **Fat Necrosis**
  - Classic location over a pressure point or bony protuberance
  - Range of appearances similar to lipoma, atypical lipomatous tumor & liposarcoma
    - Fatty mass, thickened capsule
    - May have nodular elements

LESION WITH BRIGHT T1 SIGNAL

○ Unencapsulated fat necrosis has a less mass-like appearance

• **Hemangiopericytoma**
  ○ Cannot differentiate benign hemangioma from malignant hemangiopericytoma on imaging alone
  ○ Similar appearance to hemangioma
    ▪ Mass with vessels, fat, phleboliths

• **Intervertebral Disc Calcification**
  ○ High T1 signal in disc from calcification is relatively uncommon
    ▪ Typical appearance is low T1 signal due to calcification
    ▪ T1 proton shortening may be related to surface area of calcium crystals
  ○ High T1 signal may also occur with disc ossification
    ▪ Most commonly seen with ankylosing spondylosis and multiple myeloma
  ○ Correlate with radiographs or CT for presence of calcification

• **Chondrocalcinosis**
  ○ Calcium crystal deposition in menisci may produce high T1 signal
  ○ If chondrocalcinosis reaches surface of meniscus, it may simulate meniscal tear
    ▪ Decreased sensitivity, specificity and accuracy for meniscal tear when chondrocalcinosis present
  ○ Correlate with radiographs or CT for presence of calcification
  ○ Articular cartilage chondrocalcinosis may appear as low T1 centrally with high T1 halo

• **Lipomatosis**
  ○ Exuberant, unencapsulated fat collection in anterior mediastinum and pelvis
  ○ No soft tissue elements or thickened septae
  ○ Displaces normal structures without invasion

Helpful Clues for Rare Diagnoses

• **Lipoma Arborescens, Knee**
  ○ Represents a benign intraarticular lipoma
  ○ Frond-like appearance of fatty nodules floating in synovial fluid

• **Lipomatosis, Nerve**
  ○ Fatty and fibrous nerve infiltration
  ○ Commonly affects median nerve and digital branches
    ▪ Ulnar nerve involvement second most common
  ○ Formerly known as fibrolipomatous hamartoma
  ○ Associated with macrodactyly in one third of patients
    ▪ Less commonly associated with neurofibromatosis

• **Hibernoma**
  ○ Benign, fat containing tumor
  ○ Similar appearance to lipoma on CT
    ▪ May contain vessels, nodules suggesting liposarcoma
  ○ Does not follow pure fat signal intensity on MR
    ▪ T1 signal is higher than skeletal muscle, but lower than subcutaneous fat
  ○ Biopsy or excise for definitive diagnosis

Lipoma, Soft Tissue

Coronal T1WI MR through the posterior calf shows a lobulated mass ➡ with high T1 signal, which is the same as subcutaneous fat. A few fine muscle fibers or septations ➡ flow through the mass.

Atypical Lipomatous Tumor

Axial T1WI MR shows a large fatty mass ➡ within the thigh. The large size and nodular thickening of septa ➡ make this lesion worrisome for low grade liposarcoma, but it was an atypical lipomatous tumor upon excision.

LESION WITH BRIGHT T1 SIGNAL

(Left) Axial T1WI MR shows high T1WI signal ➡ within the extensor carpi radialis longus and brevis tendon sheaths. This was subacute blood from a distal radius fracture. The tendons were normal. **(Right)** Axial T1WI MR shows a mass ➡ in the subcutaneous tissues posterior to the olecranon ⬌. Signal within the mass is relatively high on all sequences, consistent with subacute hemorrhage. This is hemorrhagic post-traumatic olecranon bursitis.

Hematoma, Subacute

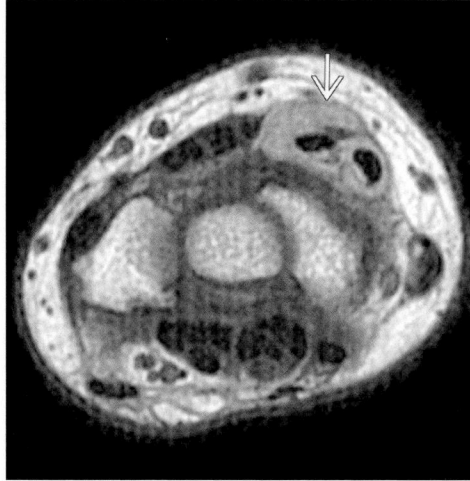

Hematoma, Subacute

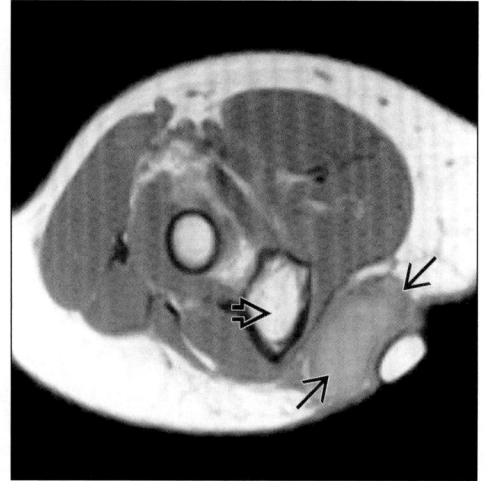

(Left) Coronal T1WI MR shows a mass in the thigh which contains fatty signal ⬌ and low signal phleboliths ➡ located anterior to the femur. Fatty stroma is usually found in soft tissue hemangiomas, along with a tangle of vessels. **(Right)** Axial T1WI MR shows a large mass ➡ located deep to the gluteus maximus muscle. The mass is predominantly high T1 signal, similar to subcutaneous fat. Thick septations ➡ suggest a malignant fatty tumor.

Hemangioma, Soft Tissue

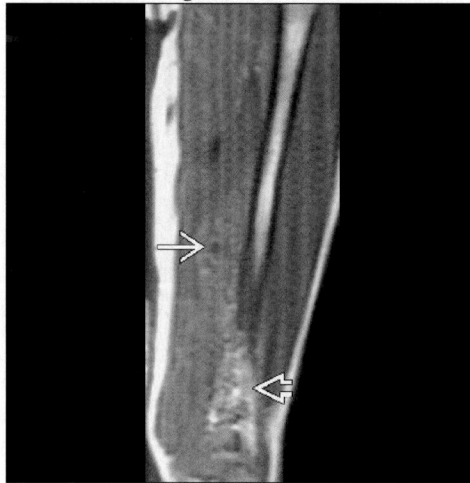

Liposarcoma, Soft Tissue

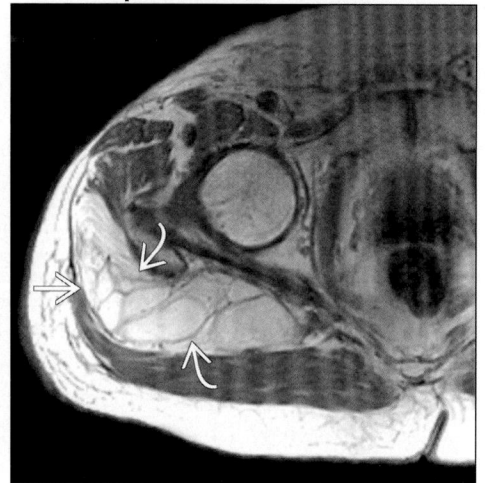

(Left) Axial T1WI MR shows a posterior thigh mass ➡ with inhomogeneous signal intensity. Areas of high T1 signal intensity ⬌ represent the lipomatous portion of the tumor, which is unusually large in this example. **(Right)** Axial T1WI MR shows a well-defined mass ➡ composed of high T1 signal, similar to subcutaneous fat, overlying the trochanteric region of the hip. This was excised due to pain, history of malignancy and thickened capsule. The location is classic for fat necrosis.

Liposarcoma, Myxoid

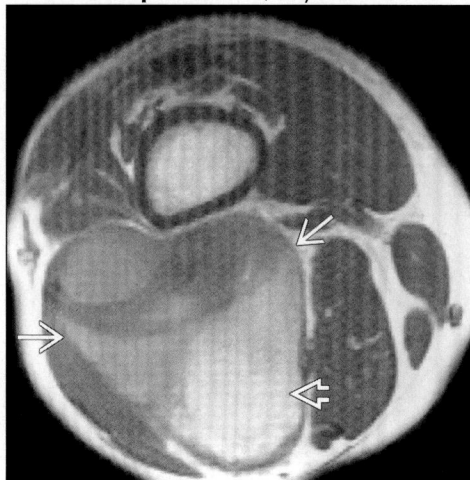

Fat Necrosis

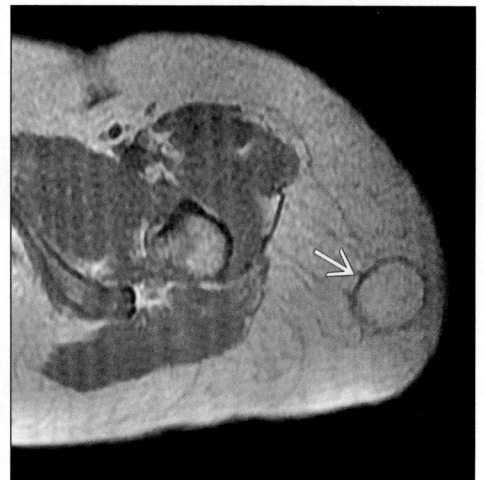

LESION WITH BRIGHT T1 SIGNAL

Fat Necrosis

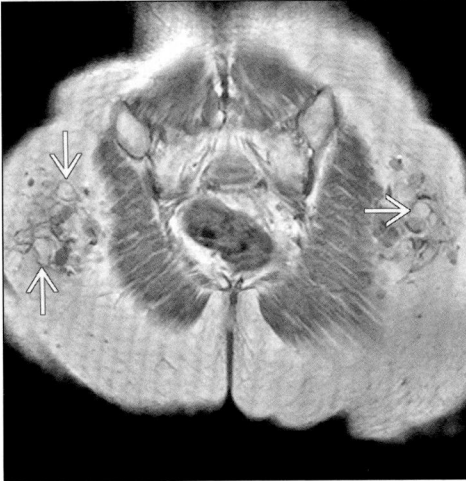

Intervertebral Disc Calcification

(Left) Coronal T1WI MR shows numerous bilateral masses in the gluteal subcutaneous fat. Some of these masses have purely fat signal intensity ➡ and represent fat necrosis from medication injection. *(Right)* Sagittal T1WI MR shows hyperintense signal within every lumbar intervertebral disc ➡. There is typical squaring of the lumbar vertebral bodies in this patient with ankylosing spondylitis.

Chondrocalcinosis

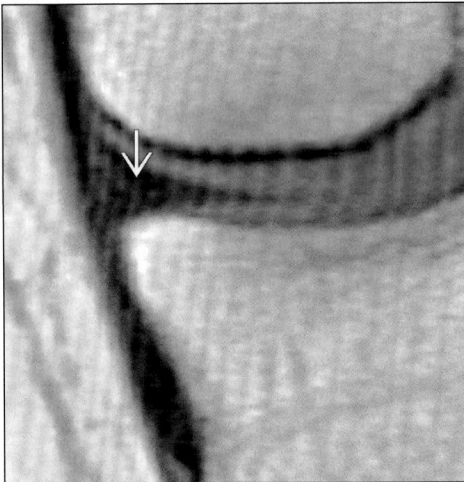

Lipoma Arborescens, Knee

(Left) Coronal T1WI MR shows a region of meniscal high signal intensity ➡ in the same region as chondrocalcinosis was identified radiographically. This may mimic a meniscal tear when the high signal extends to the meniscal surface. *(Right)* Coronal T1WI MR through the anterior knee shows a very large lobulated mass ➡ within the knee joint, having signal intensity identical to that of subcutaneus fat.

Lipomatosis, Nerve

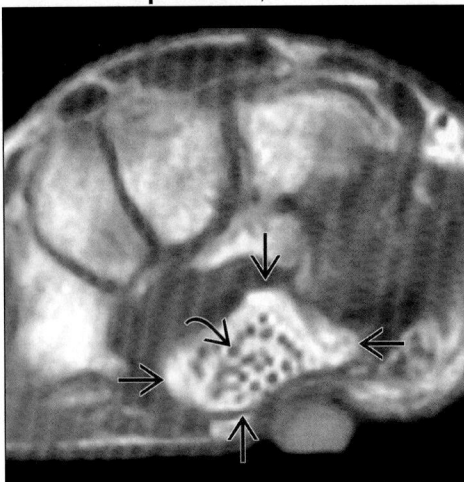

Hibernoma

(Left) Axial T1WI MR shows marked enlargement of the median nerve ➡ with fat signal filling the space between individual nerve fascicles ➡. This creates the classic "telephone cable" appearance of this condition. It caused a clinical carpal tunnel syndrome. *(Right)* Coronal T1WI MR of the elbow shows a mass ➡ with T1 signal higher than muscle, although not as high as subcutaneous fat. This is typical for the brown fat in a hibernoma.

SOFT TISSUE LESIONS WITH PREDOMINATELY LOW T1 & T2 SIGNAL

DIFFERENTIAL DIAGNOSIS

Common
- Post-Operative Changes
- Foreign Body
- Hematoma, Chronic
- Flow Voids
- Densely Calcified/Ossified Lesions
- Plantar Fibromatosis
- Gout
- Air
- Aneurysm
- Pigmented Villonodular Synovitis (PVNS)
- Giant Cell Tumor Tendon Sheath
- Arteriovenous Fistula

Less Common
- Desmoid-Type Fibromatosis
- Elastofibroma
- Fibroma of Tendon Sheath
- Metastases, Hemorrhagic
- Amyloid Deposition
- Melanoma

Rare but Important
- Infection, Calcified or Fungal
- Arteriovenous Malformation
- Cavernous Hemangioma
- Extramedullary Hematopoiesis
- Concentrated Gadolinium

ESSENTIAL INFORMATION

Key Differential Diagnosis Issues
- Radiographs and CT can help differentiate some low T1 & T2 signal entities
  ○ Ossification
  ○ Calcification
  ○ Metal
  ○ Air
- Paramagnetic substances alter MR signal
  ○ Blood products, iron, copper, melanin
  ○ Metal, gadolinium, air
  ○ Blooming signal on gradient echo images

Helpful Clues for Common Diagnoses
- **Post-Operative Changes**
  ○ Micrometallic artifact occurs from scalpel use, drilling, sawing, scraping
    ▪ Metal particles are so small they are not evident on radiographs or CT
  ○ Cement & bone graft material are apparent on radiographs & CT

- **Foreign Body**
  ○ Endless variety of material embedded in body, patient may not recall event
  ○ Often has intense surrounding inflammatory reaction
- **Hematoma, Chronic**
  ○ Acute high signal serum has resorbed leaving debris & fibrous tissue
  ○ Peripheral or central calcification often present
- **Flow Voids**
  ○ Rapidly flowing blood produces flow voids
  ○ Blood excited by 90 degree pulse has left the slice before the refocusing pulse, thus no echo (no signal)
- **Densely Calcified/Ossified Lesions**
  ○ Heterotopic ossification, synovial sarcoma, injection granulomas, extraskeletal osteosarcoma, osteosarcoma metastases, progressive systemic sclerosis, fibrodysplasia ossificans progressiva, melorheostosis
- **Gout**
  ○ Low signal seen on all sequences is typical of sodium urate deposition in tophi
  ○ Tophi have variable moderate inhomogeneous enhancement
- **Air**
  ○ Lack of protons for excitation
  ○ Causes include: Trauma, iatrogenic/post-operative, extension into soft tissues from joint, infection
- **Aneurysm**
  ○ Turbulent blood flow in aneurysm
  ○ Low signal in thrombus
  ○ Loss of phase coherence on MR
- **Pigmented Villonodular Synovitis (PVNS)**
  ○ Single or multiple masses in and around joints
    ▪ Intraarticular masses can have similar appearance to gout & amyloid deposition
  ○ Blooming signal on gradient echo imaging from hemorrhage
- **Giant Cell Tumor Tendon Sheath**
  ○ Localized form of PVNS occurring in tendon sheath, see characteristics above
  ○ Similar imaging appearance to fibroma of tendon sheath
- **Arteriovenous Fistula**
  ○ Large, tubular flow voids due to direct communication between artery & vein

SOFT TISSUE LESIONS WITH PREDOMINATELY LOW T1 & T2 SIGNAL

Helpful Clues for Less Common Diagnoses

- **Desmoid-Type Fibromatosis**
  - Low MR signal due to immobile protons in fibrous tissue
  - Enhancement helps differentiate this from other low signal lesions
- **Elastofibroma**
  - a.k.a., Elastofibroma dorsi
  - Located between scapula & rib cage
  - May mildly enhance
- **Fibroma of Tendon Sheath**
  - Isointense or hypointense to skeletal muscle on T1 & T2 images
  - May have very low signal bands of collagen within mass
  - Variable enhancement
    - 50% moderate to marked enhancement
    - 50% little to no enhancement
  - Not locally aggressive
  - Can be intraarticular
- **Metastases, Hemorrhagic**
  - Breast carcinoma, bronchogenic carcinoma, renal cell carcinoma, melanoma, thyroid carcinoma, teratoma, choriocarcinoma
  - Low signal on T2WI from blood breakdown products and/or calcification
- **Amyloid Deposition**
  - Intraarticular low signal masses are most common but can be extraarticular
  - Often a complication of multiple myeloma
- **Melanoma**
  - Low signal from paramagnetic properties of melanin
  - Metastases can be hemorrhagic, producing low signal intensity

Helpful Clues for Rare Diagnoses

- **Infection, Calcified or Fungal**
  - Aspergillosis & other fungal elements may cause low signal on T2WI
    - Edema in surrounding soft tissues
    - Enhancement of involved tissues
  - Chronic calcification also will cause low signal but is visible on radiographs & CT
- **Arteriovenous Malformation**
  - Congenital connection of arteries & veins
  - High flow lesions producing flow voids
  - Lacks a discrete soft tissue mass
- **Cavernous Hemangioma**
  - Lobulated mass with fatty septae
  - ± Phleboliths and fluid-fluid levels
  - Prominent enhancement of vessels
- **Extramedullary Hematopoiesis**
  - Paravertebral masses are common
  - Associated abnormal bone marrow signal
    - Obliterated macroscopic marrow fat, signal intensity lower than muscle on T1WI, lack of signal dropout on opposed phase imaging
- **Concentrated Gadolinium**
  - Soft tissue extravasation of IV gadolinium or inadvertent injection of non-dilute gadolinium into joint for MR arthrography

---

Post-Operative Changes

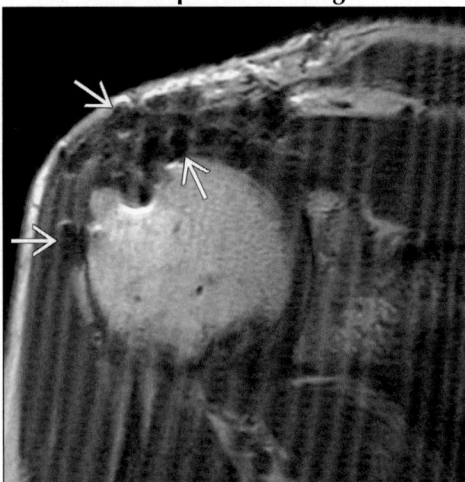

Coronal T1WI MR shows scattered low signal foci ➡ throughout the region of the distal supraspinatus tendon. These foci of low signal are micrometallic artifacts from a rotator cuff repair.

Foreign Body

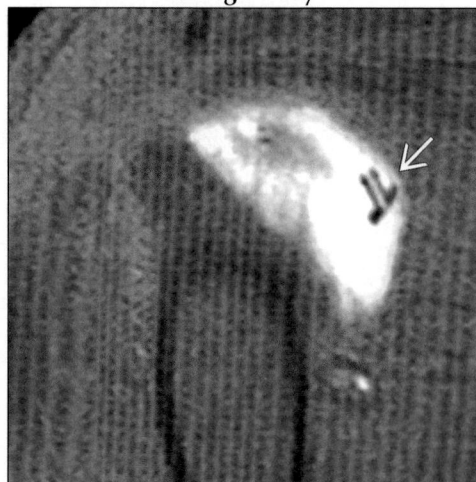

Coronal oblique MR arthrogram T1WI FS shows a low signal foreign body ➡ in the posterior shoulder joint. This is a screw which has pulled out. The hollow core is filled with fluid.

SOFT TISSUE LESIONS WITH PREDOMINATELY LOW T1 & T2 SIGNAL

(Left) Axial T1 C+ MR shows regions of low signal ➡ surrounded by areas of mild enhancement ➡ within the deltoid muscle. This is a foreign body reaction, related to the multiple injections received. *(Right)* Coronal T1WI MR shows bilateral injection granulomas ➡ in the gluteal subcutaneous fat. These low signal foci are common and are due to a variety of medications.

Foreign Body

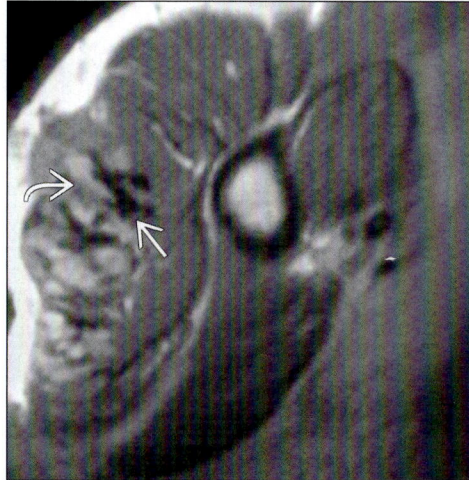

Foreign Body

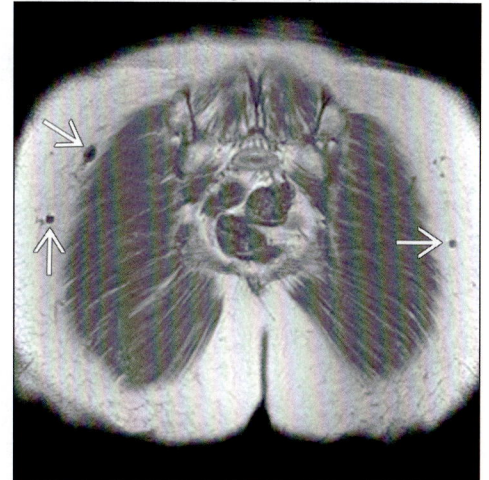

(Left) Sagittal PD FSE MR shows a focal low intensity mass ➡ in the lateral band of the plantar fascia at the level of the calcaneus. Low signal was also present on T1WI. The lesion showed mild enhancement post-contrast. *(Right)* Coronal T2WI MR shows a homogeneous low signal mass distal to the medial malleolus ➡. The mass is immediately adjacent to the bone, with the adjacent tendons displaced medially.

Plantar Fibromatosis

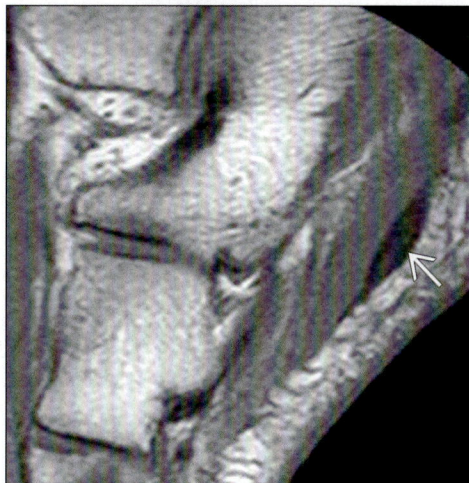

Gout

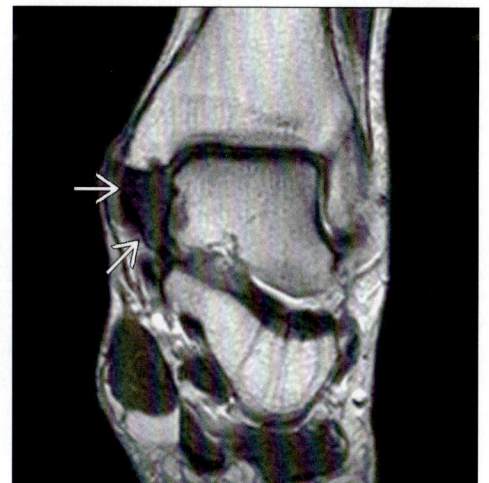

(Left) Coronal T1WI MR of the pelvis shows multiple low signal air bubbles ➡ in one of several renal cell carcinoma metastases ➡. This air was presumed due to extension from the sacroiliac joint since there was no history of biopsy and there was no clinical evidence of infection. *(Right)* Sagittal T1WI FS MR shows an unusual case of PVNS in the pes anserinus region. The mass ➡ contains nodular areas of persistently low signal, which were present both pre- and post-contrast.

Air

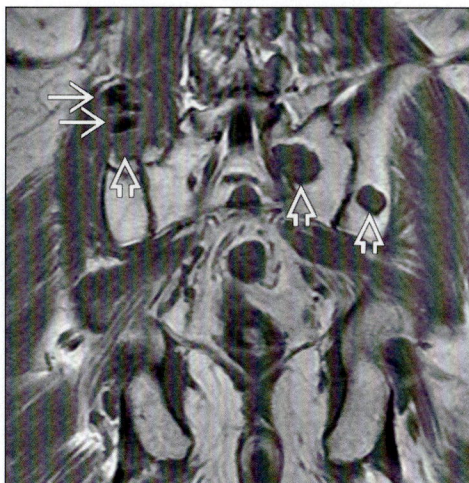

Pigmented Villonodular Synovitis (PVNS)

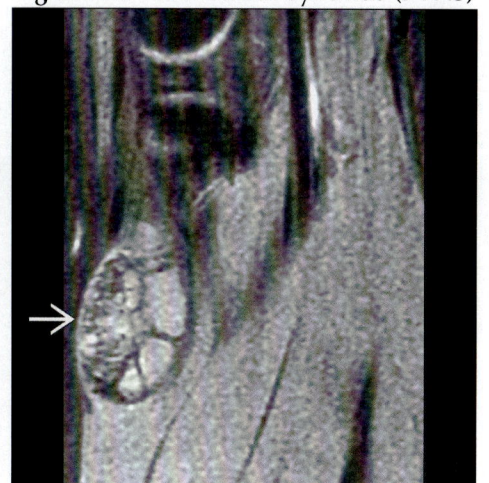

SOFT TISSUE LESIONS WITH PREDOMINATELY LOW T1 & T2 SIGNAL

Giant Cell Tumor Tendon Sheath

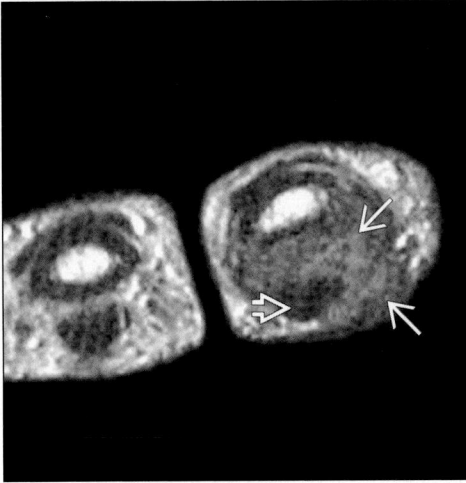

Arteriovenous Fistula

(Left) Axial T2WI MR shows a lobular mass ➡ with relatively low T2 signal that was isointense to muscle on T1WI. The mass arises deep to the flexor tendons ➡ and extends radially and volarly. A superficial location is more common. *(Right)* Sagittal T1WI MR shows an atrophic distal thoracic spinal cord ➡ caused by massively enlarged, tortuous vessels seen as prominent flow voids ➡, representing enlarged arterial feeders (posterior spinal arteries) and arterialized draining veins.

Desmoid-Type Fibromatosis

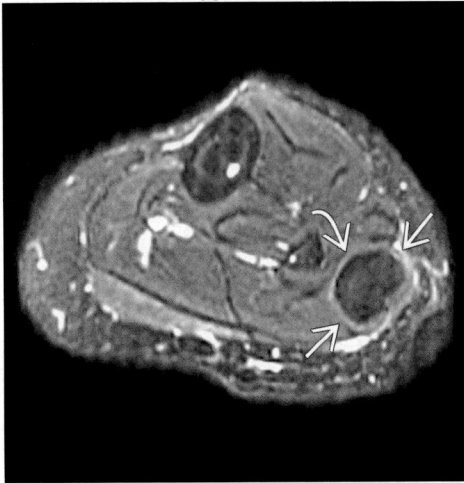

Elastofibroma

(Left) Axial T2WI FS MR shows a low signal mass ➡ within the far lateral aspect of the soleus muscle. The mass has a small amount of surrounding edema ➡ and diffusely enhanced with gadolinium administration. *(Right)* Axial T1WI MR shows a chest wall mass ➡ that is nearly isointense to muscle, located between the lower tip of the scapula ➡ and the rib cage. The mass remained similar to muscle intensity on T2WI.

Fibroma of Tendon Sheath

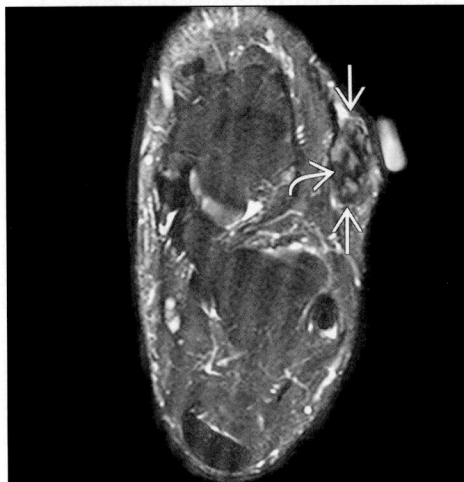

Arteriovenous Malformation

(Left) Axial T2WI FS MR shows an oval, lobulated mass ➡ in the lateral foot. The mass abuts the flexor digitorum longus tendon and has heterogeneous, predominantly low T2 signal. Undulating areas of very low signal in the mass ➡ are due to dense collagen. *(Right)* Coronal T1WI MR shows a region of tubular low signal structures ➡ in the forearm. Prominent flow voids are indicative of an arteriovenous malformation.

II

153

SOFT TISSUE LESIONS WITH FLUID/FLUID LEVELS

DIFFERENTIAL DIAGNOSIS

Common
- Hematoma
- Hemarthrosis/Lipohemarthrosis
- Vascular & Lymphatic Malformations
- Medication Injection

Less Common
- Tumoral (Idiopathic) Calcinosis
- Polymyositis/Dermatomyositis
- Malignant Neoplasm
- Non-Neoplastic Structure
- Neoplasm, Mixed Fluid Contents
- Synovial Sarcoma, Cystic
- Ganglion or Synovial Cyst
- Bursitis
- Tenosynovitis

Rare but Important
- Soft Tissue Abscess
- Myositis Ossificans
- Peripheral Nerve Sheath Tumor, Benign & Malignant
- Hemangioma, Synovial

ESSENTIAL INFORMATION

Key Differential Diagnosis Issues
- Fluid-fluid levels can be present in benign and malignant entities
- Any fluid collection in the body may contain material of different densities
  - Confluence of mucinous or cystic regions with debris
  - Blood separation into serum and cells
  - Sedimentation of necrotic tumor cells
  - Liquified fat cells in fluid

Helpful Clues for Common Diagnoses
- **Hematoma**
  - Blood products separate and layer producing fluid-fluid level
  - History of surgery, trauma or pharmaceutical anticoagulation
  - Be extremely vigilant for underlying hemorrhagic malignancy
    - Enhanced MR, with pre- and post-contrast subtraction when high T1 signal present or follow-up
- **Hemarthrosis/Lipohemarthrosis**
  - Blood in joint fluid from fracture, ligament injury, hemophilia

- Fat admixed with joint fluid and blood due to fracture
  - Superior layer is fat, central layer is fluid, dependent layer is blood cells
- **Vascular & Lymphatic Malformations**
  - Cavernous fluid-filled spaces
  - May also contain regions of fat
  - Lymphangioma does not have central enhancement like hemangioma
  - Difficult to differentiate benign hemangioma from malignant hemangioendothelioma with imaging alone
- **Medication Injection**
  - Typical distribution in subcutaneous fat of gluteal region and anterior abdomen
  - Small volume of multiple injection sites
  - May peripherally calcify
  - Steroids and illicit drugs are most likely to cause tissue irritation and complications such as abscess

Helpful Clues for Less Common Diagnoses
- **Tumoral (Idiopathic) Calcinosis**
  - Multiloculated calcific collections around large joints
  - Patients with renal disease
  - Fluid-fluid levels have milk of calcium appearance on CT
- **Polymyositis/Dermatomyositis**
  - Sheet-like calcification of muscles and fascia
  - May have coexisting findings of scleroderma
  - Fluid-fluid levels have calcific dependent layer and are relatively uncommon
- **Malignant Neoplasm**
  - Necrosis from growth beyond blood supply, radiotherapy, or chemotherapy
  - Variety of tumor types may have spontaneous hemorrhage producing fluid-fluid levels
    - Synovial sarcoma, 18-25% of all subtypes have fluid-fluid levels
    - Liposarcoma
    - Fibrosarcoma
    - Leiomyosarcoma
    - Malignant fibrous histiocytoma
    - Primitive neuroectodermal tumor
    - Angiomatoid fibrous histiocytoma
- **Non-Neoplastic Structure, Mixed Fluid Contents**

SOFT TISSUE LESIONS WITH FLUID/FLUID LEVELS

- Fluid-fluid level, often due to fat or blood, in normal or abnormal body structure
  - Hemosalpinx, hematocolpos, bladder diverticulum, bronchogenic cyst, pancreatic pseudocyst, subarachnoid hemorrhage, venous varix
  - Excreted contrast produces fluid-fluid level in urinary bladder, gallbladder
  - Iatrogenic cerebrospinal fluid leak, seroma
- **Neoplasm, Mixed Fluid Contents**
  - More common in body, rather than musculoskeletal, diagnoses
    - Endometrioma, hamartoma, ovarian teratoma, craniopharyngioma, phyllodes tumor, galactocele
- **Synovial Sarcoma, Cystic**
  - Uncommon subtype of synovial sarcoma
  - Approximately 70% have fluid-fluid levels
- **Ganglion or Synovial Cyst**
  - Ganglion and synovial cyst terminology often used interchangeably
    - Can use term synovial cyst for lesions extending from a synovial-lined space: Joint, bursa, tendon sheath
  - Very common fluid-filled lesion with uncommon fluid-fluid level
    - Hemorrhage or debris in lesion
- **Bursitis**
  - Usually a simple fluid collection with a smooth border
  - May contain layering debris producing fluid-fluid level
    - Uncommon, but most common in iliopsoas bursa

- **Tenosynovitis**
  - Fat in tendon sheath from adjacent fracture, especially around ankle
  - Debris or hemorrhage in tendon sheath is relatively uncommon

Helpful Clues for Rare Diagnoses
- **Soft Tissue Abscess**
  - Complex fluid with thick, enhancing rim
  - Contents are typically too viscous to have fluid-fluid levels
  - May have concurrent layering hemorrhage
- **Myositis Ossificans**
  - Fluid-fluid levels relatively uncommon but occur in central aspect of lesion
  - Range of appearances from early calcification to late peripheral ossification
    - Periphery is more mature than center
- **Peripheral Nerve Sheath Tumor, Benign & Malignant**
  - Very high T2 signal of mass may simulate cyst or be cystic
    - Target appearance on MR
  - Cystic regions have fluid-fluid levels from hemorrhage, necrosis or confluent cystic or mucinous regions
    - More common in large lesions
- **Hemangioma, Synovial**
  - Fluid-filled spaces similar but smaller than cavernous hemangioma
  - Very rare lesion

Hematoma

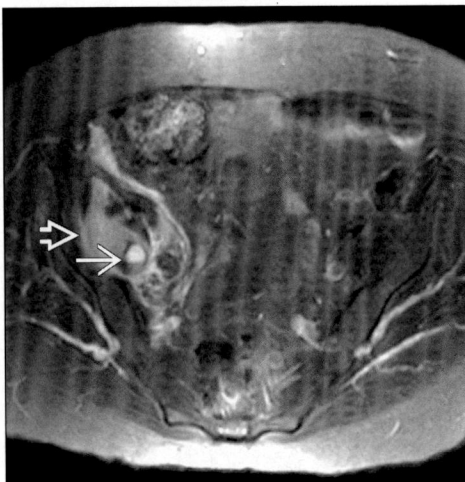

Axial T2WI FS MR shows a complex mass ➡ in the right iliopsoas muscle containing a fluid-fluid level ➡. This anticoagulated patient was carefully followed to exclude underlying malignancy.

Hematoma

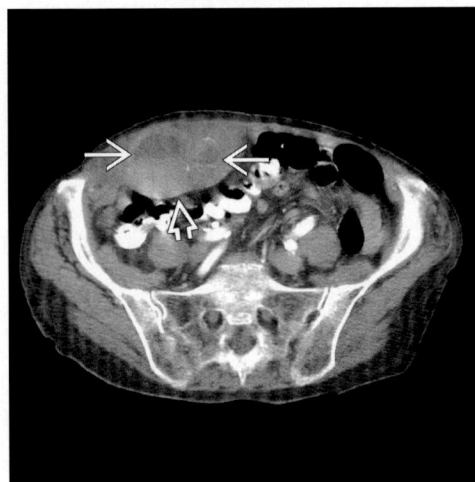

Axial CECT shows marked enlargement of the right abdominal wall musculature ➡. Fluid-fluid levels are present within the hematoma resulting from the hematocrit effect as the blood separates ➡.

SOFT TISSUE LESIONS WITH FLUID/FLUID LEVELS

(Left) Axial T2WI FS MR shows a knee lipohemarthrosis due to a tibial plateau fracture. Two fluid-fluid levels correspond to fat-fluid ➔ superficially and fluid-cells ➔ dependent in the joint. *(Right)* Axial STIR MR shows a multiloculated mass ⮞ in the right neck and submandibular space with multiple fluid-fluid levels ➔ consistent with layering blood products. The lesion lacked contrast enhancement, typical for lymphatic malformation.

Hemarthrosis/Lipohemarthrosis

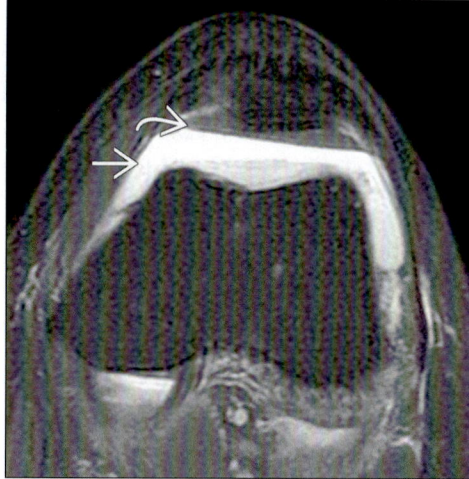

Vascular & Lymphatic Malformations

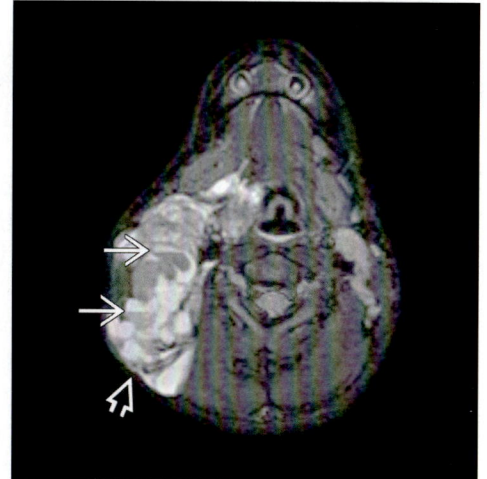

(Left) Axial T2WI FS MR shows multiple small lesions with fluid-fluid levels ➔ in the subcutaneous fat of the right gluteal region. Signal intensity varies with medication content and associated bleeding. *(Right)* Axial NECT shows a multiloculated mass ⮞ along the posterolateral chest wall. Fluid-fluid levels ➔ were subtle on MR since the dependent calcified material had low signal intensity. Prone positioning is for CT-guided biopsy.

Medication Injection

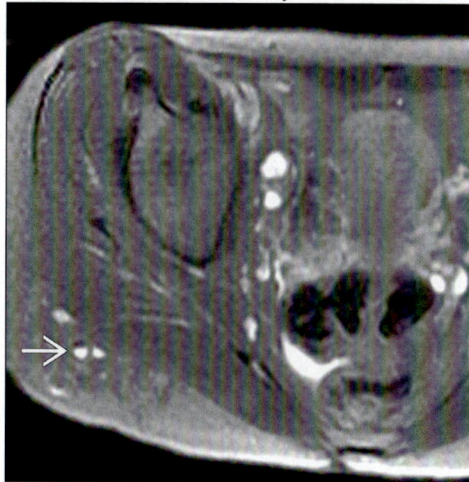

Tumoral (Idiopathic) Calcinosis

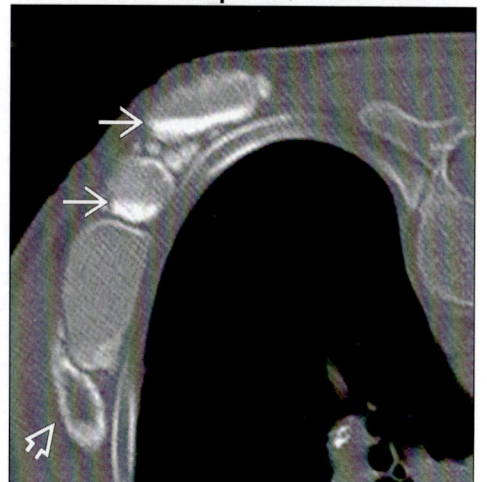

(Left) Axial NECT shows bilateral sheet-like calcification ⮞ of the muscles and fascial planes of the thighs, with scattered fluid-fluid levels ➔ due to dermatomyositis. *(Right)* Axial T2WI FS MR shows a very large, heterogeneous mass ⮞ in the posterior thigh. The mass contains areas of signal intensity higher and lower than subcutaneous fat. Fluid-fluid levels ➔ suggest hemorrhage within a portion of the mass.

Polymyositis/Dermatomyositis

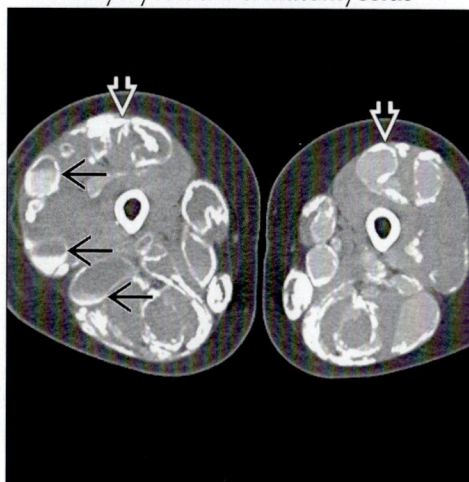

Malignant Neoplasm

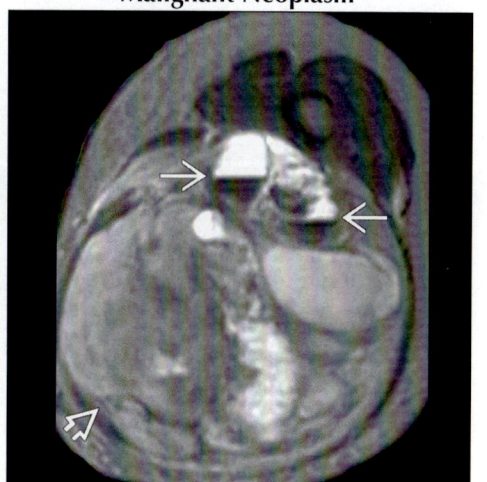

SOFT TISSUE LESIONS WITH FLUID/FLUID LEVELS

Non-Neoplastic Structure

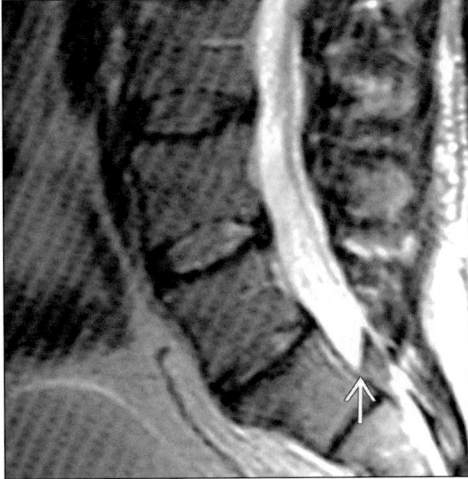

Synovial Sarcoma, Cystic

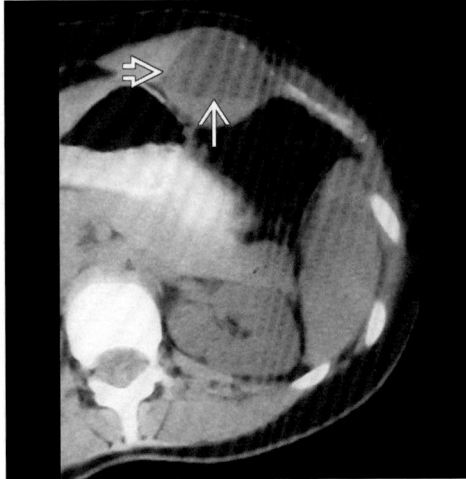

(Left) Sagittal T2WI MR shows a low signal fluid-fluid level ➜ in caudal thecal sac from subarachnoid hemorrhage. The dependent blood was relatively isointense on T1WI. *(Right)* Axial NECT shows a soft tissue mass arising in or immediately adjacent to the anterior abdominal muscles ➔. Note that there is a prominent fluid level ➜ in this synovial sarcoma.

Synovial Sarcoma, Cystic

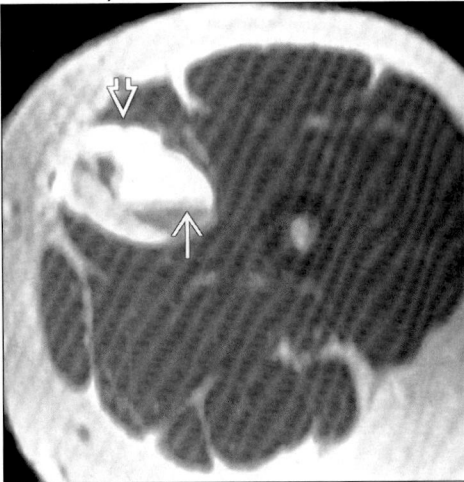

Bursitis

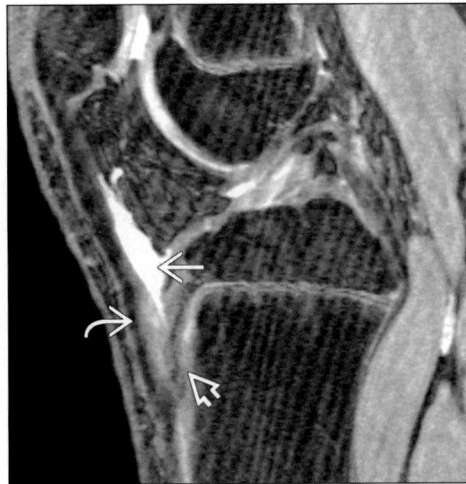

(Left) Axial T2WI MR shows a medial thigh heterogeneous mass ➔, in which a large portion of the lesion is distinctly cystic, with a fluid level ➜. The solid regions intensely enhanced. *(Right)* Sagittal FISP 3D WE MR shows increased signal in the distal patellar tendon ➔ and edema within the tibial tubercle bone marrow ➔ from Osgood-Schlatter. Bleeding into the deep infrapatellar bursa is evident by a fluid-fluid level ➜.

Soft Tissue Abscess

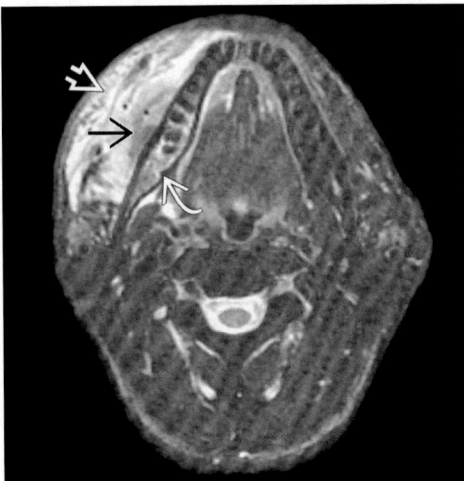

Peripheral Nerve Sheath Tumor, Benign & Malignant

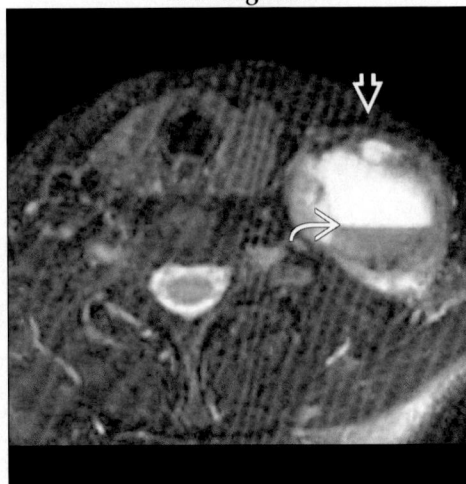

(Left) Axial T2WI FS MR shows increased signal in the right hemimandible ➔ and soft tissues ➔ due to osteomyelitis and abscess. A subtle fluid-fluid level ➜ is apparent within a focal collection in the buccal space. *(Right)* Axial T2WI FS MR shows a large mass ➔ in the posterior cervical space of the left neck. This benign schwannoma is hyperintense to muscle, markedly heterogeneous and has a fluid-fluid level ➜ suggesting hemorrhage.

TARGET LESION OF SOFT TISSUES

DIFFERENTIAL DIAGNOSIS

Common
- Neurofibroma, Cellular

Less Common
- Schwannoma, Conventional
- Centrally Calcified Mass
- Malignant Peripheral Nerve Sheath Tumor
- Metastasis
- Aneurysm

Rare but Important
- Amyloid Deposition
- Melanoma
- Epithelioid Sarcoma

ESSENTIAL INFORMATION

Key Differential Diagnosis Issues
- Target lesion = mass with low signal intensity centrally surrounded by high signal intensity (or reverse pattern)
  - Discussion limited to musculoskeletal MR
  - Radiologic target sign on radiographs, ultrasound & CT due to different entities

Helpful Clues for Common Diagnoses
- **Neurofibroma, Cellular**
  - Fusiform mass in subcutaneous tissues
  - Target sign on T2WI is classic finding
  - Diffusely involves affected nerve
  - Marked tenderness to palpation can suggest neurogenic tumor over other soft tissue masses

Helpful Clues for Less Common Diagnoses
- **Schwannoma, Conventional**
  - Target sign less common than in neurofibroma
  - Ovoid mass draped over nerve
  - Deep location & larger nerve involvement favors schwannoma over neurofibroma
- **Centrally Calcified Mass**
  - Meningioma, synovial sarcoma
  - Any soft tissue mass may calcify
- **Malignant Peripheral Nerve Sheath Tumor**
  - Can be indistinguishable from benign nerve sheath tumor on imaging
  - Ill-defined borders suggest malignancy
- **Metastasis**
  - Variable calcification or ossification can produce low signal center
- **Aneurysm**
  - Lamellated appearance due to mural thrombus + rapid or turbulent blood flow

Helpful Clues for Rare Diagnoses
- **Amyloid Deposition**
  - Paramagnetic effect may cause blooming on gradient echo sequences
  - Central calcification is rare
- **Melanoma**
  - Rim-enhancement with variable paramagnetic effect from melanin
- **Epithelioid Sarcoma**
  - Rare tumor, most common in distal upper extremity
  - Mimics appearance of peripheral nerve sheath tumor

Neurofibroma, Cellular

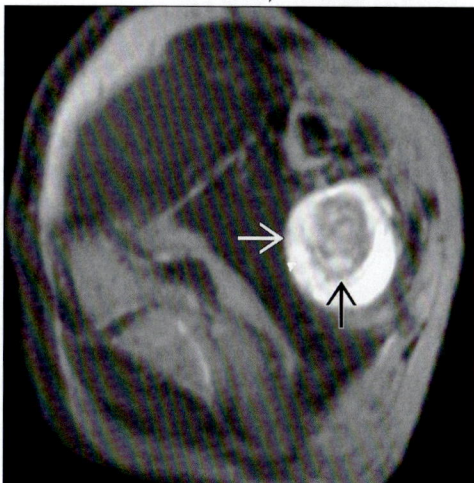

Axial T2WI MR shows a mass ➡ between brachialis muscle & biceps tendon, in the expected location of the median nerve. The mass was isointense to muscle on T1WI with a target sign ➡ on T2WI. (†MSK Req).

Schwannoma, Conventional

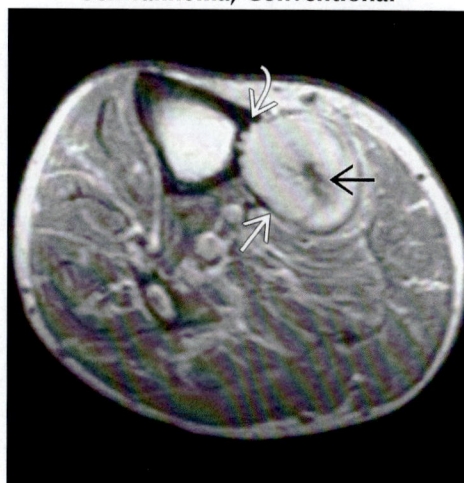

Axial T1 C+ MR shows a soft tissue mass ➡ of the lower leg, eroding the tibial cortex ➡. The lesion had low signal on T1WI, high signal on T2WI, and a target sign ➡ on T2WI and enhanced images.

TARGET LESION OF SOFT TISSUES

Schwannoma, Conventional

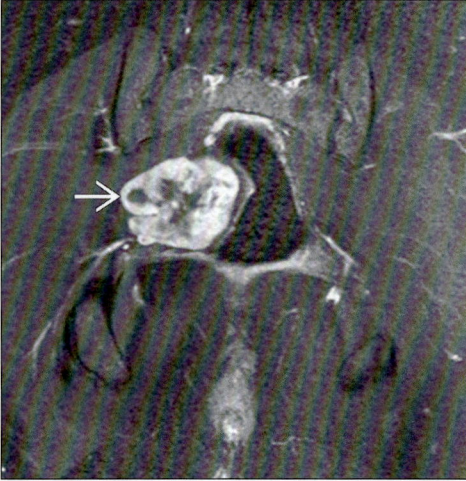

Centrally Calcified Mass

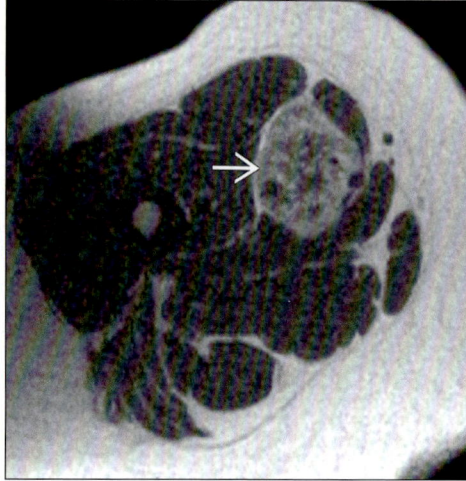

(Left) Coronal T1 C+ FS MR shows a mass ➡ in the right sciatic notch, which had low signal on T1WI and high signal on T2WI, with intense enhancement. Low signal seen centrally was more extensive than the known areas of calcification. *(Right)* Axial T2WI MR shows a mass ➡ in the medial thigh with high peripheral signal and inhomogeneous low central signal on T2WI. This was a peripheral nerve sheath tumor with central calcification.

Centrally Calcified Mass

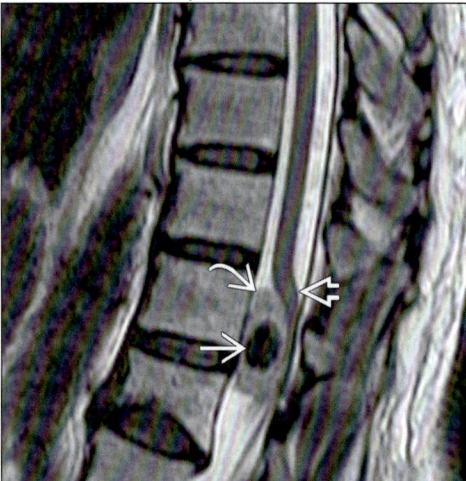

Malignant Peripheral Nerve Sheath Tumor

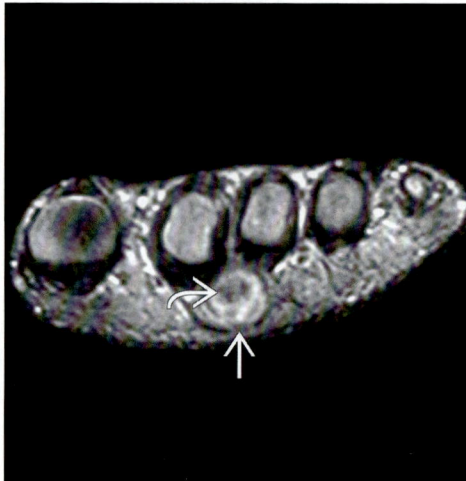

(Left) Sagittal T2WI MR shows a calcified meningioma. This well-defined intradural, extramedullary mass displaces the distal cord ➡ and has a target appearance due to enhancement ➡ and central low signal ➡ due to calcification. *(Right)* Axial T2WI MR shows a neurogenic sarcoma in an unusual location. The mass ➡ had low signal intensity on T1WI and a target sign on T2WI ➡. A longitudinally elongated contour suggested a neurogenic origin.

Aneurysm

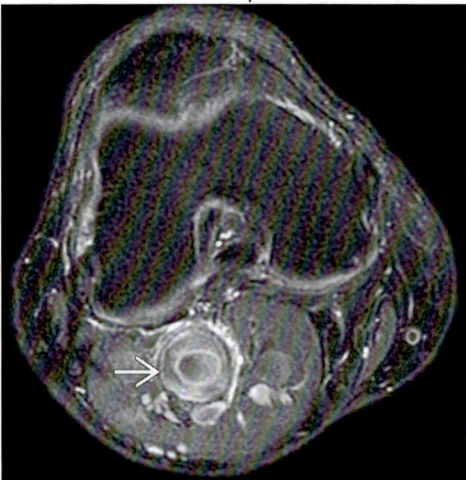

Amyloid Deposition

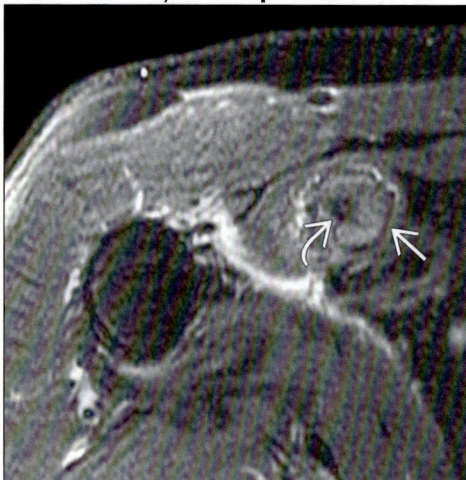

(Left) Axial T2WI FS MR shows a lamellated mass ➡ in popliteal fossa of the knee. This mass is in the expected location of the popliteal artery. Signal characteristics are due to mural thrombus and blood flow of varying speed and turbulence. *(Right)* Axial T2WI FS MR shows a round mass ➡ in the anteromedial shoulder of a patient with multiple myeloma. The mass had low to intermediate signal on T1WI and T2WI with a persistently low signal center ➡ due to calcification.

CYSTIC MASSES

DIFFERENTIAL DIAGNOSIS

Common
- Ganglion Cyst
- Synovial Cyst
  - Popliteal Cyst
  - Meniscal Cyst
  - Labral Cyst
- Sebaceous Cyst
- Soft Tissue Abscess
- Bursitis
- Hematoma
- Malignant Tumor, Necrotic
- Hemangioma, Soft Tissue

Less Common
- Lymphangioma
- Myxoma (Mimic)
- Sarcoma, Soft Tissue (Mimic)

Rare but Important
- Hydatid Cyst
- Eccrine Hidradenoma

ESSENTIAL INFORMATION

Key Differential Diagnosis Issues
- Cystic soft tissue masses have high T2WI & low T1WI signal
  - Border of lesion may enhance
  - May have complex, but nonenhancing, central contents
- Enhancement pattern is extremely important
  - Some soft tissue masses appear cystic on T1WI & T2WI images but are solid
  - Central enhancement confirms solid mass & malignancy must be excluded

Helpful Clues for Common Diagnoses
- **Ganglion Cyst**
  - Well-defined border, often multiloculated
  - Lacks synovial lining & contains viscous or mucinous fluid
  - Similar appearance to synovial cyst on imaging
- **Synovial Cyst**
  - Well-defined, smooth border
  - Connects to joint or tendon sheath
  - Has synovial lining & contains synovial fluid
  - **Popliteal Cyst**
    - Synovial cyst in popliteal fossa
    - Lies between medial head gastrocnemius & semimembranosus in popliteal fossa
    - Smooth border with teardrop to rounded shape
    - Irregular border when cyst ruptures into proximal calf or distal thigh
  - **Meniscal Cyst**
    - Intraarticular knee synovial cyst, adjacent to meniscus
    - Suggests underlying meniscal tear
  - **Labral Cyst**
    - Synovial cyst in shoulder or hip
    - Suggests underlying labral tear
- **Sebaceous Cyst**
  - Well-defined round mass in subcutaneous fat
  - Common lesion but uncommonly purely cystic
  - No central enhancement
- **Soft Tissue Abscess**
  - Ill-defined, ragged borders
  - Irregular, thick peripheral enhancement
- **Bursitis**
  - Well-defined, smooth-bordered fluid collection in region of bursa
    - Anatomic bursae around joints
    - Pseudobursa due to pressure, for example over osteochondroma
  - Presence of rice bodies suggests rheumatoid arthritis
  - May also have thickening of associated tendons
  - Greater trochanteric bursitis at hip
    - Mild amount of fluid adjacent to each greater trochanter may be asymptomatic
  - Subacromial-subdeltoid bursitis at shoulder
    - Fluid from joint may extend through full thickness rotator cuff tear
  - Pes anserine bursitis at anteromedial knee
  - Patellar bursitis at anterior knee
    - Superficial to patellar tendon
  - Iliopsoas bursitis most likely to mimic cystic neoplasm
    - Lateral to femoral vessels & iliopsoas muscle and tendon
    - Medial to the anterior inferior iliac spine
    - Extends proximally into deep pelvis & can simulate adnexal mass on ultrasound
    - May have complex internal contents (synovium, debris)

CYSTIC MASSES

- Higher incidence with prior hip surgery & hip joint disease producing large effusion
- **Hematoma**
  - Well-defined to irregular mass
  - No internal enhancement
  - Complex internal contents common
    - Acute blood causes increased T1-weighted signal
    - Can appear lamellated or septated when subacute to chronic
  - Peripheral and internal calcification chronically
  - Associated evidence of trauma
- **Malignant Tumor, Necrotic**
  - Well-defined to irregular mass
  - Thick, irregular peripheral & internal enhancement
  - Centrally located necrosis lacks enhancement
  - Sarcomas, high grade and treated
- **Hemangioma, Soft Tissue**
  - Elongated tangle of vessels
  - Enhancement varies by type of vessels producing mass
    - MR angiography can best delineate type of feeder vessels
  - Fat & phleboliths are classic findings
  - Occasional hypertrophy or periosteal thickening of adjacent bone

Helpful Clues for Less Common Diagnoses
- **Lymphangioma**

- Well-defined to infiltrative, multiloculated masses
- May erode or cause resorption of adjacent bone
- Calcifications are rare
- **Myxoma (Mimic)**
  - Well-defined, round to oval mass in muscle
  - Contains central areas of enhancement
  - Mazabraud syndrome = multiple myxomas + fibrous dysplasia
- **Sarcoma, Soft Tissue (Mimic)**
  - Signal intensity mimicking simple to complex cysts on T1WI & T2WI
    - May have cystic appearance even without necrosis
  - Presence of central or nodular enhancement makes mass suspicious for neoplasm

Helpful Clues for Rare Diagnoses
- **Hydatid Cyst**
  - Multiple, round, peripherally calcified lesions
  - Daughter cysts common
  - Organ involvement seen before soft tissue involvement
- **Eccrine Hidradenoma**
  - Benign sweat gland tumor
  - Enhancing mural nodule (gland which produces fluid portion of mass)
  - Located in subcutaneous fat adjacent to skin

Ganglion Cyst

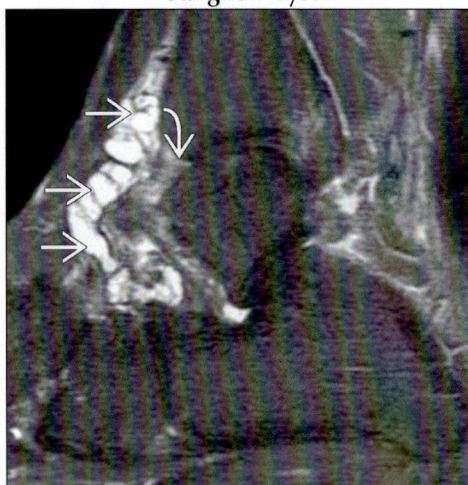

Sagittal STIR MR demonstrates a multiloculated mass ➤ and adjacent thickened synovium ➤ with minimal adjacent joint space narrowing of the tibiotalar joint. This cyst produced anterolateral ankle impingement.

Ganglion Cyst

Sagittal T2WI FS MR shows a cyst ➤ on the dorsum of the wrist, with homogeneously high signal intensity and a connecting tail ➤ which tracks proximally and deep, into the radio-carpal joint, from which it probably arose.

CYSTIC MASSES

(Left) Coronal T2WI FS MR demonstrates a well-defined fluid collection ⇒ lateral to the abductor pollicis longus and extensor pollicis brevis tendons ⇒. A marker ⇒ indicates that this was a site of pain. *(Right)* Axial PD FSE FS MR shows a high signal collection ⇒ extending between the semimembranosus ⇒ and medial head of the gastrocnemius ⇒ tendons in the classic location for a popliteal or Baker cyst.

Synovial Cyst

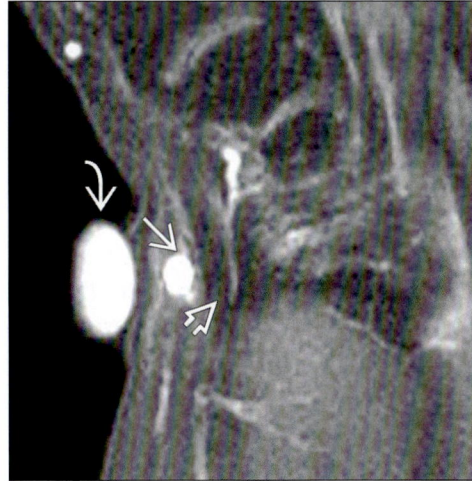

Popliteal Cyst

Popliteal Cyst

(Left) Axial PD FSE FS MR shows high signal fluid ⇒ dissecting through the posterior soft tissues of the knee. This collection merged into the popliteal cyst *(shown on previous image)*. A ruptured popliteal cyst can look somewhat infiltrative at the point of rupture. *(Right)* Coronal T2WI MR shows a meniscal tear ⇒, as well as a meniscal cyst ⇒. Medial meniscal cysts often migrate further from the meniscal tear than is seen with lateral meniscal cysts.

Meniscal Cyst

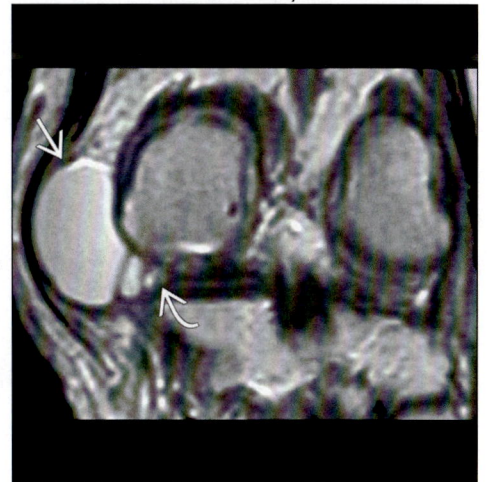

Labral Cyst

(Left) Axial T2WI MR shows a typical posterior shoulder paralabral cyst ⇒. The posterior and inferior labral tear which connects to the cyst is seen ⇒. In this case, there is no associated muscle atrophy. *(Right)* Axial T1WI FS MR shows the torn anterior hip labrum ⇒, extending into a paralabral cyst ⇒. Note in addition the thickened pulvinar occupying space within the joint, typical of DDH ⇒.

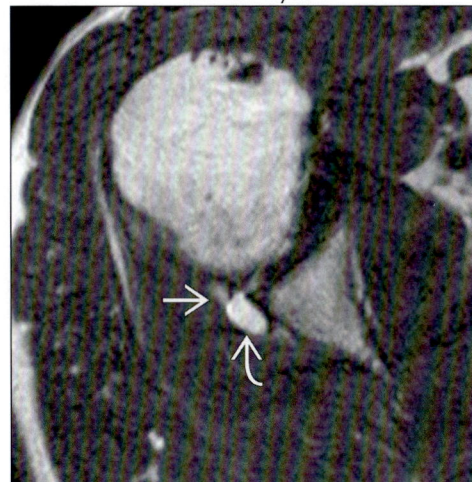

Labral Cyst

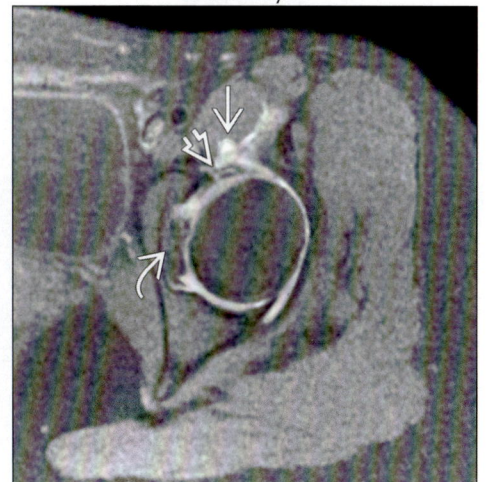

CYSTIC MASSES

Soft Tissue Abscess

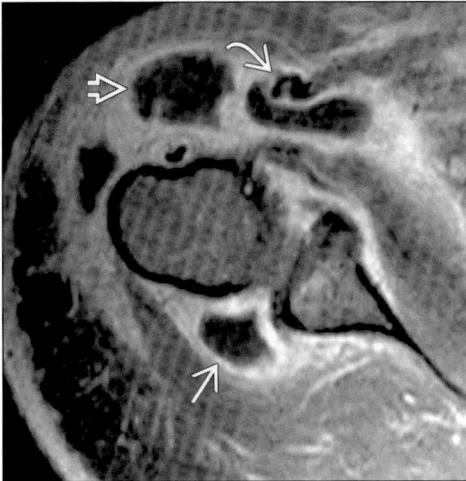

Soft Tissue Abscess

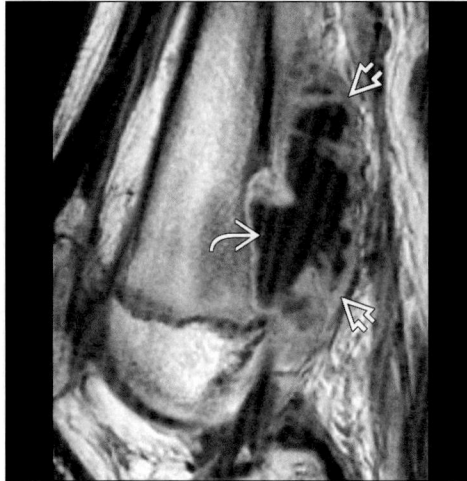

(Left) Axial T1 C+ FS MR shows a thick enhancing rind surrounding fluid within the glenohumeral joint ➡. There is also an abscess within the anterior deltoid muscle ➡, as well as an abscess surrounding the ruptured pectoralis major tendon ➡. *(Right)* Sagittal T1 C+ MR shows a large soft tissue mass ➡ with central fluid contents ➡ extending from a subtle defect in the posterior femur. This was an abscess with adjacent osteomyelitis from Yersinia pestis.

Bursitis

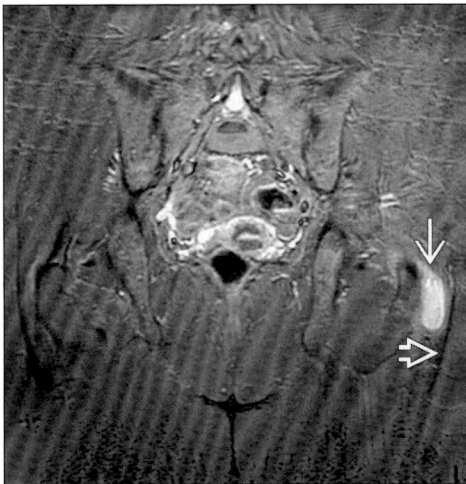

Bursitis

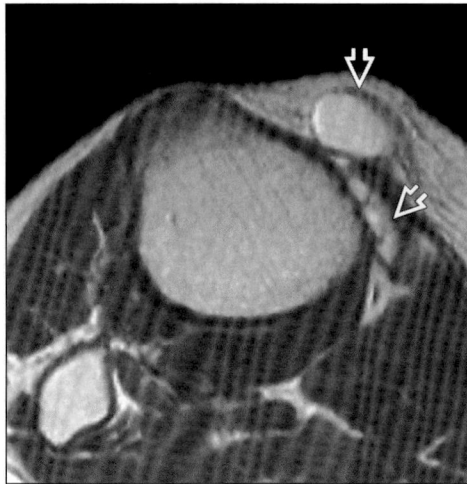

(Left) Coronal T2WI FS MR demonstrates a fluid collection ➡ lateral to the left greater femoral trochanter, consistent with greater trochanteric bursitis. The iliotibial band ➡ is located just lateral to the inflamed bursa. *(Right)* Axial T2WI MR shows a cyst ➡ adjacent to the pes anserinus, wrapping around the tibia. There were several components of the cyst, involving all three tendons of the pes anserinus.

Bursitis

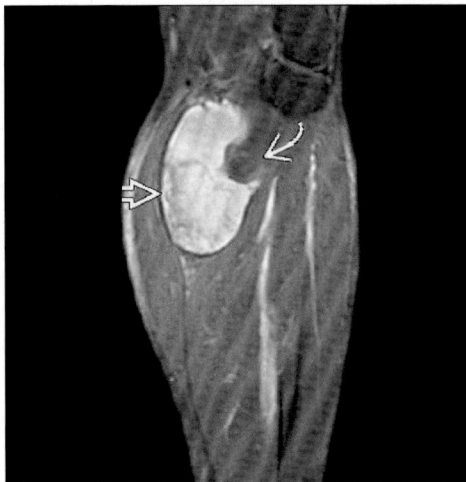

Bursitis

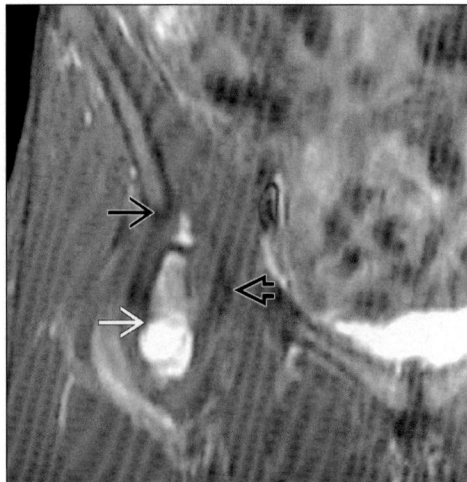

(Left) Coronal T2WI FS MR shows a large bursa ➡ complicating an osteochondroma ➡. The bursa is high in signal intensity and contains inhomogeneous areas. The periphery of the bursa enhanced. *(Right)* Coronal PD FSE FS MR shows the typical tear-drop-shaped fluid collection within the iliopsoas bursa ➡ extending proximally, traveling medial to the anterior inferior iliac spine ➡ and lateral to the iliopsoas muscle and tendon ➡.

CYSTIC MASSES

(Left) *Axial T2WI FS MR shows a heterogeneous mass* ➡ *lying between the medial head of the gastrocnemius and the soleus due to plantaris tendon rupture. Increased signal within the medial head of the gastrocnemius muscle* ➡ *is consistent with partial thickness tearing.* **(Right)** *Axial T2WI FS MR shows a hyperintense collection* ➡ *extending from a defect at the site of the medial gastrocnemius rupture. The plantaris tendon has ruptured and retracted.*

Hematoma

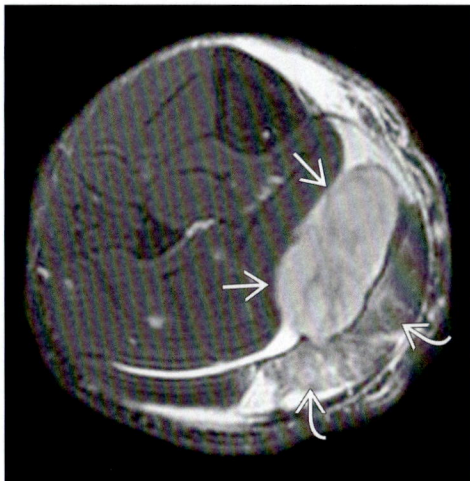

Hematoma

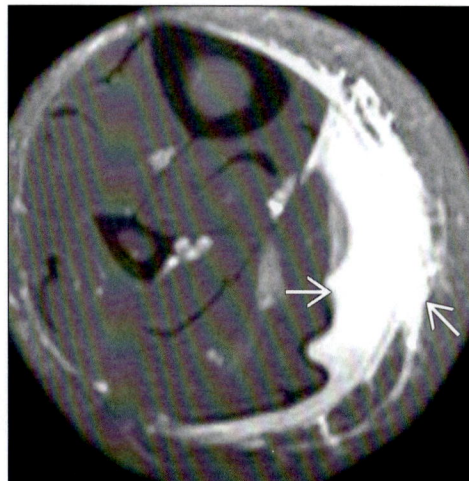

(Left) *Axial T1 C+ FS MR shows an inhomogeneous mass* ➡ *with predominantly peripheral enhancement in the adductor brevis muscle. This is a typical case of a soft tissue fibrosarcoma with central necrosis* ➡. **(Right)** *Axial T1 C+ FS MR shows fibrosarcoma involvement of all of the muscles in the anterior compartment* ➡ *and irregular regions within the mass that lack enhancement* ➡, *consistent with necrosis.*

Malignant Tumor, Necrotic

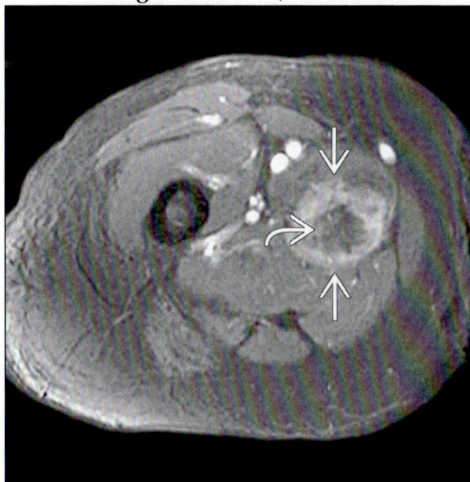

Malignant Tumor, Necrotic

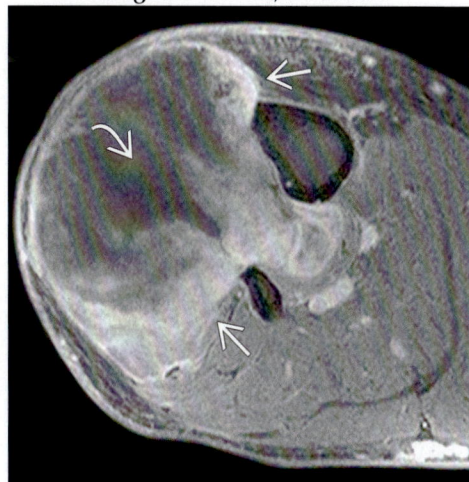

(Left) *Coronal T2WI MR shows a high signal, lobulated soft tissue mass* ➡ *in the thigh. A phlebolith* ➡ *was low signal on all sequences. Fatty stroma is usually found in soft tissue hemangiomas, along with the tangle of vessels.* **(Right)** *Axial STIR MR shows a perineural cyst* ➡ *located immediately adjacent to the normal tibial nerve* ➡. *Lack of enhancement as well as normal tibial nerve make a nerve sheath tumor unlikely. The cystic structure is an elongated lymphangioma.*

Hemangioma, Soft Tissue

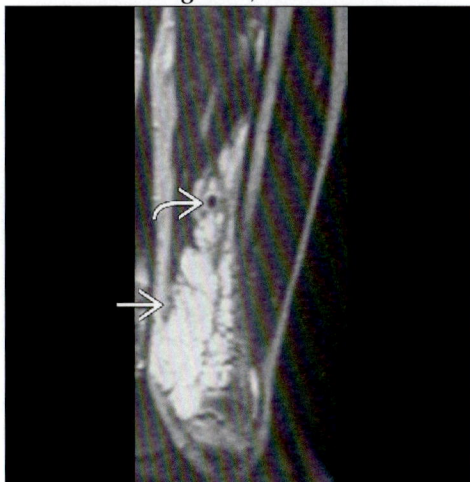

Lymphangioma

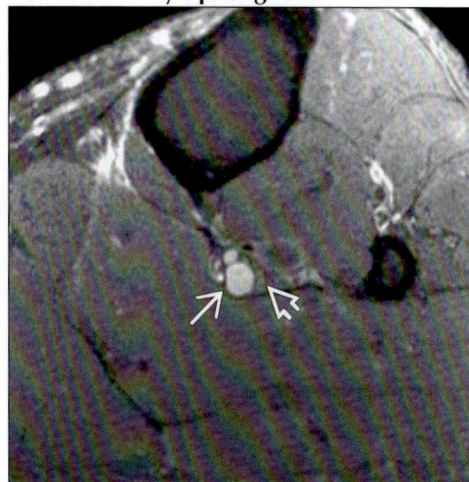

CYSTIC MASSES

Myxoma (Mimic)

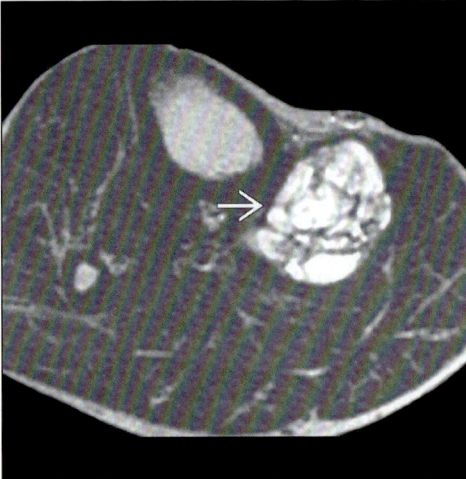

Myxoma (Mimic)

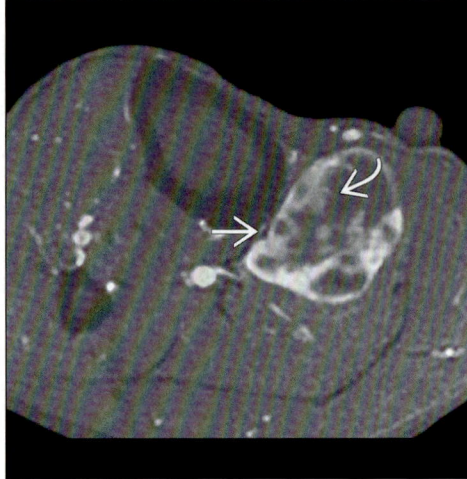

(Left) Axial T2WI MR shows a solitary, high signal intramuscular mass ➡ with septae. *(Right)* Axial T1 C+ FS MR in the same patient as previous image, shows areas of irregular enhancement ➡ within the lesion ➡. Histologically these lesions consist of myxoid matrix and spindle-shaped stromal cells. Multiple intramuscular myxomas suggests Mazabraud syndrome.

Sarcoma, Soft Tissue (Mimic)

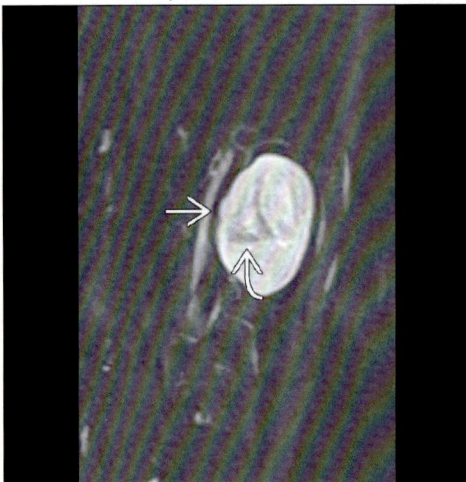

Sarcoma, Soft Tissue (Mimic)

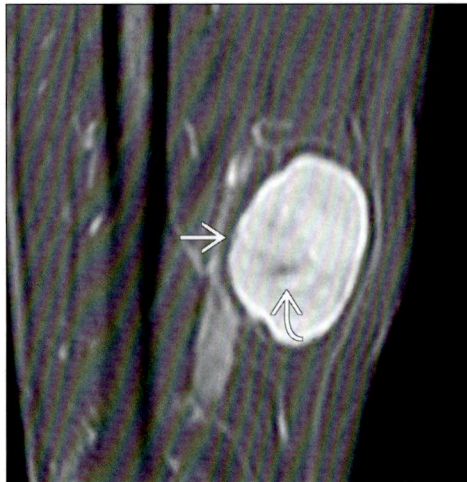

(Left) Coronal STIR MR shows a myxoid liposarcoma ➡ with the majority of the lesion of high signal, but internal foci of fat ➡ have low signal. The mass solidly enhanced, except for the fatty tissue. *(Right)* Coronal T1 C+ FS MR shows the same myxoid liposarcoma ➡ as the prior image, composed of high signal central enhancement with central low signal fat ➡.

Sarcoma, Soft Tissue (Mimic)

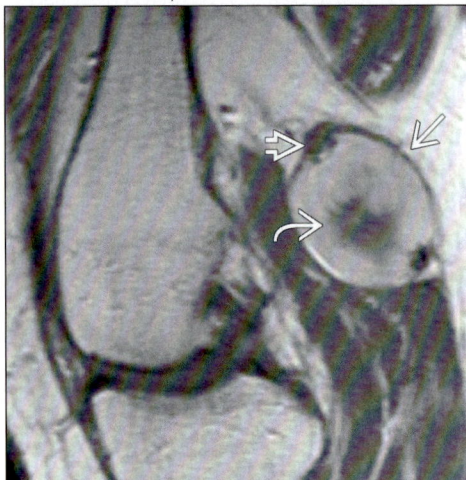

Eccrine Hidradenoma

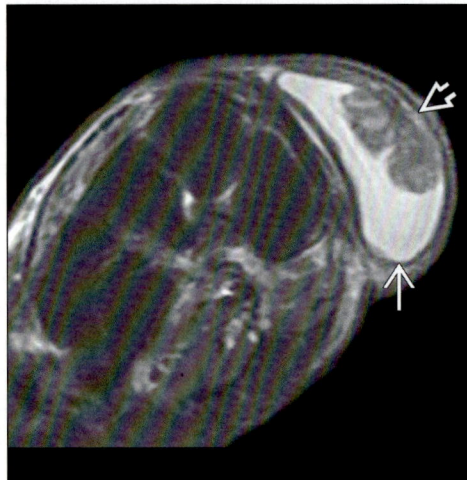

(Left) Sagittal T1 C+ MR shows a round soft tissue mass ➡ with calcification ➡ and thick peripheral enhancement, with the exception of a central cystic region ➡. It is important to consider the diagnosis of synovial sarcoma when calcification is present in a soft tissue mass. *(Right)* Coronal T2WI MR shows a nodule with inhomogeneous low signal ➡ intimately associated with the skin and surrounding fluid ➡, secreted by this eccrine hydradenoma.

SUBCUTANEOUS MASS

DIFFERENTIAL DIAGNOSIS

Common
- Sebaceous Cyst
- Varicose Veins
- Hematoma
- Lipoma, Soft Tissue
- Adenopathy
- Abscess
- Fat Necrosis
- Foreign Body
- Gout
- Epidermoid Inclusion Cyst
- Glomus Tumor
- Neurofibromatosis
- Melanoma
- Malignant Fibrous Histiocytoma
- Desmoid-Type Fibromatosis
- Vascular Malformation

Less Common
- Lymphoma
- Atypical Lipomatous Tumor
- Liposarcoma, Soft Tissue
- Metastases, Subcutaneous
- Tumor Recurrence
- Dermatofibrosarcoma Protuberans
- Venom Induced Complications
- Synovial Sarcoma
- Spindle Cell Lipoma
- Leiomyoma
- Lipodystrophy
- Kaposi Sarcoma

Rare but Important
- Multiple Myeloma
- Squamous Cell Carcinoma
- Merkel Cell Carcinoma
- Pilomatrixoma/Pilomatrix Carcinoma
- Mycosis Fungoides (T-Cell Lymphoma)
- Spindle Cell Sarcoma
- Angiosarcoma of Soft Tissue
- Granuloma Annulare
- Myxofibrosarcoma
- Fibrous Hamartoma of Infancy
- Angiomatoid Fibrous Histiocytoma
- Periosteal Chondroma
- Soft Tissue Chondroma
- Heterotopic Ossification
- Eccrine Hidradenoma

ESSENTIAL INFORMATION

Key Differential Diagnosis Issues
- Extensive differential diagnosis for subcutaneous masses
- Many entities are not possible to differentiate from each other on the basis of imaging alone
- Benign and malignant masses can have an identical appearance on MR
  - Imaging should not dissuade from biopsy or excision unless the mass is clearly a blood vessel or simple lipoma
    - Subcutaneous location allows safe & easy excisional procedures

Helpful Clues for Common Diagnoses
- **Sebaceous Cyst**
  - a.k.a., Epidermoid cyst, keratinous type
  - Slightly hyperintense to muscle on T1WI
  - High signal on T2WI + may contain angular low signal foci
  - Lacks central enhancement
- **Varicose Veins**
  - Tubular configuration is easily identifiable as a blood vessel
  - Enhancement characteristics altered if vessels are thrombosed
- **Hematoma**
  - Correlate with history of trauma
  - Must be vigilant to exclude underlying hemorrhagic malignancy
    - Lack of enhancement and/or interval follow-up
- **Lipoma, Soft Tissue**
  - Follows fat signal intensity on all sequences ± low signal capsule
  - May have thin septations measuring less than 2 mm in diameter
- **Adenopathy**
  - Typical location of lymph nodes
  - Enlargement & obliterated fatty hilum suggests neoplastic involvement
- **Fat Necrosis**
  - a.k.a., Post-traumatic pseudolipoma
  - Follows fat signal intensity on all sequences similar to lipoma
  - May contain fibrosis & septations suggesting an atypical lipoma or liposarcoma
  - Predominantly located over pressure points or bony protuberances in the body

SUBCUTANEOUS MASS

- **Foreign Body**
  - Low signal intensity foreign material surrounded by intense inflammatory reaction & enhancement
- **Gout**
  - Soft tissue tophi
    - Low to intermediate signal on T1WI
    - Variable low to high signal on T2WI
  - Associated with juxtaarticular erosions having overhanging edges
- **Epidermoid Inclusion Cyst**
  - History of trauma causing implantation of dermal elements into subcutaneous tissues or bone
- **Glomus Tumor**
  - Mass associated with the nail bed
  - May erode underlying bone
- **Neurofibromatosis**
  - Mass follows course of nerve
  - May demonstrate classic target sign on T2WI & enhanced images
- **Melanoma**
  - Metastases tend to vary in size ± surrounding edema
  - Heterogeneous T1 signal on MR depends on melanin content
- **Malignant Fibrous Histiocytoma**
  - Large masses with heterogeneous enhancement and a necrotic center are more suggestive of malignancy

Helpful Clues for Less Common Diagnoses
- **Atypical Lipoma & Liposarcoma**
  - Non-fatty elements including thickened, enhancing septae (> 2 mm) or nodules help differentiate from simple lipoma
- **Metastases & Tumor Recurrence**
  - Correlate with clinical history of malignancy & site of primary lesion resection
- **Lipodystrophy**
  - Term refers to abnormal collections of fat or atrophy of fat
  - Lumps or atrophy from repeated injection of medication in same site
  - HIV-related accumulation of fat in abdominal, axillary, dorsocervical regions & loss of fat in face, buttocks, extremities
- **Kaposi Sarcoma**
  - Local extension from skin may erode underlying bone & cause periosteal reaction

Helpful Clues for Rare Diagnoses
- **Multiple Myeloma**
  - Extramedullary involvement is rare
  - Subcutaneous mass can be a solitary plasmacytoma
- **Pilomatrixoma/Pilomatrix Carcinoma**
  - Solid skin appendage tumor involves dermis & may contain calcification
- **Fibrous Hamartoma of Infancy**
  - Suspect diagnosis when patient is less than 2 years old
- **Eccrine Hidradenoma**
  - Mass with solid peripheral nodule & surrounding nonenhancing fluid

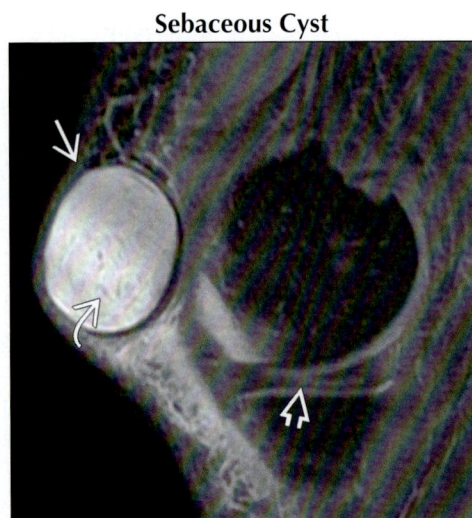

Sebaceous Cyst

Sagittal PD FSE FS MR shows a well-defined subcutaneous mass ➡ adjacent to the knee joint. Note the low signal debris ➡ within the predominately T2 hyperintense lesion. A meniscal tear ➡ is also visible.

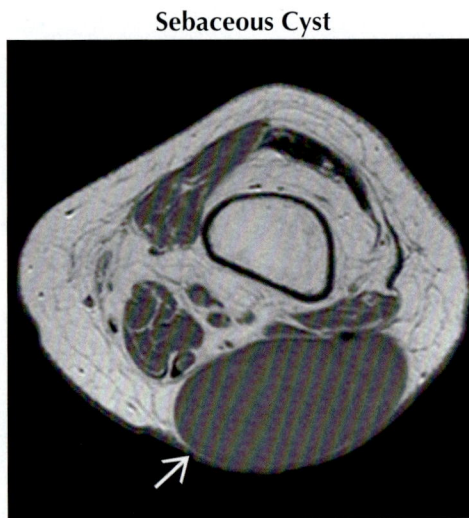

Sebaceous Cyst

Axial T1WI MR shows a subcutaneous mass ➡ in the distal thigh, which is mildly hyperintense to muscle and lacked central enhancement. This lesion also had internal low signal foci on T2WI, as seen on prior case.

SUBCUTANEOUS MASS

Varicose Veins

Hematoma

(Left) Coronal CECT shows numerous subcutaneous, tubular masses ➡ involving the right flank. These collateral vessels developed due to occlusion of the IVC and thrombosis of the subsequently placed IVC-femoral graft ➡. *(Right)* Axial T1WI MR shows a subcutaneous mass ➡ lateral to the hip. The mass had low T1 signal, high T2 signal and lacked central enhancement. This hematoma occurred after significant blunt trauma.

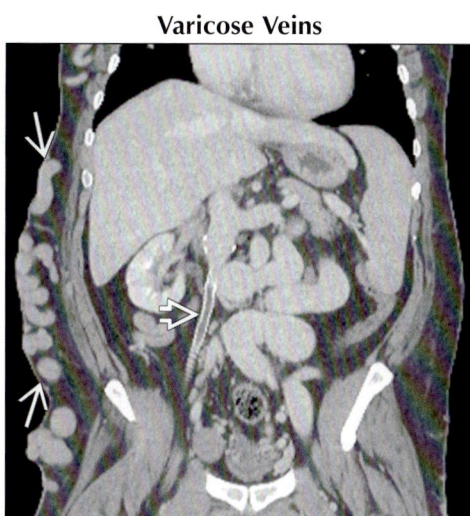

Lipoma, Soft Tissue

Abscess

(Left) Axial T1WI MR shows an encapsulated subcutaneous mass ➡ in the medial elbow. The mass followed the signal intensity of subcutaneous fat on all sequences, consistent with a simple lipoma. There were no aggressive features. *(Right)* Axial T1 C+ FS MR shows multiple peripherally enhancing abscesses ➡ in the gluteal subcutaneous fat and musculature, associated with sacral osteomyelitis ➡. A few low signal foci of air are present in the most superficial abscess ➡.

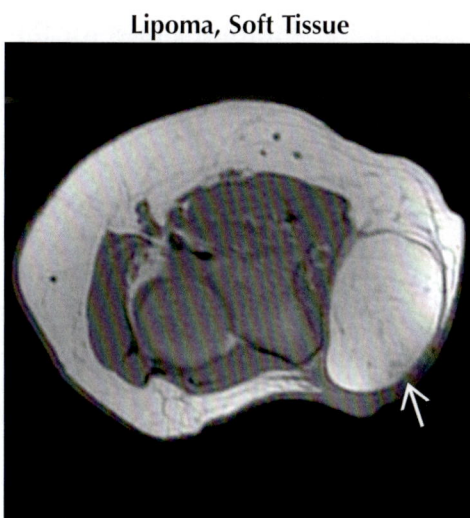

Fat Necrosis

Foreign Body

(Left) Coronal T1WI MR shows a subcutaneous mass ➡ having a very similar appearance to a lipoma. The diagnosis of fat necrosis was made after excision and is suggested on imaging by the thick surrounding capsule and location over the greater trochanter. *(Right)* Coronal T1 C+ FS MR shows two foreign bodies with surrounding intense enhancement ➡, located beneath the metatarsal heads. This was due to embedded glass shards.

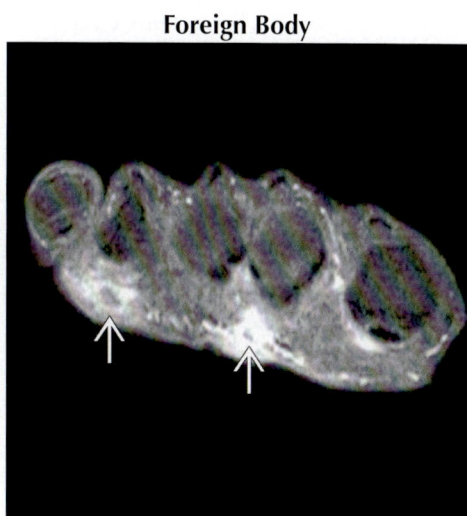

SUBCUTANEOUS MASS

Glomus Tumor

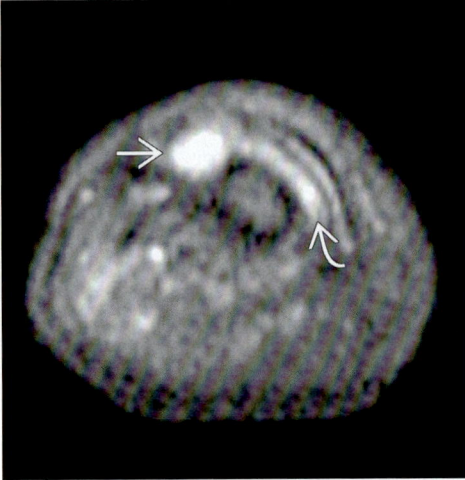

Neurofibromatosis

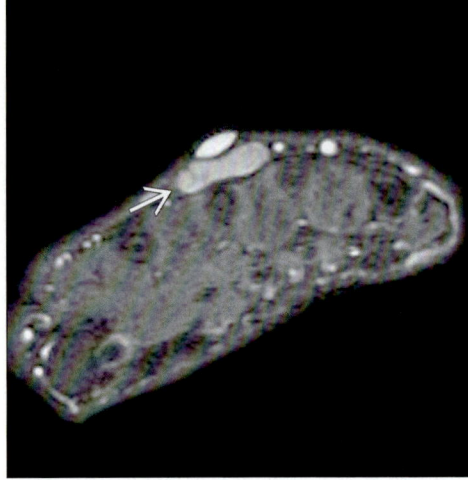

(Left) Axial T1 C+ FS MR shows a small, round, homogeneously enhancing mass ➡ along the radial side of the index finger. The mass had high signal on T2WI and enhanced slightly more prominently than the adjacent nail bed ➡. (Right) Axial T2WI FS MR shows an oval subcutaneous mass ➡ along the dorsum of the hand. The mass has fairly homogeneous high signal on T2WI but lacks the classic target sign of benign peripheral nerve sheath tumors.

Melanoma

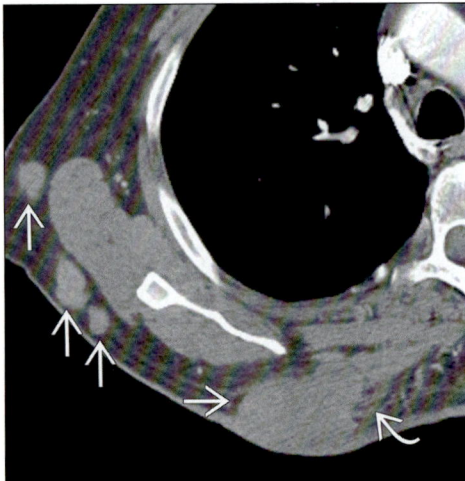

Malignant Fibrous Histiocytoma

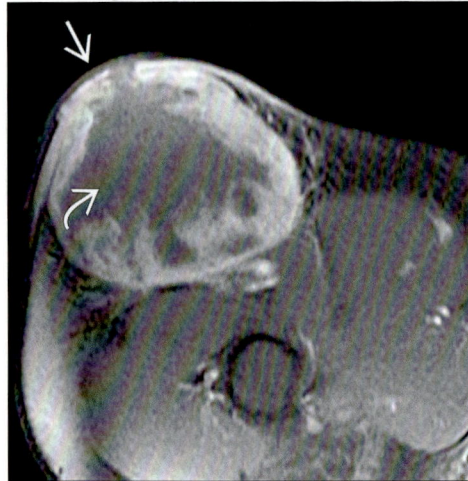

(Left) Axial CECT shows multiple subcutaneous masses ➡ in the posterolateral chest wall. These masses vary in size and have surrounding inflammatory changes in the fat ➡. The appearance is nonspecific but suggests a neoplastic process. (Right) Axial T1 C+ FS MR shows a large subcutaneous mass ➡ in the upper arm. There is irregular, thick peripheral enhancement and central necrosis ➡. Signal intensity was high on T2WI and low on T1WI.

Vascular Malformation

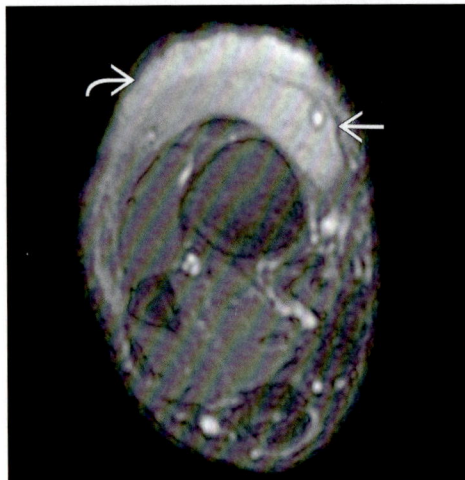

Lymphoma

(Left) Axial T2WI FS MR shows a mass ➡ in the lower leg that had been present since childhood. The mass involves the skin ➡ causing marked thickening. An MR angiogram showed very slow filling of this vascular malformation. (Right) Axial T1 C+ FS MR shows an enhancing nodular mass ➡ in the anteromedial thigh with surrounding edema ➡. Lymphoma was suspected based on the patient history, but otherwise the appearance of the lesion is nonspecific.

SUBCUTANEOUS MASS

(Left) Axial T2WI MR shows a subcutaneous mass ➡ in the left paraspinous region with heterogeneous increased signal on T2WI. This mass had low signal on T1WI and enhanced diffusely. Pathology revealed metastatic high grade gastrointestinal carcinoma. (Right) Axial NECT shows an irregular subcutaneous mass ➡ in the anterior chest wall. This was recurrent breast carcinoma in the mastectomy surgical site.

Metastases, Subcutaneous

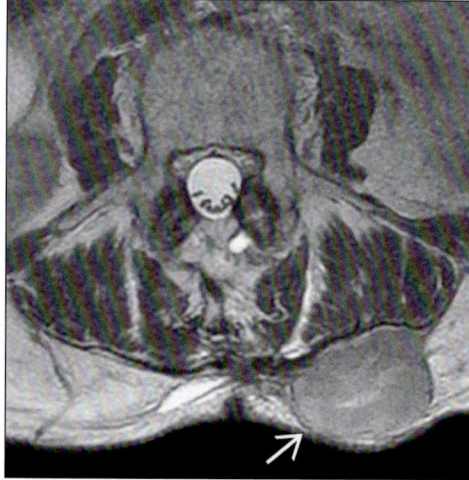

Tumor Recurrence

(Left) Axial T1WI MR shows superficial mass ➡ with a low signal capsule surrounding a central region of increased signal ➡. On T2WI, the peripheral portion remained low signal and the central portion had higher signal. The entire lesion diffusely enhanced. (Right) Axial T2WI FS MR shows a heterogeneous, high signal intensity subcutaneous mass ➡ in the posterolateral knee. The lesion had mild heterogeneous enhancement.

Dermatofibrosarcoma Protuberans

Spindle Cell Lipoma

(Left) Axial T1 C+ FS MR shows an oval subcutaneous mass ➡ in the lateral ankle that had minimally enlarged over 6 years. The target sign ➡, a low signal center on T2WI and enhanced images, gives this mass a similar appearance to a nerve sheath tumor. (Right) Coronal T2WI FS MR shows a heterogeneous mass ➡ along the medial aspect of the elbow. This was excised and found to be squamous cell carcinoma, metastatic to the medial epitrochlear lymph node.

Leiomyoma

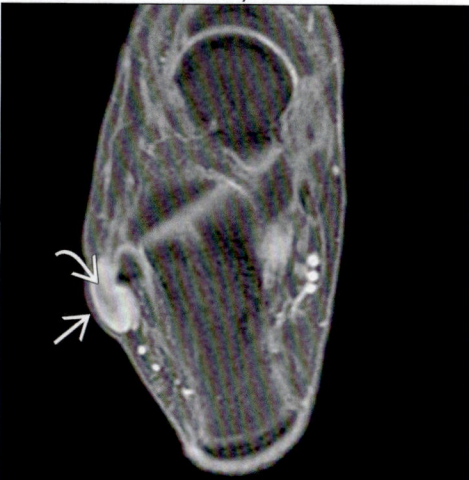

Squamous Cell Carcinoma

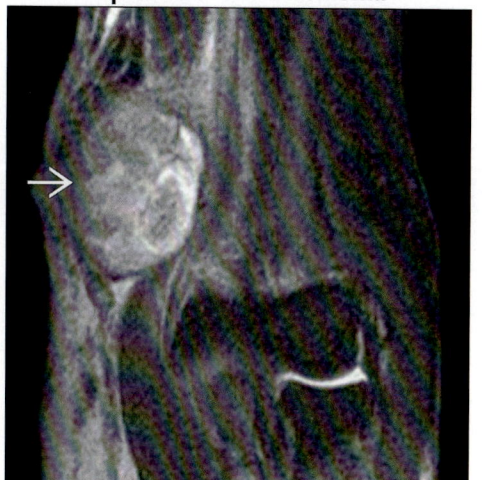

SUBCUTANEOUS MASS

Pilomatrixoma/Pilomatrix Carcinoma

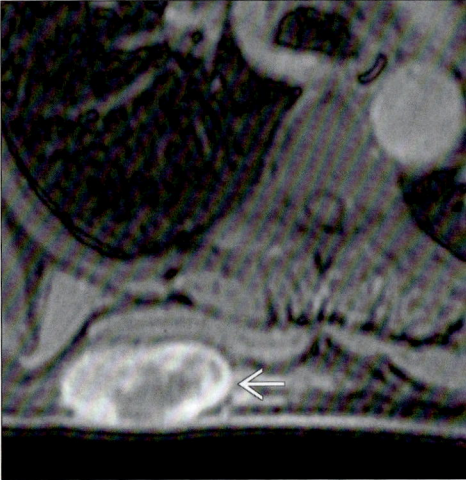

Mycosis Fungoides (T-Cell Lymphoma)

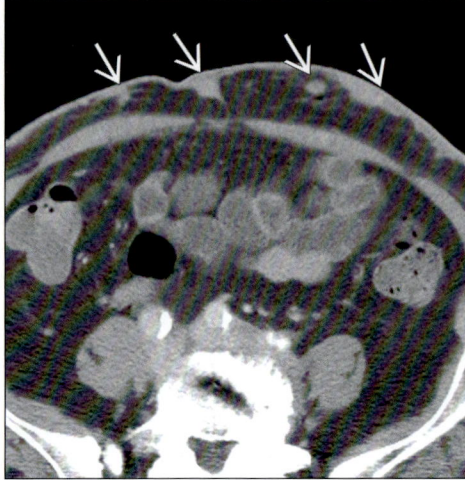

(Left) Axial T1 C+ FS MR shows a heterogeneously enhancing subcutaneous mass ➡ in the back. The mass had nonspecific low signal on T1WI and high signal on T2WI. This was excised and found to be a pilomatrix carcinoma. *(Right)* Axial CECT shows irregular subcutaneous nodules and skin thickening ➡ along the anterior abdominal wall. This diagnosis was clinically apparent as purple plaques and ulcerated masses.

Spindle Cell Sarcoma

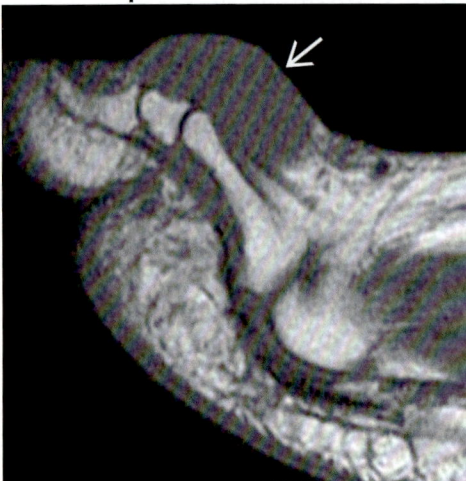

Myxofibrosarcoma

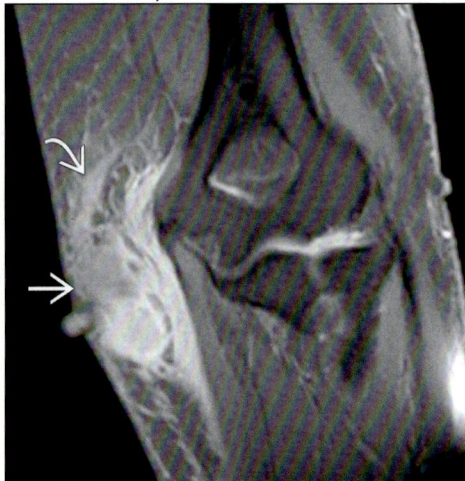

(Left) Sagittal T1WI MR shows a subcutaneous mass ➡ along the dorsum of the toe. Signal intensity was low on T1WI, high on T2WI and showed diffuse enhancement. Other etiologies such as giant cell tumor of tendon sheath or fibroma of tendon sheath could have this appearance. *(Right)* Coronal T1 C+ FS MR shows an ill-defined, diffusely enhancing mass ➡ in the subcutaneous fat of the medial elbow. There is a marked surrounding edema, which is nonspecific ➡.

Angiomatoid Fibrous Histiocytoma

Eccrine Hidradenoma

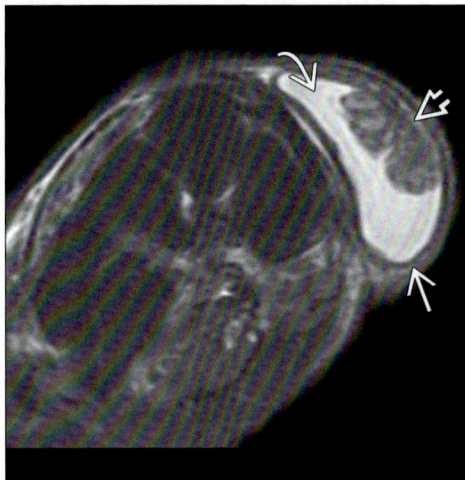

(Left) Axial T1 C+ FS MR shows a multilobulated enhancing mass ➡ in the posteromedial thigh. The mass had nonspecific low signal on T1WI and high signal on T2WI. The more superficial component ➡ had lower signal intensity on all sequences. *(Right)* Axial T2WI MR shows a mass ➡ in the subcutaneous tissues of the midfoot with a peripheral, solid nodule ➡ and a large amount of surrounding fluid ➡, which is produced by this sweat gland tumor.

ENLARGED MUSCLE

DIFFERENTIAL DIAGNOSIS

Common
- Exercise Induced Muscle Hypertrophy
- Hematoma
- Compensatory Muscle Hypertrophy

Less Common
- Diabetes: MSK Complications (Myonecrosis)
- Pyomyositis
- Rhabdomyolysis
- Compartment Syndrome
- Denervation Hypertrophy
- Intramuscular Neoplasm
  - Lymphoma
  - Malignant Fibrous Histiocytoma
  - Liposarcoma
  - Hemangioma, Soft Tissue
  - Lymphangioma
  - Rhabdomyoma
  - Rhabdomyosarcoma, Soft Tissue

Rare but Important
- Fibromatosis Colli
- Muscular Dystrophy
- Pseudotumor, Orbit
- Graves Disease, Orbit

ESSENTIAL INFORMATION

Key Differential Diagnosis Issues
- Important features
  - Clinical presentation
    - Presence or absence of pain
  - Muscles involved
    - Single muscle
    - All muscles in compartment
    - Contiguous muscles
  - Morphology of muscle enlargement
    - Generalized: Involves entire muscle
    - Partial: Involves segments of muscle, no discrete mass
    - Focal: Mass
  - Architectural distortion: Preservation or disruption internal fat distribution
  - Imaging characteristics
    - MR preferred imaging modality

Helpful Clues for Common Diagnoses
- **Exercise Induced Muscle Hypertrophy**
  - Asymptomatic
  - Typically all muscles of an extremity
  - Generalized enlargement
  - Normal architecture & MR appearance
- **Hematoma**
  - Pain, history of trauma, anti-coagulation
  - Random muscle involvement
    - Rectus abdominus, rectus femoris, hamstring muscles common
  - Partial or focal enlargement
  - Architectural distortion
  - Fluid-fluid levels (US, CT or MR)
  - MR appearance
    - Bright T1WI signal is specific finding
    - Low T2WI signal rim (hemosiderin)
- **Compensatory Muscle Hypertrophy**
  - Trauma, surgery, denervation of associated muscles
  - Single muscle or muscle group
  - Otherwise identical to exercise induced hypertrophy

Helpful Clues for Less Common Diagnoses
- **Diabetes: MSK Complications (Myonecrosis)**
  - Pain, history of poorly controlled diabetes
  - Random muscle/muscles involved
    - Anterior compartment thigh classically involved
  - Partial or generalized enlargement
  - Early
    - Normal architecture
    - Bright T2WI signal, enhancement
  - Late
    - Architecture distortion
    - Necrotic muscle mimics fluid
    - Limited generalized enhancement
    - Periphery of necrotic muscle may enhance
- **Pyomyositis**
  - Pain, history of soft tissue injury/injection
  - Single muscle
    - May extend to contiguous muscles
  - Focal enlargement
  - Architecture distortion around abscess
  - MR: Fluid signal mass with rim enhancement
- **Rhabdomyolysis**
  - Pain, weakness, fever
  - Elevated CK, myoglobin, potassium; acidosis; renal failure
  - Random muscle involvement
  - Partial or generalized enlargement
  - Imaging changes identical to myonecrosis
    - See above for imaging characteristics

ENLARGED MUSCLE

- **Compartment Syndrome**
  - Pain, paresthesia, diminished/absent pulses
  - All muscles in compartment
  - Generalized enlargement
  - Leads to myonecrosis (see above for imaging characteristics)
- **Denervation Hypertrophy**
  - Lumbar spine disease most common cause
  - Painless
  - Generalized enlargement
  - Single muscle
    - Tensor fascia lata, semimembranosus muscle common
  - True hypertrophy: Normal architecture
  - Pseudohypertrophy: Increased internal fat
  - MR appearance
    - Normal T1WI signal
    - Increased T2WI signal
- **Intramuscular Neoplasm**
  - ± Pain
  - Single muscle
    - May extend to contiguous muscles
  - Focal enlargement
  - Architectural distortion
  - Abnormal nonspecific MR appearance

Helpful Clues for Rare Diagnoses
- **Fibromatosis Colli**
  - Neonatal torticollis
  - Partial enlargement lower 1/3 sternocleidomastoid muscle
  - Hyperintense T2WI signal
    - May have linear low signal 2° collagen

- **Muscular Dystrophy**
  - Under 20 years of age
  - Painless, profound progressive weakness
  - Calf musculature only
    - Posterior compartment: Especially soleus
  - Generalized enlargement
  - Architecture: Increased internal fat (pseudohypertrophy)
  - MR appearance reflects increased fat
- **Pseudotumor, Orbit**
  - Clinical
    - Pain, diplopia, proptosis
    - Conjunctivitis, lid swelling
  - Extra-ocular muscles
    - Superior complex, medial rectus commonly involved
    - Bilateral in 1/3
  - Generalized enlargement
    - Involves tendon insertion
    - Bulging inner margin of muscle
  - Normal architecture
  - MR appearance
    - Intramuscular hyperintense T2 signal
    - Inflammatory changes adjacent fat
- **Graves Disease, Orbit**
  - Painless
  - Exophthalmos, lid retraction, limited motion of globe
  - Bilateral asymmetric involvement extra-ocular muscles
  - Generalized enlargement, spares tendon insertion
  - Normal architecture
  - MR: Hyperintense T2WI signal

Hematoma

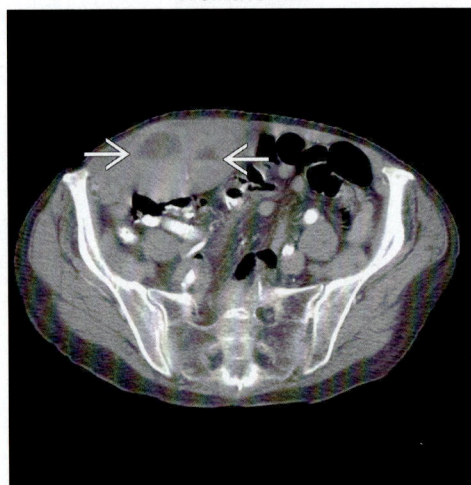

Axial CECT shows enlargement of the right rectus abdominis muscle with internal fluid-fluid levels ➡ consistent with hematoma. The bleeding was secondary to anti-coagulation.

Compensatory Muscle Hypertrophy

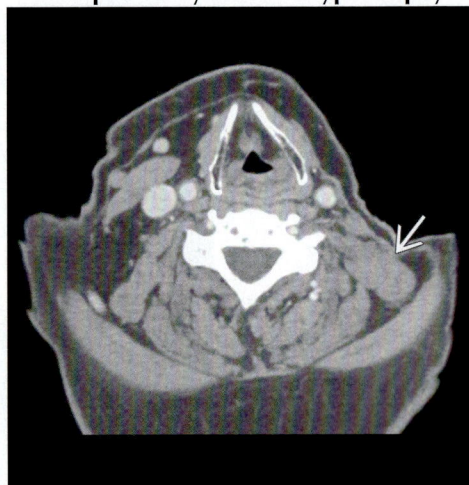

Axial CECT shows true hypertrophy of the levator scapulae muscle ➡ following radical neck dissection. The muscle is enlarged but otherwise identical to the surrounding musculature.

ENLARGED MUSCLE

Diabetes: MSK Complications (Myonecrosis)

Pyomyositis

(Left) Axial T2WI MR shows enlargement with myonecrosis and fatty replacement of the medial gastrocnemius and both heads of the soleus in this patient with diabetic myonecrosis. *(Right)* Axial CECT shows a low density lesion with a thin enhancing rim causing enlargement of the deltoid muscle ➡ consistent with pyomyositis following recent intramuscular injection.

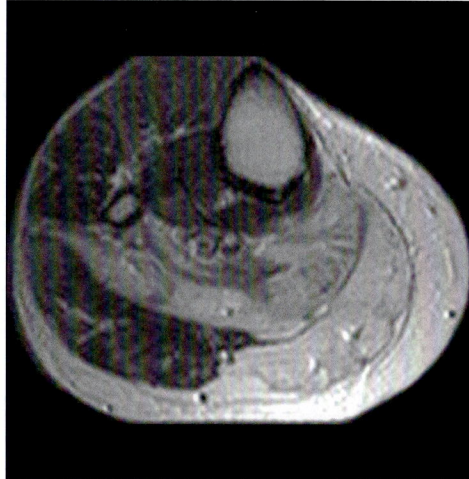

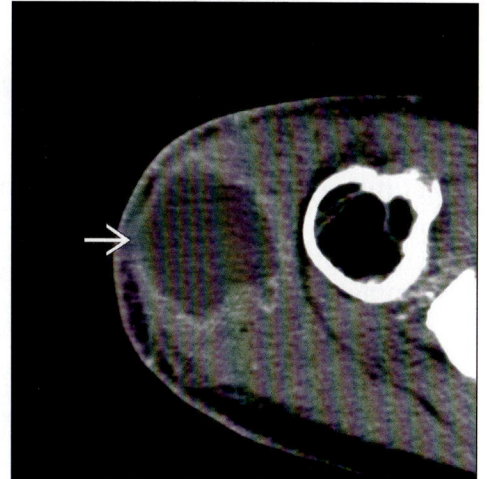

Rhabdomyolysis

Compartment Syndrome

(Left) Axial T2WI MR shows enlarged left paraspinal musculature ➡ with hyperintense signal secondary to rhabdomyolysis due to prolonged surgical positioning. *(Right)* Axial T2WI FS MR shows marked enlargement of the anterior tibialis muscle ➡ with edema in the adjacent extensor hallucis longus muscle ➡ and bowing of the interosseous membrane ➡ resulting in compartment syndrome.

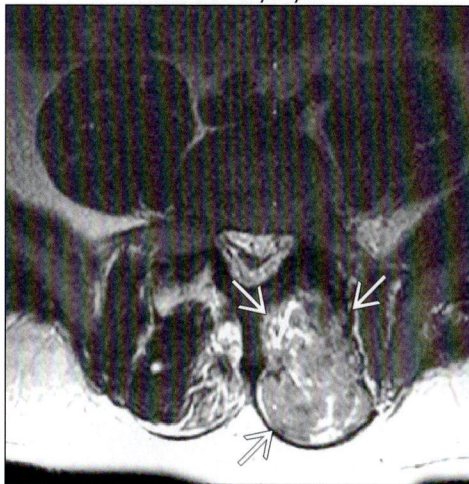

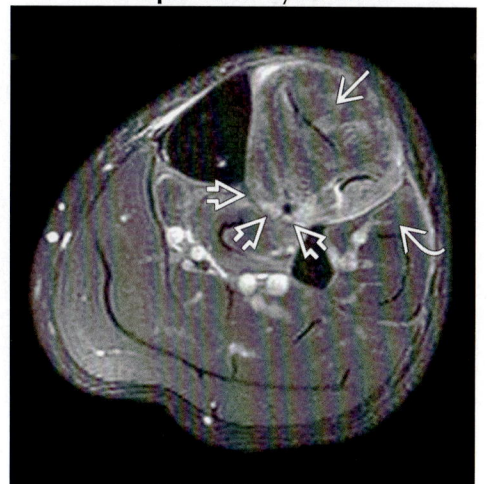

Denervation Hypertrophy

Lymphoma

(Left) Coronal T1 C+ MR shows enlargement of the gastrocnemius muscle ➡ with mild diffuse enhancement and mild increase in intramuscular fat resulting from denervation hypertrophy. *(Right)* Coronal T1WI MR shows primary soft tissue lymphoma enlarging the right gluteus minimus and gluteus medius muscles with distortion of the internal muscle architecture.

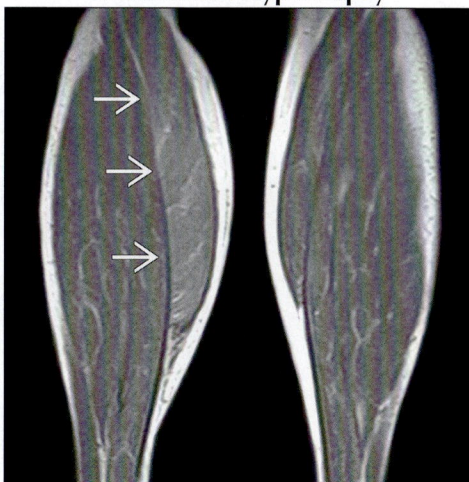

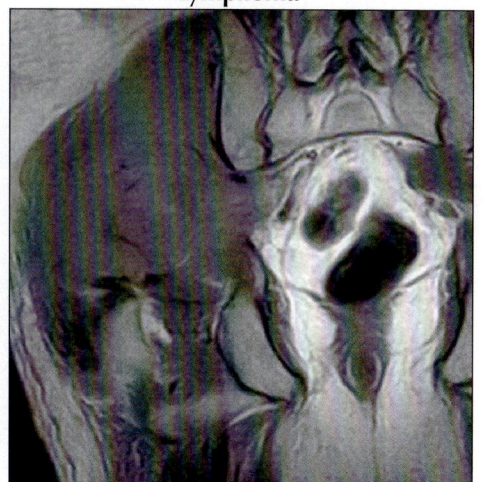

ENLARGED MUSCLE

Malignant Fibrous Histiocytoma

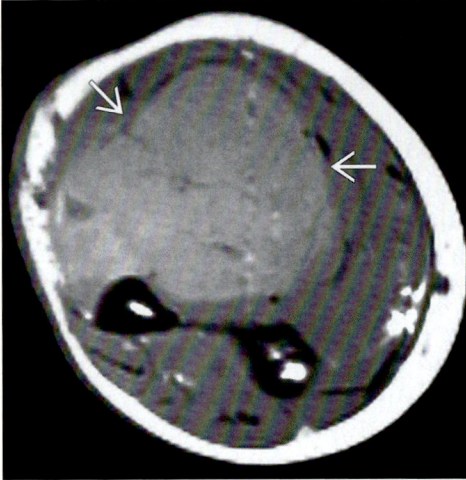

Liposarcoma

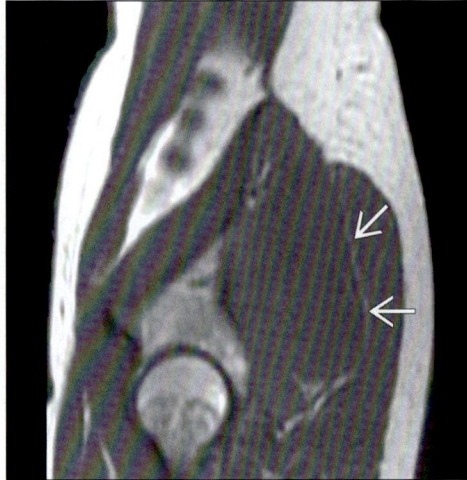

(Left) Axial T1WI MR shows a malignant fibrous histiocytoma creating focal enlargement of the anterior forearm musculature as a large infiltrating mass which is nearly isointense with muscle on T1 imaging ➡. *(Right)* Sagittal T1WI MR shows a nice example of a poorly differentiated liposarcoma ➡ which contains no fat. The mass causes marked enlargement of the gluteus medius muscle. Remember that high grade liposarcoma often contains little or no fat.

Hemangioma, Soft Tissue

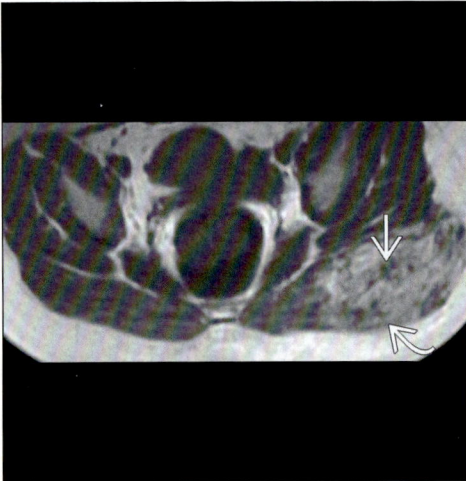

Rhabdomyosarcoma, Soft Tissue

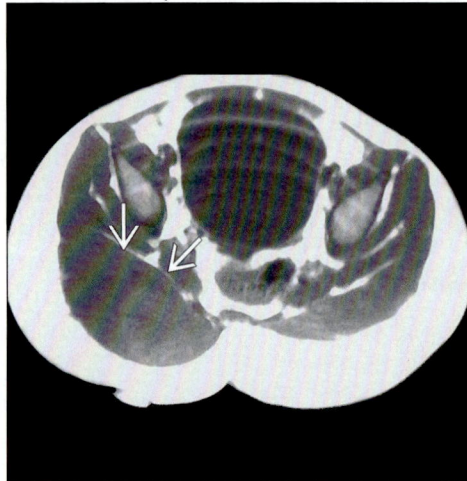

(Left) Axial T2WI FS MR shows a nice example of intramuscular hemangioma. Tubular structures ➡ are present within a background of fatty stroma ➡. *(Right)* Axial T1WI MR shows marked enlargement of the right gluteus maximus muscle ➡ with heterogeneous internal signal secondary to rhabdomyosarcoma.

Fibromatosis Colli

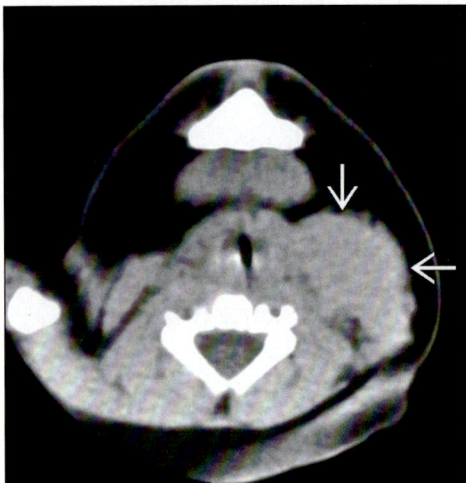

Pseudotumor, Orbit

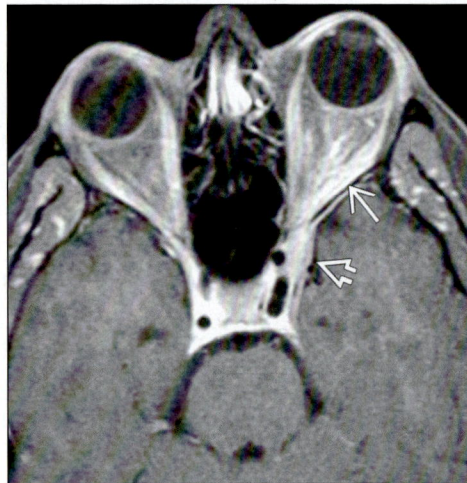

(Left) Axial NECT shows typical CT appearance of fibromatosis colli with generalized enlargement of the left sternocleidomastoid muscle ➡; density remains typical of normal muscle. *(Right)* Axial T1 C+ FS MR shows typical MR example of pseudotumor with enhancing tissue involving the left orbital apex and lateral rectus muscle ➡ with contiguous involvement of the ipsilateral anterior cavernous sinus ➡.

MUSCLE ATROPHY

DIFFERENTIAL DIAGNOSIS

Common
- Post-Operative
- Immobilization
- Tendon, Injury
- Spinal Cord Injury
- Peripheral Nerve Injury
- Neuropathy
- Complications of Steroids
- Diabetes: MSK Complications

Less Common
- Muscle Injury
- Neurofibromatosis
- Cushing Disease
- Muscular Dystrophy
- Thermal Injury, Burns
- Charcot-Marie-Tooth Disease
- Amyotrophic Lateral Sclerosis
- Guillain-Barré Syndrome
- Meningomyelocele

Rare but Important
- Polio
- Spondyloepiphyseal Dysplasia (Pseudoachondroplasia)
- Tethered Cord Syndrome
- Arthrogryposis
- Werdnig-Hoffmann Disease
- Farber Disease
- Progeria

ESSENTIAL INFORMATION

Key Differential Diagnosis Issues
- Replacement of muscle fibers by fat produces high signal on T1WI and low signal on fat-suppressed sequences
  - Muscle atrophy may also present as a decrease in muscle volume without interdigitating fat
- High signal on T2WI FS MR in the remaining atrophic muscle may represent ongoing denervation or inflammation
- Distribution, history and associated findings are most helpful for differentiating etiologies

Helpful Clues for Common Diagnoses
- **Post-Operative**
  - Associated with micrometallic artifact or other evidence of surgical intervention

- Atrophy, such as in the rotator cuff, may have preceded surgery
- **Immobilization**
  - Muscle atrophy begins after 10 days of immobilization
    - Correlate findings with time of injury
  - Atrophy from prolonged immobilization (> 4 months) may be irreversible, especially in elderly patients
- **Tendon, Injury**
  - Common involving the rotator cuff and gluteus minimus tendons
    - Full thickness tendon tear results in atrophy of the associated muscle
- **Spinal Cord Injury**
  - Rapid muscle atrophy below level of injury
    - 18-46% decrease in muscle cross sectional area 6 weeks post injury
  - Associated findings: Cord atrophy, cord disruption, tethered cord, myelomalacia, syrinx
- **Peripheral Nerve Injury**
  - Often possible to identify the abnormal nerve based on muscle denervation pattern
- **Neuropathy**
  - Associated neuropathic changes in joints include distention, debris, disorganization, deformity, dislocation
- **Complications of Steroids**
  - Myopathy with high-dose steroid therapy
  - Weakening of bone leads to increased fractures with resultant immobilization
- **Diabetes: MSK Complications**
  - Multiple potential causes for atrophy
    - Neuropathy, muscle infarction, increased incidence of fracture leading to immobilization, infection

Helpful Clues for Less Common Diagnoses
- **Muscle Injury**
  - Myonecrosis
    - Compartment syndrome
    - Diabetic myonecrosis
    - Trauma
- **Neurofibromatosis**
  - Peripheral neuropathies associated with involvement of large nerve root and subcutaneous neurofibromas
- **Cushing Disease**
  - Proximal muscles more severely affected than distal

- Associated clinical findings: Cushingoid facial appearance, truncal obesity, skin atrophy
  - MR to assess for pituitary, adrenal or ectopic corticotropin-producing tumor
- **Muscular Dystrophy**
  - MR imaging of thighs and calves can be used to assess the extent and pattern of muscle atrophy
  - Least affected muscles in thigh include gracilis, semimembranosus, semitendinosus and sartorius
- **Thermal Injury, Burns**
  - Necrosis of muscle, peripheral neuropathy, skin contractures
- **Charcot-Marie-Tooth Disease**
  - Also known as hereditary motor sensory neuropathy
  - Different types, all with lower extremity muscle wasting
  - Associated findings: Stork leg or inverted champagne bottle appearance of leg, pes cavus, scoliosis
- **Amyotrophic Lateral Sclerosis**
  - Adult onset motor neuron disease may initially involve the upper or lower limbs
  - Brain imaging reveals T2WI hyperintense corticospinal tracts, from corona radiata to brainstem
- **Guillain-Barré Syndrome**
  - Spine imaging reveals thick nerve roots and enhancing cauda equina
  - History of ascending, symmetric paralysis
- **Meningomyelocele**
  - Associated findings: Posterior spinal defect (or post-operative repair), low lying spinal cord

Helpful Clues for Rare Diagnoses
- **Polio**
  - Virtual eradication of new cases in the Western hemisphere
  - Symmetric or asymmetric atrophy in affected limb(s)
- **Spondyloepiphyseal Dysplasia (Pseudoachondroplasia)**
  - Delayed, irregular ossification centers
  - Platyspondyly
  - Odontoid hypoplasia or os odontoideum
  - Horizontal acetabular roofs
  - Short, broad, tubular bones
- **Arthrogryposis**
  - Contracted distal joints, limb shortening, decreased muscle mass, abnormal tendon attachments, absent patella, missing or extra carpal and tarsal bones
- **Werdnig-Hoffmann Disease**
  - Also known as spinal muscular atrophy, type 1
  - Extensive muscle degeneration, flexed abducted hips, flexed knees
  - Unable to move extremities except fingers and toes
- **Progeria**
  - Accelerated aging with associated findings of atherosclerotic disease, osteoporosis, arthritis, acroosteolysis & muscle atrophy in young patient with normal bone age

Post-Operative

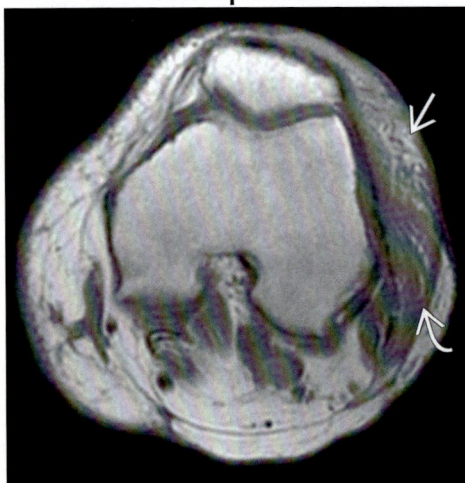

Axial T1WI MR shows fatty atrophy ➡ of a gastrocnemius muscle flap ➡. This was placed after sarcoma resection. The normal muscle undergoes atrophy due to altered biomechanics (disuse).

Immobilization

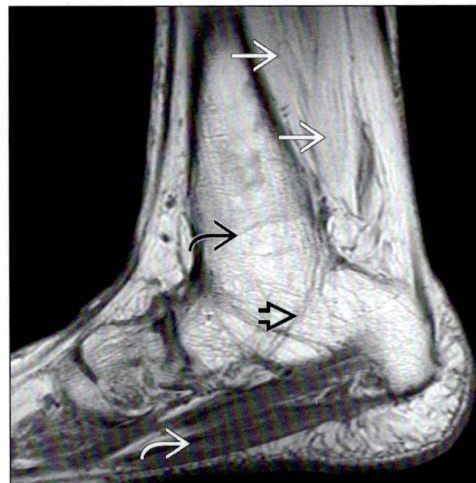

Sagittal T1WI MR shows chronic fatty atrophy ➡ of the calf flexor muscles. Atrophy is secondary to surgical arthrodesis of the ankle ➡ and subtalar ➡ joints. The foot musculature ➡ is normal.

MUSCLE ATROPHY

(Left) Coronal T1WI MR shows bilateral gluteus minimus muscle atrophy ➡ due to bilateral gluteus minimus tendon tears. This is a relatively common injury in older patients that can cause chronic pain. *(Right)* Axial T1WI MR shows chronic atrophy ➡ of the left flexor hallucis longus muscle demonstrated by high signal fat interdigitating with the muscle fibers. The tendon was normal suggesting a nerve branch injury as the etiology.

Tendon, Injury

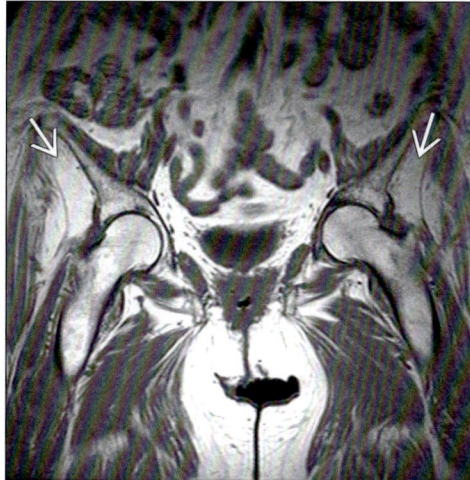

Peripheral Nerve Injury

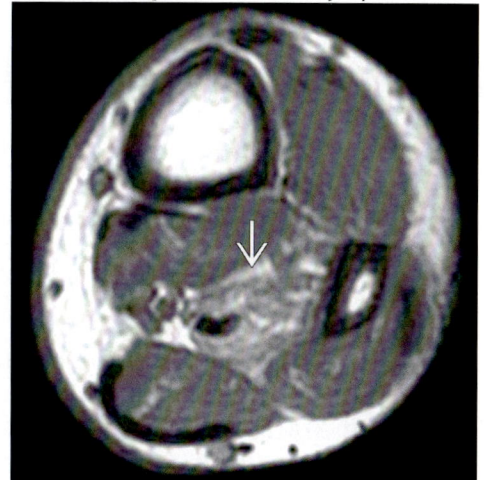

(Left) Axial T1WI MR shows the sequelae of quadrilateral space syndrome with disproportionate fatty atrophy ➡ of the teres minor muscle without tendon tear. The adjacent infraspinatus muscle ➡ is normal. *(Right)* Coronal T1WI MR shows enlarged medial ➡ and lateral ➡ plantar branches of the posterior tibial nerve. Muscle atrophy ➡ is present. Nerve entrapment in this case is probably due to scarring and thickening of the retinaculum ➡.

Peripheral Nerve Injury

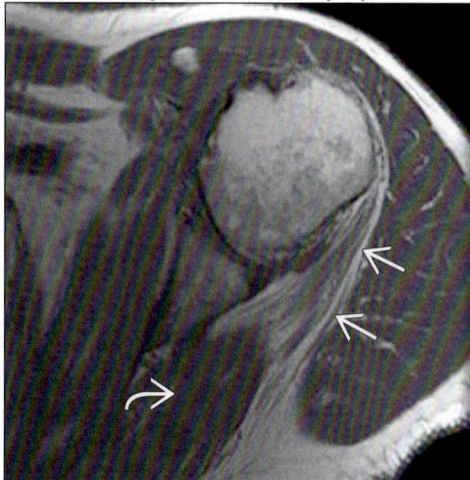

Peripheral Nerve Injury

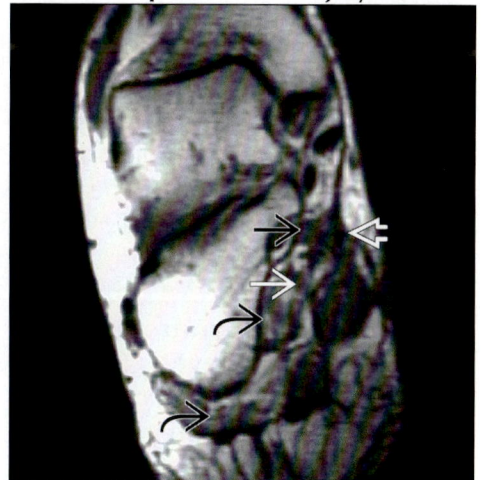

(Left) Axial T1WI MR shows mild fat atrophy ➡ in the supinator muscle, a sign of denervation of the radial nerve. This is consistent with a high radial neuropathy likely related to remote trauma. The other muscles demonstrate normal bulk and signal. *(Right)* Sagittal T1WI MR shows prominent fatty atrophy involving the calf muscles ➡ and, less prominently, the foot muscles ➡. A combination of neuropathy and disuse are likely etiologies in this diabetic patient.

Peripheral Nerve Injury

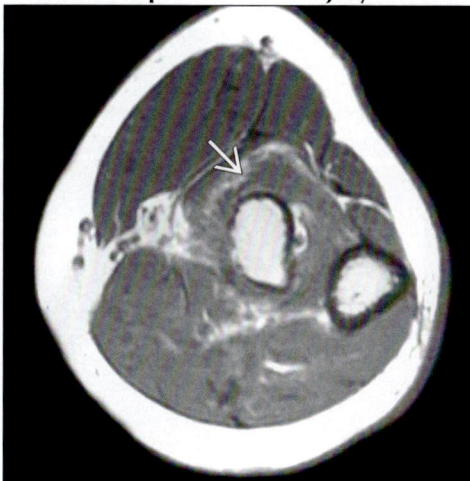

Diabetes: MSK Complications

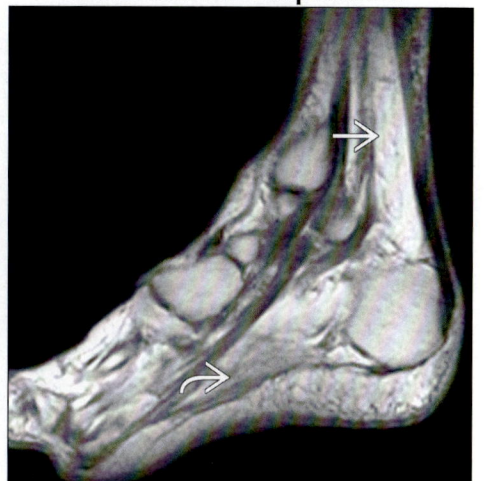

MUSCLE ATROPHY

Muscle Injury

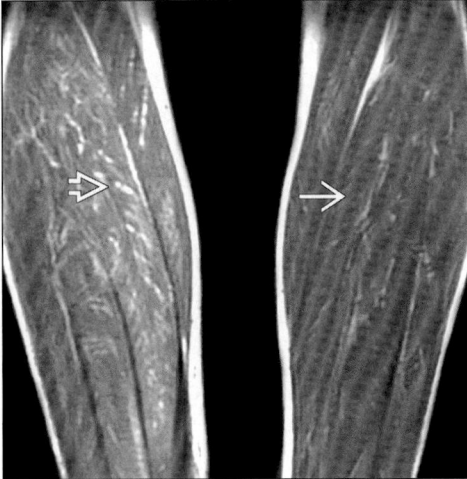

Neurofibromatosis

(Left) Coronal T1WI MR shows fatty infiltration ⇨ of the right calf musculature due to subacute gastrocnemius soleus strain. Compare the pattern of "marbling" seen in the normal left leg ➡ with the abnormal right leg. *(Right)* Axial T1WI MR shows marked fatty atrophy ➡ of posterior calf muscles in a patient with neurofibromatosis and multiple prior thigh surgeries. Peripheral neuropathy and post-operative changes likely contribute to atrophy.

Muscular Dystrophy

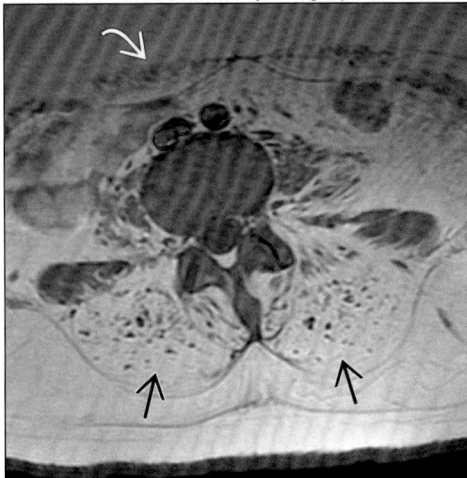

Muscular Dystrophy

(Left) Axial T1WI MR shows marked atrophy of all visualized muscles, including the paraspinal muscles ➡ and abdominal wall ➡, with extensive fatty infiltration. This is caused by muscular dystrophy. *(Right)* Sagittal PD FSE MR shows severe fatty replacement of the majority of the muscles about the knee, typical of muscular dystrophy. The atrophy is not uniform; the vastus medialis ➡ and semimembranosus ➡ muscles show some residual muscle fibers.

Meningomyelocele

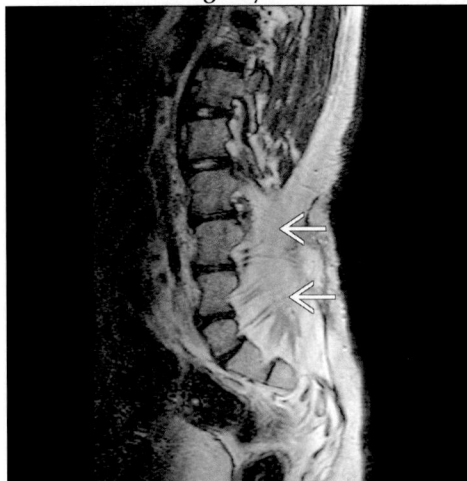

Polio

(Left) Sagittal T2WI MR shows profound chronic fatty atrophy ➡ of the paraspinal muscles in a patient with a repaired meningomyelocele. The atrophy is due to severe chronic denervation. *(Right)* Axial T2WI MR of both thighs shows near complete replacement of the right thigh musculature with hyperintense fat ➡. The appearance of the left thigh ➡ is normal. Chronic denervation and atrophy of the right thigh is due to a remote history of polio.

INTERMUSCULAR EDEMA

DIFFERENTIAL DIAGNOSIS

Common
- Trauma
- Intramuscular Injection
- Venous Insufficiency
- Popliteal Cyst, Rupture
- Tendon Tear
- Bursitis
- Deep Venous Thrombosis

Less Common
- Soft Tissue Abscess
- Syndesmosis Sprain
- Infectious Myositis
- Polymyositis/Dermatomyositis
- Soft Tissue or Bone Neoplasm
- Radiation-Induced Non-Neoplastic Soft Tissue Abnormalities
- Complications of Iodinated Contrast
- Diabetes: MSK Complications
- Compartment Syndrome

Rare but Important
- Necrotizing Fasciitis
- Nephrogenic Systemic Fibrosis

ESSENTIAL INFORMATION

Key Differential Diagnosis Issues
- Look for an underlying cause and evaluate for pertinent history to differentiate similar appearing etiologies
- Intermuscular and intramuscular edema often coexist

Helpful Clues for Common Diagnoses
- **Trauma**
  - Edema and hemorrhage tracks along facial planes from injury site
  - Intermuscular edema can be located proximal, distal and at the injury site
  - Edema associated with fracture is obvious
  - Injury with hematoma may simulate neoplasm especially if injury is not remembered by patient
    - Necessitates follow-up to exclude hemorrhagic malignancy
- **Intramuscular Injection**
  - Commonly has linear edema extending from skin surface due to needle tract
  - Medication will diffuse within muscle and along fascial planes

- **Venous Insufficiency**
  - Best diagnosed with ultrasound examination
    - Venous flow reversal, enlarged deep to superficial perforating vessels
  - Range of soft tissue changes from mild subcutaneous edema to soft tissue ulceration
- **Popliteal Cyst, Rupture**
  - Classic location of popliteal cyst between medial head of gastrocnemius and semimembranosus in popliteal fossa
  - Ruptured fluid may track proximally and distally in leg
  - Symptomatic and often associated with underlying knee pathology
  - **Hint:** If the fluid is not contiguous with a popliteal cyst, evaluate for venous thrombosis
- **Tendon Tear**
  - Inflammatory fluid from tendon tear tracks along the fascial planes of the associated and surrounding muscles
- **Bursitis**
  - Fluid in unexpected areas may still represent an obscure or pseudo-bursa
  - Fluid extends along fascial planes from location of bursa when ruptured
- **Deep Venous Thrombosis**
  - Marked edema within and between muscles and soft tissues
  - Can produce pain and be clinically unsuspected
  - May involve dominant deep venous structure or intramuscular plexus
    - Examine vessels for lack of ↑ T2 signal
    - Peripheral enhancement of thrombus

Helpful Clues for Less Common Diagnoses
- **Soft Tissue Abscess**
  - Thick, enhancing rind of tissue around abscess
    - Surrounding inflammatory fluid may track beyond extent of infection
    - Central, nonenhancing necrotic center
- **Syndesmosis Sprain**
  - Tear or partial tear of ankle syndesmotic ligaments
    - Anterior and posterior tibiofibular ligaments, transverse tibiofibular ligament, interosseous membrane
  - Widened tibiofibular space (diastasis)

INTERMUSCULAR EDEMA

- **Infectious Myositis**
  - Intramuscular and intermuscular edema with a nonspecific appearance
  - Wide range of etiologies produces a wide range of severity
    - Viral, bacterial, fungal, parasitic
- **Polymyositis/Dermatomyositis**
  - Abnormal muscle & subcutaneous fat from inflammation, edema & calcification
  - Typical sheet-like involvement of muscles and subcutaneous tissues with calcification evident on radiographs/CT
- **Soft Tissue or Bone Neoplasm**
  - Any bone or soft tissue malignancy may induce an inflammatory response, with adjacent edema in soft tissues
- **Radiation-Induced Non-Neoplastic Soft Tissue Abnormalities**
  - High T2 signal involving soft tissues in region of radiation therapy
  - Lack of enhancement and non mass-like appearance differentiates from residual or recurrent tumor
- **Complications of Iodinated Contrast**
  - Extravasation of IV contrast material into soft tissues is almost always apparent at time of imaging
  - Instruct patient to report signs of persistent or increasing pain, skin blistering, numbness, tingling, or increased swelling → surgical consult
- **Diabetes: MSK Complications**
  - Muscle ischemia and infarction due to diabetes is uncommon

- Low T1 and high T2 signal edema is present within and between muscles
- Enhancement is present with muscle ischemia and absent with infarction
- Commonly bilateral & involving thighs
- Difficult to differentiate from traumatic, infectious or inflammatory muscle conditions on imaging alone
- **Compartment Syndrome**
  - High T2 signal and enlargement of all muscles in compartment
  - Lower extremity (calf, foot) most commonly involved
  - Muscle herniation may be present
  - Findings necessitate clinical measurement of compartment pressures

Helpful Clues for Rare Diagnoses
- **Necrotizing Fasciitis**
  - Gas tracking along fascial planes is classic
  - Thickened deep and superficial fascia
  - Fascial enhancement is patchy or uniform
  - Is a clinical diagnosis, although imaging can be suggestive
- **Nephrogenic Systemic Fibrosis**
  - Low T1 and high T2 signal in skeletal muscle, intermuscular fascia and skin
  - Correlate with history of relatively recent gadodiamide administration (within 3 months) and renal insufficiency
  - Similar appearance to polymyositis
  - Severe muscle swelling can mimic necrotizing fasciitis

Trauma

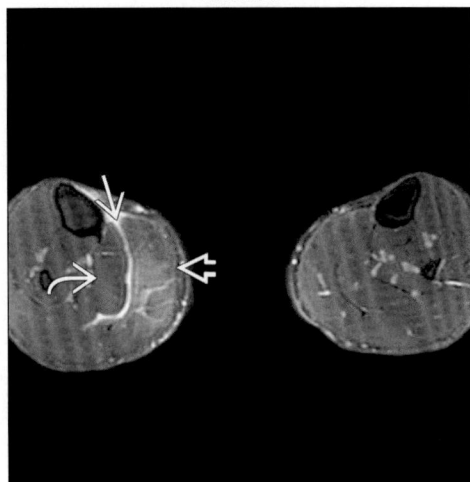

Axial STIR MR shows edema along the deep fascial plane ➡ and within the fibers of the medial head of the gastrocnemius ➤ muscle. The soleus muscle ➤ is normal. This is a grade I gastrocnemius muscle strain.

Popliteal Cyst, Rupture

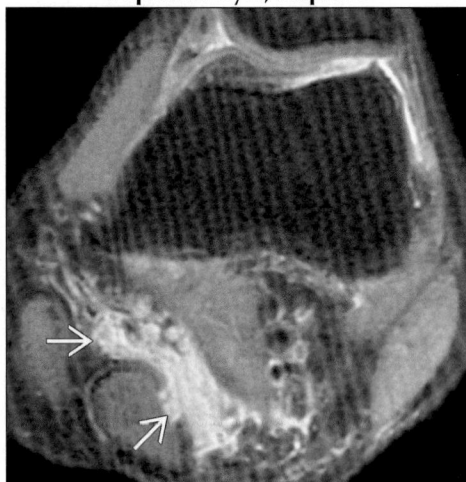

Axial PD FSE FS MR shows high signal edema ➡ dissecting through the popliteal fossa soft tissues. Note that there is not a mass-like configuration. This fluid merged distally with a classic popliteal cyst.

INTERMUSCULAR EDEMA

Tendon Tear

Bursitis

(Left) Axial T2WI FS MR shows intermuscular edema ➡ and a hematoma ⇒ in the posterior calf due to plantaris tendon rupture. Increased signal within the medial head of the gastrocnemius muscle is due to partial thickness tearing ➡. *(Right)* Axial T2WI FS MR shows a distended bicipital radial bursa ➡ arising between the radius ⇒ and biceps tendon ➡. The biceps have changes of tendinosis with mild surrounding soft tissue edema ➡.

Deep Venous Thrombosis

Soft Tissue Abscess

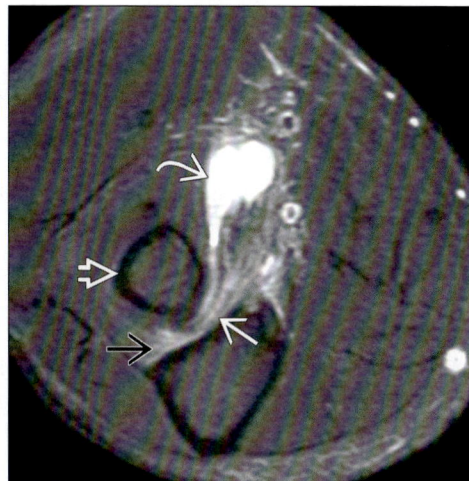

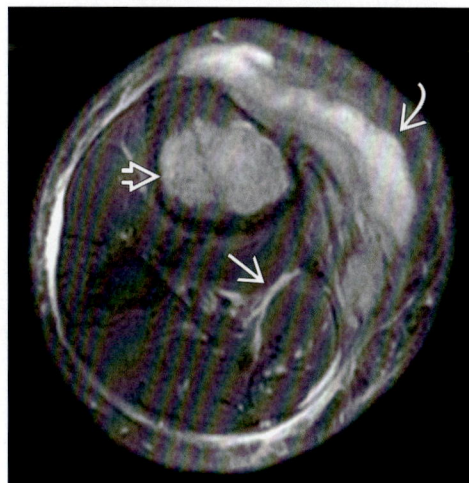

(Left) Axial T2WI FS MR shows edema ➡ in the musculature surrounding the left hip. Deep venous thrombosis ⇒ is seen as low T2 signal intensity in the vessel and has caused edema throughout the adjacent musculature. The thrombosis extended from the common iliac artery to the common femoral artery. *(Right)* Axial T2WI FS MR shows intermuscular edema ➡ due to a soft tissue abscess ➡ and osteomyelitis ⇒. The infecting agent was mycobacterium tuberculosis.

Syndesmosis Sprain

Polymyositis/Dermatomyositis

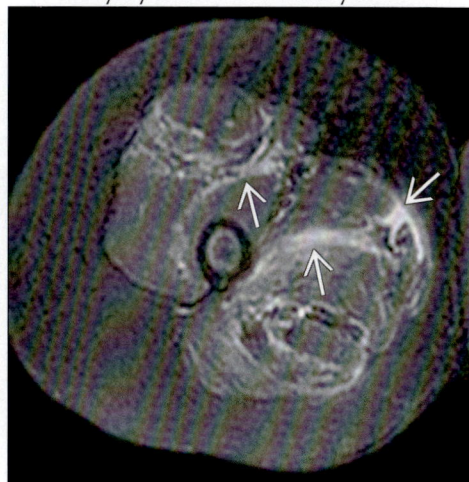

(Left) Coronal STIR MR shows disruption of the ankle syndesmosis, including not only the anterior tibiofibular ligament but also the interosseous membrane ➡. There was extensive surrounding edema ➡ in the subcutaneous fat and between the muscles, without evidence of a fracture. *(Right)* Axial T2WI FS MR shows high T2 signal from edema ➡ both in and around the thigh muscles in a dermatomyositis patient. CT showed these areas to be partially calcified.

INTERMUSCULAR EDEMA

Soft Tissue or Bone Neoplasm

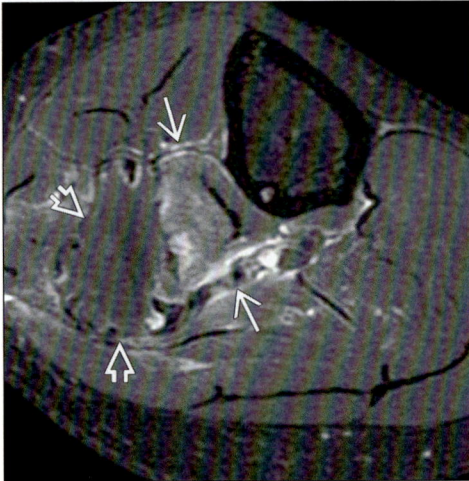

Radiation-Induced Non-Neoplastic Soft Tissue Abnormalities

(Left) Axial T2WI FS MR shows a low signal mass ⇨ expanding the proximal fibula, with edema ➡ tracking between the adjacent muscles. This was a desmoplastic fibroma but any neoplasm may incite inflammatory fluid. (Right) Axial T2WI FS MR shows intermuscular edema ⇨ in the posterior thigh. The patient had a prior medial thigh sarcoma resection that was treated with radiation. Lack of enhancement made recurrence or metastasis unlikely.

Complications of Iodinated Contrast

Diabetes: MSK Complications

(Left) Axial T2WI FS MR shows increased signal ⇨ in the soft tissues adjacent to the extensor pollicis brevis tendon ➡. This could be mistaken for de Quervain tenosynovitis, but corresponding high T1 signal confirmed contrast infiltration into the soft tissues. (Right) Axial T2WI FS MR shows bilateral intra- ⇨ and inter- ⇨ muscular edema in this diabetic patient. Lack of enhancement in the affected muscles suggests muscle ischemia or myonecrosis.

Compartment Syndrome

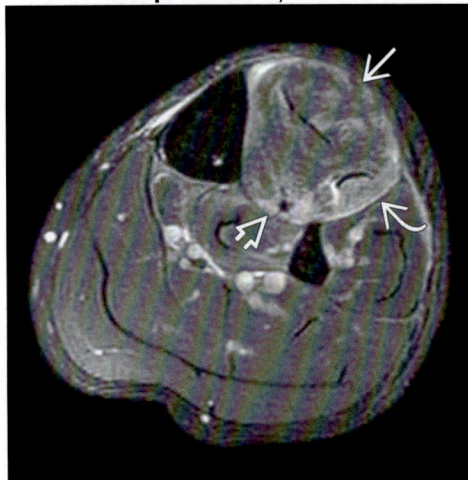

Necrotizing Fasciitis

(Left) Axial T2WI FS MR shows edema and swelling of the anterior compartment ⇨ with adjacent intermuscular edema ➡. The bowed interosseous membrane ⇨ compromises neurovascular structures. (Right) Sagittal STIR MR shows edema ⇨ extending along the gastrocnemius muscle. The longitudinal distribution of the collection suggests fasciitis and a more rounded posterior fluid collection ⇨ had a thin enhancing rim suggesting abscess.

TENOSYNOVITIS/TENOSYNOVIAL FLUID

DIFFERENTIAL DIAGNOSIS

Common
- Normal Variant
- Tendon, Injury
- Arthritis

Less Common
- Repetitive Trauma
- Infection
- Iatrogenic

Rare but Important
- Giant Cell Tumor, Tendon Sheath
- Synovial Osteochondromatosis
- Fibroma of Tendon Sheath

ESSENTIAL INFORMATION

Key Differential Diagnosis Issues
- All tendons covered by sheath except Achilles tendon
- Evaluate by X-ray, ultrasound, CT or MR
- Stenosing tenosynovitis: Adhesions restrict tendon & fluid motion in sheath

Helpful Clues for Common Diagnoses
- **Normal Variant**
  - A small amount of fluid is normal
  - Tendons communicating with joint may have sheath fluid reflecting joint effusion (e.g., long head biceps & shoulder joint or flexor hallucis longus and tibiotalar joint)
- **Tendon, Injury**
  - Look for tendon thickening, thinning or complete disruption

- Sheath fluid without synovial thickening
- **Arthritis**
  - Most common: Inflammatory (RA), crystalline (gout) or seronegative
  - Look for associated arthropathy features (e.g., erosions, osteophytes, osteopenia)

Helpful Clues for Less Common Diagnoses
- **Repetitive Trauma**
  - Variable sheath fluid; ± normal tendon
  - Correlate with mechanism of injury (e.g., FHL in ballet dancers)
- **Infection**
  - Pyogenic, fungal or tuberculous
  - Look for co-existing medical problems, immunocompromise, etc.
  - Extensive fluid, often in multiple sheaths & joints; thick enhancing synovium
- **Iatrogenic**
  - History of recent injection, or prior surgery which may result in tenosynovitis

Helpful Clues for Rare Diagnoses
- **Giant Cell Tumor, Tendon Sheath**
  - Multiple heterogeneous nodules; variable enhancement; normal tendon; fluid rare
  - Hemosiderin may cause GRE "blooming"
- **Synovial Osteochondromatosis**
  - Extensive sheath fluid with multiple small ovoid bodies
- **Fibroma of Tendon Sheath**
  - Ovoid hypodense enhancing intrasheath mass < 2.5 cm; fluid rare
  - Mild adjacent osseous erosion

Normal Variant

Sagittal PD FSE FS MR shows a small amount of fluid in the flexor hallucis longus tendon sheath ➡. This is normal. Note the intimate relationship with the tibiotalar joint ➡.

Tendon, Injury

Axial T2WI FS MR shows a complete tear of the posterior tibial tendon with associated tenosynovitis ➡. The adjacent FDL ➡ & FHL ➡ tendons & sheaths are normal.

TENOSYNOVITIS/TENOSYNOVIAL FLUID

Arthritis

Repetitive Trauma

(Left) Axial PD FSE FS MR shows thickened extensor tendon sheaths with extensive synovial pannus ⊳ & a small tendon sheath effusion (hyperintense rim) ➔ in 30 year old female with rheumatoid arthritis. *(Right)* Sagittal PD FSE FS MR shows tenosynovitis in a 10 year old ballerina learning to dance on toe. The FHL is normal but surrounded by fluid which is restricted behind the talus resulting in stenosing tenosynovitis.

Infection

Iatrogenic

(Left) Axial STIR MR shows fluid ➔ in flexor tendon sheaths, ECU & distal radioulnar joint with synovial pannus & debris ➔ in this steroid dependent woman infected with Mycobacterium marinum. *(Right)* Coronal STIR MR shows ulnar "mass" which is the ECU ➔ tendon sheath filled with fluid and debris ➔ related to wrist arthroplasty failure ➔ & foreign body reaction.

Giant Cell Tumor, Tendon Sheath

Synovial Osteochondromatosis

(Left) Oblique T2WI MR shows hypodense, multinodular mass ➔ eroding the 1st MCP ➔. It encases the flexor tendon & enhances moderately (not shown), representing giant cell tumor of tendon sheath. *(Right)* Sagittal T1 C+ FS MR shows popliteus tendon sheath ➔ involvement in this multinodular process. Minimal enhancement in & around multiple small bodies ➔ (seen as punctate bodies on radiograph), represents synovial osteochondromatosis.

ENLARGED PERIPHERAL NERVES

DIFFERENTIAL DIAGNOSIS

Common
- Neurofibromatosis
- Tunnel Syndromes (Carpal, Ulnar, Tarsal)
- Trauma
- Morton Neuroma
- Traumatic Neuroma
- Benign Peripheral Nerve Sheath Tumor (Benign PNST)
- Malignant Peripheral Nerve Sheath Tumor (MPNST)

Less Common
- Lipomatosis, Nerve (Fibrolipomatous Hamartoma)
- Macrodystrophia Lipomatosa
- Charcot Marie Tooth

Rare but Important
- Cystic Lymphangioma (Mimic)
- Neurogenic Sarcoma
- Perineurioma, Intraneural
- Acromegaly

ESSENTIAL INFORMATION

Key Differential Diagnosis Issues
- Anatomy & morphology should alert you to neural origin of these lesions
  - Any lesion in or adjacent to a neurovascular bundle should make a neural lesion a consideration
  - **Hint**: Neural lesions tend to be elongated, or oval/teardrop-shaped
  - **Hint**: The associated nerve is often seen entering or exiting lesion
  - **Hint**: "Target" sign should raise suspicion for tumor of neurogenic origin
    - Target seen as low signal centrally surrounded by high SI on T2 imaging
    - Target highly suggestive of neural tumor, but not exclusive to this type of lesion
    - Target sign originally described in neurofibroma
    - Target sign may be seen in neurofibroma, schwannoma, or MPNST; not specific
  - **Hint**: Watch for associated muscle abnormalities (know innervation patterns)
    - Denervation hypertrophy
    - Muscle atrophy
    - Hyperintense muscle

- Clinical symptoms should alert you to possibility of nerve mass or disturbance
  - "Shocking" sensation is elicited when a neurogenic tumor is tapped
  - Similar sensation is found with entrapped nerves (signs elicited for tunnel syndromes)
  - Percutaneous biopsy of a neurogenic tumor is exquisitely painful
- Hints for MR imaging of nerves "neurograms"
  - T1 without fat-saturation is extremely helpful in locating the course of the nerve
    - Perform at least one T1 sequence without fat-saturation; axial often most useful
  - Fluid sensitive sequences are useful in identifying enlargement and/or hyperintensity of nerve
  - Post-contrast imaging is useful in identifying an irritated nerve; normal nerves do not enhance
  - Imaging planes deserve attention; choose plane that will best follow the course of nerve of interest
    - Sciatic nerve with reference to piriformis: Sagittal plane especially useful
    - Sciatic nerve roots: Angled coronal of sacrum shows all nerve roots
    - Nerves following a curved course around a joint (e.g., peroneal around fibular neck or ulnar through ulnar tunnel of elbow): Axial plane may be most useful

Helpful Clues for Common Diagnoses
- **Neurofibromatosis**
  - Generalized longitudinal enlargement of nerve fascicles may be seen
  - Any nerve may be involved
  - May have additional "beaded" appearance due to focal neurofibromas
- **Tunnel Syndromes (Carpal, Ulnar, Tarsal)**
  - Tunnels with transiting nerves, restricted by retinacula, are at risk
  - Nerves may be compressed by lipoma, ganglion cyst, displaced fractures most frequently
    - Nerves usually are compressed but less frequently may be enlarged, hyperintense, and enhance with contrast
- **Trauma**
  - Direct trauma may transect nerve

- If not transected, nerve may swell & become hyperintense
- **Morton Neuroma**
  - Perineural fibrosis causes enlargement of interdigital nerve
  - 2nd & 3rd intertarsal spaces most common; short axis (coronal) imaging shows best; prone positioning may help
  - Teardrop-shaped, location specific; low signal on T1 with surrounding fat
  - Slightly hyperintense on T2, enhances intensely
- **Traumatic Neuroma**
  - Focal enlargement of nerve at site of trauma
  - Hypointense rim on T2 images is frequently seen
- **Benign Peripheral Nerve Sheath Tumor (Benign PNST)**
  - Intimately involved with nerve; tends to be elongated with nerve seen entering or exiting mass
  - Often shows target sign on T2 sequence
  - Size helps differentiate malignant from benign; other features not helpful

Helpful Clues for Less Common Diagnoses
- **Lipomatosis, Nerve (Fibrolipomatous Hamartoma)**
  - Median nerve most frequently involved; radial & ulnar nerve involvement have been reported
  - With median nerve involvement, presents with carpal tunnel symptoms & volar mass

- Some degree of macrodactyly is present in 2/3 of patients
- MR is characteristic & pathognomonic
  - Cable-like longitudinal configuration of enlarged nerve fascicles within surrounding fatty stroma
  - Each fascicle is enlarged to approximately 2-3 mm due to perineural fibrosis
  - Fascicles are low signal on all sequences; surrounding stroma follows fat signal on all sequences
- **Macrodystrophia Lipomatosa**
  - Localized giantism, particularly involving a portion of the hand or foot
  - Adjacent digits involved, generally following the distribution of a nerve
  - All mesenchymal elements are involved
    - Bones & soft tissue proportionately ↑
    - Lipomatous hypertrophy predominates
    - Involved nerve may show focal ↑ in size
- **Charcot Marie Tooth**
  - Denervation edema, hyperintense & enlarged nerve

Helpful Clues for Rare Diagnoses
- **Cystic Lymphangioma (Mimic)**
  - Single or multiple cystic masses, may mimic adjacent nerve enlargement
  - Cystic nature is demonstrated by lack of contrast-enhancement
  - Normal nerve (in size and signal characteristics) seen adjacent; may be compressed and develop symptoms

Neurofibromatosis

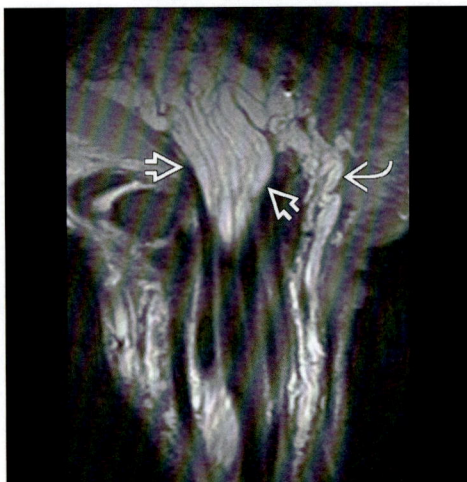

Coronal PD FSE FS MR shows massive enlargement of the fascicles of the median nerve ➡ and ulnar nerve ➡, seen in a patient with neurofibromatosis.

Tunnel Syndromes (Carpal, Ulnar, Tarsal)

Coronal PD FS MR shows hyperintensity of an enlarged posterior tibial nerve ➡. There is atrophy of quadratus plantae & abductor digiti minimi ➡. This patient had an unsuccessful tarsal tunnel release 1 year prior.

ENLARGED PERIPHERAL NERVES

(Left) Coronal STIR MR shows thickening of the posterior cord of the brachial plexus ➡. This resulted from direct trauma; the patient had a luxatio erecta (inferior) shoulder dislocation 4 weeks earlier. *(Right)* Coronal T1WI FS MR reveals a teardrop-shaped, intensely enhancing, plantar mass ➡ arising between the 2nd and 3rd MT heads. Altered weight-bearing, related to a silicone implant in the 1st MT ➡, likely contributed to the development of the neuroma.

Trauma

Morton Neuroma

(Left) Axial T1WI MR shows a significantly enlarged sural nerve ➡ located in the posterior subcutaneous tissues of the leg. A marker ➡ was placed at the site where pressure elicits an exquisitely painful shocking sensation. *(Right)* Axial T1WI MR shows a more proximal cut in the same patient as previous image. At this level, the sural nerve ➡ is only slightly enlarged. Note its relationship to the lesser saphenous vein ➡. This patient sustained a blow to the region 6 months earlier.

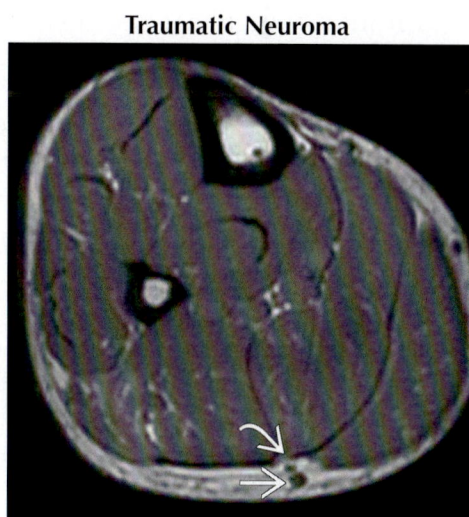

Traumatic Neuroma

Traumatic Neuroma

(Left) Coronal T1WI MR shows a mass in the location of peroneal nerve ➡, with nerve extending distally from it ➡. Mass deviates the gastrocnemius ➡. By location & appearance, this is a benign PNST. *(Right)* Coronal T2WI FS MR shows a large, inhomogeneous mass in the posterior thigh ➡, which proved to be a MPNST of the sciatic nerve. Note the enlargement and nodularity of the proximal & distal nerves, representing multiple neurofibromas ➡. (†MSK Req).

Benign Peripheral Nerve Sheath Tumor (Benign PNST)

Malignant Peripheral Nerve Sheath Tumor (MPNST)

Malignant Peripheral Nerve Sheath Tumor (MPNST)

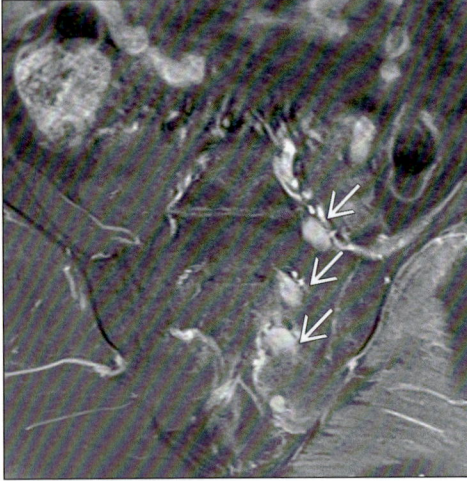

Lipomatosis, Nerve (Fibrolipomatous Hamartoma)

(Left) Coronal oblique T1 C+ FS MR shows enhancement & enlargement of multiple sacral nerve roots ➡ in a patient who had a sciatic MPNST resected 6 months earlier. This represents recurrence extending proximally up all the contributing nerve roots. *(Right)* Axial T1WI MR shows mild enlargement of the individual fascicles of the median nerve ➡, with surrounding lipomatous stroma. The mass displaces the flexor tendons ➡. The appearance is typical.

Macrodystrophia Lipomatosa

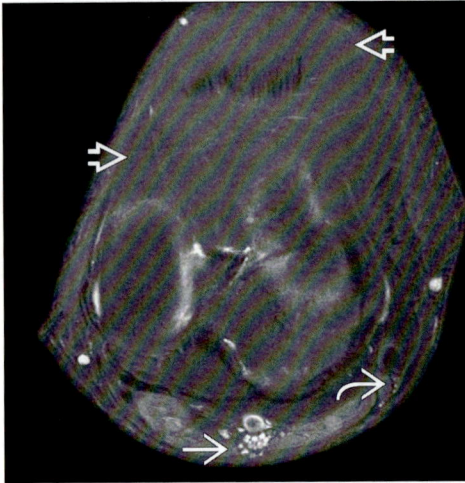

Charcot Marie Tooth

(Left) Axial T2WI FS MR shows tremendous lipomatous overgrowth both intra- and extra-articularly ➡. There is hyperintensity and enlargement of fascicles in the tibial ➡ and peroneal nerves ➡, all typical of macrodystrophia lipomatosa. *(Right)* Axial PD FSE FS MR shows enlargement of the tibial nerve ➡, as well as denervation edema of the muscles of the posterior compartment of the leg. The patient had a cavus foot deformity, typical of Charcot Marie Tooth.

Cystic Lymphangioma (Mimic)

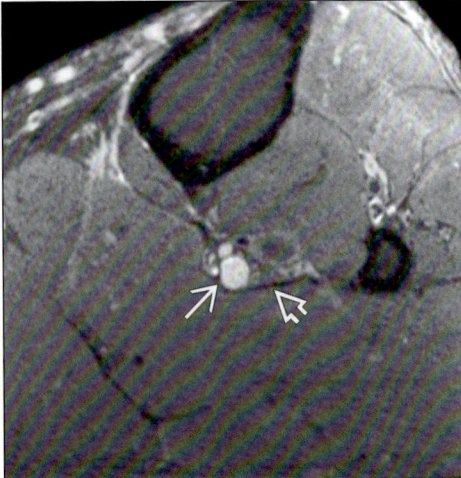

Neurogenic Sarcoma

(Left) Axial STIR MR shows multiple perineural cysts ➡ located adjacent to the tibial nerve ➡, which itself is normal in size. The cysts did not enhance, proving their cystic nature, and their mimicking of tibial nerve enlargement. *(Right)* Axial T1WI MR shows a tubular subcutaneous mass ➡, deviating the flexor tendons, which proved to be quite elongated. It became invasive at one point. This is an example of a rare lesion, neurogenic sarcoma.

189

INTRAARTICULAR LOW SIGNAL MATERIAL, ALL SEQUENCES

DIFFERENTIAL DIAGNOSIS

Common
- Metallic Foreign Bodies
- Loose Bodies
- Synovitis
- Gout
- Silastic Implant
- Synovial Osteochondromatosis
- Pigmented Villonodular Synovitis (PVNS)
- Intraarticular Gas

Less Common
- Hemophilic Arthropathy
- Nodular Synovitis
- Amyloid Deposition

ESSENTIAL INFORMATION

Key Differential Diagnosis Issues
- Clinical information may be useful
  - Monoarticular vs. pauciarticular vs. polyarticular process
    - Of those entities listed, synovitis is the most likely to be polyarticular (inflammatory arthropathies)
    - Of those entities listed, gout, hemophilic arthropathy, and amyloid deposition are most likely to be pauciarticular
    - Of those entities listed, loose bodies, synovial osteochondromatosis, PVNS, & nodular synovitis are most likely to be monoarticular
- Consider adding a gradient echo sequence if suspect an entity which would show blooming (PVNS, hemophilic arthropathy)

Helpful Clues for Common Diagnoses
- **Metallic Foreign Bodies**
  - Depending on composition, may show susceptibility artifact
  - Some metal, particularly titanium, is visualized without distorting artifact
- **Loose Bodies**
  - If an osteochondral body is secondary to delamination, it may be oblong & curvilinear in shape, matching the defect (often a convex surface)
  - Long-standing loose bodies tend to be more round or oval in shape
  - MR signal reflects composition of body
    - Cortical bone is low signal on all sequences
    - Cortical bone with attached cartilage shows a stripe of low signal (cortex) associated with a stripe of slightly higher signal (cartilage)
    - Mature loose body with trabeculae follows normal bone signal, high on T1 and low with fat suppression
- **Synovitis**
  - Inflammatory arthritic cases usually polyarticular
  - Small innumerable nodular masses lining the entire synovium of joint
  - Low signal nodularity is outlined well by high signal effusion on T2 sequences
  - Synovium often thick, showing uniform enhancement
- **Gout**
  - Monoarticular or pauciarticular
  - May be juxtaarticular as well as intraarticular
  - Frequent associated erosions; may have soft tissue tophi which mimic the intraarticular deposition signal characteristics
  - T2 sequences often have admixed low and high signal, varying according to amount of density of sodium urate deposition
  - Enhances with contrast, also with varying regions of low signal, depending on amount of density of sodium urate deposition
  - At-risk population: Elderly males, Polynesians, patients with underlying disease with rapid metabolic turnover (end stage renal disease, multiple myeloma)
- **Silastic Implant**
  - Implant is low signal on all sequences, often surrounded by synovitis
- **Synovial Osteochondromatosis**
  - Bodies show varying MR signal, depending on size, maturity, & composition
    - Cartilaginous bodies have different characteristics than osseous bodies
    - Small immature osseous bodies have different characteristics than larger mature bodies, which follow the signal of normal bone on all sequences
  - May present as conglomerate mass, rarely extending into adjacent soft tissues
    - Soft tissue extension, though rare, may be highly invasive

INTRAARTICULAR LOW SIGNAL MATERIAL, ALL SEQUENCES

- **Pigmented Villonodular Synovitis (PVNS)**
  - Nodular deposits may be scattered throughout joint, or focally conglomerate
  - Deposits may escape through capsular perforations to extraarticular locations
  - May cause large erosions & cysts
  - Low signal on T1, varying low to high signal on T2
  - Generally enhances significantly
  - Iron deposition in synovium results in "blooming" on gradient echo imaging
- **Intraarticular Gas**
  - Non-dependent portions of joint
  - Low signal on all sequences, blooms on gradient echo
  - Generally small round bubbles; larger amount may conform to shape of confining articular tissues

Helpful Clues for Less Common Diagnoses
- **Hemophilic Arthropathy**
  - Iron deposition from repeated bleeds results in low signal synovium which blooms on gradient echo
  - May have mixed low & high signal on T2 and post-contrast due to synovitis
- **Nodular Synovitis**
  - Same signal characteristics as generalized synovitis or PVNS
  - Nodular pattern, most frequently located in Hoffa fat pad
- **Amyloid Deposition**
  - Low signal deposition in bone, tendon, or synovium

- May have some high signal components on T2 and post-contrast
- Primary or secondary (particularly in end stage renal disease or myeloma)

Alternative Differential Approaches
- Intraarticular low signal masses, all sequences (without exception)
  - Metallic Foreign Bodies or silastic implants
  - Intraarticular Gas
- Intraarticular masses which are usually low signal, but which have exceptions or might show regions of high signal on fluid sensitive sequences or with contrast
  - Loose Bodies: Signal depends on composition
  - Synovitis: Enhances with contrast
  - Gout: May have high signal areas mixed with low signal on T2; enhances
  - Synovial Osteochondromatosis: Signal of bodies depends on composition (mature bone versus cartilage)
  - Pigmented Villonodular Synovitis: Mixed low and high T2 signal, usually enhances
  - Hemophilic Arthropathy: Usually deposits are low signal on all sequences; may enhance if synovitis is active
  - Nodular Synovitis: Mixed T2 SI, enhances
  - Amyloid Deposition: Synovitis enhances
- Processes which "bloom" on gradient echo
  - Metallic Foreign Bodies
  - Pigmented Villonodular Synovitis (PVNS)
  - Intraarticular Gas
  - Hemophilic Arthropathy

Metallic Foreign Bodies

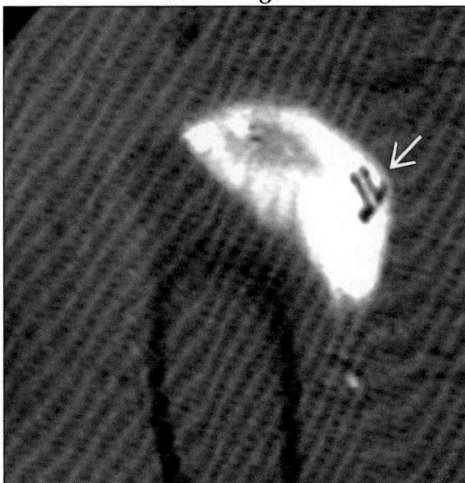

Coronal oblique MR arthrogram T1WI FS shows a screw (with hollow core) located posteriorly in the shoulder joint ➡. This screw is metallic, and is low signal on all sequences.

Metallic Foreign Bodies

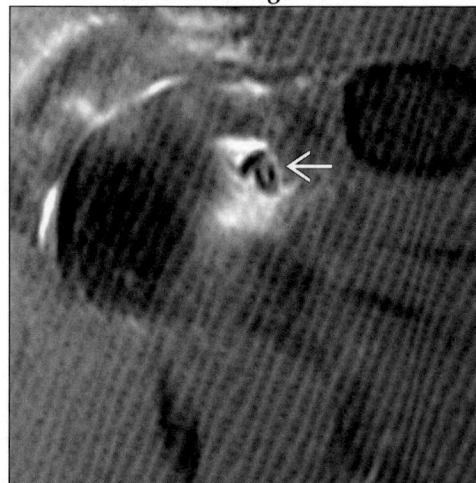

Coronal oblique T2WI FS MR shows a loose screw located far anteriorly within the joint ➡ following capsular repair. The screw is low signal, with fluid entering its hollow center.

INTRAARTICULAR LOW SIGNAL MATERIAL, ALL SEQUENCES

(Left) Coronal oblique T2WI FS MR shows a large loose body floating in the knee effusion ➡. The body has a strip of very low signal and another of moderately low signal, representing the cortex and cartilage, respectively. **(Right)** Sagittal T2WI FS MR shows diffuse nodularity of the synovium ➡, which remains low signal on all sequences, though it may enhance. This patient has rheumatoid arthritis.

Loose Bodies

Synovitis

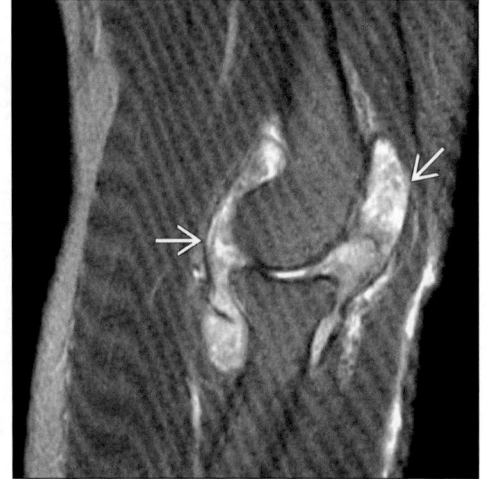

(Left) Sagittal T1WI MR shows a low signal intraarticular mass surrounding & distal to the medial malleolus ➡. The appearance is nonspecific on T1 imaging but was also low signal on T2 & proved to be gout. **(Right)** Sagittal T1 C+ FS MR shows a silastic implant placed in the subtalar joint ➡, surrounded by synovitis. This was placed several years earlier for coalition. The implant is low signal on all sequences.

Gout

Silastic Implant

(Left) Coronal T1WI MR shows a large fluid collection within the subdeltoid bursa ➡ which appears to contain many tiny low signal bodies. Radiograph was normal. **(Right)** Coronal T2WI FS MR (same case as previous image) confirms the multiple low signal bodies, & the diagnosis of synovial chondromatosis. In this case, the bodies remained low signal on all sequences. In other cases, they may acquire other signal, depending on how much cartilage/bone they contain.

Synovial Osteochondromatosis

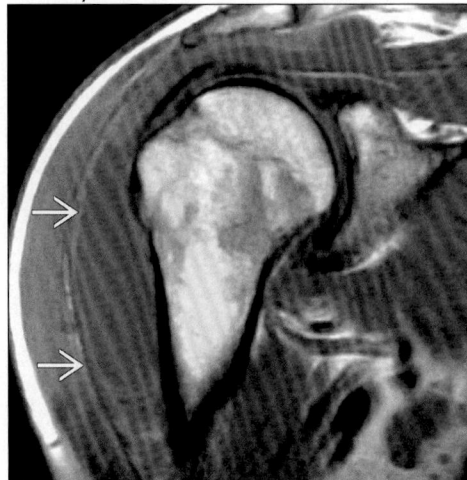

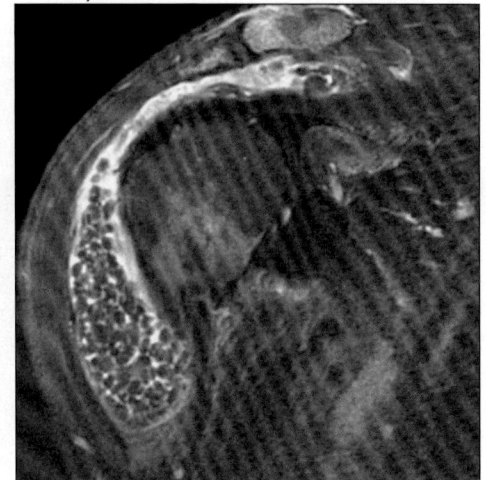

Synovial Osteochondromatosis

INTRAARTICULAR LOW SIGNAL MATERIAL, ALL SEQUENCES

Pigmented Villonodular Synovitis (PVNS)

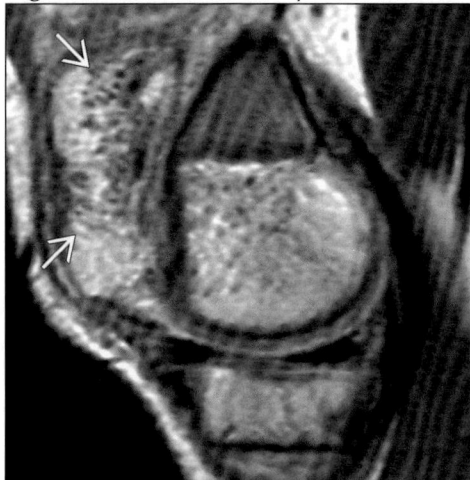

Pigmented Villonodular Synovitis (PVNS)

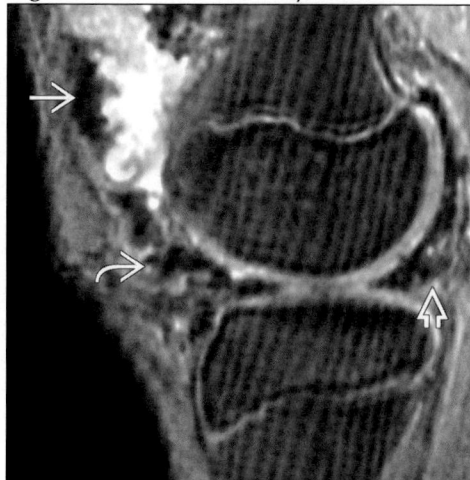

(Left) Sagittal PD FSE MR shows a large effusion containing multiple nodular bodies ➡. The radiograph was normal. These bodies remained low signal on T1 and T2WI. *(Right)* Sagittal T2* GRE MR (same knee as previous image) shows "blooming" of the areas of low signal, now seen to be lining the suprapatellar bursa ➡, Hoffa fat pad ➡, & posterior capsule ➡. This wide articular distribution, as well as the blooming effect on GRE confirms the diagnosis of PVNS.

Intraarticular Gas

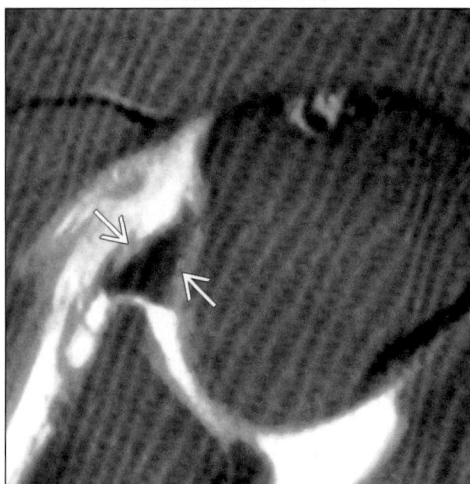

Hemophilic Arthropathy

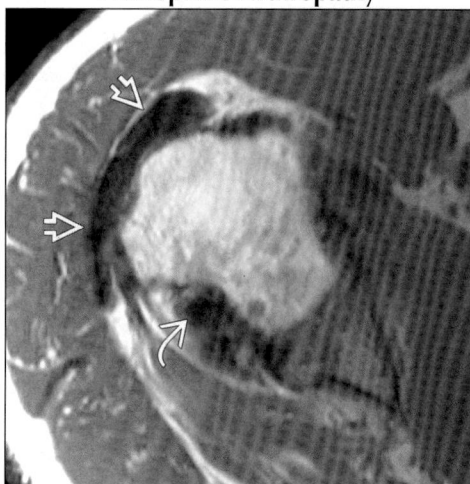

(Left) Axial MR arthrogram T1WI FS shows air which has assumed a triangular shape ➡, trapped between the glenohumeral ligament & humeral head; it was inadvertently injected during the arthrogram. Air is low signal on all sequences. *(Right)* Axial PD FSE MR shows low signal collections within the subdeltoid bursa ➡ & glenohumeral joint ➡ in a patient with a history of hemophilic bleeds. With chronicity, iron is deposited in the synovium, resulting in low signal masses.

Nodular Synovitis

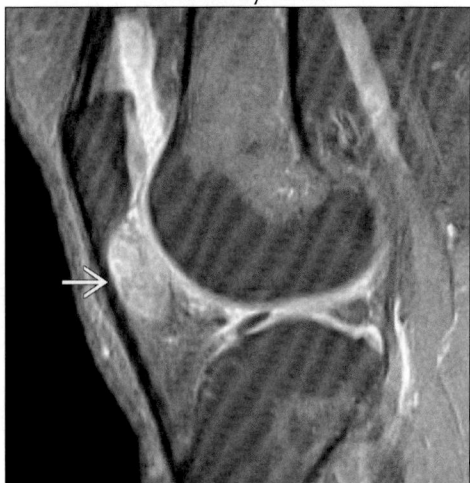

Amyloid Deposition

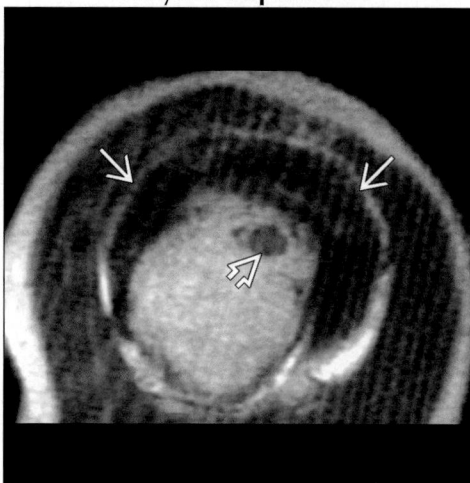

(Left) Sagittal T2WI FS MR shows predominantly low signal within a discrete mass adjacent to Hoffa fat pad ➡. This signal characteristic, along with the location, make the diagnosis of nodular synovitis highly probable. *(Right)* Sagittal T2WI MR shows low signal material within an erosion/subchondral cyst ➡, as well as densely & diffusely thickened rotator cuff tendons ➡. This patient has end stage renal disease; the imaging is typical of amyloid.

ANECHOIC MASS

DIFFERENTIAL DIAGNOSIS

Common
- Ganglion Cyst
- Synovial Cyst
- Joint Effusion (Mimic)
- Bursitis
- Tenosynovitis (Mimic)
- Hematoma
- Soft Tissue Abscess
- Muscle Injury (Mimic)

Less Common
- Aneurysm (Mimic)
- Pseudoaneurysm
- Seroma
- Lymphocele

Rare but Important
- Myxoma
- Hemophilic Pseudotumor

ESSENTIAL INFORMATION

Key Differential Diagnosis Issues
- Anechoic: Minimal echoes, + thru-transmission & posterior enhancement

Helpful Clues for Common Diagnoses
- **Ganglion Cyst**
  - Ovoid or lobulate; thin-walled; ± septations
  - Synovial cysts communicate with joint & ganglia do not
- **Joint Effusion (Mimic)**
  - Synovium thickness variable depending on chronicity, underlying cause
- **Bursitis**
  - Acute: Thin wall, anechoic (chronic becomes more echogenic)
- **Tenosynovitis (Mimic)**
  - Fluid surrounding tendon; ± synovial thickening; ± tendon injury
- **Hematoma**
  - Acute: Hyperechoic
  - Subacute (3+ days): Anechoic
  - Subacute (organizing): Echogenic
  - Chronic (liquifying): Anechoic
- **Soft Tissue Abscess**
  - Thickened, irregular wall
- **Muscle Injury (Mimic)**
  - Partial: Irregular cavity, accentuated with muscle contraction
  - Complete: Muscle retracted, hematoma creates "mass"

Helpful Clues for Less Common Diagnoses
- **Aneurysm (Mimic)**
  - Saccular or fusiform, ± luminal thrombus
  - Pseudoaneurysm: History of catheterization
- **Seroma/Lymphocele**
  - History of prior surgery

Helpful Clues for Rare Diagnoses
- **Myxoma**
  - Discrete hypoechoic mass, ± cystic areas
- **Hemophilic Pseudotumor**
  - Masses may be anechoic or more complex
  - Follows pattern of hematoma

Ganglion Cyst

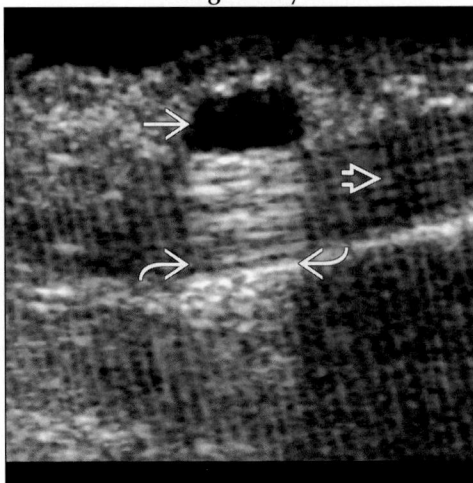

Transverse ultrasound shows a discrete anechoic mass ➡ with posterior enhancement ➡ superficial to the index finger flexor digitorum tendon ➡. This is a ganglion cyst.

Synovial Cyst

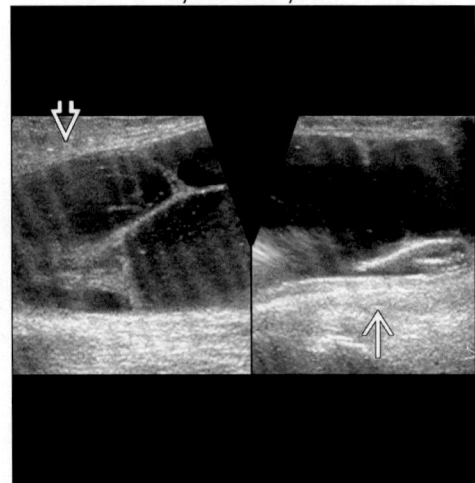

Dual ultrasound shows a thin-walled, multiseptate, anechoic mass interposed between the medial head of the gastrocnemius ➡ & the semimembranosus ➡, representing a Baker cyst.

ANECHOIC MASS

Joint Effusion (Mimic)

Tenosynovitis (Mimic)

(Left) Dual ultrasound shows joint effusion ➡ near the medial humeral condyle ➡ in rheumatoid arthritis with associated synovial proliferation ➡. (Right) Transverse ultrasound of the biceps tendon ➡ with associated tenosynovitis. Note the anechoic halo ➡ surrounding the long head biceps. Longitudinal ultrasound (not shown) delineated linear tendon fibers.

Hematoma

Soft Tissue Abscess

(Left) Transverse ultrasound shows a well-defined anechoic mass ➡ displacing the muscle belly ➡. This is a chronic hematoma with a remote history of trauma. (Right) Longitudinal ultrasound shows an irregular abscess cavity ➡ with marked thickening of the margin ➡. Note the adjacent tendon ➡.

Muscle Injury (Mimic)

Myxoma

(Left) Transverse ultrasound shows an irregular anechoic mass ➡, just superficial to the femur ➡, defining this as a quadriceps partial tear. (Right) Transverse ultrasound at the mid femur shows a discrete anechoic cyst ➡ which is, in fact, within a more solid mass ➡ in this myxoma [misinterpreted as a ganglion by MR (not shown)]. Note the adjacent femoral cortex ➡.

PHOTOPENIC LESIONS & FALSE NEGATIVE SCANS

DIFFERENTIAL DIAGNOSIS

Common
- Overlying Metallic Object
- Arthroplasty/Hardware
- Artifact: Post Processing to Remove Bladder Activity
- Cement & Bone Fillers
- Bone Graft
- Osteomyelitis, Early
- Post-Radiation
- Surgical Resection
- Multiple Myeloma
- Breast Metastases
- Osteonecrosis (Especially Femoral Head)
- Vascular Compromise

Less Common
- Anaplastic & Aggressive Tumors

ESSENTIAL INFORMATION

Key Differential Diagnosis Issues
- Mechanisms
  - Disruption of blood supply leading to poor delivery of radioisotope
  - Limited bone response to destructive process
- Correlation with radiographs should be confirmatory

Helpful Clues for Common Diagnoses
- **Overlying Metallic Object**
  - Pacemaker, electrical stimulation devices
  - Bladder shield
- **Arthroplasty/Hardware**
  - Characteristic shapes
    - Radiographs not usually required
- **Cement & Bone Fillers and Bone Graft**
  - Bone fillers & graft initially create defect
    - As incorporate, defect may disappear
- **Osteomyelitis, Early**
  - Prior to bone destruction
  - Radiographs negative, MR marrow edema
- **Post-Radiation**
  - Geographic photopenic defect, may involve several bones
  - Due to poor vascular supply
- **Surgical Resection**
  - Amputation, resection, curettage
- **Multiple Myeloma**
  - Usually false negative
- **Breast Metastases**
  - See Aggressive & Anaplastic Metastases below
- **Osteonecrosis (Especially Femoral Head)**
  - Disruption of blood supply → round osteopenic focus in angiographic phase
- **Vascular Compromise**
  - Prohibits delivery of radiopharmaceutical

Helpful Clues for Less Common Diagnoses
- **Anaplastic & Aggressive Tumors**
  - Limited response to destructive process
  - Uptake often patchy, diminished, or nl
  - Ill-defined lytic or permeative lesions
  - Tumors: Renal, thyroid, oat cell, neuroblastoma, sarcoma (both primary & metastatic)

Arthroplasty/Hardware

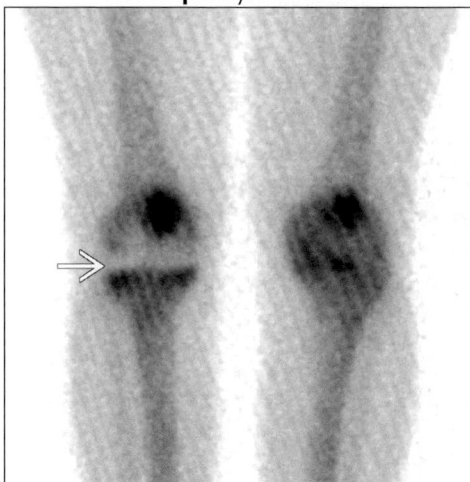

Anterior bone scan centered over the knees shows a right knee replacement which creates a photopenic defect in the expected location of the femorotibial articulation ➡.

Artifact: Post Processing to Remove Bladder Activity

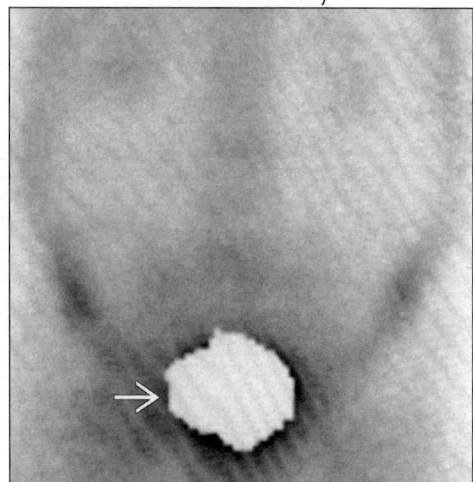

Anterior bone scan shows the photopenic defect ➡ created when activity from the bladder is electronically subtracted.

PHOTOPENIC LESIONS & FALSE NEGATIVE SCANS

Post-Radiation

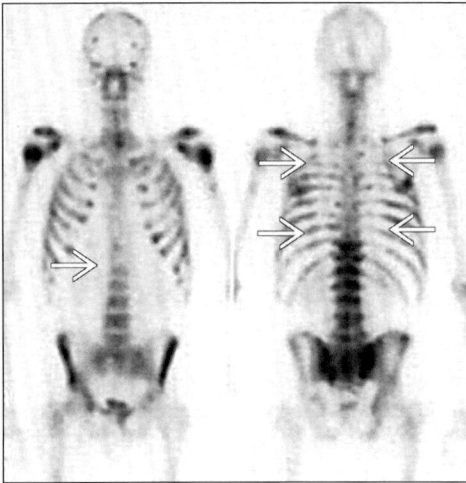

Multiple Myeloma

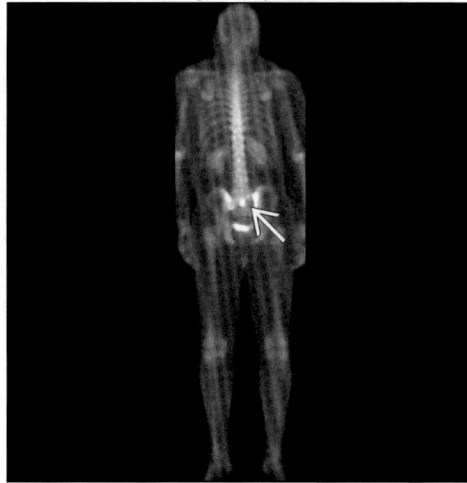

(Left) Anterior and posterior bone scans demonstrate geographic defect involving several thoracic vertebral bodies and adjacent ribs ➡ corresponding to previous radiation port. Note the sharp zone of transition. *(Right)* Posterior bone scan shows a photopenic defect in the right sacral ala ➡ which is much smaller than the corresponding defect on CT scan in this patient with multiple myeloma. Note the tiny defect in the left sacral ala.

Multiple Myeloma

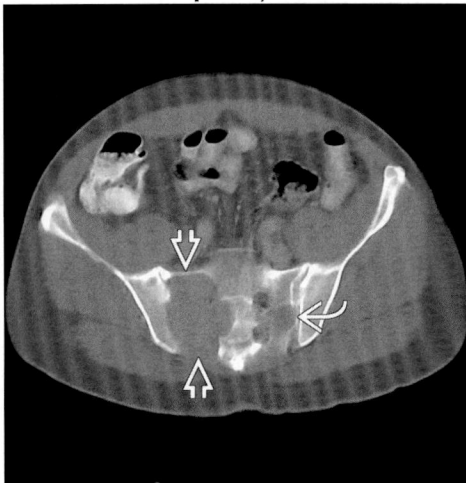

Osteonecrosis (Especially Femoral Head)

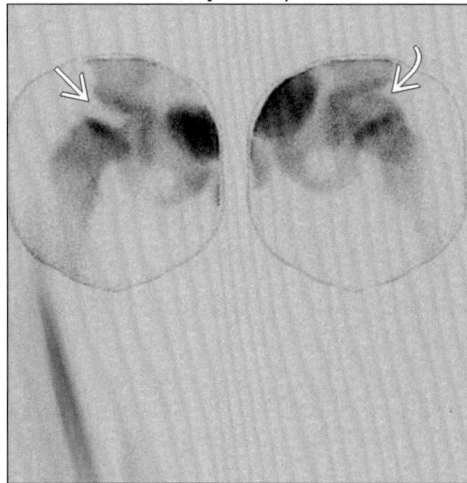

(Left) Axial bone CT (same patient as previous) shows a large lytic lesion with nonsclerotic geographic margins in the right sacral ala ➡. On the bone scan the majority of the lesion is photopenic. A second smaller lesion is present in the left ala ➡. *(Right)* Anterior pin-hole images of each hip from a bone scan shows absent activity within the right femoral head ➡ compared to normal activity on the left ➡ in this patient with Legg-Calve-Perthes disease.

Anaplastic & Aggressive Tumors

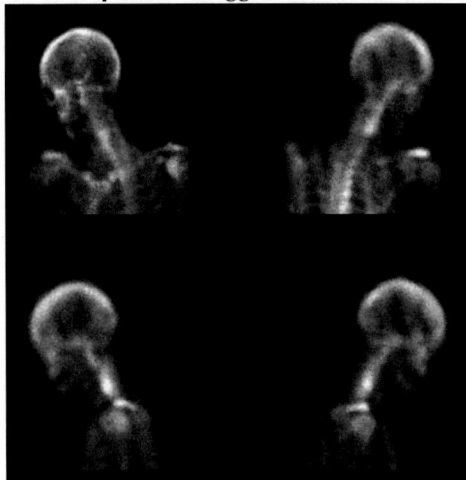

Anaplastic & Aggressive Tumors

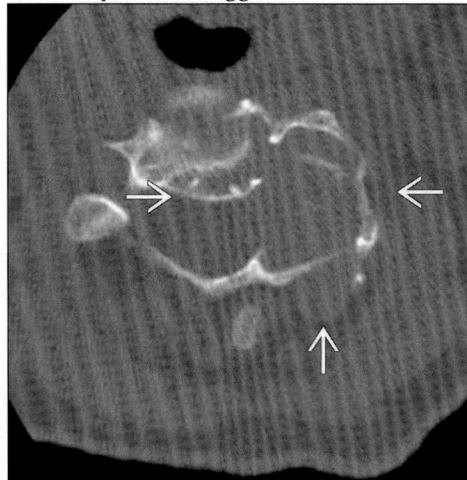

(Left) Oblique and lateral bone scan images fail to demonstrate the expansile lytic thyroid metastasis seen on a CT examination. *(Right)* Axial NECT (same patient as previous) shows classic appearance of thyroid metastasis with expansile lytic lesion of the left side of the C3 vertebral body and neural arch ➡. No corresponding lesion is seen on the bone scan.

SOFT TISSUE UPTAKE ON BONE SCAN

DIFFERENTIAL DIAGNOSIS

Common
- Injection Site (Mimic)
- Urine Contamination (Mimic)
- Camera Contamination (Mimic)
- Dilated Pelvicaliceal System (Mimic)
- Gastric Secretion of Free Pertechnetate (Mimic)
- Myocardial Infarction
- Amyloid Deposition, Especially Cardiac
- Sickle Cell Anemia, Spleen
- Calcification within Neoplasm
- Breast with Breast Cancer
- Generalized Soft Tissue from Poor Radiopharmaceutical Preparation
- Renal Failure

Less Common
- Brain Infarct
- Malignant Pleural Effusion
- Malignant Ascites
- Dystrophic Calcification, Any Cause
- Synovial Osteochondromatosis
- Malignant Pericardial Effusion
- Heterotopic Ossification
- Infarcted Tissue, Other
- Soft Tissue Ossification, Any Cause
- Neuroblastoma
- Metastatic Calcification, Especially Stomach, Liver, Kidney, Peri-articular Soft Tissues
- Pericarditis
- Myonecrosis

Rare but Important
- Osteosarcoma

ESSENTIAL INFORMATION

Key Differential Diagnosis Issues
- **Hint**: Nonpathologic mimics are most common
  - Always exclude urine contamination; hands can touch anywhere & spread urine droplets
    - Not always perineal or lower extremity
    - Clean site then re-image
    - One reason to check all scans before patient leaves department
- SPECT scanning may aid in localization
- Injection site should always be identified
- **Hint**: Correlation with radiographs & CT may be useful

  - Calcification is not always radiographically apparent
- Mechanisms of soft tissue abnormalities leading to radiopharmaceutical uptake
  - Dystrophic calcification
  - Metastatic calcification
  - Calcinosis
  - Ossification, neoplastic & nonneoplastic

Helpful Clues for Common Diagnoses
- **Amyloid Deposition, Especially Cardiac**
  - Heart most common site radiopharmaceutical uptake
  - Associated findings
    - Bilateral symmetric arthritis with subchondral cysts, erosions, joint spaces normal to widened
    - Soft tissue masses
- **Sickle Cell Anemia, Spleen**
  - Calcified spleen may be apparent
  - Associated findings
    - Osteoporosis, coarse trabecula
    - Multiple infarcts & AVN, H-shaped vertebra
    - Osteomyelitis, septic arthritis, dactylitis
    - Widened diploic space sparing skull base
- **Breast with Breast Cancer**
  - Not all uptake in breast is malignant
  - Correlate with mammogram
- **Renal Failure**
  - May lead to diffuse renal uptake
  - May have Superscan
  - Leads to metastatic calcification
  - Associated renal osteodystrophy (combination osteomalacia & HPTH)
    - HPTH: Bone resorption subperiosteal, subchondral, subligamentous, subtendinous, cortical tunneling; osteoporosis, brown tumors
    - Osteomalacia: Coarse ill-defined trabecula, Looser's zones, pseudofractures, metaphyseal cupping & fraying (child)
    - Neostosis, Rugger jersey spine

Helpful Clues for Less Common Diagnoses
- **Synovial Osteochondromatosis**
  - Primary or secondary to arthritis
  - Multiple intraarticular osteocartilaginous bodies
- **Neuroblastoma**
  - Uptake typically within primary in adrenal gland

SOFT TISSUE UPTAKE ON BONE SCAN

- Patient under 2 years old
- **Myonecrosis**
  - Associated with prior trauma, compartment syndrome, diabetic rhabdomyolysis, snake venom, infection especially anaerobic

Helpful Clues for Rare Diagnoses
- **Osteosarcoma**
  - Both extraskeletal primary & metastases
  - Lungs common site of metastases

Alternative Differential Approaches
- Discussion of the various causes is best focused around the mechanism of radiopharmaceutical uptake
- List presented below includes many specific sites & etiologies typically seen although there are many potential causes
- Dystrophic calcification
  - Occurs at sites of previous tissue damage with random sites of involvement
  - Hematoma, abscess, trauma, necrosis, infarction, tuberculosis, vascular abnormalities
- Ossification
  - Neoplastic ossification occurs in osteosarcoma, may be primary extraskeletal or metastatic disease
  - Nonneoplastic ossification
    - Wide differential diagnosis for heterotopic ossification
    - Wide differential diagnosis for soft tissue ossification
    - Idiopathic pulmonary ossification

- Calcinosis
  - Collagen vascular disease, idiopathic tumoral calcinosis
  - Commonly peri-articular
- Metastatic calcification
  - Any condition leading to hypercalcemia
    - Common etiologies: Renal osteodystrophy, HPTH, hypoparathyroidism, cases of extensive bone destruction
  - Common sites include GI tract especially stomach, kidney, lungs, peri-articular soft tissues
- Neoplasm with calcification
  - Primarily adenocarcinomas, especially mucinous
  - Mechanisms not always clear
    - May be dystrophic
    - Psammomatous
    - Enchondral (chondroid tumors)
  - Colon, breast, ovary (mucinous), GI, neuroblastoma, endometrial
  - Soft tissue chondroid tumors
  - Primary tumor and metastases can calcify
    - Calcified metastases most commonly seen in liver
  - Wide differential diagnosis for soft tissue neoplasm containing calcification

Injection Site (Mimic)

Anterior bone scan shows linear accumulation of activity within the antecubital fossa ➔ at the injection site. This activity is the result of poor flushing after radioisotope injection.

Urine Contamination (Mimic)

Posterior bone scan shows focal area of radioisotope uptake adjacent to the right scapula ➔. No mass was present. The uptake is from urine contamination which can occur anywhere on the skin surface.

SOFT TISSUE UPTAKE ON BONE SCAN

(Left) Anterior bone scan shows an amorphous accumulation of activity in the perineal region and upper thigh consistent with urine contamination ➡. **(Right)** Anterior and posterior bone scan shows accumulation of radioisotope within a dilated left pelvocaliceal system ➡ and normal activity within the right renal parenchyma ➡.

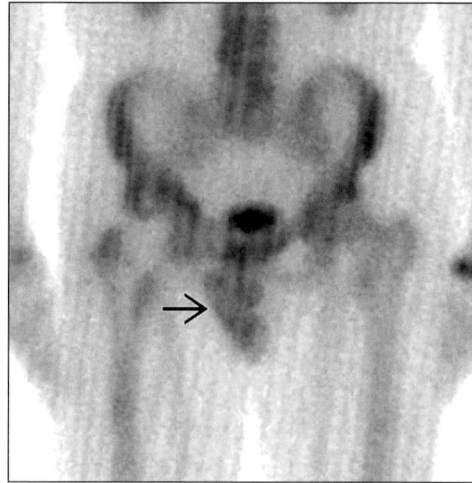

Urine Contamination (Mimic)

Dilated Pelvicaliceal System (Mimic)

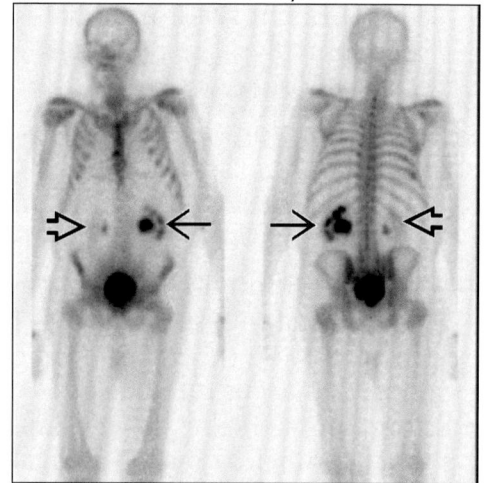

(Left) Anterior bone scan shows activity within the stomach traveling through the proximal jejunum ➡. With a poor radioisotope tag free pertechnetate is secreted by the stomach. **(Right)** Anterior bone scan shows doughnut-shaped uptake in the left hemithorax ➡ consistent with myocardial uptake resulting from an MI. The uptake is quite extensive and consistent with a severe myocardial insult.

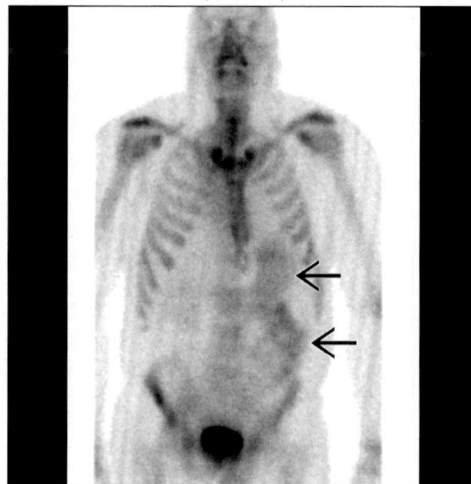

Gastric Secretion of Free Pertechnetate (Mimic)

Myocardial Infarction

(Left) Anterior bone scan shows accumulation of activity within the myocardium of all four chambers of the heart ➡ secondary to amyloid deposition. (Courtesy K. Morton, MD). **(Right)** Posterior bone scan shows intense uptake in the left upper quadrant ➡. The shape of the uptake indicates that it is within the spleen in this child with sickle cell anemia.

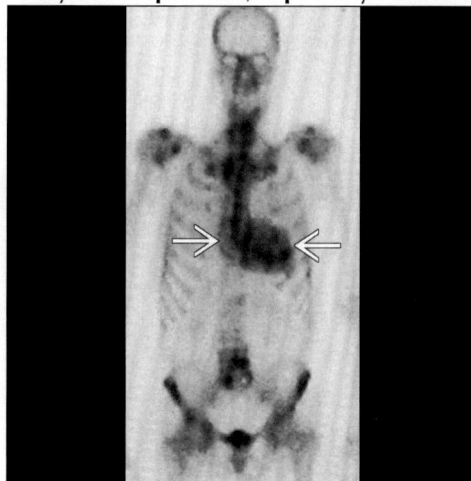

Amyloid Deposition, Especially Cardiac

Sickle Cell Anemia, Spleen

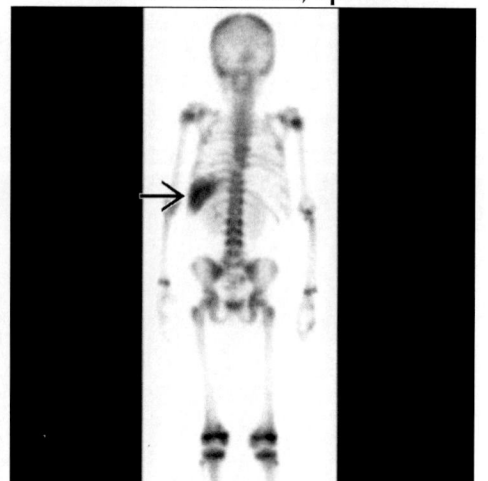

SOFT TISSUE UPTAKE ON BONE SCAN

Calcification within Neoplasm

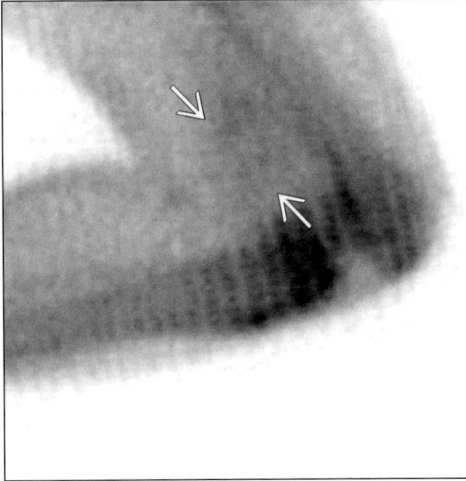

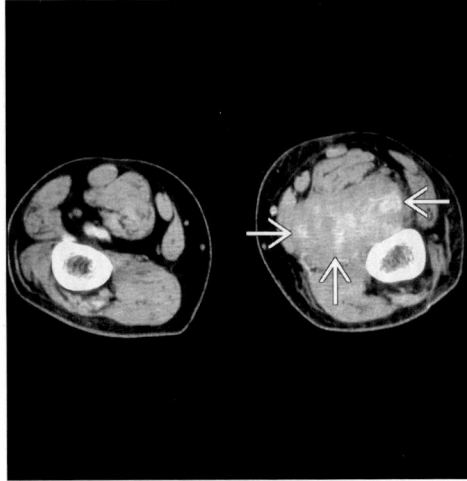

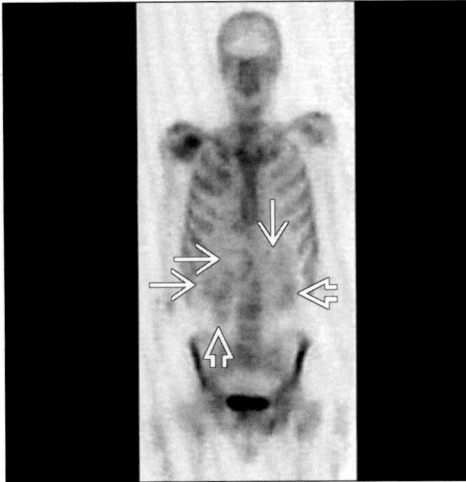

Calcification within Neoplasm

(Left) Lateral bone scan centered over the knee demonstrates uptake in the distal thigh ➡. The orthogonal view helped to confirm that the activity was located in the soft tissue & not osseous. (Courtesy K. Morton, MD). *(Right)* Axial CECT in the prone position of the same patient shows soft tissue sarcoma with multiple foci of calcification ➡; this results in focal accumulation of activity on bone scan.

Calcification within Neoplasm

Breast with Breast Cancer

(Left) Anterior bone scan shows multiple ring-like areas of activity in the RUQ in the region of the liver ➡. This patient has metastatic colon cancer, one of the most frequent neoplasms to form calcific deposits in metastases. This activity should not be confused with normal renal activity ➡. *(Right)* Anterior bone scan shows diffuse uptake in right breast ➡ as well as a relatively large intense focus within same breast ➡. This patient has breast cancer. (Courtesy K. Morton, MD).

Brain Infarct

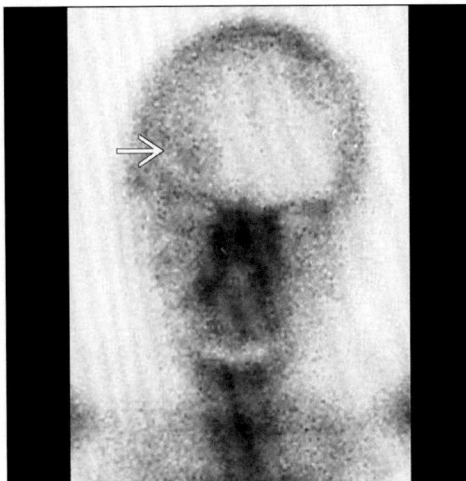

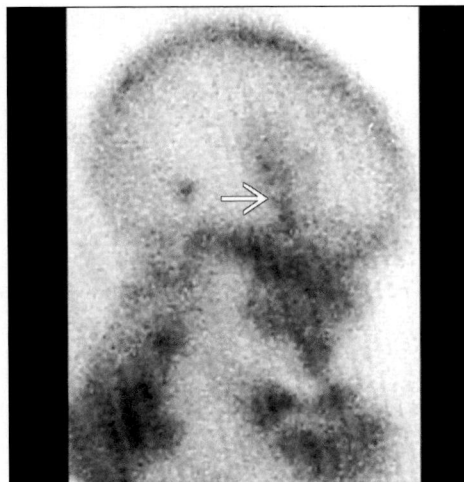

Brain Infarct

(Left) Anterior bone scan reveals focal uptake in the right hemisphere in this patient with a stroke ➡. (Courtesy K. Morton, MD). *(Right)* Lateral bone scan shows focal activity within the frontal region of the brain, consistent with an acute infarct ➡. (Courtesy K. Morton, MD).

SOFT TISSUE UPTAKE ON BONE SCAN

(Left) Posterior bone scan reveals asymmetric activity within the hemithoraces with greater activity on the right ➡. The uptake is not focal and is consistent with a malignant pleural effusion. (Right) Anterior bone scan shows a protuberant abdomen ➡ containing amorphous activity. This patient has malignant ascites. Note the negative defect of the bowel within the ascites ➡. (Courtesy K. Morton, MD).

Malignant Pleural Effusion

Malignant Ascites

(Left) Anterior bone scan centered over the right forearm shows lobulated uptake involving the forearm ➡ and fingers ➡. This patient has Maffucci syndrome with extensive soft tissue hemangiomas and multiple phleboliths. (Right) Posteroanterior radiograph of the right hand in the same patient reveals a spectacular example of Maffucci syndrome with multiple hemangiomas with widespread phleboliths. (Courtesy K. Morton, MD).

Dystrophic Calcification, Any Cause

Dystrophic Calcification, Any Cause

(Left) Anterior bone scan shows activity in the central chest in the configuration of the cardiac silhouette ➡ which is due to a malignant pericardial effusion. (Courtesy K. Morton, MD). (Right) Anterior bone scan shows extensive uptake in both thighs and in the region of the left hemipelvis ➡ in this patient with extensive heterotopic ossification. (Courtesy K. Morton, MD).

Malignant Pericardial Effusion

Heterotopic Ossification

SOFT TISSUE UPTAKE ON BONE SCAN

Soft Tissue Ossification, Any Cause

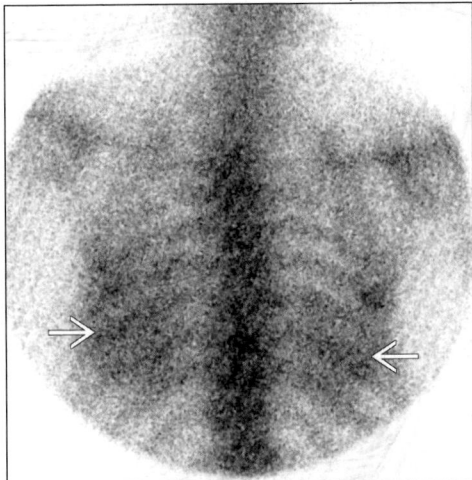

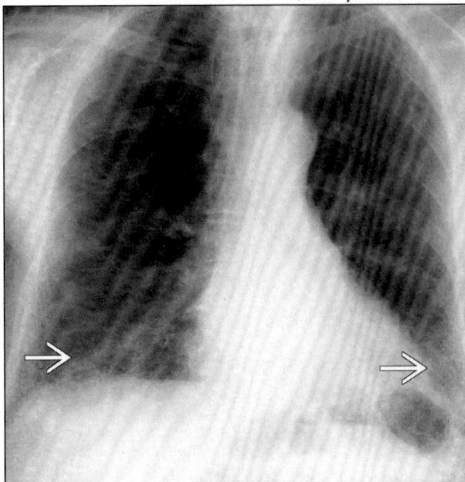

Soft Tissue Ossification, Any Cause

(Left) Posterior bone scan shows amorphous foci of uptake within both hemithoraces, especially at the lung bases →. This patient has idiopathic pulmonary ossification. (Right) Posteroanterior radiograph in the same patient as previous image, shows density at both lung bases → secondary to idiopathic pulmonary ossification.

Neuroblastoma

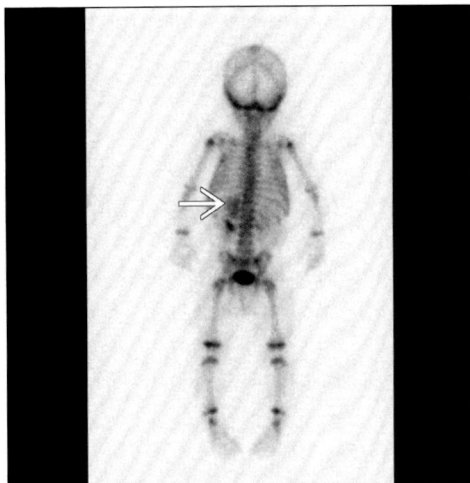

Osteosarcoma

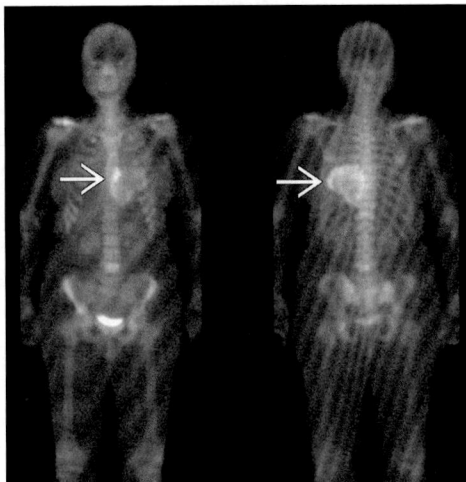

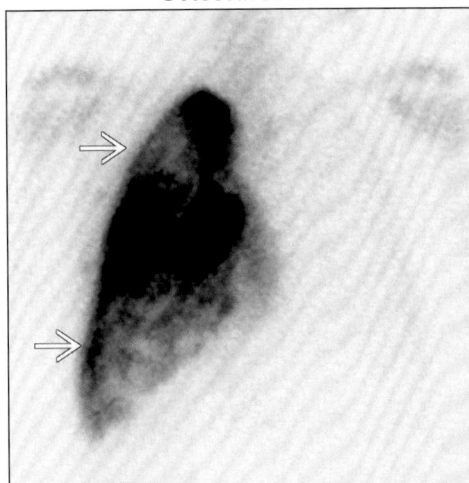

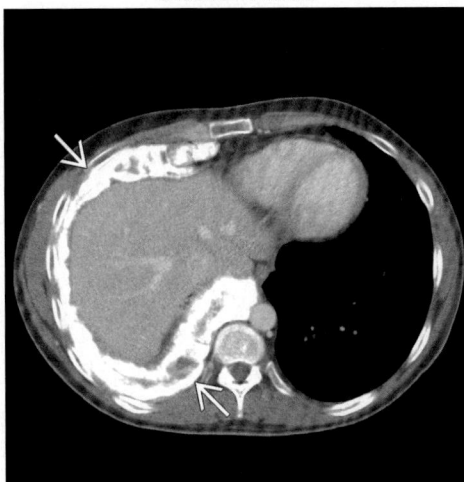

(Left) Posterior bone scan shows uptake in a right adrenal mass → most likely related to microcalcifications in this patient with neuroblastoma. (Right) Anterior and posterior bone scan shows a case of metastatic osteosarcoma with radioisotope uptake within a left lower lobe mass →. A calcified mass was evident on chest x-ray. In this case the uptake mimics cardiac uptake.

Osteosarcoma

Osteosarcoma

(Left) Anterior bone scan shows intense activity throughout the right hemithorax → mimicking the shape of the lung due to a large osteosarcomatous mass within the pleural space. (Courtesy K. Morton, MD). (Right) Axial CECT shows a large osteosarcoma which has arisen in the pleural space →. (Courtesy K. Morton, MD).

SUPERSCAN

DIFFERENTIAL DIAGNOSIS

Common
- Metastases, Diffuse

Less Common
- Renal Osteodystrophy
- Myelofibrosis
- Hyperparathyroidism (HPTH)
- Hyperthyroidism
- Mastocytosis

Rare but Important
- Aplastic Anemia
- Leukemia
- Lymphoma
- Osteopetrosis

ESSENTIAL INFORMATION

Key Differential Diagnosis Issues
- Superscan: Diffuse, intense skeletal uptake
  - Little/no activity in kidneys & soft tissues
- Clinical history usually diagnostic
- MR will have nonspecific abnormal marrow except in cases of metabolic disease

Helpful Clues for Common Diagnoses
- **Metastates, Diffuse**
  - Prostate, breast, lung
  - Widespread blastic or lytic lesions

Helpful Clues for Less Common Diagnoses
- **Renal Osteodystrophy**
  - Combination of HPTH & osteomalacia
  - HPTH (see below)

- Osteomalacia/rickets
  - Coarse ill-defined trabecula, Looser zones, pseudofractures, cortical tunneling, metaphyseal cupping & fraying
- **Myelofibrosis**
  - Osteoporosis early then diffuse sclerosis
  - MR: Fibrotic marrow
- **Hyperparathyroidism (HPTH)**
  - Bone resorption: Subperiosteal, subchondral, subtendinous, subligamentous, cortical tunneling
  - Osteoporosis, soft tissue calcium deposition, Brown tumors
- **Hyperthyroidism**
  - Osteoporosis
  - Rapid bone turnover with cortical tunneling
- **Mastocytosis**
  - Osteoporosis
  - Characteristic cutaneous involvement

Helpful Clues for Rare Diagnoses
- **Aplastic Anemia**
  - MR: Increased marrow fat
- **Leukemia**
  - Osteoporosis, lucent metaphyseal bands, periostitis, permeative lytic lesions
- **Lymphoma**
  - Variable radiographic appearance
- **Osteopetrosis**
  - Diffuse osteosclerosis

Metastases, Diffuse

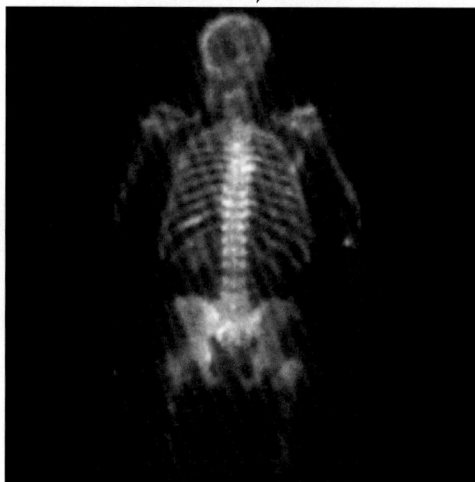

Posterior bone scan shows diffuse uptake throughout the skeleton. Minimal renal uptake is present. This is a superscan in a patient with diffuse blastic prostatic metastases.

Metastases, Diffuse

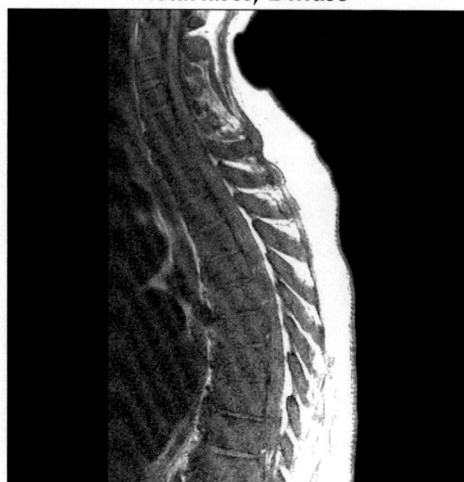

Sagittal T1WI MR shows extensive blastic prostate carcinoma with diffuse marrow involvement. Such disease correlates with a superscan appearance on bone scan.

Renal Osteodystrophy

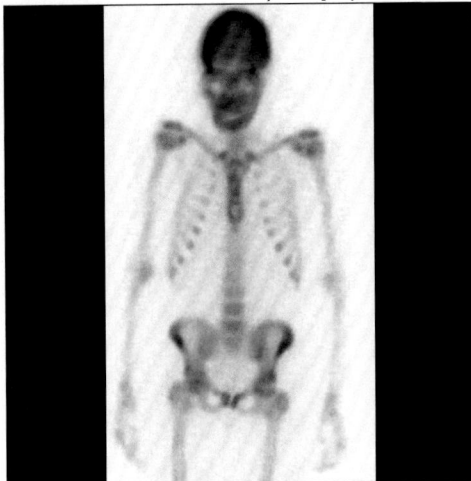

Renal Osteodystrophy

(Left) Anterior bone scan shows intense uptake in the skull which is characteristic of secondary HPTH. The intensity of skeletal uptake appears relatively normal which can be misleading but note how the uptake is seen even within the fingers. This is not normal. *(Right)* Lateral radiograph shows a pattern of trabecular resorption of mixed lytic and dense areas which has been termed "salt and pepper". This correlates with the intense uptake in the skull on bone scan.

Mastocytosis

Leukemia

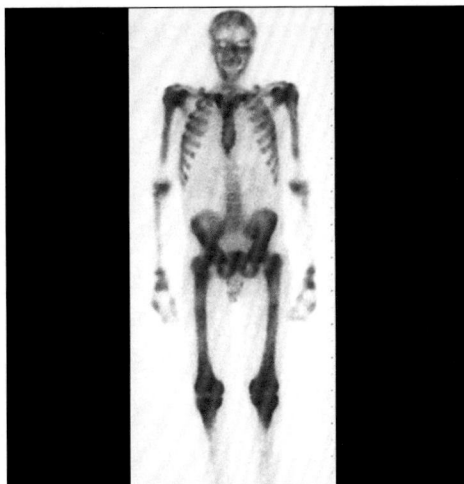

(Left) Bone scan shows the nonspecific appearance of a superscan in this patient with mastocytosis. *(Right)* Anterior bone scan shows extremely intense uptake throughout the skeleton. The limited renal activity helps to put the skeletal uptake into perspective in this patient with CML blast crisis.

Osteopetrosis

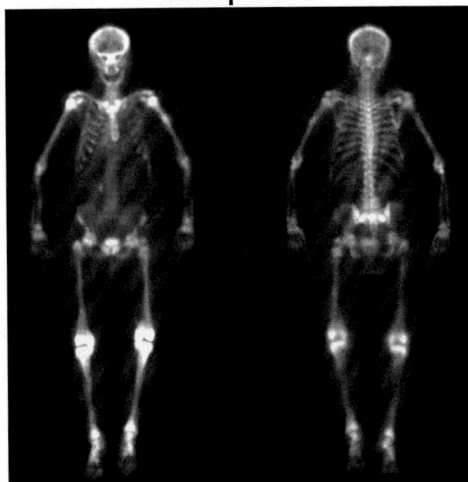

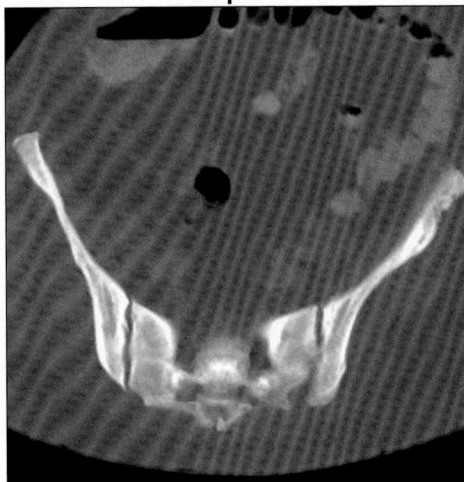

Osteopetrosis

(Left) Anterior and posterior bone scan shows diffuse intense uptake throughout the axial and appendicular skeleton in this patient with osteopetrosis. *(Right)* Axial bone CT shows a typical case of osteopetrosis with diffuse sclerosis throughout the entire skeleton including the pelvis as shown here. It is easy to appreciate the diffuse skeletal uptake on bone scan seen in these patients.

PART III
Clinically Based

Shoulder Girdle and Upper Arm
Elbow and Forearm
Wrist and Hand
Pelvis, Hip, and Thigh
Knee and Leg
Ankle and Foot
Spine
Systemic Disease

PAINFUL OR ENLARGED STERNOCLAVICULAR JOINT

DIFFERENTIAL DIAGNOSIS

Common
- Osteoarthritis
- Post-Traumatic
- Dislocation

Less Common
- Septic Joint
- Metastatic Calcification
- Ankylosing Spondylitis
- Psoriatic Arthritis
- Rheumatoid Arthritis
- Osteitis Condensans of Clavicle
- Sternoclavicular Hyperostosis/SAPHO

Rare but Important
- Mucopolysaccharidoses
- Tumoral (Idiopathic) Calcinosis
- Ischemic Necrosis of the Clavicle

ESSENTIAL INFORMATION

Helpful Clues for Common Diagnoses
- **Osteoarthritis**: Joint space narrowing, subchondral sclerosis & cysts, osteophytes
- **Post-Traumatic**: Clavicular head fx may lead to malunion, unilateral osteoarthritis
- **Dislocation**: Majority anterior; if posterior concern for trachea, neurovascular injury

Helpful Clues for Less Common Diagnoses
- **Septic Joint**
  - Unilateral, peri-articular osteoporosis, joint space narrowing, bone destruction

- **Metastatic Calcification**: Peri-articular calcium deposition, unilateral or bilateral, underlying hypercalcemia
- **Ankylosing Spondylitis**
  - Bilateral symmetric, ranges from enthesopathy to ankylosis
- **Psoriatic Arthritis**: Bilateral asymmetric, joint space narrowing, erosions, periostitis, enthesopathy
- **Rheumatoid Arthritis**
  - Bilateral symmetric erosive arthritis
- **Osteitis Condensans of Clavicle**
  - Unilateral, seen in middle aged women
  - **Hint**: Sclerosis in inferior aspect clavicular head, inferomedial osteophyte
- **Sternoclavicular Hyperostosis/SAPHO**
  - Synovitis, Acne, Pustulosis, Hyperostosis, Osteitis
  - Older teenagers & adults, primarily men
  - Unilateral or bilateral sclerosis clavicle, sternum or both, enthesitis
  - ± Manubriosternal, & 1st, 2nd costochondral articulations
  - Chronic recurrent multifocal osteoarthritis (CRMO) is variant seen in children, adolescents; bone destruction, extensive sclerosis leads to enlarged clavicle

Helpful Clues for Rare Diagnoses
- **Mucopolysaccharidoses**: Wide clavicles
- **Tumoral (Idiopathic) Calcinosis**
  - Peri-articular calcium deposition
- **Ischemic Necrosis of Clavicle**: Clavicular head sclerosis in children 2° trauma, emboli

Post-Traumatic

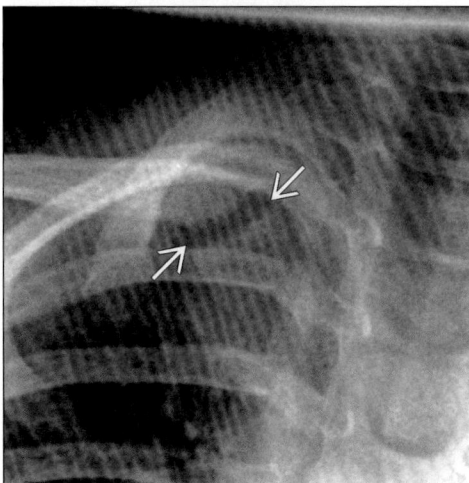

Anteroposterior radiograph shows fracture of the medial head of the clavicle ➡ with inferior displacement which presented as a painful lump.

Dislocation

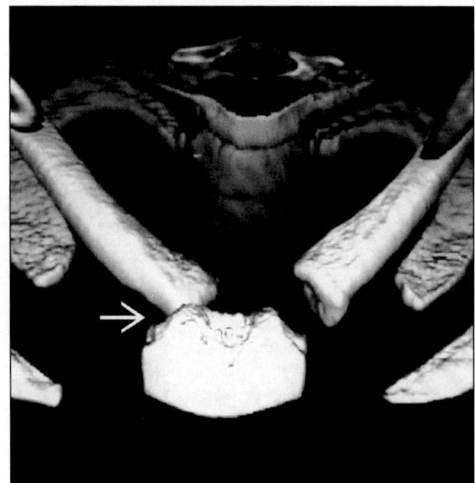

Frontal bone CT with 3D reconstruction shows a posterior dislocation of the right clavicle ➡ relative to the manubrium. The vascular structures are at risk in this dislocation.

PAINFUL OR ENLARGED STERNOCLAVICULAR JOINT

Septic Joint

Ankylosing Spondylitis

(Left) Axial STIR MR shows abnormal signal within the distal clavicle ➡ along with an effusion ➡ in this drug abuser with septic arthritis of the right sternoclavicular joint. *(Right)* Axial bone CT shows erosive change at the sternoclavicular joints ➡ and complete fusion at the costovertebral ➡ and costochondral ➡ joints in this patient with ankylosing spondylitis.

Osteitis Condensans of Clavicle

Osteitis Condensans of Clavicle

(Left) Anteroposterior radiograph shows the characteristic appearance of osteitis condensans of the clavicle with sclerosis involving the inferior medial aspect of the left clavicle head ➡. *(Right)* Axial bone CT shows diffuse sclerosis within the medial aspect of the left clavicle ➡. No periostitis or soft tissue mass is seen in this patient with osteitis condensans of the clavicle.

Sternoclavicular Hyperostosis/SAPHO

Sternoclavicular Hyperostosis/SAPHO

(Left) Axial bone CT shows sclerosis (hyperostosis) of the left first rib ➡ and the left side of the manubrium ➡. The clavicles and sternoclavicular joint are both normal ➡ in this patient who fits the criteria for SAPHO. *(Right)* Coronal NECT shows dense sclerosis (hyperostosis) involving the left side of the sternum ➡ and marked increased density within the left first costochondral articulation (osteitis) ➡ in this patient with sternoclavicular hyperostosis.

ROTATOR CUFF SYMPTOMS

DIFFERENTIAL DIAGNOSIS

Common
- Rotator Cuff Tendinosis/Tear
- Cervical Radiculopathy
- Suprascapular Neuropathy
- Subacromial Bursitis
- Shoulder Subluxation/Dislocation
- Osteonecrosis
- Fracture
- AC Joint Separation
- Arthritis
  - Osteoarthritis (OA)
  - Rheumatoid Arthritis (RA)
  - Hydroxyapatite Deposition Disease (HADD) (a.k.a., Milwaukee Shoulder)
  - Ankylosing Spondylitis (AS)
  - Polymyalgia Rheumatica

Less Common
- Septic Joint
- Adhesive Capsulitis, Shoulder
- Intraosseous Neoplasm

Rare but Important
- Myopathies
- Myocardial Infarction

ESSENTIAL INFORMATION

Key Differential Diagnosis Issues
- Most common signs/symptoms: Pain with impingement testing
- Insidious, continuously increasing pain, weakness, loss of shoulder motion
- Clinical signs are non-specific enough that there may be many etiologies
- **Hint**: MR is frequently required, but always evaluate radiograph
  - Calcification
  - Neoplasm
  - Erosions/osteophytes/fracture

Helpful Clues for Common Diagnoses
- **Rotator Cuff Tendinosis/Tear**
  - Spectrum of tendinosis → complete RCT
  - Tendinosis
    - Thickening of tendon; higher signal, especially on proton density
    - Watch for calcification within tendon, often easier to see on radiograph than MR (usually low signal, ± tendon edema)
  - Similar insidious pain, weakness, loss of range of motion as complete tear
  - Partial rotator cuff tear
    - Pain with impingement test; may be more painful than full thickness tear
    - May be on articular surface, bursal surface, or intrasubstance (interstitial)
  - Full thickness rotator cuff tear
    - Full thickness insertional tear within rotator crescent
    - ± Complete tear (complete anterior to posterior extent of tendon)
    - ± Retraction & degeneration tendon
    - ± Fatty atrophy of muscles
- **Cervical Radiculopathy**
  - Combination of facet & uncovertebral joint arthropathy, disk disease, & listhesis
  - **Hint**: Before ascribing shoulder pain to cervical radiculopathy, be certain there are no abnormalities at the cervicothoracic junction which could be causative
    - Cervical ribs or Pancoast tumor
- **Suprascapular Neuropathy**
  - Suprascapular nerve generally impinged at spinoglenoid notch
  - Most common etiology: Paraglenoid cyst, usually associated with labral tear
  - Supraspinatus and/or infraspinatus
    - Muscle may appear normal
    - Muscle may show high T2 signal and/or enhancement
    - Muscle eventually shows fatty atrophy
  - Clinically, presents with pain & weakness, similar to rotator cuff tear
- **Subacromial Bursitis**
  - Presents clinically as subacromial impingement
    - Pain to palpation of rotator cuff within the range of extension
    - Pain and weakness like rotator cuff injury, but ROM often preserved
  - Compression of supraspinatus tendon by productive changes or morphological abnormality at AC joint
    - Bursal fluid forms in subacromial region; may extend to subdeltoid bursa
    - Watch for partial bursal rotator cuff tear
- **Shoulder Subluxation/Dislocation**
  - Generally have symptoms of instability
    - May present with pain and weakness, similar to rotator cuff injury

- Following dislocation, may have (reverse) Hill Sachs and/or (reverse) Bankart injuries
  - May result in subtle subluxation; watch for this on axial MR imaging
  - Watch for capsular redundancy
- **Osteonecrosis**
  - Presents with generalized shoulder pain prior to collapse of subchondral bone
  - Radiograph: Subchondral fracture, increased density weight-bearing portion (superomedial head)
  - MR: Subchondral, ± serpiginous double line sign of osteonecrosis
- **Fracture**
  - Direct impact or related to dislocation
  - Greater tuberosity fracture (nondisplaced) may be occult radiographically
  - Presents with limited range of motion & pain; often present for MR as presumed rotator cuff injury
- **AC Joint Separation**
  - Pain and limited range of motion (ROM), but generally should be differentiated from rotator cuff symptoms
  - Grade II: AC joint widened; grade III: AC and coracoclavicular joints widened
- **Osteoarthritis (OA)**
  - Slowly progressive pain and limited ROM
  - Often antecedent trauma
    - If no such history, consider deposition etiologies (HADD or pyrophosphate)
  - Typical findings of OA: Cartilage thinning, subchondral cysts

- Ring osteophyte around glenoid; ring osteophyte at anatomic humeral neck margin, largest inferiorly
- **Rheumatoid Arthritis (RA)**
  - Pain, swelling, morning stiffness
  - Osteopenia, subchondral cysts, erosions
  - Synovitis, sometimes with rice bodies
  - Chronic rotator cuff tear
    - Elevation of humeral head → mechanical erosion medial humeral neck → at risk for surgical neck fracture
- **Hydroxyapatite Deposition Disease (HADD) (a.k.a., Milwaukee Shoulder)**
  - Aggressive joint destruction otherwise mimicking osteoarthritis
  - Consider with shoulder appearance of OA but without history of trauma
- **Ankylosing Spondylitis (AS)**
  - When peripheral joints are involved, it tends to be hip or shoulder
  - Osteoporotic, erosive ± productive
- **Polymyalgia Rheumatica**
  - Pain, weakness, & stiffness, especially hip and shoulder; no structural abnormalities

Helpful Clues for Less Common Diagnoses
- **Septic Joint**
  - Swelling, abscess, effusion, ± bone & cartilage destruction
- **Adhesive Capsulitis, Shoulder**
  - Painful limited ROM; mimics RCT disease
  - Thickened & edematous inferior capsule
  - Restricted capsule with arthrography, no filling of axillary or subscapularis bursae

Rotator Cuff Tendinosis/Tear

Coronal oblique T2WI FS MR shows calcific deposits within the supraspinatus tendon ➡ with surrounding edema ➡. The tendon is intact, but weakened. In this case, the calcifications were visible on radiograph.

Rotator Cuff Tendinosis/Tear

Coronal T1 FS MR arthrogram shows a full thickness tear in the supraspinatus portion of the rotator cuff ➡. Though the tear is full thickness, it was not complete, as residual fibers were seen in other images.

ROTATOR CUFF SYMPTOMS

(Left) *Sagittal PD FSE MR shows higher signal than expected within the supraspinatus and infraspinatus tendons* ⮕ *as well as thickening of the tendon. Findings are of tendinosis.* **(Right)** *Axial T1 C+ FS MR shows a large spinoglenoid notch cyst* ➡ *with rim-enhancement crossing the pathway of the suprascapular nerve. Note the mild enhancement of infraspinatus* ⮕*. Depending on the location of the cyst, supraspinatus, infraspinatus, or both may be involved.*

Rotator Cuff Tendinosis/Tear

Suprascapular Neuropathy

(Left) *Coronal T2WI MR shows fluid in the subacromial bursa* ➡*. A slightly more posterior coronal image showed an abnormal morphology of the acromion & associated tendinopathy.* **(Right)** *Axial PD FSE MR shows Hill Sachs lesion* ➡ *indicating prior anterior dislocation. Note the anterior subluxation of the humeral head, which is chronic, and the redundancy of the posterior capsule* ➡*. This is an unstable shoulder.*

Subacromial Bursitis

Shoulder Subluxation/Dislocation

(Left) *Anteroposterior radiograph shows a subchondral fracture* ➡ *in the weight-bearing portion of the humeral head. This is a typical appearance of osteonecrosis; the patient used steroids for asthma.* **(Right)** *Coronal T1WI MR shows bone marrow edema* ⮕ *& linear fracture line* ➡ *in the greater tuberosity. This nondisplaced fracture was radiographically occult; MR was requested to evaluate for rotator cuff tear. The cuff and remainder of the shoulder were normal.*

Osteonecrosis

Fracture

ROTATOR CUFF SYMPTOMS

AC Joint Separation

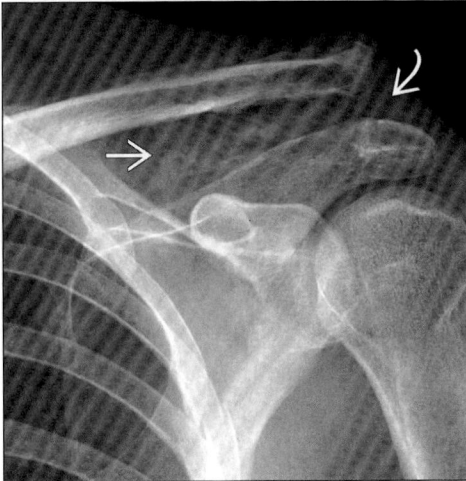

Osteoarthritis (OA)

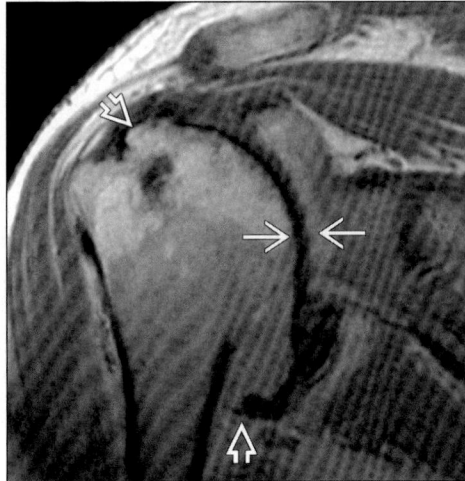

(Left) Anteroposterior radiograph shows grade 3 AC separation ➡. Heterotopic bone is formed between the clavicle and coracoid ➡, indicating coracoclavicular ligament injury. *(Right)* Coronal T1WI MR shows complete cartilage loss ➡ and huge osteophytes ringing the margin of the joint ➡; this ring osteophyte is particularly large inferomedially. The rotator cuff remains intact.

Rheumatoid Arthritis (RA)

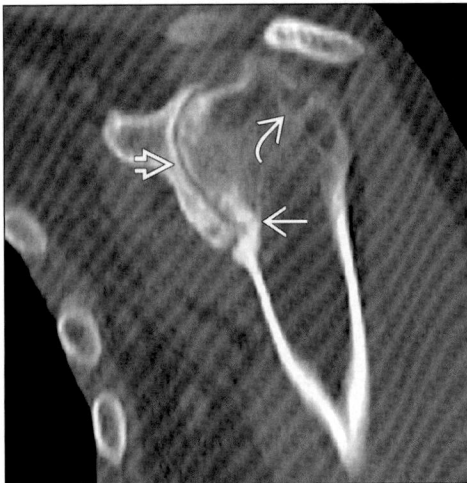

Septic Joint

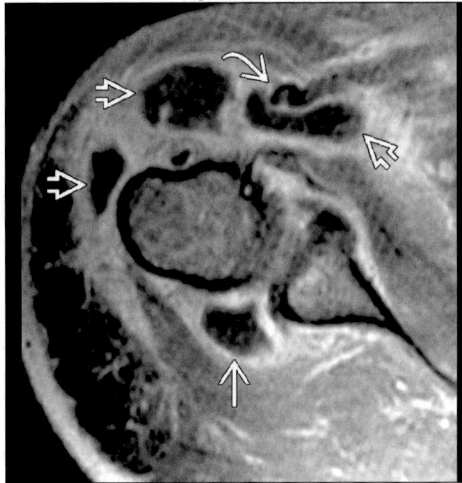

(Left) Coronal bone CT shows uniform cartilage loss without osteophytes ➡. Subchondral cysts & erosions ➡ are typical of RA. The elevated humeral head shows a chronic rotator cuff tear & there is a mechanical erosion of the medial humeral neck ➡. *(Right)* Axial T1 C+ FS MR shows glenohumeral joint fluid with thick rind of enhancing tissue ➡ & subdeltoid bursa abscesses ➡. Note that with this massive septic joint & bursa, the pectoralis muscle is ruptured & retracted ➡.

Adhesive Capsulitis, Shoulder

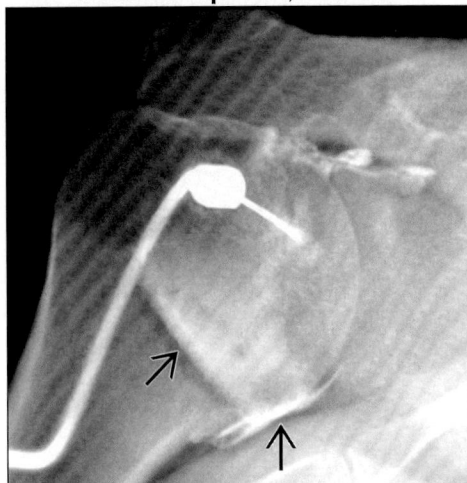

Intraosseous Neoplasm

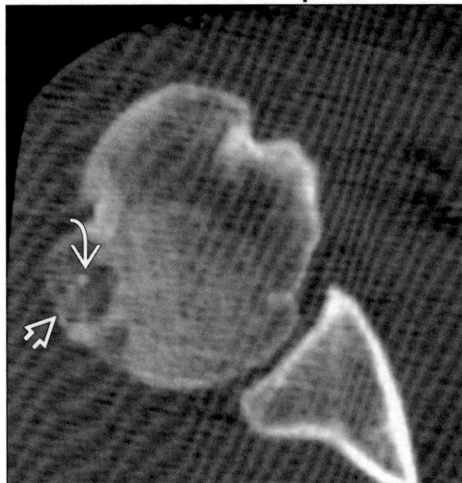

(Left) AP radiograph obtained during arthrogram injection shows effacement of the subscapularis & axillary bursae. Only 5 cc of fluid could be injected into this very tight shoulder capsule ➡. This is typical of adhesive capsulitis. *(Right)* Axial bone CT shows an eccentric slightly expanded humeral head lesion ➡ containing a small amount of chondroid matrix ➡. Chondroblastoma was diagnosed, but not before two arthroscopies for the patient's pain & popping.

SHOULDER INSTABILITY

DIFFERENTIAL DIAGNOSIS

Common
- Rotator Cuff Tear (RCT)
- Labral Tear
- Capsular Laxity
- Humeral Head Fracture
- Glenohumeral Ligament Tear

Less Common
- Glenoid Fracture
- Biceps Tendon Tear
- Inflammatory Arthropathy
- Crystalline Arthropathy
- Glenoid Malformation

Rare but Important
- Charcot, Neuropathic
- Axillary Nerve Injury
- Humeral Head Retroversion
- Neuromuscular Causes: Cerebral Palsy
- Ehlers Danlos
- Marfan Syndrome
- Intraarticular Neoplasm

ESSENTIAL INFORMATION

Key Differential Diagnosis Issues
- Shoulder is inherently unstable
  - Ball & socket joint, with very small area of osseous contact
  - Integrity of joint largely maintained by soft tissues: Labrum, tendon, capsule & related glenohumeral ligaments
- Instability may be related to osseous morphological abnormalities
  - **Hint:** Always be aware of size, shape, & alignment of glenoid & humeral head
- Instability is rarely related to inflammation
  - **Hint:** Watch for patulous capsule with synovitis & ligamentous damage
- Most frequently instability is related to traumatically-induced soft tissue injury
  - **Hint:** Soft tissue injury leading to instability is often multifactorial; examine all supporting soft tissues carefully
- **Hint:** Subtle soft tissue injury may be seen on routine MR, but often best seen with MR arthrogram
  - Distension with arthrogram is useful, especially when there is a rotator cuff tear which decompresses the natural effusion

Helpful Clues for Common Diagnoses
- **Rotator Cuff Tear (RCT)**
  - Subscapularis tear frequently results from dislocation, either anterior or posterior
  - Subscapularis is important to integrity of anterior shoulder joint
  - Tear may be either of subscapularis plus fibers crossing bicipital groove, or isolated to subscapularis
- **Labral Tear**
  - Labrum functions to significantly increase the surface area of glenohumeral articulation
  - When secondary to dislocation, tear is usually anteroinferior or posterior; humeral head subluxates accordingly
  - Labral tear may be isolated, but when secondary to dislocation may be associated with other injuries
  - May have associated IGHL disruption (Bankart), periosteal sleeve stripping (Perthes) or disruption with rotation (ALPSA)
  - Often has adjacent articular cartilage defect (GLAD)
- **Capsular Laxity**
  - Patulous capsule, distended by fluid
  - May have associated stripping of periosteum from scapula
  - Related to prior dislocations; increased risk for recurrent dislocations
  - Rarely is isolated
    - Usually glenohumeral ligament disruption, other injuries
- **Humeral Head Fracture**
  - Hill Sachs (posterolateral) impaction fracture with anterior dislocation
  - Reverse Hill Sachs (anteromedial) impaction with posterior dislocation
  - Both put patient at significant increased risk for recurrent dislocations
  - Remember these fractures occur above the equator of the humeral head
- **Glenohumeral Ligament Tear**
  - Often results from anterior shoulder dislocation (occurs in up to 50%)
  - Rare as an isolated lesion
    - Associated capsular stretching or tear
    - Often associated Hill Sachs and Bankart or labral tear

SHOULDER INSTABILITY

○ Anterior inferior glenohumeral band of ligament (IGHL) is most important portion assisting in stability

Helpful Clues for Less Common Diagnoses

- **Glenoid Fracture**
  - ○ Usually Bankart (anteroinferior) or reverse Bankart (posteroinferior), related to anterior or posterior dislocation
  - ○ Makes the surface area of osseous contact even more deficient; leads to instability
  - ○ Subluxation seen on axillary lateral radiograph or axial MR
- **Biceps Tendon Tear**
  - ○ Role of biceps in stability is debated
  - ○ Biceps dislocation/tear most frequently is associated with subscapularis tendon tear, which in turn is strongly associated with instability
- **Inflammatory Arthropathy**
  - ○ Rheumatoid arthritis (less frequently psoriatic or ankylosing spondylitis)
  - ○ Synovitis distends joint; frequent RCT; ligamentous laxity → instability
- **Crystalline Arthropathy**
  - ○ Hydroxyapatite deposition disease (HADD): Calcific deposits & often impressive destruction
  - ○ Pyrophosphate arthropathy: Deposition, usually with more degenerative change than destruction of joint
- **Glenoid Malformation**
  - ○ Glenoid may be hypoplastic, usually posteriorly & inferiorly

○ Makes an already small osseous articulation even more insufficient

Helpful Clues for Rare Diagnoses

- **Charcot, Neuropathic**
  - ○ Destructive articular process
    - ▪ Dislocation, highly unstable
    - ▪ Destruction humeral head (often with straight cut-off at humeral neck)
    - ▪ Debris: Subscapularis & axillary bursa
    - ▪ Often RCT, so debris extends into subdeltoid bursa
    - ▪ Clinical presentation is with shoulder mass due to huge distension
  - ○ Etiology usually is syringomyelia
- **Axillary Nerve Injury**
  - ○ Very rare etiology of drooping shoulder
- **Humeral Head Retroversion**
  - ○ Glenohumeral joint is normally anteverted; a retroverted head predisposes to posterior instability
- **Neuromuscular Causes: Cerebral Palsy**
  - ○ Fixed spasticity during skeletal growth → glenohumeral malformation
- **Ehlers Danlos**
  - ○ Ligamentous laxity → instability
- **Marfan Syndrome**
  - ○ Connective tissue disorder; phenotypic heterogeneity
  - ○ Ligamentous laxity may lead to instability
- **Intraarticular Neoplasm**
  - ○ Distortion of humeral head/glenoid or truly intraarticular mass could lead to subluxation

Rotator Cuff Tear (RCT)

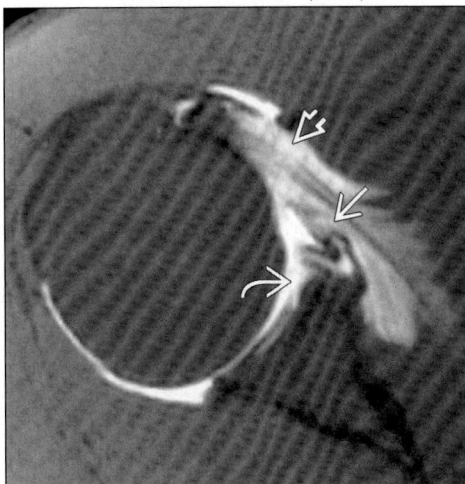

Axial T1WI FS MR arthrogram shows a subscapularis tendon tear ➡, with fluid imbibed by the muscle fibers. There is also a tear of MGHL ➡ and a glenolabral articular defect ➡; all contribute to anterior instability.

Labral Tear

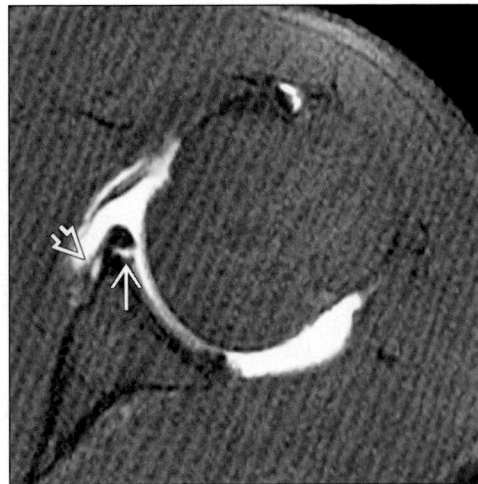

Axial T1WI FS MR arthrogram shows an anterior labral tear ➡, extending as a periosteal sleeve avulsion ➡, termed a Perthes lesion. This is one of the forms of labral injury which may contribute to instability.

SHOULDER INSTABILITY

(Left) ABER T1WI FS MR arthrogram shows an inferior labral tear ➡ as well as glenoid articular cartilaginous defect (GLAD) ➡ in a patient who presented with instability. *(Right)* Axial CT arthrogram shows an anterior-inferior labral tear, distracted with external rotation ➡. A Hill Sachs impaction was seen more proximally at the posterolateral humeral head. The combination typically results from anterior shoulder dislocation, and predisposes to recurrent dislocation.

Labral Tear

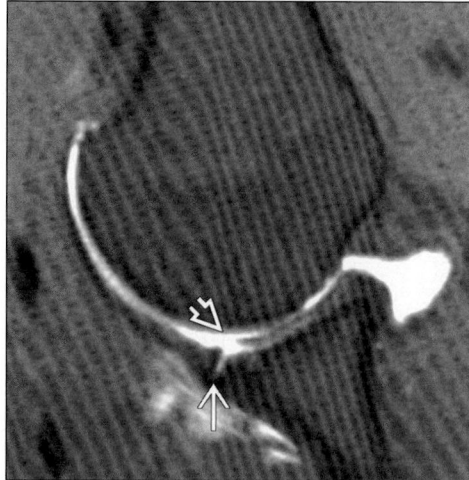

Labral Tear

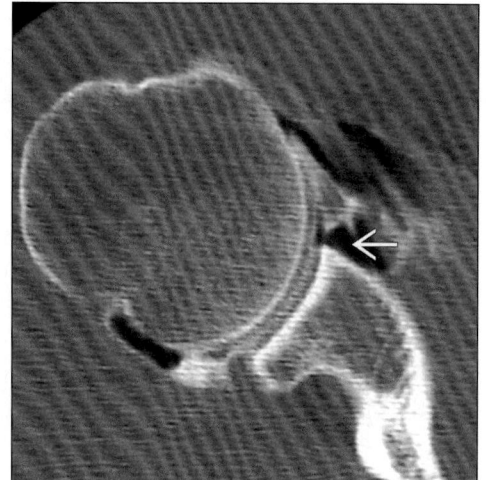

(Left) Axial T1WI FS MR arthrogram shows labral tear with periosteal stripping anteriorly. This has resulted in a significantly patulous anterior capsule ➡; this redundancy leads to instability. Note additionally the partial subscapularis tear with biceps dislocation ➡. *(Right)* Axial PD FSE MR shows Hill Sachs impaction fracture of the posterolateral humeral head ➡. Note the patulous posterior capsule ➡ and anterior labral tear ➡. The head is subluxated anteriorly.

Capsular Laxity

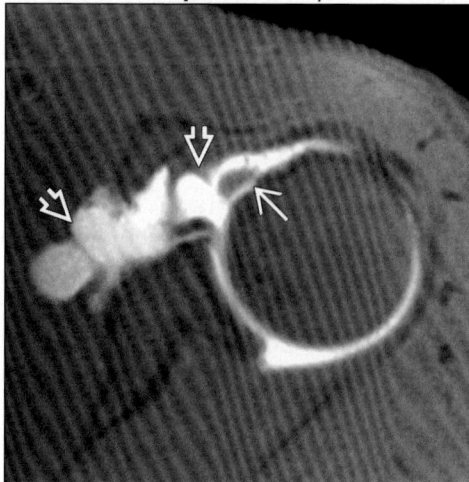

Humeral Head Fracture

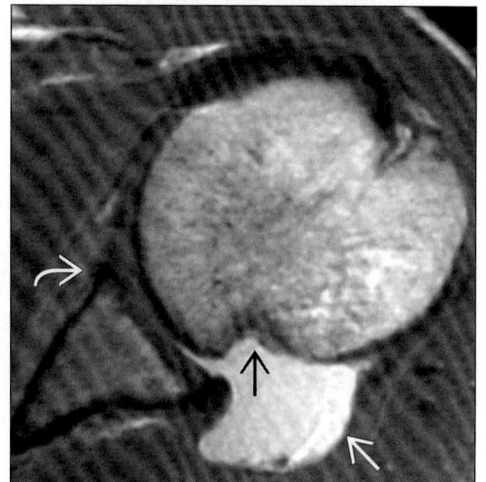

(Left) Sagittal T1WI FS MR arthrogram shows an intact MGHL ➡ but imbibition of contrast into a partial subscapularis tear ➡. The posterior capsule is extremely redundant ➡ and contains wavy fibers which are part of the torn IGHL ➡. The patient had multidirectional instability. *(Right)* Sagittal T1WI FS MR arthrogram shows a redundant rotator interval ➡ & wavy disrupted IGHL ➡, with a patulous joint capsule. It is not surprising that instability is multidirectional.

Glenohumeral Ligament Tear

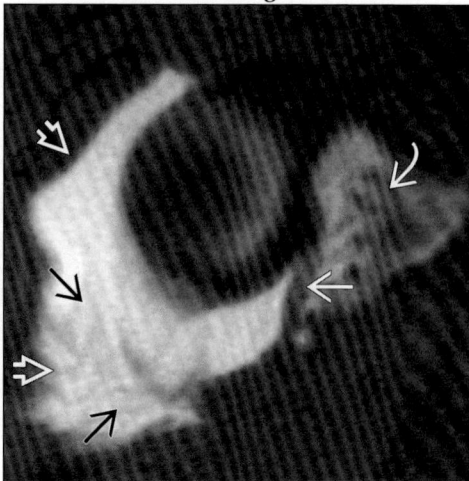

Glenohumeral Ligament Tear

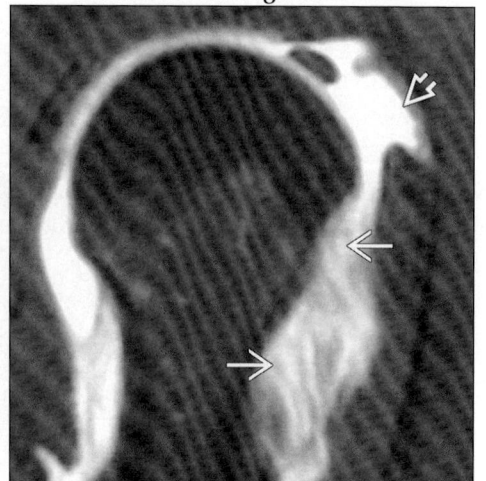

SHOULDER INSTABILITY

Glenoid Fracture

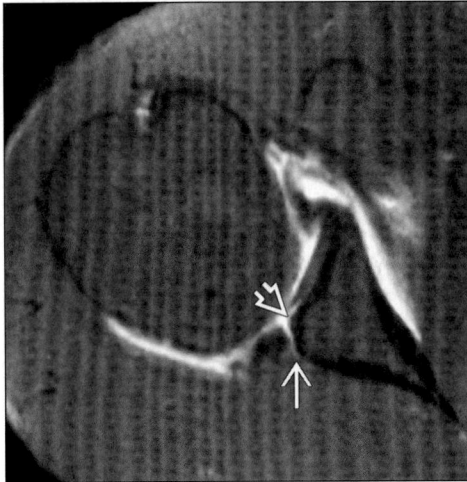

Biceps Tendon Tear

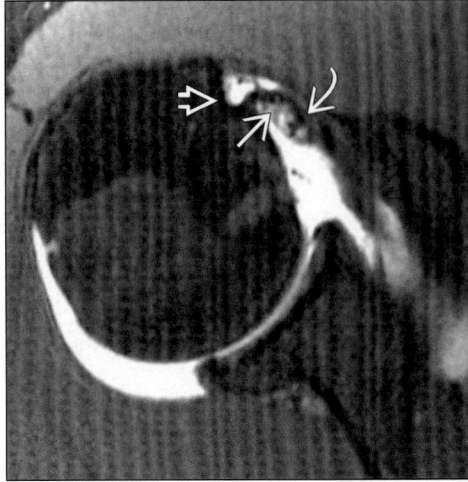

(Left) Axial T1WI FS MR shows reverse bony Bankart fracture ⮕. Note the cartilage disruption as well ⮕. The humeral head is posteriorly subluxated, indicating at least a posterior instability. *(Right)* Axial T1WI FS MR arthrogram shows a partial biceps tear ⮕ with dislocation into partial undersurface tear of the subscapularis tendon ⮕. Note the empty bicipital groove ⮕. The biceps dislocation and subscapularis injury contribute to anterior instability.

Inflammatory Arthropathy

Crystalline Arthropathy

(Left) Coronal PD FSE FS MR in a patient with rheumatoid arthritis shows a rotator cuff tear ⮕, patulous joint ⮕, & extensive synovitis with rice bodies. The combination may lead to instability. *(Right)* Anteroposterior radiograph shows pyrophosphate arthropathy, with a chronic RCT and degenerative change. HADD (Milwaukee shoulder) often shows more destruction as well as calcific deposits than is seen here and is more likely to be unstable.

Glenoid Malformation

Charcot, Neuropathic

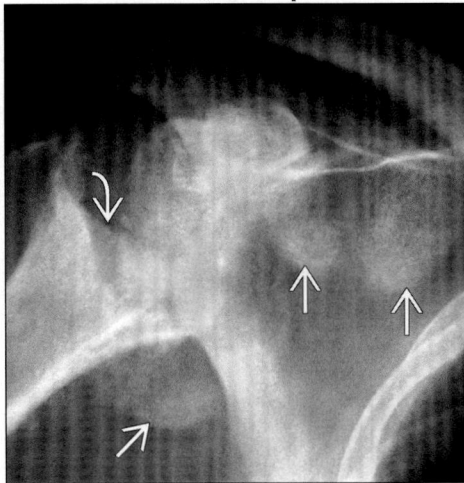

(Left) Lateral radiograph shows posterior hypoplasia of the glenoid ⮕. The glenoid was hypoplastic inferiorly as well. This decreases the already small area of osseous contact, leading to further instability. *(Right)* Anteroposterior radiograph shows unstable, dislocated humeral head with "cut-off" sign at the humeral neck ⮕. There is osseous debris within axillary & subscapularis bursae ⮕ showing these structures to be distended. This is typical of Charcot shoulder.

ANTEROINFERIOR LABRAL/CAPSULE INJURY

DIFFERENTIAL DIAGNOSIS

Common
- Bankart Lesion
- GLAD Lesion

Less Common
- ALPSA Lesion
- Perthes Lesion
- HAGL Lesion

Rare but Important
- Congenital Hypermobility Syndrome

ESSENTIAL INFORMATION

Key Differential Diagnosis Issues
- **Hint**: Watch for radiographic abnormality
  - Hill-Sachs impaction deformity
  - Glenoid fracture fragments
- CT: Malalignment, glenoid hypoplasia
- MR: Marrow and soft tissue edema, labral tears; sensitivity/specificity (S/S): 80/45-80%
- MR/CT with intra-articular contrast: ↑ conspicuity; S/S: 95/86%
- **AB**duction **E**xternal **R**otation (ABER) view
  - Inferior glenohumeral labroligamentous (IGHL) structures taut for improved visibility, eliminates magic angle
  - Position gently to avoid re-dislocation
- Young adult dislocation: Bankart, variants
- Older adult dislocation = 1/3 supraspinatus tear; 1/3 greater tuberosity fracture; 1/3 subscapularis/capsular avulsion

Helpful Clues for Common Diagnoses
- **Bankart Lesion**
  - Anteroinferior labroligamentous avulsion from glenoid & periosteal sleeve tear; ± adjacent glenoid fracture
  - Acute: Discrete or fragmented tear across labral base
  - Chronic: Fibrotic medial "mass"
- **GLAD Lesion**
  - Glenoid Labrum Articular Disruption
  - Labrum partial tear & adjacent cartilage damage

Helpful Clues for Less Common Diagnoses
- **ALPSA Lesion**
  - Anterior Labroligamentous Periosteal Sleeve Avulsion
  - Bankart but periosteal sleeve intact
  - Acute: Torn labroligamentous complex rolls medial & inferior
  - Chronic: Fibrotic medial "mass"
- **Perthes Lesion**
  - Bankart & intact but redundant periosteal sleeve
- **HAGL Lesion**
  - Humeral Avulsion of Glenohumeral Ligament
  - Capsule avulsion of IGHL from humeral attachment without subscapularis tear; no age predilection

Helpful Clues for Rare Diagnoses
- **Congenital Hypermobility Syndrome**
  - Diagnosis of exclusion

Bankart Lesion

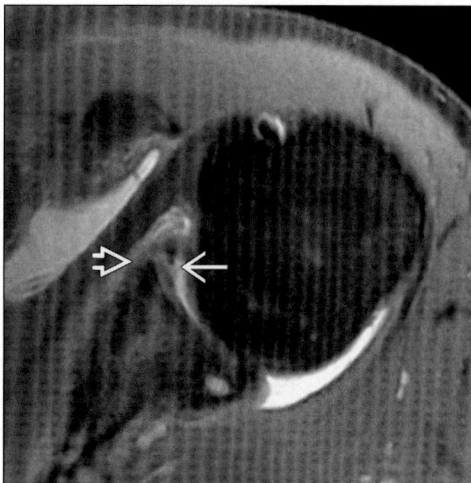

Axial T1 C+ FS MR shows complete disruption of the anteroinferior labrum ➡ & periosteal sleeve ⮞ with ↑ SI crossing the labral base in a patient with recent dislocation.

Bankart Lesion

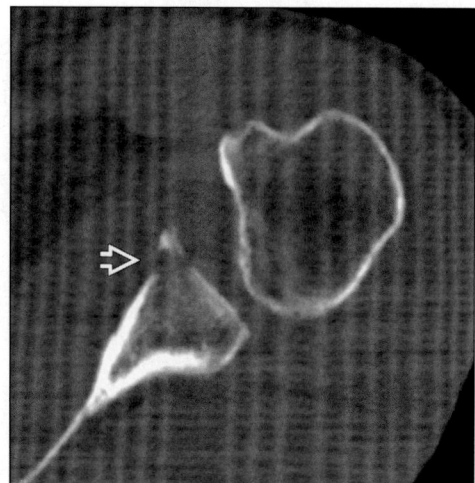

Axial NECT in the same patient as previous image shows a concomitant fracture ⮞ (osseous Bankart) along the anteroinferior osseous glenoid.

ANTEROINFERIOR LABRAL/CAPSULE INJURY

Bankart Lesion

Bankart Lesion

(Left) Axial CECT double-contrast arthrogram in external rotation shows a soft tissue Bankart lesion with air passing through the anteroinferior labral tear ➡. Note the completely disrupted fragment ➡ displaced medially. Similar information can be obtained with a single contrast CT arthrogram. (Right) ABER T1 C+ FS MR shows a complete labral tear ➡ (Bankart lesion) with the abduction external rotation (ABER) position placing tension across the inferior capsule.

GLAD Lesion

ALPSA Lesion

(Left) Axial T1 C+ FS MR shows a partial tear ➡ of the anteroinferior labrum with adjacent cartilage damage ➡ of a GLAD lesion. Note biceps medial subluxation ➡ into a subscapularis tear. (Right) Axial T1 C+ FS MR shows an anterior labral tear with anterior & medial displacement of the fragment ➡ with intact scapular periosteum ➡ forming an ALPSA lesion. This is an acute injury with an accompanying Hill-Sachs lesion (not shown).

Perthes Lesion

HAGL Lesion

(Left) Axial T1 C+ FS MR shows an anteroinferior labral tear ➡ & intact periosteal sleeve ➡ (Perthes lesion). The labral fragment is not medially displaced & the periosteal sleeve is slightly redundant, distinguishing this from an ALPSA lesion. (Right) ABER T1 C+ FS MR shows avulsion of the anterior band inferior glenohumeral ligament's humeral attachment ➡ (HAGL lesion) with extensive intrasubstance ➡ (partial tear) of the anterior band itself.

NERVE ENTRAPMENT, SHOULDER

DIFFERENTIAL DIAGNOSIS

Common
- Thoracic Outlet Synd. (Brachial Plexus)
- Suprascapular Nerve Entrapment

Less Common
- Parsonage-Turner Syndrome
- Quadrilateral Space Synd. (Axillary N.)

Rare but Important
- Long Thoracic Nerve Syndrome
- Saturday Night Palsy (Radial Nerve)

ESSENTIAL INFORMATION

Key Differential Diagnosis Issues
- Entrapment neuropathy: Nerve function altered by compression, often at predictable site of anatomic narrowing
- Symptoms: Muscle weakness, paresthesias, muscle atrophy
- MR: Look for nerve course & contour; muscle signal intensity (SI) & distribution
- Look for: Ganglia, tumors, inflammation, post-trauma, scarring, edema, anomalies
- Muscle SI in entrapment
  - Acute (< 1 mo): T1 normal; STIR ↑ SI; enhancement: +
  - Subacute (1-6 mos): T1 ± normal; STIR ↑ SI; enhancement: ±
  - Chronic (> 6 mos): T1 ↑ SI; STIR ↓ SI; enhancement - none

Helpful Clues for Common Diagnoses
- **Thoracic Outlet Synd. (Brachial Plexus)**
  - Compression sites: Anterior scalene, costoclavicular, or pectoralis minor
  - F > M; compression may be neurogenic or vascular
  - X-ray: Cervical ribs, clavicle deformity
    - CT or MR angiography: Vascular injury
    - Image with arms in neutral & hyperextended position to highlight compression
- **Suprascapular Nerve Entrapment**
  - Compression sites/muscles affected
    - At suprascapular notch: Supraspinatus, infraspinatus muscles
    - At spinoglenoid notch: Infraspinatus m.

Helpful Clues for Less Common Diagnoses
- **Parsonage-Turner Syndrome**
  - Acute brachial neuritis; M > F
  - Patchy muscle involvement with supraspinatus, infraspinatus, deltoid most common
- **Quadrilateral Space Synd. (Axillary N.)**
  - Compression site: Space bounded by triceps (medial), teres minor (superior), teres major (inferior), humerus (lateral)
  - Muscles affected: Teres minor, deltoid

Helpful Clues for Rare Diagnoses
- **Long Thoracic Nerve Syndrome**
  - Compression site: Serratus anterior between clavicle & 1st rib
  - Winged scapula; seen with crutches, sports
- **Saturday Night Palsy (Radial Nerve)**
  - Compression site: Proximal radial groove
  - Muscles affected: Triceps, anconeus

Thoracic Outlet Synd. (Brachial Plexus)

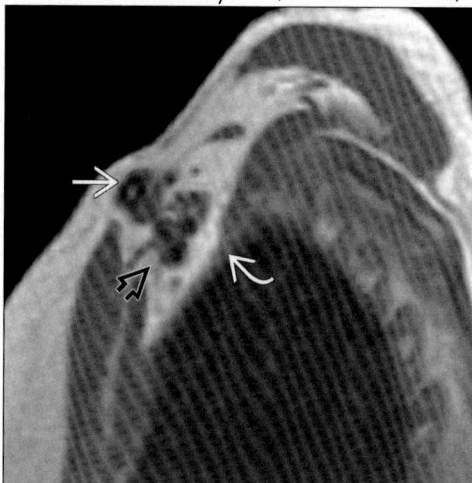

Sagittal T1WI MR with arms in neutral position shows the neurovascular bundle ⇾ passing between the clavicle ➡ & the 1st rib ➡ with no compression in 50 year old female.

Thoracic Outlet Synd. (Brachial Plexus)

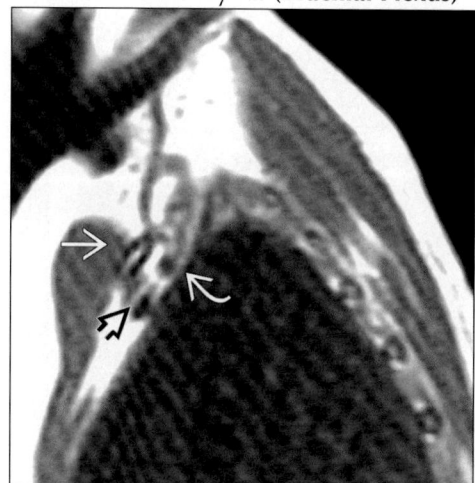

Sagittal T1WI MR with arms hyperabducted in the same patient shows flattening of the neurovascular bundle ⇾ with compression of the brachial plexus between the clavicle ➡ & 1st rib ➡.

Suprascapular Nerve Entrapment

Suprascapular Nerve Entrapment

(Left) Coronal T2WI FS MR shows a paralabral cyst ⇨ extending into the suprascapular notch ➔ & compressing the suprascapular nerve, resulting in edema of the supraspinatus & infraspinatus muscles (not shown). *(Right)* Sagittal PD FSE FS MR shows a multiseptate cyst ➔ compressing the infraspinatus branch of the suprascapular nerve as it passes through the spinoglenoid notch ➔ with resultant infraspinatus weakness.

Parsonage-Turner Syndrome

Quadrilateral Space Synd. (Axillary N.)

(Left) Sagittal T2WI FS MR shows edema in the supraspinatus ➔, infraspinatus ➔, & deltoid ➔ muscles in a male with acute onset shoulder pain in early stage Parsonage-Turner syndrome. *(Right)* Coronal oblique T1WI MR shows fatty atrophy of the teres minor ➔ & deltoid ➔ muscles due to axillary nerve neuropathy in quadrilateral space syndrome (quadrilateral space ➔). No compressive lesion is seen; fibrous bands may account for the neuropathy.

Quadrilateral Space Synd. (Axillary N.)

Quadrilateral Space Synd. (Axillary N.)

(Left) Sagittal T1WI MR shows the normal relationship of the axillary nerve ➔ to the adjacent joint structures including the humerus ➔, subscapularis ➔, & teres minor ➔ muscles. *(Right)* Sagittal T1 C+ FS MR shows the axillary nerve ➔ being compressed superiorly toward the normal shoulder structures including the humeral head ➔ by a large heterogeneous liposarcoma presenting with fatty ➔ & solid ➔ components.

ELBOW DEFORMITIES IN CHILDREN AND YOUNG ADULTS

DIFFERENTIAL DIAGNOSIS

Common
- Complication of Fracture Healing
- Physeal Bar

Less Common
- Juvenile Idiopathic Arthritis (JIA)
- Hemophilia
- Nontraumatic Radial Head Dislocation

Rare but Important
- Radiation-Induced Growth Deformities
- Radiation Osteonecrosis
- Congenital Cubitus Valgus
- Radius & Ulna, Aplasia/Hypoplasia

ESSENTIAL INFORMATION

Helpful Clues for Common Diagnoses
- **Complication of Fracture Healing**
  - Malunion & nonunion
  - Cubitus valgus: Lateral condyle fracture
    - Pain, instability, limited ROM, delayed onset ulnar nerve palsy
  - Cubitus varus: Malrotated supracondylar fracture, leads to ulnar nerve subluxation, cosmetic rather than functional deformity
  - Fishtail deformity: Gap between capitellum & trochlea
- **Physeal Bar**
  - Following trauma, infection, radiation
  - CT or MR may be required to detect
    - Appears as osseous bridge across physis
    - Location more important than size

Helpful Clues for Less Common Diagnoses
- **Juvenile Idiopathic Arthritis (JIA)**
  - Epiphyseal overgrowth, especially radius; peri-articular osteoporosis, uniform joint space narrowing, marginal erosions, periosteal new bone formation
- **Hemophilia**
  - Epiphyseal overgrowth (may result in deformity), especially radius; peri-articular osteoporosis, uniform cartilage loss, subchondral cysts, dense effusion
- **Nontraumatic Radial Head Dislocation**
  - Congenital: Hypoplastic capitellum, radial neck elongated, radial head domed-shaped & dislocated posteriorly; painless, decreased extension & supination
    - Always associated anomalies such as Fong disease; never unilateral & isolated
  - Developmental: Neuromuscular conditions such as cerebral palsy, Ehlers Danlos
  - Hereditary multiple exostoses, Ollier disease

Helpful Clues for Rare Diagnoses
- **Radiation-Induced Growth Deformities**
  - Regional osteoporosis & osseous underdevelopment, ± physeal bar
- **Radiation Osteonecrosis**
  - Regional osteoporosis, articular surface collapse & fragmentation
- **Congenital Cubitus Valgus**
  - Turner & Noonan syndromes
- **Radius & Ulna, Aplasia/Hypoplasia**
  - VACTERL syndrome, TAR syndrome

Complication of Fracture Healing

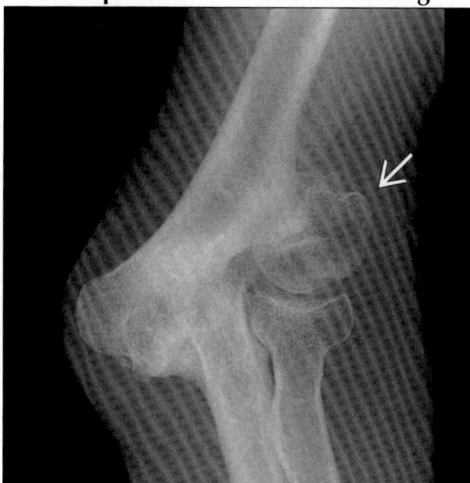

Anteroposterior radiograph shows a fracture of the lateral condyle ➡ with proximal displacement, resulting in a cubitus valgus deformity. Reformatted CT (not shown) demonstrated nonunion.

Physeal Bar

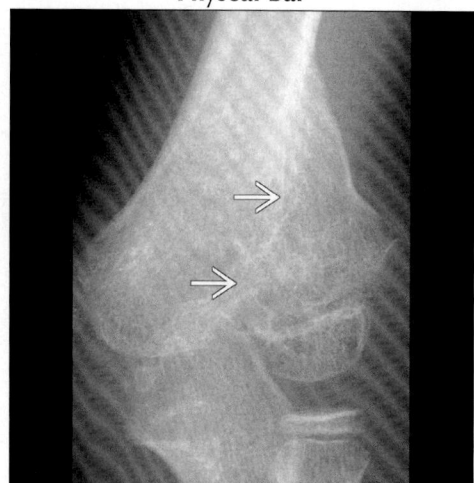

AP radiograph shows old Salter IV fracture of the lateral condyle ➡, with proximal displacement of the fragment. The displaced fragment allowed formation of a physeal bar, resulting in a cubitus valgus deformity.

ELBOW DEFORMITIES IN CHILDREN AND YOUNG ADULTS

Juvenile Idiopathic Arthritis (JIA)

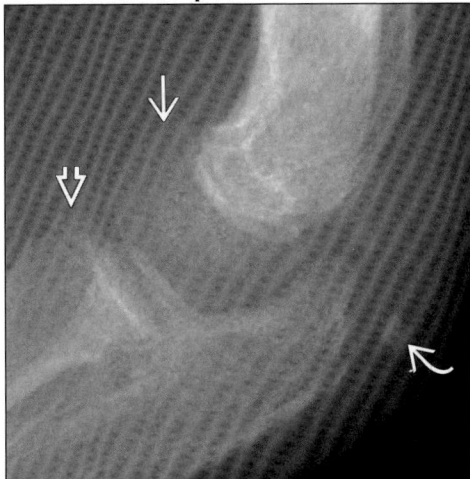

Hemophilia

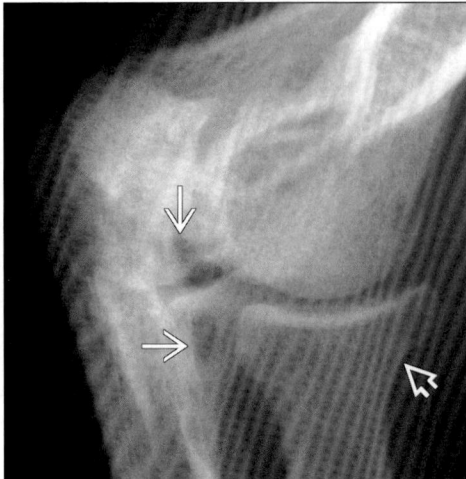

(Left) Lateral radiograph shows osteoporosis & overgrowth of capitellum ➡. When compared to the opposite side there is advanced maturation of radius ➡ & olecranon ➡ in this patient with JIA. (†MSK Req). *(Right)* Oblique radiograph shows overgrowth of the radial head epiphysis ➡, peri-articular osteoporosis, & subchondral cysts ➡ in this individual with hemophilia. Asymmetric overgrowth may result in alignment abnormalities.

Nontraumatic Radial Head Dislocation

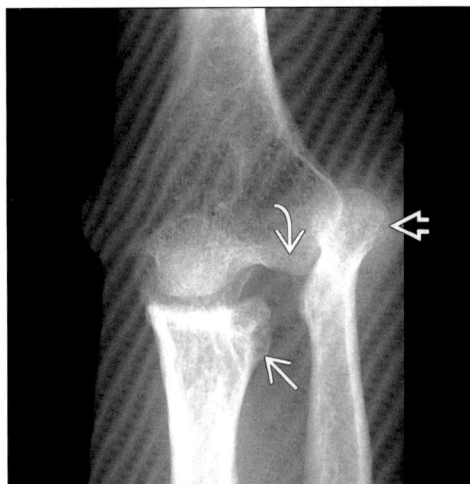

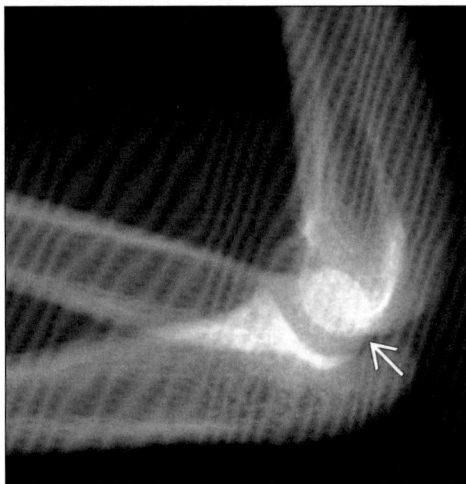

Nontraumatic Radial Head Dislocation

(Left) Anteroposterior radiograph shows exostosis of the proximal ulna ➡. The capitellum is hypoplastic ➡ & the radial head is dome-shaped & dislocated ➡ in this child with radial head dislocation associated with multiple hereditary exostoses. *(Right)* Lateral radiograph shows characteristic congenital radial head dislocation. The head has a convex contour & is dislocated posteriorly ➡. Additionally, the radial head is overgrown & is long relative to the ulna.

Radius & Ulna, Aplasia/Hypoplasia

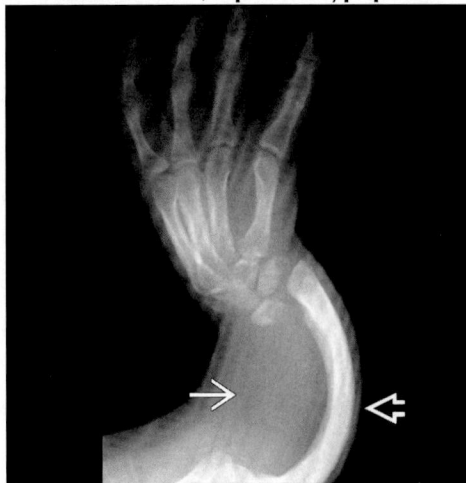

Radius & Ulna, Aplasia/Hypoplasia

(Left) Oblique radiograph shows a hypoplastic radial head ➡ which resulted in an increased carrying angle in this patient with nail-patella syndrome or Fong disease. *(Right)* Posteroanterior radiograph shows phocomelia, with predominance of radial-sided abnormalities. The ulna is short and bowed ➡, and the radius is nearly completely aplastic ➡. Other associated anomalies helped to make the diagnosis of VACTERL syndrome.

LATERAL ELBOW PAIN

DIFFERENTIAL DIAGNOSIS

Common
- Lateral Epicondylitis
- Radial Head/Neck Fracture
- Radial Head Dislocation
- Capitellar Osteochondritis
- Capitellar Osteonecrosis
- Lateral Condylar Fracture
- Common Extensor Mechanism Injury

Less Common
- Capitellum Fracture
- Lateral Collateral Ligament Injury
- Radial Head Subluxation (Nursemaid Elbow)
- Neoplasm, Bone
- Neoplasm, Soft Tissue

Rare but Important
- Radial Neuropathy
- Synovial Fringe

ESSENTIAL INFORMATION

Key Differential Diagnosis Issues
- Clinical history of trauma or overuse helpful for directing workup
- Presence of significant effusion favors fracture (even when not visible) or an inflammatory etiology

Helpful Clues for Common Diagnoses
- **Lateral Epicondylitis**
  - a.k.a., "tennis elbow"
  - Radiographs demonstrate soft tissue swelling or are normal
  - Thickening & increased signal of the common extensor tendon on MR
    - Extensor carpi radialis brevis most susceptible to tearing/degeneration
    - Fluid signal intensity is consistent with partial thickness tearing
  - ± Tearing & degeneration of lateral ulnar collateral ligament complex
  - CT arthrography shows contrast extravasation if capsule is disrupted
- **Radial Head/Neck Fracture**
  - Joint effusion almost invariably present
    - Anterior fat pad elevated, "sail sign"
    - Posterior fat pad visible
  - Lucent fracture line(s) on radiographs
  - Low signal fracture line with high signal surrounding edema on MR
  - Anterolateral head vulnerable to fracture due to less supporting bone
  - CT to assess for occult fracture or associated fractures
    - Fall on outstretched hand may also be associated with scaphoid fracture
  - Radial head fracture is common in adults
    - Fracture of the radial neck is more common in children & teenagers
  - Essex-Lopresti fracture
    - Radial head or neck fracture
    - Disrupted forearm interosseous membrane
    - Unstable distal radioulnar joint
- **Radial Head Dislocation**
  - Posterior dislocation
    - ± Lateral ligament & common extensor tendon tears
    - ± Capitellar or coronoid fracture
    - Capsular disruption
    - Hemorrhage
  - Secondary osteoarthritis occurs late
- **Capitellar Osteochondritis**
  - Focal lucency in the capitellum on radiographs
  - Flattened capitellar articular surface
  - Loose bodies in joint
  - Check for bilaterality (20%)
  - Variable signal intensity on MR
    - May have internal & surrounding edema
    - Hyperintense fluid deep to lesion on T2WI indicates a loose fragment
  - Teenage athletic patients
- **Capitellar Osteonecrosis**
  - Sclerosis of capitellum in younger patient than osteochondritis
  - More likely to involve the entire capitellum than osteochondritis
  - Less likely than osteochondritis to have intraarticular loose bodies
- **Lateral Condylar Fracture**
  - Pediatric: Second most common elbow fracture
    - Attached common extensor tendon may produce distal retraction of fracture fragment
    - MR to evaluate physeal injury
  - Adult: Lateral condyle fracture involves capitellum ± lateral trochlea
    - May have disruption of lateral collateral ligament & common extensor tendon

○ Positive fat pad sign due to effusion
- **Common Extensor Mechanism Injury**
  ○ Degeneration or tear of common extensor tendon components
    ▪ Extensor carpi radialis brevis has most lateral location & is injured most often

Helpful Clues for Less Common Diagnoses
- **Capitellum Fracture**
  ○ Fracture usually in the coronal plane
    ▪ Best seen on sagittal images
    ▪ Variable anterior displacement of capitellar fracture fragment
  ○ Positive fat pad sign
  ○ Very uncommon in children
  ○ Evaluate for associated radial head fracture
- **Lateral Collateral Ligament Injury**
  ○ Components: Radial collateral ligament & lateral ulnar collateral ligament
  ○ History of trauma or chronic overuse
  ○ Radiographs may be normal or show malalignment to dislocation
    ▪ Fractures of coronoid process, capitellum and/or radial head
  ○ Arthrography demonstrates extravasation via lateral capsular defect
  ○ MR shows disruption of ligament fibers
- **Radial Head Subluxation (Nursemaid Elbow)**
  ○ Radiographs are usually normal
    ▪ Radial head subluxation or joint widening is uncommon

○ Radial head slips beneath the annular ligament, which normally lies over the radial neck, becoming trapped between the radial head & capitellum
○ Clinically, the joint is held fixed in pronation
○ Imaging is not typically necessary for reduction (often occurs with supination)
- **Neoplasm, Bone**
  ○ Lesions in or near the end of bone
    ▪ Giant cell tumor, chondroblastoma, aneurysmal bone cyst, osteoid osteoma, chondrosarcoma, metastasis, myeloma
- **Neoplasm, Soft Tissue**
  ○ Synovial sarcoma, nerve sheath tumors, malignant fibrous histiocytoma

Helpful Clues for Rare Diagnoses
- **Radial Neuropathy**
  ○ Look for denervation edema or atrophy in muscles supplied by radial nerve
    ▪ Increased signal on T2WI
  ○ Associated symptoms of radial tunnel syndrome
    ▪ Pain anterolateral proximal forearm (no sensation deficit or weakness)
    ▪ May be an early posterior interosseous nerve syndrome
  ○ ± Fracture of the humerus
- **Synovial Fringe**
  ○ Thickened triangular synovial fold (plica) between radial head & capitellum on MR
  ○ Radiographs & CT may show associated capitellar lucency or sclerosis

Lateral Epicondylitis

Coronal T2WI FS MR shows increased signal within a diffusely thickened common extensor tendon origin ➡ at the lateral humeral epicondyle. There is no fluid signal within the origin to indicate focal tear.

Radial Head/Neck Fracture

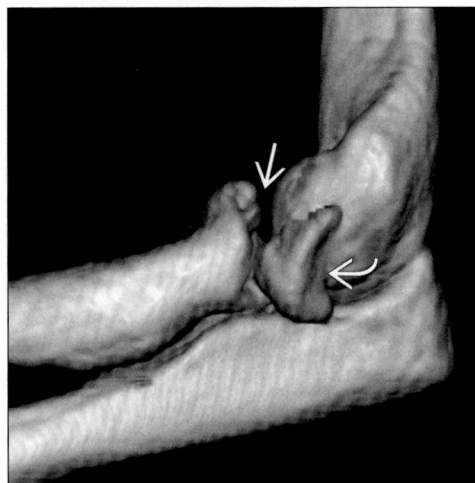

NECT 3D VRT shows a fracture of the radial head and neck ➡. The dominant fracture fragment ➡ is rotated and displaced into the lateral gutter of the joint.

LATERAL ELBOW PAIN

(Left) Oblique radiograph shows a comminuted fracture of the radial head/neck with displacement and impaction ➡. This is an Essex-Lopresti injury, associated with a disrupted interosseous membrane and an unstable distal radioulnar joint. **(Right)** Lateral radiograph shows posterior dislocation of the radial head ➡. There is an obliquely oriented fracture of the proximal ulna ➡. This combination of injuries is termed a Monteggia fracture dislocation.

(Left) Anteroposterior radiograph shows a focal lucent region ➡ in the capitellum without collapse of the articular surface. This area of lucency was enlarging in a teenaged throwing athlete. **(Right)** Sagittal T1WI FS MR arthrogram in the same patient as the prior image shows the osteochondral lesion ➡ in the capitellum. It is located slightly anterior along the articular surface. The lack of fluid extending beneath the lesion indicates that it is stable.

(Left) Coronal NECT shows sclerosis and fragmentation ➡ of the entire capitellum. Small fracture fragments ➡ are loose in the joint. Osteonecrosis began before the patient was a teenager. **(Right)** Anteroposterior radiograph shows a fracture ➡ involving the lateral condyle of the humerus. These fractures can be difficult to detect and it can be helpful to obtain radiographs of the opposite elbow.

Radial Head/Neck Fracture

Radial Head Dislocation

Capitellar Osteochondritis

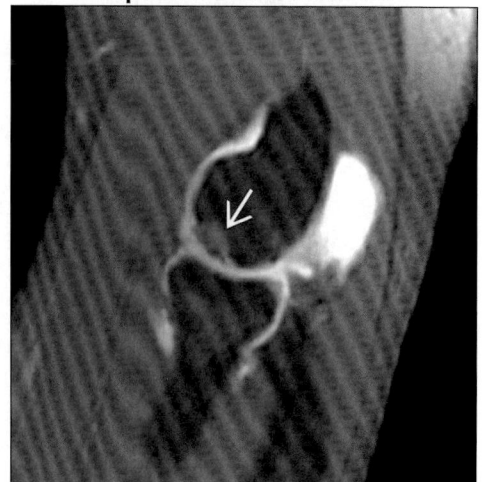

Capitellar Osteochondritis

Capitellar Osteonecrosis

Lateral Condylar Fracture

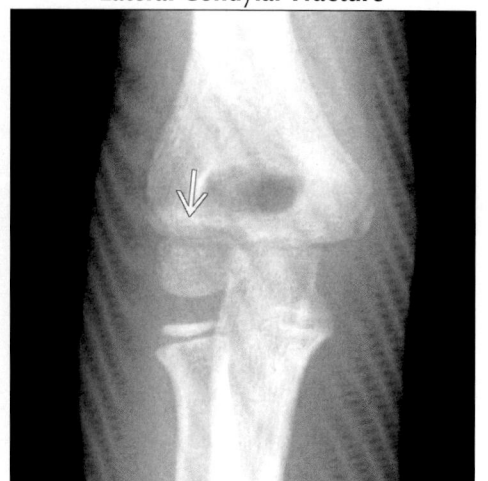

LATERAL ELBOW PAIN

Common Extensor Mechanism Injury

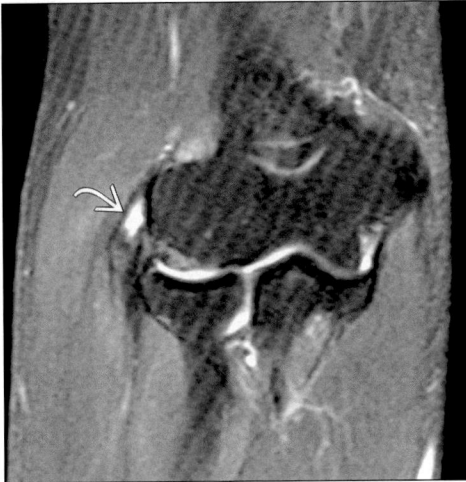

Capitellum Fracture

(Left) Coronal T2WI FS MR shows a focus of high signal ➡ in the common extensor tendon near the origin on the lateral epicondyle. Fluid signal within the tendon indicates a partial thickness tear. *(Right)* NECT reformatted 3D VRT shows a fracture of the capitellum ➡. The dominant fracture fragment ➡ has flipped anterior to the radial head.

Lateral Collateral Ligament Injury

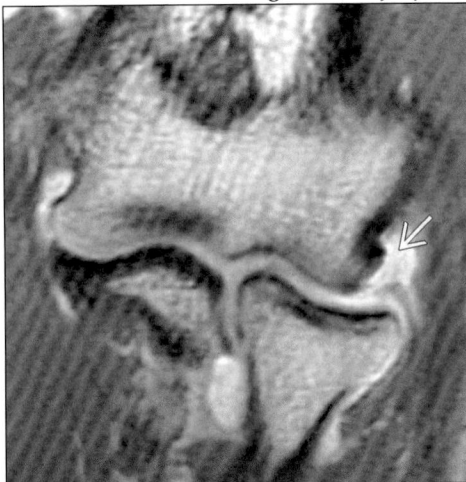

Neoplasm, Bone

(Left) Coronal T2WI MR shows complete disruption of both the lateral ulnar collateral ligament as well as the lateral collateral ligament ➡. Slightly more posteriorly, there was an extensive partial thickness tear of the common extensor tendon origin. *(Right)* Oblique radiograph shows a lytic, mildly expansile lesion ➡ in the radial head and neck. In an adult, the differential diagnosis includes giant cell tumor, metastasis, myeloma and lymphoma.

Radial Neuropathy

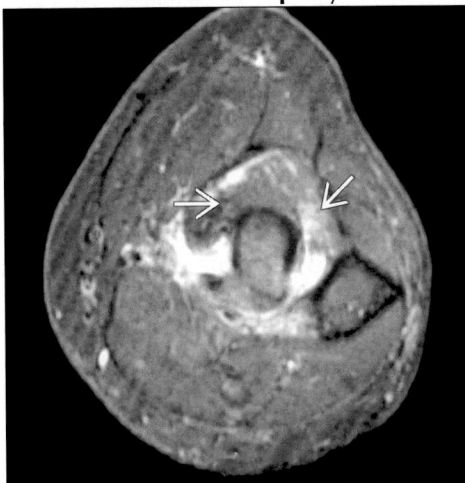

Synovial Fringe

(Left) Axial T2WI FS MR shows moderate edema ➡ in the supinator muscle, a sign of denervation of the radial nerve. This is a high radial neuropathy likely related to remote trauma, with mild atrophic changes in the supinator. *(Right)* Coronal T2WI FS MR shows a large meniscoid structure ➡ extending into the radiocapitellar joint, consistent with a synovial fringe. In this case it was symptomatic; the pain ceased once it was surgically removed.

MEDIAL ELBOW PAIN

DIFFERENTIAL DIAGNOSIS

Common
- Medial Epicondylitis
- Medial Collateral Ligament (MCL) Injury
- Olecranon Fracture
- Common Flexor Mechanism Injury
- Medial Epicondyle Avulsion, Pediatric
- Coronoid Process Fracture
- Medial Condylar Fracture
- Ulnar Neuropathy
- Little Leaguer's Elbow
- C8-T1 Radiculopathy (Mimic)
- Median Neuropathy

Less Common
- Triceps Tendon Rupture
- Anconeus Epitrochlearis

Rare but Important
- Cat Scratch Disease

ESSENTIAL INFORMATION

Key Differential Diagnosis Issues
- Common mechanism is valgus stress
  - **Hint:** In skeletally immature athlete injury to physis most common; in adult one sees injury to medial (ulnar) collateral ligament (MCL) and/or flexor-pronator muscle group
  - UCL injuries and injuries to flexor-pronator group often co-exist
- Typically present with medial elbow pain, may also have loss of grip strength
- Usually in dominant upper extremity
- Flexor-pronator group: Common tendon origin arising from the medial epicondyle
  - Flexor carpi radialis, flexor carpi ulnaris, flexor digitorum superficialis, palmaris longus, pronator teres muscles

Helpful Clues for Common Diagnoses
- **Medial Epicondylitis**
  - Valgus stress overuse injury of flexor-pronator group
    - Golf, baseball, tennis
  - Range: Acute inflammation to tendinosis
    - May progress to common flexor partial or full thickness tear
  - Associated ulnar neuropathy
  - MR: Multitude of appearances
    - Intermediate T1WI signal

- Peritendon inflammation
- Epicondyle marrow edema
- Intermediate to bright T2WI signal within tendon
- Tendon thickening
- **Medial Collateral Ligament (MCL) Injury**
  - Chronic repetitive trauma
  - Injury to anterior bundle most common, most significant; anterior bundle most important stabilizer in valgus stress
  - Radiographs
    - Ossification late finding
  - MR
    - Periligamentous edema
    - Bright T2WI signal within ligament
    - Ligament thickening or discontinuity
    - Ossification
  - MR arthrography
    - "T" sign (extension of contrast between MCL and coronoid process), though may be normal
    - Intraligamentous contrast or extravasation indicative of tear
  - US with valgus stress demonstrates instability with medial joint widening
  - Avulsion of sublime tubercle
    - Attachment site of anterior band of medial collateral ligament on coronoid process
- **Olecranon Fracture**
  - Fall on outstretched hand with flexed elbow or direct blow
    - Triceps pull creates distraction forces at fracture site & may require internal fixation
- **Common Flexor Mechanism Injury**
  - Sequelae of overuse injury and tendonitis/inflammation within the flexor-pronator group
  - Ranges from partial to full thickness tears
  - MR
    - Peritendon edema
    - Intratendinous bright T2WI signal
    - Discontinuity, wavy fibers, gap
  - MR arthrography not useful
  - Ultrasound may identify tear
- **Medial Epicondyle Avulsion, Pediatric**
  - Ossification center appears age 4-6 years
  - 50% associated with elbow dislocation
  - Other mechanism: Sudden forceful contraction with onset of pain

- **Hint**: When fragment displaced into joint, mimics trochlear ossification center
  - Always identify epicondyle ossification center when evaluating pediatric elbow
  - Requires transient joint widening
  - May be manifestation of Little Leaguer's elbow
- **Coronoid Process Fracture**
  - Often seen with dislocation
  - Unstable when > 50% coronoid involved
- **Medial Condylar Fracture**
  - Fall with angular force or direct blow
  - Extension lateral to capitellotrochlear groove leads to instability
- **Ulnar Neuropathy**
  - a.k.a. tarda ulnar palsy, cubital tunnel syndrome
  - Entrapment at multiple sites in elbow region: Intermuscular septum, epicondylar region, ulnar groove, cubital tunnel
  - May complicate fracture, dislocation, overuse injuries
  - Clinical
    - Tingling elbow to hand especially fingers 4 & 5, inability to abduct fingers 4 & 5, muscle atrophy
  - MR: Nerve may appear normal or may be enlarged, have bright T2WI signal within, or perineural inflammation
- **Little Leaguer's Elbow**
  - Injury during rapid growth, age 9-14 years
    - Has resulted in pitching restrictions in little league

- Irregular ossification or overgrowth of medial epicondyle apophysis; widening, irregularity, edema in growth plate
- **C8-T1 Radiculopathy (Mimic)**
  - Degenerative disc disease, disc herniation, impingement in neural foramina
- **Median Neuropathy**
  - Tingling/aching in fingers sparing little finger, extending proximally especially base of thumb
  - Weakness of flexor pollicis longus, pronator teres, pronator quadratus, flexor carpi radialis
  - MR changes: See ulnar neuropathy

Helpful Clues for Less Common Diagnoses
- **Triceps Tendon Rupture**
  - May be post-traumatic or associated with underlying conditions such as rheumatoid arthritis, hyperparathyroidism
  - Tears range from small intrasubstance tears to full thickness tears with retraction
- **Anconeus Epitrochlearis**
  - Accessory muscle: Origin medial olecranon, insertion medial epicondyle
  - Compresses ulnar n. in cubital tunnel

Helpful Clues for Rare Diagnoses
- **Cat Scratch Disease**
  - Painful adenopathy following cat scratch
  - Mild constitutional symptoms
  - Enlarged medial epitrochlear lymph node characteristic but not common
    - MR imaging may show an enlarged lymph node with adjacent inflammation

Medial Epicondylitis

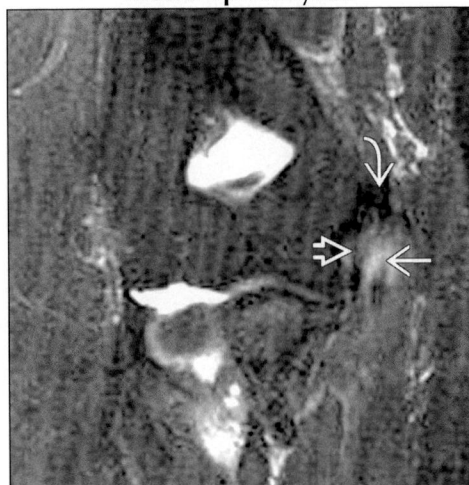

Coronal T2WI FS MR shows edema in the proximal flexor/pronator muscle bundle ➔ in the medial forearm, superficial to the ulnar collateral ligament ➔. The proximal flexor tendon origin ➔ is intact.

Medial Epicondylitis

Axial PD FSE MR shows intermediate to bright signal indicative of moderate tendinopathy of the flexor/pronator tendon origin ➔ at the medial humeral epicondyle.

MEDIAL ELBOW PAIN

(Left) Coronal T2WI FS MR shows edema and irregularity around the humeral attachment of the anterior band of the ulnar collateral ligament ➡ consistent with a partial tear. (Right) Coronal T2WI FS MR shows poor definition of the anterior band of the MCL consistent with disruption ➡. There is diffuse surrounding soft tissue edema, and mild marrow edema in the medial humeral condyle ➡, possibly related to chronic traction forces.

Medial Collateral Ligament (MCL) Injury

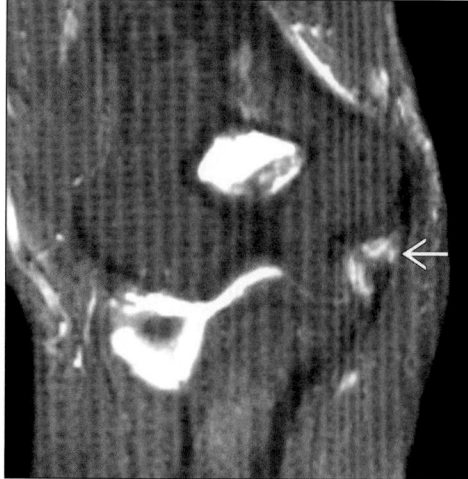

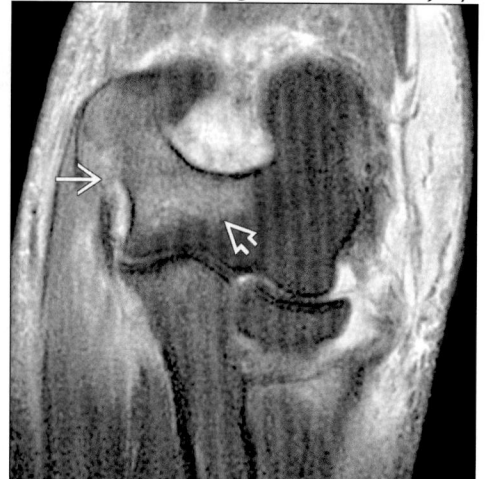

Medial Collateral Ligament (MCL) Injury

(Left) Lateral radiograph shows a fracture of the olecranon process ➡. Swelling of the olecranon bursa ➡ accompanies this injury. (Right) Coronal T2WI FS MR shows a partial tear of the origin of the forearm flexors from the medial epicondyle ➡.

Olecranon Fracture

Common Flexor Mechanism Injury

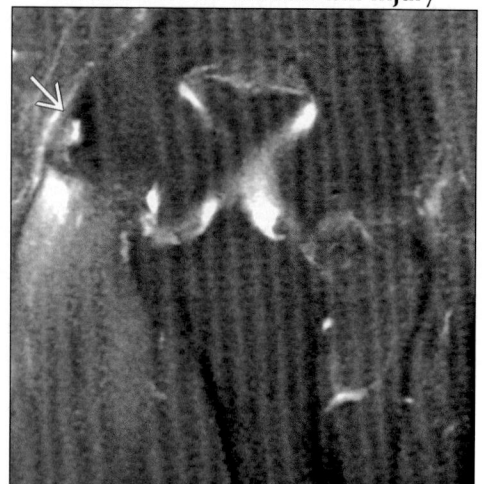

(Left) Coronal T2WI FS MR shows partial displacement of the medial humeral epicondylar ossification center ➡ from the medial condyle ➡. There is edema in the marrow of both osseous structures, as well as diffusely in the surrounding soft tissues ➡. (Right) Anteroposterior radiograph shows the apophysis of the medial epicondyle avulsed from the medial humeral metaphysis and entrapped within the joint ➡ where it may be misinterpreted as a different ossification center.

Medial Epicondyle Avulsion, Pediatric

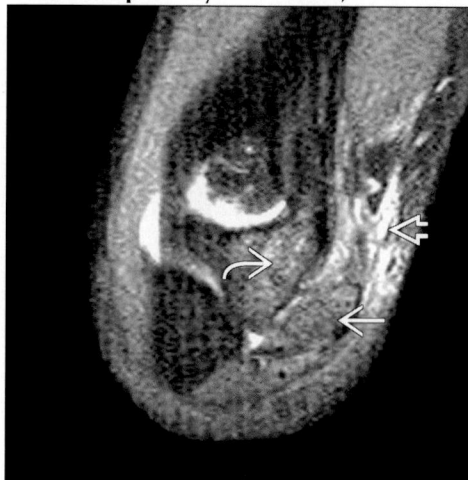

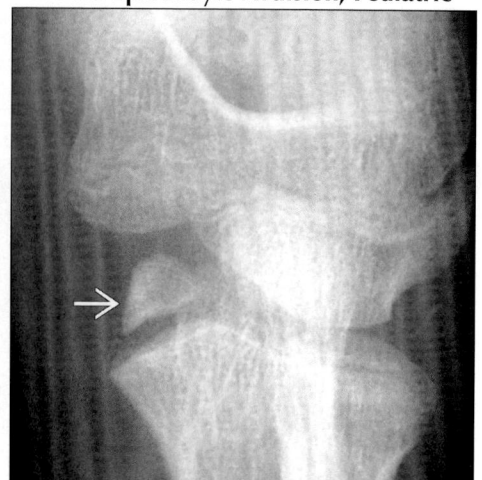

Medial Epicondyle Avulsion, Pediatric

MEDIAL ELBOW PAIN

Coronoid Process Fracture

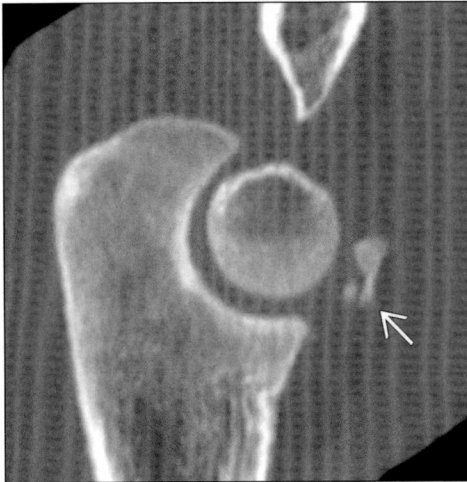

Medial Condylar Fracture

(Left) Sagittal bone CT shows a coronoid process fracture ➡ which frequently results from a dislocation. The fragment is fairly small and the joint should remain stable. *(Right)* Anteroposterior radiograph shows distal humerus fracture with a large medial condyle fragment ➡ which is displaced and impacted.

Ulnar Neuropathy

Median Neuropathy

(Left) Axial T2WI MR shows mild edema in the subcutaneous fat ➡ adjacent to the cubital tunnel. The ulnar nerve ➡ is subluxed medially and it is slightly enlarged in this patient with ulnar neuropathy. *(Right)* Axial T2WI FS MR shows mild elevated signal indicating edema in the pronator teres muscle ➡, a finding due to median nerve impingement by a high humeral fracture.

Triceps Tendon Rupture

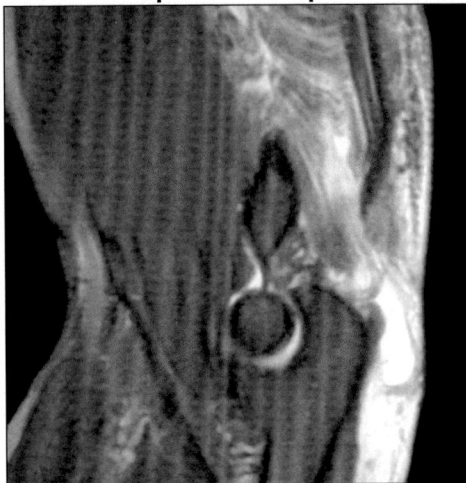

Anconeus Epitrochlearis

(Left) Sagittal T2WI FS MR shows increased signal intensity within the distal triceps tendon as well as retraction and surrounding hemorrhage, consistent with a complete tear. *(Right)* Axial T2WI MR shows large anconeus epitrochlearis muscle found incidentally on MR imaging ➡. The muscle overlies the cubital tunnel. The ulnar nerve is normal in caliber ➡.

III

25

OLECRANON BURSITIS

DIFFERENTIAL DIAGNOSIS

Common
- Post-Traumatic
- Wire/Cerclage Fixation
- Infectious Bursitis
- Gout
- Rheumatoid Arthritis

Less Common
- Rheumatoid Nodule (Mimic)
- Tophus (Mimic)
- Xanthoma (Mimic)

Rare but Important
- Triceps Tendon Rupture
- Calcific Bursitis

ESSENTIAL INFORMATION

Helpful Clues for Common Diagnoses
- **Post-Traumatic**
  - Acute or chronic repetitive trauma
  - Dialysis elbow: Chronic repetitive trauma from pressure on elbow during dialysis
  - With acute trauma may or may not have fracture; bursitis may be hemorrhagic
- **Wire/Cerclage Fixation**
  - Irritation → bursal inflammation
- **Infectious Bursitis**
  - Unilateral
  - Often has preceding history of trauma
    - Commonly related to direct puncture
- **Gout**
  - Commonly bilateral

- May see marginal, peri-articular, nonarticular erosions which are well-defined, with sclerotic margin & overhanging edges; < 15% calcify
- **Rheumatoid Arthritis**
  - Commonly bilateral
  - Nodules within bursa may be palpable
  - ± Arthritic changes: Uniform joint space narrowing, marginal erosions, osteoporosis

Helpful Clues for Less Common Diagnoses
- **Rheumatoid Nodule (Mimic)**
  - Firm, smooth, mobile, painless
  - May cause pressure erosions, rarely calcify
  - ± Arthritic changes
  - MR: Nonspecific low to intermediate T1, bright T2, enhances, ± cystic component
- **Tophus (Mimic)**
  - MR: Low to intermediate T1WI, variable on T2WI, diffusely enhance; ± Erosions
- **Xanthoma (Mimic)**
  - Usually bilateral
  - Familial hypercholesterolemia, cerebrotendinous xanthomatosis
  - US: Hypoechoic lesions
  - MR: Stippled/speckled signal ± tendon enlargement

Helpful Clues for Rare Diagnoses
- **Triceps Tendon Rupture**
  - Hemorrhage may extend into bursa
  - Tendon fibers thickened, wavy; ± gap
- **Calcific Bursitis**
  - Hydroxyapatite deposition disease
  - Triceps rupture uncommon complication

Post-Traumatic

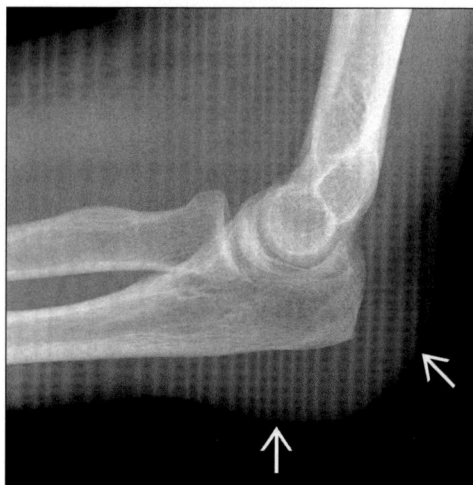

Lateral radiograph shows soft tissue prominence ➡ over the olecranon consistent with olecranon bursitis. Given the history of trauma, this likely represents hemorrhagic bursitis.

Infectious Bursitis

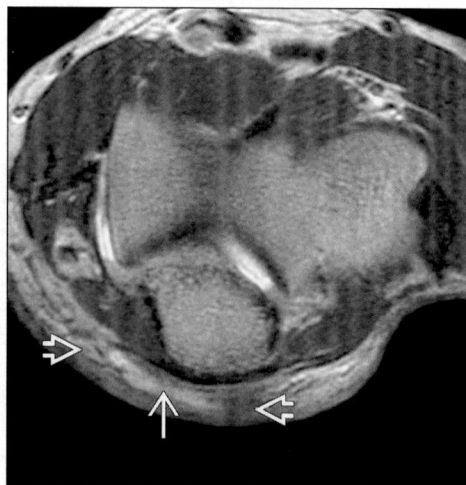

Axial T2WI MR shows infectious olecranon bursitis with an irregular fluid collection in the olecranon bursa ➡ and infiltrative changes in the adjacent fat ➡.

OLECRANON BURSITIS

Gout

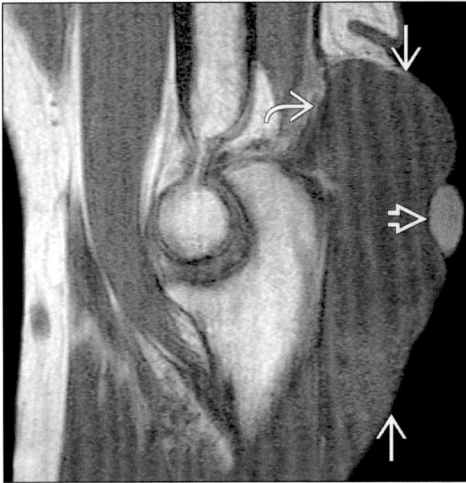

Rheumatoid Arthritis

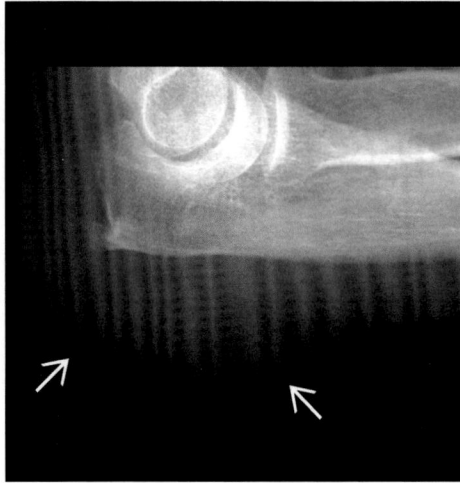

(Left) Sagittal T1WI FS MR shows a predominantly fluid-signal mass posterior to the olecranon ➡. The triceps tendon is seen anterior to the bursa ➡ in this patient with olecranon bursitis secondary to gout. Marker is seen posteriorly ➡. *(Right)* Lateral radiograph shows soft tissue swelling in the region of the olecranon bursa ➡ consistent with bursitis, a typical site of involvement in rheumatoid arthritis.

Tophus (Mimic)

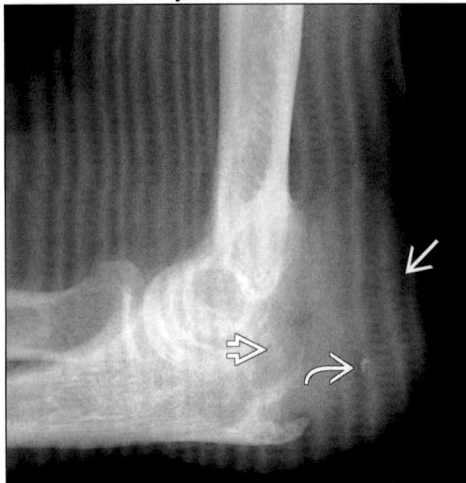

Xanthoma (Mimic)

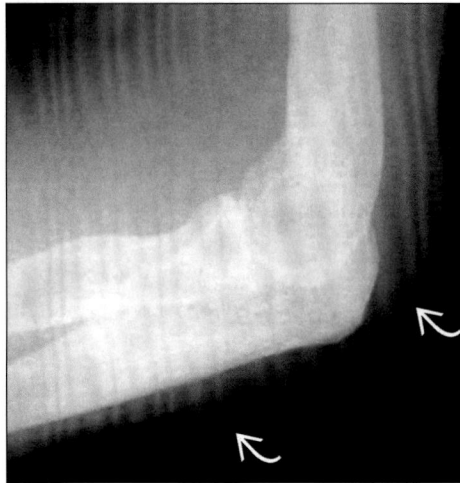

(Left) Lateral radiograph shows a large soft tissue mass posterior to the elbow ➡ in this patient with tophaceous gout. The mass has eroded the olecranon ➡ and has calcified ➡, an uncommon finding. *(Right)* Lateral radiograph with soft tissue windowing, shows a subtle soft tissue mass along the extensor surface of the elbow ➡. This is a common location for xanthoma (an uncommon lesion itself, which was proven in this case).

Triceps Tendon Rupture

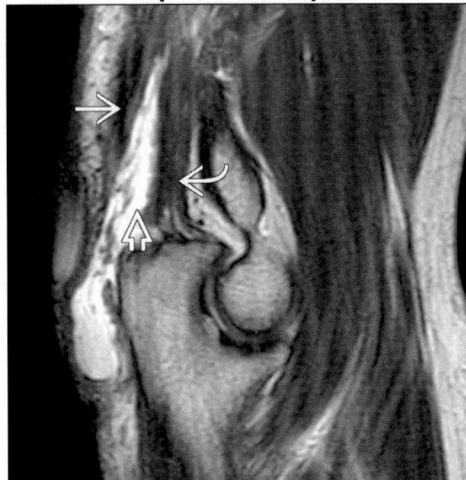

Calcific Bursitis

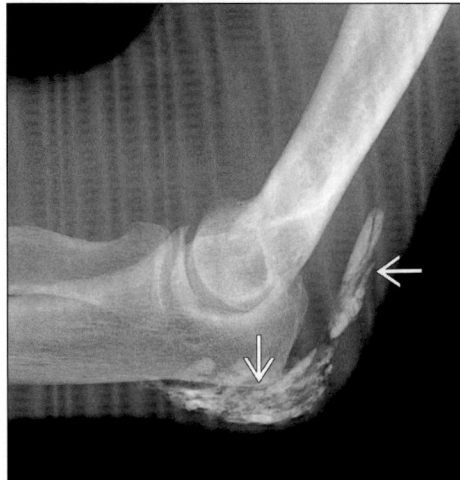

(Left) Sagittal T2WI MR shows partial tear of the posterior fibers of the triceps tendon with hematoma ➡ interposed between the torn ➡ and intact ➡ portions of the tendon, mimicking olecranon bursitis. *(Right)* Lateral radiograph shows extensive dense mineralization in the region of the olecranon bursa ➡ indicative of hydroxyapatite deposition disease.

Clinically Based: Elbow and Forearm

III

27

DIFFERENTIAL DIAGNOSIS

Common
- Carpal Tunnel Syndrome
- Cubital Tunnel Syndrome

Less Common
- Pronator Syndrome
- Radial Entrapment Neuropathy
  - Radial Tunnel Syndrome
  - Posterior Interosseous Nerve Syndrome
- Ulnar Tunnel Syndrome

Rare but Important
- Wartenberg Syndrome
- Kiloh Nevin Syndrome

ESSENTIAL INFORMATION

Key Differential Diagnosis Issues
- Entrapment neuropathy: Short segment nerve compression at a specific site, often while passing through fibroosseous tunnel, muscle or fibrous tissue
- Symptoms: Muscle weakness, paresthesias, atrophy
- MR appearance: Look for nerve signal, course & contour (adjacent vessels may provide landmarks); muscle signal intensity (SI) & distribution
- Look for: Ganglia, tumors, inflammation, post-trauma, scarring, edema, anomalies
- Muscle SI in entrapment/denervation
  - Acute (< 1 month): T1 - normal; STIR - ↑ SI; enhancement: +
  - Subacute (1-6 months): T1 - ± normal; STIR - ↑ SI; enhancement: ±
  - Chronic (> 6 months): T1 - ↑ SI; STIR - ↓ SI; enhancement - none

Helpful Clues for Common Diagnoses
- **Carpal Tunnel Syndrome**
  - Median nerve at wrist; most common upper extremity entrapment
  - Symptoms
    - Radial-sided (1st - radial 4th fingers) numbness, tingling; thenar muscle wasting
  - MR & ultrasound useful but specificity limited
  - Entrapment site
    - Transverse carpal ligament (flexor retinaculum)
  - MR: Median nerve enlargement ± flattening, ↑ SI; flexor retinacular bowing
  - Post-operative findings
    - Symptom free: Flexor retinaculum completely disrupted with palmar migration of tunnel contents
    - Recurrent symptoms: Look for incomplete release, post-op scarring, nerve enlargement, tenosynovitis
- **Cubital Tunnel Syndrome**
  - Ulnar nerve at elbow; 2nd most common upper extremity entrapment
  - Symptoms
    - Pain/paresthesias radiating from forearm to 4/5th fingers & aggravated by prolonged elbow flexion
  - Entrapment sites
    - Struthers arcade, intermuscular septum medial edge, thickened arcuate ligament, anconeus epitrochlearis, deep flexor aponeurosis
  - MR: ↑ SI & nerve enlargement; ± ulnar nerve subluxation
  - Denervation patterns: Flexor carpi ulnaris, flexor digitorum profundus muscles; interossei muscle wasting

Helpful Clues for Less Common Diagnoses
- **Pronator Syndrome**
  - Median nerve at elbow
  - Symptoms
    - Volar forearm pain, worse with exercise; thenar muscle weakness; radial-sided (1st - radial 4th fingers) paraesthesias
  - Entrapment sites
    - Supracondylar process, Struthers arcade, lacertus fibrosis (bicipital aponeurosis), pronator teres, proximal arch of flexor digitorum superficialis
  - Denervation pattern: Pronator teres, flexor carpi radialis, palmaris longus, flexor digitorum superficialis
- **Radial Entrapment Neuropathy**
  - Radial nerve at elbow
  - Symptoms
    - Deep forearm pain, weakness; loss of extension at fingers & wrist
  - Entrapment sites
    - Fibrous bands arising from radiocapitellar joint
    - Tendinous edge of extensor carpi radialis brevis (2nd most common)

- Radial recurrent artery & branches (leash of Henry)
- Arcade of Frohse (most common)
- Fibrous band at distal supinator muscle
  ○ Syndromes named for symptom pattern
  ○ **Radial Tunnel Syndrome**
    - Posterior interosseous nerve (PIN) compression with sensory symptoms but no motor deficits
  ○ **Posterior Interosseous Nerve Syndrome**
    - PIN compression with primary motor symptoms
    - Denervation patterns: Isolated supinator > > supinator & extensors
- **Ulnar Tunnel Syndrome**
  ○ Ulnar nerve at wrist; known as Guyon canal syndrome
  ○ Symptoms
    - 4/5 digit pain & paresthesias, cold intolerance; results from blunt trauma (neurologic counterpart to hypothenar hammer syndrome)
  ○ Compression may occur at
    - Zone 1 (proximal palmar carpal ligament to ulnar nerve bifurcation) - results in combined motor/sensory deficits
    - Zone 2 (ulnar nerve bifurcation to hypothenar muscle fibrous arch, radial to hamate hook) - pure motor deficits (least common)
    - Zone 3 (parallels zone 2, ulnar to hamate hook) - pure sensory deficits

  ○ Affected muscles: Palmaris brevis, hypothenar, lateral lumbrical , interossei, adductor pollicis, flexor, profundus brevis, abductor digiti minimi

Helpful Clues for Rare Diagnoses
- **Wartenberg Syndrome**
  ○ Superficial radial nerve at distal forearm; known as watch strap or handcuff neuropathy
  ○ Symptoms
    - Pain/paraesthesias around distal radial forearm & dorsal radial hand
  ○ Most commonly due to tight cast or postop scarring
  ○ Entrapment sites
    - Nerve in subcutaneous tissue as it exits between brachioradialis & ECR longus tendons
- **Kiloh Nevin Syndrome**
  ○ Median nerve, anterior interosseous branch at elbow
  ○ Symptoms
    - Pure motor deficits of flexor pollicis longus, 2nd flexor digitorum profundus, pronator quadratus
    - Distinguished from pronator syndrome by complete absence of sensory deficit
  ○ Entrapment sites
    - Flexor muscle along interosseous membrane
  ○ **Hint:** Image elbow & forearm to fully evaluate

Carpal Tunnel Syndrome

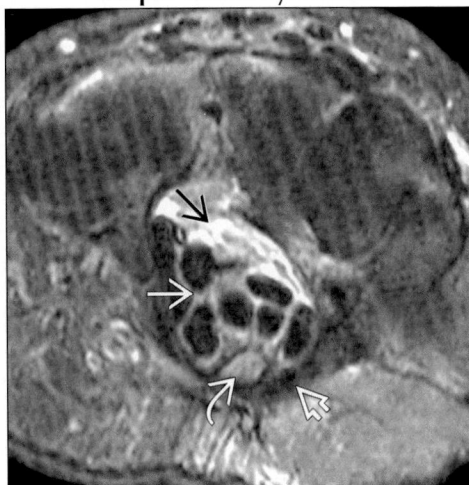

Axial T2WI FS MR shows flexor retinaculum bowing ➡ & peritendinous thickening ➡ in carpal tunnel syndrome. Deep soft tissue edema ➡ contributes to symptoms. Median nerve ➡ is normal.

Carpal Tunnel Syndrome

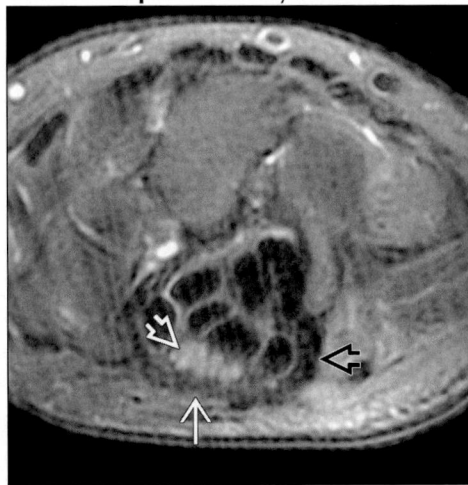

Axial T2WI FS MR shows carpal tunnel release ➡ with palmar migration of tendons with residual scarring near hamate hook ➡. Median nerve ➡ is mildly enlarged with normal SI.

NERVE ENTRAPMENT, ELBOW & WRIST

(Left) Axial T1WI MR shows a lipoma ➡ within the carpal tunnel, displacing the tendons, & median nerve flattening ➡ with radial-sided palm & finger numbness, typical of carpal tunnel syndrome. **(Right)** Axial T1WI MR shows a carpal tunnel mass ➡ due to fatty stroma interdigitating with median nerve fascicles ⤵. This is a fibrolipomatous hamartoma. Note tendon displacement & retinaculum bowing.

Carpal Tunnel Syndrome

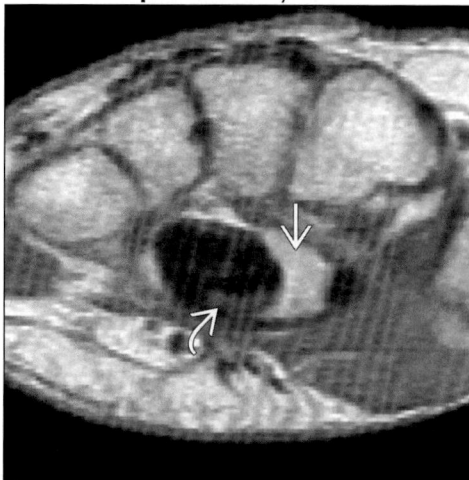

Carpal Tunnel Syndrome

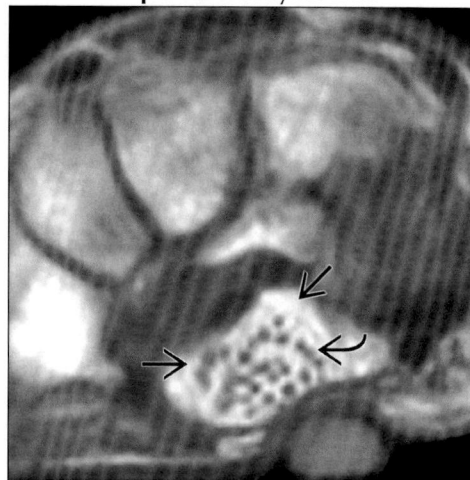

(Left) Sagittal STIR MR shows marked flexor tenosynovitis ➡ with fluid displaced proximally & distally by pressure of the flexor retinaculum ➡. Median nerve ➡ is palmarly displaced & slightly enlarged in this mycobacterium avium tenosynovitis. **(Right)** Axial T2WI FS MR shows ulnar nerve ↑ SI & enlargement ➡ in this cubital tunnel syndrome resulting from direct blow injury to the posteromedial elbow. Note surrounding soft tissue edema ⤵.

Carpal Tunnel Syndrome

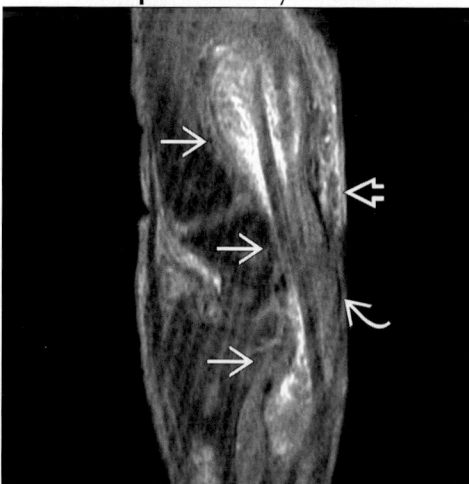

Cubital Tunnel Syndrome

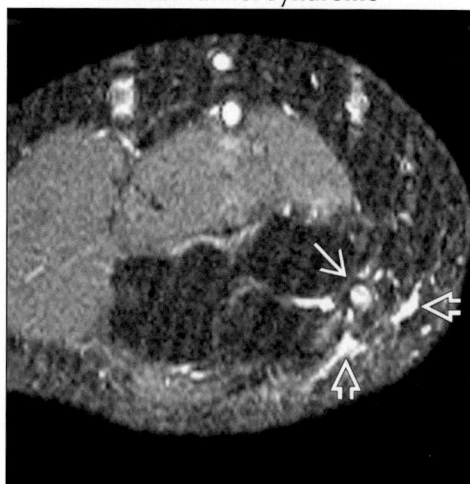

(Left) Axial T2WI MR shows a large anconeus epitrochlearis muscle ➡ over the cubital tunnel. This could create cubital tunnel entrapment of ulnar nerve ➡, particularly when the elbow is flexed. **(Right)** AP radiograph shows a supracondylar process ("avian spur") as a corticated osseous excrescence ➡. The ligament of Struthers may arise from this, creating potential median nerve entrapment ➡ as the pronator teres contracts.

Cubital Tunnel Syndrome

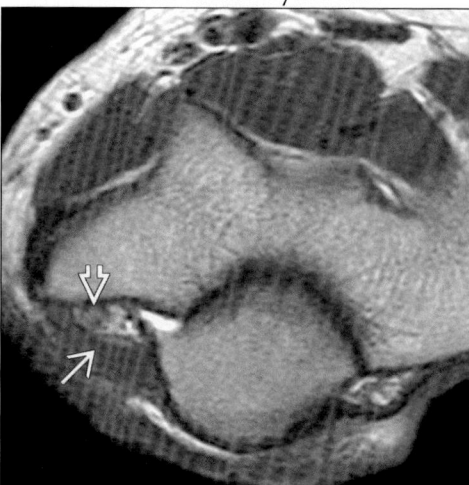

Pronator Syndrome

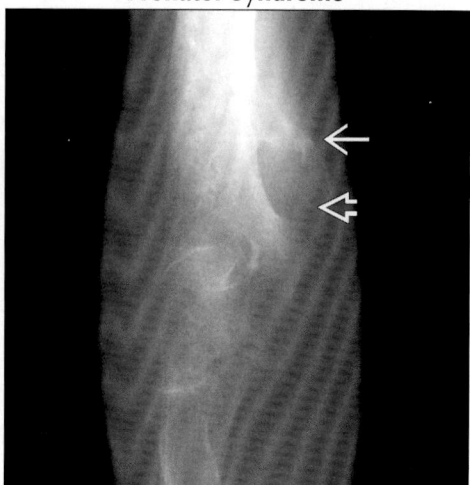

NERVE ENTRAPMENT, ELBOW & WRIST

Pronator Syndrome

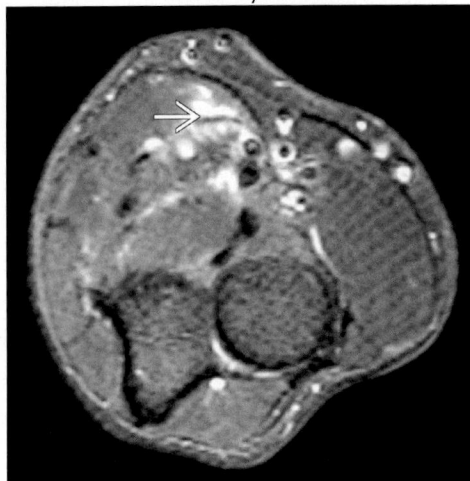

Radial Entrapment Neuropathy

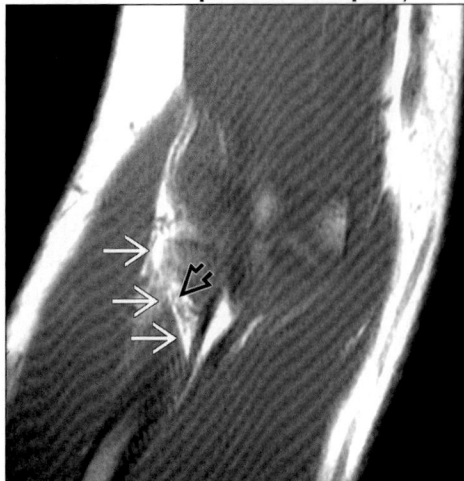

(Left) Axial T2WI FS MR shows pronator teres edema ➔ in a patient with pronator syndrome due to median nerve entrapment following humerus fracture. There is no muscle atrophy on T1WI, suggesting a reversal neuropathy. *(Right)* Coronal T1WI MR shows the normal sharp proximal margin of the supinator, the arcade of Frohse ➔, under which the radial nerve, deep branch, ⇨ must pass. This is a frequent site of radial nerve entrapment.

Posterior Interosseous Nerve Syndrome

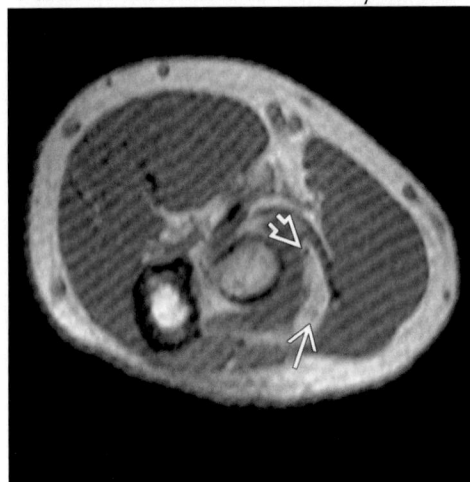

Posterior Interosseous Nerve Syndrome

(Left) Axial T1WI MR shows posterior interosseous nerve ➔ engulfed by a compressive lipoma ➔, resulting in posterior interosseous nerve syndrome with motor weakness involving the supinator & wrist extensors. *(Right)* Axial T1WI MR shows mild fatty atrophy ➔ of the supinator, typical of chronic posterior interosseous nerve syndrome due to remote trauma. There is mild edema in this same distribution on STIR imaging (not shown).

Ulnar Tunnel Syndrome

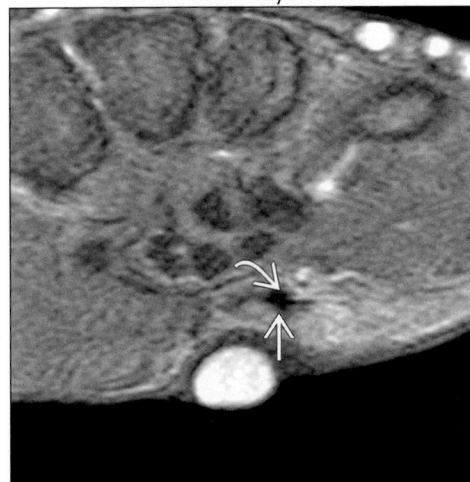

Ulnar Tunnel Syndrome

(Left) Axial T2WI FS MR shows post-traumatic thickening of palmar aponeurosis ➔ causing ulnar tunnel syndrome with impingement of the ulnar nerve ➔ in distal Guyon canal. *(Right)* Axial T1WI MR shows ulnar tunnel syndrome at Guyon canal due to hamate hook fracture nonunion ➔. The fragment ➔ impinges on Guyon canal ⇨ in zone 1, resulting in both motor & sensory deficits.

WRIST CLICKING/CLUNKING/INSTABILITY

DIFFERENTIAL DIAGNOSIS

Common
- Triangular Fibrocartilage Tear
- Scapholunate Ligament Tear
- Lunotriquetral Instability
- Carpal Instabilities
  - Dorsal Intercalated Segment Instability
  - Volar Intercalated Segment Instability
  - Palmar Midcarpal Instability
- Perilunate Instability
- Osteonecrosis

Less Common
- Tendon, Injury
- Ganglion Cyst, Wrist
- Fracture, Malunion
- Hardware Complications
- Distal Radioulnar Joint Instability

Rare but Important
- Carpal Translocation
- Madelung Deformity

ESSENTIAL INFORMATION

Key Differential Diagnosis Issues
- Instability - joint malalignment may be static or dynamic
- Due to trauma, chronic attenuation of supporting ligaments, arthritis
- Click/clunk may be audible/palpable; ± painful
- Imaging techniques
  - Radiography should include neutral & stress views
  - Videofluoroscopy to evaluate motion of proximal, distal carpal rows through range of motion (ROM)
  - Arthrography (± digital subtraction) to evaluate ligament integrity
  - CT to evaluate fractures; alignment
  - MR ± arthrography to evaluate ligament, tendon integrity; alignment

Helpful Clues for Common Diagnoses
- **Triangular Fibrocartilage Tear**
  - May be traumatic or attritional ranging from mild wear to full tear with ulnocarpal abutment
  - Ulnocarpal abutment: Ulnar positive (plus) variant, triangular fibrocartilage (TFC) tear, lunate/triquetral edema, cyst, osteophytes

- **Scapholunate Ligament Tear**
  - Arthrography: Visible contrast through scapholunate (SL) space; ± SL widening > 4 mm
  - MR or CT arthrography: Sensitivity for complete & partial tears - 80-95%; MR without arthrography ~ 70%
  - May have tear without malalignment or symptoms due to degenerative attrition
  - SL dissociation with scaphoid rotatory subluxation
    - Widening of SL space, scaphoid volar tilt creates a "ring" of distal scaphoid pole
- **Lunotriquetral Instability**
  - Lunotriquetral (LT) tear contributes to several carpal instability patterns
  - Arthrography: Visible contrast flow between lunate & triquetrum
  - MR or CT arthrography: Sensitivity 70-90%; MR without arthrography 45%
- **Carpal Instabilities**
  - **Dorsal Intercalated Segment Instability**
    - (DISI): Seen in SL tear, RA, CPPD, scaphoid fracture
    - Lunate dorsal tilt > 20°; SL angle > 70°; capitolunate (CL) angle > 20°; lunate triangular on AP X-ray
  - **Volar Intercalated Segment Instability**
    - (VISI): Seen in LT tear, RA, CPPD
    - Lunate volar tilt > 20°; SL angle < 30°; CL angle > 20°; lunate rounded on AP x-ray
  - **Palmar Midcarpal Instability**
    - Distal carpal row translated volarly while proximal row stays flexed; extreme ulnar deviation → proximal row snaps back
    - Failure of volar (arcuate, triquetrohamate, capitolunate) & dorsal (radiotriquetral) ligaments
  - Other instability patterns: Triquetrohamate, triquetrolunate related to stabilizing ligament disruption
- **Perilunate Instability**
  - Fracture/dislocations disrupt key perilunate ligaments in predictable order
  - 1: SL tear ± scaphoid rotatory subluxation
  - 2: Radiocapitate tear; perilunate dislocation
  - 3: Volar radiotriquetral, dorsal radiocarpal tears; midcarpal dislocation
  - 4: Dorsal radiocarpal tear; lunate dislocation

WRIST CLICKING/CLUNKING/INSTABILITY

- **Osteonecrosis**
  - Scaphoid osteonecrosis (AVN) may occur after scaphoid fracture
  - Lunatomalacia (Kienbock disease) associated with ulnar minus variant, trauma
  - Clicking/clunking seen in advanced stage AVN with collapse resulting in proximal capitate migration, SL dissociation

Helpful Clues for Less Common Diagnoses
- **Tendon, Injury**
  - Ranges from tendinosis (thickening & intrasubstance ↑ SI) to complete disruption (tear or avulsion)
  - Tenosynovitis results from trauma, arthritis, infection in tendon sheath, ± tendon injury
    - De Quervain tenosynovitis: Abductor pollicis longus (APL), extensor pollicis brevis (EPB) inflammation
    - Extensor carpi ulnaris (ECU) subluxation/dislocation: Occurs with tear of fibrous subsheath that normally holds tendon in ulnar groove through ROM
- **Ganglion Cyst, Wrist**
  - Thin-walled ± septations, usually solitary; commonly dorsal near SL ligament
- **Fracture, Malunion**
  - Contributes to instability patterns, both at time of injury with accompanying ligament injury & with subsequent malalignment
- **Hardware Complications**
  - Misplacement, hardware fracture, loosening
- **Distal Radioulnar Joint Instability**
  - Associated with trauma or arthritis; associated TFC tear often present
  - Dorsal instability most common (unable to supinate); volar less common (unable to pronate)
  - X-ray: Prominent ulnar head ± widened joint
  - Axial CT/MR: Evaluate subtle instability
    - Acquire in supination & pronation to accentuate abnormalities
    - Image both wrists simultaneously for comparison

Helpful Clues for Rare Diagnoses
- **Carpal Translocation**
  - Defined as ulnar shift of entire carpus relative to radius
  - Most common: Ulnar translocation associated with rheumatoid arthritis
  - Dorsal & palmar carpal translocation may also occur, associated with distal radial trauma
- **Madelung Deformity**
  - Radius: Dorsal/ulnar curvature; decreased radius length; triangular radial epiphysis
  - Ulna: Dorsal subluxation, ulnar head enlargement
  - Carpals wedged between radius & ulna with lunate at apex

Triangular Fibrocartilage Tear

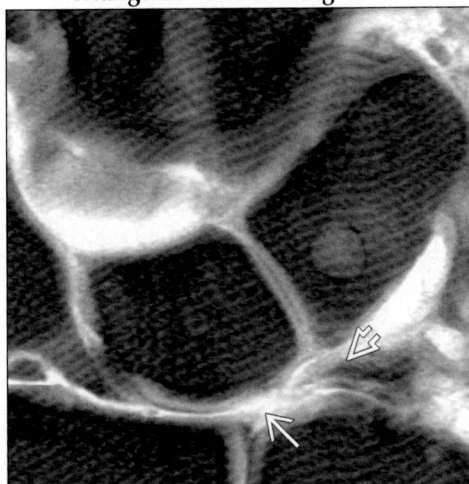

Coronal T1WI FS MR arthrogram shows disruption ➡ of radial aspect of TFC articular disc ➡. Contrast flows through the disruption into both the distal radioulnar joint and radiocarpal joint.

Triangular Fibrocartilage Tear

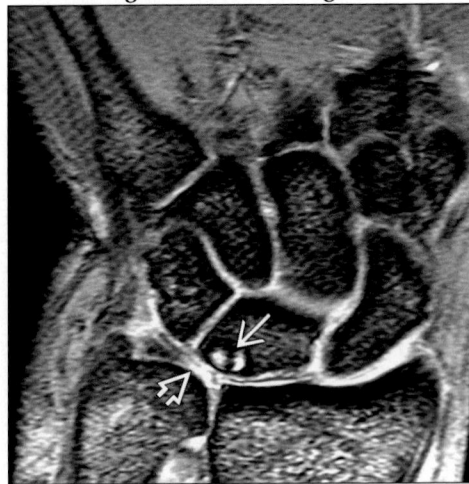

Coronal T2 GRE MR shows triangular fibrocartilage tear ➡ with secondary osteoarthritis characterized as cartilage loss & subchondral cyst formation ➡, representing ulnocarpal abutment.*

(Left) Anteroposterior radiograph shows scapholunate interval widening > 4 mm ➡ when hand is fisted & radially deviated, consistent with SL ligament tear. *(Right)* Coronal T2* GRE MR following a radiocarpal arthrogram shows contrast flowing into the midcarpal compartment through a defect in the SL ligament ➡. The TFC is intact ➡.

Scapholunate Ligament Tear

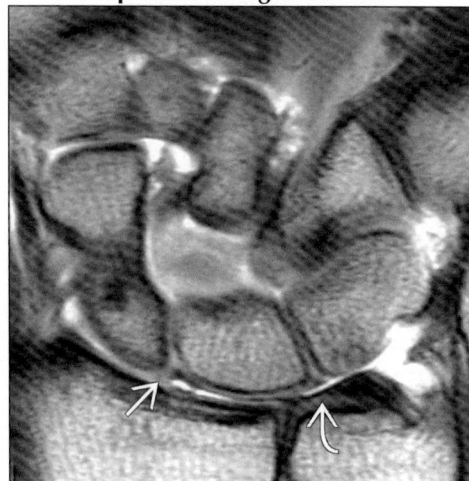

Scapholunate Ligament Tear

(Left) Coronal T1WI MR shows a flap tear of the lunate triquetral ligament ➡, with contrast crossing from the radiocarpal joint into the midcarpal joint. There is also ulnar positive variance, & an associated TFC tear ➡. *(Right)* Lateral radiograph shows dorsal intercalated segmental instability, or alternatively dorsiflexion carpal instability. Lunate ➡ is dorsiflexed relative to capitate ➡ with a CL angle which is > 20° & SL angle > 70°.

Lunotriquetral Instability

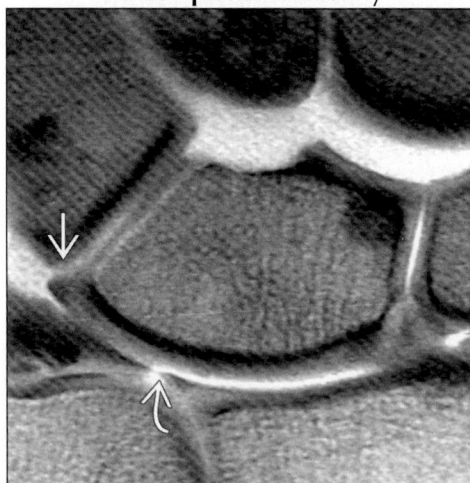

Dorsal Intercalated Segment Instability

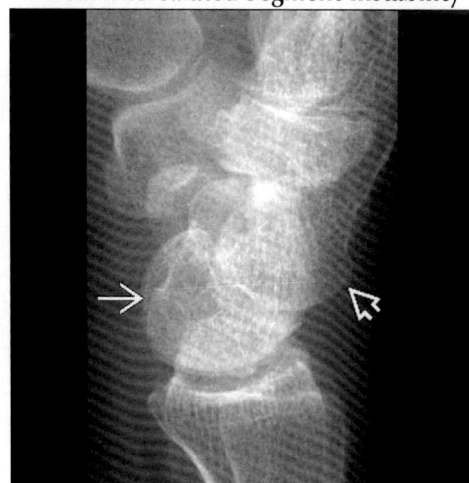

(Left) Lateral radiograph shows volar intercalated segmental instability (VISI). Lunate ➡ is volar flexed relative to capitate ➡ & scaphoid ➡ with CL angle > 20 ° & SL angle < 30°. Note osteopenia related to RA. *(Right)* Lateral radiograph shows lunate ➡ maintaining normal articulation with radius ➡ while capitate ➡ is dorsally dislocated from the lunate. This is a perilunate dislocation. Note remainder of carpus moves dorsally with capitate.

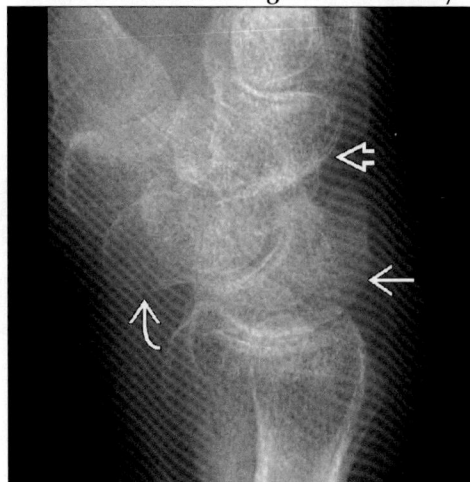

Volar Intercalated Segment Instability

Perilunate Instability

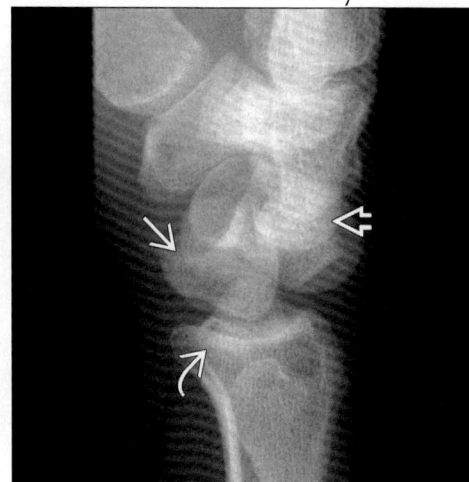

WRIST CLICKING/CLUNKING/INSTABILITY

Osteonecrosis

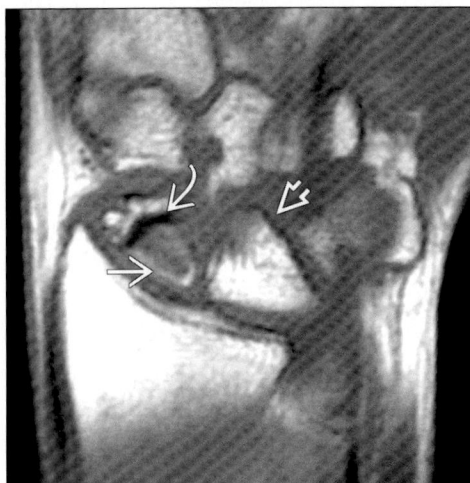

Tendon, Injury

(Left) Coronal T1WI MR shows scaphoid osteonecrosis ➡ (↓ SI with flattening & early collapse) from prior midwaist scaphoid fracture ➡. Note the triangular lunate contour ➡ due to associated DISI deformity. *(Right)* Axial PD FSE FS MR shows marked tendon thickening & ↑ SI of APL & EPB (1st extensor compartment) ➡ with surrounding edema, typical of De Quervain tendinitis/tenosynovitis. ECU tenosynovitis ➡ is also present.

Tendon, Injury

Ganglion Cyst, Wrist

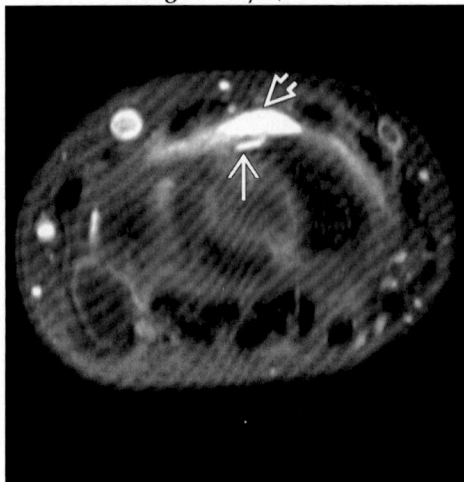

(Left) Axial PD FSE FS MR shows DRUJ effusion ➡ with fluid in ECU tendon sheath as well. The ECU is torn longitudinally ➡ & subluxated from the ulnar groove ➡ due to disruption of the fibrous subsheath that normally maintains ECU position through ROM. *(Right)* Axial PD FSE FS MR shows a thin-walled dorsal ganglion ➡ with a small tail ➡ directed toward the scapholunate joint in this 14 year old who complained of wrist clicking with joint rotation.

Hardware Complications

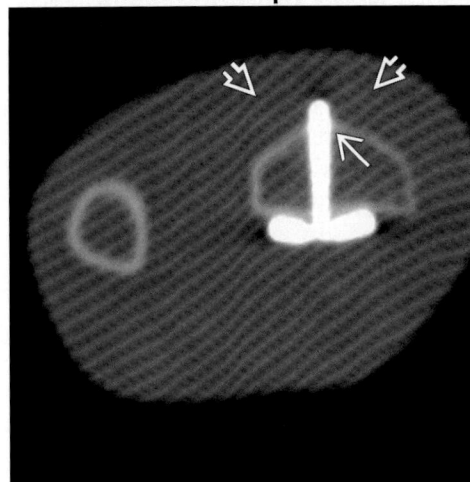

Carpal Translocation

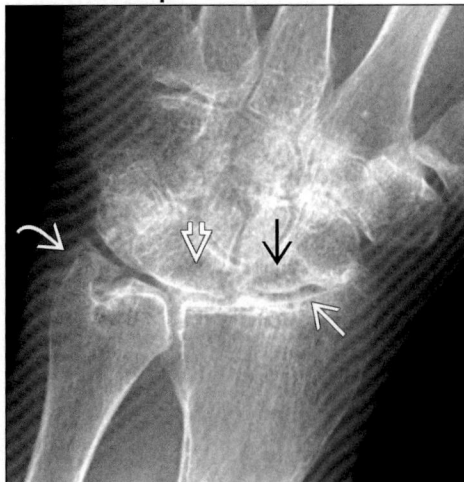

(Left) Axial NECT shows a bicortical screw, used to secure a volar plate that stabilizes a distal radial fracture. The screw extends beyond the radial dorsal cortex ➡ & impinges 2nd & 3rd extensor compartment tendons ➡ during normal ROM. *(Right)* PA radiograph shows carpal ulnar translocation, defined as lunate articulating > 50% with ulna ➡. Radiocarpal joint space loss ➡, scaphoid rotation & erosion ➡, ulnar capping ➡ & osteopenia are typical of RA.

ULNAR SIDED WRIST PAIN

DIFFERENTIAL DIAGNOSIS

Common
- Arthritis
- Triangular Fibrocartilage Tear
- Lunotriquetral Instability
- Ulnocarpal Abutment

Less Common
- Tendon Injury
- Fractures
- Carpal Dislocations
- Osteonecrosis
- Infection

Rare but Important
- Vascular Abnormalities
- Osseous Neoplasm
- Soft Tissue Neoplasm
- Madelung Deformity

ESSENTIAL INFORMATION

Key Differential Diagnosis Issues
- Ulnar & radial wrist pain etiologies often overlap

Helpful Clues for Common Diagnoses
- **Arthritis**
  - Rheumatoid arthritis
    - Early: Symmetric swelling, juxta-articular osteopenia, subtle erosions
    - Late: Diffuse osteopenia, joint space loss, large erosions, ulnar carpal translocation, ulnar capping
    - Contrast-enhanced MR: Effusions, synovitis, synovial hypertrophy, active (enhancing) & inactive (nonenhancing) erosions
  - Osteoarthritis
    - Normal bone density, joint space loss, subchondral sclerosis, osteophytes; typically due to trauma
  - Pyrophosphate arthropathy
    - Multiple well-defined intraosseous cysts, radiocarpal & capitolunate joint space narrowing, TFCC chondrocalcinosis
  - Gout
    - Normal bone density, soft tissue swelling & calcifications, punched-out erosions with sclerotic borders, especially in CMCs
  - Juvenile idiopathic arthritis

- Early: Juxta-articular osteopenia, soft tissue swelling
- Later: Diffuse osteopenia, accelerated maturation, enlarged carpals with irregular margins (crenulation), ankylosis

- **Triangular Fibrocartilage Tear**
  - Traumatic: Hyperrotation, distraction or axial loading; associated with distal forearm fractures
  - Degenerative: Ranges from mild wear to full tear with ulnocarpal abutment; many are asymptomatic
  - X-ray: Look for ulnar plus variant
  - Arthrography (± digital subtraction): Visible contrast flow through TFCC
  - MR or CT arthrography: Sensitivity 80-95%; MR without arthrography 30-45%
- **Lunotriquetral Instability**
  - Tears due to trauma with hyperextension & radial deviation
  - Volar intercalated segment instability (VISI) results in volar flexed lunate, scapholunate angle < 30°, capitolunate angle > 20°
  - Arthrography (± digital subtraction): Visible contrast flow between lunate & triquetrum
  - MR or CT arthrography: Sensitivity 70-90%; MR without arthrography 30-45%
- **Ulnocarpal Abutment**
  - Swelling & tenderness localized to TFCC, LT joint
  - X-ray: Ulnar plus variant, triquetral & lunate cysts, sclerosis, osteophytes
  - MR: TFCC tear, triquetral & ulnar side of lunate chondromalacia, edema, cysts

Helpful Clues for Less Common Diagnoses
- **Tendon Injury**
  - Ranges from tendinosis (thickening & intrasubstance ↑ SI) to complete disruption (tear or avulsion)
  - Tenosynovitis results from trauma, arthritis, or infection in tendon sheath
  - Extensor carpi ulnaris (ECU) tendinitis/tenosynovitis: Thickened tendon ± sheath fluid
  - ECU subluxation: Occurs in supination due to ECU subsheath tear; tendon displaced ulnarward out of ulnar groove
- **Fractures**
  - Triquetrum: Commonly fractured

- Joint capsule avulsion or ulnar styloid impaction results in small dorsal fragment best seen on lateral X-ray
  - Body fractures typically associated with other injuries, e.g., perilunate transtriquetral fracture dislocation
- Hamate
  - Hook: Direct blow or repetitive stress, e.g., carpenters, golfers, racquet sports; best seen on carpal tunnel view or CT
  - Body: Rare; often associated with 4th, 5th CMC fractures
- Ulnar styloid: Isolated or in combination with other injuries
  - Nonunion common but rarely symptomatic
  - If fracture at styloid base & TFCC disrupted, distal radioulnar joint may be unstable
- **Carpal Dislocations**
  - Occur in combination with fractures as an ulnarward extension of scapholunate (SL) instability/trauma
- **Osteonecrosis**
  - Lunate: Kienbock disease (lunatomalacia); associated with ulnar minus, trauma
  - Stage 1: X-ray-normal; MR T1 ↓ SI & T2 ↑ SI
  - Stage 2: X-ray-sclerosis; MR T1 ↓ & T2 ↑ SI
  - Stage 3: X-ray-collapse, proximal capitate migration, SL dissociation, scaphoid rotatory subluxation; MR T1 & T2 ↓ SI
  - Stage 4: X-ray-secondary osteoarthritis of surrounding carpus MR T1 & T2 ↓ SI
- **Infection**

- History of diabetes, inflammatory arthritis, immunocompromise, puncture wounds, open fracture
- Septic joint: Extensive effusion of one or more compartments, ± carpal edema
- Osteomyelitis: Marked osteopenia; cortical loss, joint malalignment

Helpful Clues for Rare Diagnoses
- **Vascular Abnormalities**
  - Hypothenar hammer syndrome: Thrombosis, spasm, or aneurysm of ulnar artery due to repetitive trauma; may compress adjacent ulnar nerve
  - Arteriography: Narrowing, occlusion, or aneurysm of ulnar artery adjacent to hamate hook
- **Osseous Neoplasm**
  - Benign: Giant cell tumor, enchondroma, osteoid osteoma
  - Malignant: Squamous cell metastases
- **Soft Tissue Neoplasm**
  - Benign: Ganglion, GCTTS, hemangioma, tendon sheath fibroma, neurogenic tumor
  - Malignant: MFH, synovial sarcoma, angiosarcoma, fibrosarcoma
- **Madelung Deformity**
  - Radius: Dorsal/ulnar curvature; decreased radius length; triangular radial epiphysis
  - Ulna: Dorsal subluxation, ulnar head enlargement
  - Carpals wedging between radius & ulna with lunate at apex

Arthritis

Posteroanterior radiograph shows rheumatoid arthritis with diffuse osteopenia and joint space loss ➔, erosions ➔ & carpal ulnar translocation. Ulnar capping ➔ (osseous lip around distal ulna) is present.

Arthritis

Coronal T1 C+ FS MR shows an enhancing ulnarward hamate erosion ➔ & synovitis ➔ in this 59 year old woman with rheumatoid arthritis.

Arthritis

Arthritis

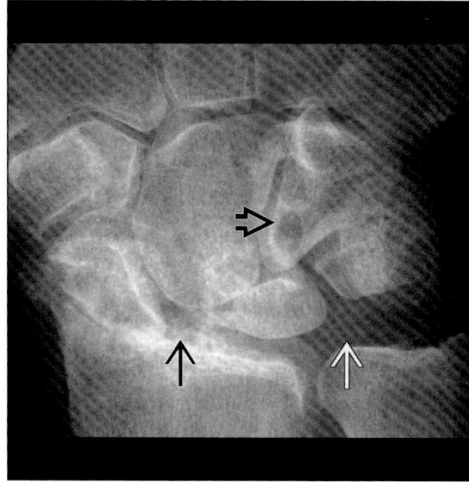
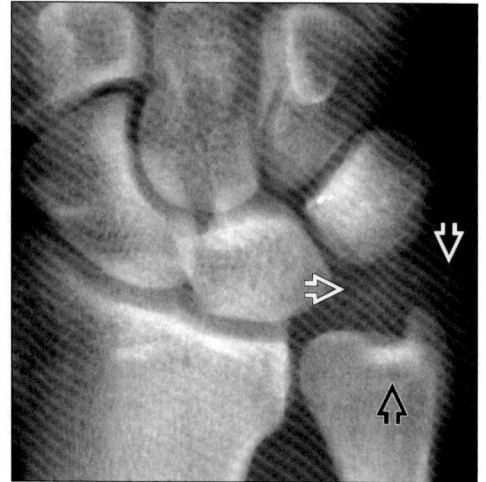

(Left) PA radiograph shows triangular fibrocartilage chondrocalcinosis ➡ in this pyrophosphate arthropathy as well as multiple intraosseous cysts ⮞. A scapholunate advanced collapse (SLAC) wrist deformity is present ➡. (Right) PA radiograph shows nodular soft tissue calcification surrounding ulnar styloid ⮞ (atypical for chondrocalcinosis), representing a gouty tophus in this young Polynesian man. Note the small ulnar erosion ⮞.

Arthritis

Arthritis

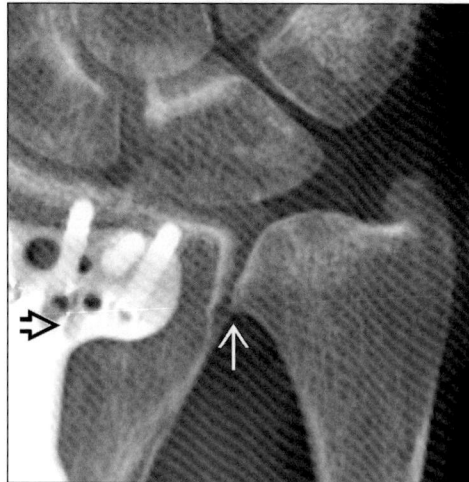
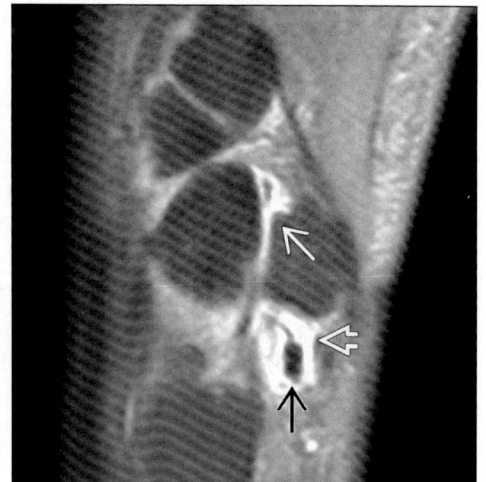

(Left) Posteroanterior radiograph shows osteoarthritis with distal radioulnar joint space narrowing & a small osteophytic ridge ➡ along the proximal ulnar head in this patient with prior distal radial fracture treated by ORIF ⮞. (Right) Sagittal PD FSE FS MR shows pisotriquetral osteoarthritis with joint space narrowing and a small osteophytic ridge ➡, as well as joint effusion ⮞ & a small loose body ➡ in the proximal capsular recess.

Triangular Fibrocartilage Tear

Triangular Fibrocartilage Tear

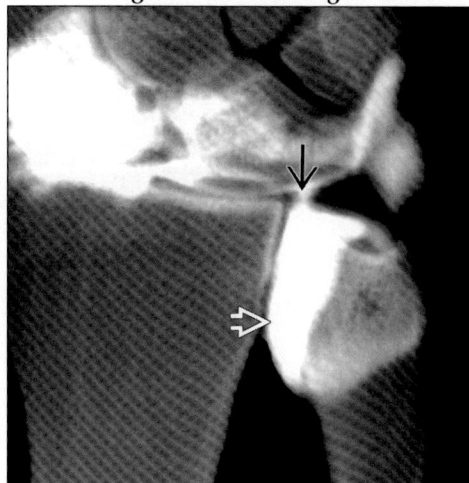

(Left) Anteroposterior radiograph arthrogram shows typical triangular fibrocartilage tear, highlighted by radiocarpal contrast flowing through the tear ➡ and filling the distal radioulnar joint ⮞. (Right) Coronal T2 GRE MR shows a central triangular fibrocartilage tear ⮞. This is well-visualized, in part due to effusions in all three wrist compartments ➡.*

III

ULNAR SIDED WRIST PAIN

Lunotriquetral Instability

Lunotriquetral Instability

(Left) Anteroposterior radiograph arthrogram shows flow of radiocarpal contrast between the lunate & triquetrum ➔ into the midcarpal compartment through the torn lunotriquetral ligament. *(Right)* Coronal MR arthrogram (T1WI FS) in the same patient shows gadolinium extending through the lunotriquetral ligament ➔ & into midcarpal compartment. The scapholunate ligament ➔ & triangular fibrocartilage ➔ are intact.

Ulnocarpal Abutment

Ulnocarpal Abutment

(Left) Anteroposterior radiograph shows ulnar plus variance ➔ (ulna longer than radius) resulting in impaction of ulna on lunate. This leads to sclerosis & cyst formation ➔ at point of impact. *(Right)* Coronal T1WI MR shows ulnocarpal abutment with a central triangular fibrocartilage tear ➔ in combination with ulnar plus variance. The ulnarward lunate shows subchondral low SI ➔, representing cyst &/or sclerosis from impaction.

Tendon Injury

Tendon Injury

(Left) Axial PD FSE FS MR shows a distal radioulnar joint effusion ➔ & tenosynovitis ➔ surrounding extensor carpi ulnaris (ECU). ECU is flattened with a split-type intrasubstance tear ➔ & ulnarward tendon subluxation. *(Right)* Axial T1 C+ FS MR shows marked synovial hypertrophy ➔ with small accompanying tendon sheath effusions ➔ of all extensor compartments in 33 year old woman with new onset rheumatoid arthritis & extensor tenosynovitis.

III

39

ULNAR SIDED WRIST PAIN

Fractures

Fractures

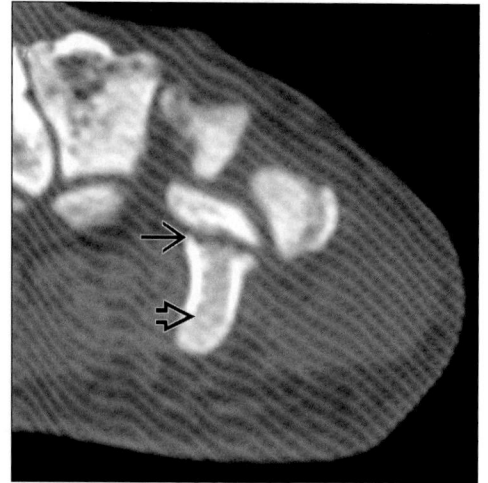

(Left) Lateral radiograph shows dorsal soft tissue swelling & a small fracture fragment from the dorsal triquetrum ➡. This may result from capsular avulsion or direct impact of the ulna on the triquetrum. *(Right)* Axial NECT shows an acute fracture ➡ of the hamate hook ➡. This is a nondisplaced fracture & may result from direct impact during activities such as golf (impact from club hitting the turf).

Fractures

Fractures

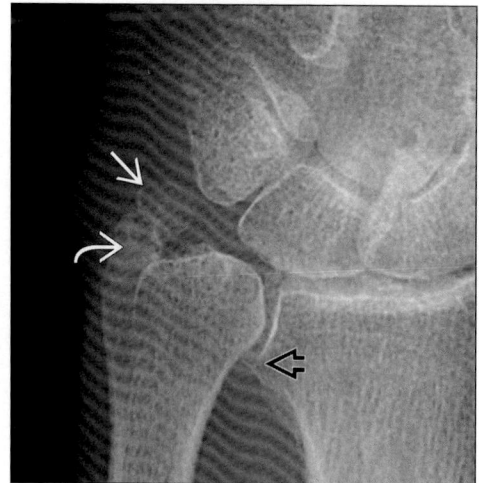

(Left) Anteroposterior radiograph shows comminuted intraarticular 5th metacarpal base fracture ➡ with slight ulnarward subluxation. CT (not shown) confirmed this as an isolated fracture. *(Right)* Anteroposterior radiograph shows a well-corticated osseous fragment ➡ near the ulnar styloid ➡, representing a chronic non-union. Mild osteoarthritis of the adjacent distal radiocarpal joint is present with a small osteophytic ridge ➡.

Carpal Dislocations

Carpal Dislocations

(Left) Posteroanterior radiograph shows a transradial, transscaphoid, transtriquetral perilunate fracture dislocation with fractures of radius ➡, scaphoid ➡, & triquetrum ➡ as well as loss of normal lunate contour ➡. *(Right)* Lateral radiograph in the same patient confirms a perilunate dislocation with dorsal dislocation of the capitate ➡ but intact radial-lunate articulation ➡ in this complex fracture dislocation.

ULNAR SIDED WRIST PAIN

Osteonecrosis

Osteonecrosis

(Left) Anteroposterior radiograph shows increased density of the lunate ⊳ with no contour abnormality or fragmentation. This is stage 2 Kienbock disease. *(Right)* Coronal T1WI MR shows grade 3 Kienbock disease with partial collapse ⊲ of the lunate. The scapholunate ligament is still intact, but the cortical fragmentation → indicates more advanced disease.

Infection

Vascular Abnormalities

(Left) Coronal STIR MR shows Mycobacterium avium septic arthritis/osteomyelitis with extensive erosion of the ulnar styloid ⊳, disruption of the distal radioulnar joint →, & joint effusion with associated synovial hypertrophy →. *(Right)* PA angiogram with digital subtraction shows an ulnar artery aneurysm ⊳ just distal to the hamate hook ⊳ in 50 year old auto repairman, who pounds out fender dents with his palm. This is hypothenar hammer syndrome.

Osseous Neoplasm

Madelung Deformity

(Left) Anteroposterior radiograph shows multiple enchondromatosis (Ollier disease) with a markedly foreshortened distal ulna with chondroid calcification of the bulbous ulnar head ⊳. Note the multiple enchondromas → of the fingers as well. *(Right)* Posteroanterior radiograph shows Madelung deformity with distal radial bowing ⊳, distal radioulnar joint dislocation →, & dorsal displacement of the ulnar head →. The carpals are wedge-shaped.

RADIAL SIDED WRIST PAIN

DIFFERENTIAL DIAGNOSIS

Common
- Fracture
- Arthritis
- Ganglion Cyst, Wrist
- Tendon, Injury
- Scapholunate Ligament Tear

Less Common
- Carpal Instabilities
- Carpal Dislocations
- Osteonecrosis, Wrist (Scaphoid & Lunate)
- Infection

Rare but Important
- Osseous Neoplasm
- Soft Tissue Neoplasm
- Madelung Deformity

ESSENTIAL INFORMATION

Key Differential Diagnosis Issues
- Radial & ulnar wrist pain etiologies often overlap

Helpful Clues for Common Diagnoses
- **Fracture**
  - Fall on an outstretched hand (FOOSH)
    - 4-10: Distal radial metaphysis buckle
    - 11-16: Distal radius Salter II
    - 17-40: Scaphoid, ± triquetrum
    - 40: Colles fracture, distal radius
  - Scaphoid: Most common carpal fracture
    - Early: X-ray - loss of scaphoid fat pad, subtle cortical irregularity; MR - ↑ SI edema; more sensitive
    - Healing: Midwaist/proximal pole fracture complications-AVN, delayed or non-union
    - Delayed/non-union: Sclerosis, cysts, scapholunate (SL) widening, OA
  - Fractures of other radialward carpals rare
  - Radial styloid: Due to ligament avulsion or direct blow; look for other fractures
  - 1st CMC: Look for subtle volar lip (Bennett) fracture
- **Arthritis**
  - Rheumatoid arthritis
    - Early: Symmetric soft tissue swelling, juxta-articular osteopenia, subtle erosions

- Late: Diffuse osteopenia, joint space loss, large erosions, ulnar carpal translocation
    - Contrast-enhanced MR: Effusions, synovitis, synovial hypertrophy, active (enhancing) & inactive (nonenhancing) erosions
  - Osteoarthritis
    - Normal bone density, joint space loss, subchondral sclerosis, osteophytes; particularly in 1st CMC, scaphoid-trapezium area
    - Carpal boss: Prominent dorsal ridge 2nd CMC best seen on CT; ± symptomatic
  - Pyrophosphate arthropathy
    - Multiple well-defined carpal cysts, radiocarpal & capitolunate joint space loss
    - Scapholunate advanced collapse (SLAC) wrist: SL dissociation, lunate dorsiflexion, radioscaphoid joint loss, capitate between scaphoid & lunate
  - Gout
    - Normal bone density, soft tissue swelling & calcifications, punched-out erosions with sclerotic borders, especially in CMCs
  - Juvenile idiopathic arthritis
    - Early: Juxta-articular osteopenia, STS
    - Later: Diffuse osteopenia, accelerated maturation, enlarged carpals, irregular margins, ankylosis
- **Ganglion Cyst, Wrist**
  - Thin-walled ± septations, usually solitary; commonly dorsal near SL ligament
- **Tendon, Injury**
  - Ranges from tendinosis (thickening & intrasubstance ↑ SI) to complete disruption (tear or avulsion)
  - Tenosynovitis results from trauma, arthritis or infection in tendon sheath
  - De Quervain tenosynovitis: Abductor pollicis longus (APL), extensor pollicis brevis (EPB) inflammation
  - Intersection syndrome: Extensor carpi radialis longus/brevis inflammation at musculotendinous junction; may also involve APL/EPB
- **Scapholunate Ligament Tear**
  - Arthrography (± digital subtraction): Visible contrast through SL interspace; ± SL widening > 4 mm

○ MR or CT arthrography: Sensitivity for complete & partial tears - 80-95%; MR without arthrography - 40-70%

Helpful Clues for Less Common Diagnoses

• **Carpal Instabilities**
  ○ Volar intercalated segment instability (VISI): Seen in LT tear, RA, CPPD
    ▪ Lunate volar tilt > 20°; SL angle < 30°; CL angle > 20°; lunate rounded on AP
  ○ Dorsal intercalated segment instability (DISI): Seen in SL tear, RA, CPPD
    ▪ Lunate dorsal tilt > 20°; SL angle > 70°; CL angle > 20°; lunate triangular on AP
• **Carpal Dislocation**
  ○ Stages due to perilunate ligament injury; look for accompanying fractures
    ▪ 1: SL tear ± scaphoid rotatory subluxation
    ▪ 2: Radiocapitate tear; perilunate dislocation
    ▪ 3: Volar radiotriquetral, dorsal radiocarpal tears; midcarpal dislocation
    ▪ 4: Dorsal radiocarpal tear; lunate dislocation
• **Osteonecrosis, Wrist (Scaphoid & Lunate)**
  ○ Scaphoid proximal pole AVN due to trauma
  ○ Lunate: Kienbock disease (lunatomalacia); associated with ulnar minus, trauma
    ▪ Stage 1: X-ray - normal; MR - T1 ↓ SI, T2 ↑ SI
    ▪ Stage 2: X-ray - sclerosis; MR - T1 ↓ SI, T2 ↑ SI

▪ Stage 3: X-ray-collapse, proximal capitate migration, SL dissociation, scaphoid rotatory subluxation; MR - T1 & T2 ↓ SI
▪ Stage 4: X-ray-secondary OA; MR - T1 & T2 ↓ SI

• **Infection**
  ○ History of diabetes, inflammatory arthritis, immunocompromise, puncture wounds, open fracture
  ○ Septic joint: Extensive effusion of one or more compartments, ± carpal edema
  ○ Osteomyelitis: Marked osteopenia; cortical loss, joint malalignment

Helpful Clues for Rare Diagnoses

• **Osseous Neoplasm**
  ○ Benign: Giant cell tumor, enchondroma, osteoid osteoma
  ○ Malignant: Squamous cell metastases
• **Soft Tissue Neoplasm**
  ○ Benign: Ganglion, giant cell tumor of tendon sheath, hemangioma, tendon sheath fibroma, lipoma
  ○ Malignant: MFH, synovial sarcoma, angiosarcoma, liposarcoma, fibrosarcoma
• **Madelung Deformity**
  ○ Radius: Dorsal/ulnar curvature; decreased radius length; triangular radial epiphysis
  ○ Ulna: Dorsal subluxation, ulnar head enlargement
  ○ Carpals wedging between radius & ulna with lunate at apex

Fracture

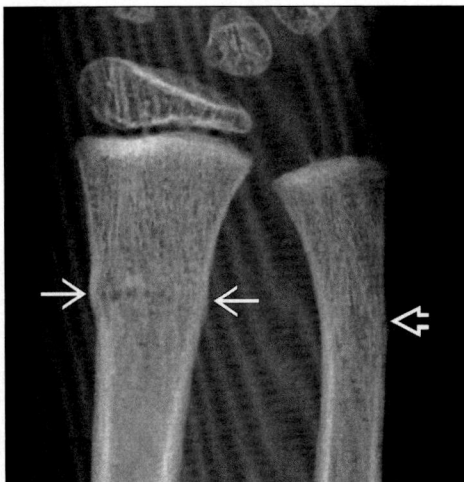

Anteroposterior radiograph shows an incomplete buckle fracture ➡ of distal radial metaphysis in a 7 year who fell on an outstretched hand. A subtle distal ulnar fracture is also present ➡.

Fracture

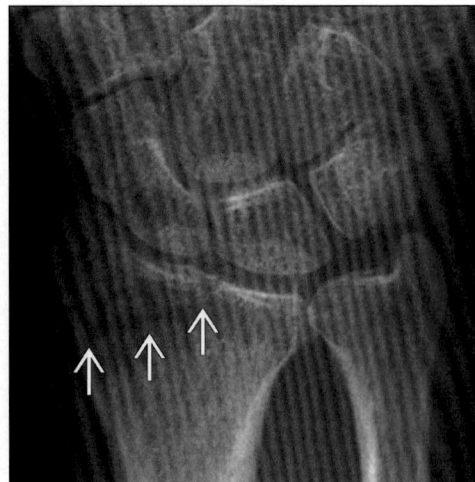

Anteroposterior radiograph shows a subtle fracture line ➡ crossing the radial styloid base & extending into the radiocarpal joint in this 55 year old female who struck her wrist against a wall.

RADIAL SIDED WRIST PAIN

Fracture

Fracture

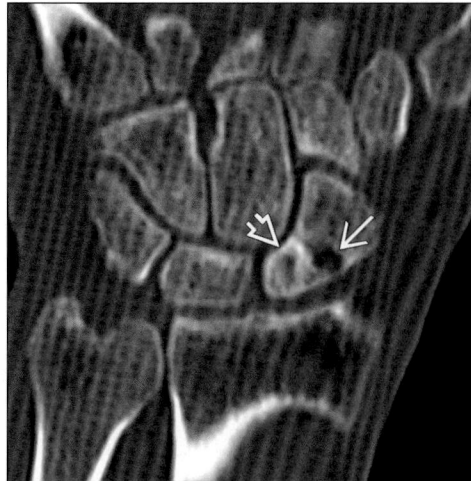

(Left) Coronal CT reformation shows midwaist scaphoid fracture with cystic margins ➡ & proximal pole sclerosis ➡ 8 months following acute fracture. While there is not malalignment, sclerosis suggests underlying AVN. (Right) Coronal T1WI MR in the same patient shows focal ↓ SI ➡ in the scaphoid proximal pole on both T1 & STIR (not shown), consistent with osteonecrosis following scaphoid fracture.

Arthritis

Arthritis

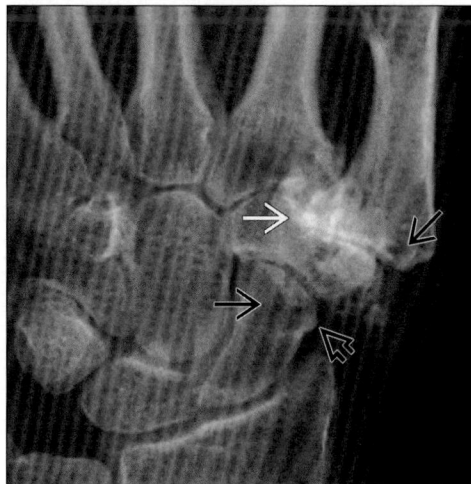

(Left) Anteroposterior radiograph shows scaphoid-trapezium-trapezoid & 1st CMC joint space narrowing ➡ & osteophytic ridges ➡ with small subchondral cysts ➡. This is classic osteoarthritis. (Right) Coronal STIR MR shows osteoarthritis with scaphoid-trapezium-trapezoid & 1st CMC joint space loss ➡, small joint effusions ➡ & subchondral reactive marrow edema (↑ SI) ➡.

Arthritis

Arthritis

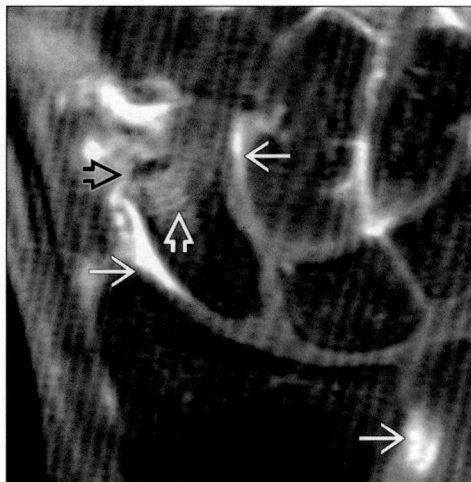

(Left) Coronal T1 C+ FS MR shows an enhancing distal scaphoid erosion ➡ with surrounding osteitis ➡ as well as joint effusions ➡ in the midcarpal, radiocarpal & distal radioulnar joints in 59 year old with rheumatoid arthritis. (Right) Posteroanterior radiograph shows long-standing rheumatoid arthritis with diffuse soft tissue swelling ➡, osteopenia, midcarpal & radiocarpal joint space loss ➡, & proximal carpal row collapse ➡.

RADIAL SIDED WRIST PAIN

Arthritis

Arthritis

(Left) Coronal T1 C+ FS MR shows scapholunate dissociation ➡ with capitate ⏩ moving toward distal radius, resulting in scapholunate advanced collapse (SLAC). This deformity occurs in pyrophosphate arthropathy or post-trauma. *(Right)* Posteroanterior radiograph shows juvenile idiopathic arthritis with profound diffuse osteopenia, carpal enlargement & ankylosis ➡. Irregular/eroded distal radial ⏩ & trapezium ➡ cortices are also present.

Ganglion Cyst, Wrist

Tendon, Injury

(Left) Sagittal T2WI FS MR shows a ganglion cyst with a tail ➡ tracking to the wrist near the lunate ⏩. This thin-walled multiseptate mass is homogeneous ↑ SI & insinuates between the extensor tendons. *(Right)* Axial T1WI MR shows extensor pollicis brevis tendinosis (thickened, mass-like) ⏩, & high grade partial tears of abductor pollicis longus ➡ & flexor carpi radialis (markedly attenuated) ⏩ with associated tenosynovitis ➡.

Tendon, Injury

Tendon, Injury

(Left) Axial T2WI FS MR shows De Quervain tenosynovitis involving both abductor pollicis longus ➡ & extensor pollicis brevis ⏩ tendons, the first extensor compartment. This is caused by repetitive motion and microtrauma. Note the adjacent joint effusion ➡. *(Right)* Axial T1 C+ FS MR shows tenosynovitis ⏩ of all extensor compartments with enhancement of thickened synovium in this 33 year old female newly diagnosed with rheumatoid arthritis.

RADIAL SIDED WRIST PAIN

Scapholunate Ligament Tear

Carpal Instabilities

(Left) PA fluoroscopic digital subtraction radiograph shows a needle ➡ in the radiocarpal joint ➡ with injected contrast outlining the scaphoid ➡ & flowing through the disrupted scapholunate ligament ➡. *(Right)* Anteroposterior radiograph shows scapholunate interval widening ➡ of 5 mm, indicating disruption of the scapholunate ligament.

Carpal Instabilities

Carpal Instabilities

(Left) Lateral radiograph shows volar intercalated segment instability (VISI) in this diffusely osteoporotic rheumatoid arthritis patient. The scaphoid ➡ is flexed & lunate ➡ angled volarly. The scapholunate angle is < 20° & capitolunate angle > 80°. *(Right)* Sagittal T1WI MR shows dorsal intercalated segment instability (DISI) in patient with scaphoid fracture nonunion & SL angle > 80° (not shown). Dorsally tilted lunate ➡ creates a capitolunate angle > 30°.

Carpal Dislocations

Carpal Dislocations

(Left) Lateral radiograph shows a perilunate dislocation with the lunate ➡ maintaining normal articulation with radius while the capitate ➡ is dislocated dorsal to the distal lunate articular surface. The remaining carpals ➡ move with the capitate. *(Right)* Lateral radiograph shows a midcarpal dislocation with lunate subluxated volarly ➡ with respect to the distal radius ➡ as the fully dislocated capitate ➡ moves proximally, displacing the lunate palmarward.

RADIAL SIDED WRIST PAIN

Carpal Dislocations

Osteonecrosis, Wrist (Scaphoid & Lunate)

(Left) Lateral radiograph shows lunate dislocation with the lunate ⮊ displaced into the volar soft tissue & the capitate ⮊ approaching the radius articular surface ⮊. There is an associated scaphoid fracture ⮕, resulting in a transcaphoid lunate fracture dislocation. *(Right)* Anteroposterior radiograph shows multiple bone osteonecrosis related to steroid use. There is scaphoid sclerosis ⮊ with collapse ⮊ as well as lunate sclerosis ⮕.

Infection

Osseous Neoplasm

(Left) Coronal T1 C+ FS MR shows Mycobacterium avium septic arthritis/osteomyelitis with extensive erosion of scaphoid ⮊, trapezium, trapezoid, & ulnar styloid ⮕. There is radial shaft marrow edema (↑ SI) ⮊. Extensive joint effusion & synovial hypertrophy ⮊ is also present. *(Right)* AP radiograph shows a giant cell tumor with an expansile lytic subchondral distal radius lesion ⮊ with pseudotrabeculations ⮊ in this young adult.

Soft Tissue Neoplasm

Madelung Deformity

(Left) Coronal oblique PD FSE FS MR shows a discrete ↑ SI mass ⮊ eccentric to but arising from median nerve ⮊. This fusiform mass was exquisitely tender to the touch & was pathologically proven to be a schwannoma. *(Right)* Anteroposterior radiograph shows a classic Madelung deformity with a shortened curved radius ⮕, a longer (& dislocated) ulna ⮊ & a V-shaped radiocarpal articulation with the lunate ⮊ forming the leading edge.

GROIN/HIP PAIN

DIFFERENTIAL DIAGNOSIS

Common
- Fracture
- Arthritis
- Osteonecrosis, Hip
- Muscle Strain, Hip
- Tendon, Injury
- Labral Tear, Hip
- Bursitis

Less Common
- Hardware Failure
- Transient Bone Marrow Edema
- Infection
  ○ Septic Joint
  ○ Osteomyelitis
  ○ Soft Tissue Abscess
- Intraosseous Neoplasm
- Osteitis Pubis
- Hip Malformation
- Sciatica

Rare but Important
- Soft Tissue Neoplasm
- Kidney Stones
- Testicular/Scrotal Pathology
- Adnexal Pathology
- Nerve Entrapment

ESSENTIAL INFORMATION

Key Differential Diagnosis Issues
- X-rays: Essential for initial evaluation
- CT: Best for bone detail
- MR: Best for marrow, soft tissues
- Bone scan: Useful for screening

Helpful Clues for Common Diagnoses
- **Fracture**
  ○ Avulsion: Common in skeletally immature
    ▪ Common locations: Adductor & hamstring origins
    ▪ X-rays: Thin curvilinear fragment
    ▪ MR: Marrow & soft tissue edema mask fragment
  ○ Stress: Abnormal stress → normal bone
    ▪ Common locations: Medial femoral neck, subtrochanter, symphysis
  ○ Insufficiency: Normal stress → abnormal bone
    ▪ Common locations: Symphysis, pubic rami, acetabulum, femoral head & neck

- If anterior pelvic fractures are seen, look for sacral fractures
  ○ **Hint**: Marrow edema may mask fracture line; use T1 to identify fracture line
- **Arthritis**
  ○ Osteoarthritis
    ▪ Asymmetric joint space loss (usually superior), articular flattening, subchondral sclerosis & cyst formation, ± loose bodies
  ○ Inflammatory: Rheumatoid, ankylosing spondylitis, psoriatic
    ▪ Uniform joint loss, ± erosions or osteophytes, ± rice bodies
  ○ Crystalline: Gout, CPPD
    ▪ Chondrocalcinosis, joint space loss symmetric or asymmetric, osteophytes
- **Osteonecrosis, Hip**
  ○ X-rays: Focal sclerosis, crescentic subchondral lucency (fracture), flattened articular surface
  ○ MR: Serpentine "double line" sign with the paralleling ↓/↑ SI of reparative & necrotic tissue, crescentic subcortical fluid (fracture), flattened joint surface
- **Muscle Strain, Hip**
  ○ Muscle injury ranges from minimal fiber tear (grade 1) to complete fiber disruption (grade 3) with retraction & edema
  ○ Hematoma
    ▪ Acute (< 48 hrs): T1 isodense to muscle
    ▪ Subacute (< 30 days): ↑ SI on T1 & T2 (methemoglobin)
    ▪ Chronic (> 30 days): Heterogeneous; ↓ SI if hemosiderin deposition
- **Tendon, Injury**
  ○ Most common: Adductors, pectineus, obturators, hamstrings
  ○ Range from tendinosis (thickening & intrasubstance signal) to complete tear (tendon disruption & retraction)
  ○ Sports hernia: Rectus abdominus/adductor aponeurosis avulsion from anterior pubis periosteum
- **Labral Tear, Hip**
  ○ MR arthrography with dilute gadolinium (1:200) facilitates diagnosis
  ○ Ranges from blunting of labrum through intrasubstance signal & tear to detachment
  ○ Paralabral cyst indicates labral tear
- **Bursitis**

- ○ ↑ SI on fluid sensitive sequences in potential spaces between tendons, ligaments, bony protuberances
- ○ Common sites: Iliopsoas, obturator canal

Helpful Clues for Less Common Diagnoses
- **Hardware Failure**
  - ○ Loosening, subsidence, foreign body reaction, polyethylene failure
- **Transient Bone Marrow Edema**
  - ○ Acute onset focal pain; middle-age men
  - ○ X-rays - osteopenia; MR - intense ↑ SI edema without collapse or fracture
  - ○ Also known as transient osteoporosis
- **Infection**
  - ○ **Septic Joint**
    - ▪ Focal osteopenia; large effusion
    - ▪ Requires aspiration for confirmation
    - ▪ Transient synovitis (ages 3-10) mimics septic joint but noninfectious, a diagnosis of exclusion
  - ○ **Osteomyelitis**
    - ▪ Cortical disruption, ± periostitis & soft tissue involvement
  - ○ **Soft Tissue Abscess**
    - ▪ Mass with thick, irregular walls; ± sinus tracts & bone destruction or reaction
- **Intraosseous Neoplasm**
  - ○ Metastases & multiple myeloma > > > primary neoplasms
  - ○ May be lytic, sclerotic or mixed
  - ○ **Hint**: Lesions in lesser trochanter should raise the possibility of metastases
- **Osteitis Pubis**

- ○ Painful symphysis; related to GU surgery, pregnancy, infection
- ○ X-ray: Irregular symphyseal cortex with resorption, subchondral eburnation
- ○ MR: Marrow edema; ± effusion
- ○ Aspiration needed to exclude infection
- **Hip Malformation**
  - ○ Malformation from developmental dysplasia, SCFE, fracture malunion, etc. results in secondary osteoarthritis, abnormal gait
- **Sciatica**
  - ○ Referred pain from neural impingement at L2 or L3

Helpful Clues for Rare Diagnoses
- **Soft Tissue Neoplasm**
  - ○ Benign: Lipoma, neurofibroma, hemangioma, myxoma
  - ○ Malignant: MFH, lymphoma, liposarcoma, fibrosarcoma, synovial sarcoma
- **Kidney Stones, Testicular/Scrotal/Adnexal Pathology**
  - ○ Referred pain
- **Nerve Entrapment**
  - ○ Referred pain from entrapped nerves including ilioinguinal, genitofemoral, obturator nerves

Alternative Differential Approaches
- **Pubalgia**
  - ○ Fracture, muscle tendon injury, osteitis pubis, sports hernia, GU abnormalities, ilioinguinal neuralgia

Fracture

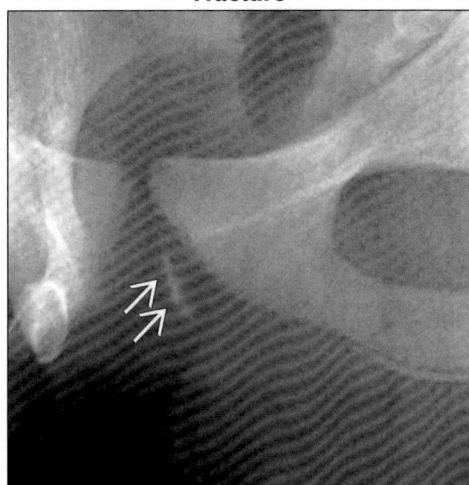

Anteroposterior oblique radiograph shows a small avulsion fragment ➡ at the adductor brevis origin in this 14 year old soccer player.

Fracture

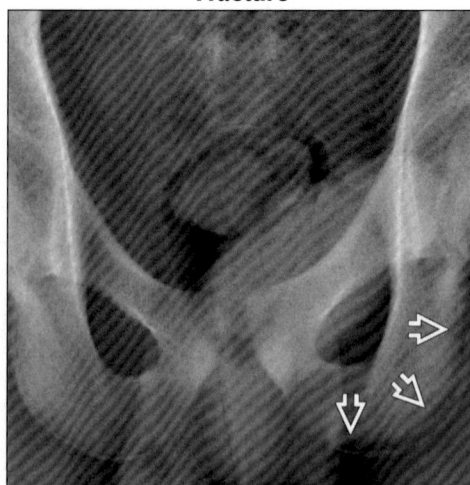

Anteroposterior radiograph shows widening of the left ischial growth plate ➡ in this young patient with chronic hamstring apophyseal stress injury.

49

GROIN/HIP PAIN

Fracture

Fracture

(Left) Sagittal T1WI MR shows ↓ SI in a broad band across the femoral neck which represents edema surrounding & obscuring an underlying subcapital fracture ➡. *(Right)* Coronal STIR MR in a distance runner shows an incomplete fatigue fracture (↓ SI ➡) surrounded by edema (↑ SI ➡) in the basicervical region.

Fracture

Fracture

(Left) Coronal STIR MR in this elderly female shows extensive linear ↑ SI ➡ of a transcervical incomplete insufficiency fracture with edema (↓ SI ➡)in the femoral head. *(Right)* Axial NECT shows a non-displaced posterior rim fracture ➡ in this patient who had a recent transient posterior dislocation. Note the small intracapsular loose fragment ➡.

Arthritis

Arthritis

(Left) Coronal PD FSE FS MR shows osteoarthritis characterized by joint space loss with flattening of the articular surface ➡, subchondral edema & cyst formation ➡. Note the medial femoral neck osteophyte ➡. *(Right)* Anteroposterior radiograph shows severe uniform cartilage loss ➡ & diffuse osteopenia. Note the lack of osteophyte development in this patient with psoriatic arthritis. The right SI joint (not shown) is fused.

Osteonecrosis, Hip

Muscle Strain, Hip

(Left) Coronal STIR MR shows a serpentine double line with ↑ SI ➡ paralleling ↓ SI ➡, representing the interface between necrotic & reparative tissue in this 55 year old male with prednisone-induced osteonecrosis. *(Right)* Coronal PD FSE FS MR shows a subtle fracture(↓ SI ➡) of the superior pubic ramus with surrounding marrow edema (↑ SI ➡). The obturator externus edema ➡ indicates muscle strain in the 65 year old.

Muscle Strain, Hip

Tendon, Injury

(Left) Sagittal PD FSE FS MR shows extensive ↑ SI in an iliopsoas partial muscle tear (grade 2) ➡ with associated acute (↑ SI) hematoma ➡. A posterior femoral head marrow contusion is present ➡. *(Right)* Coronal STIR MR shows bilateral semimembranosus partial tears with ↑ SI of edema/blood in the area of disruption ➡. Additional injury to the right conjoined tendon (biceps femoris/semitendinosus) ➡ is also present.

Labral Tear, Hip

Labral Tear, Hip

(Left) Coronal T1WI FS MR shows labral tear of the superior acetabular labrum with contrast ➡ interposed between the acetabular rim & the torn labrum ➡. *(Right)* Sagittal PD FSE FS MR shows a thin-walled multiseptate paralabral cyst ➡ tracking along the superior acetabulum is this patient with a small associated anterior labral tear (not shown).

Bursitis

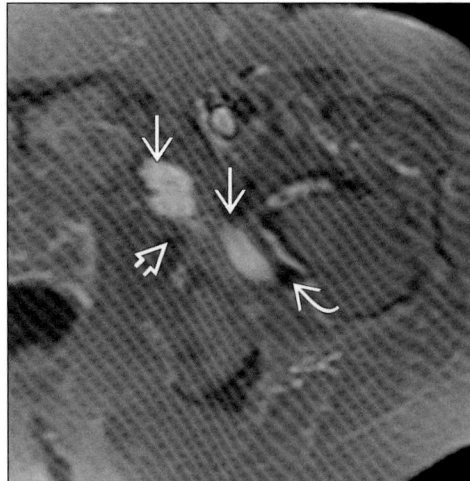

Hardware Failure

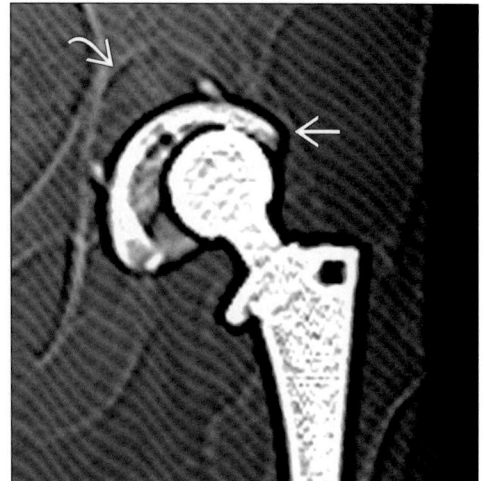

(Left) Axial PD FSE FS MR shows obturator externus bursitis with a multiloculate fluid collection ➡ interposed between the obturator externus ⊟ & the ischiofemoral capsular ligament ⊟. *(Right)* AP CT scanogram demonstrates failure of a left THA with eccentric polyethylene wear ➡ & a large lytic lesion ➡ in the acetabulum confirmed to be foreign body osteolysis at surgery.

Transient Bone Marrow Edema

Transient Bone Marrow Edema

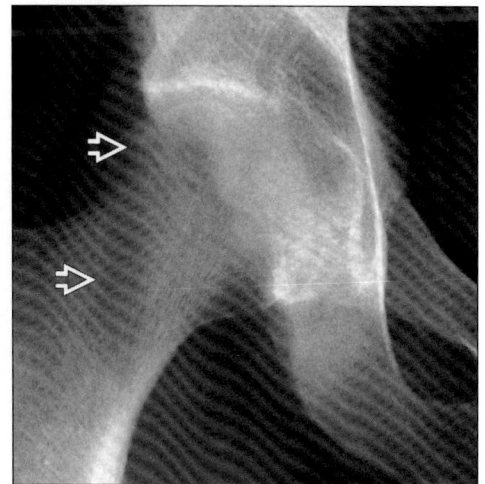

(Left) Coronal STIR MR shows intense right femoral head & neck bone marrow edema ⊟ in this 47 year old male with abrupt onset of hip pain. Attempts at aspiration yielded no fluid. Pain resolved over a 4 month period. *(Right)* Anteroposterior radiograph in a middle-aged male reveals femoral head & neck osteoporosis ⊟ while the adjacent acetabulum & joint are normal. This is the radiographic pattern seen in transient bone marrow edema syndrome.

Infection

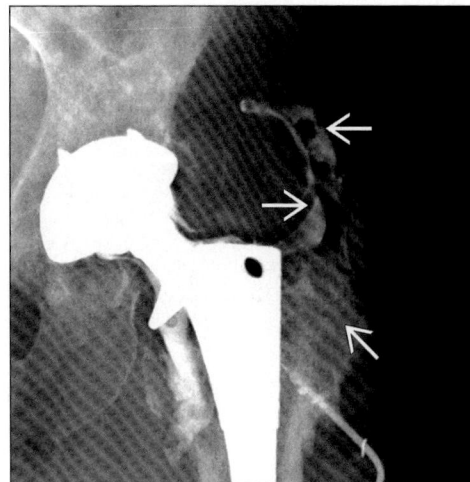

Septic Joint

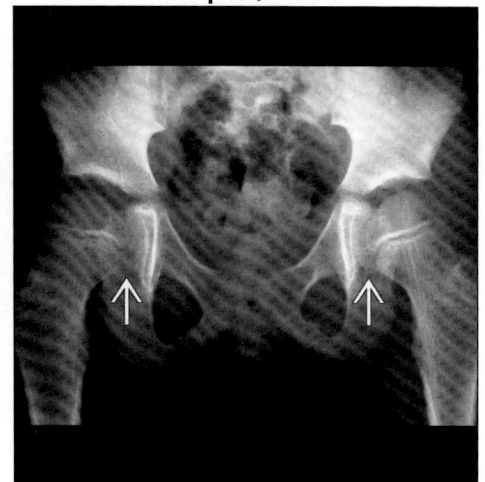

(Left) AP radiograph during arthrogram/aspiration reveals contrast flowing into an abscess cavity laterally ➡. The greater trochanter has a moth-eaten appearance of osteomyelitis in this female with E. Coli osteomyelitis. *(Right)* Anteroposterior radiograph shows subtle widening of right "teardrop" distance ➡ in this 6 year old with right hip pain. Septic joint must be considered. Aspiration yielded normal synovial fluid & patient recovered uneventfully from transient synovitis.

GROIN/HIP PAIN

Soft Tissue Abscess

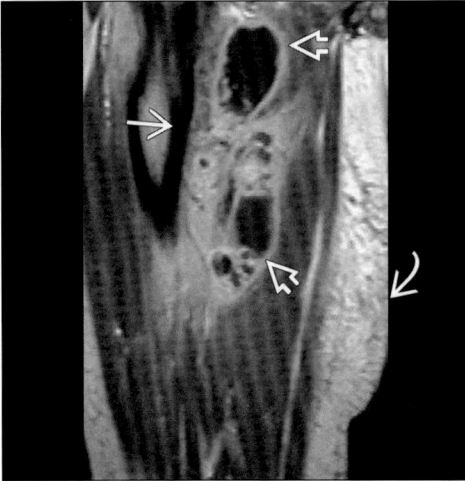

Intraosseous Neoplasm

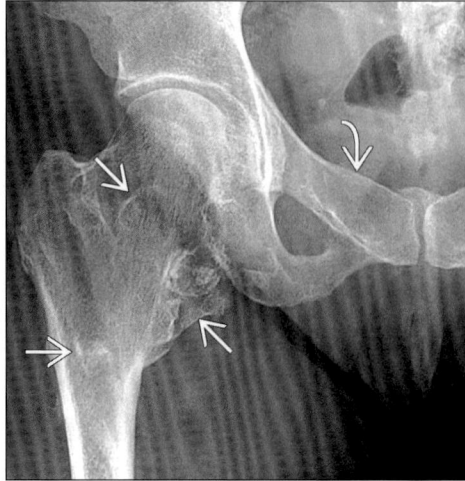

(Left) Coronal T1 C+ MR shows multiloculated abscess in the thigh ⇒ with adjacent cortical reaction in the femur ⇒ and cellulitis ⇒. This patient had slowly worsening groin pain and swelling over several months. *(Right)* Anteroposterior radiograph shows multiple hereditary exostoses with both pedunculated ⇒ & sessile ⇒ lesions which deform the hip contours, resulting in mechanical impingement. Malignant degeneration occurs in up to 20% of patients.

Intraosseous Neoplasm

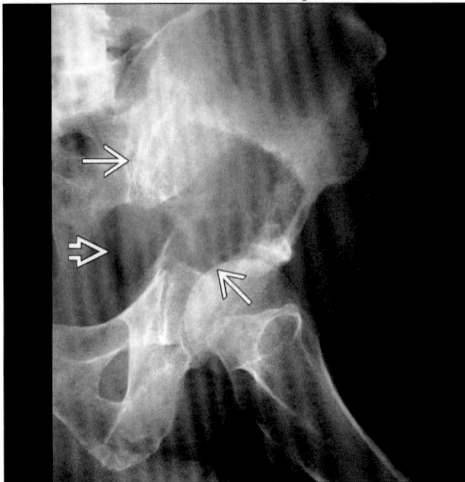

Osteitis Pubis

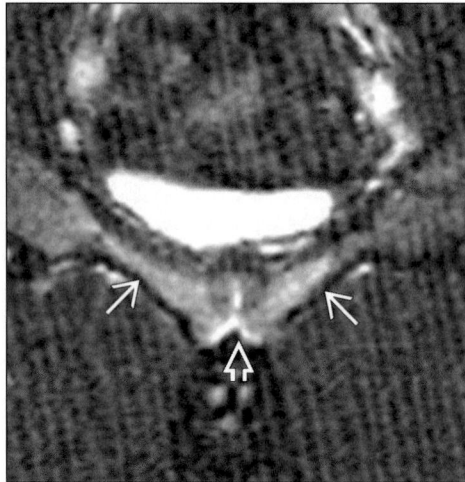

(Left) Frogleg lateral radiograph shows an aggressive lytic lesion extending to the joint surfaces of the hip & SI joint ⇒. There is no internal matrix. Cortical breakthrough & soft tissue mass ⇒ are seen medially. This is a plasmacytoma. *(Right)* Coronal STIR MR shows intense ↑ SI of the symphysis pubis & bilateral superior pubic rami ⇒ with minimal fluid in the joint ⇒. This is a traumatic osteitis pubis in this young male athlete.

Hip Malformation

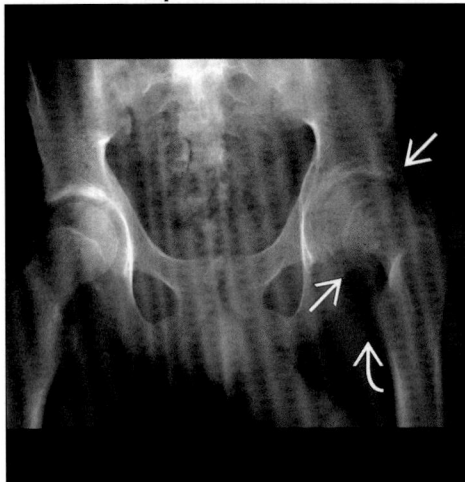

Soft Tissue Neoplasm

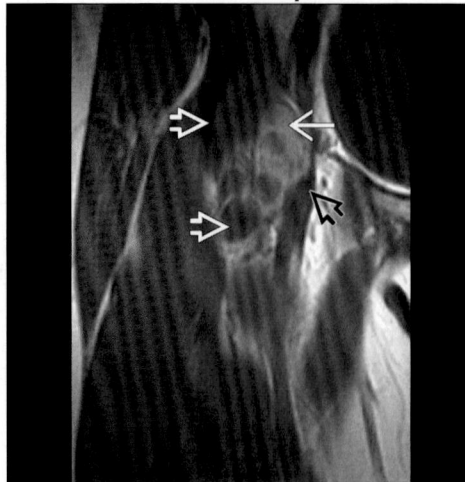

(Left) Anteroposterior radiograph in this 15 year old reveals the medial & posterior rotation of a slipped capital femoral epiphysis ⇒ with limb shortening (note the lesser trochanter position ⇒). *(Right)* Coronal T1WI MR shows a myxoid liposarcoma as a heterogeneous soft tissue mass anterior to the hip, containing fatty (↑ SI ⇒) & myxoid (↓ SI ⇒) elements. It abuts the neurovascular bundle ⇒.

III

LATERAL HIP PAIN

DIFFERENTIAL DIAGNOSIS

Common
- Bursitis
- Tendon, Injury
- Muscle Strain, Hip
- Arthritis
- Labral Tear, Hip

Less Common
- Fracture
- Hardware Failure
- Soft Tissue Hematoma
- Sacroiliac Dysfunction
- Sciatica - L4, L5

Rare but Important
- Developmental Dysplasia of the Hip
- Soft Tissue Abscess
- Intraosseous Neoplasm
- Soft Tissue Neoplasm
- Meralgia Paresthetica (Lateral Femoral Nerve)

ESSENTIAL INFORMATION

Key Differential Diagnosis Issues
- Soft tissue injury is the most common explanation for lateral hip pain
- **Hint**: Don't let satisfaction of search stop you from looking for all causes of lateral hip pain

Helpful Clues for Common Diagnoses
- **Bursitis**
  - Inflammation of potential spaces between tendons, ligaments, bony protuberances
  - Common hip bursae include greater trochanter, subgluteus medius, subgluteus minimus
  - May have accompanying pathology such as tendon/muscle tear, hematoma
  - May be seen in acute or chronic trauma, arthritis, infection
  - Results in bursal effusion, ± thickened synovium
- **Tendon, Injury**
  - Most common: Gluteus maximus & medius (rotator cuff of the hip)
  - Partial: Disruption of some tendon fibers with minimal retraction & associated edema

- Complete: Complete disruption of tendon with significant retraction & edema/hematoma
  - Fatty atrophy of associated muscle bellies may occur over time
- **Muscle Strain, Hip**
  - Muscle injury ranges from minimal fiber tear (grade 1) to complete disruption of muscle (grade 3) with retraction & extensive ↑ SI of edema/hemorrhage
  - May evolve to atrophy with fatty infiltration with loss of muscle bulk
- **Arthritis**
  - Lateral hip pain is referred
  - May originate from osteoarthritis, inflammatory, crystalline or infectious arthropathy
  - Look for joint space narrowing, subchondral sclerosis, edema & cyst formation
- **Labral Tear, Hip**
  - May present as pain referred to lateral hip though labral tear symptoms usually include catching & clicking
  - Irregular ↑ SI in acetabular labrum ± adjacent cartilage damage
  - Signal may involve articular surface of labrum or extend through the full labral thickness
  - MR arthrography is imaging study of choice

Helpful Clues for Less Common Diagnoses
- **Fracture**
  - Look for avulsion fractures
    - Sartorius avulsion of anterior superior iliac spine
    - Rectus femoris avulsion of anterior inferior iliac spine
    - Gluteal avulsion of greater trochanter
  - Acute traumatic fracture: Look for appropriate mechanism of injury
  - Insufficiency: Look for lateral basicervical fracture line
  - Poorly reduced fractures may result in altered mechanics including impingement or gait alteration
- **Hardware Failure**
  - Look for loosening, subsidence, hardware or periprosthetic fracture, stress shielding
  - Comparison with prior studies important to identify early changes

LATERAL HIP PAIN

- **Soft Tissue Hematoma**
  - Intramuscular or subcutaneous
  - Acute (48 hrs): T1 isointense to muscle
  - Subacute (< 30 days): ↑ SI on T1 & T2 (methemoglobin)
  - Chronic (> 30 days): Heterogeneous; ↓ SI if hemosiderin
  - May evolve to a seroma, particularly in the subcutaneous tissue superficial to tensor fascia lata
- **Sacroiliac Dysfunction**
  - Referred pain
  - Sacroiliac joint pain more commonly presents as low back pain but may present as lateral hip pain
- **Sciatica - L4, L5**
  - Referred pain
  - Neural impingement in lateral recess, neural foramina or central stenosis at L4 &/or L5

Helpful Clues for Rare Diagnoses
- **Developmental Dysplasia of the Hip**
  - Altered hip conformation may result in direct impingement or pain from 2° OA
  - Acetabular labral pathology may accompany hip deformity
- **Soft Tissue Abscess**
  - Soft tissue mass with central fluid surrounded by thickened, irregular wall; ± intralesional gas; ± sinus tract
  - ± Involvement of adjacent bones
  - Surrounding soft tissue inflammation with stranding of the fat

- May be difficult to distinguish from necrotic neoplasm
- **Intraosseous Neoplasm**
  - Metastases & multiple myeloma are most common neoplasms
  - Look for aggressive features including cortical breakthrough, periosteal reaction & soft tissue mass
  - Adolescent: Ewing sarcoma, osteosarcoma, periosteal osteoid osteoma
  - Adult: MFH, PNET, fibrosarcoma
- **Soft Tissue Neoplasm**
  - Appearance of neoplasms tend to be nonspecific with ↓ SI on T1 & ↑ SI on T2 except lipomas
  - Lipomas: ↑ SI on T1; intermediate SI on T2; follows fatty signal on all sequences
  - Common adult tumors
    - Benign: Lipoma, neurogenic tumors, hemangioma
    - Malignant: Liposarcoma, MFH, lymphoma, synovial sarcoma, fibrosarcoma
- **Meralgia Paresthetica (Lateral Femoral Nerve)**
  - Lateral femoral cutaneous nerve entrapment with anterolateral thigh paresthesias
  - May result from mass of retroperitoneal space proximal to inguinal ligament or as nerve passes under ligament
  - Seen in diabetics, pregnancy, obesity, tight clothing

Bursitis

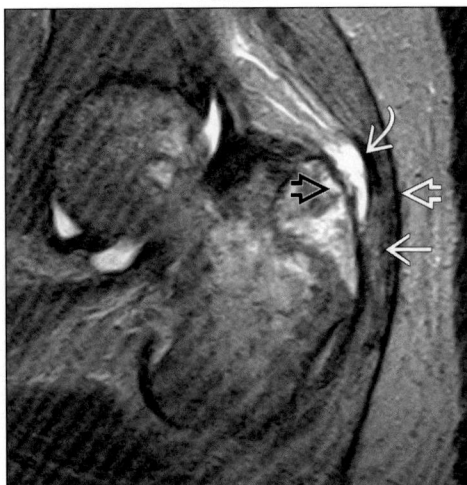

Coronal T2WI FS MR shows fluid ➡ in the bursa between gluteus medius ➡ & greater trochanter ➡. There is tendinosis ➡. Marrow infiltration from metastatic disease is incidentally noted.

Bursitis

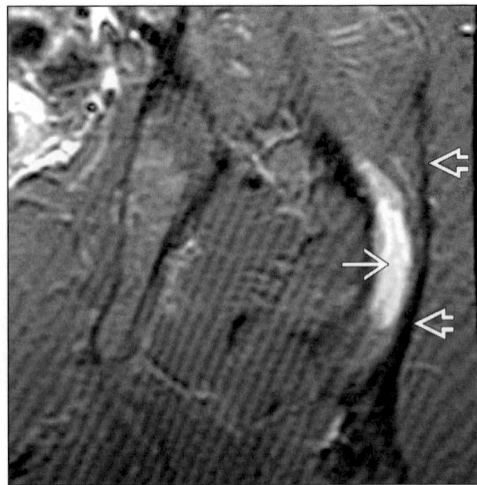

Coronal T2WI FS MR demonstrates a fluid collection ➡ lateral to the left greater femoral trochanter, consistent with greater trochanteric bursitis. The iliotibial band ➡ is located just lateral to the inflamed bursa.

LATERAL HIP PAIN

(Left) Coronal STIR MR shows thickening & partial tear of gluteus medius ⇨ with tendinosis of minimus ⇨ as well. Note fluid within & surrounding the hip rotator cuff. **(Right)** Sagittal PD FSE FS MR shows complete tear of the gluteus medius ⇨ & dorsal portion of the gluteus minimus ⇨ with retraction of the torn tendon from the greater trochanter ⇨.

Tendon, Injury

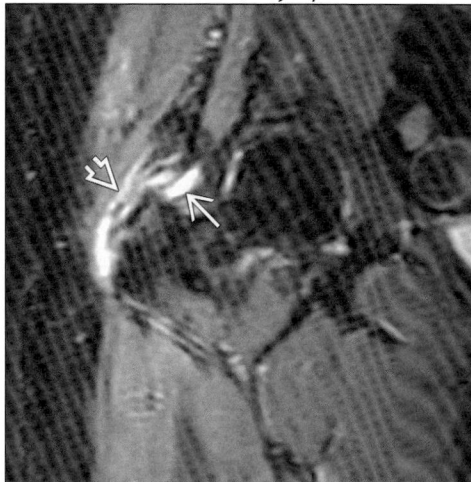

Tendon, Injury

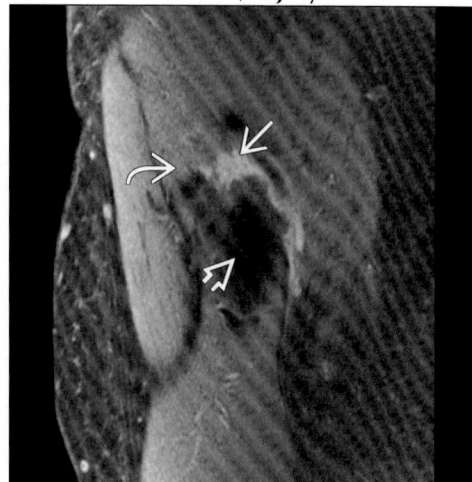

(Left) Axial T2WI FS MR shows edema & hemorrhage of grade 2 muscle strain in the gluteus maximus ⇨ & medius ⇨ as well as the adjacent fascial planes. **(Right)** Anteroposterior radiograph shows osteoarthritis with severe joint space loss ⇨, subchondral eburnation of both sides of joint & extensive cyst formation including an Egger cyst ⇨.

Muscle Strain, Hip

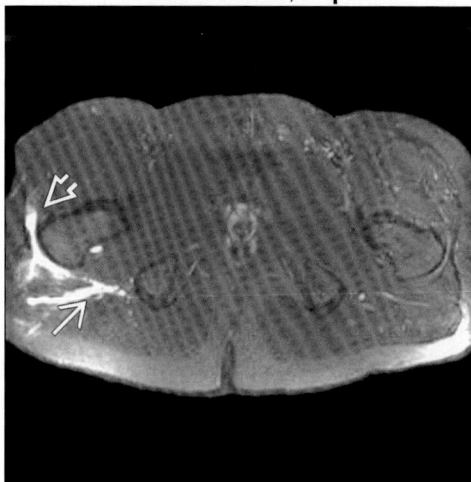

Arthritis

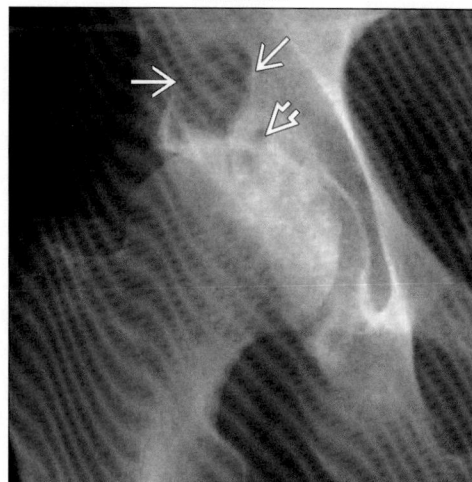

(Left) Coronal T1WI FS MR shows an irregular superior labral tear ⇨ with loss of the adjacent articular cartilage ⇨. Note the accompanying lateral femoral dysplastic "bump" ⇨ of femoroacetabular impingement. **(Right)** Coronal bone CT shows a subtle minimally displaced greater trochanteric fracture ⇨ in this osteoporotic patient. MR (not shown) revealed an intertrochanteric component to this fracture, requiring pinning.

Labral Tear, Hip

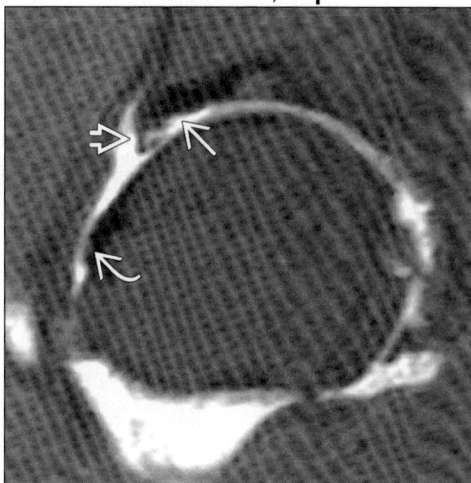

Fracture

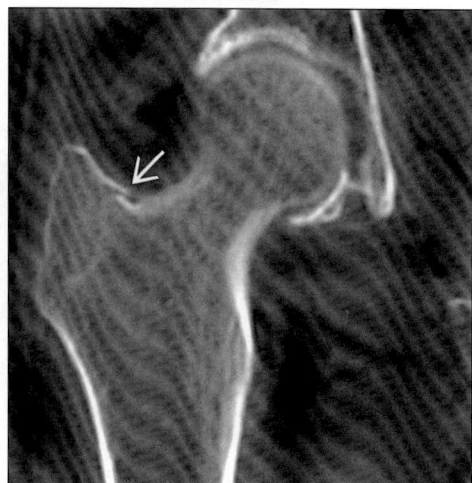

Hardware Failure

Soft Tissue Hematoma

(Left) Anteroposterior radiograph demonstrates 3 retracted cannulated lag screws (Knowles pins) ➜ projecting into the lateral soft tissues. The pins had been placed for subcapital fracture, which has collapsed, resulting in femoral head/neck nonunion ➜, proven by CT. *(Right)* Coronal STIR MR shows focal curvilinear ↑ SI ➜ in subcutaneous fat superficial to greater trochanter. This hematoma resulted after a recent fall on the left hip in an anticoagulated patient.

Sacroiliac Dysfunction

Developmental Dysplasia of the Hip

(Left) Oblique coronal T1WI MR shows ↓ SI on both sides of left sacroiliac joint ➜ which enhanced with IV contrast (not shown) in this HIV patient with septic arthritis. Sacroiliac joint disease may present with lateral hip pain rather than the more usual buttock or groin pain. *(Right)* Anteroposterior radiograph shows DDH with coxa magna ➜, superolateral femoral head subluxation, medial acetabular wall overgrowth ➜, & greater trochanteric deformity ➜.

Intraosseous Neoplasm

Soft Tissue Neoplasm

(Left) Anteroposterior radiograph shows a mildly expanded, partially well-circumscribed lytic lesion in the acetabulum ➜ without associated matrix, which proved to be breast metastasis. Note a slightly more sclerotic lesion in the ischium ➜. *(Right)* Axial T2WI FSE MR shows an intermediate SI mass enlarging the gluteus minimus ➜ & medius ➜ & displacing the maximus ➜. It extends through the sciatic notch ➜. This is a non-Hodgkin lymphoma.

SNAPPING HIP

DIFFERENTIAL DIAGNOSIS

Common
- Tendon Impingement

Less Common
- Loose Bodies, Hip
- Labral Tear, Hip
- Synovial Osteochondromatosis
- Osteochondroma

Rare but Important
- Osteonecrosis, Hip
- Ligamentum Teres Tear

ESSENTIAL INFORMATION

Key Differential Diagnosis Issues
- Difficult to demonstrate dynamic problem with static imaging
  - Ultrasound: Excellent dynamic imaging
  - Bursography: Indirect visualization
  - CT/MR: Soft tissue/bony abnormalities

Helpful Clues for Common Diagnoses
- **Tendon Impingement**
  - Restriction due to bony prominences, bursitis, cysts or masses
  - Iliopsoas tendon (IPT)
    - In flexion-abduction-external rotation, IPT lateral & anterior to IP muscle
    - As hip brought to neutral, IPT glides back medial & posterior to IP muscle resting on superior pubic ramus

- IPT may "catch" on iliopectineal eminence, anteroinferior iliac spine, lesser trochanter or on IP muscle medial margin
- Ultrasound best for dynamic evaluation of IP tendon motion/restriction
  - Iliotibial band/gluteus maximus: Moves anteriorly in flexion; snaps back over greater trochanter when hip straightened
  - Biceps femoris: Snaps over ischial tuberosity
  - Iliofemoral ligament: Snaps over anterior femoral head
  - Bursitis & tendonitis/tenosynovitis may be a cause or a result of impingement

Helpful Clues for Less Common Diagnoses
- **Loose Bodies, Hip**
  - May be calcified, ossified or cartilaginous
- **Labral Tear, Hip**
  - Unstable flap tear may act as loose body
  - Anterior paralabral cyst may impinge IPT
- **Synovial Osteochondromatosis**
  - Multiple intraarticular bodies; ± calcified
- **Osteochondroma**
  - Femoral head & neck deformities may impinge surrounding tendons

Helpful Clues for Rare Diagnoses
- **Osteonecrosis, Hip**
  - Look for classic serpentine "double line" sign; rarely causes snapping
- **Ligamentum Teres Tear**
  - Best seen with joint distension, MR arthrography

Tendon Impingement

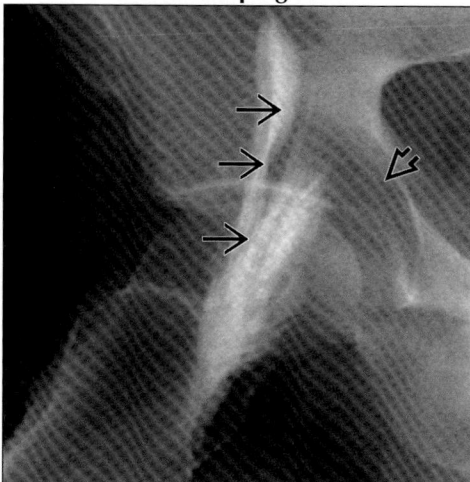

Bursography in flexion, abduction & external rotation shows IPT position as a filling defect ➔ lateral to the iliopectineal eminence ➔. Snapping may occur in this area as the hip is moves to neutral.

Tendon Impingement

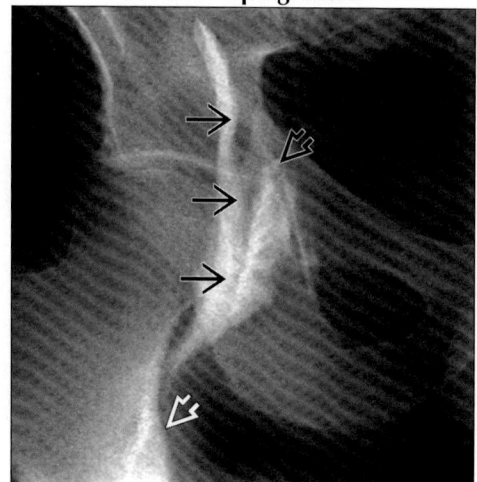

Bursography in neutral position in the same patient shows the medial motion of the IPT ➔. Its relationship to the iliopectineal eminence ➔ or lesser trochanter ➔ may restrict motion.

Tendon Impingement

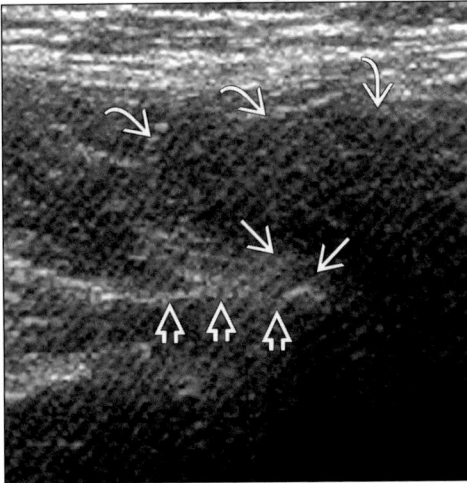

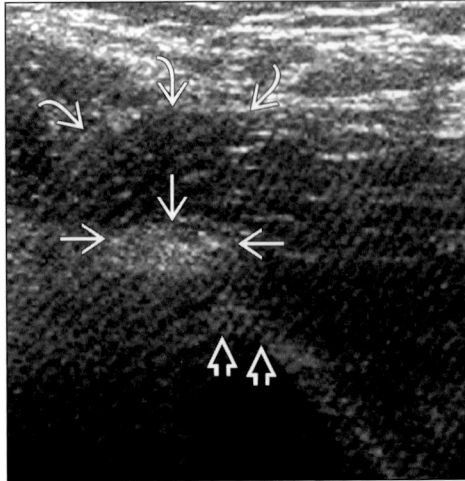

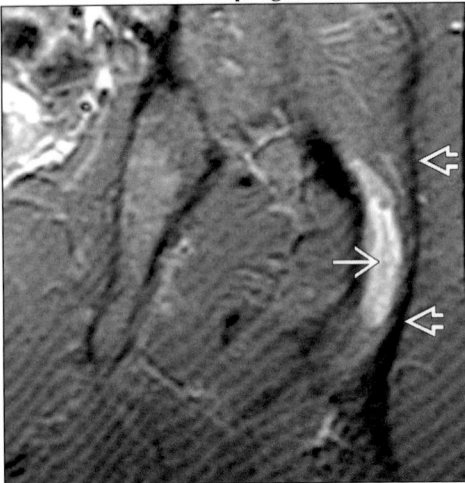

Tendon Impingement

(Left) Transverse ultrasound in flexion, abduction, external rotation shows the IPT ➡ lying lateral to the iliopectineal eminence ⊳. Note the slightly hypoechoic iliac muscle ➜ superficial to the tendon. (Right) Transverse ultrasound in neutral position in same patient shows IPT ➡ medial to the eminence ⊳. Dynamic imaging shows abrupt tendon snap as patient moves to neutral position. Note the iliac muscle belly ➜.

Tendon Impingement

Loose Bodies, Hip

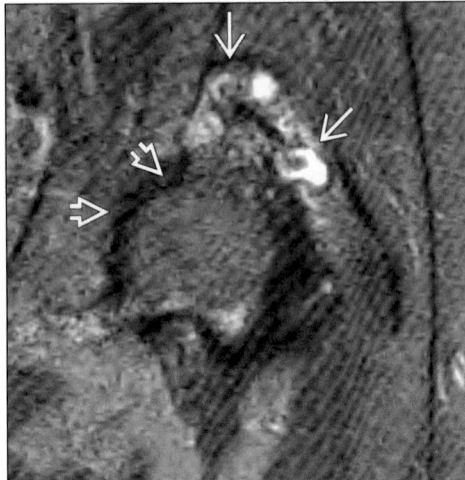

(Left) Coronal T2WI FS MR shows greater trochanteric bursitis causing external snapping hip syndrome. Note the thickened iliotibial band ⊳ as it courses over the greater trochanteric bursitis ➡. (Right) Coronal T2WI FS MR shows multiple irregular filling defects ➡ of intraarticular loose bodies in this patient with advanced osteoarthritis ⊳. Hip snapping may due to the hip malformation or the loose bodies.

Synovial Osteochondromatosis

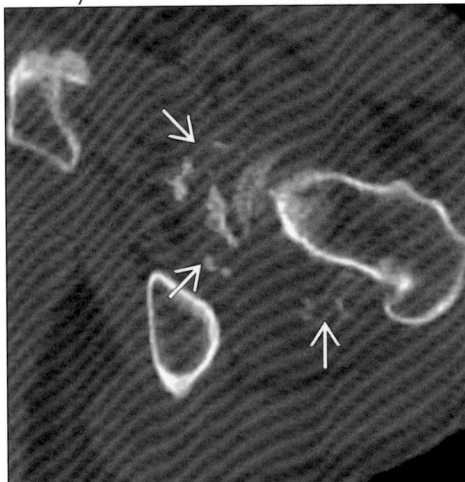

Osteochondroma

(Left) Axial NECT shows multiple mineralized intra-articular bodies ➡ in this 45 year old male with advanced secondary osteoarthritis. Synovial osteochondromatosis was confirmed at surgery. (Right) Anteroposterior radiograph shows multiple sessile ➜ & pedunculated (cauliflower) ➡ osteochondromas in this young adult with multiple hereditary exostoses. The masses may impinge the surrounding tendons through normal range of motion.

THIGH PAIN

DIFFERENTIAL DIAGNOSIS

Common
- Acute Fracture
- Stress Reaction
- Muscle Injury
  - Delayed Onset Muscle Soreness
  - Compartment Syndrome
- Hematoma
- Tendon, Injury
- Arthritis (Hip or Knee)
- Neurogenic Claudication
- Sciatica
- Metastases

Less Common
- Hardware Complications
- Fracture, Malunion
- Osteonecrosis
- Septic Arthritis
- Osteomyelitis

Rare but Important
- Complications of Statins
- Nerve Entrapment
- Polymyositis/Dermatomyositis
- Thrombophlebitis
- Leriche Syndrome
- Soft Tissue Neoplasm
- Intraosseous Neoplasm

ESSENTIAL INFORMATION

Key Differential Diagnosis Issues
- Consider both primary and referred sources when evaluating thigh pain

Helpful Clues for Common Diagnoses
- Fracture
  - **Acute Fracture**
    - MR-most sensitive; CT-best bone detail
  - **Stress Reaction**
    - Grade 1: X-ray -; bone scan +; MR periosteal edema ↑ SI (signal intensity)
    - Grade 2: X-ray -; bone scan +; MR periosteal/endosteal edema ↑ SI STIR
    - Grade 3: X-ray ± periosteal reaction; bone scan +; MR ↑ SI on T1 & STIR
    - Grade 4: X-ray + fracture; bone scan +; MR fracture + ↑ SI edema
    - Hint: Edema may be so extensive that it obscures the underlying fracture
- **Muscle Injury**
  - Grading of muscle injury
    - Grade 1: Minimal fiber tear; diffuse ↑ SI
    - Grade 2: Tear of < 50% of fibers; ↑ SI in tear defect
    - Grade 3: Complete tear; ↑ SI with large defect & muscle retraction
  - Muscle atrophy
    - Decreased bulk; ± edema; ± fatty infiltration
  - **Delayed Onset Muscle Soreness**
    - Muscle soreness & tenderness occurs 1-3 days after exertion
    - Follows a grade I muscle strain pattern
  - **Compartment Syndrome**
    - MR/CT: Swelling, loss of normal fat/fascial planes; stranding of adjacent fat planes; muscle ↑ SI
    - May lead to myonecrosis in acute setting
- **Hematoma**
  - Intramuscular or along fascial planes; resulting from direct blow, muscle or tendon tear
  - Acute (< 48 hrs): T1 isointense to muscle
  - Subacute (< 30 days): ↑ SI on T1 & T2 (methemoglobin)
  - Chronic (> 30 days): Heterogeneous; ↓ SI if hemosiderin
  - May evolve to heterotopic ossification
- **Tendon, Injury**
  - Tendinosis: Tendon thickening, ± intrasubstance ↑ SI
  - Partial tear: Partial fiber tear, ↑ SI ± surrounding edema
  - Complete tear: Full fiber tear with retracted tendons
  - ± Associated muscle injury
- **Arthritis (Hip or Knee)**
  - Arthritic complaints related to hip or knee may present as thigh pain
  - Hint: Look for joint narrowing, subchondral cysts, joint effusion
- **Neurogenic Claudication**
  - Central spinal stenosis at L3-4 &/or L4-5
- **Sciatica**
  - Possible neural impingement in lateral recesses, neural foramina, particularly at L3, L4, &/or L5
- **Metastases**
  - Hint: Look for bone marrow replacement, particularly near the lesser trochanter

Helpful Clues for Less Common Diagnoses
- **Hardware Complications**
  - Look for loosening or subsidence of hardware; fractured screws or plates; subtle fractures
- **Fracture, Malunion**
  - Malalignment results in altered gait resulting in thigh pain or aggravate arthritis in adjacent joints/spine
- **Osteonecrosis**
  - Metadiaphyseal bone infarctions may be acutely painful
  - History of sickle cell anemia, Gaucher disease common
  - Initial: nl X-rays; ↑ marrow edema
  - Evolves to typical circumscribed heterogeneous lesion
- **Septic Arthritis**
  - Effusion, synovial thickening, avid enhancement of hip or knee joint
- **Osteomyelitis**
  - Often associated with hardware, prior trauma
  - Look for marrow edema, cortical loss, periosteal reaction, enhancement

Helpful Clues for Rare Diagnoses
- **Complications of Statins**
  - Ranges from myalgias to rhabdomyolysis
    - Myalgia: Pain, ± weakness; normal creatine kinase (CK); normal MR
    - Myositis: Pain, weakness; ↑ CK; ↑ SI
    - Rhabdomyolysis: Pain, weakness; ↑ CK > 10x, myoglobinuria; ↑↑ SI

- **Nerve Entrapment**
  - Look for mass, retraction, restriction, post surgical changes
  - Lateral femoral cutaneous nerve: Anterolateral thigh paraesthesias
  - Femoral nerve: Anterior thigh, proximal leg dysesthesia
  - Saphenous nerve: Deep aching pain in thigh, knee
  - Obturator nerve: Medial thigh pain
- **Polymyositis/Dermatomyositis**
  - Symmetric proximal muscle weakness, tenderness in adults
  - MR: Diffuse edema, fatty atrophy
  - **Hint**: MR limited for diagnosis; good to evaluate disease progress
- **Thrombophlebitis**
  - Ultrasound: Distended, noncompressive vessel lumen
  - CT venography & MR: Vessel filling defects, distension
- **Leriche Syndrome**
  - Aortoiliac occlusive vascular disease; vascular claudication
- **Soft Tissue Neoplasm**
  - Benign: Lipoma, myxoma, hemangioma, neurogenic tumors
  - Malignant: Liposarcoma, MFH, synovial sarcoma, fibrosarcoma
- **Intraosseous Neoplasm**
  - Adolescent: Ewing sarcoma, osteosarcoma, osteoid osteoma
  - Adult: Metastases, myeloma far exceed primary tumors

Acute Fracture
Anteroposterior radiograph shows a linear longitudinal fracture ➡ in the distal femoral diaphysis. CT (not shown) confirmed periosteal reaction and cortical break in this athlete.

Acute Fracture
Anteroposterior radiograph shows a displaced transverse fracture ➡, suggesting high energy injury or pathologic process. This fracture occurred in patient on bisphosphonate treatment for osteopenia.

THIGH PAIN

Stress Reaction

(Left) Sagittal PD TSE FS shows a grade 4 stress reaction/fracture with a cortical break and low signal linear band ➡, periosteal ➡ and endosteal/medullary edema ➡. *(Right)* Axial PD FSE FS MR shows heterogeneous high signal and swelling of a partial (grade 2) vastus medialis muscle tear. This high signal represents a combination of edema (↑ SI) ➡ and hemorrhage (↓ SI) ➡.

Muscle Injury

Delayed Onset Muscle Soreness

(Left) Axial STIR MR shows edema of the biceps femoris within the muscle belly ➡ and along the musculotendinous junction ➡. This is typical of a grade 1 muscle injury with edema but no definitive fiber tear. *(Right)* Axial T1WI MR shows herniation of a part of vastus lateralis ➡. Exercise-induced compartment syndrome is sometimes related to such muscle herniations.

Compartment Syndrome

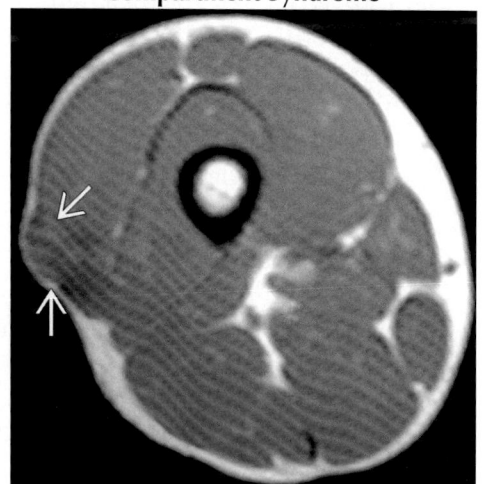

Hematoma

(Left) Sagittal STIR MR shows large fluid collection ➡ in posterior thigh of an 80 year old male (on aspirin) who fell while rollerblading. In the acute phase, this hematoma appears as simple fluid (↑ SI). Note the torn hamstring ➡. *(Right)* Coronal STIR MR shows ↑ SI of edema/hemorrhage ➡ at the hamstring origin with a high grade partial tear ➡ and retraction of tendon fibers. Note the subtle edema ➡ in the ischial tuberosity.

Tendon, Injury

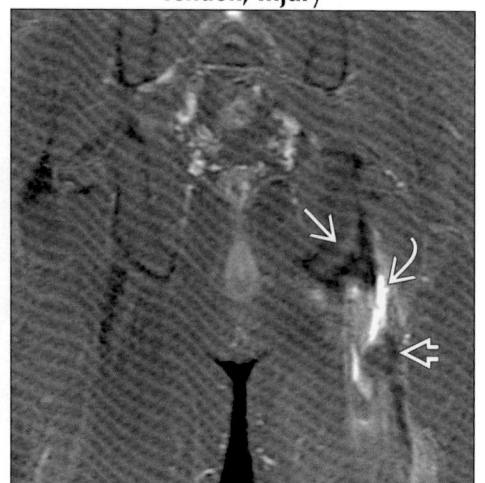

Metastases

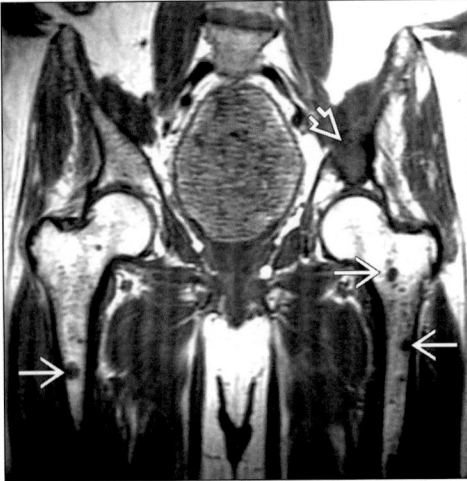

Hardware Complications

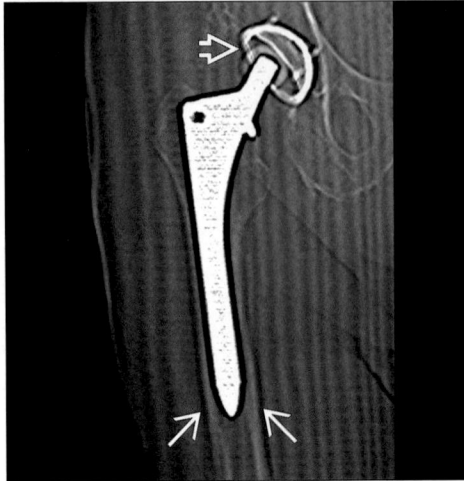

(Left) Coronal T1WI MR shows multiple punctate foci ➜ of marrow replacement (representing breast metastases) on the background of normal fatty marrow. A larger lesion is located in the left ilium ➜. *(Right)* NECT scanogram shows a cementless THA in patient with persistent thigh pain. Note eccentric femoral head position related to polyethylene wear ➜ and subtle endosteal remodeling ➜ near the femoral stem, indicative of loosening.

Osteonecrosis

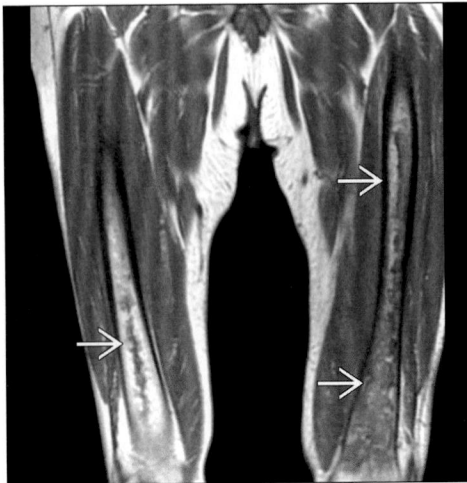

Osteomyelitis

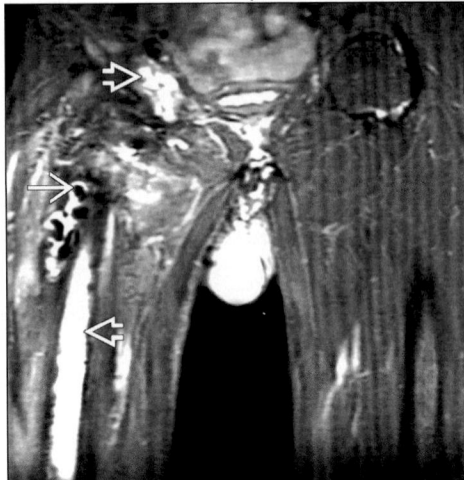

(Left) Coronal PD FSE FS MR shows diffuse serpentine heterogeneous signal ➜ in the bilateral metadiaphyses (left > right), representing medullary osteonecrosis in patient with Gaucher disease. *(Right)* Coronal STIR MR shows a Girdlestone arthroplasty resulting from infection of a THA. The metal prosthesis is removed and replaced with antibiotic-impregnated beads ➜. There is extensive marrow ↑ SI ➜ of femur and acetabulum due to ongoing osteomyelitis.

Polymyositis/Dermatomyositis

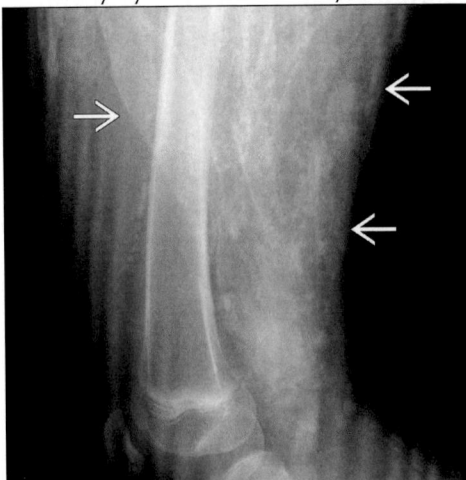

Soft Tissue Neoplasm

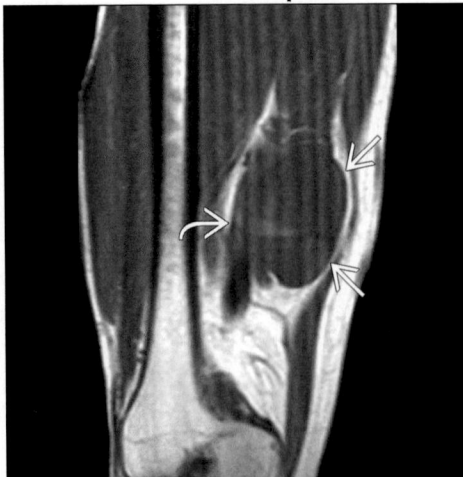

(Left) Lateral radiograph shows extensive, sheet-like calcification ➜ of muscles and fascial planes in this adolescent with profound proximal muscle weakness and dermatomyositis. *(Right)* Coronal oblique T1WI FSE MR shows a large soft tissue mass displacing rather than infiltrating the surrounding soft tissues ➜. An area of subtle ↑ SI ➜ in the mass represents fatty tissue within this liposarcoma.

NERVE ENTRAPMENT, LOWER EXTREMITY

DIFFERENTIAL DIAGNOSIS

Common
- Peroneal Tunnel Syndrome
- Morton Neuroma

Less Common
- Sciatic Neuropathy
- Iliacus Muscle Syndrome
- Meralgia Paresthetica
- Saphenous Nerve Syndrome
- Tarsal Tunnel Syndrome
- Superficial Peroneal Nerve Entrapment
- Anterior Tarsal Tunnel Syndrome

Rare but Important
- Piriformis Syndrome
- Obturator Tunnel Syndrome
- Popliteal Entrapment Syndrome
- Sural Nerve Syndrome
- Calcaneal Nerve Entrapment
- Jogger's Foot
- Jogger's Heel

ESSENTIAL INFORMATION

Key Differential Diagnosis Issues
- Entrapment neuropathy: Short segment nerve compression at a specific site, often while passing through fibroosseous tunnel, muscle or fibrous tissue
- Symptoms: Muscle weakness, paresthesias, muscle atrophy
- MR appearance: Look for nerve signal & contour, adjacent vessels may serve as landmark; muscle signal intensity (SI) & distribution
- Look for: Ganglia, tumors, inflammation, post-trauma, scarring, edema, anomalies
- Muscle SI in entrapment/denervation
  - Acute (< 1 mo): T1 - normal; STIR - ↑ SI; enhancement: +
  - Subacute (1-6 mos): T1 - ± normal; STIR - ↑ SI; enhancement: ±
  - Chronic (> 6 mos): T1 - ↑ SI; STIR - ↓ SI; enhancement: None

Helpful Clues for Common Diagnoses
- **Peroneal Tunnel Syndrome**
  - Common peroneal at knee
  - Symptoms: Foot drop with loss of ankle/toe inversion/eversion, sensory deficits in lateral leg, dorsal & plantar foot
  - Entrapment site: Fibular neck or as nerve pierces peroneus longus (PL)
  - Denervation: Leg, anterior & lateral compartments
- **Morton Neuroma**
  - Interdigital nerve fibrotic nodule, 2nd or 3rd intermetatarsal space most common
  - Entrapment site: Transverse metatarsal ligament
  - MR: Ovoid mass centered on nerve & plantar to transverse metatarsal ligament, T1 & T2 ↓ SI, ± enhancement; ± bursitis

Helpful Clues for Less Common Diagnoses
- **Sciatic Neuropathy**
  - Sciatic nerve at pelvis
  - Symptoms: Flail leg with foot drop, loss of ankle/toe inversion/eversion, sensory deficits in lateral leg, dorsal & plantar foot; after trauma including iatrogenic (i.e., hip surgery)
  - Entrapment site: Sciatic notch, hip
  - Denervation: Anterior tibialis (AT), peroneus longus (PL) & brevis (PB)
- **Iliacus Muscle Syndrome**
  - Femoral nerve at pelvis
  - Symptoms: Decreased hip flexion, absent knee jerk, pain &/or paresthesias in anteromedial thigh, medial knee, calf, foot; seen after trauma including iatrogenic (i.e., femoral artery catheterization, hip surgery)
  - Entrapment site: Iliacus tunnel formed by iliac bone/iliopsoas (floor) & iliopectineal arch/inguinal ligament (roof)
  - Denervation: Quadriceps, iliopsoas
- **Meralgia Paresthetica**
  - Lateral femoral cutaneous nerve at pelvis
  - Symptoms: Burning pain, paresthesia of proximal lateral thigh; seen with trauma including iatrogenic (i.e., iliac crest bone-graft harvest)
  - Entrapment sites: Inguinal ligament at anterosuperior iliac spine or as nerve penetrates fascia lata
  - Denervation: None, purely sensory
- **Saphenous Nerve Syndrome**
  - Femoral nerve at distal thigh
  - Symptoms: Numbness & paraesthesias in medial distal thigh & knee down to medial leg/foot

- Due to compression, masses, trauma including iatrogenic (i.e., knee arthroscopy)
  - Entrapment site: Adductor canal
  - Denervation: None, purely sensory
- **Tarsal Tunnel Syndrome**
  - Tibial nerve at ankle
  - Symptoms: Sharp pain worsened with activity; paraesthesia along plantar foot
  - Entrapment site: Tarsal tunnel formed by talus, calcaneus & flexor retinaculum
  - Denervation: Minimal; sensory deficits most common
- **Superficial Peroneal Nerve Entrapment**
  - Superficial peroneal nerve at distal leg
  - Symptoms: Lower leg, dorsal foot numbness, tingling
  - Entrapment site: Lateral compartment fascia ~ 10-15 cm above ankle
  - Denervation: PL/PB
- **Anterior Tarsal Tunnel Syndrome**
  - Deep peroneal nerve at ankle
  - Symptoms: Dorsal foot aching pain, numbness into 1st web space
  - Entrapment site: Superior/inferior extensor retinaculum distal margin, extensor hallucis longus (EHL) tendon
  - Denervation: Extensor digitorum brevis & longus, AT, EHL, peroneus tertius

Helpful Clues for Rare Diagnoses
- **Piriformis Syndrome**
  - Sciatic nerve at sciatic notch
  - Controversial; diagnosis of exclusion

  - MR: Image pelvis for side-to-side comparison; look for asymmetry
  - Symptoms: Buttock pain, aggravated by sitting, squatting, gluteal weakness
  - Entrapment site: Sciatic notch
  - Denervation: Hamstrings, adductor magnus
- **Obturator Tunnel Syndrome**
  - Obturator nerve at pelvis
  - Symptoms: Groin or medial thigh pain, adductor weakness, seen in trauma including iatrogenic (i.e., hip replacement)
  - Entrapment site: Obturator canal formed by pubic bone & obturator muscles
  - Denervation: Pectineus, gracilis, adductor longus, brevis, ± magnus
- **Popliteal Entrapment Syndrome**
  - Tibial nerve at knee
  - Symptoms: Plantar & invertor, intrinsic foot muscles weakness; heel sensory loss
  - Entrapment site: Popliteal fossa
- **Sural Nerve Syndrome**
  - Tibial nerve branch at distal leg
  - Symptoms: Pain, paraesthesias, lateral foot tenderness; chronic calf pain
  - Entrapment sites: Lower leg, lateral malleolus
  - Denervation: None, pure sensory nerve
- Foot Entrapment Syndromes
  - **Calcaneal Nerve Entrapment**: Medial calcaneal nerve
  - **Jogger's Foot**: Medial calcaneal nerve
  - **Jogger's Heel**: First branch of lateral plantar nerve

Peroneal Tunnel Syndrome

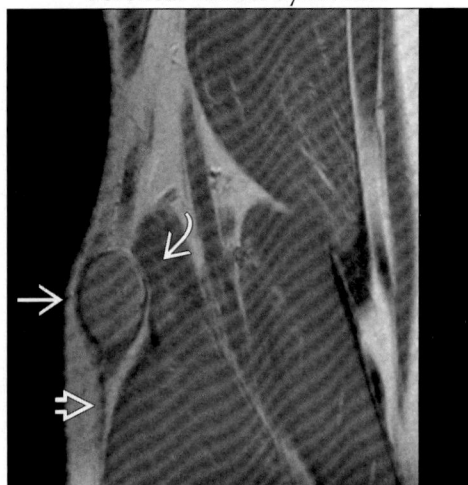

Coronal T1WI MR shows an elongated mass in the peroneal nerve, deviating the gastrocnemius lateral head. This schwannoma caused peroneal tunnel syndrome with lateral leg & foot paresthesias.

Peroneal Tunnel Syndrome

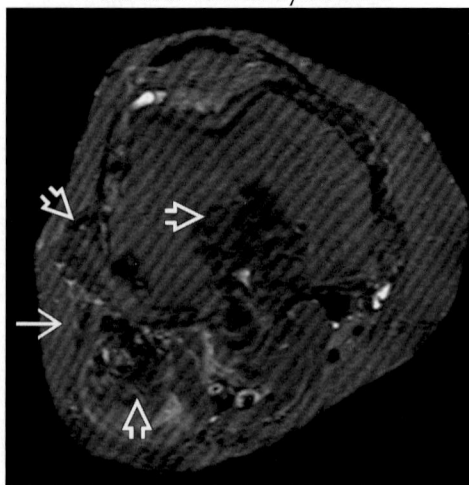

Axial PD FSE FS MR shows multiple heterogeneous ↓ SI masses of pigmented villonodular synovitis displacing the peroneal nerve anteriorly. Symptoms included knee pain & lateral leg numbness.

NERVE ENTRAPMENT, LOWER EXTREMITY

(Left) Coronal T1WI MR shows a typical Morton neuroma ➡ arising between the 3rd & 4th metatarsal heads plantar to the transverse metatarsal ligament ➡. This ↓ SI nodule presented with burning, point tender pain. **(Right)** Coronal T2WI FS MR in the same patient, shows a tear-drop-shaped Morton neuroma ➡ as ↓ SI with fat suppression. There was minimal enhancement following gadolinium administration (not shown).

Morton Neuroma

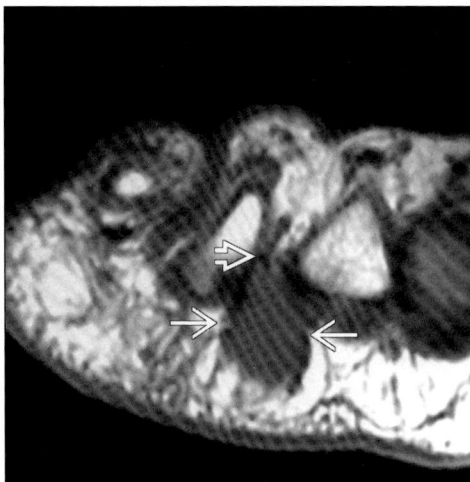

Morton Neuroma

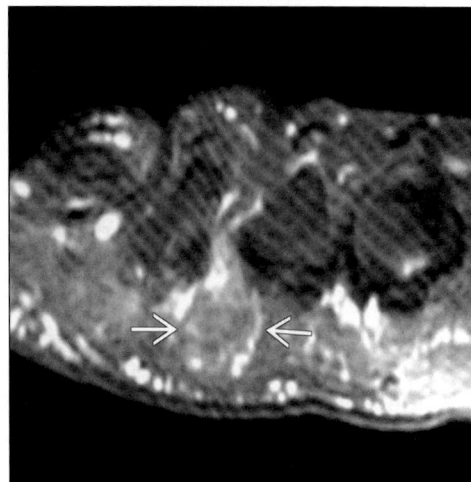

(Left) Coronal T2WI FS MR shows a Morton neuroma ➡ at the 2nd-3rd intermetatarsal space with slight increased SI. Note the silastic 1st MTP prosthesis ➡. Altered weight-bearing may contribute to interdigital neuroma development. **(Right)** Axial PD FSE FS MR shows a hamstring tear with tendon retraction ➡ & hematoma ➡. Note adjacent sciatic nerve & surrounding soft tissues edema ➡. This 80 year old has acute onset foot drop from sciatic neuropathy.

Morton Neuroma

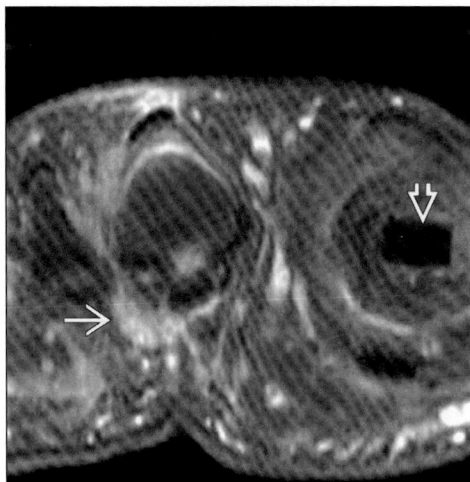

Sciatic Neuropathy

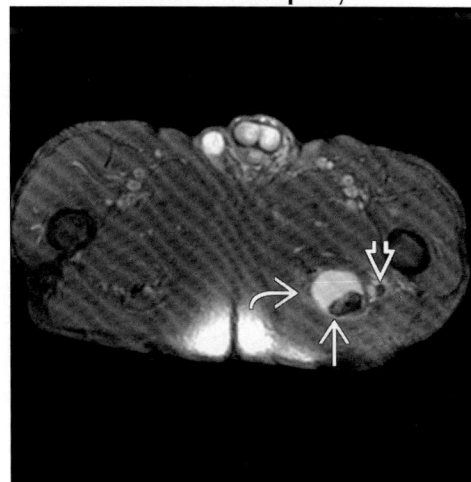

(Left) Coronal PD FSE FS MR shows intense iliacus muscle edema ➡ in this patient status post left total hip arthroplasty ➡ with decreased hip flexion and anteromedial thigh pain, typical of iliacus muscle syndrome. **(Right)** Sagittal T2WI FS MR shows fluid in subtalar joint ➡ extending medially & inferiorly into the tarsal tunnel creating tunnel constriction with resultant venous distension ➡ & associated plantar neurologic symptoms.

Iliacus Muscle Syndrome

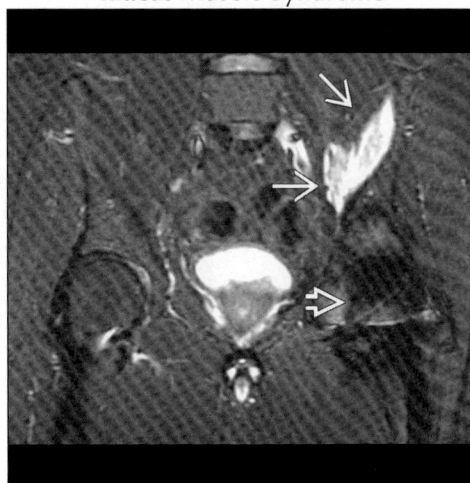

Tarsal Tunnel Syndrome

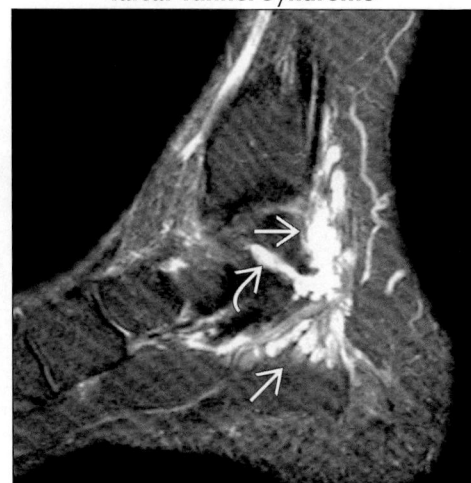

Tarsal Tunnel Syndrome

Superficial Peroneal Nerve Entrapment

(Left) Coronal T1WI MR shows that the posterior tibial nerve ➡ is enlarged & surrounded by amorphous scar tissue. There is atrophy of the quadratus plantae ⮕ & abductor digiti minimi ➡, muscles innervated by lateral plantar nerve. (Right) Axial T1WI MR shows superficial peroneal nerve thickening ➡ in the subcutaneous fat just distal to its point of emerging through the lower leg fascia in this dancer with lateral leg numbness & tingling with exertion.

Anterior Tarsal Tunnel Syndrome

Piriformis Syndrome

(Left) Coronal oblique T1WI MR at the talonavicular joint shows the normal deep peroneal nerve, medial ⮕, & lateral ➡ branches separated by the dorsalis pedis vessels ➡ which serve as a landmark for the nerve. (Right) Axial PD FSE FS MR shows a venous varix ➡ at the sciatic notch, resulting in piriformis syndrome with left buttock pain when sitting. This "mass" impinges the sciatic nerve & adjacent piriformis muscle ⮕.

Obturator Tunnel Syndrome

Sural Nerve Syndrome

(Left) Coronal PD FSE FS MR shows a fluid-filled ganglion ➡ in the obturator tunnel, impinging the obturator nerve in this patient with persistent groin pain. Note the mild edema in the obturator externus ⮕. Aspiration relieved the symptoms. (Right) Axial T1WI MR shows an enlarged sural nerve ➡ due to neuroma. This nerve is located midline & superficial in mid calf, becoming more posterolateral near the ankle. Skin marker ⮕ caused tingling pain.

HIP PAIN, ELDERLY PATIENT

DIFFERENTIAL DIAGNOSIS

Common
- Fracture
- Arthritis
- Tendon, Injury
- Bursitis
- Muscle Strain, Hip
- Metastases, Bone Marrow

Less Common
- Osteonecrosis, Hip
- Hardware Failure
- Hematoma
- Infection
  - Septic Joint
  - Osteomyelitis, Adult
  - Soft Tissue Abscess
- Fracture, Malunion
- Sciatica
- Osteoarthritis, Knee

Rare but Important
- Soft Tissue Neoplasm
- Intrapelvic Mass
- Testicular/Scrotal Pathology

ESSENTIAL INFORMATION

Key Differential Diagnosis Issues
- Patients with painful hips tend to hold hip in flexion & external rotation
- **Hint**: Don't let satisfaction of search keep you from seeing all abnormalities

Helpful Clues for Common Diagnoses
- **Fracture**
  - Osteoporosis: Leading cause of hip fractures in elderly
  - Radiographs: Look for subtle trabecular pattern & cortical margins
    - Garden classification: I-incomplete or impacted; II-complete, nondisplaced; III-complete, partially displaced; IV-markedly displaced
  - CT: High resolution thin section imaging (< 1 mm) essential for subtle fractures
  - MR: Fluid sensitive sequences emphasize edema (↑ SI) associated with fracture but may obscure fracture lines; T1 better to identify fracture line
  - Combining MR (to direct the search) & CT (fracture delineation) may be useful
  - Bone scan useful but takes up to 24 hrs to be positive
  - Know where to look
    - Femoral head: May mimic AVN or OA; look for articular surface collapse
    - Femoral neck: Subcapital, transcervical or basicervical; fracture tends to propagate from lateral to medial
    - Trochanteric: Infrequent, related to direct blow or avulsion often due to fall; evaluate for intertrochanteric extension
    - Intertrochanteric: Complete or incomplete; single discrete fracture without displacement or comminuted
    - Subtrochanteric/proximal femoral shaft: Atypical fractures may be seen in patients treated with bisphosphonates
    - Pelvis fractures: Symphysis, superior/inferior pubic rami
    - Look for additional fractures in sacrum if anterior pelvic ring fractured & vice versa
    - Superior acetabular: Insufficiency fracture horizontal to 1° trabecula
- **Arthritis**
  - Osteoarthritis: Asymmetric joint space narrowing, usually superior, subchondral sclerosis & cyst formation; osteophytes, ± loose bodies
  - Inflammatory arthritis
    - Rheumatoid: Diffuse osteopenia, uniform joint space loss, ± erosions, ± rice bodies
    - Ankylosing spondylitis: Uniform joint space loss, ± osteophytes, SI joint likely fused if hip joint is involved
  - Crystalline: Chondrocalcinosis, symmetric or asymmetric joint space loss, osteophytes
- **Tendon, Injury**
  - Commonly injured tendons: Hamstrings, hip rotator cuff, abductors, iliopsoas
  - Injury ranges from tendinosis with thickening & internal intermediate SI to complete tear of tendon with retraction & edema/hematoma
  - Fatty atrophy of associated muscle
- **Bursitis**
  - Inflammation/fluid in potential space between tendons, ligaments, bony protuberances
  - ↑ SI on fluid sensitive sequences, often crescentic in shape

- Commonly involved bursae: Greater trochanteric, subgluteus medius, subgluteus minimus
- Look for associated tendon/muscle injury
- **Muscle Strain, Hip**
  - Ranges from minimal fiber tear (grade 1) to complete disruption of muscle (grade 3) with retraction
  - Fatty atrophy of associated muscle
- **Metastases, Bone Marrow**
  - Metastases & multiple myeloma common in this age group
  - Radiographs: Lytic, sclerotic or mixed; ± cortical disruption
  - MR: Typically ↓ SI on T1WI, ↑ SI on fluid sensitive sequences; ± cortical disruption

Helpful Clues for Less Common Diagnoses
- **Osteonecrosis, Hip**
  - Radiograph: Focal sclerosis; crescentic subchondral lucency (fracture); flattened joint surface
  - MR: Serpentine heterogeneous wedge-shaped lesion; crescentic subchondral fluid (fracture); flattened joint surface
- **Hardware Failure**
  - Loosening, subsidence, foreign body reaction, polyethylene failure
- **Hematoma**
  - Develop with relatively little trauma
  - Acute (48 hrs): T1 isointense to muscle
  - Subacute (< 30 days): ↑ SI on T1 & T2 (methemoglobin)

- Chronic (> 30 days): Heterogeneous; ↓ SI if hemosiderin
- **Infection**
  - **Septic Joint**
    - Large effusion; focal osteopenia
    - Requires aspiration to confirm infection
  - **Osteomyelitis, Adult**
    - Cortical disruption, ± periostitis & soft tissue involvement
  - **Soft Tissue Abscess**
    - Mass with thick, irregular walls; ± sinus tracts & bone involvement
- **Fracture, Malunion**
  - Malunion results in abnormal gait, mechanics
- **Sciatica**
  - Referred pain
  - Lateral recess, neural foramina or central stenosis at L3, L4, L5, or S1
- **Osteoarthritis, Knee**
  - Referred pain

Helpful Clues for Rare Diagnoses
- **Soft Tissue Neoplasm**
  - Benign: Lipoma, neurofibroma, myxoma, schwannoma, hemangioma
  - Malignant: Lymphoma, MFH, liposarcoma, fibrosarcoma, MPNST
- **Intrapelvic Mass**
  - Referred pain from mass arising from uterine or adnexal pathology
- **Testicular/Scrotal Pathology**
  - Referred pain from testicular or scrotal pathology including inguinal hernia

Fracture

Coronal STIR MR shows the linear ↑ SI in the lateral femoral neck ➡ of an incomplete (Garden type I) fracture in this 77 year old female. Note diffuse edema of the femoral head ➡.

Fracture

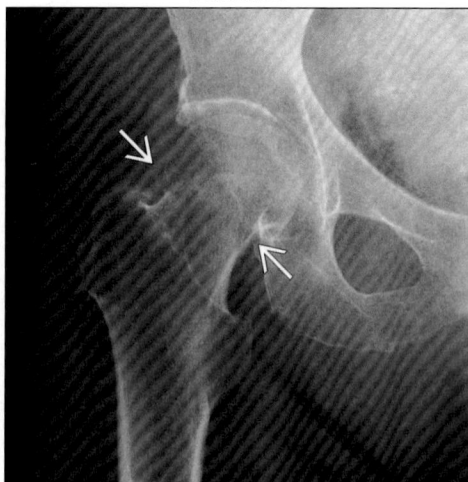

Anteroposterior radiograph shows a transcervical femoral neck fracture with subtle disruption of medial & lateral cortices ➡ This is a Garden III fracture with valgus alignment across the fracture.

HIP PAIN, ELDERLY PATIENT

Fracture

Fracture

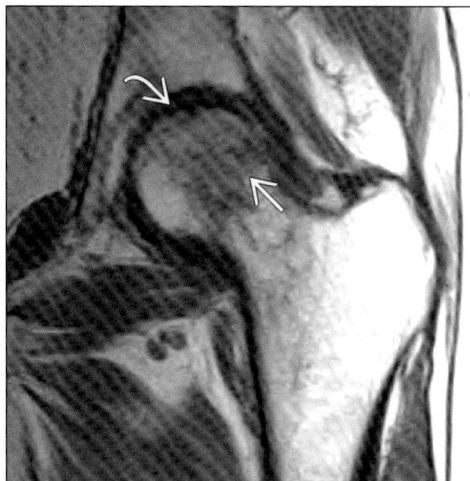

(Left) Coronal T1WI MR shows a comminuted femoral head fracture with subcapital & femoral head ➡ components. T1WI allows for better fracture line conspicuity as surrounding marrow edema may obscure the fracture. Note the slight articular surface flattening ➡. *(Right)* Coronal T1WI MR shows an incomplete intertrochanteric fracture ➡ originating at the greater trochanter & extending distally across the intertrochanteric line.

Fracture

Fracture

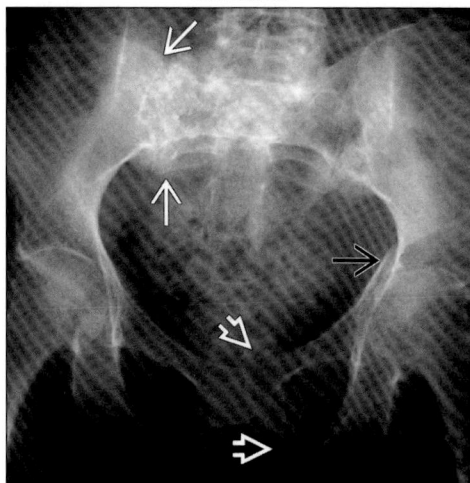

(Left) Anteroposterior radiograph shows multiple fractures sustained in ground level fall including left symphysis, inferior pubic ramus ➡ & acetabulum ➡, as well as a vertical right sacral body fracture ➡. *(Right)* Coronal bone CT shows bilateral subacute transverse incomplete subtrochanteric fractures ➡ in this 70 year old female being treated with bisphosphonates for osteopenia. This site is typical for bisphosphonate related fractures.

Arthritis

Arthritis

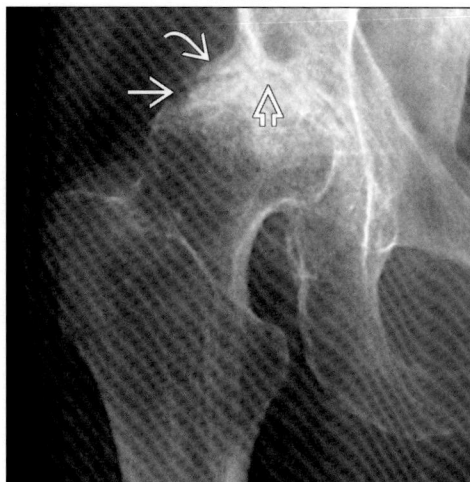

(Left) Anteroposterior radiograph shows superior joint space loss ➡, subchondral sclerosis, & femoral head flattening ➡, as well as acetabular osteophytes ➡, along with diffuse osteopenia in this elderly patient with osteoarthritis. *(Right)* Coronal STIR MR shows typical MR appearance of osteoarthritis with bilateral superior joint space loss from subtle cartilage thinning ➡ & acetabular subchondral cysts ➡. There is a minimal right hip effusion ➡.

HIP PAIN, ELDERLY PATIENT

Arthritis

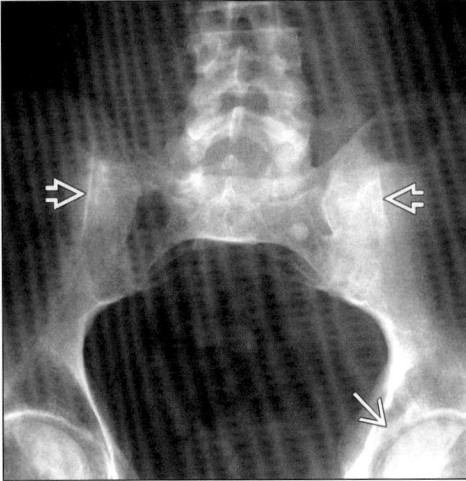

Arthritis

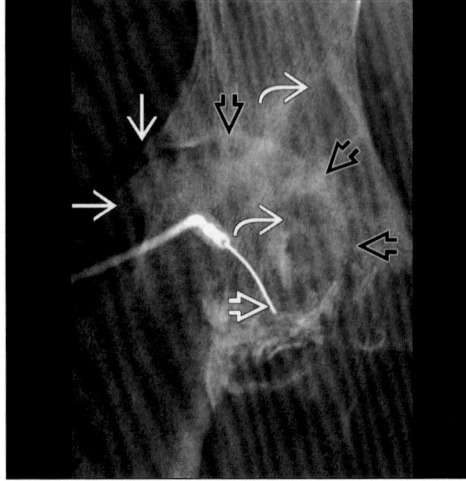

(Left) Anteroposterior radiograph shows ankylosing spondylitis with fusion of bilateral SI joints ➡. Note the rather uniform joint space narrowing of the left hip ➡. (Right) Anteroposterior radiograph after a hip arthrogram (needle in place ➡) in a patient with known rheumatoid arthritis. Uniform cartilage loss ➡ is accompanied by large acetabular & femoral erosions ➡. Osteophytes ➡ represent secondary osteoarthritis.

Tendon, Injury

Tendon, Injury

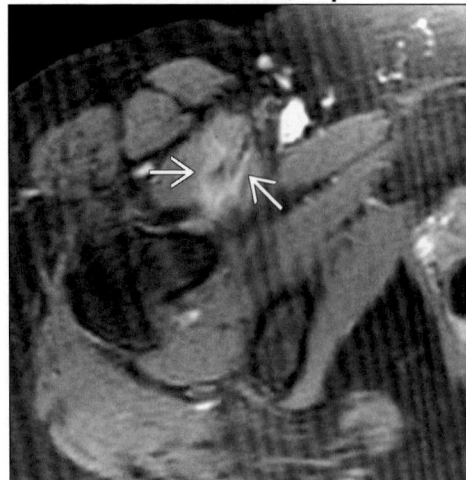

(Left) Coronal STIR MR shows partial left hamstring tear with ↑ SI & disruption of the semimembranosus portion of the tendon ➡ in this 76 year old male with acute onset pain. Note the ischial marrow edema ➡. (Right) Axial STIR MR shows complete iliopsoas tendon tear in this 86 year old female. There is retraction of tendon fibers & associated edema/hematoma ➡ near the tendon insertion.

Bursitis

Muscle Strain, Hip

(Left) Coronal STIR MR shows small crescentic fluid collections in the subgluteus minimus ➡ & subgluteus medius bursae ➡. There is mild thickening of the gluteus minimus tendon near the trochanteric insertion ➡. (Right) Axial PD FSE FS MR shows ↑ SI in the central iliopsoas muscle belly representing a grade I muscle strain ➡ in this 77 year old patient after injury during a yoga class.

HIP PAIN, ELDERLY PATIENT

Metastases, Bone Marrow

Metastases, Bone Marrow

(Left) Anteroposterior radiograph shows sclerosis of the lesser trochanter with cortical disruption ➡ in this elderly patient with prostate metastasis. A more subtle lesion is located in the ischium ⮕. *(Right)* Coronal T1WI MR shows multiple small ↓ SI lesions in the proximal femurs ➡ with a larger lesion in the left ilium ⮕ in this patient with breast metastases.

Osteonecrosis, Hip

Osteonecrosis, Hip

(Left) Coronal T1WI MR shows the classic serpentine heterogeneous focus of femoral head avascular necrosis ⮕ with surrounding edema (↓ SI) of the head & neck ➡. There is no articular collapse. *(Right)* Coronal STIR MR shows a circumscribed subchondral focus of ↓ SI (osteonecrosis) ➡ with surrounding edema ⮕ in the right femoral head with a smaller but similar lesion in the left femoral head ➡.

Hardware Failure

Hematoma

(Left) Coronal CT reformation shows a lucency ➡ in the periprosthetic ilium & acetabulum related to foreign body osteolysis from polyethylene wear characterized by slight narrowing of polyethylene liner ⮕. *(Right)* Axial T2WI FS MR shows a crescentic heterogeneous "mass" ➡ superficial to the left gluteus maximus in this elderly patient who takes aspirin & recently sustained a fall. This was an acute hematoma & completely resolved with time.

HIP PAIN, ELDERLY PATIENT

Septic Joint

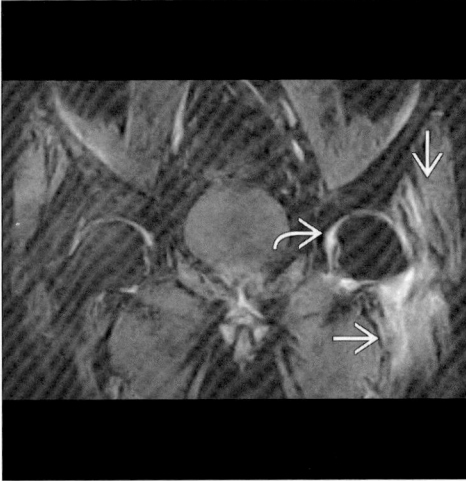

Osteomyelitis, Adult

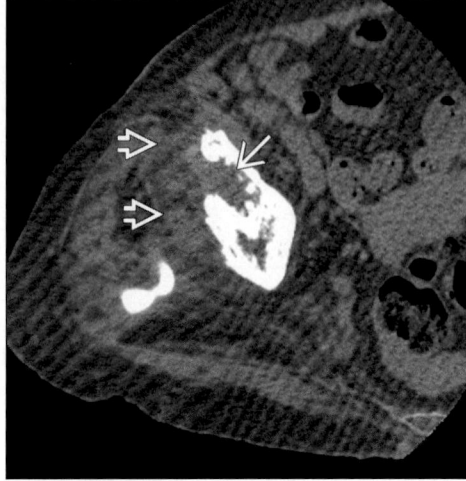

(Left) Coronal STIR MR shows early MR appearance of septic arthritis of the hip with a joint effusion ➡ and surrounding soft tissue edema ➡. Aspiration confirmed infection in this 80 year old male. *(Right)* Axial bone CT shows right acetabulum cortical destruction ➡ with soft tissue swelling ➡ in this 85 year old female who had increasing hip pain several months following hip arthroplasty. This proved to be osteomyelitis at surgery.

Soft Tissue Abscess

Soft Tissue Neoplasm

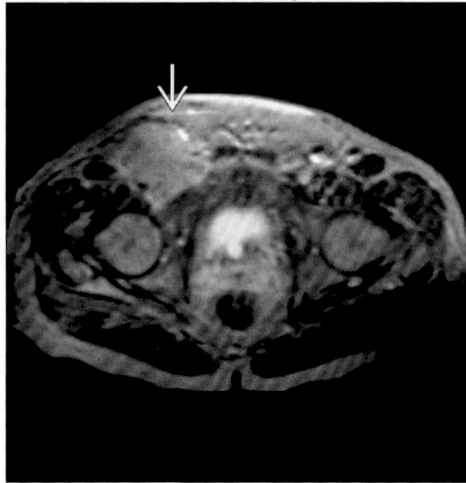

(Left) Coronal CT scanogram obtained following arthrogram demonstrates extensive soft tissue contrast collections ➡ within the multiple soft tissue abscesses resulting from an E. coli infection. Note the associated sinus tract ➡. *(Right)* Axial T2WI MR shows a soft tissue mass in the right groin ➡ which infiltrates the obturator internus. It is ↓ SI T1WI (not shown) & ↑ SI T2WI in a nonspecific pattern & proved to be lymphoma at biopsy.

Intrapelvic Mass

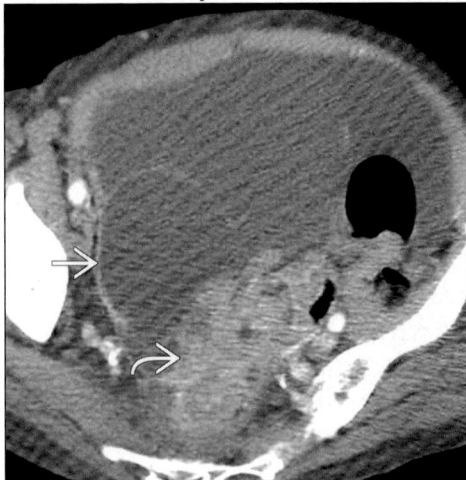

Testicular/Scrotal Pathology

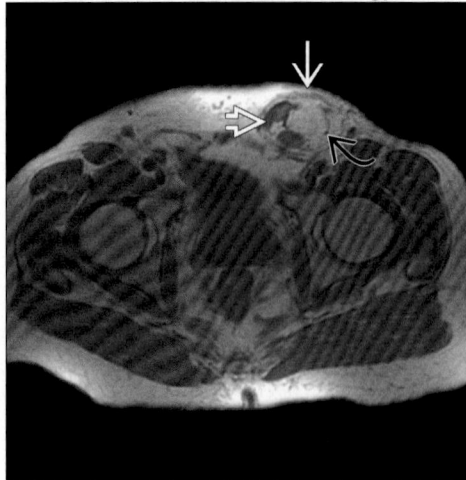

(Left) Axial CECT shows a large cystic adnexal mass ➡, representing primary ovarian carcinoma in this 65 year old female who presented with hip pain. Extensive soft tissue density tumor is noted along the dependent surfaces of the peritoneal cavity ➡. *(Right)* Axial T1WI MR shows a large left inguinal hernia ➡ with loops of small bowel ➡ & peritoneal fat ➡ within the hernia in this 83 year old male with left hip pain.

III

73

DIFFERENTIAL DIAGNOSIS

Common
- Arthroplasty Loosening
- Arthroplasty Dislocation
- Component Malposition
- Septic Joint
- Arthroplasty Component Wear
- Particle Disease/Massive Osteolysis
- Stress Shielding (Mimic)
- Heterotopic Ossification

Less Common
- Arthroplasty Hardware Failure
- Periprosthetic Fracture
- Iliopsoas Bursitis

ESSENTIAL INFORMATION

Key Differential Diagnosis Issues
- Total hip arthroplasty (THA) complications are common but may be subtle initially
- To avoid missing subtle complications, must compare image with both
  - Index radiograph (initial post-operative image)
  - Most recent comparison radiograph
- Make use of transischial line as baseline for measuring angulation of acetabular component & relative limb length (generally compare level of lesser trochanters)

Helpful Clues for Common Diagnoses
- **Arthroplasty Loosening**
  - For cemented components, 2 mm lucency at bone-cement interface surrounding component is diagnostic
  - For cementless components, 2 mm lucency at bone-component interface (usually with surrounding sclerotic line) surrounding component is diagnostic
  - For any component, change in position is diagnostic
    - Positional change may be a new tilt or angulation of component
    - Acetabular components tend to subside superiorly
    - Femoral components tend to subside inferiorly down shaft
  - To evaluate subtle change in position, compare with index radiograph and use transischial line as reference
    - Measure angle of lateral cup opening

- Choose landmarks to measure for superior or inferior subsidence of either component
- **Arthroplasty Dislocation**
  - Femoral head dislocation is obvious; must look for component malposition as underlying etiology (see Component Malposition below)
- **Component Malposition**
  - May result in pain and/or dislocation
  - Lateral opening of cup should be 40° ± 10°; excess in either direction puts at risk for dislocation
  - Limb lengths should be equal (usually assessed by measuring distance of lesser trochanter to transischial line and comparing to contralateral side)
    - If component placement results in over-lengthening, at risk for spasm and dislocation
    - If component placement results in shortening, muscles are inefficient
  - Cup should be anteverted 15° ± 10°; this is evaluated on groin lateral radiograph
    - Retroversion puts patient at risk for dislocation
    - Excessive anteversion puts patient at risk for dislocation
  - Cup should not be placed excessively laterally; if center of rotation is lateral to iliopsoas tendon as it crosses joint, flexion places it at risk for dislocation
- **Septic Joint**
  - Usually no radiographic signs; if septic joint is suspected, must aspirate
  - Rarely, serpiginous tracking and periosteal reaction are seen (late findings)
  - Occasionally fluffy, amorphous heterotopic bone formation heralds infection
- **Arthroplasty Component Wear**
  - Wear generally occurs in polyethylene liner
  - Wear is on most frequent weight-bearing portion of liner (superolateral)
  - Wear is visualized by femoral head placement within the cup; if the head is asymmetric and superolateral, that indicates polyethylene liner wear
- **Particle Disease/Massive Osteolysis**

- Debris of a critical size triggers cascade effect
  - Inflammatory reaction with macrophage and foreign body giant cells → osteolysis → loosening or fracture
- Debris may be of multiple origins
  - Most frequent: Polyethylene particles from wear (particles not directly visualized)
  - Metallic beads from component surface may abrade and stimulate massive osteolysis
  - Less commonly, osseous or cement debris may contribute to osteolysis
- Degree of lysis may be impressive; differential includes metastasis, plasmacytoma, or primary bone tumor
  - **Hint:** With lytic lesion adjacent to THA, look for possible sources of particles
- **Stress Shielding (Mimic)**
  - With altered weight-bearing on THA, some areas of proximal femur have less stress
    - Bone is resorbed, leading to an osteopenic region which may be confused with osteolysis
    - Most frequent region affected is proximal femoral metaphysis, particularly in region extending into greater trochanter
  - Identify by location and fact that bone is resorbed rather than destroyed
    - This will avoid misdiagnosis of massive osteolysis or tumor
  - Because of bone resorption, bone is at risk for insufficiency periprosthetic fracture

- **Heterotopic Ossification**
  - Frequent around femoral neck
  - Matures into normal bone
    - Rarely is massive enough to cause obstruction or significant symptoms

Helpful Clues for Less Common Diagnoses
- **Arthroplasty Hardware Failure**
  - Femoral stem may fracture; generally subtle since non-displaced
  - Cup may fracture, but generally only when there is already failure due to loosening
  - Liner rarely may displace from cup
- **Periprosthetic Fracture**
  - Most frequently femoral shaft
    - Watch for fracture extending from tip of femoral component
    - Do not confuse with nutrient artery
    - Most likely with a long-stem revision femoral component: The long stiff stem fractures through the anteriorly bowed femoral cortex (visualize on lateral view)
  - Fractures around acetabulum less frequent, though with loosening or lysis, medial wall may erode
  - Regions of osteolysis or stress shielding are at risk for pathologic or insufficiency fracture; watch these carefully
- **Iliopsoas Bursitis**
  - Large hip effusion may decompress into the iliopsoas bursa
  - Presents as a hard anterior groin mass
  - May be drained through large bore needle; generally very gelatinous

Arthroplasty Loosening

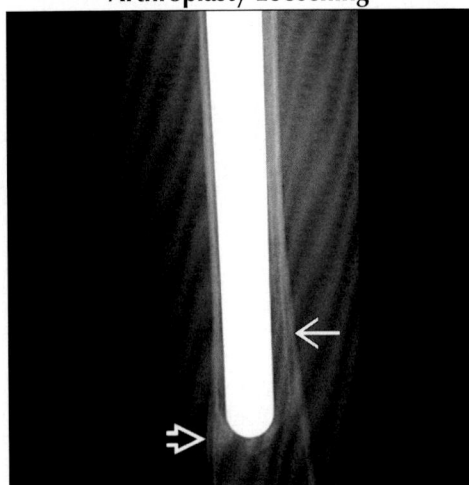

AP radiograph shows a wide lucency at the bone-component interface ➡, surrounding most of the femoral shaft prosthesis. Endosteal & periosteal bone production ➡ indicates toggling at tip. (†MSK Req).

Arthroplasty Loosening

AP radiograph shows superior subsidence of the acetabular component (subsided over the distance between ➡). Additionally, there is abnormal tilt of the cup ➡, another indication of gross loosening.

PAINFUL HIP REPLACEMENT

(Left) AP radiograph shows a wide bone-component interface lucency ➡. Note that the femoral component has subsided inferiorly by approximally 2 cm. Subsidence, even without the obvious lucency at the component interface, indicates loosening. (Right) AP radiograph shows 2 mm bone-component interface lucency surrounding the acetabular cup ➡. There is also a 3 mm lucency at the bone-cement interface of the femoral component ⏩. Both are loose.

Arthroplasty Loosening

Arthroplasty Loosening

(Left) AP radiograph shows dislocation of the total hip. There is no obvious malalignment of the components predisposing to the dislocation. (Right) Groin lateral radiograph of the same hip as previous image, following relocation, shows retroversion of the cup ➡. A retroverted acetabular component puts the patient at risk for dislocation, as in this case. Note that this malposition is seen only on this view.

Arthroplasty Dislocation

Arthroplasty Dislocation

(Left) AP radiograph shows dislocation of the total hip. Although the cup does not have an abnormal lateral opening angle, it does show significant opening in the antero-posterior plane (note the anterior & posterior rims delineated by ➡). (Right) Groin lateral radiograph on the same patient as previous image, shows exaggerated anteversion of the cup ➡. Although retroversion is a greater concern, excessive anteversion also predisposes to dislocation.

Arthroplasty Dislocation

Arthroplasty Dislocation

PAINFUL HIP REPLACEMENT

Arthroplasty Dislocation

Component Malposition

(Left) AP radiograph shows no loosening, but dislocation of the component. Note the prominent lateral opening of the cup ➡; this puts the hip at risk for dislocation. *(Right)* AP postoperative radiograph shows abnormally decreased lateral opening of the cup ➡. This puts the hip at risk for dislocation since the neck of the shaft may catch and torque on the lateral cup.

Component Malposition

Septic Joint

(Left) AP radiograph shows a total hip placed with asymmetric lengthening of the limb. Note the position of the lesser trochanter ➡ on the left relative to the right and to the intertrochanteric line. Abnormal length predisposes to dislocation. *(Right)* AP radiograph shows irregular serpiginous lucency throughout the acetabulum ➡. This indicates septic joint with osteomyelitis.

Septic Joint

Arthroplasty Component Wear

(Left) AP radiograph shows irregular and prominent lucency about the tip of the femoral component ➡. Additionally, there is focal and very thick endosteal and periosteal reaction ➡. The appearance is too irregular for simple loosening and represents infection. *(Right)* AP radiograph shows offset of the femoral head within the cup. Note that the distance between head and edge of cup superiorly ➡ is significantly less than inferiorly ➡, indicating wear of the polyethylene.

PAINFUL HIP REPLACEMENT

(Left) AP radiograph shows offset of the head within the cup, indicating polyethylene wear. Additionally, there is massive osteolysis in the surrounding bone ➡. This osteolysis develops due to polyethylene particles.
(Right) AP radiograph shows massive osteolysis in the acetabulum ➡. There is no polyethylene wear. However, there are tiny metallic microspheres ➡ which have rubbed off the cup; they are of the optimal size to cause osteolysis.

Particle Disease/Massive Osteolysis

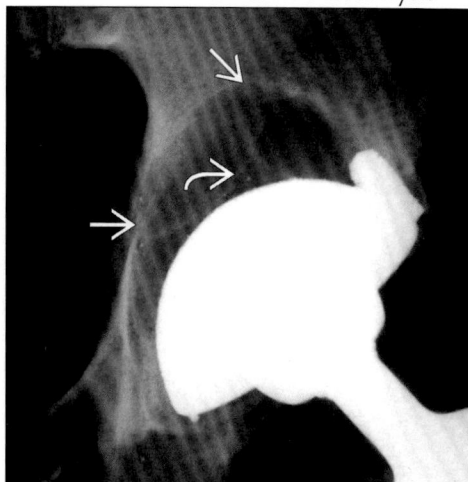

Particle Disease/Massive Osteolysis

(Left) CT coronal reformat shows polyethylene wear (note offset of femoral head in cup) & extensive osteolysis, not only in the acetabulum ➡, but in the proximal femur as well. CT can be a valuable asset in determining bone stock.
(Right) AP radiograph shows lucency in the proximal metaphysis ➡ due to stress shielding. The focal loss of bone density is secondary to altered weight-bearing and is considered normal. Note a subtle insufficiency fracture ➡.

Particle Disease/Massive Osteolysis

Stress Shielding (Mimic)

(Left) AP radiograph shows fluffy heterotopic ossification (HO) ➡ surrounding an arthroplasty. HO frequently forms superolaterally without consequence. In this case, there is air ➡ in the soft tissues as well, indicating infection. *(Right)* Frogleg lateral radiograph shows metallic wedges ➡ which have loosened from the polyethylene liner, representing cup failure. There is also fracture of the component ➡ and resultant dislocation of the hip.

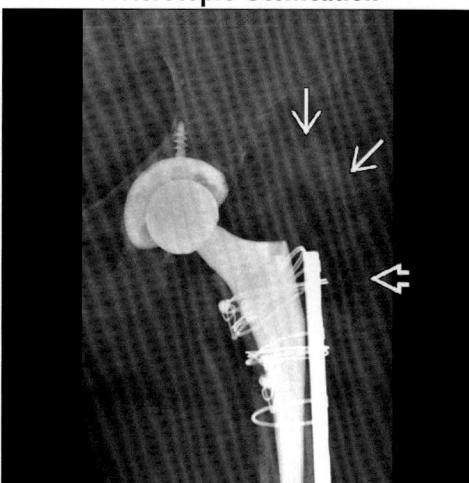

Heterotopic Ossification

Arthroplasty Hardware Failure

PAINFUL HIP REPLACEMENT

Arthroplasty Hardware Failure

Arthroplasty Hardware Failure

(Left) AP radiograph shows fracture of the femoral component ➡. The femur shows massive osteolysis and loosening; this can put the hardware at risk for fracture. *(Right)* AP radiograph shows gross loosening of the cup ➡ with subsidence. This loosening has resulted in fracture of the acetabular component ➡.

Periprosthetic Fracture

Periprosthetic Fracture

(Left) AP radiograph shows a wide lucency at the bone-cement interface ➡ in this femoral component, indicating loosening. With a grossly loose component, the osteopenic bone is put at risk for fracture, as has occurred here ➡. *(Right)* Post-operative lateral radiograph shows a long-stem femoral prosthesis to have fractured the anterior femoral cortex ➡. Longer stems put the femur at risk for periprosthetic fracture because of the normal anterior bowing of the femur.

Iliopsoas Bursitis

Iliopsoas Bursitis

(Left) Anteroposterior radiograph shows total hip without malposition. However, lucency is seen, thinning the iliac wing ➡. Concern was for a destructive lesion. *(Right)* CT in the same patient, above the level of the arthroplasty shows significant thinning of the iliac wing ➡, explaining the radiographic appearance of a "lytic lesion". Aspiration of the iliac bursal mass (note needle in position) showed thick synovial fluid, decompressed from the arthroplasty.

ANTERIOR KNEE PAIN

DIFFERENTIAL DIAGNOSIS

Common
- Patellofemoral Syndrome
- Meniscal Tear
- Meniscal Cyst
- Arthritis

Less Common
- Transient Patellar Dislocation
- Patellar Fracture
- Patellar Malalignment
  - Patellar Subluxation
  - Patella Alta
  - Patella Baja
- Bursitis
- Patellar Tendon Tears & Tendinosis
- Quadriceps Tendon Tear
- Infection
- Medial Plica Syndrome
- Pigmented Villonodular Synovitis (PVNS)
- Post-Operative Fibrosis

Rare but Important
- Synovial Osteochondromatosis
- Intraarticular Chondroma
- Osgood-Schlatter Disease
- Sinding Larsen Johansson Disease
- Hoffa Disease
- Lipoma Arborescens, Knee
- Intraosseous Neoplasm
- Soft Tissue Neoplasm

ESSENTIAL INFORMATION

Helpful Clues for Common Diagnoses
- **Patellofemoral Syndrome**
  - Patellar &/or femoral trochlea cartilage damage; ± patellar tracking abnormalities
  - Radiograph/CT: Subchondral irregularity, sclerosis
  - MR: Cartilage damage, subchondral edema, cyst formation
  - Chondromalacia grading
    - I: Swelling & softening
    - II: Fissuring
    - III: Deeper, broader damage
    - IV: Full thickness loss
- **Meniscal Tear**
  - Anterior horn lateral > medial
- **Meniscal Cyst**
  - Multiloculated cysts arise from meniscal tear

- **Arthritis**
  - Osteoarthritis: Cartilage loss, subchondral cysts, osteophytic ridging, ± osteopenia
  - Crystalline
    - Pyrophosphate arthropathy: Chondrocalcinosis, cartilage loss - patellofemoral > tibiofemoral, ± osteopenia
    - Gouty arthropathy: Patellar erosion, ± osteopenia
  - Inflammatory: Effusion, synovial hypertrophy, osteopenia

Helpful Clues for Less Common Diagnoses
- **Transient Patellar Dislocation**
  - Medial patella & anterolateral femoral bone bruise
  - Look for impaction or avulsion fractures
  - May sprain medial retinaculum or sprain vastus medialis
- **Patellar Fracture**
  - Fracture patterns: Transverse, marginal, osteochondral, vertical
  - Evaluate articular surface congruity, extensor mechanism
  - Distinguish normal variants
    - Bi- or multipartite patella; dorsal defect
    - Typically superolateral; overlying cartilage intact
- **Patellar Subluxation**
  - Lateral subluxation: Common
  - Related to patellar tendinopathy; patella or trochlea dysplasia; arthritis
  - Patellar tracking difficult to assess in static imaging
- **Patella Alta**
  - High-riding patella
  - Lateral radiograph: Tendon length (TL)/patellar length (PL) ratio > 1.2
  - Sagittal MR: TL/PL > 1.5
- **Patella Baja**
  - Low-riding patella
  - Lateral radiograph: TL/PL < 0.8
  - Sagittal MR: TL/PL < 0.74
- **Bursitis**
  - Synovial-lined potential space irritation from trauma, infection, arthropathy
  - Prepatellar: Housemaid knee from kneeling in a forward position
  - Infrapatellar: Parson's knee from kneeling in upright position
- **Patellar Tendon Tears & Tendinosis**

- Tendon thickening & ↑ SI; ± tendon fiber tear; ± distal patellar edema
- Jumper's knee: Proximal tendinopathy in jumping athletes
- **Quadriceps Tendon Tear**
  - Occurs with eccentric quad contraction with planted foot, flexed knee
  - Predisposition: Degenerative tendon; co-existing disease such as chronic renal failure, diabetes, RA, SLE, steroids
  - MR best defines extent of tear
- **Infection**
  - Septic arthritis: Effusion, synovial thickening ± osteopenia, bone marrow edema
  - Osteomyelitis: Osteopenia, cortical loss, bone marrow edema, effusion
- **Medical Plica Syndrome**
  - Thickened media plicae impinges medial femoral condyle; due to trauma, inflammation
- **Pigmented Villonodular Synovitis (PVNS)**
  - Focal or diffuse villonodular synovial thickening; effusion; ± bone erosion; variable enhancement
  - ± ↓ SI due to hemosiderin deposition
- **Post-Operative Fibrosis**
  - Hoffa fat pad scarring with linear ↓ SI stranding & retraction of normal fat pad contours

Helpful Clues for Rare Diagnoses
- **Synovial Osteochondromatosis**
  - Synovial metaplasia resulting in multiple small ovoid intraarticular bodies ± ossification
- **Intraarticular Chondroma**
  - Ossifying cartilaginous metaplasia in Hoffa fat pad
  - Heterogeneous mass with cartilage (↑ SI) & calcification/ossification (↓ SI)
- **Osgood-Schlatter Disease**
  - Traction apophysitis at tibial tubercle in adolescents
  - Fragmentation at apophysis with soft tissue swelling ± bone edema
- **Sinding Larsen Johansson Disease**
  - Traction apophysitis at inferior patella in adolescents
  - Fragmentation at apophysis with soft tissue swelling ± bone edema
- **Hoffa Disease**
  - Inflammation of Hoffa fat pad from acute or repetitive trauma
  - Results in hemorrhage & edema; may evolve to fibrosis
- **Lipoma Arborescens, Knee**
  - Villous synovial proliferation with lipomatous hypertrophy; predilection for suprapatellar pouch
  - **Hint**: Synovial hypertrophy is "fatty" signal on MR sequences
- **Intraosseous Neoplasm**
  - Giant cell tumor, chondroblastoma, osteoblastoma, SBC, hemangioma
- **Soft Tissue Neoplasm**
  - Synovial sarcoma, MFH, hemangioma

Patellofemoral Syndrome

Axial T2WI MR shows full thickness cartilage loss along the lateral patellar facet with adjacent subchondral reactive marrow edema ➡ as well as edema in the lateral femoral sulcus ➡.

Patellofemoral Syndrome

Sagittal PD FSE FS MR shows full thickness cartilage loss ➡ with subchondral cyst formation & adjacent subchondral edema.

ANTERIOR KNEE PAIN

Patellofemoral Syndrome

Meniscal Tear

(Left) Sagittal PD FSE MR shows a chondral fracture ⮊ with undercutting ➡ of the surface, creating a chondral flap. *(Right)* Sagittal PD FSE MR shows a macerated tear ➡ of the lateral meniscus anterior horn. Note the adjacent femoral trochlear cartilage loss ⮊.

Meniscal Cyst

Arthritis

(Left) Axial PD FSE MR shows a multilobulated parameniscal cyst ➡ arising from a lateral meniscus anterior horn tear ⮊ and extending into Hoffa fat pad ⮊. *(Right)* Lateral radiograph shows erosion ⮊ of patella and a small osteophytic ridge ➡. There is chondrocalcinosis in the menisci (not shown). The pattern of predominant patellofemoral disease (mixed erosive/productive) and chondrocalcinosis is typical of pyrophosphate arthropathy.

Arthritis

Transient Patellar Dislocation

(Left) Merchant view radiograph shows marked prepatellar soft tissue swelling ⮊, a joint effusion ➡ & ventral erosions ➡ with a poorly-defined pathologic fracture of the lateral patella ➡. *(Right)* Axial PD FSE FS MR shows the typical bone bruise of a transient lateral patellar dislocation, involving lateral femoral condyle ➡ & medial patella ⮊. Note the irregularity of the patellar surface due to impaction fracture.

ANTERIOR KNEE PAIN

Patellar Fracture

Patellar Subluxation

(Left) Sagittal PD FSE FS MR shows a horizontal fracture ➡ of the patella and articular cartilage. Note effusion extending into horizontal ➡ and vertical clefts ➡ in Hoffa fat pad. *(Right)* Axial PD FSE FS MR shows lateral patellar subluxation with associated articular cartilage damage ➡ and subchondral reactive marrow edema ➡.

Patella Alta

Patella Baja

(Left) Lateral radiograph shows patella alta with an elongated tendon ➡ and high-riding patella ➡ due to prior trauma. The TL/PL is > 1.2. *(Right)* Sagittal PD FSE MR shows patella baja ➡ in this patient status post ACL reconstruction ➡. The TL/PL is < 0.74. Note Hoffa post-operative fibrosis ➡ which may contribute to the tendon shortening.

Bursitis

Bursitis

(Left) Sagittal STIR MR shows a well-circumscribed fluid collection ➡ contained within the bursa superficial to the patella resulting from a fall 5 months earlier. Aspiration revealed sterile sero-sanguinous fluid. *(Right)* Sagittal PD FSE FS MR shows fluid in the deep infrapatellar bursa ➡, resulting from recent trauma.

ANTERIOR KNEE PAIN

Patellar Tendon Tears & Tendinosis

Quadriceps Tendon Tear

(Left) Sagittal PD FSE MR shows thickening of the proximal patellar tendon ➡ with high tendon signal ➡ in this young volleyball player, consistent with patellar tendinosis (jumper's knee). *(Right)* Sagittal PD FSE MR shows a high grade partial tear of the quadriceps tendon with minimal retraction. There is fluid ➡ in the gap created by the tendon fiber disruption ➡.

Medial Plica Syndrome

Pigmented Villonodular Synovitis (PVNS)

(Left) Sagittal MRA shows a thickened medial plica ➡ which snaps & pops, causing pain, particularly when climbing stairs, as it catches on the anteromedial femoral condyle ➡. *(Right)* Sagittal T1 C+ FS MR shows a suprapatellar minimally enhancing synovial nodule ➡. There is a large effusion with thickened synovium ➡. The mass is biopsy-proven PVNS & is atypical in that it has minimal hemosiderin.

Synovial Osteochondromatosis

Intraarticular Chondroma

(Left) Lateral radiograph shows synovial osteochondromatosis, presenting a conglomerate of small faintly calcified bodies ➡ in the suprapatellar pouch just above the patella ➡. *(Right)* Sagittal T2WI FSE MR shows a rounded heterogeneous mass ➡, expanding & displacing Hoffa fat pad. This is an intraarticular chondroma. Radiographs (not shown) reveal rounded fat pad calcifications, corresponding to low signal areas ➡.

Osgood-Schlatter Disease

Sinding Larsen Johansson Disease

(Left) Lateral radiograph shows tibial tubercle fragmentation ➡ & soft tissue swelling ➡ corresponding to the area of tenderness in this 13 year old male with Osgood-Schlatter disease. *(Right)* Sagittal PD FSE FS MR shows edema in the distal patella ➡ and adjacent tendon as well as Hoffa fat pad ➡ in this 12 year old with acute onset pain at the inferior patella without known trauma.

Lipoma Arborescens, Knee

Lipoma Arborescens, Knee

(Left) Sagittal PD FSE FS MR shows numerous suprapatellar pouch filling defects ➡ in a moderate joint effusion. These are, in fact, villous in nature and are low signal with fat suppression. *(Right)* Sagittal T1WI MR in the same patient as previous image, shows the "filling defects" ➡ to be fatty on T1WI, typical of villous synovitis and subsynovial fat hypertrophy of lipoma arborescens.

Intraosseous Neoplasm

Soft Tissue Neoplasm

(Left) Lateral radiograph shows giant cell tumor presenting as a lytic patellar lesion ➡ without effusion, cortical disruption or matrix. *(Right)* Sagittal STIR MR shows a cystic mass involving Hoffa fat pad ➡ as well as the prepatellar subcutaneous fat ➡. It is somewhat tubular and multi-septate, proving to be a cavernous hemangioma at excision.

MEDIAL KNEE PAIN

DIFFERENTIAL DIAGNOSIS

Common
- Medial Collateral Ligament Sprain
- Medial Meniscus Tear
  - Medial Meniscal Cyst
- Arthritis
  - Osteoarthritis
  - Rheumatoid Arthritis
  - Pyrophosphate Arthropathy
- Insufficiency Fracture
- Acute Trauma, Fracture
- Hardware Failure, Post-Operative

Less Common
- Pes Anserine Bursitis
- Medial Collateral Ligament Bursitis
- Osteochondritis Dissecans
- Osteonecrosis
- Medial Plica Syndrome
- Septic Joint
- Pigmented Villonodular Synovitis (PVNS)
- Synovial Osteochondromatosis
- Hip Pathology

Rare but Important
- Soft Tissue Neoplasm
- Intraosseous Neoplasm
- Nerve Impingement (Saphenous Neuritis)

ESSENTIAL INFORMATION

Key Differential Diagnosis Issues
- Diagnoses may occur in combination
- **Hint**: Don't let satisfaction of search keep you from looking for all the possible causes of medial knee pain

Helpful Clues for Common Diagnoses
- **Medial Collateral Ligament Sprain**
  - Most commonly injured ligament
  - Composed of deep & superficial layers
    - Superficial layer originates from medial femoral epicondyle; inserts tibial metaphysis 4-5 cm distal to joint line
    - Deep layer attaches to medial meniscus body with meniscofemoral ligament proximally & meniscotibial ligament distally
  - Ligament sprain grading
    - 1: Few torn fibers; structurally intact
    - 2: Incomplete tear; no joint laxity
    - 3: Complete tear; joint laxity
  - Pellegrini Stieda: Ossification at femoral origin; indicates prior injury
- **Medical Meniscus Tear**
  - Medial tears are most common
  - Orientations: Horitzontal, horizontal oblique, radial, vertical longitudinal
- **Medial Meniscal Cyst**
  - Medial parameniscal cysts are most common
  - Typically multiloculated mucin-filled cyst
  - Look for the associated meniscal tear
- **Arthritis**
  - Osteoarthritis: Cartilage loss, subchondral cysts, osteophytic ridging, loose bodies, ± osteopenia
    - Loose bodies range in size, shape, appearance
  - Inflammatory arthritis: Effusion, synovial hypertrophy, osteopenia, rice bodies
    - Rice bodies are small, regular
  - Crystalline arthritis: Effusion, subchondral edema, soft tissue chondrocalcinosis, usually not osteopenic until endstage
- **Insufficiency Fracture**
  - Acute pain with no trauma; osteopenia
  - Linear low signal subchondral band parallels articular surface with extensive surrounding edema
  - May be located at mid femoral condyle (formerly discussed as spontaneous osteonecrosis of knee)
  - May be located at medial proximal tibial condyle
- **Acute Trauma, Fracture**
  - Appropriate mechanism of injury
  - Look for associated injuries in ligaments, menisci, cartilage
- **Hardware Failure, Post-Operative**
  - Look for lucency at bone-cement-prosthesis interfaces; fractures; ± effusion

Helpful Clues for Less Common Diagnoses
- **Pes Anserine Bursitis**
  - Bursa between MCL & distal sartorius, gracilis, semitendinosus tendons as they insert on anteromedial tibia
  - Seen in distance runners
- **Medial Collateral Ligament Bursitis**
  - Bursa between deep & superficial MCL layers

- Vertical elongate fluid collection paralleling superficial MCL
- **Osteochondritis Dissecans**
  - Fragmentation ± separation of a part of articular surface
  - Most common in the lateral aspect of medial femoral condyle
  - May be cartilage, cartilage & bone, or bone alone
- **Osteonecrosis**
  - Serpentine, demarcated heterogeneous lesions in metadiaphysis may extend to subchondral epiphyses
  - Look for risk factors: Steroids, alcohol, sickle cell anemia, Gaucher disease, trauma
- **Medial Plica Syndrome**
  - Thickened medial plica results from fibrosis & impinges the medial femoral condyle causing pain with normal range of motion
  - Due to inflammation from trauma, OCD, inflammatory arthritis
- **Septic Joint**
  - Effusion, synovial thickening, avid enhancement
- **Pigmented Villonodular Synovitis (PVNS)**
  - Focal or diffuse villous &/or nodular synovial thickening; effusion; bone erosion
  - May have marked low signal due to hemosiderin deposition
  - Heterogeneous enhancement
- **Synovial Osteochondromatosis**
  - Cartilaginous metaplasia

- Multiple small ovoid intra-articular bodies ± ossification
- **Hip Pathology**
  - Referred pain pattern

Helpful Clues for Rare Diagnoses
- **Soft Tissue Neoplasm**
  - May be difficult to distinguish benign from malignant
  - Evaluate patient age, tumor size, location, imaging characteristics, enhancement patterns
  - MR/CT allows delineation of involved anatomy, especially the neurovascular bundle
- **Intraosseous Neoplasm**
  - Pain tends to be gradual and insidious
  - Acute onset pain, look for pathologic fracture
  - Benign
    - Epiphyseal/subchondral: Giant cell tumor, chondroblastoma
    - Metaphyseal: Enchondroma, exostosis, nonossifying fibroma, fibrous dysplasia
  - Malignant
    - Secondary neoplasm is most common & includes metastasis, multiple myeloma
    - Primary neoplasm is less common & includes osteosarcoma, chondrosarcoma, Ewing sarcoma
- **Nerve Impingement (Saphenous Neuritis)**
  - May result from impingement at the adductor canal
  - Mimics medial meniscus tear or arthritis

Medial Collateral Ligament Sprain

Coronal PD FSE FS MR shows a grade 1 MCL sprain with minimal fiber disruption. Edema outlines the superficial fibers ➡ & is interposed between the ligament's deep & superficial layers ➡ as well.

Medial Collateral Ligament Sprain

Coronal PD FSE MR shows a grade 3 MCL tear with retraction of the superficial fibers ➡ as well as complete tears of the meniscofemoral ➡ & meniscotibial ➡ portions of the deep fibers.

MEDIAL KNEE PAIN

(Left) *Anteroposterior radiograph shows ossification* ➡ *of the MCL at the femoral origin. This ossification, termed Pellegrini-Stieda, is indicative of MCL sprain at some time in the past.* **(Right)** *Coronal PD FSE MR through the mid knee shows a truncated medial meniscus* ➡ *resulting in bucket handle tear with a large fragment* ➡ *displaced into the intercondylar notch.*

Medial Collateral Ligament Sprain

Medial Meniscus Tear

(Left) *Coronal PD FSE FS MR shows a typical nondisplaced horizontal oblique tear* ➡ *of the medial meniscus body, extending to the inferior articular surface.* **(Right)** *Coronal STIR MR shows a thin-walled multilobulated cystic mass* ➡ *arising from the capsular surface of a horizontal medial meniscus tear* ➡, *just posterior to the MCL* ➡.

Medial Meniscus Tear

Medial Meniscal Cyst

(Left) *Anteroposterior radiograph shows joint space narrowing* ➡, *subchondral eburnation* ➡ *& osteophytic ridging* ➡, *typical of osteoarthritis. Osteoarthritis often, but not invariably, presents in the medial compartment of the knee. Diffuse osteopenia is present due to patient age & gender.* **(Right)** *AP radiograph shows a large erosion* ➡ *of the medial tibial plateau in this patient with long-standing RA. Note the accompanying osteopenia & diffuse narrowing of joint space.*

Osteoarthritis

Rheumatoid Arthritis

MEDIAL KNEE PAIN

Pyrophosphate Arthropathy

Insufficiency Fracture

(Left) AP radiograph shows chondrocalcinosis ➡, normal bone density, & a large subchondral cyst within the medial tibial condyle ➡ in a patient with pyrophosphate arthropathy. (Right) Coronal STIR MR shows medial femoral condylar subchondral insufficiency fracture ➡ in a 72 year old female with acute onset medial joint line tenderness. Note the extensive bone edema. This fracture may remain radiographically occult until it develops collapse.

Acute Trauma, Fracture

Hardware Failure, Post-Operative

(Left) Coronal PD FSE MR shows an impaction fracture ➡ of the medial tibial plateau with minimal displacement of the fragment in this 15 year old soccer player. Such fractures may be radiographically occult. (Right) Anteroposterior radiograph shows a total knee arthroplasty complicated by a fracture ➡ along the medial femoral condyle with resultant loosening of the femoral component.

Pes Anserine Bursitis

Pes Anserine Bursitis

(Left) Sagittal PD FSE FS MR shows fluid in the pes anserine bursa ➡, paralleling distal sartorius & gracilis. This bursa is located anterior & medial to the usual Baker cyst location. Note the unassociated medial meniscus body tear ➡. (Right) Coronal PD FSE FS MR in the same patient, shows a crescent-shaped medial fluid collection ➡, intimate with the medial tibial cortex typical of pes anserine bursitis.

MEDIAL KNEE PAIN

(Left) Coronal STIR MR shows fluid ➡ interposed between the superficial portion of the MCL ➡ & the adjacent proximal tibial metaphysis, representing medial collateral ligament bursitis. *(Right)* Sagittal PD FSE MR shows a medial OCD lesion ➡ in a 14 year old. The discrete fragment is covered by intact cartilage ➡ & does not appear loose, though the cystic changes at the margin are concerning. Careful scrutiny in multiple planes is important.

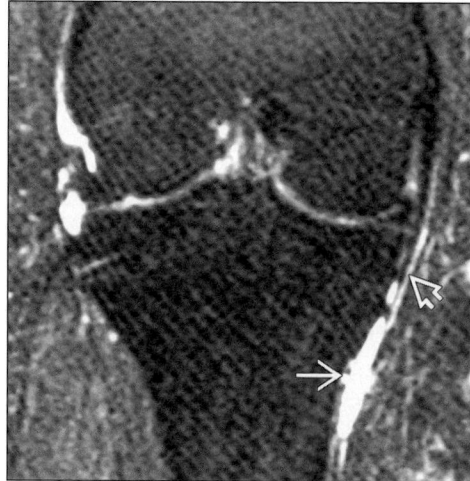

Medial Collateral Ligament Bursitis

Osteochondritis Dissecans

(Left) Coronal PD FSE FS MR shows an OCD in the typical lateral aspect of the medial femoral condyle with fluid ➡ between the fragment & the condyle, indicating a loose fragment in this 52 year old. *(Right)* Coronal PD FSE MR shows a heterogeneous tibial lesion extending to the subchondral medial tibial plateau in this Gaucher patient. This osteonecrosis has the typical serpentine margin ➡ demarcating the extent of the bone infarction.

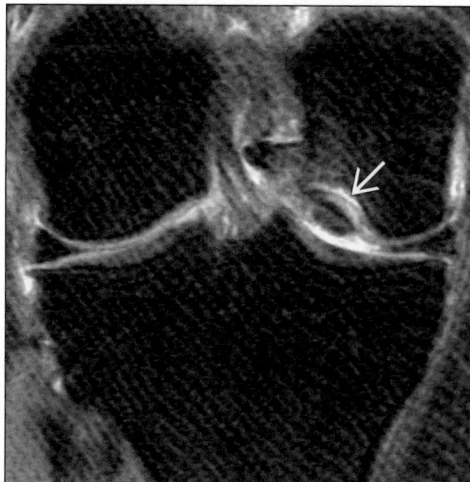

Osteochondritis Dissecans

Osteonecrosis

(Left) Axial T1 C+ FS MR shows a slightly thickened medial plica ➡ in a 42 year old who reports pain & snapping when extending knee. The plica impinges on the medial femoral condyle ➡. *(Right)* Axial T1 C+ FS MR shows thickened, avidly enhancing synovitis ➡ with adjacent reactive femoral condylar osteitis ➡ in this patient with gram positive cocci septic arthritis.

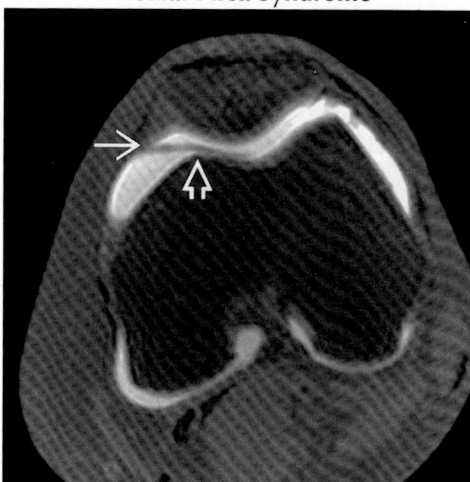

Medial Plica Syndrome

Septic Joint

Pigmented Villonodular Synovitis (PVNS)

Pigmented Villonodular Synovitis (PVNS)

(Left) Coronal T2* GRE MR shows nodular synovial thickening ➡ in this 13 year old with a large joint effusion. On GRE, the nodules are low signal with "blooming" artifact, typical of hemosiderin deposit & classic for PVNS. (Right) Sagittal PD FSE MR shows a discrete intracapsular slightly heterogeneous mass ➡. This is biopsy proven PVNS but without the typically more prominent hemosiderin deposition.

Synovial Osteochondromatosis

Soft Tissue Neoplasm

(Left) Axial PD FSE FS MR shows a large effusion with innumerable small round bodies ➡, particularly in Hoffa fat pad, corresponding to ossific densities on radiograph (not shown). The appearance is typical of synovial chondromatosis. (Right) Coronal T1WI MR shows an extraarticular soft tissue mass ➡ along the medial joint line. This is a synovial sarcoma in this young adult. Age and location should suggest the diagnosis.

Intraosseous Neoplasm

Intraosseous Neoplasm

(Left) Anteroposterior radiograph shows an eccentric lytic geographic lesion, typical for giant cell tumor ➡. The lesion is metaphyseal, approaches the subchondral bone & expands the medial cortex. (Right) Lateral radiograph shows a nonaggressive matrix-forming epiphyseal lesion ➡ in the posteromedial tibia which is low signal intensity on T2 MR (not shown). Note the associated periosteal reaction ➡ incited by this chondroblastoma.

DIFFERENTIAL DIAGNOSIS

Common
- Fracture
- Popliteal Cyst
- Muscle Injury
  - Muscle Strain
  - Compartment Syndrome
  - Calcific Myonecrosis
- Hematoma
- Arthritis of Knee or Ankle
- Sciatica
- Neurogenic Claudication

Less Common
- Tendon, Injury
- Vascular Abnormalities
  - Arterial Insufficiency
  - Deep Venous Thrombosis
  - Venous Insufficiency
- Infection
- Fracture, Malunion

Rare but Important
- Intraosseous Neoplasm
- Soft Tissue Neoplasm
- Nerve Entrapment

ESSENTIAL INFORMATION

Helpful Clues for Common Diagnoses
- **Fracture**
  - May result from high energy trauma or repetitive stress (abnormal stress on normal bone) or from insufficient bone (normal stress on abnormal bone)
  - Radiographs/CT delineate fracture alignment, healing & potential complications
  - Bone scintigraphy useful for identifying injury but poor resolution
  - MR sensitive to early stress response, surrounding soft tissue injury
  - Stress response grading
    - Grade 1: Periosteal edema; ↑ SI T2/STIR
    - Grade 2: Endosteal/periosteal edema; ↑ SI T2/STIR
    - Grade 3: Endosteal/periosteal edema; ↑ SI T2/STIR & ↓ SI T1
    - Grade 4: Discrete cortical fracture perpendicular to long bone surface
- **Popliteal Cyst**
  - Baker cyst most common; arises from posterior medial capsule between semimembranosus & gastrocnemius (medial head) tendons
  - Simple or complex with multiple septations; ± loose bodies
  - May decompress into surrounding soft tissues with symptoms mimicking DVT
  - DVT may co-exist in ~ 10% of symptomatic patients
- **Muscle Injury**
  - **Muscle Strain**
    - Ranges from mild edema (grade 1) to complete fiber disruption (grade 3) with retraction
  - **Compartment Syndrome**
    - Elevated pressure in confined space may irreversibly damage muscle & nerves
    - MR or CT: Swelling, edema, loss of normal muscle markings
  - **Calcific Myonecrosis**
    - History of trauma; residua of compartment syndrome & nerve injury; anterior compartment most common
    - Fusiform mass with plaque-like amorphous calcifications
- **Hematoma**
  - Acute (< 48 hours): T1 isointense to muscle
  - Subacute (< 30 days): ↑ SI on T1 & T2 (methemoglobin)
  - Chronic (> 30 days): Heterogeneous; ↓ SI if hemosiderin present
- **Arthritis of Knee or Ankle**
  - Referred pain
- **Sciatica**
  - Referred pain; neural impingement at L4, L5 &/or S1
- **Neurogenic Claudication**
  - Referred pain from central stenosis at L4, L5 or S; typically bilateral & symmetric pain

Helpful Clues for Less Common Diagnoses
- **Tendon, Injury**
  - Most common: Achilles, plantaris
  - Range from tendinosis (thickening & intrasubstance signal) to complete tear (tendon disruption & retraction) with associated hematoma
- **Vascular Abnormalities**

○ Duplex ultrasound (Duplex = 2D US combined with Doppler flow detection) highly sensitive to vessel disease
○ Radiograph: Look for arterial calcification, phleboliths
○ CT/MR angiography highly sensitive with advanced imaging techniques
○ **Arterial Insufficiency**
  ▪ Artery occlusion from peripheral vascular disease or direct vessel impingement
  ▪ Angiography remains gold standard for evaluation vessel disease/obstruction
  ▪ Popliteal entrapment: Artery impingement from extrinsic source such as aberrant muscles or cystic adventitial disease
○ **Deep Venous Thrombosis**
  ▪ US: Look for incompressibility of vessels, loss of flow augmentation when vessels distal to obstruction are compressed, intraluminal mass or obstruction
  ▪ US of vessels distal to popliteal artery is less sensitive
  ▪ CT/MR venography used for direct visualization of intraluminal defect
○ **Venous Insufficiency**
  ▪ Radiographs: ± Phleboliths, varicosities as elongate masses, long bone periosteal thickening
• **Infection**
  ○ Osteomyelitis
    ▪ X-ray: Lytic, permeative with cortical disruption, ± periostitis & soft tissue edema; ± sinus tracts

▪ MR will better delineate osseous & soft tissue involvement
○ Brodie abscess
  ▪ Subacute osteomyelitis, variable presentation; classic appearance = discrete, lytic metaphyseal lesion; ± periostitis
○ Soft tissue abscess
  ▪ Mass with thick, irregular walls; ± sinus tracts & bone destruction
• **Fracture, Malunion**
  ○ Abnormal alignment (including rotation malalignment) may alter gait, limb length

Helpful Clues for Rare Diagnoses
• **Intraosseous Neoplasm**
  ○ Pain tends to be gradual, insidious
  ○ Benign: Enchondroma, exostosis, fibrous dysplasia, Paget disease
  ○ Malignant: Lymphoma, osteosarcoma, chondrosarcoma, Ewing sarcoma
• **Soft Tissue Neoplasm**
  ○ Benign: Hemangioma, fibromatosis, neurofibroma, myxoma
  ○ Malignant: Synovial sarcoma, MFH, liposarcoma, MPNST
• **Nerve Entrapment**
  ○ May be entrapped by mass, hardware, scarring
  ○ Commonly entrapped nerves
    ▪ Common peroneal
    ▪ Tibial nerves

Fracture

Coronal T1WI MR shows ↓ SI in the proximal tibial diaphyseal medullary space ➔ at the area of point tenderness in this 40 year old distance runner with a grade 3 stress response.

Fracture

Coronal STIR MR in the same patient shows ↑ SI of extensive medullary ➔ & periosteal ➔ edema which extends far beyond the primary focus ➔ of developing fracture seen in T1WI.

CALF PAIN

Fracture

Fracture

(Left) Axial STIR MR shows subtle ↑ SI of the periosteum ➡ & a crescent of ↑ SI in the endosteum ➡ of the mid tibia in this athlete with intermittent "shin" pain. This is a grade 2 stress injury. (Right) Anteroposterior radiograph shows an incomplete insufficiency fracture of the proximal medial tibial metadiaphysis with sclerosis ➡ at the fracture site & adjacent subtle periostitis ➡ due to healing.

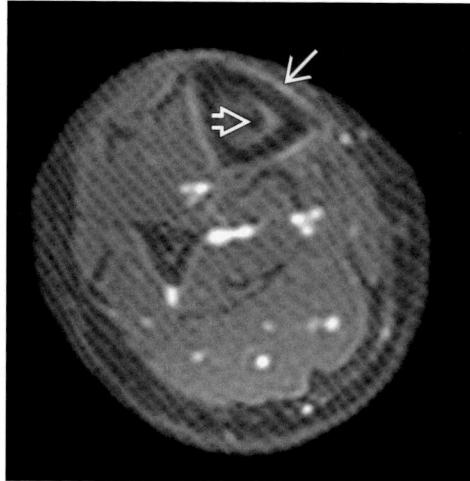

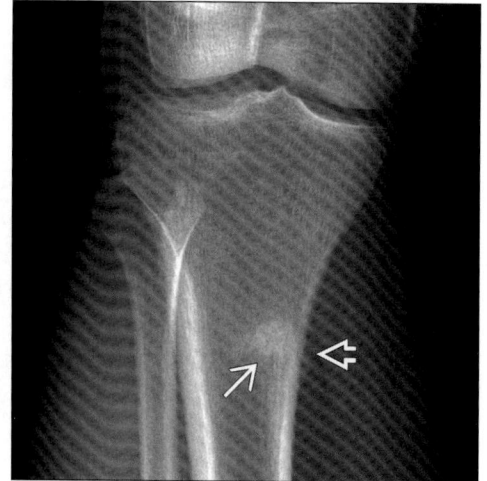

Popliteal Cyst

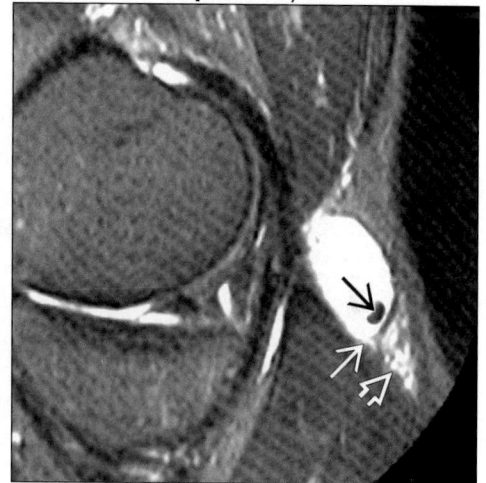

Popliteal Cyst

(Left) Sagittal PD FSE FS MR shows typical multiseptate synovial cyst ➡ tracking along the semimembranosus tendon ➡. It follows the gastrocnemius (medial head) ➡ as well as dissecting into its muscle belly ➡. (Right) Sagittal PD FSE FS MR shows a discrete thin-walled cyst which has partially decompressed ➡ into the adjacent subcutaneous soft tissues ➡ along the gastrocnemius. Note the small loose body ➡ in the popliteal cyst.

Popliteal Cyst

Muscle Strain

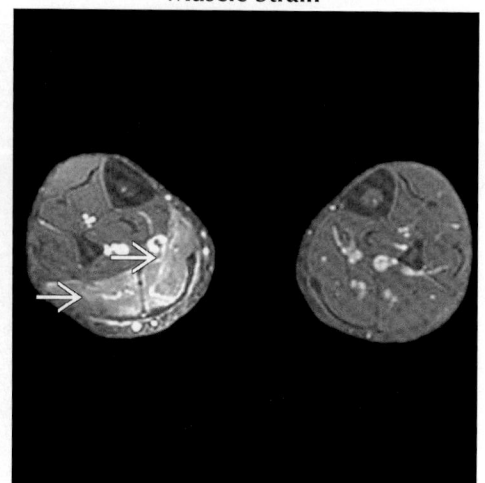

(Left) Two contiguous longitudinal views of the posterior medial knee/calf demonstrate a large, thin-walled multiseptate ➡ chronic Baker cyst with dissection along the superficial fascial of the gastrocnemius ➡. (Right) Axial STIR MR shows a typical case of gastrocnemius soleus strain with a pattern of diffuse muscle edema ➡ without clear pattern of myofibril disruption, consistent with grade 1 muscle strain.

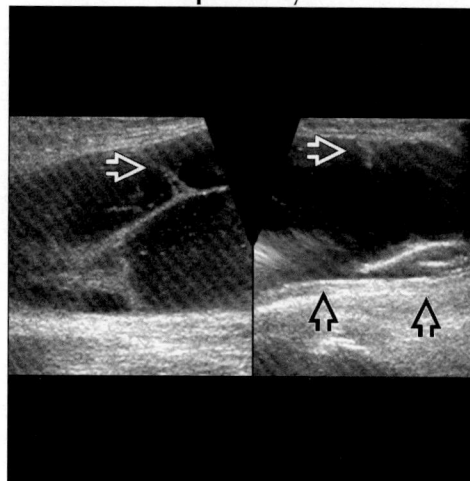

CALF PAIN

Compartment Syndrome

Calcific Myonecrosis

(Left) Axial T1 C+ FS MR shows patchy enhancement (↑ SI) of the swollen anterior tibialis ⇢ & extensor hallucis longus ⇢ with interosseous membrane bowing ⇢ in this compartment syndrome. The enhancement suggests some remaining viability of the injured muscle. *(Right)* Anteroposterior radiograph shows calcific myonecrosis of lower leg anterior compartment with diffuse amorphous plaque-like calcifications ⇢ in areas of necrosis & prior hemorrhage.

Hematoma

Tendon, Injury

(Left) Coronal STIR MR shows a complex mass in right medial gastrocnemius. ↑ SI of edema ⇢ surrounds a mass of intermediate & ↓ SI typical of subacute/chronic hemorrhage with methemoglobin ⇢ & hemosiderin ⇢. *(Right)* Axial T2WI FS MR shows plantaris tendon rupture ⇢ with focal heterogeneous mass between deep & superficial posterior compartments, representing hematoma. Grade 1 soleus strain ⇢ is also present.

Tendon, Injury

Arterial Insufficiency

(Left) Sagittal STIR MR shows complete Achilles tendon rupture ⇢ at musculotendinous junction with acute hemorrhage (↑ SI) ⇢ & retraction of muscle. There is underlying tendinosis with marked thickening & heterogeneity ⇢. *(Right)* CT angiogram (aortic runoff) shows occlusion of left popliteal artery ⇢ with extensive distal collateral flow ⇢ in this 82 year old with intermittent claudication. Note normal right leg runoff ⇢.

CALF PAIN

Arterial Insufficiency

Arterial Insufficiency

(Left) Axial T2WI FSE MR shows popiteal artery entrapment due to a large aberrant slip of the medial head of gastrocnemius ➡ lateral to popliteal neurovascular bundle ➡ & a smaller slip ➡ medial to the vessels. (Right) Coronal MRA shows deviation of the popliteal artery ➡; the medial displacement results from an aberrant slip of the medial head of the gastrocnemius. The patient had symptoms of claudication in the calf.

Deep Venous Thrombosis

Venous Insufficiency

(Left) Transverse ultrasound shows distended posterior tibial veins ➡ which do not compress with applied pressure ➡. Note the adjacent slightly compressible posterior tibial artery ➡. (Right) Lateral radiograph shows chronic, calcified venous thrombus with a serpentine calcified calf mass ➡ corresponding to a previously documented venous thrombus. Signs of venous insufficiency including varicose veins ➡ & phleboliths ➡ are also present.

Infection

Infection

(Left) Coronal STIR MR shows a Brodie abscess in this skeletally immature patient with a meta-epiphyseal ↑ SI well-defined fluid-filled lesion ➡ with intense surrounding edema ➡ including periosteal edema ➡. (Right) Sagittal T1 C+ FS MR shows avidly enhancing anterior subperiosteal soft tissue ➡ lifting the periosteum ➡. Adjacent intramedullary edema ➡ is present as well as a soft tissue abscess with a thickened, shaggy rim ➡.

CALF PAIN

Infection

Infection

(Left) Lateral radiograph shows tuberculosis osteomyelitis with an ill-defined lytic lesion ➡ in the proximal tibial metaphysis with minimal soft tissue swelling ➡. Mineralization is normal. (Right) Sagittal T1 C+ FS MR in the same patient, shows the true extent of this tuberculosis osteomyelitis. There is heterogeneous interosseous enhancement ➡ surrounding necrotic bone ➡. There is also a soft tissue abscess with thickened irregular walls ➡.

Intraosseous Neoplasm

Intraosseous Neoplasm

(Left) Sagittal CT reformation shows a permeative distal fibular lesion ➡ originally diagnosed as stress fracture. However, delayed healing with aggressive periostitis ➡ led to biopsy, confirming lymphoma. (Right) Anteroposterior radiograph shows an aggressive lytic lesion of the proximal fibular metaphysis with extensive periosteal reaction ➡. There is bone expansion, cortical breakthrough ➡ & a large soft tissue mass ➡. This is Ewing sarcoma.

Soft Tissue Neoplasm

Soft Tissue Neoplasm

(Left) Axial T2WI MR shows a lesion in the gastrocnemius (lateral head) of a child who had spasm of the calf muscles. The heterogeneous mass ➡ reveals multiple serpentine channels with interdigitating fat, typical of a hemangioma. (Right) Axial T1 C+ MR shows a heterogeneous ↓ SI mass ➡ which is tender to palpation. Its signal ➡ suggests fibrous, mineralized or hemorrhagic content. This was a low grade malignant peripheral nerve sheath tumor at biopsy.

III

97

PAINFUL KNEE REPLACEMENT

DIFFERENTIAL DIAGNOSIS

Common
- Arthroplasty Loosening
- Knee Instability
- Component Malpositioning
- Arthroplasty Dislocation
- Septic Joint
- Stress Shielding (Mimic)
- Arthroplasty Component Wear
- Particle Disease/Massive Osteolysis
- Arthroplasty Hardware Failure
- Periprosthetic Fracture

Less Common
- Quadriceps Tendon Tear
- Soft Tissue Impingement
- Stress Fracture of Fabella
- Peroneal Nerve Injury

ESSENTIAL INFORMATION

Key Differential Diagnosis Issues
- Many abnormalities are subtle & must be carefully sought; index radiographs for comparison are essential

Helpful Clues for Common Diagnoses
- **Arthroplasty Loosening**
  - Of all the components, tibial is most likely to show loosening
  - Usually begins at medial portion of tibial tray, with lucency at bone-cement or bone-component interface
    - Following lucency, bone may show impaction & component may shift (tilt)
    - Eventual subsidence, usually into medial tibial cancellous bone
    - Eventually, lucency surrounding component, > 2 mm at interface
    - Progression may be subtle; may need to compare with multiple earlier radiographs, not just the most recent
  - Patellar button may subside superiorly
  - Femoral component rarely loosens
- **Knee Instability**
  - TKA usually not hinged or mechanically constrained; stability depends on
    - Posterior cruciate usually retained
    - Medial and lateral soft tissue constraints are retained and may be tightened

- If medial and lateral collateral ligaments are stretched, may use a wider polyethylene spacer on tibial tray to eliminate soft tissue slack
  - Stability also conferred by concave shape of polyethylene spacer, which partially conforms to the femoral component
- **Component Malpositioning**
  - TKA placement designed to duplicate the normal knee
    - Femoral component placed without angulation on distal femur
    - Tibial component positioned to produce 7° ± 3° valgus angulation overall
    - Mechanical axis through center knee
    - On lateral, expect to see 10° posterior tilt on tibial side, mimicking normal tibial tilt (may be provided either by tibial tray tilt or a differential thickness of polyethylene liner)
    - Patellar button centrally placed
  - Watch for malrotation of tibial component relative to femoral component
- **Arthroplasty Dislocation**
  - Dislocation of patella may occur with soft tissue imbalance
  - Dislocation of polyethylene occurs; may be more subtle to note
    - Tibial polyethylene dislocation: Watch for lucency with concave shape displaced in any direction; with dislocation, may develop gapping of joint, mimicking soft tissue imbalance
    - Patellar button dislocation: Watch for lucency with convex shape dislocated relative to patella; may carry cement or part of metal backing with the polyethylene
  - With polyethylene dislocation, there may be abrasion of the adjacent metal
    - Abraded metal often shifts within joint to line either synovium or polyethylene
    - Linear collections of abraded metal termed "metallosis"
- **Septic Joint**
  - Radiographic manifestations of septic joint (other than large effusion) are rare
    - Clinical manifestations are generally obvious and diagnosis made before osseous destruction occurs
  - Diagnosis made by aspiration of joint

PAINFUL KNEE REPLACEMENT

- **Stress Shielding (Mimic)**
  - Weight-bearing through knee is altered with TKA, with less anteriorly and more posteriorly through femoral metaphysis
    - With less anterior weight-bearing, bone is resorbed anteriorly in femur
    - With more posterior weight-bearing, bone is produced along a line from posterior cortex across to posterior femoral component or peg; linear sclerosis is seen
    - Lucency and sclerosis may be progressive
  - Resorption anteriorly in femur is so prominent that it might be mistaken for osteolysis or osseous lytic lesion
  - Not associated with pain, loosening, or other complication
  - Pattern is constant; recognize as normal
- **Arthroplasty Component Wear**
  - Wear occurs in tibial polyethylene liner; need to observe joint line in tangent to evaluate thinning
- **Particle Disease/Massive Osteolysis**
  - Source of particles is polyethylene, metal (bead shedding), and less frequently, fractured cement or bone
  - Particle disease seen most frequently in patella or tibia
    - If tibial component has screws extending into cancellous bone, particles may track through screw holes & develop osteolysis which appears separate from the TKA
  - CT useful in determining extent of lysis & visualizing associated pathologic fractures

- **Arthroplasty Hardware Failure**
  - Fracture of femoral or tibial hardware rare
  - Fracture of metal-backed patellar buttons may occur & may contribute to metallosis
- **Periprosthetic Fracture**
  - Patella is at great risk for fracture
    - Generally transverse; may displace or not
    - Risk increased because of osteotomy for preparation of button placement: Patella is thinned & vascular supply altered
  - Tibial periprosthetic fractures are subtle
    - Watch for thin linear sclerosis
    - Increased risk with osteoporosis (rheumatoid arthritis; patients on steroids)
    - Increased risk when patient has had prior tibial apophyseal transfer

Helpful Clues for Less Common Diagnoses
- **Quadriceps Tendon Tear**
  - Occurs in patients at risk for this injury
    - Rheumatoid arthritis or connective tissue disease, especially on steroids
    - End stage renal disease
- **Soft Tissue Impingement**
  - Generally a clinical diagnosis
- **Stress Fracture of Fabella**
  - Subtle complication; may be detected on radiograph, but CT more reliable
- **Peroneal Nerve Injury**
  - If the pre-operative knee is in severe chronic valgus & the position is corrected by TKA, the peroneal nerve is stretched and patient may develop foot-drop

Arthroplasty Loosening

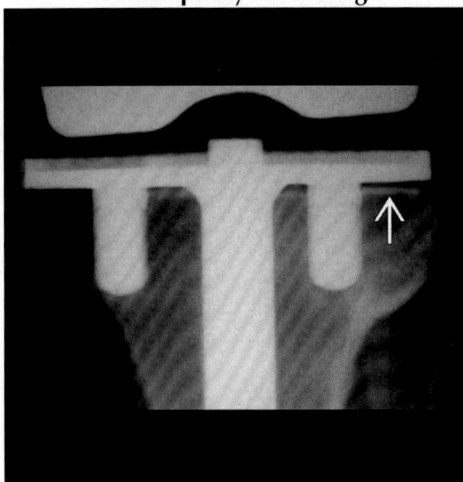

AP radiograph shows a 2 mm lucency at the bone-component interface ➡. This represents early loosening, and is likely to progress. Of the three components, the tibial is the most likely to loosen.

Arthroplasty Loosening

AP radiograph shows impaction at the medial tibial plateau ➡, where there is progressive loosening. Even without gross lucency at the site, progressive impaction and shift of the component indicates loosening.

PAINFUL KNEE REPLACEMENT

(Left) Lateral radiograph shows posterior subluxation of the tibia relative to the femur. This indicates posterior cruciate ligament insufficiency, and a deficit of one of the important stabilizers of a knee arthroplasty. *(Right)* Anteroposterior radiograph shows the femoral component to be in normal position, but the tibial component is malpositioned. It is rotated relative to the femoral component. The patient cannot achieve full extension.

Knee Instability

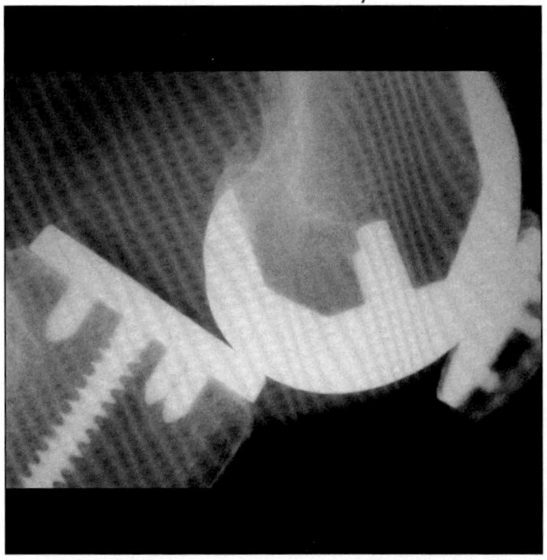

Component Malpositioning

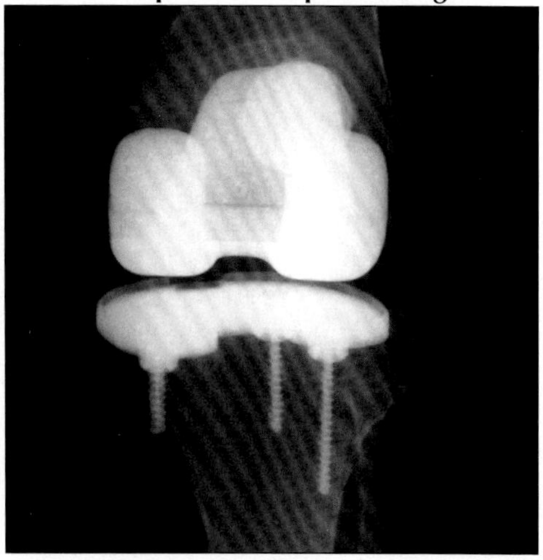

(Left) Lateral radiograph shows a lucent body located inferior to the patella ➡. This lucency is the polyethylene patellar "button", which has dislocated from the patella. *(Right)* Sunrise view shows the lucent polyethylene patellar "button" ➡, with its cement, which has dislocated laterally from the patella. The patellar component is the most frequent of the three to fail.

Arthroplasty Dislocation

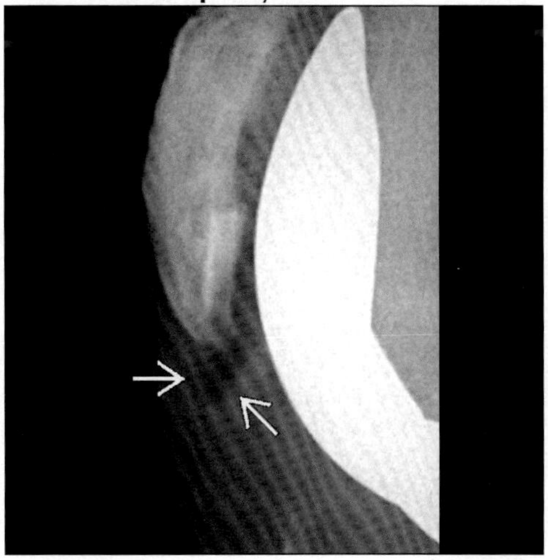

Arthroplasty Dislocation

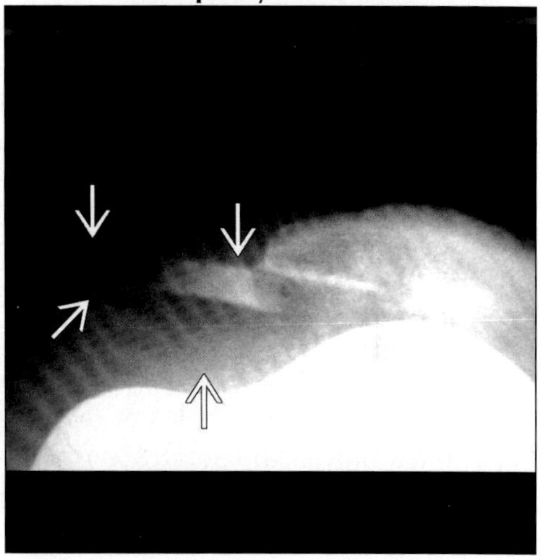

(Left) Anteroposterior radiograph shows gapping at the medial joint line ➡. While instability with medial collateral insufficiency might initially be considered the diagnosis, the answer is seen on the lateral view (next image). *(Right)* Lateral radiograph shows the tibial polyethylene liner ➡ to have dislocated anteriorly from the tibial tray. The polyethylene can be seen if the radiograph is carefully scrutinized.

Arthroplasty Dislocation

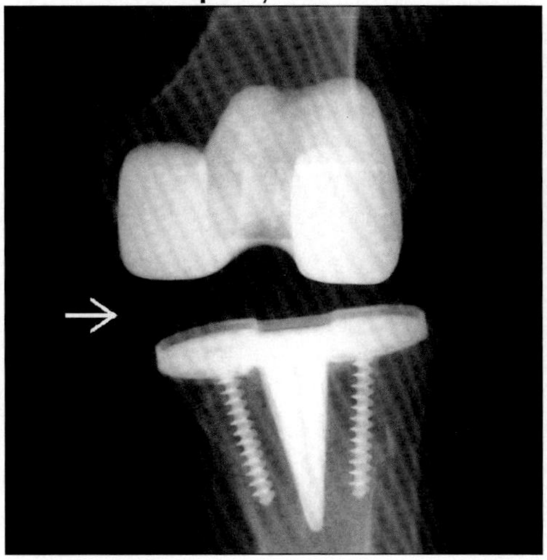

Arthroplasty Dislocation

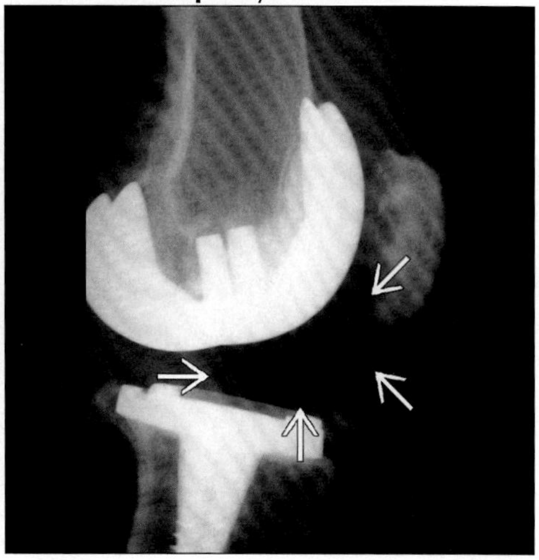

PAINFUL KNEE REPLACEMENT

Stress Shielding (Mimic)

Stress Shielding (Mimic)

(Left) Lateral radiograph shows a relative lucency in the anterior metaphysis ⇨ of this patient who is not symptomatic. This is expected in knee arthroplasties, and should be followed as stress shielding. (Right) Lateral radiograph of the same patient 1 year later, shows more pronounced lucency ⇨, and increased bone density streaming posteriorly from the femoral peg to the posterior cortex ➡. Stress shielding occurs because of altered weight-bearing.

Arthroplasty Component Wear

Arthroplasty Component Wear

(Left) Anteroposterior radiograph shows a unicondylar arthroplasty, with metal-on-metal, due to complete wearing down of the polyethylene component which should be seen on the tibial tray. This component should normally be visible. (Right) Anteroposterior radiograph shows thinning of the medial portion of the polyethylene component ➡ compared with the lateral ⇨, indicating asymmetric wear. Note that, additionally, there is osteolysis ➡, related to particle disease.

Particle Disease/Massive Osteolysis

Particle Disease/Massive Osteolysis

(Left) Sunrise radiograph shows a patellar button which demonstrates bead shedding ➡, along with severe osteolysis ⇨. The metallic beads are of the size required to produce this massive osteolysis. (Right) Anteroposterior radiograph shows massive osteolysis involving the tibia ➡. The particles, likely from polyethylene wear, have moved down the medial screw to elicit the reactive osteolysis.

PAINFUL KNEE REPLACEMENT

Particle Disease/Massive Osteolysis

Particle Disease/Massive Osteolysis

(Left) Coronal CT reformat shows the extent of massive osteolysis ➡ in this patient who had polyethylene wear. The large region of osteolysis puts the patient at risk for fracture. *(Right)* Coronal CT reformat in the same patient, obtained more posteriorly, shows healing attempt of pathologic fracture ➡ due to the large region of osteolysis. The fracture was not seen on radiographs.

Arthroplasty Hardware Failure

Arthroplasty Hardware Failure

(Left) Anteroposterior radiograph shows the metallic patellar button to be breaking up and dissociating from the patella ➡. The patellar hardware is the most likely of the components to have metallic failure. *(Right)* Lateral radiograph shows an angular deformity at the superior patellar button ➡ where it has fractured. Additionally, free metal particles line the polyethylene component ➡; this has been termed "metallosis".

Arthroplasty Hardware Failure

Arthroplasty Hardware Failure

(Left) Anteroposterior radiograph shows a ring of metal ➡ located superior to the patella, corresponding to a portion of the patellar button which has fractured and displaced. *(Right)* Lateral radiograph shows a metallic ring of the patellar button ➡ which has fractured and displaced.

PAINFUL KNEE REPLACEMENT

Periprosthetic Fracture

Periprosthetic Fracture

(Left) Lateral radiograph shows fracture of the superior pole of the patella ➡. It is important to protect this patella, so that it does not displace. *(Right)* Lateral radiograph shows fracture and displacement of the superior pole of the patella ➡. Note that, at this point, the patellar button can still be seen to be attached normally ➡ to the remainder of the patella.

Periprosthetic Fracture

Periprosthetic Fracture

(Left) Anteroposterior radiograph shows linear sclerosis ➡, indicating subacute fracture. Periprosthetic fractures are subtle but important to identify. Note the screws ➡, located in a position which indicates that the patient had a tibial tubercle transfer. *(Right)* Lateral radiograph shows linear sclerosis of a periprosthetic fracture ➡ in a patient who had a prior tibial tubercle transfer. That procedure reportedly places the patient at additional risk for fracture.

Periprosthetic Fracture

Periprosthetic Fracture

(Left) Anteroposterior radiograph shows linear sclerosis ➡ typical of an incomplete periprosthetic fracture. Note the patient's osteoporosis, resulting from underlying rheumatoid arthritis, placing her at risk for fracture. *(Right)* Anteroposterior radiograph shows an angular deformity ➡ in the femoral metaphysis. This is not normal, and was changed relative to prior exams. It is the only indication in this patient of a periprosthetic fracture.

ANTERIOR ANKLE PAIN/IMPINGEMENT

DIFFERENTIAL DIAGNOSIS

Common
- Anterior Impingement
- Anterolateral Impingement
- Syndesmosis Sprain

Less Common
- Stress Fracture, Tibia
- Stress Fracture, Talus
- Tibialis Anterior Tendinosis
- Tibialis Anterior Tendon Tear
- Avascular Necrosis (AVN) of the Talus
- Osteochondral Lesion of the Talus
- Navicular Fractures
- Loose Body
- Talus Fractures

ESSENTIAL INFORMATION

Key Differential Diagnosis Issues
- Difficult to differentiate on physical examination
- Clinical history will help narrow the differential diagnosis
- Begin imaging evaluation with radiographs
- MR preferred for advanced imaging

Helpful Clues for Common Diagnoses
- **Anterior Impingement**
  - Symptoms worse in dorsiflexion
  - Result of chronic repetitive trauma with talus impinging upon anterior tibia
    - Repetitive impingement leads to osteophyte formation along anterior tibia
  - Osteophytes best seen on lateral view and in sagittal plane
  - MR may show marrow edema at impaction sites
- **Anterolateral Impingement**
  - Chronic pain
    - Pain over lateral gutter & anterior talofibular ligament (ATFL)
  - History of inversion injury (acute sprain)
  - Injury leads to inflammation, thickening of ATFL & formation of meniscoid lesion
    - Meniscoid lesion: Hyalinized tissue extending into joint from talofibular ligament
- **Syndesmosis Sprain**
  - Chronic pain, history of ankle sprain

- Anterior tibiofibular ligament thickened or discontinuous
  - Injury may extend into interosseous ligament

Helpful Clues for Less Common Diagnoses
- **Stress Fracture, Tibia & Talus**
  - Insufficiency fractures: Poor quality bone such as osteoporosis, normal stress
  - Fatigue fractures: Normal bone, excessive stress such as overuse
  - MR appearance can be divided into stress response & stress fracture
    - Stress response: Focal area of marrow edema in typical location & appropriate history; may have generalized linear configuration
    - Stress fracture: Low signal fine line within focus of marrow edema; sequence on which the line is visible varies between patients
  - Radiographs show ill-defined, somewhat thickened, linear region of sclerosis
  - Periostitis not seen on talus, rarely seen on distal tibia
  - Tibia
    - Fatigue fracture at base of medial malleolus
    - Insufficiency fracture occurs in distal metaphysis
- **Tibialis Anterior Tendonosis**
  - Pain with dorsiflexion
  - Overuse injury, especially in runners
  - MR: Thickened tendon with intermediate signal
- **Tibialis Anterior Tendon Tear**
  - Inability to coordinate normal foot motion, especially dorsiflexion (major function) & inversion
  - Mechanism
    - Laceration (most common mechanism)
    - Sudden onset of pain after forced plantarflexion
  - MR: Tendon usually thickened with heterogeneous bright signal
    - May be discontinuous, wavy, retracted or have longitudinal split
- **Avascular Necrosis (AVN) of the Talus**
  - Multitude of causes including previous talar neck fracture

ANTERIOR ANKLE PAIN/IMPINGEMENT

- May occur entirely within body or extend to talar dome with subsequent articular surface fragmentation & collapse
- MR: Range from nonspecific marrow edema to typical serpiginous low signal periphery, central fat
- **Osteochondral Lesion of the Talus**
  - Pain worse with activity
  - History of inversion injury
  - Equal distribution between medial & lateral talar dome
  - Evaluate stability with CT arthrography, MR or MR arthrography
  - Stable: Overlying articular cartilage intact
  - Unstable: Displaced fragment, contrast or fluid signal at margin of fragment
    - See Loose Body below
- **Navicular Fractures**
  - Avulsion fractures most common, most from superior surface
    - If acute, donor site may be visible, margin of avulsed fragment ill-defined & not corticated, overlying soft tissue swelling
    - If remote, fragments well-corticated; need to continue search for acute source of pain
  - Body fractures often radiographically occult; orientation is sagittal; moderate energy trauma
  - Tuberosity fractures coronally oriented
    - Result from forefoot abduction with avulsion of posterior tibial tendon insertion

- **Loose Body**
  - Pain, locking
  - Underlying conditions include osteochondral injury, osteoarthritis, trauma
  - Fragments reside in anterior & posterior recesses of joint or in osteochondral defect
  - Synovial osteochondromatosis
    - Leads to multiple osteocartilaginous bodies of uniform size
    - Many but not all will be "loose"; others remain attached to synovium
- **Talus Fractures**
  - Pain, swelling, difficulty bearing weight
  - History of trauma
  - Neck: Most common site
    - May lead to AVN
    - Hawkins sign (lucency beneath talar dome) excludes AVN
  - Body: Includes lateral process, posterior process, dome, central body
    - Posterior & lateral process fractures unlikely to cause anterior pain
    - Central body fracture results from high impact injury such as MVA or fall from height; coronally oriented; commonly have associated dislocation
    - Dome: See Osteochondral Fracture above
  - Head: Includes small avulsion fractures
    - Most common from superior surface
    - Avulsions: See Navicular Fractures above

Anterior Impingement

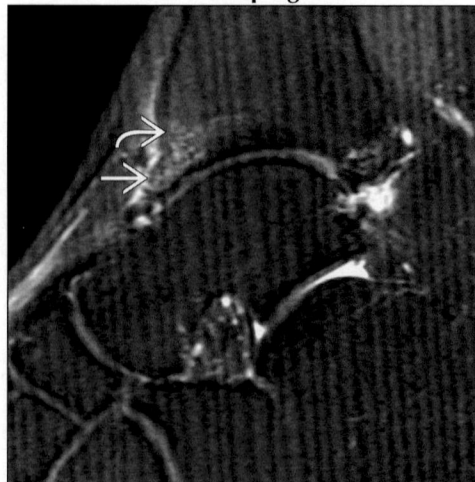

Sagittal NECT shows a case of anterior impingement due to prominent tibial ➡ and talar ➡ osteophytes.

Anterior Impingement

Sagittal T2WI FS MR shows anterior ankle impingement due to a large osteophyte ➡ arising from the anterior edge of the distal tibia. Adjacent marrow edema ➡ and soft tissue edema are present.

ANTERIOR ANKLE PAIN/IMPINGEMENT

(Left) Axial T2WI FS MR shows a typical example of a meniscoid lesion in the anterolateral gutter of the ankle ➡ deep to the talofibular ligament ➡ in this patient with anterolateral impingement. (Right) Oblique PD FSE FS MR shows typical appearance of an isolated, anterior, inferior, tibiofibular ligament disruption. A small remnant of the ligament is visible ➡. Extension of fluid beyond the anterolateral corner of the tibia is an indicator of disruption of this ligament.

Anterolateral Impingement

Syndesmosis Sprain

(Left) Anteroposterior radiograph shows an insufficiency type of stress fracture of the distal tibia. The fracture appears as an ill-defined, sclerotic, linear abnormality in the metaphysis ➡. (Right) Sagittal T1WI MR shows discrete fracture lines within the neck of the talus ➡ and adjacent bone marrow edema ➡ in this patient with a stress fracture.

Stress Fracture, Tibia

Stress Fracture, Talus

(Left) Axial STIR MR shows a subtle MR appearance of anterior tibialis tendinosis ➡. The tendon is slightly enlarged without intrinsic signal abnormality. (Right) Sagittal PD FSE MR shows a rupture of the tibialis anterior tendon ➡. The tendon fibers are wavy and thickened with diffuse intermediate signal.

Tibialis Anterior Tendinosis

Tibialis Anterior Tendon Tear

ANTERIOR ANKLE PAIN/IMPINGEMENT

Avascular Necrosis (AVN) of the Talus

Osteochondral Lesion of the Talus

(Left) Oblique radiograph shows a classic case of subchondral bone collapse ➡ following avascular necrosis of the talus. Note the extensive sclerosis throughout the talar dome ➡. *(Right)* Sagittal bone CT shows an osteochondral lesion with small osseous fragments within the defect ➡. The margin of the defect is sclerotic with small cysts ➡.

Osteochondral Lesion of the Talus

Navicular Fractures

(Left) Sagittal T2WI FS MR shows a rounded lesion ➡ located posteromedially on the dome of the talus which has the typical appearance of an osteochondral injury. There is no overlying articular cartilage defect or ossific fragment. *(Right)* Oblique radiograph shows a vertical navicular body fracture ➡. The fracture was not visible on the AP or lateral views.

Loose Body

Talus Fractures

(Left) Anteroposterior radiograph shows an ossific body projecting along the medial aspect of the joint ➡. This body is the result of an unstable osteochondral injury. On the lateral view it was still partially located within the defect. *(Right)* Sagittal STIR MR shows a typical appearance of a coronally oriented talar body fracture ➡. This particular fracture is complicated by a non-union of the fracture fragments.

MEDIAL ANKLE PAIN

DIFFERENTIAL DIAGNOSIS

Common
- Tendon, Injury
- Tenosynovitis
- Osteochondral Lesion of the Talus
- Arthritis
- Fracture

Less Common
- Hardware Failure
- Infection
- Tarsal Coalition
- Os Trigonum Syndrome
- Tarsal Tunnel Syndrome

Rare but Important
- Transient Bone Marrow Edema
- Osteonecrosis
- Deltoid Ligament Sprain
- Intraosseous Neoplasm
- Soft Tissue Neoplasm

ESSENTIAL INFORMATION

Helpful Clues for Common Diagnoses
- **Tendon, Injury**
  - Tendinopathy: Intrasubstance signal, thickening, central or delaminating
  - Tear patterns may seen on ultrasound (US) & MR
    - Type 1: Partial with contour hypertrophy
    - Type 2: Partial with contour attenuation
    - Type 3: Complete with retraction
  - Medial (flexor) tendons: Posterior tibialis (PTT), flexor hallucis longus (FHL), flexor digitorum longus (FDL), anterior tibialis (ATT)
  - May see marrow edema (↑ SI) at or near tendon attachments
- **Tenosynovitis**
  - Inflammation due to trauma, arthritis or infection in tendon sheath ± visible tendon pathology
  - Small amount of fluid normal in tendon sheaths
  - FHL communicates with tibiotalar joint & may have fluid related to joint effusions; look for ↑ fluid volume out of proportion to joint fluid
  - Stenosing tenosynovitis
    - Due to adhesions between sheath and tendon; limits tendon movement
    - Imaging shows fluid restricted to one portion of tendon sheath
- **Osteochondral Lesion of the Talus**
  - Entity is traumatic or atraumatic (including osteochondritis dissecans, thought to be due to ischemic necrosis)
    - Trauma history in 85%; often with ligament laxity
  - Represents variable articular cartilage & subchondral bone fracture injury
  - Staged as follows
    - Stage 1: Articular cartilage injury only
    - Stage 2: Cartilage injury + subchondral fracture
    - Stage 3: Detached (but nondisplaced) fragment
    - Stage 4: Detached & displaced fragment
    - Stage 5: Subchondral cyst formation
- **Arthritis**
  - Osteoarthritis: Joint space narrowing, osteophytes, subchondral sclerosis & cysts, ± effusions
  - Rheumatoid arthritis: Juxta-articular osteoporosis, symmetric joint space narrowing, erosions, effusions
  - Gout: Corticated erosions, soft tissue masses, relatively normal mineralization
  - Neuropathic: Joint dissolution, debris, dislocation, subluxation, distention; occurs in diabetics
- **Fracture**
  - Traumatic: Look for appropriate mechanism of injury
  - Insufficiency: Osteoporosis, fracture line perpendicular to major trabeculae/cortex
  - Symptomatic accessory navicular synchondrosis: Edema/inflammation due to PTT traction or direct impingement (ill-fitting shoes, etc.)

Helpful Clues for Less Common Diagnoses
- **Hardware Failure**
  - Look for lucency surrounding hardware, loosening & withdrawal, failure of fusion or fracture healing
- **Infection**
  - Osteomyelitis
    - Lytic lesions, cortical loss, periosteal reaction, ± sinus tracts
  - Septic arthritis

MEDIAL ANKLE PAIN

- ▪ Juxta-articular osteopenia, effusion, synovial thickening, + synovial enhancement, ± sinus tracts
- o Soft tissue abscess
  - ▪ Often have thickened, irregular walls & multiple sinus tracts
  - ▪ Look for foreign body
- **Tarsal Coalition**
  - o Most common: Calcaneonavicular & talocalcaneal (medial facet)
  - o Look for broad, flat, irregular articular surfaces; may be osseous, fibrous or cartilaginous; 20% are bilateral
  - o May develop secondary signs such as talar beak, horizontal sustentaculum, ball-and-socket tibiotalar joint
- **Os Trigonum Syndrome**
  - o Seen in athletes with extreme plantar flexion movements, (e.g., ballet)
  - o Irregular synchondrosis margins, marrow edema of talus & os trigonum, FHL tenosynovitis ± stenosis
- **Tarsal Tunnel Syndrome**
  - o Tibial nerve compression at ankle flexor retinaculum
  - o Pain & paresthesias in medial ankle & foot
  - o Look for ganglion, venous or other vascular malformation, mass, bony prominence, prior trauma

Helpful Clues for Rare Diagnoses
- **Transient Bone Marrow Edema**
  - o Diagnosis of exclusion; abrupt onset pain

- o Transient osteopenia involving a single tarsal; may involve other tarsal bones over time
- o Patchy or diffuse bone marrow edema of an isolated tarsal with recovery of normal signal over time; second episode likely involves a different bone
- **Osteonecrosis**
  - o Look for underlying cause: Trauma, alcoholism, steroids, sickle cell anemia, Gaucher disease, etc.
  - o Regional sclerosis ± articular collapse; serpentine ↑/↓ SI lesion most common in talus, navicular
- **Deltoid Ligament Sprain**
  - o Strongest capsuloligament complex; medial malleolus usually fractures before deltoid fails
  - o Edema ± discrete disruption of deep or superficial ligaments
- **Intraosseous Neoplasm**
  - o Benign: Lipoma, osteoid osteoma, SBC, ABC, osteoblastoma, chondroblastoma
  - o Malignant: Chondrosarcoma, Ewing sarcoma, osteosarcoma
- **Soft Tissue Neoplasm**
  - o Benign: Lipoma, hemangioma, neurofibroma, chondroma, fibromatosis
  - o Malignant: Synovial sarcoma, clear cell sarcoma, fibrosarcoma, dermatofibrosarcoma protuberans, MFH, liposarcoma

Tendon, Injury

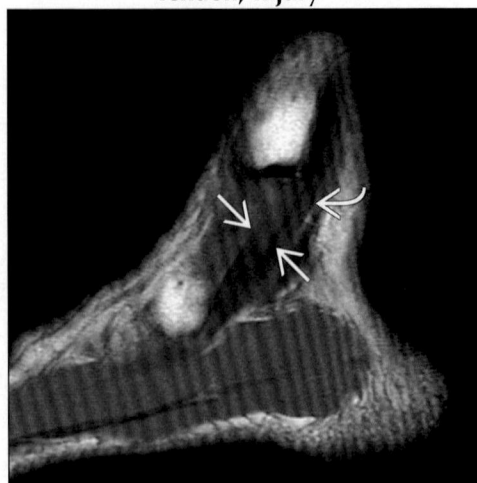

Axial PD FSE FS MR shows marked thickening and ↑ SI in posterior tibial tendon (PTT) ➡ as it passes behind the medial malleolus ➡. Note the normally contoured adjacent flexor digitorum longus tendon ➡.

Tendon, Injury

Sagittal T1WI MR in the same patient shows the grade 1 intrasubstance partial tear with "hypertrophy" of the tendon contour ➡. The normally contoured FDL ➡ is proximal & posterior to PTT.

MEDIAL ANKLE PAIN

(Left) Axial T2WI FS MR shows FHL tenosynovitis. Fluid (↑ SI) ➡ surrounds the normally contoured tendon ➡. Fluid volume in the tendon sheath is out of proportion to volume of fluid in the joint ➡. (Right) Axial PD FSE FS MR shows ATT tenosynovitis with excessive tendon sheath fluid ➡ encircling the normal tendon. Note the constriction of tendon as it passes under the extensor retinaculum ➡.

Tenosynovitis

Tenosynovitis

(Left) Sagittal PD FSE FS MR shows FHL ➡ tenosynovitis with a large volume of tendon sheath fluid ➡. Note tendon sheath constriction ➡ at the calcaneocuboid joint, representing stenosing tenosynovitis. (Right) Oblique radiograph shows a medial talus osteochondral lesion ➡ with lucency surrounding a detached but nondisplaced fragment (stage 3).

Tenosynovitis

Osteochondral Lesion of the Talus

(Left) Sagittal CT reformation shows typical talar osteochondral lesion with cartilage disruption ➡ & a fracture fragment surrounded by small osseous cysts ➡. There is no articular surface flattening. (Right) Coronal STIR MR shows a small ↑ SI area in the medial talar subchondral bone ➡ with subtle hyaline cartilage irregularity ➡ representing osteochondral lesion of the talus at stage 2.

Osteochondral Lesion of the Talus

Osteochondral Lesion of the Talus

Arthritis

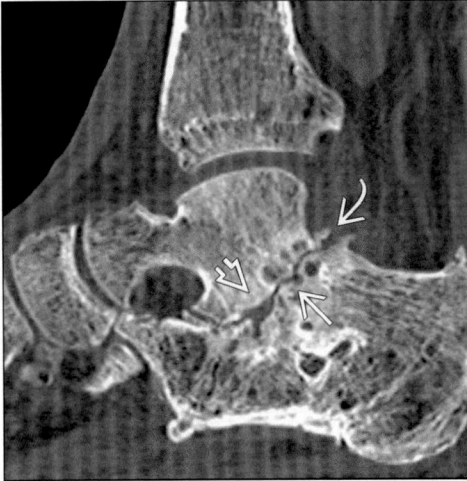

Arthritis

(Left) Sagittal CT reformation shows marked posterior subtalar joint space narrowing ➡ with small subchondral cysts ➡ & osteophytic ridging ➡ as well as profound osteopenia in this posttraumatic osteoarthritis. *(Right)* Sagittal T1 C+ FS MR shows a moderate joint effusion ➡, joint space narrowing with an enhancing erosion ➡ & periarticular bone marrow edema ➡ in rheumatoid arthritis. The contralateral ankle had similar findings.

Arthritis

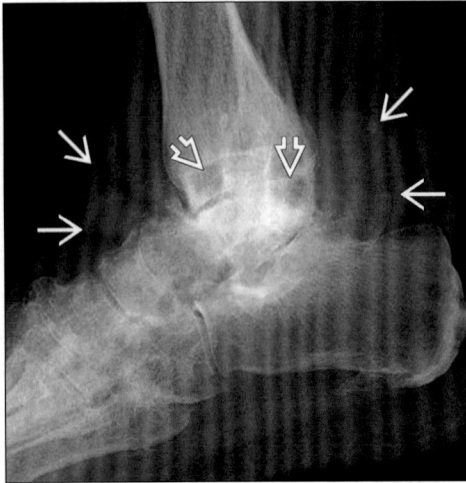

Arthritis

(Left) Lateral radiograph shows a large & radiodense soft tissue mass ➡ in the tibiotalar joint representing tophaceous gout with large associated erosions ➡ in the tibiotalar, subtalar & intertarsal joints. *(Right)* Lateral radiograph shows a typical neuropathic (Charcot) joint in a diabetic patient with distention ➡, disorganization ➡, debris ➡, & joint dislocation ➡ (talonavicular). Aspiration may be necessary to exclude infection.

Fracture

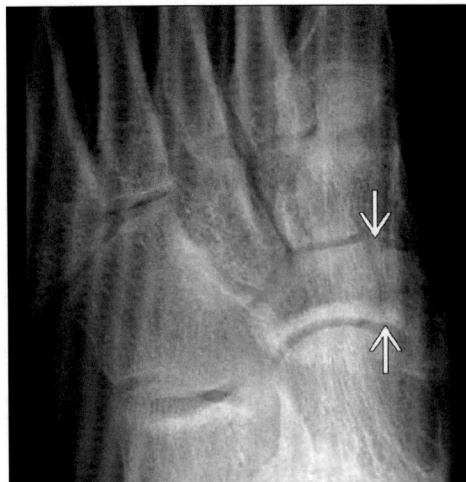

Fracture

(Left) Oblique radiograph shows a nondisplaced vertical navicular fracture ➡. The lateral & AP radiographs (not shown) appeared completely normal. This may occur in athletes in jumping & sprinting sports. *(Right)* Coronal oblique T1WI MR shows an incomplete insufficiency fracture ➡ of the posterior medial plantar calcaneus with surrounding edema ➡ in this 39 year old anorexic female runner.

MEDIAL ANKLE PAIN

Fracture

Hardware Failure

(Left) Axial T2WI FS MR shows a symptomatic accessory navicular with ↑ SI in both the navicular ➡ & the accessory navicular ➡ with a small amount of fluid in the synchondrosis ➡. *(Right)* Sagittal CT reformation shows a dome-shaped metal trabecular ingrowth implant ➡, initially placed to facilitate tibiotalar arthrodesis. Instead, the metal has become a wedge-inhibiting fusion ➡ and requires removal.

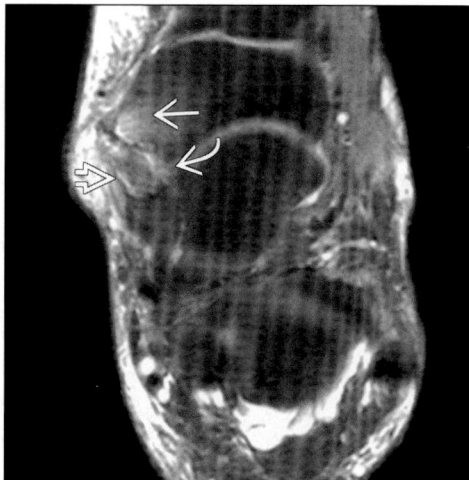

Infection

Tarsal Coalition

(Left) Coronal CT reformation shows failed tibiotalar arthrodesis due to infection. Lucency at the screw-bone interface ➡ indicates loosening. Note the periosteal reaction ➡ & surrounding soft tissue swelling ➡. *(Right)* Axial NECT shows talocalcaneal tarsal coalition, which is one of the most common coalition patterns. Note widened & slightly irregular left middle subtalar facet ➡ compared to the normal right facet ➡. (†MSK Req).

Os Trigonum Syndrome

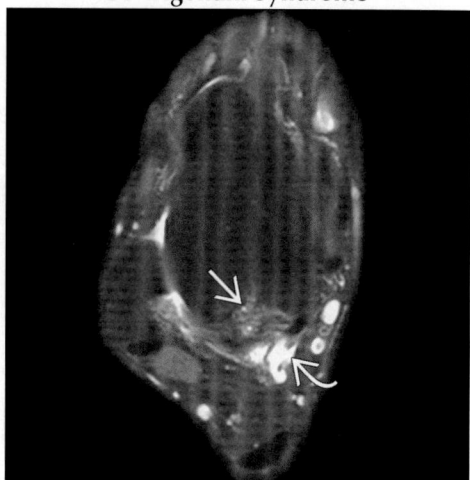

Os Trigonum Syndrome

(Left) Sagittal T1WI MR shows an irregular & sclerotic (↓ SI) os trigonum ➡ & the adjacent talus with a small subtalar joint effusion. This young woman is a ballerina with pain when in plantar flexion. *(Right)* Axial PD FSE FS MR in the same patient shows edema (↑ SI) in the talus & os trigonum ➡ with FHL tenosynovitis (fluid out of proportion to joint effusion) ➡ in this instance of os trigonum syndrome.

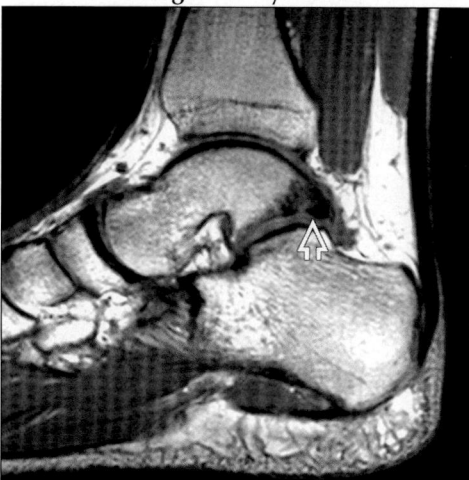

MEDIAL ANKLE PAIN

Tarsal Tunnel Syndrome

Transient Bone Marrow Edema

(Left) Axial T2WI FS MR shows a ganglion cyst ➡ in the tarsal tunnel, deep to the flexor retinaculum, impinging on the neurovascular bundle ➡ with resultant pain in the medial ankle. *(Right)* Sagittal PD FSE FS MR shows mild diffuse navicular edema ➡. The patient has had similar episodes of isolated edema in the talus & medial cuneiform, which spontaneously resolved. This represents transient regional bone marrow edema.

Osteonecrosis

Deltoid Ligament Sprain

(Left) Sagittal PD FSE FS MR shows heterogeneous serpentine ↑ SI (edema) ➡ & ↓ SI (preserved marrow fat) ➡ throughout the talus & subtle articular surface flattening ➡. This patient's primary risk factor for osteonecrosis was alcohol abuse. *(Right)* Coronal STIR MR shows edema (↑ SI) within the posterior tibiotalar ➡ & tibiocalcaneal ➡ portions of deltoid ligament as well as medial malleolar marrow edema ➡ resulting from an acute pronation eversion injury.

Intraosseous Neoplasm

Soft Tissue Neoplasm

(Left) Coronal STIR MR shows an intracortical nidus (↓ SI) ➡ surrounded by intense edema ➡ in the talus in this 14 year old soccer player with an osteoid osteoma. *(Right)* Axial PD FSE MR shows a discrete ↑ SI mass ➡ medial & superficial to the abductor hallucis muscle ➡. Fat suppression (not shown) confirmed this mass to be a lipoma. While a lipoma does not typically cause pain, this patient's medial ankle was painful due to pressure from her shoes.

LATERAL ANKLE PAIN

DIFFERENTIAL DIAGNOSIS

Common
- Anterior Talofibular Ligament Tear
- Fracture, Base 5th Metatarsal
- Traumatic Fracture, Fibula
- Fracture, Anterior Process Calcaneus
- Cuboid Fracture
- Calcaneofibular Ligament Tear
- Peroneal Tendinosis/Tear/Tenosynovitis
- Subtalar Arthritis
- Insufficiency Fracture, Fibula
- Osteochondral Lesion of the Talus
- Extensor Digitorum Brevis Avulsion

Less Common
- Tarsal Coalition
- Anterolateral Impingement
- Tillaux Fracture
- Peroneal Tendon Subluxation
- Sinus Tarsus Syndrome
- Fracture, Lateral Process of Talus

Rare but Important
- Peroneus Quartus Muscle
- Syndesmosis Sprain
- Syndesmotic Impingement

ESSENTIAL INFORMATION

Key Differential Diagnosis Issues
- Common features to many of the entities
  - Chronic pain, varying degrees instability
  - History of inversion injury, "ankle sprain"
  - Typical sequence of injury in ankle sprain: Anterior talofibular ligament (ATFL), calcaneofibular ligament, posterior talofibular ligament

Helpful Clues for Common Diagnoses
- **Anterior Talofibular Ligament Tear**
  - Weakest of lateral ankle ligaments
  - Ligament thick, thin, wavy or discontinuous
  - Adjacent edema if acute
- **Fracture, Base 5th Metatarsal**
  - May mimic ankle sprain
    - Base of fifth metatarsal should always be included on ankle films
  - Tuberosity avulsion by peroneus brevis: Longitudinal or oblique orientation of fracture

- Jones (dancer's) fracture: Transverse thru proximal shaft, nonunion common
- **Traumatic Fracture, Fibula**
  - Weber classification aids in surgical decision making
    - Weber A: Below tibiotalar joint, typically avulsion of tip of lateral malleolus
    - Weber B: At level of the tibiotalar joint
    - Weber C: Above the tibiotalar joint
- **Fracture, Anterior Process Calcaneus**
  - Avulsion of bifurcate ligament
  - Seen on lateral view
- **Cuboid Fracture**
  - Usually small fractures from lateral margin
    - Direct blow or nutcracker fracture resulting from forefoot abduction
- **Calcaneofibular Ligament Tear**
  - Tear in association with ATFL tear more common than isolated tear
  - Tear usually midsubstance
- **Peroneal Tendinosis/Tear/Tenosynovitis**
  - Tendinosis: Tendon thickened, intermediate internal signal
  - Tear: Tendon thinned, wavy, or discontinuous
    - Peroneus brevis split: Longitudinal tear or tendon fraying
    - Peroneus longus tear usually transverse
  - Tenosynovitis: Fluid signal surrounding tendon, small amounts of fluid are within realm of normal
- **Subtalar Arthritis**
  - Causes include previous trauma, osteoarthritis, rheumatoid arthritis
- **Insufficiency Fracture, Fibula**
  - Normal stresses on poor quality bone
  - Radiographs may show ill-defined linear sclerosis
  - MR appearance ranges from stress response to stress fracture
    - Stress response: Focal area of marrow edema, may have linear configuration
    - Stress fracture: Fine low signal intensity line within area of marrow edema, sequence which demonstrates line is variable
- **Osteochondral Lesion of the Talus**
  - Equal distribution between medial & lateral talar dome
  - Evaluate stability with CT arthrography, MR, MR arthrography

LATERAL ANKLE PAIN

- ○ Stable: Overlying articular cartilage intact
- ○ Unstable: Displaced fragment, bright signal or contrast at fragment margin
- **Extensor Digitorum Brevis Avulsion**
  - ○ Small flake of bone from lateral margin of calcaneus near anterior process
  - ○ Seen on AP, mortise views

Helpful Clues for Less Common Diagnoses
- **Tarsal Coalition**
  - ○ Flatfoot, pain especially after activity
  - ○ Talocalcaneal or calcaneonavicular
  - ○ Fibrous, cartilaginous, or osseous
  - ○ Lateral pain due to spasm of peroneals
- **Anterolateral Impingement**
  - ○ Injury leads to inflammation, thickening of ATFL, formation of meniscoid lesion
    - ■ Meniscoid lesion: Hyalinized tissue extending into joint from ATFL
- **Tillaux Fracture**
  - ○ Avulsion of anterior tibiofibular ligament from anterior tibia
    - ■ Variant: Wagstaffe-LeFort fracture, avulsion of ligament from fibula
  - ○ Juvenile Tillaux: Salter III tibial fracture occurs at stage where medial physis closed, lateral physis open, around age 14
- **Peroneal Tendon Subluxation**
  - ○ Creates snapping sensation
  - ○ Retinaculum avulsion from posterolateral margin of lateral malleolus may create small osseous fragment
- **Sinus Tarsus Syndrome**

- ○ Trauma most common cause, also gout, osteoarthritis
- ○ MR shows sinus edema/inflammation
- ○ Talocalcaneal & cervical ligaments may be edematous or disrupted
- ○ Late findings are subchondral sclerosis & cysts in adjacent talus
- **Fracture, Lateral Process of Talus**
  - ○ Commonly seen in snowboarders
  - ○ Best seen on mortise view
  - ○ Vertically oriented fracture
  - ○ Fragment of variable size
    - ■ May involve subtalar articular surface

Helpful Clues for Rare Diagnoses
- **Peroneus Quartus Muscle**
  - ○ Variable origin & insertion
  - ○ Crowds peroneus longus, brevis in retromalleolar groove leading to tendinosis, tears, subluxation
- **Syndesmosis Sprain**
  - ○ Abduction, external rotation, dorsiflexion
  - ○ Anterior tibiofibular ligament thickened or discontinuous
  - ○ Injury may extend into interosseous ligament
  - ○ Adjacent edema if acute
- **Syndesmotic Impingement**
  - ○ Sequelae of syndesmotic sprain
  - ○ ATFL, posterior tibiofibular ligament, interosseous membrane involved in isolation or combination
  - ○ Ligamentous thickening, synovial proliferation responsible for symptoms

Anterior Talofibular Ligament Tear

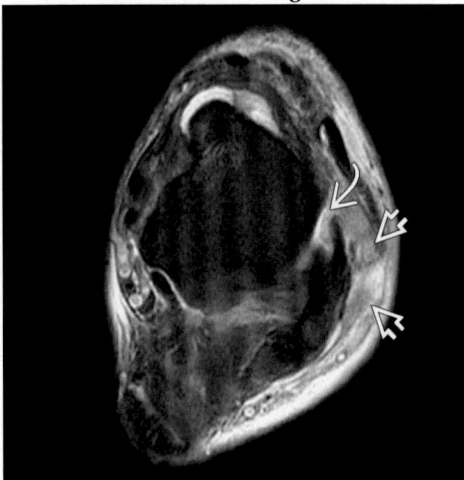

Axial T2WI FS MR shows acute traumatic rupture of the anterior talofibular ligaments near its talar attachment ➡. Extensive surrounding edema ➡ is consistent with an acute injury.

Fracture, Base 5th Metatarsal

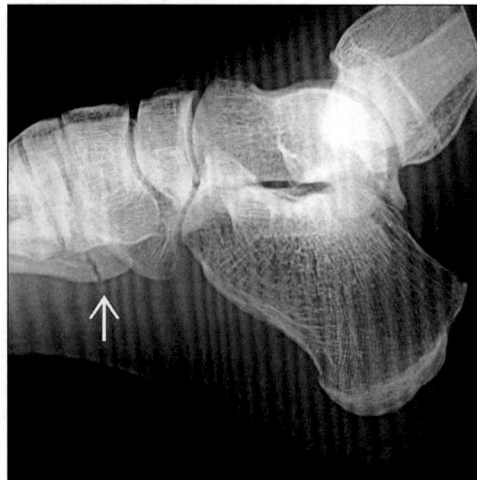

Lateral radiograph shows a nondisplaced fracture through the base of the fifth metatarsal ➡ following an inversion injury.

LATERAL ANKLE PAIN

Fracture, Anterior Process Calcaneus

Fracture, Anterior Process Calcaneus

(Left) Sagittal PD FSE FS MR shows bright signal at the anterosuperior process of the calcaneus ➡ consistent with a small anterosuperior process avulsion by the bifurcate ligament. *(Right)* Sagittal NECT shows a fracture through the anterior process of the calcaneus ➡. The posterior third of the fracture appears healed ➡.

Cuboid Fracture

Cuboid Fracture

(Left) Oblique radiograph shows cortical irregularity of the cuboid on this oblique radiograph ➡ consistent with a nondisplaced fracture. *(Right)* Sagittal T2WI FS MR shows marrow edema within the cuboid ➡. Close inspection reveals irregularity of the cortex ➡ and a small osseous fragment ➡ indicative of a fracture.

Calcaneofibular Ligament Tear

Calcaneofibular Ligament Tear

(Left) Coronal PD FSE MR shows acute traumatic rupture of the calcaneofibular ligament ➡. The ligament is discontinuous and abnormally oriented. *(Right)* Axial PD FSE FS MR shows a classic case of partial tear of the calcaneofibular ligament. A few intact ligament fibers are present but the majority of the ligament is replaced by increased signal ➡ in the typical position of the ligament between the calcaneus and the adjacent peroneal tendons.

LATERAL ANKLE PAIN

Peroneal Tendinosis/Tear/Tenosynovitis

Peroneal Tendinosis/Tear/Tenosynovitis

(Left) Axial PD FSE FS MR shows a typical case of the peroneus brevis split form of tendon tear. The peroneus brevis tendon (typically the more anterior tendon) is divided ➡ and wraps around the peroneus longus tendon ➡. (Right) Sagittal T2WI FS MR shows focal inflammatory change in the peroneus longus tendon ➡ and marrow edema within the os peroneum ➡ in this patient with peroneus longus tendonitis and painful os peroneum syndrome.

Subtalar Arthritis

Insufficiency Fracture, Fibula

(Left) Coronal reformatted CT shows significant degenerative change at the posterior (lateral) facet of the subtalar joint ➡. Note the associated soft tissue swelling ➡, centered distal to the fibula. (Right) Anteroposterior radiograph shows moderately severe osteopenia in this patient with rheumatoid arthritis. An insufficiency fracture is present in the fibular diaphysis ➡.

Osteochondral Lesion of the Talus

Extensor Digitorum Brevis Avulsion

(Left) Coronal STIR MR shows a classic appearance of an osteochondral lesion of the talus with cyst formation ➡, adjacent edema ➡, and ill-definition of the overlying subchondral bone and articular cartilage. (Right) AP radiograph shows an osseous fragment adjacent to the anterolateral portion of the calcaneus ➡ with associated soft tissue swelling. This extensor digitorum brevis avulsion may also be seen on an AP view of the ankle, 2 cm distal to the tip of fibula.

LATERAL ANKLE PAIN

(Left) *Coronal PD FSE FS MR shows typical MR appearance of a talocalcaneal coalition. The middle facet is hypoplastic* ⮊ *and the joint is narrowed without definite osseous bridging* ➡. *(Right) Lateral radiograph shows a large talar beak* ⮊ *which results from constant traction by the talonavicular ligament. The C sign is a continuous curve from the talar dome to the sustentaculum tali* ➡. *It is an insensitive but specific sign of talocalcaneal coalition.*

Tarsal Coalition

Tarsal Coalition

(Left) *Axial PD FSE FS MR shows a typical case of anterolateral impingement with marked thickening and intrasubstance intermediate signal of the anterior talofibular ligament* ⮊ *and intermediate signal in the anterolateral gutter representing synovitis* ➡. *(Right) Coronal NECT shows a juvenile Tillaux fracture resulting from injury during a specific stage of physeal maturation with closure medially and incomplete fusion laterally.*

Anterolateral Impingement

Tillaux Fracture

(Left) *Axial T2WI FS MR shows a split in the peroneus longus, with subluxation of the anterior fibers of the split* ⮊ *located lateral to the fibula, while the posterior fibers* ⮊ *are in a normal position, posterior to the fibula. The superior peroneal retinaculum is stretched* ➡. *(Right) Sagittal PD FSE FS MR shows extensive soft tissue edema replacing normal fat signal typically seen in the sinus tarsus* ⮊ & *ill-definition of the cervical ligament* ➡ *in this patient with sinus tarsus syndrome.*

Peroneal Tendon Subluxation

Sinus Tarsus Syndrome

LATERAL ANKLE PAIN

Fracture, Lateral Process of Talus

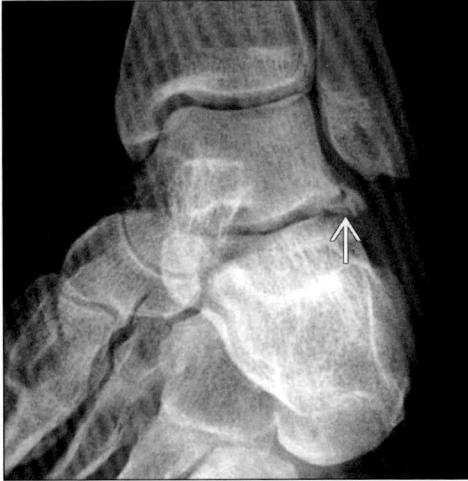

Peroneus Quartus Muscle

(Left) Anteroposterior, mortise view radiograph shows a fracture of the lateral process of the talus with a small nondisplaced fragment ➡. *(Right)* Axial T2WI FSE MR shows a peroneus quartus muscle ➡. The peroneus brevis tendon has a normal appearance ➡ and the peroneus longus tendon is seen divided into two fragments by a longitudinal split tear ➡.

Syndesmosis Sprain

Syndesmosis Sprain

(Left) Axial PD FSE FS MR shows a typical case of injury to the anterior tibiofibular ligament. The ligament is thickened with intermediate signal within ➡ and surrounding soft tissue edema. *(Right)* Coronal STIR MR shows a typical MR appearance of an acute syndesmotic sprain. The injury not only involved the anterior tibiofibular ligament but extended up into the interosseous ligament ➡.

Syndesmotic Impingement

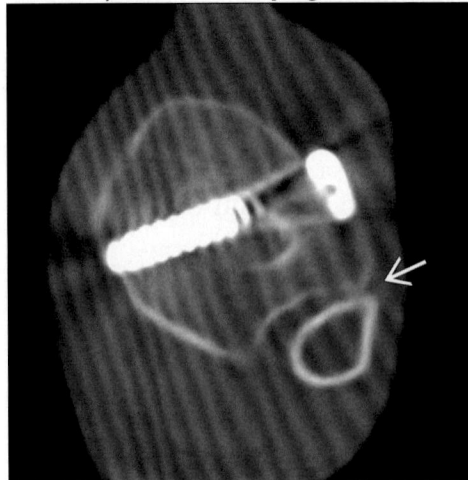

Syndesmotic Impingement

(Left) Axial NECT shows bony impingement of the anterior aspect of the distal tibiofibular syndesmosis. There is anterior subluxation of the fibula, with resultant narrowing anteriorly and frank bony impingement of the tibia and fibula ➡. *(Right)* Axial T2WI MR shows synovitis and chronic fibrosis around an old tear of the anterior inferior tibiofibular (syndesmotic) ligament ➡.

HEEL PAIN

DIFFERENTIAL DIAGNOSIS

Common
- Plantar Fasciitis
- Calcaneal Insufficiency Fracture
- Calcaneal Stress Fracture
- Calcaneal Fracture, Traumatic
- Achilles Tendon Tear & Tendinopathy
- Osteomyelitis

Less Common
- Retrocalcaneal or Retro-Achilles Bursitis
- Plantar Fascia Rupture
- Tarsal Tunnel Syndrome
- Haglund Syndrome
- Foreign Body
- Heel Pad Atrophy
- Chronic Reactive Arthritis (CRA)
- Rheumatoid Arthritis
- Sever Disease
- Psoriatic Arthritis (PSA)

Rare but Important
- Inflammatory Bowel Disease Arthritis (IBD)
- Sarcoidosis
- Neoplasm, Bone
- Tarsal Coalition
- Paget Disease
- Traumatic Neuroma
- Bone Infarct
- Hemophilic Pseudotumor
- Radiation Osteonecrosis

ESSENTIAL INFORMATION

Helpful Clues for Common Diagnoses
- **Plantar Fasciitis**
  - Intermediate to high signal in the normally low signal plantar fascia
  - Continuum from thickening & degeneration to partial thickness tear
  - Most commonly involves the medial band plantar fascia near calcaneal attachment
  - May have reactive edema in the calcaneus & surrounding soft tissue edema
- **Calcaneal Insufficiency Fracture**
  - Oriented perpendicular to the bone trabeculae/long axis of bone
  - Most common location: Posterior tubercle
  - Second most common location parallels the subtalar joint
  - Variant: Diabetic calcaneal insufficiency avulsion fracture
    - Avulsed posterior tubercle of calcaneus
    - May see associated vascular calcifications
- **Calcaneal Stress Fracture**
  - Similar appearance as calcaneal insufficiency fractures
  - Differentiate by clinical presentation
    - Stress fx: Younger patient, overuse
    - Insufficiency fx: Older, osteopenic
- **Calcaneal Fracture, Traumatic**
  - Several classification schemes; Sanders classification most often used
  - Key features for classification
    - Intraarticular or extraarticular
    - Extension into subtalar joint
    - Number of fracture fragments in subtalar joint on coronal images
    - Medial to lateral location of the subtalar joint fractures
- **Achilles Tendon Tear & Tendinopathy**
  - Tendon thickening appears as round configuration on axial images
  - Increased signal on T1WI & T2WI
  - Watershed area 2-6 cm proximal to calcaneal insertion is prone to tear
  - Location of tear, cross-sectional area involvement & extent are important for surgical planning
- **Osteomyelitis**
  - Abnormal bone marrow edema & enhancement on MR
  - Progressive destruction of bone seen on serial radiographs
  - Look for abscess or sinus tract extending from skin surface to bone

Helpful Clues for Less Common Diagnoses
- **Retrocalcaneal or Retro-Achilles Bursitis**
  - Focal collections of fluid around the calcaneus & Achilles tendon
  - Retrocalcaneal bursa located at posterosuperior aspect of calcaneus, dorsally bordered by Achilles tendon
  - Retro-Achilles bursa located dorsal to Achilles tendon, deep to subcutaneous fat
- **Plantar Fascia Rupture**
  - High signal, fluid-filled gap along the course of plantar fascia
  - Rupture at proximal or mid portion
- **Tarsal Tunnel Syndrome**
  - Mass or scar along course of posterior tibial nerve, deep to flexor retinaculum
  - Edema in tarsal tunnel on MR

HEEL PAIN

- Associated clinical findings of pain & muscle weakness
- **Haglund Syndrome**
  - Enlarged calcaneal tuberosity
    - a.k.a., "pump bump"
  - Retrocalcaneal & retro-Achilles bursitis
- **Foreign Body**
  - Wide variety of foreign bodies may be embedded in heel during walking
  - Foreign object may not be visible on imaging, especially organic material
  - Surrounding edema on MR
- **Heel Pad Atrophy**
  - Atrophy of the subcutaneous fat
  - May have history of steroid injections
  - Associated with plantar fascia rupture
- **CRA, PSA, IBD Arthritis**
  - Calcaneus involved in 50% of cases CRA
  - Erosions & reactive spurring at Achilles tendon and plantar aponeurosis
- **Rheumatoid Arthritis**
  - Erosions involving the calcaneus are located near the plantar aponeurosis & Achilles tendon attachments
  - Look for classic rheumatoid erosions in metacarpal & metatarsal heads
- **Sever Disease**
  - Calcaneal apophysitis in preteen patients
  - Sclerosis & fragmentation of the calcaneal apophysis on radiographs is somewhat unreliable due to anatomic variation
  - Calcaneal apophysis edema on MR

Helpful Clues for Rare Diagnoses
- **Sarcoidosis**
  - Bilateral heel pain with or before arthritis
- **Neoplasm, Bone**
  - Some neoplastic entities are not painful unless bone cortex is traversed or associated with pathologic fracture
  - Simple bone cyst, intraosseous lipoma, Ewing sarcoma, metastases, chondroblastoma, chondrosarcoma, osteosarcoma
- **Tarsal Coalition**
  - Talocalcaneal or calcaneonavicular may cause hindfoot pain
  - Bony, cartilaginous or fibrous fusion
- **Paget Disease**
  - Sclerotic stage has thickened cortex & coarsened trabeculae
  - Calcaneal involvement in 3-10% of cases
- **Traumatic Neuroma**
  - Focal mass along course of nerve
  - Area of amputation or trauma
- **Bone Infarct**
  - Serpiginous sclerosis within bone
  - Predilection for posterior half of the calcaneus
- **Hemophilic Pseudotumor**
  - Calcaneus one of 3 top locations
- **Radiation Osteonecrosis**
  - Delineated by location of radiation port
  - Mixed lytic and sclerotic changes in bone may mimic an aggressive entity

Plantar Fasciitis

Sagittal T2WI FS MR shows thickening and increased signal in the medial head of the plantar fascia ➡, with surrounding soft tissue edema and marrow edema in the calcaneal origin ➡.

Calcaneal Insufficiency Fracture

Sagittal T1WI MR shows an oblique low intensity fracture ➡ extending posterosuperior to anteroinferior across the posterior calcaneus, perpendicular to the primary trabecular struts.

HEEL PAIN

Calcaneal Insufficiency Fracture

Calcaneal Stress Fracture

(Left) Lateral radiograph shows a calcaneal insufficiency avulsion fracture of the calcaneus in a diabetic patient. Note the vascular calcification ⇒. The fracture pattern is across the posterior tubercle of the calcaneus ⇒, with the Achilles tendon elevating the fracture fragment. *(Right)* Sagittal T1WI MR shows an incomplete, low signal intensity fracture line ⇒ is present in the body of the calcaneus, with mild surrounding bone marrow edema.

Calcaneal Fracture, Traumatic

Achilles Tendon Tear & Tendinopathy

(Left) Axial bone CT shows a calcaneal shear fracture, divided into anteromedial ⇒ and posterolateral ⇒ fragments. The anteromedial fragment maintains alignment with the talus, while the posterolateral fragment is angulated and depressed ⇒. *(Right)* Sagittal T2WI FS MR shows marked thickening, increased signal and partial thickness tearing of the distal Achilles tendon ⇒. A mild amount of fluid is present in the retro-Achilles bursa ⇒.

Achilles Tendon Tear & Tendinopathy

Osteomyelitis

(Left) Sagittal T2WI FS MR shows a thickened distal Achilles tendon ⇒. Intermediate signal is consistent with tendinopathy. Bursal fluid is present in both retrocalcaneal ⇒ and retro-Achilles ⇒ regions. *(Right)* Coronal T1WI FS MR shows extensive enhancement within the marrow of the calcaneus ⇒. A sinus tract ⇒ is clearly depicted extending to bone. There is loss of the cortical margin where the sinus tract abuts the calcaneus.

HEEL PAIN

Plantar Fascia Rupture

Tarsal Tunnel Syndrome

(Left) Sagittal T2WI FS MR shows disruption in the plantar fascia ➜ with mild surrounding soft tissue edema. The torn fascia ends are thickened either due to the tear with mild retraction or due to pre-existing plantar fasciitis. (Right) Sagittal T2WI FS MR shows a round fluid signal mass in the tarsal tunnel ➜, located just posterior to the tibial nerve ➜. This is a ganglion cyst in the tarsal tunnel which resulted in clinical tarsal tunnel syndrome.

Haglund Syndrome

Foreign Body

(Left) Sagittal T2WI FS MR shows tremendous thickening of the distal Achilles tendon ➜. There is an enthesophyte arising at the tendon insertional site ➜ and an increased amount of fluid within the retrocalcaneal bursa ➜. (Right) Oblique radiograph shows a subtle linear lucency ➜ in the soft tissues of the heel. The round skin entrance site ➜ of the embedded golf tee is better seen.

Chronic Reactive Arthritis (CRA)

Chronic Reactive Arthritis (CRA)

(Left) Lateral radiograph shows dense reactive change with ➜ enthesopathy and effacement of the normal pre-Achilles fat pad. This is not pathognomonic of chronic reactive arthritis, but that is the most likely diagnosis for this appearance. (Right) Lateral radiograph shows severe erosive disease of the posterior calcaneus in a patient with chronic reactive arthritis ➜. Note the normal bone density. CRA may be erosive, productive, or mixed, depending on stage.

HEEL PAIN

Rheumatoid Arthritis

Rheumatoid Arthritis

(Left) Lateral radiograph shows severe erosive disease ⇒ as well as soft tissue swelling & obliteration of the pre-Achilles fat pad. Though this could represent any inflammatory arthritis, it is rheumatoid arthritis in this case. **(Right)** Lateral radiograph shows erosions ⇒ involving the plantar aspect of the calcaneus adjacent to the attachment of the plantar aponeurosis, as well as soft tissue inflammation ⇒, all secondary to rheumatoid arthritis.

Sever Disease

Psoriatic Arthritis (PSA)

(Left) Sagittal T2WI FS MR shows inflammatory change with edema in the calcaneal apophysis ⇒ and metaphysis ⇒. Retrocalcaneal bursitis ⇒ and retro-Achilles edema are present in this child with Sever disease, or calcaneal apophysitis. **(Right)** Lateral radiograph shows mixed erosive ⇒ and productive ⇒ change involving the posterior calcaneus. This patient has psoriatic arthritis with involvement of the heel.

Inflammatory Bowel Disease Arthritis (IBD)

Neoplasm, Bone

(Left) Lateral radiograph shows subtle filling in of the pre-Achilles fat pad ⇒, indicating an inflammatory process in this child who refuses to walk and had a several month history of diarrhea. This represents inflammatory bowel disease arthropathy. **(Right)** Sagittal T2WI FS MR shows a mass ⇒ involving the posterior calcaneus. The normal low signal marrow is obliterated. Both primary and malignant tumors should be considered in this region. Biopsy showed metastatic melanoma.

HEEL PAIN

Neoplasm, Bone

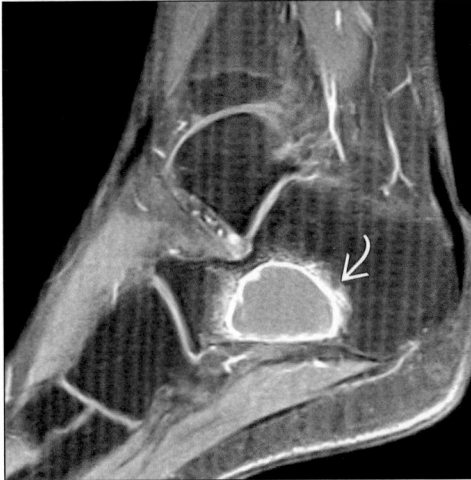

Neoplasm, Bone

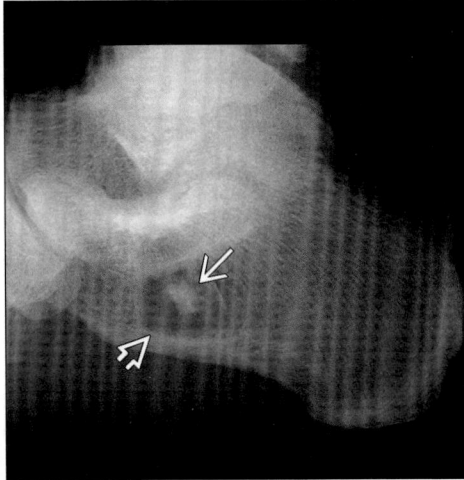

(Left) Sagittal T1 C+ FS MR shows rim-enhancement around a unicameral bone cyst ➡. This is a common location for this lesion; it becomes painful if a pathologic fracture develops. *(Right)* Lateral radiograph shows a lytic lesion ➡ involving the portion of the calcaneus typically seen with intraosseous lipoma or unicameral bone cyst. The central calcific density ➡ proves the former diagnosis. This lesion may be asymptomatic unless it develops pathologic fracture.

Tarsal Coalition

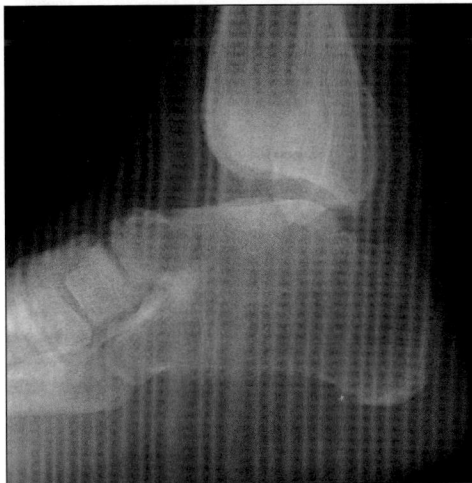

Bone Infarct

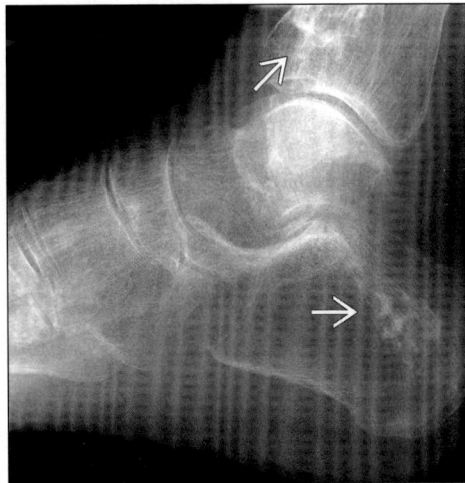

(Left) Lateral radiograph shows extensive coalition at the talocalcaneal, talonavicular, and calcaneocuboid joints. This results in a painful hindfoot and ball-and-socket tibiotalar joint. *(Right)* Lateral radiograph shows typical serpiginous bone infarcts in the calcaneus and distal tibia ➡. This patient had no known risk for infarction.

Hemophilic Pseudotumor

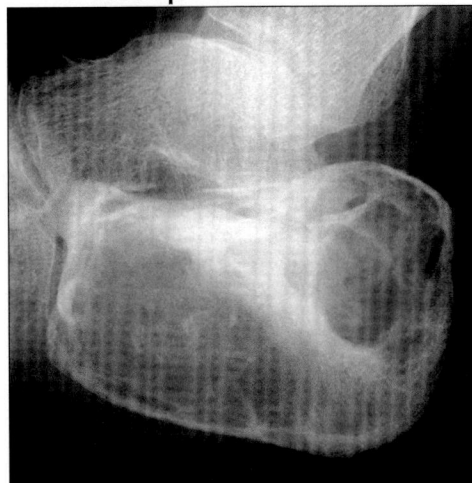

Radiation Osteonecrosis

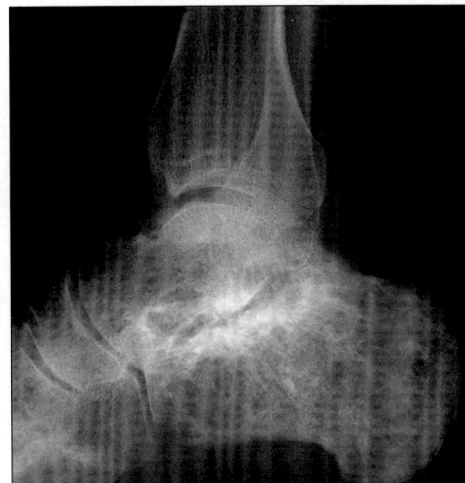

(Left) Lateral radiograph shows a bubbly appearance replacing the entire calcaneus. This young male has hemophilia and this lesion has developed slowly over the course of several years. It developed secondary to subperiosteal and intraosseous bleeds. *(Right)* Lateral radiograph shows a port-like distribution of mixed lytic & sclerotic bone density involving the entire calcaneus and the plantar portion of the talus. The patient was treated 10 years earlier for PNET.

PAIN IN THE BALL OF THE FOOT

DIFFERENTIAL DIAGNOSIS

Common
- High Impact Activities
- Obesity
- Improperly Fitting Shoes
- High Heel Shoes
- Osteoarthritis
- Aging
- Acute Trauma
- Stress Fracture
- Hallux Valgus Deformity & Other Malalignment Deformities
- Morton Neuroma
- Vascular Insufficiency
- Gout
- Cellulitis/Ulcer/Abscess
- Osteomyelitis & Septic Arthritis
- Diabetes: MSK Complications
- Bursitis

Less Common
- Freiberg Infarction
- Rheumatoid Arthritis (RA)
- Sesamoiditis
- Foreign Body
- Plantar Plate Rupture
- Neuralgia
- Psoriatic Arthritis
- Chronic Reactive Arthritis
- High Arch
- Plantar Fibromatosis
- Heel Cord Contracture

Rare but Important
- Coalition

ESSENTIAL INFORMATION

Key Differential Diagnosis Issues
- Underlying factors include excessive activity, abnormal forces or altered foot mechanics
- Many entities on the list are clinical only, may cause pain without imaging abnormality or may predispose to other conditions with imaging abnormalities

Helpful Clues for Common Diagnoses
- **Osteoarthritis**
  - Especially 1st MTP & sesamoids
  - Joint space narrowing, subchondral sclerosis, cysts, osteophytes
- **Acute Trauma**

- Especially phalangeal, MT neck fractures
- **Stress Fracture**
  - Especially 2, 3, 4 metatarsals
    - Sesamoids less commonly involved
  - Radiographs, CT may be negative
  - MR shows soft tissue & marrow edema ± fracture line
- **Hallux Valgus Deformity & Other Malalignment Deformities**
  - Requires weight-bearing views to diagnose
  - Hallux valgus angle: Angle between long axis 1st metatarsal & 1st proximal phalanx, abnormal > 15°
  - Associated bunion, 1st MTP osteoarthritis, sesamoid subluxation
    - Bunion: Bone proliferation or bursa over medial eminence 1st metatarsal head
  - Morton toe: Short 1st metatarsal, long 2nd toe alters mechanics
  - Hammertoe: MTP neutral/extended, PIP flexion
  - Claw toe: MTP extension, PIP & DIP flexion
- **Morton Neuroma**
  - Perineural fibrosis plantar digital nerve
  - Intermittent pain
  - Common site is third web space
  - MR: Low to intermediate on T1 & T2WI, most conspicuous on T1, diffusely enhances
- **Gout**
  - Synovitis in acute phase, early disease
  - May develop 2° osteoarthritis
  - Tophi: Soft tissue or intra-osseous
    - Create erosions which may be marginal, peri-articular, nonarticular; have sclerotic margins, overhanging edges; < 15% calcify
    - MR intermediate to low on T1WI, variable on T2WI, diffuse enhancement
- **Cellulitis/Ulcer/Abscess**
  - Diabetics: Vascular insufficiency
  - Cellulitis: Subcutaneous edema
  - Ulcer: Soft tissue defect, may contain air
  - Abscess: Rim-enhancing fluid collection
- **Osteomyelitis & Septic Arthritis**
  - Diabetics: Vascular insufficiency
  - Direct spread from soft tissue infection
  - Over pressure points especially 1st, 5th metatarsal heads

PAIN IN THE BALL OF THE FOOT

- ○ Radiographs: Osteopenia, bone destruction, joint space narrowing, air
- ○ MR: Marrow & soft tissue edema, bone destruction, effusion, sinus tract
- **Diabetes: MSK Complications**
  - ○ Changes related to infection, vascular insufficiency or Charcot disease, may lead to other deformities such as hammer toe
- **Bursitis**
  - ○ Intermetatarsal, plantar surface metatarsal heads, within bunion

Helpful Clues for Less Common Diagnoses
- **Freiberg Infarction**
  - ○ 2nd & 3rd MT heads; common in women
  - ○ Radiographs: Subchondral fracture, fragmentation, articular surface flattening
  - ○ MR
    - ■ Early: Nonspecific edema
    - ■ Late: Dark on fluid sensitive sequence
- **Rheumatoid Arthritis (RA)**
  - ○ Bilateral symmetric erosive arthritis, peri-articular osteopenia, MTP joints common
- **Sesamoiditis**
  - ○ Causes the following
    - ■ Periosteal inflammation
    - ■ AVN: Dark marrow signal T1 & T2WI
    - ■ Fracture: Trauma or stress; high rate of nonunion; medial > lateral
- **Foreign Body**
  - ○ US, CT, MR for nonradiopaque objects
  - ○ Soft tissue edema, foreign body granuloma, osseous pseudotumor

- **Plantar Plate Rupture**
  - ○ 2-5 MTP joints (particularly 2nd); F > M
  - ○ Radiographs, CT normal
  - ○ MR: Edema base metatarsal head; edema, thinning or discontinuity of plate
  - ○ Turf Toe: 1st MTP hyperextension injury
    - ■ Male, kicking on artificial turf
    - ■ Complete rupture may result in malpositioned sesamoids
- **Psoriatic Arthritis**
  - ○ Bilateral asymmetric erosive arthritis, periostitis, ankylosis
  - ○ DIP, PIP, MTP joints
  - ○ Sausage digit
  - ○ Ivory digit (distal phalanx great toe)
  - ○ Hands more common than feet
- **Chronic Reactive Arthritis**
  - ○ Imaging identical to psoriasis
  - ○ Feet more common than hands
- **High Arch**
  - ○ Cavus deformity on weight-bearing view
  - ○ Increases pressure on ball of foot
- **Plantar Fibromatosis**
  - ○ Variable size soft tissue mass(es) arise in plantar fascia
  - ○ Pain not common
  - ○ MR: Intermediate to low T1, variable mainly intermediate T2

Helpful Clues for Rare Diagnoses
- **Coalition**
  - ○ Isolated or with other anomalies
    - ■ Midfoot rare relative to hindfoot

Osteoarthritis

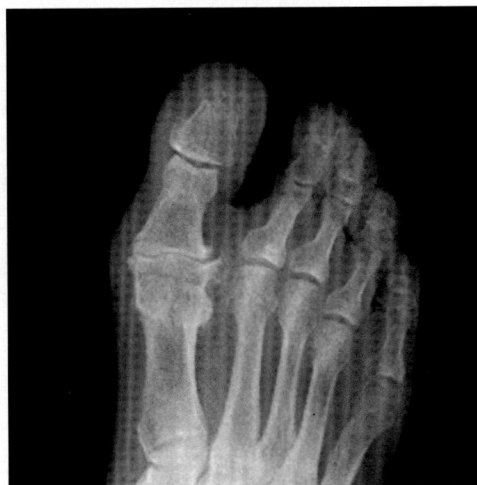

Anteroposterior radiograph shows classic osteoarthritis of the first MTP joint with joint space narrowing, subchondral sclerosis and osteophyte formation.

Osteoarthritis

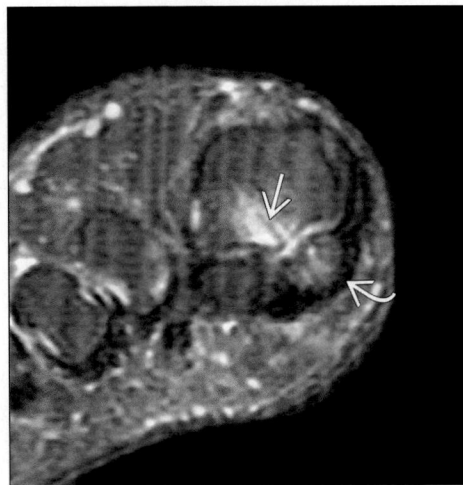

Coronal T2WI FS MR shows degenerative arthritis of the hallux-sesamoid joint. The cartilage space is narrowed and subchondral signal changes are present in the metatarsal ➡ and the tibial sesamoid ➡.

PAIN IN THE BALL OF THE FOOT

Acute Trauma

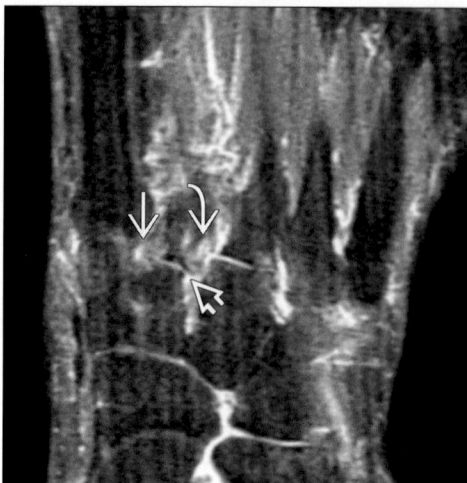

Stress Fracture

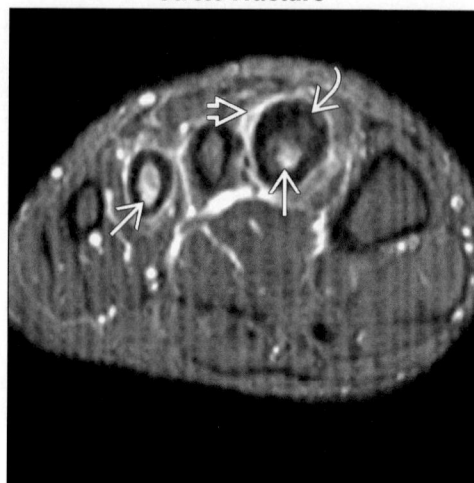

(Left) Axial STIR MR shows marrow edema in the base of the second metatarsal ➡. The Lisfranc ligament is disrupted near its medial cuneiform attachment ➡ in this patient with a Lisfranc dislocation. Note the lateral subluxation of the second metatarsal ➡. *(Right)* Coronal STIR MR shows second & fourth metatarsal stress fractures with marrow edema ➡ and adjacent soft tissue edema ➡. Cortical thickening of the second metatarsal ➡ is also present.

Hallux Valgus Deformity & Other Malalignment Deformities

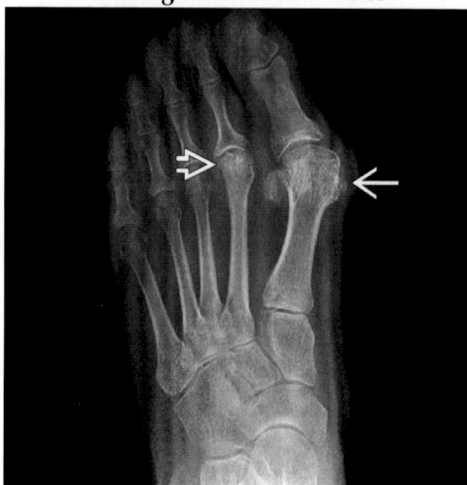

Hallux Valgus Deformity & Other Malalignment Deformities

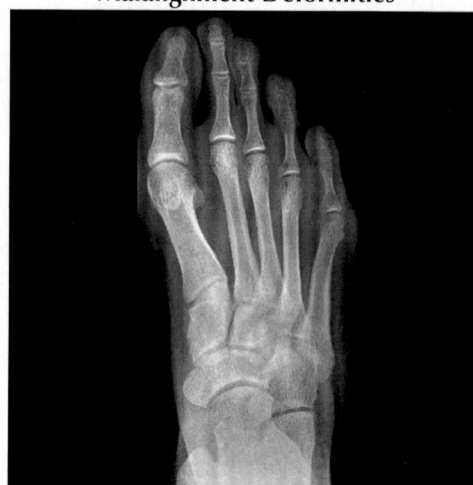

(Left) Anteroposterior radiograph shows a hallux valgus deformity. Bone proliferation is present on the medial eminence of the 1st metatarsal head consistent with bunion ➡. Altered mechanics has lead to Freiberg infarction of the 2nd metatarsal head ➡. *(Right)* Anteroposterior radiograph shows a Morton toe configuration. The first metatarsal is short and the second toe is longer than the first. A mild hallux valgus deformity is present as well.

Morton Neuroma

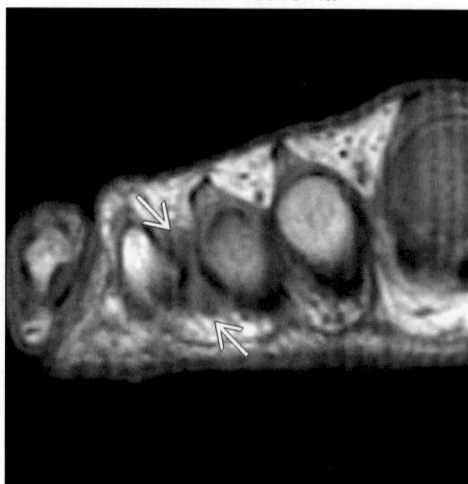

Morton Neuroma

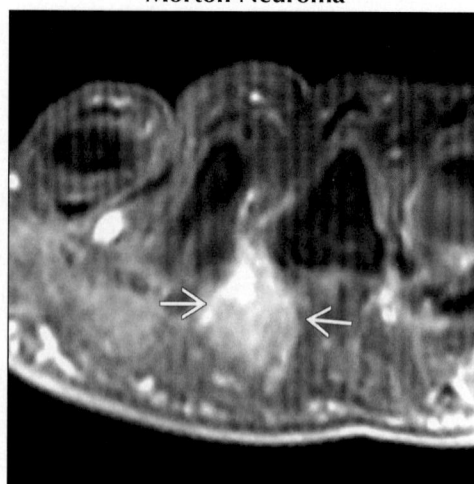

(Left) Coronal T1WI MR shows an intermediate signal bulbous soft tissue mass ➡ between the third and fourth metatarsal heads extending slightly plantarward. Slight widening between the third and fourth metatarsals is also present in this patient with a Morton neuroma. *(Right)* Axial T1 C+ FS MR shows typical example of a Morton neuroma appearing as a mass with heterogeneous enhancement ➡ between the third and fourth metatarsals.

PAIN IN THE BALL OF THE FOOT

Gout

Gout

(Left) Anteroposterior radiograph shows typical changes of gout in the foot. Osseous erosions from tophi are seen within the articular surface of the proximal phalangeal head and along the shaft ➡. The 3rd toe is also involved ➡. *(Right)* Sagittal T2WI MR shows severe circumferential destruction of the neck of the 1st metatarsal with an associated soft tissue mass ➡. The mass shows low signal on this T2 weighted image, typical of a tophus.

Cellulitis/Ulcer/Abscess

Osteomyelitis & Septic Arthritis

(Left) Coronal T1 C+ MR shows soft tissue abscess formation along the dorsum of the foot ➡ complicating septic arthritis of the great toe in this diabetic patient. Note the extensive phlegmon surrounding the metatarsal neck ➡. *(Right)* Oblique radiograph shows severe periarticular osteopenia, osseous destruction along the articular surfaces of the proximal and distal phalanx ➡ in this patient with diabetes complicated by septic arthritis and osteomyelitis.

Diabetes: MSK Complications

Bursitis

(Left) Oblique radiograph shows typical case of soft tissue infection with gas forming organism and associated Charcot changes. Extensive soft tissue air is present and the articulation between the navicular and the medial cuneiform is disrupted ➡. *(Right)* Coronal T1 C+ MR shows a large bursa beneath the first MTP joint ➡. No enhancement is seen within the wall. The mass had been present for several months and was becoming increasingly painful.

PAIN IN THE BALL OF THE FOOT

(Left) *Anteroposterior radiograph shows Freiberg infraction involving both the second and third metatarsal heads* ➡. *Findings include subchondral fracture and articular surface collapse.* **(Right)** *Axial inversion recovery FSE MR shows erosion involving the fifth metatarsal head* ➡ *and surrounding synovitis* ➡ *in this young patient with newly diagnosed rheumatoid arthritis. The 5th metatarsal is often the earliest site of involvement in the foot by RA.*

Freiberg Infraction

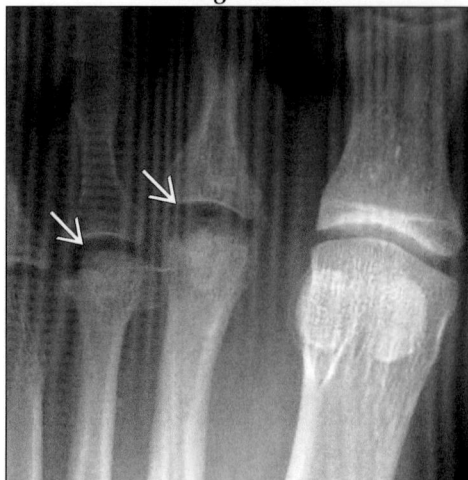

Rheumatoid Arthritis (RA)

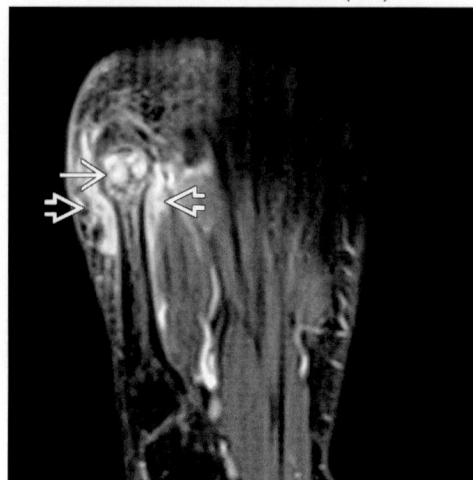

(Left) *Coronal T1WI MR shows an acute fracture of the medial sesamoid. Diffuse marrow edema is present in the tibial sesamoid* ➡. *The fracture line was seen on other images.* **(Right)** *Coronal T1WI MR shows avascular necrosis of the lateral hallux sesamoid* ➡, *with sclerosis and resultant low signal intensity of the marrow on all imaging sequences.*

Sesamoiditis

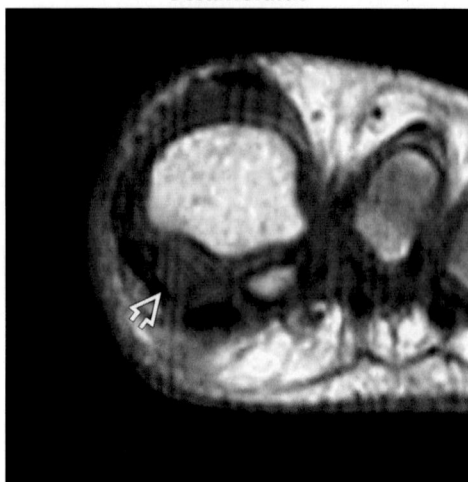

Sesamoiditis

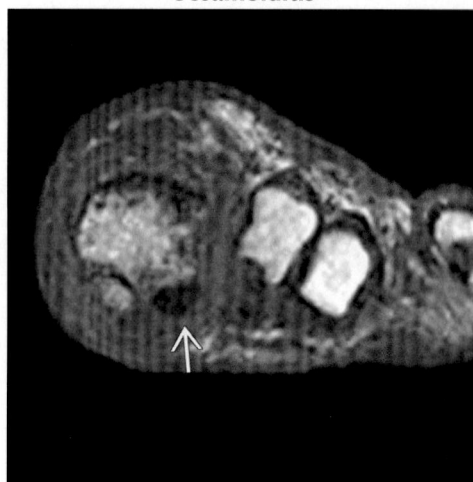

(Left) *Coronal T1 C+ FS MR shows low signal foreign bodies* ➡ *surrounded by inflammatory reaction. This patient had stepped on glass, but the foreign bodies were not demonstrable by radiograph.* **(Right)** *Coronal bone CT demonstrates widening between the first metatarsal head and the tibial sesamoid* ➡. *The sesamoids are laterally subluxated which can only result from loss of the stabilizing medial collateral ligament and medial portion of the plantar plate.*

Foreign Body

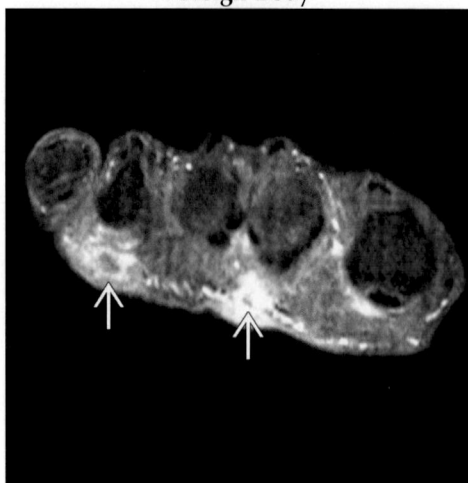

Plantar Plate Rupture

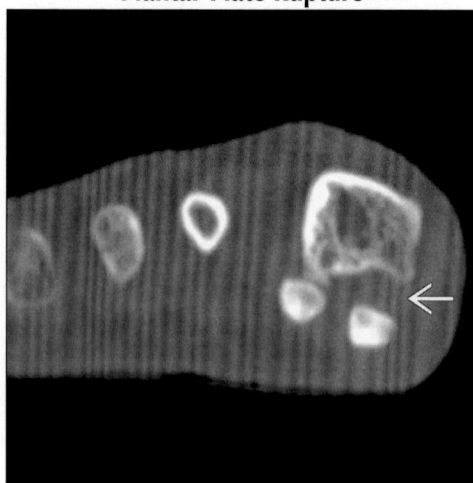

PAIN IN THE BALL OF THE FOOT

Plantar Plate Rupture

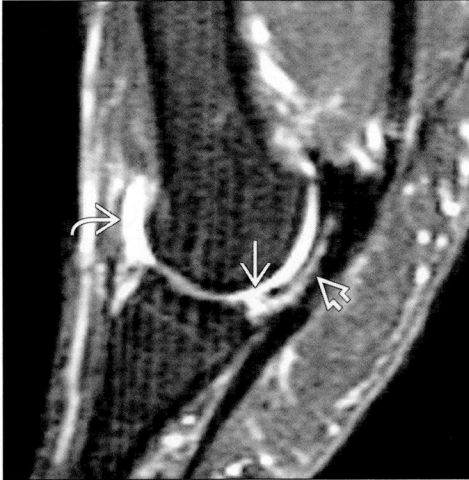

Psoriatic Arthritis

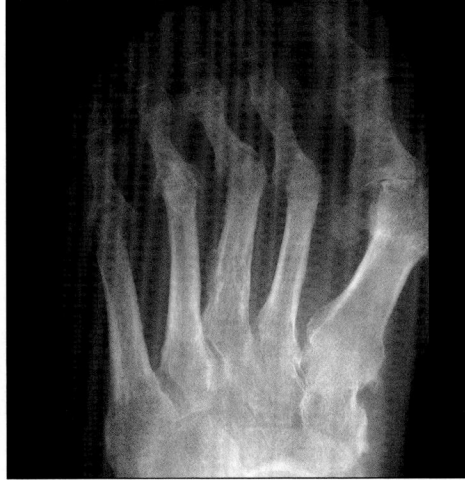

(Left) Sagittal T2WI FS MR shows disruption of the plantar plate of the great toe with discontinuity ➡ and diffuse internal signal ➡. A joint effusion is also present ➡. *(Right)* Anteroposterior radiograph shows diffuse MTP erosive change, with early pencil-in-cup erosions typical of psoriatic arthritis. Note the periostitis; psoriatic arthritis often shows mixed erosive and productive changes.

Chronic Reactive Arthritis

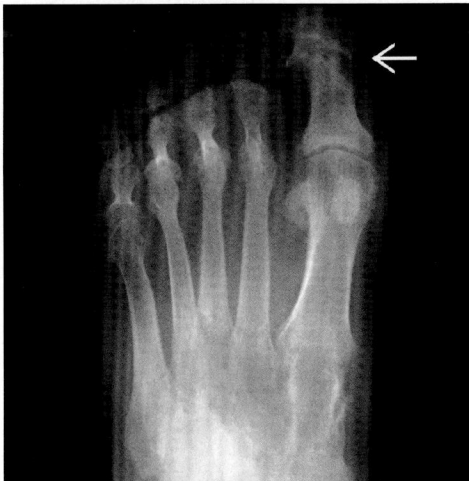

High Arch

(Left) Anteroposterior radiograph shows predominantly erosive change at the IP joint of the great toe ➡ with adjacent whiskering in this patient with chronic reactive arthritis. *(Right)* Lateral radiograph shows pes cavovarus in a patient with Charcot Marie Tooth. This malalignment may result in added pressure on the ball of the foot, resulting in pain.

Plantar Fibromatosis

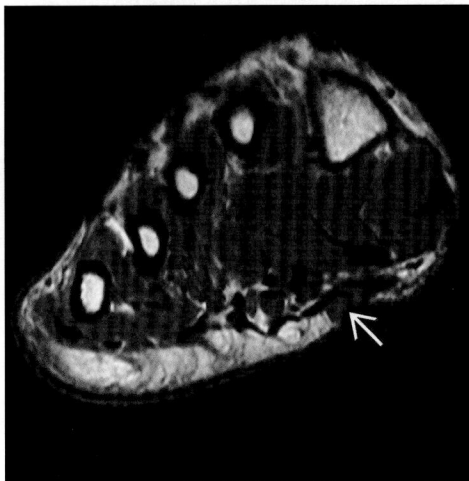

Coalition

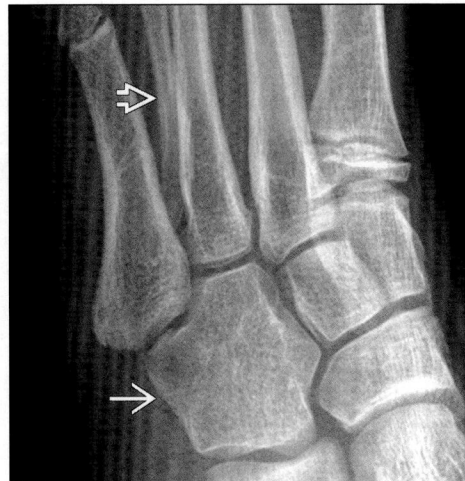

(Left) Coronal T1WI MR shows a small mass with intermediate signal arising from the plantar fascia ➡. The mass had intermediate signal on all sequences consistent with plantar fibromatosis. *(Right)* Oblique radiograph shows a cubocuneiform coalition ➡ accompanied by a hypoplastic 4th metatarsal ➡. This is an uncommon form of tarsal coalition.

PES PLANO VALGUS (FLATFOOT)

DIFFERENTIAL DIAGNOSIS

Common
- Pes Planus (Mimic)
- Pes Planovalgus (Flexible Flatfoot)
- Tibialis Posterior Tendon Tear
- Diabetic Foot
- Traumatic Lisfranc Ligament Disruption

Less Common
- Tarsal Coalition
- Congenital Vertical Talus (Rocker Bottom Foot)

Rare but Important
- Marfan Syndrome
- Ehlers Danlos
- Rheumatoid Arthritis

ESSENTIAL INFORMATION

Key Differential Diagnosis Issues
- Terminology of "flatfoot deformity" is variable & confusing
  - Pes planus, pes valgus, congenital hypermobile flatfoot, talipes calcaneovalgus, compensated talipes equinus, collapsing pes valgo planus
- Multiple etiologies are recognized & even more are theorized
- Clinically, the foot is recognized as having some or all of the following
  - Everted heel
  - Abduction of forefoot on hindfoot
  - Collapse of medial column
  - Flexibility of foot with reducibility of deformity
- Support of arch depends on several factors, both dynamic & static
  - Osseous architecture
  - Intrinsic & extrinsic musculature/tendons
  - Fascia & ligaments
- Basic definitions and measurements
  - Hindfoot valgus: ↑ Talocalcaneal angle
    - On lateral, T-C angle normally 25-55°
    - On AP, T-C angle normally 15-40°
  - Calcaneal pitch angle: 20-30°
  - Forefoot pronation: On AP, metatarsals do not converge at bases
  - Forefoot pronation on lateral: Angle of inclination decreases for metatarsals 1-4

Helpful Clues for Common Diagnoses
- **Pes Planus (Mimic)**
  - "Low arch foot"
  - Not synonymous with unstable hypermobile pes valgus deformity
  - Not necessarily a pathologically pronating foot & may have no other morphological abnormalities
  - Generally does not require treatment
- **Pes Planovalgus (Flexible Flatfoot)**
  - Common abnormality
  - Requires weight-bearing radiographs to make the diagnosis
    - Hindfoot shows valgus deformity (increased talocalcaneal angle on both AP and lateral weight-bearing radiographs)
    - Forefoot shows pronation/valgus deformity (on lateral, metatarsals are superimposed, with ↓ inclination angle 1st MT; on AP, ↓ convergence at bases of metatarsals
    - No equinus
  - Flexible (non-fixed) deformity: Non-weight-bearing radiographs are completely normal
- **Tibialis Posterior Tendon Tear**
  - Most common etiology of new onset flatfoot deformity in middle-aged to elderly women
  - Tibialis posterior tendon characteristics leading to flatfoot deformity
    - Tibialis posterior tendon has the longest lever arm & is the most efficient supinator of foot
    - Arch-stabilizing effect also attributed to its extensive ligamentous support provided by its many deep insertions
    - Damaged tendon prevents normal resupination of foot when walking → leads to pronated foot & flexible pes planovalgus
  - MR appearance of tear may be variable
    - Complete rupture w/retraction is unusual
    - Altered morphology: Usually enlargement of the tendon, but may be thin (note, tibialis posterior tendon is normally twice as large in diameter as flexor digitorum)
    - Increased signal within tendon
- **Diabetic Foot**

PES PLANO VALGUS (FLATFOOT)

○ Neuropathic joints generally result in collapse of longitudinal arch
  - Lisfranc (tarso-metatarsal joints)
  - Mid-tarsal joints
  - Chopart articulation (midfoot-hindfoot: Calcaneocuboid & talonavicular)
○ Associated abnormalities
  - Vascular calcifications
  - Fragmentation & dislocation of joints
  - Large fluid collections
- **Traumatic Lisfranc Ligament Disruption**
  ○ If Lisfranc ligament disruption is not detected and treated
    - Progressive disruption of the tarso-metatarsal joints
    - Develops pronation of forefoot, with collapse of the longitudinal arch

Helpful Clues for Less Common Diagnoses
- **Tarsal Coalition**
  ○ Also termed "spastic peroneal flatfoot"
  ○ Most common etiology of painful flatfoot in 2nd & 3rd decades
  ○ Most frequent coalitions are talocalcaneal and calcaneonavicular
  ○ Coalition decreases motion in hindfoot; in turn, other tarsal joints increase their motion to retain flexibility
  ○ "Flatfoot" occurs due to spastic peroneal contraction, pulling the forefoot/midfoot into pronation
  ○ Watch for
    - Direct sign of calcaneonavicular coalition: Seen on oblique radiograph
    - Indirect sign of coalition: Talar beak
    - Indirect sign of calcaneonavicular coalition: "Anteater" extension of anterior calcaneus on lateral
    - Indirect sign of talocalcaneal coalition: "C" sign of subtalar sclerosis on lateral radiograph
- **Congenital Vertical Talus (Rocker Bottom Foot)**
  ○ Rigid flatfoot deformity
  ○ Four required abnormalities
    - Plantarflexed talus, dislocated from navicular
    - Hindfoot valgus (increased talocalcaneal angle on both AP and lateral)
    - Forefoot pronation & valgus (lateral shows superimposition of metatarsals, with angle of inclination significantly decreased for first MT; AP shows decreased convergence at bases of MTs)
    - Hindfoot equinus

Helpful Clues for Rare Diagnoses
- **Marfan Syndrome**
  ○ Ligamentous laxity results from defect in collagen synthesis
  ○ Foot structure stretches & relaxes; develops hypermobility
- **Ehlers Danlos:** Similar to Marfan
- **Rheumatoid Arthritis**
  ○ As in the hand, ligamentous stretching & disruption may result in abnormal motion at the osseous articulations, with collapse of the arch

Pes Planus (Mimic)

Lateral radiograph shows a low arch, but no evidence of hindfoot valgus and no suggestion of pronation. This is the full extent of the abnormalities in this patient, and does not need surgical treatment.

Pes Planovalgus (Flexible Flatfoot)

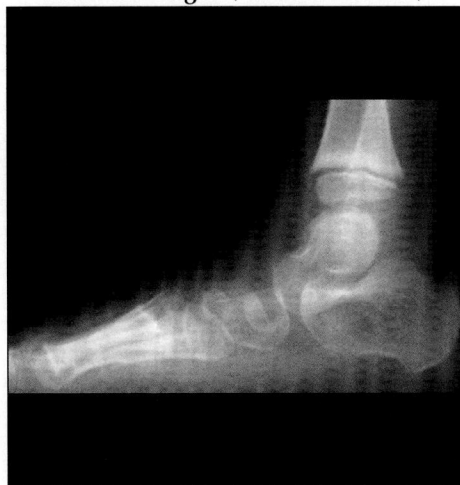

Lateral weight-bearing radiograph shows a valgus hindfoot (↑ talocalcaneal angle) and pronated forefoot (superimposed metatarsals, decreased metatarsal inclination angle). This is a flexible flatfoot deformity.

PES PLANO VALGUS (FLATFOOT)

Pes Planovalgus (Flexible Flatfoot)

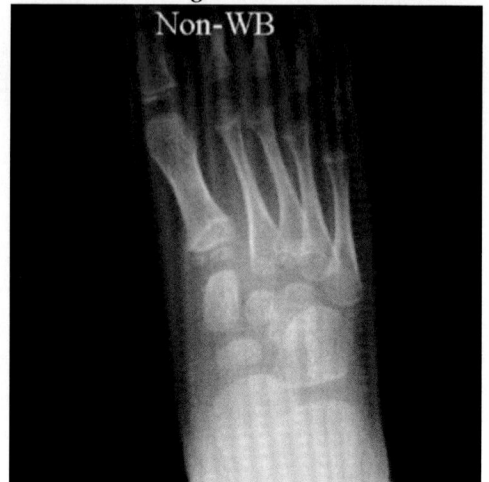

WB

Pes Planovalgus (Flexible Flatfoot)

Non-WB

(Left) AP weight-bearing radiograph shows increased talocalcaneal angle, indicating valgus hindfoot. The metatarsals do not show normal convergence at the bases, indicating pronation. *(Right)* AP non-weight-bearing radiograph of the same patient, taken on the same day as the prior image, shows the flexible nature of this deformity. The hindfoot valgus as well as forefoot pronation have completely reduced.

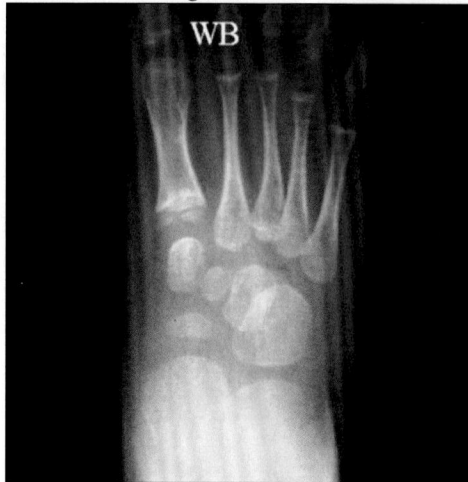

Tibialis Posterior Tendon Tear

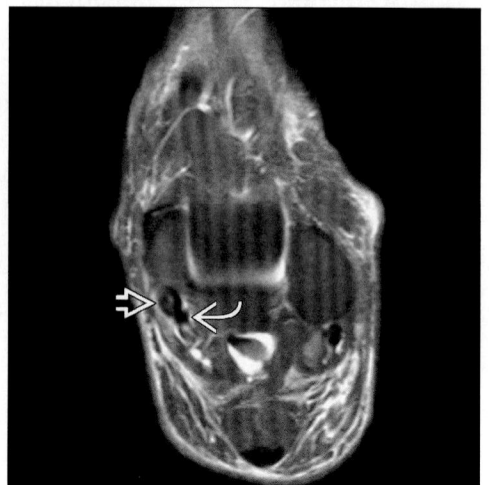

Tibialis Posterior Tendon Tear

(Left) Lateral radiograph shows a mild valgus hindfoot, with early collapse of the midfoot. Note that the articulations of the talus, navicular & cuneiform articular surfaces are not as parallel as expected ➡. *(Right)* Axial PD FSE FS MR in the same patient shows the tibialis posterior tendon to be enlarged ➡ relative to flexor digitorum ➡. It also contains central high signal. These morphologic changes indicate tendon tear.

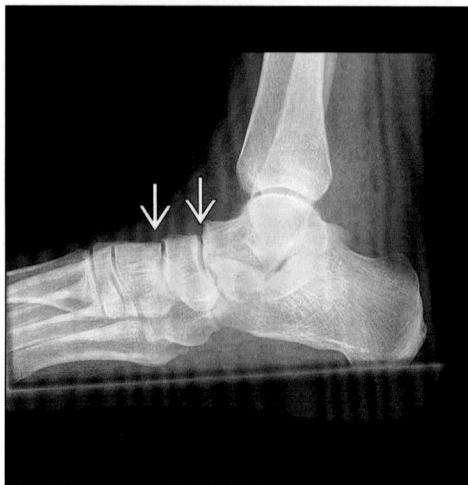

Diabetic Foot

Diabetic Foot

(Left) Lateral radiograph shows collapse and resorption of the talus, deformity of the calcaneus, and subluxation of the Chopart (hindfoot-midfoot) articulation, resulting in loss of the normal longitudinal arch. This patient is diabetic and the findings result from Charcot joint changes. *(Right)* AP radiograph of the same patient confirms the destruction at the calcaneocuboid joint and talonavicular dislocation, typical of neuropathic Chopart joint.

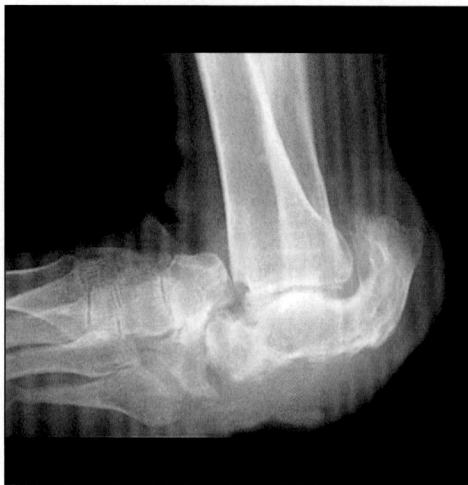

PES PLANO VALGUS (FLATFOOT)

Traumatic Lisfranc Ligament Disruption

Traumatic Lisfranc Ligament Disruption

(Left) AP weight-bearing radiograph shows a chronic untreated Lisfranc disruption. Note particularly the offset at the second ➡️ and third ➡️ tarsometatarsal joints. There is also significant pronation; note the lack of overlap at the metatarsal bases. *(Right)* Lateral radiograph in the same patient shows collapse of the midfoot ➡️, a typical long-term effect of untreated Lisfranc injury. The forefoot is pronated; note the abnormal MT inclination angles.

Tarsal Coalition

Tarsal Coalition

(Left) Lateral weight-bearing radiograph shows flattening of the longitudinal arch. There is prominence & elongation of the anterior process of the calcaneus ➡️, termed the "anteater sign", indicating calcaneonavicular coalition. *(Right)* Oblique radiograph of the same patient as previous image, confirms the calcaneonavicular coalition ➡️. Tarsal coalition results in flatfoot deformity due to peroneal muscle spasticity & resultant pronation.

Congenital Vertical Talus (Rocker Bottom Foot)

Marfan Syndrome

(Left) Lateral weight-bearing radiograph shows plantarflexed talus ➡️, dislocated from the navicular, as well as hindfoot equinus, valgus, and forefoot valgus/pronation. This is typical of congenital vertical talus. *(Right)* AP radiograph shows valgus hindfoot (increased talocalcaneal angles) and valgus, pronated forefoot (lack of convergence of metatarsal bases), bilaterally. There is also arachnodactyly; the patient has Marfan syndrome.

CAVUS FOOT DEFORMITY

DIFFERENTIAL DIAGNOSIS

Common
- Idiopathic
- Charcot-Marie-Tooth Disease
- Cerebral Palsy
- Fracture, Malunion
- Muscular Dystrophy
- Spina Bifida

Less Common
- Stroke
- Compartment Syndrome
- Thermal Injury, Burns
- Spinal Cord Injury
- Spinal Cord Tumor
- Syringomyelia
- Meningocele
- Friedreich Ataxia
- Polio
- Spinal Dysraphism
- Arthrogryposis

Rare but Important
- Bound Foot

ESSENTIAL INFORMATION

Key Differential Diagnosis Issues
- Radiographic findings are diagnostic but nonspecific as to cause
  - Anteroposterior view = normal or forefoot adduction & supination
  - Lateral view, standing
    - Increased talocalcaneal angle (high calcaneal pitch)
    - Unusual profile view of talus
    - Mid talus-first metatarsal lines form angle with apex upward (first ray plantarflexed)
    - Hindfoot varus or valgus (less common)
    - Claw toe deformities
- Pes cavus & hindfoot varus are commonly associated findings
- Findings are typically due to imbalance of intrinsic & extrinsic muscles ± contraction of plantar fascia & soft tissues

Helpful Clues for Diagnoses
- **Charcot-Marie-Tooth Disease**
  - Classic neuromuscular cause of pes cavus
  - Forefoot pronation, first metatarsal pronation & plantar flexion
- **Fracture, Malunion**
  - Hindfoot-midfoot deformity
  - Talar neck fracture malunion with varus rotation of talar head
- **Compartment Syndrome**
  - Deep posterior compartment of calf
    - Muscle atrophy & calcification
  - May occur in foot after calcaneal fracture
  - May have evidence of prior tibia, fibula, hindfoot or midfoot fracture
- **Polio**
  - Increased calcaneal pitch angle due to gastrocnemius-soleus complex weakness
  - ± Normal forefoot alignment

Idiopathic

Lateral radiograph shows an abnormally high longitudinal arch ➡ of the foot. Hindfoot varus produces the nonstandard appearance of the talus ➡.

Charcot-Marie-Tooth Disease

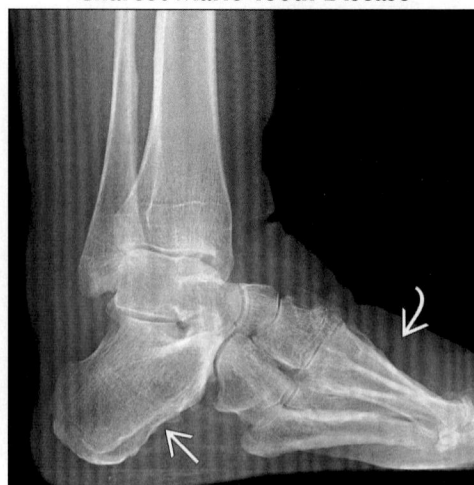

Lateral radiograph shows a cavus foot with excessive calcaneal dorsiflexion ➡ and forefoot varus ➡. This combination suggests spasticity.

CAVUS FOOT DEFORMITY

Cerebral Palsy

Muscular Dystrophy

(Left) Lateral radiograph shows valgus and mild equinus of the hindfoot ➡. The forefoot shows supination and varus ➡, which is quite severe. The combination of varus and valgus is usually seen in a spastic foot, and is not otherwise specific. *(Right)* Lateral radiograph shows a cavus foot deformity and diffuse osteopenia. Note the high calcaneal pitch ➡ and atrophied soft tissues in this child with muscular dystrophy.

Spinal Cord Injury

Meningocele

(Left) Lateral radiograph shows a high arch and claw toe ➡ deformities. Note that the talonavicular and calcaneocuboid joints appear stacked ➡ and almost the entire subtalar joint ➡ is visible. *(Right)* Anteroposterior radiograph shows foot asymmetry due to an occult intrasacral meningocele with tethered spinal cord. In addition to the smaller size of the foot, the metatarsals are mildly adducted ➡ due to forefoot varus and claw toe deformities are present ➡.

Polio

Bound Foot

(Left) Lateral radiograph shows cavus with a valgus hindfoot (↑ talocalcaneal angle) ➡, flattened midfoot ➡, & varus forefoot ➡. This odd combination is only seen in spastic feet, here due to polio. *(Right)* Lateral radiograph shows cavus in a Chinese bound foot. Note the indentation of soft tissue ➡ where the foot was folded upon itself. These patients are at risk for infection from tissue necrosis developed during the deforming procedure. (†MSK Req).

CONGENITAL FOOT DEFORMITY

DIFFERENTIAL DIAGNOSIS

Common
- Metatarsus Adductus
- Pes Planovalgus (Flexible Flatfoot)
- Club Foot (Talipes Equinovarus)
- Tarsal Coalition

Less Common
- Congenital Vertical Talus (Rocker Bottom Foot)
- Pes Cavus (Mimic)
- Polio (Mimic)
- Cerebral Palsy (Mimic)

Rare but Important
- Metaphyseal Bar

ESSENTIAL INFORMATION

Key Differential Diagnosis Issues
- **Hint**: Do not attempt to diagnosis foot deformities without weight-bearing films
- **Hint**: Most congenital foot deformities can be diagnosed by evaluation of three relationships
  - Hindfoot equinus or calcaneus
    - On lateral radiograph, normal angle between lines bisecting calcaneus and tibia ranges between 60° and 90°
    - Hindfoot equinus: Tibiocalcaneal angle > 90° (excessive plantarflexion of calcaneus)
    - Hindfoot calcaneus: Tibiocalcaneal angle < 60° (excessive dorsiflexion of calcaneus); also termed "cavus"
  - Hindfoot varus or valgus
    - On lateral radiograph, normal angle between lines bisecting talus and calcaneus ranges between 25° and 55° (termed Kite angle, or lateral talocalcaneal angle)
    - On AP radiograph, normal angle between lines bisecting talus and calcaneus ranges between 15° and 40°
    - Varus hindfoot: Decreased talocalcaneal angle (bones approach parallel), < 25° on lateral and < 15° on AP
    - Valgus hindfoot: Increased talocalcaneal angle (bones diverge): > 55° on lateral and > 40° on AP
  - Forefoot varus or valgus
    - On lateral radiograph, metatarsals normally are moderately superimposed, with 5th in plantar-most position; angle of inclination of metatarsals gradually increases from 5° for the 5th to 20° for the 1st
    - On AP radiograph, metatarsals normally show moderate convergence of the bases
    - Varus forefoot: Inversion and supination; on lateral, decreased superimposition of metatarsals (ladder-like) with 5th MT in plantar-most position; on AP, increased overlap of MT bases
    - Valgus forefoot: Eversion & pronation; on lateral, increased superimposition of metatarsals with 1st MT in plantar-most position; on AP, decreased convergence of MT bases
- **Hint**: Most congenital foot deformities match the type of hindfoot & forefoot deformities
  - Varus hindfoot with varus forefoot
  - Valgus hindfoot with valgus forefoot
- **Hint**: If hindfoot and forefoot deformities are unmatched (i.e., varus hindfoot and valgus forefoot or valgus hindfoot and varus forefoot), it is usually due to a spastic foot

Helpful Clues for Common Diagnoses
- **Metatarsus Adductus**
  - Most common structural foot abnormality of infants
  - Adduction of metatarsals; normal hindfoot
  - Rarely imaged, since it is a flexible deformity and self-correcting
- **Pes Planovalgus (Flexible Flatfoot)**
  - Common (4% of population)
  - Note: It is **flexible**; non-weight-bearing radiographs are normal
  - Abnormalities on weight-bearing radiographs
    - Hindfoot valgus
    - Forefoot valgus
    - **No equinus**
- **Club Foot (Talipes Equinovarus)**
  - Incidence 1:1,000 births
  - Male > female 2-3: 1
  - Constant structural abnormalities
    - Hindfoot equinus
    - Hindfoot varus
    - Forefoot varus
- **Tarsal Coalition**

CONGENITAL FOOT DEFORMITY

- ○ Painful flatfoot: Persistent or intermittent spasm of peroneal muscles
- ○ Usually secondary to congenital lack of segmentation of bones of hindfoot
- ○ Symptoms begin in late first or second decade
- ○ Secondary signs
  - Talar beak: Due to excessive motion at talonavicular joint because of rigid subtalar joint
  - "Ball and socket" tibiotalar joint: Conversion of this hinge joint to a rounded articulation; generally due to an unusually extensive subtalar coalition
- ○ Calcaneonavicular coalition
  - Anterior process of calcaneus extends and broadens at the union with navicular
  - Directly visualized on oblique radiograph
- ○ Talonavicular coalition
  - Generally mid subtalar joint (sustentaculum tali) and not directly visualized
  - Diagnosed by CT or MR where this portion of subtalar joint is directly visualized on radiographs
  - Rarely will involve posterior and/or anterior subtalar facets
- ○ 25% bilaterality

Helpful Clues for Less Common Diagnoses
- **Congenital Vertical Talus (Rocker Bottom Foot)**
  - ○ Rigid flatfoot

- ○ Isolated, or part of several syndromes (frequently associated with meningomyelocele)
- ○ Constant structural abnormalities
  - Hindfoot equinus
  - Hindfoot valgus
  - Plantarflexed talus, dislocated from navicular
  - Forefoot valgus
- **Pes Cavus (Mimic)**
  - ○ Multiple etiologies; none are strictly congenital, hence the "mimic" designation
    - Upper motor neuron lesions (Friedrich ataxia)
    - Lower motor neuron lesions (poliomyelitis)
    - Vascular ischemia
    - Charcot Marie Tooth
    - Chinese bound foot
- **Polio (Mimic) & Cerebral Palsy (Mimic)**
  - ○ Spastic abnormalities, often with mismatch of hindfoot and forefoot abnormalities (varus-valgus)
  - ○ Soft tissues show muscle atrophy

Helpful Clues for Rare Diagnoses
- **Metaphyseal Bar**
  - ○ Rare congenital link between the proximal and distal epiphyses of the first metatarsal
  - ○ Link is on the medial side, resulting in a curved 1st MT, concave medially
  - ○ Clinical appearance is of metatarsus adductus, but the deformity is rigid

Pes Planovalgus (Flexible Flatfoot)

Lateral radiograph shows increased plantarflexion of the talus ➡, forming hindfoot valgus. There is also pronation of the forefoot, with superimposition of the metatarsals & decreased inclination angle of MT 1-3 ➡.

Pes Planovalgus (Flexible Flatfoot)

AP radiograph, same patient, shows a wide T-C angle (hindfoot valgus), with lack of convergence at the metatarsal bases ➡ (forefoot pronation/valgus). The abnormalities reduce on non-weightbearing.

CONGENITAL FOOT DEFORMITY

Club Foot (Talipes Equinovarus)

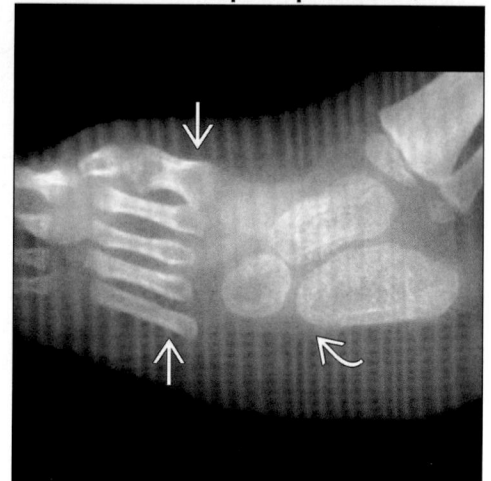

Club Foot (Talipes Equinovarus)

(Left) AP radiograph shows near superimposition of talus → & calcaneus → (decreased talocalcaneal angle, hindfoot varus). There is increased convergence at the bases of the metatarsals →, typical of forefoot supination/varus. *(Right)* Lateral radiograph in the same patient, shows equinus of the calcaneus →. The calcaneus & talus are nearly parallel, confirming hindfoot varus. The forefoot shows severe supination, with the metatarsals → appearing stacked, typical of clubfoot.

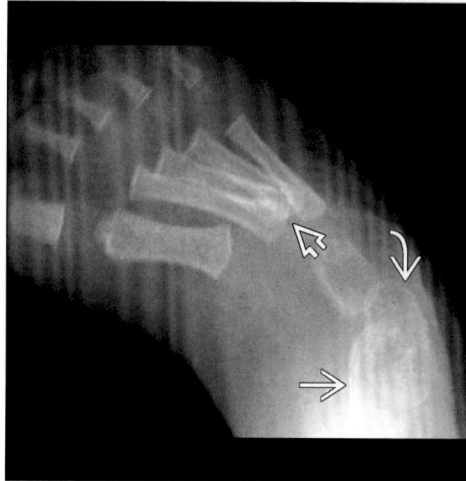

Tarsal Coalition

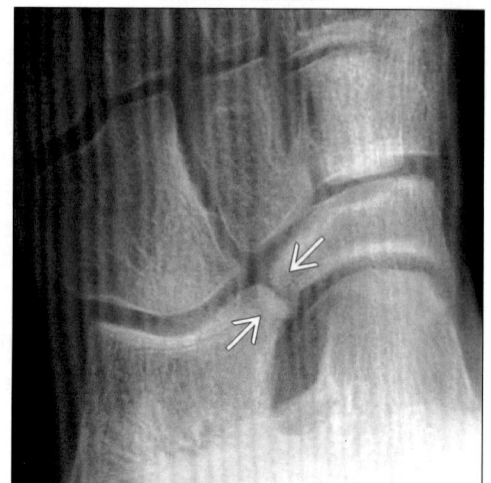

Tarsal Coalition

(Left) Lateral radiograph shows the "anteater sign" of an elongated anterior process of the calcaneus →. This long process extends to the navicular and is highly suggestive of calcaneonavicular coalition. In this case there is no talar beak. *(Right)* Oblique radiograph confirms the calcaneonavicular coalition →. This type of coalition can usually be diagnosed with oblique radiograph. If there is further question, CT is confirmatory.

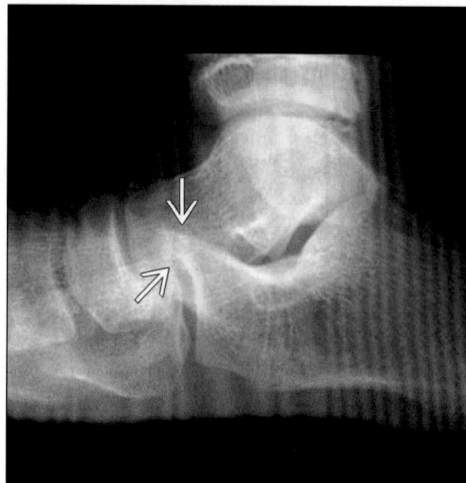

Tarsal Coalition

Tarsal Coalition

(Left) Lateral radiograph shows a large talar beak →, a secondary sign of tarsal coalition. The coalition itself is not seen, but there is a sclerotic "C sign" in the region of the subtalar joint →, which is highly suggestive. *(Right)* Angled axial bone CT shows the broad and sclerotic talocalcaneal coalition at the middle facet →, compared with the normal left side →. Talocalcaneal coalitions most frequently involve this portion of the subtalar joint.

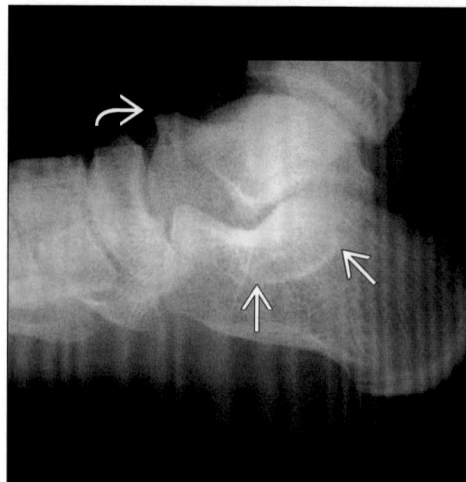

CONGENITAL FOOT DEFORMITY

Congenital Vertical Talus (Rocker Bottom Foot)

Congenital Vertical Talus (Rocker Bottom Foot)

(Left) Lateral radiograph shows all the elements of congenital vertical talus, including calcaneal equinus ➡ & hindfoot valgus. Note the severe plantarflexion of the talus ➡, contributing to the valgus. The forefoot is severely pronated ➡. *(Right)* AP radiograph in same patient shows ↑ talocalcaneal angle, with severe medial angulation of the talus ➡. There is pronation/valgus of the forefoot, with lack of convergence at the MT bases ➡.

Pes Cavus (Mimic)

Polio (Mimic)

(Left) Lateral radiograph shows abnormal dorsiflexion of the calcaneus ➡ and varus deformity of the forefoot. This cavovarus pattern is typically seen in Charcot Marie Tooth, as in this case, but may be seen with other spastic conditions as well. *(Right)* Lateral radiograph shows a mixed pattern of hindfoot valgus (increased talocalcaneal angle) and forefoot varus/supination. This unusual combination is seen in spastic conditions, including polio.

Cerebral Palsy (Mimic)

Metaphyseal Bar

(Left) Lateral radiograph shows equinus of the calcaneus, valgus hindfoot, and supinated forefoot. This is another pattern of a spastic foot, this time in a patient with cerebral palsy. *(Right)* Axial T1WI MR shows bridging bone extending from the proximal to distal epiphysis, across the diaphysis of the first metatarsal ➡. It is bilaterally symmetric, and causes bowing and shortening of the bone. It results in overall fixed metatarsus adductus.

DIABETIC FOOT COMPLICATIONS

DIFFERENTIAL DIAGNOSIS

Common
- Ulceration/Cellulitis/Soft Tissue Abscess
- Osteomyelitis, Adult
- Charcot, Neuropathic
- Insufficiency Fracture, Tarsal & Metatarsal
- Calcaneal Insufficiency Fracture

ESSENTIAL INFORMATION

Key Differential Diagnosis Issues
- All complications of the diabetic foot are common
- Watch for vascular calcification in foot as a hint of underlying diabetic condition
- Many may be subtle; knowledge of expected sites of complication should allow early detection
  - Charcot sites in foot: Lisfranc (tarsal metatarsal) > talonavicular > Chopart (hindfoot/midfoot)
  - Insufficiency fractures (isolated, not associated with Charcot) most frequently seen in metatarsals & posterior calcaneal tubercle; tarsals less common
- Ulcers and cellulitis are common
  - Must differentiate from osteomyelitis
  - Osseous structures may show reactive edema which simulates osteomyelitis
- It may not be possible to distinguish an uncomplicated Charcot joint from one complicated by osteomyelitis; both may have similar features

Helpful Clues for Common Diagnoses
- **Ulceration/Cellulitis/Soft Tissue Abscess**
  - Plantar aspect, or at the site of any deformity of foot
  - May have foreign bodies present without patient's knowledge
  - Air seen in sinus tract, outlined by enhancing tissue
  - Surrounding cellulitis is common, as are soft tissue abscesses
- **Osteomyelitis, Adult**
  - If sinus tract is demonstrated extending to osseous destruction, diagnosis is secure
  - Otherwise, may have reactive osseous edema to adjacent soft tissue abscess or ulceration which is not truly osteomyelitis
    - "Confluent" rather than "reticulated" low signal on T1 imaging may help differentiate osteomyelitis from reaction
    - Either osteomyelitis or osseous reaction will be hyperintense and enhance with contrast; again, confluence of MR abnormality may make osteomyelitis a stronger consideration
- **Charcot, Neuropathic**
  - Fragmentation, debris (though may be atrophic in diabetic foot), large soft tissue fluid collections, disruption of joint
  - Because of abnormal mechanics, there is osseous hyperintensity & enhancement
  - May be impossible to differentiate uncomplicated from infected Charcot joint

Ulceration/Cellulitis/Soft Tissue Abscess

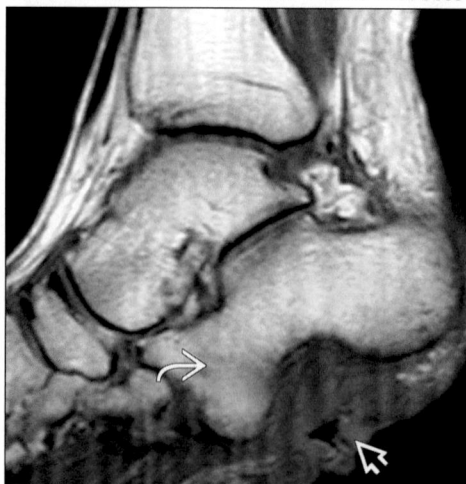

Sagittal T1WI MR shows air in a sinus tract ➡ extending towards a calcaneus (deformed from surgery several years earlier). There is fine reticulated low signal within the calcaneus ➡, but no confluence of signal.

Ulceration/Cellulitis/Soft Tissue Abscess

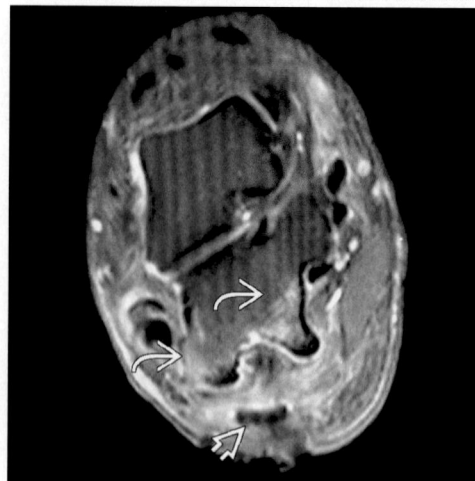

Coronal T1 C+ FS MR shows enhancement of the sinus tract ➡ (same patient). There is reactive edema in the calcaneus ➡, but no confluence of signal; this was soft tissue abscess without osteomyelitis.

DIABETIC FOOT COMPLICATIONS

Osteomyelitis, Adult

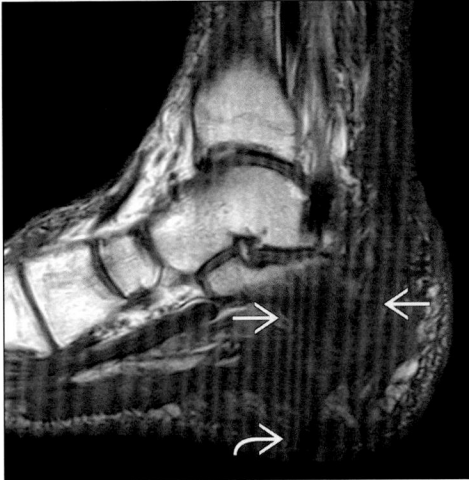

Osteomyelitis, Adult

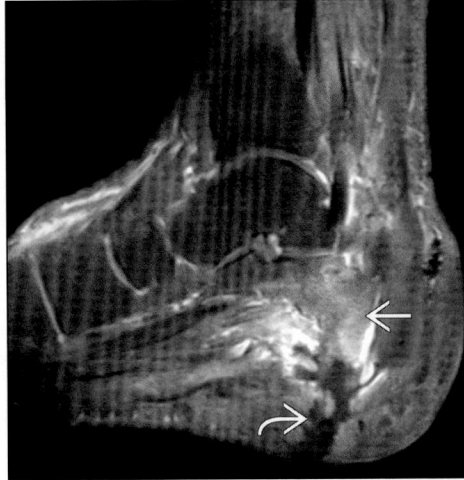

(Left) Sagittal T1WI MR shows low signal in a sinus tract with surrounding edema ➡. There is confluent low signal occupying the majority of the calcaneus ➡; this confluent pattern is highly suspicious for osteomyelitis. (Right) Coronal T1 C+ FS MR shows air within the sinus tract ➡ (same patient) extending from the plantar aspect of the heel, all the way to the calcaneus. The calcaneus enhances ➡ diffusely, indicating osteomyelitis.

Charcot, Neuropathic

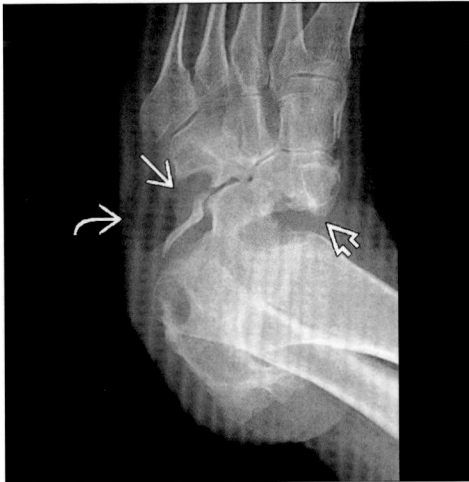

Charcot, Neuropathic

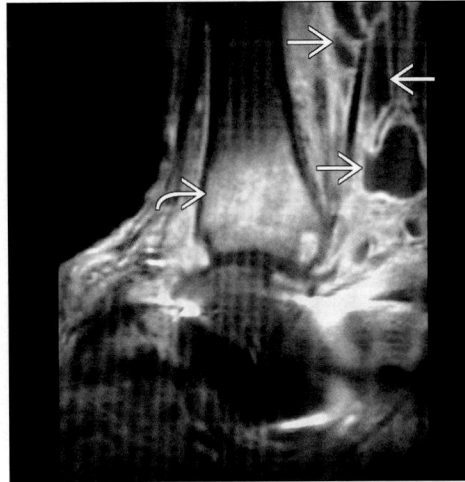

(Left) AP radiograph shows a neuropathic joint at the Chopart joint (hindfoot/midfoot junction). Destruction & fragmentation is seen at the calcaneocuboid joint ➡, as well as dislocation at the talonavicular joint ➡. Air is seen in an adjacent ulcer ➡. (Right) Sagittal T1 C+ FS MR shows large fluid collections ➡, tenosynovitis, & enhancement of the distal tibia ➡. Patient had Charcot joint but was not infected; the metallic artifact is due to failed subtalar arthrodesis.

Insufficiency Fracture, Tarsal & Metatarsal

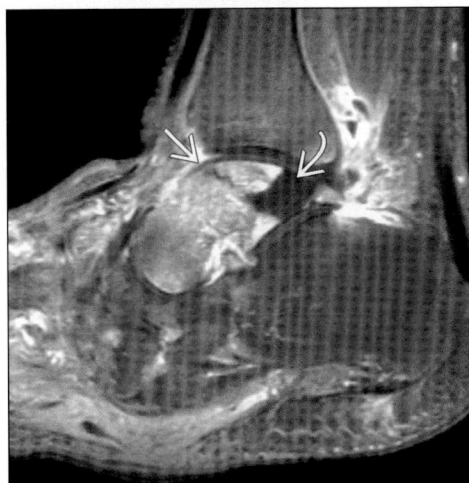

Calcaneal Insufficiency Fracture

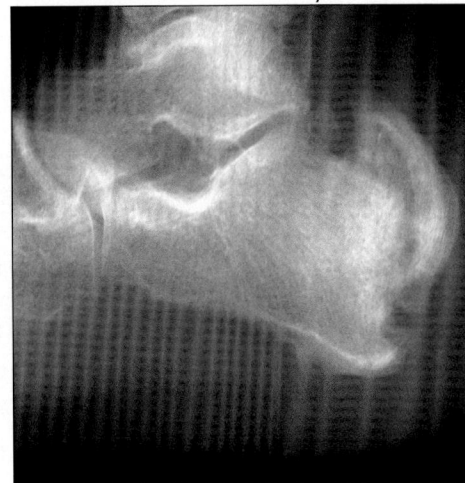

(Left) Sagittal T1 C+ FS MR shows an insufficiency fracture of the talar body ➡ with surrounding edema. There is also a wedge-shaped unenhanced region of the posterior talus ➡ which represents avascular necrosis. (Right) Lateral radiograph shows fracture of the posterior tubercle of the calcaneus, with proximal displacement of the fragment. This is a fracture which is typically seen only in diabetic patients. It does not heal well.

DIFFERENTIAL DIAGNOSIS

Common
- Degenerative
- Vertebral Body Osteomyelitis
- Epidural Abscess
- Iliopsoas Abscess
- Osteoid Osteoma
- Epidural Hematoma
- Asymmetric Vertebral Body Fracture

Less Common
- Spinal Fatigue Syndrome
- Paraspinal Muscle Injury
- Ewing Sarcoma
- Osteoblastoma
- Intraspinal Tumors
- Metastases, Bone Marrow
- High Thoracic Scoliosis: Neurofibromatosis

Rare but Important
- Septic Facet Joint

ESSENTIAL INFORMATION

Key Differential Diagnosis Issues
- **Hint**: Lesion along concavity of the curve
- **Hint**: In adult history is critical; infection, trauma, long standing (degenerative)
- **Hint**: Child, osteoid osteoma most common

Helpful Clues for Common Diagnoses
- **Degenerative**
  - Long history of pain
  - Most common cause in adult
- **Vertebral Body Osteomyelitis**
  - Presentation
    - Acute onset, severe unrelenting pain
    - Fever, chills, elevated WBC
    - No neurologic deficits unless associated epidural abscess
  - Radiographs & CT negative early in disease
    - Late: Adjacent endplate edema & destruction, cysts, sclerosis; differentiate from mechanical disc destruction
  - Gallium scans preferred to labeled white cell scans
  - MR preferred imaging modality
    - Endplate marrow edema & soft tissue edema, gadolinium enhancement of disc
  - May have iliopsoas and/or epidural abscess
- **Epidural Abscess**
  - Isolated or 2° vertebral body osteomyelitis

- See "Presentation" above
  - Variable neurologic manifestations include incontinence, paralysis
- Radiographs, CT, nuclear medicine studies negative in early & isolated disease
- MR preferred imaging examination
  - Epidural mass with rim-enhancement
  - Difficult to identify without gadolinium
  - Mass effect not always present
- **Iliopsoas Abscess**
  - Usually 2° vertebral osteomyelitis
    - See "Presentation" above
  - Typically unilateral, may be bilateral
  - MR preferred, CT may be useful
    - Rim enhancing fluid-filled mass
    - Near infected disc
- **Osteoid Osteoma**
  - Pain worse at night, after activity, relieved by aspirin
  - Commonly located in posterior elements
    - Most lesions based in cortex
  - Radiographs & CT
    - Sclerotic pedicle, non-rotational scoliosis
    - Central lucent nidus, variable central mineralization
    - Nidus may only be seen on CT or MR, rarely greater than 1.5 cm
  - Intense uptake on bone scan
  - MR: Nidus: Isointense T1WI, slightly more intense T2WI
    - Peripheral low signal rim all sequences
    - Adjacent marrow & soft tissue edema
- **Epidural Hematoma**
  - Surgical emergency
  - Focal back pain ± radiculopathy, incontinence
    - May rapidly progress to paralysis
  - History often includes anticoagulation or recent spine procedure
    - Trauma usually has fractures
    - Underlying AVM may be cause
  - Radiographs, nuclear scans not helpful
  - CT limited: Epidural soft tissue mass
  - MR preferred imaging modality
    - T1WI: Epidural soft tissue mass, diffuse bright signal if acute, peripheral bright rim if subacute
- **Asymmetric Vertebral Body Fracture**
  - History of trauma with lateral compression

Helpful Clues for Less Common Diagnoses
- **Spinal Fatigue Syndrome**

PAINFUL SCOLIOSIS

- ○ Underlying idiopathic scoliosis
- ○ Due to paraspinal muscle strain
- ○ Position dependent, relieved by rest
- ○ No imaging findings, image to exclude other causes
- **Paraspinal Muscle Injury**
  - ○ Trauma, surgery (retractor injury)
  - ○ Radiographs, CT, bone scan negative
  - ○ MR: Bright intramuscular signal T2WI
- **Ewing Sarcoma**
  - ○ Less common in axial than appendicular skeleton, but a relatively common tumor
  - ○ Asymmetric vertebral body destruction results in scoliosis
- **Osteoblastoma**
  - ○ Pain, weak association with activity
  - ○ Some consider giant osteoid osteoma but
    - Slightly older patient
    - Milder pain, not relieved by aspirin
    - Larger lesions (over 2 cm), less sclerosis
  - ○ Most common in spine, especially sacrum
    - Posterior elements
  - ○ Variable radiographic & CT appearance from aggressive lysis to expansile well corticated heavily mineralized lesion
    - Classic appearance is expansile lytic lesion with well-defined margins and irregular mineralization
    - Soft tissue mass common
  - ○ MR appearance: See osteoid osteoma
  - ○ Aggressive variant acts like osteosarcoma
- **Intraspinal Tumors**
  - ○ Long history of pain, worse at night

- ○ Variable neurologic symptoms especially paresthesias
- ○ Associated scoliosis more common in child
- ○ Commonly astrocytoma, adult also may have ependymomas
- ○ Radiographs & CT likely negative
  - May see interpediculate widening or posterior vertebral body scalloping
- ○ MR: Enlarged spinal cord, syrinx, mass with variable enhancement
- **Metastases, Bone Marrow**
  - ○ Pain ± radiculopathy
  - ○ Solitary or multiple lesions
  - ○ Lytic or sclerotic
  - ○ Breast, lung, prostate, multiple myeloma
- **High Thoracic Scoliosis: Neurofibromatosis**
  - ○ Angular deformity commonly convex right
  - ○ Foraminal widening, posterior vertebral body scalloping, neurofibromas, Lisch nodule, mesodermal dysplasia, optic glioma

Helpful Clues for Rare Diagnoses
- **Septic Facet Joint**
  - ○ Presentation similar to vertebral body osteomyelitis (see above)
  - ○ Risk factor: Steroid injection
  - ○ Radiographs likely negative
  - ○ CT shows joint effusion, destruction (late)
  - ○ Bone scan: Nonspecific, identifies site
  - ○ MR: Joint effusion, subchondral edema & destruction, edema adjacent paraspinal muscles, enhancement

Vertebral Body Osteomyelitis

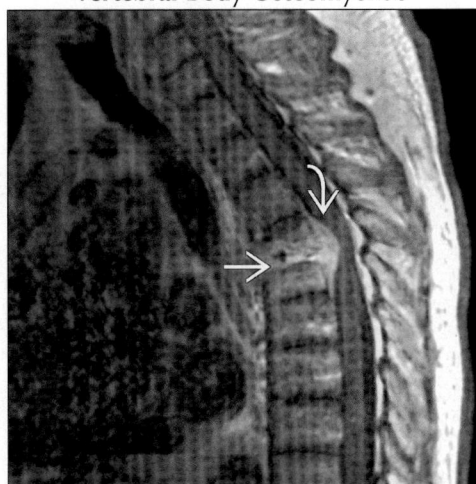

Sagittal T1 C+ MR shows diffuse enhancement within the disc space ➡, enhancement within the adjacent vertebra and an epidural phlegmon ➡ in this patient with vertebral body osteomyelitis & scoliosis.

Epidural Abscess

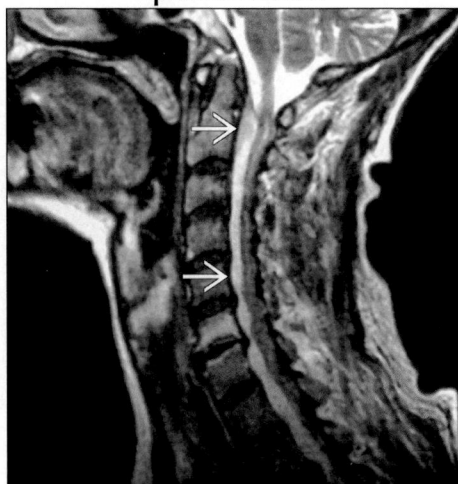

Sagittal T2WI MR shows a ventral epidural high signal intensity collection consistent with epidural abscess ➡ extending from C2 into upper thoracic spine compressing the cord posteriorly.

PAINFUL SCOLIOSIS

Iliopsoas Abscess

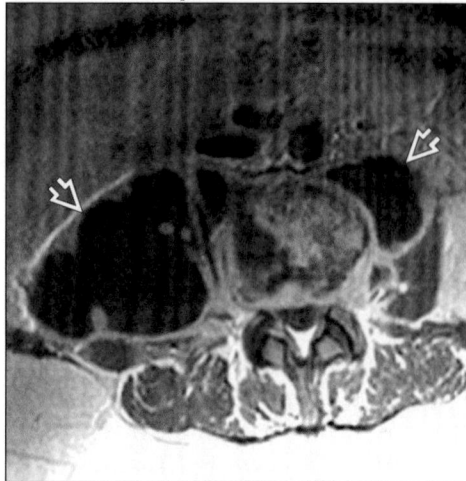

Osteoid Osteoma

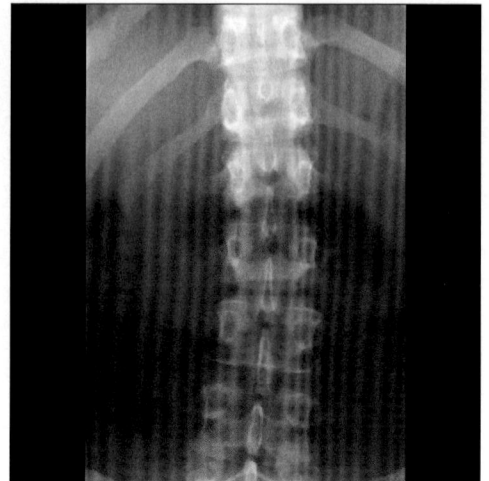

(Left) Axial T1 C+ MR shows rim enhancing abscesses in both psoas muscles ➡. Enhancement is present within the adjacent disc space indicative of vertebral body osteomyelitis. (Right) Anteroposterior radiograph shows a long thoracolumbar scoliosis, convex left, without associated rotation. This is the classic curve associated with osteoid osteoma. The lytic nidus may be impossible to identify on radiograph, so suspicion must be high.

Osteoid Osteoma

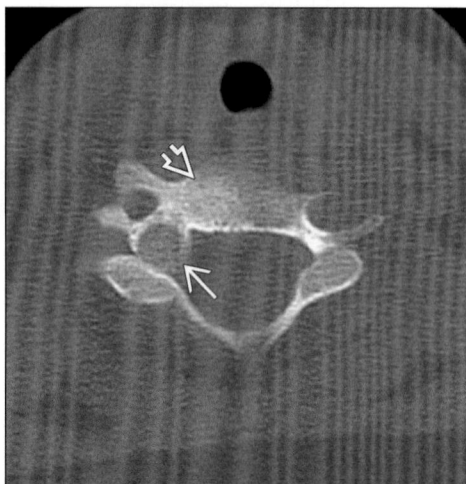

Epidural Hematoma

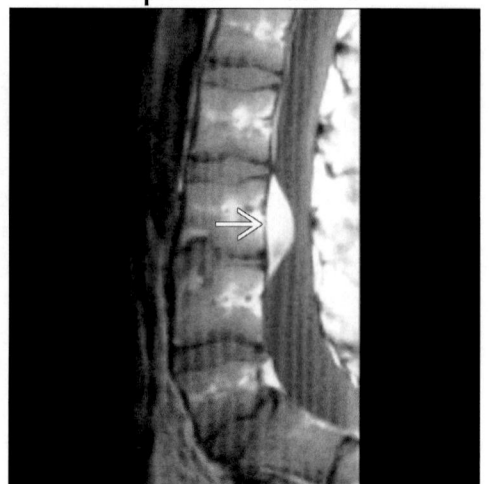

(Left) Axial bone CT shows classic location of osteoid osteoma ➡ in the pedicle with ill-defined sclerosis in the adjacent bone ➡. This caused a painful scoliosis; concave on the side with the osteoid osteoma nidus. (Right) Sagittal T1WI MR shows lentiform-shaped mass ➡ which creates moderate canal stenosis. The mass is diffusely bright, indicative of an acute epidural hematoma. This may be a surgical emergency, depending on location & extent.

Paraspinal Muscle Injury

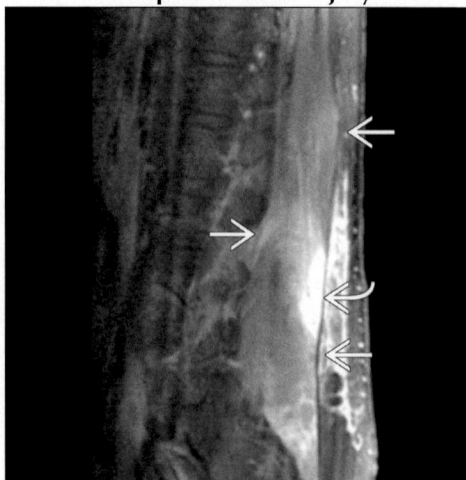

Ewing Sarcoma

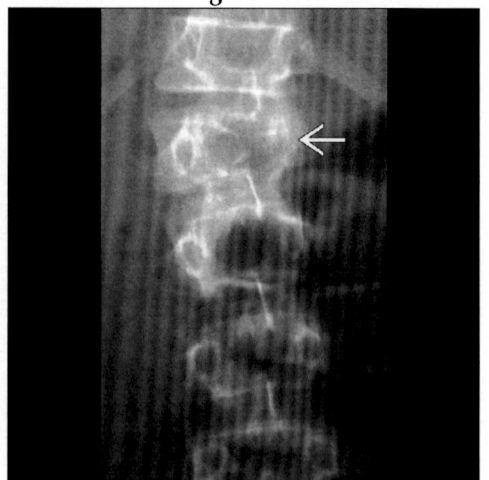

(Left) Sagittal STIR MR shows diffuse edema within the paraspinal musculature ➡ with associated hematoma ➡ in this patient with paraspinal muscle injury resulting from motor vehicle accident. Painful splinting creates a scoliosis. (Right) AP radiograph shows a mild scoliosis concave left. There is destruction of a pedicle ➡ and asymmetric compression of the vertebral body due to a lytic lesion. This 13 year old proved to have Ewing sarcoma.

PAINFUL SCOLIOSIS

Osteoblastoma

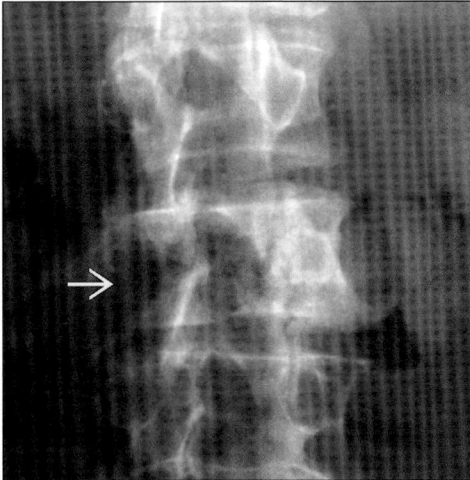

Osteoblastoma

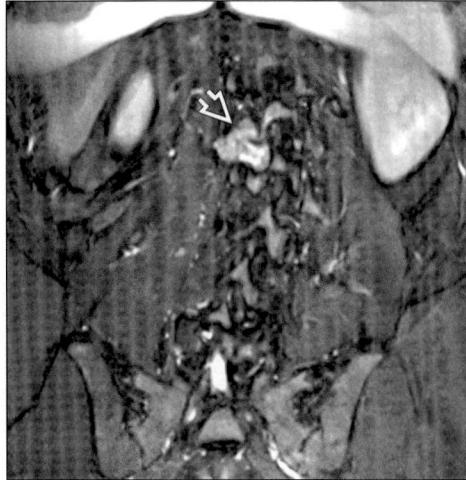

(Left) Anteroposterior radiograph shows destruction of the right vertebral body cortex and pedicle ➡ in this patient with an osteoblastoma. Note the location of the lesion along the concavity of a mild leftward curve. *(Right)* Coronal T2WI MR shows osteoblastoma ⮞ of the right L2 lamina along the concavity of a leftward curve. The lesion is a heterogeneous moderately enhancing mass expanding the lamina.

Intraspinal Tumors

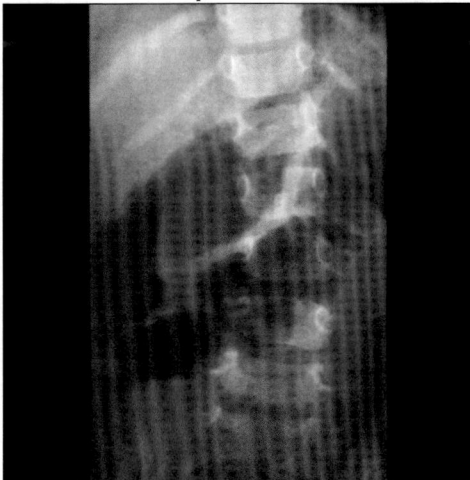

Metastases, Bone Marrow

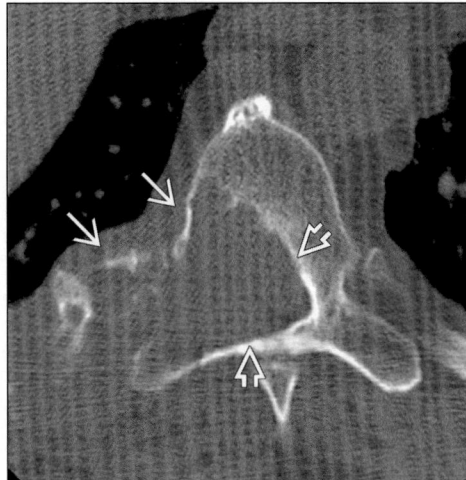

(Left) Anteroposterior radiograph demonstrates a leftward lumbar curve in this child with back pain. No focal osseous lesion is seen. MR revealed spinal cord astrocytoma. *(Right)* Axial NECT from a patient with renal cell carcinoma and severe back pain reveals and expansile lytic metastases within the right pedicle ➡. Large soft tissue mass nearly fills the spinal canal ⮞. The patient presented with a painful scoliosis.

High Thoracic Scoliosis: Neurofibromatosis

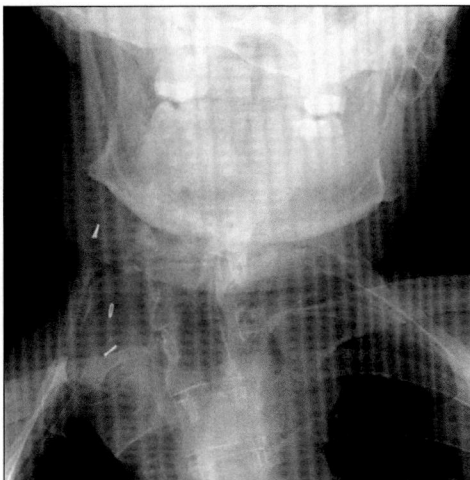

Septic Facet Joint

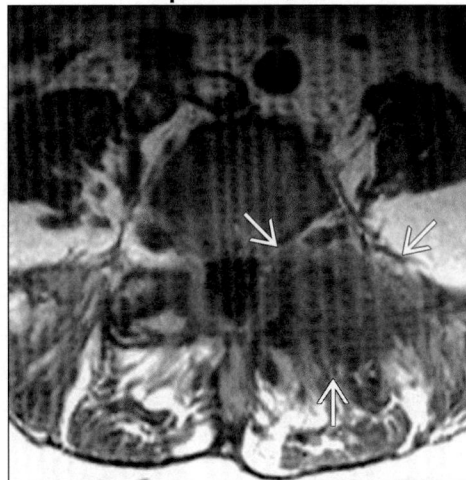

(Left) Anteroposterior radiograph shows focal rightward curve at cervicothoracic junction in a patient w/neurofibromatosis type 1. *(Right)* Axial T1WI MR shows destruction of left facet joint, with inflammatory soft tissue extending into adjacent paraspinal musculature ➡ as a result of facet joint septic arthritis. It is not surprising that the presentation is with a painful scoliosis secondary to splinting towards abnormal side.

III

ARTHRITIS IN A TEENAGER

DIFFERENTIAL DIAGNOSIS

Common
- Juvenile Idiopathic Arthritis (JIA)
- Ankylosing Spondylitis
- Psoriatic Arthritis
- Septic Joint
- Pigmented Villonodular Synovitis (PVNS)
- Femoral Acetabular Impingement (FAI)
- Developmental Dysplasia of the Hip

Less Common
- Hemophilia: MSK Complications
- Synovial Osteochondromatosis
- Legg-Calvé-Perthes, Secondary Changes
- Chronic Reactive Arthritis
- Inflammatory Bowel Disease Arthritis
- Osteoid Osteoma of Hip, 2° Changes

Rare but Important
- Congenital Insensitivity/Indifference to Pain

ESSENTIAL INFORMATION

Key Differential Diagnosis Issues
- Surprising number of arthridities originate during childhood or teenage years
- Early & accurate diagnosis is important to initiate treatment & avoid later debilitating joint disease

Helpful Clues for Common Diagnoses
- **Juvenile Idiopathic Arthritis (JIA)**
  - May have one of several manifestations
    - 5% appear indistinguishable from adult rheumatoid arthritis (RA): Most become seropositive
    - 40% are pauciarticular, affecting the knee, elbow & ankle most frequently; seronegative; 25% develop iridocyclitis
    - 20% have Still disease: Acute systemic disease with fever, anemia, hepatosplenomegaly; 25% of these have polyarticular destructive arthritis, affecting small and large joints alike
    - 25% have seronegative polyarticular disease, symmetric & widespread in adult distribution; no systemic complaints & seronegative
  - Specific features generally distinguishing JIA from other teenage arthridities

- Enlarged metaphyses & epiphyses ("balloon joints") due to overgrowth secondary to hyperemia from inflammatory process
    - Cartilage narrowing & widened notches related to pannus formation & erosion
    - Often asymmetric
  - Other distinguishing features
    - Periostitis may be first manifestation in a young child
    - Fusion frequently occurs in the carpals
    - Interbody fusion in the cervical spine limits growth of vertebral bodies, giving the "waisted" appearance
- **Ankylosing Spondylitis**
  - Earliest manifestations (clinical & radiographic) occur during teenage years
  - Spinal manifestations initiate the radiographic disease process
    - Osteitis at the anterior corners of vertebral bodies
    - SI joint widening & erosions; may be asymmetric initially
    - Teenagers normally have wide SI joints with indistinct cortices; do not overcall!
  - Appendicular disease most frequently is in large proximal joints, particularly hips; may be erosive or productive
  - **Inflammatory Bowel Disease Arthritis**
    - Less frequent, but manifestations are similar to AS
- **Psoriatic Arthritis**
  - 30-50% of psoriatic patients develop spondyloarthropathy
    - Bilateral asymmetric erosive disease; may eventually fuse
  - 20% of psoriatic patients develop arthropathy prior to skin and nail changes
  - Distinguishing features
    - May have sausage digit with periostitis
    - DIP disease predominates; hands > feet
    - Aggressive erosive disease (pencil-in-cup) & eventual fusion
  - **Chronic Reactive Arthritis**
    - Rare compared with psoriatic arthritis; appendicular manifestations usually foot/ankle
- **Septic Joint**
  - Monostotic; cartilage damage and osseous deformity eventually leads to secondary OA

- If longstanding & slow process in a child (especially tuberculous or fungal septic joint), hyperemia leads to overgrowth of epiphyses & metaphyses: "Balloon" joint
- **Pigmented Villonodular Synovitis (PVNS)**
  - Monoarticular; nodular mass or nodules lining synovium
  - Causes erosion if longstanding
  - Large effusion; iron deposition results in foci of low signal which bloom on GRE
- **Femoral Acetabular Impingement (FAI)**
  - Often bilateral abnormalities, though complaints usually begin unilaterally
  - Morphologic abnormalities of femoral head, neck, or acetabulum → impingement
    - Lateral femoral neck "bump", limiting the normal head/neck cutback: Cam type
    - Acetabular rim overgrowth or retroversion: Pincer type
    - Multiple etiologies: Trauma, DDH, SCFE
    - → Labral tear & cartilage damage; → early osteoarthritis
    - Onset of complaints 2nd or 3rd decade
- **Developmental Dysplasia of the Hip**
  - Multiple types of dysplasia
    - Shallow acetabulum
    - Femoral varus or valgus
    - Acetabular or femoral retroversion
  - Develop labral hypertrophy; with shear stress, the labrum tears; eventual cartilage damage & early osteoarthritis

Helpful Clues for Less Common Diagnoses
- **Hemophilia: MSK Complications**
  - Similar appearance to JIA, with "balloon" overgrowth of epiphyses/metaphyses due to hyperemia
  - Pauciarticular; knee > elbow > ankle
  - Hemosiderin deposits lead to low signal on MR, blooming on GRE sequence
- **Osteoid Osteoma of Hip, 2° Changes**
  - Intraarticular OO elicits synovitis → subluxation of joint → altered weight bearing & development of osteophytes

Alternative Differential Approaches
- Consider number of joints involved (some diagnoses belong in more than one)
  - Monoarticular
    - Septic joint
    - Pigmented villonodular synovitis (PVNS)
    - Synovial osteochondromatosis
    - Osteoid osteoma of hip, 2° changes
  - Pauciarticular
    - Juvenile idiopathic arthritis (JIA)
    - Ankylosing spondylitis
    - Psoriatic arthritis
    - Femoral acetabular impingement (FAI)
    - Developmental dysplasia of the hip
    - Hemophilia: MSK complications
    - Legg-Calvé-Perthes, secondary changes
    - Chronic reactive arthritis
    - Inflammatory bowel disease arthritis
    - Congenital insensitivity/indifference to pain
  - Polyarticular
    - Juvenile idiopathic arthritis (JIA)
    - Psoriatic arthritis

Juvenile Idiopathic Arthritis (JIA)

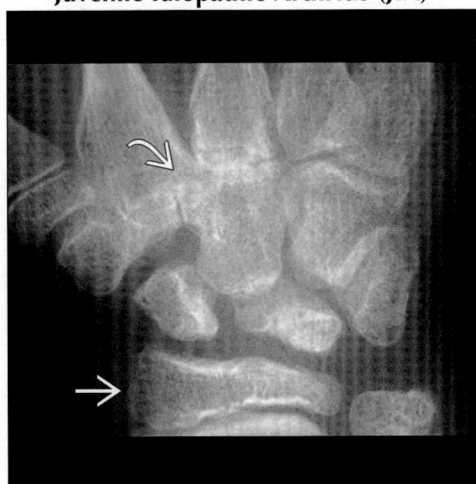

AP radiograph shows a combination of overgrowth of the radial epiphysis ➡, and erosions with fusion at the carpometacarpal joint ➡. This combination indicates hyperemia plus an inflammatory arthritis, typical of JIA.

Ankylosing Spondylitis

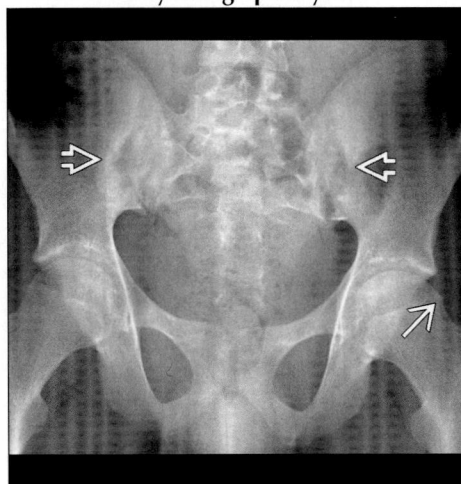

AP radiograph shows bilateral widening & erosion of the sacroiliac joints ➡, as well as a small osteophyte on the femoral neck ➡. This 18 year old male has had back pain for 3 years; findings are typical of AS.

ARTHRITIS IN A TEENAGER

Psoriatic Arthritis

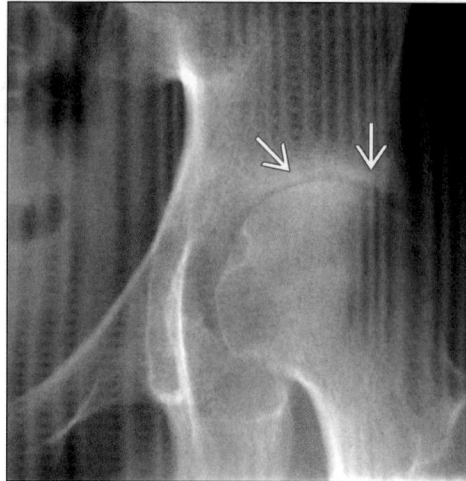

Septic Joint

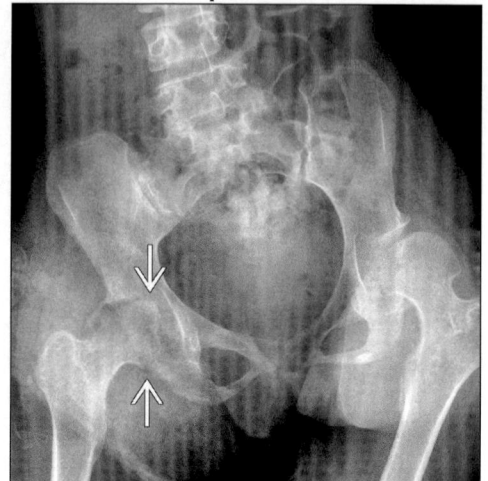

(Left) AP radiograph shows near complete loss of cartilage in this 17 yo female's hip ➡, with mild erosive change. There were hand and foot erosions, but also one site of periostitis and unilateral sacroiliitis. The patient developed psoriatic skin changes within a year. *(Right)* AP radiograph shows a chronic septic hip ➡ in a teenager with L2 paraplegia and chronic decubitus ulcer leading to the hip joint. There is complete cartilage destruction, with associated osseous deformity.

Pigmented Villonodular Synovitis (PVNS)

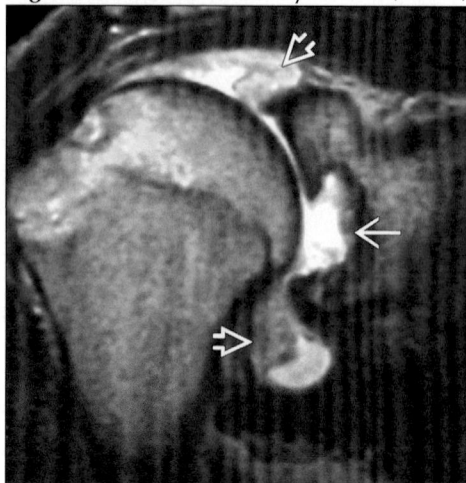

Femoral Acetabular Impingement (FAI)

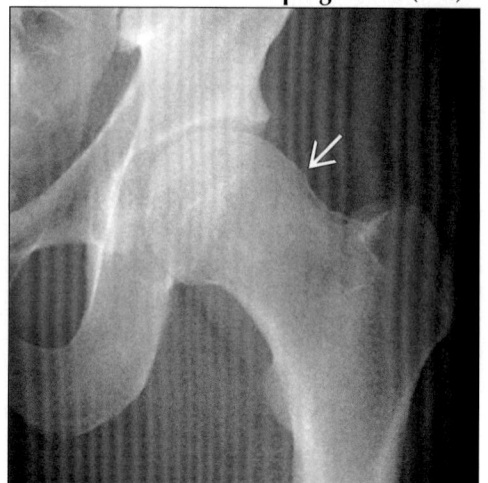

(Left) Coronal T2WI MR shows a huge glenoid erosion ➡ in a 15 yo. Also note nodular synovial masses scattered throughout joint ➡. Appearance is typical for PVNS, proven at biopsy. *(Right)* AP radiograph shows a bump at the lateral femoral junction of the head and neck ➡, eliminating the normal cutback at this site. This configuration puts patient at risk for cam-type FAI; this 20 yo already had a labral tear and cartilage damage, despite minimally abnormal appearance.

Developmental Dysplasia of the Hip

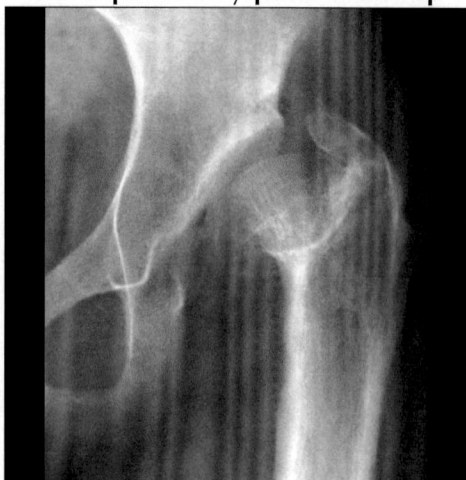

Hemophilia: MSK Complications

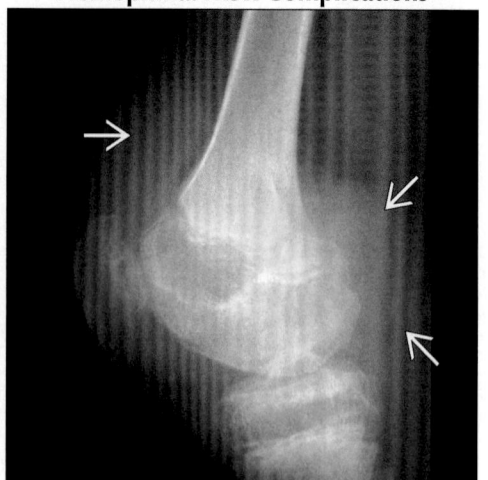

(Left) AP radiograph in a 15 yo shows severe DDH, with a shallow acetabulum, superolateral subluxation of the femoral head, and coxa magna deformity. Patient is developing a painful arthritis. *(Right)* Lateral radiograph shows a large dense effusion ➡. There is erosive change throughout the joint. Note the overgrowth of the epiphyses, particularly the femoral condyles and patella. This overgrowth is due to chronic hyperemia from multiple hemophilic bleeds.

ARTHRITIS IN A TEENAGER

Synovial Osteochondromatosis

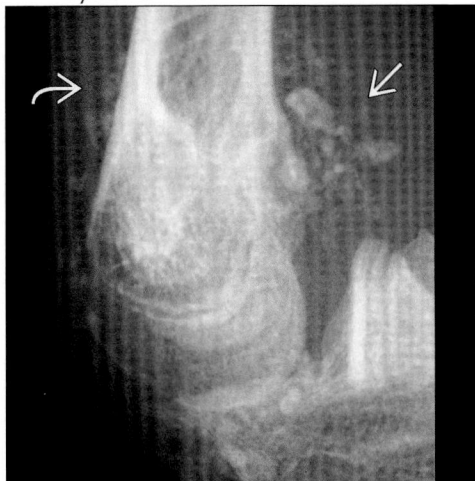

Legg-Calvé-Perthes, Secondary Changes

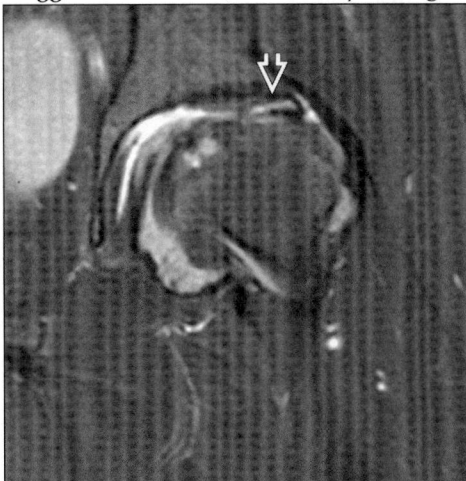

(Left) Lateral radiograph shows multiple loose bodies within a distended elbow joint of a 12 yo. Note the bodies distending the anterior ➡ as well as posterior ➡ fat pads. Synovial osteochondromatosis is unusual in children, but not rare. *(Right)* Coronal T2WI FS MR in this 15 yo with LCP shows findings of secondary arthritis, with a large labral tear ➡, subchondral cysts, and diffuse cartilage loss. This is a severely damaged hip.

Chronic Reactive Arthritis

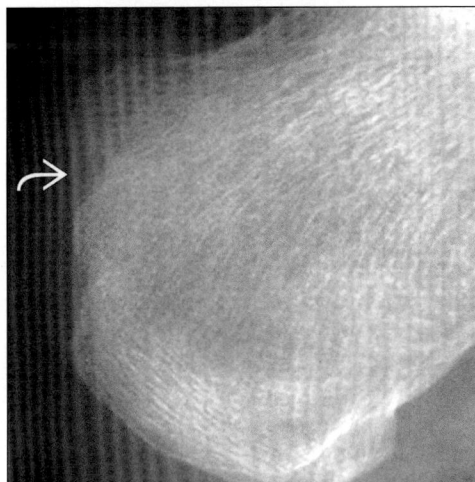

Inflammatory Bowel Disease Arthritis

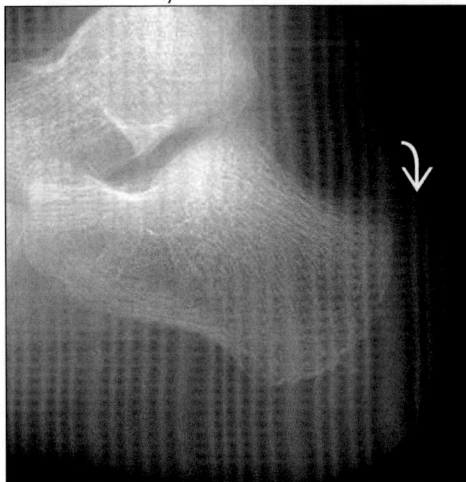

(Left) Lateral radiograph shows early erosion of the posterior calcaneus ➡. There is also soft tissue inflammatory change which obliterates the pre-Achilles fat pad. These are early heel changes in a 19 yo with chronic reactive arthritis. *(Right)* Lateral radiography shows soft tissue swelling and inflammatory change at the posterior calcaneus ➡ in a 10 yo who had diarrhea for 3 months. The heel is so painful that he cannot walk. This is inflammatory bowel disease arthropathy.

Osteoid Osteoma of Hip, 2° Changes

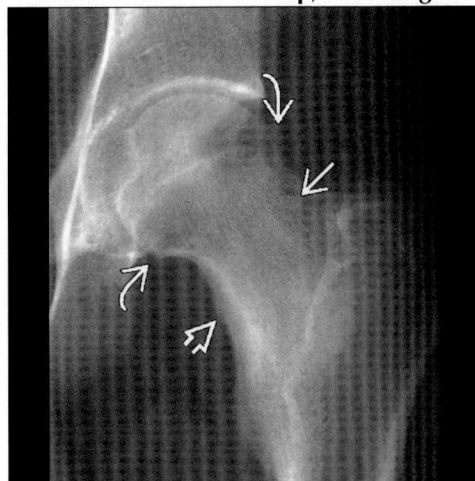

Congenital Insensitivity/Indifference to Pain

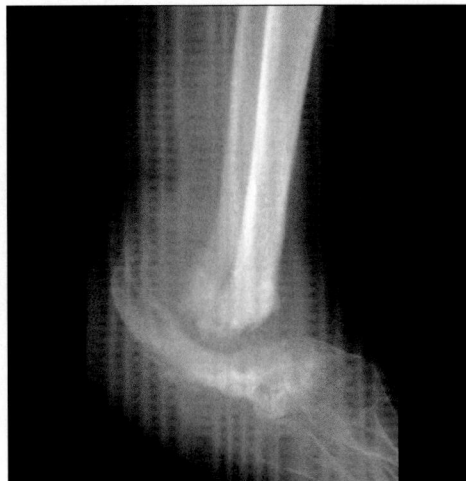

(Left) AP radiograph in a 17 yo shows surprising findings of femoral neck osteophytes ➡ & calcar buttressing ➡. These relate to the chronic synovitis developed in conjunction with an intraarticular osteoid osteoma, faintly seen in the neck ➡. (†MSK Req). *(Right)* Lateral radiograph in a 16 yo shows severe destruction of the foot & ankle. He had congenital indifference to pain; (he felt pain with ambulation, but continued to walk on it, destroying the joints).

ANEMIA WITH MUSCULOSKELETAL MANIFESTATIONS

DIFFERENTIAL DIAGNOSIS

Common
- Iron or Vitamin Deficiency Anemia
- Chronic Renal Disease
- Anemia of Chronic Disease
- Sickle Cell Anemia

Less Common
- Lead Poisoning
- Myelofibrosis
- Thalassemia
- Hypothyroidism
- Polycythemia Vera
- Aplastic Anemia

Rare but Important
- Osteopetrosis
- Down Syndrome (Trisomy 21)
- Erythroblastosis Fetalis
- Engelmann Disease (Engelmann-Camurati)
- Fanconi Anemia

ESSENTIAL INFORMATION

Key Differential Diagnosis Issues
- Musculoskeletal findings are often unrelated to anemia but are associated with the underlying disease state, thus are helpful for imaging differential diagnosis

Helpful Clues for Common Diagnoses
- **Iron or Vitamin Deficiency Anemia**
  - Most common cause of anemia
  - Red bone marrow reconversion involves central to peripheral skeleton
    - Can be confluent, patchy or mass-like
  - Reconverted red marrow tends to preserve some fatty marrow signal producing higher signal than muscle on T1WI
  - Red marrow shows signal drop out on opposed phase imaging
  - Red marrow lower signal than intervertebral disc on T1WI
  - Gadolinium enhancement not definitive for differentiating benign from malignant bone marrow infiltration since both have variable enhancement
- **Chronic Renal Disease**
  - Deranged erythropoietin production
  - Musculoskeletal findings are related to the disease state, not the anemia

- Associated findings of renal osteodystrophy
  - Rugger jersey spine
  - Osteosclerosis or osteopenia
- Associated findings of hyperparathyroidism
  - Subperiosteal bone resorption
  - Cortical thinning
  - Erosion of endplates, sacroiliac joints, entheses
  - Brown tumors
- **Anemia of Chronic Disease**
  - Any chronic disease may produce anemia
    - Rheumatoid arthritis, HIV, cirrhosis, malignancy
  - Musculoskeletal findings are specific to the underlying disease & unrelated to anemia unless inducing red marrow reconversion
- **Sickle Cell Anemia**
  - Bone infarcts = serpiginous low signal on T1WI & high signal on T2WI
  - Avascular necrosis = double line around necrotic region in weight-bearing region
    - Femoral head & humeral head are most commonly involved
  - Red bone marrow reconversion = fatty marrow signal replaced by low signal on T1WI
  - "H-shaped" vertebral body = collapse of central portion of vertebral endplates
  - Autosplenectomy = absent spleen allows bowel to collect in left upper quadrant of abdomen
  - Dactylitis = periosteal reaction can mimic osteomyelitis

Helpful Clues for Less Common Diagnoses
- **Lead Poisoning**
  - Anemia caused by a variety of mechanisms
  - Musculoskeletal findings unrelated to anemia
  - Dense metaphyseal lines at ends of bones
    - Involvement of the fibula favors lead poisoning over physiologic dense metaphyseal bands
  - May identify ingested flakes of lead paint on abdominal imaging
  - Erlenmeyer flask deformities
  - Undertubulation of bone diaphyses, late
  - Separation of cranial sutures
- **Myelofibrosis**

ANEMIA WITH MUSCULOSKELETAL MANIFESTATIONS

- ○ Osteosclerosis from replacement of the fatty marrow with fibrous tissue
  - Lower marrow signal intensity on T1WI than red marrow
- ○ No cortical thickening
- ○ Extramedullary hematopoiesis
- **Thalassemia**
  - ○ "Squaring" of bones due to marrow packing
  - ○ Hair-on-end appearance of skull
  - ○ Thinning of the endosteal cortex
  - ○ Coarse trabecular pattern
  - ○ Obliteration of paranasal sinuses
  - ○ Biconcave vertebral bodies are rare
  - ○ Extramedullary hematopoiesis
- **Hypothyroidism**
  - ○ Congenital hypothyroidism findings are unrelated to anemia
    - Kyphosis
    - Flattened vertebral bodies
    - Wedge or hook shape upper lumbar vertebral body - "sail vertebra"
    - Increased intervertebral disc spaces
  - ○ Associated with autoimmune diseases
    - Rheumatoid arthritis, lupus, ulcerative colitis, IDDM
- **Polycythemia Vera**
  - ○ Myelofibrosis may be precursor to polycythemia
  - ○ Red marrow reconversion
    - Apophyseal regions more resistant to reconversion
- **Aplastic Anemia**

- ○ Skeletal manifestations are related to the cause of aplastic anemia
  - Chemotherapy, infection, radiation, toxic exposure

Helpful Clues for Rare Diagnoses
- **Osteopetrosis**
  - ○ Autosomal recessive types are associated with hematological derangement
    - Increased fractures & infections
    - Malignant infantile type = death at young age without bone marrow transplant
  - ○ Autosomal dominant forms do not cause anemia & may be entirely asymptomatic
- **Down Syndrome (Trisomy 21)**
  - ○ Atlantoaxial subluxation
  - ○ Short humerus & femur
  - ○ Flared iliac wing
  - ○ Flattened acetabular roof
  - ○ Absent or hypoplastic nasal bone
- **Erythroblastosis Fetalis**
  - ○ Transverse metaphyseal bands
  - ○ Diffuse diaphyseal sclerosis
- **Fanconi Anemia**
  - ○ Short stature
  - ○ Absent, malformed or hypoplastic thumbs
  - ○ Absent or hypoplastic radius
  - ○ Dysplastic ulna
  - ○ Microcephaly
  - ○ Micrognathia
  - ○ Scoliosis
  - ○ Developmental hip dysplasia
  - ○ Malformed toes

Iron or Vitamin Deficiency Anemia

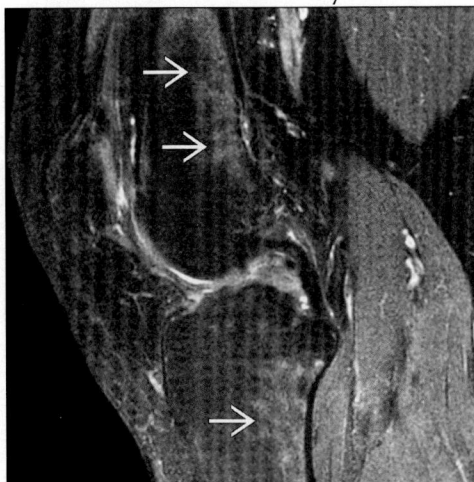

Sagittal T1WI FS MR shows areas of increased signal in the distal femoral and proximal tibial marrow space due to red bone marrow reconversion ➡ in this young, anemic female patient.

Chronic Renal Disease

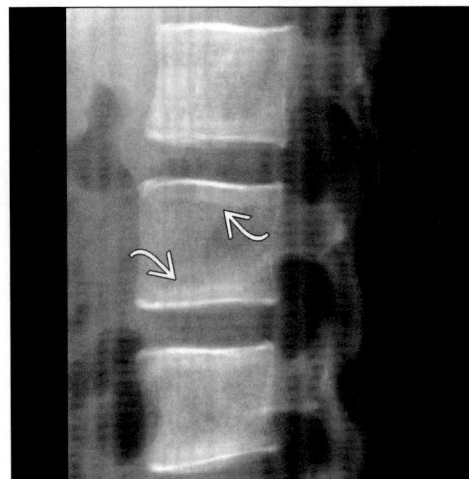

Lateral radiograph shows dense lines at the vertebral endplates ➡ due to osteoblastic activity, which occurs in addition to osteoclastic activity, producing the so called rugger jersey appearance.

ANEMIA WITH MUSCULOSKELETAL MANIFESTATIONS

(Left) Sagittal T1WI MR shows diffuse low signal in the marrow in a patient with HIV. Other sequences did not suggest infiltrating tumor. HIV may have a dysplasia affecting one of the blood cell lines resulting in anemia. *(Right)* Lateral radiograph shows normal vertebral body height in the anterior and posterior aspects but an abrupt loss of height ➡ in the mid portion of the body, producing the classic "H-shape" ➡. There is biconcavity of the remaining vertebral bodies.

Anemia of Chronic Disease

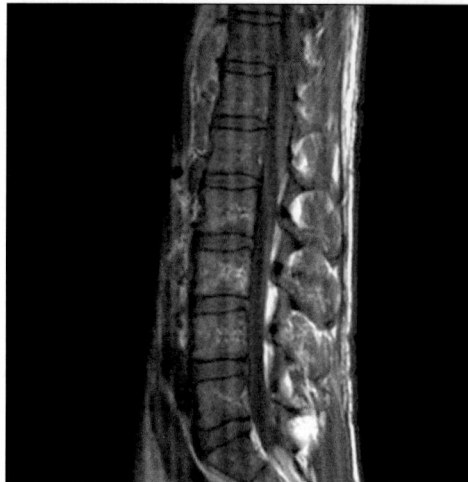

Sickle Cell Anemia

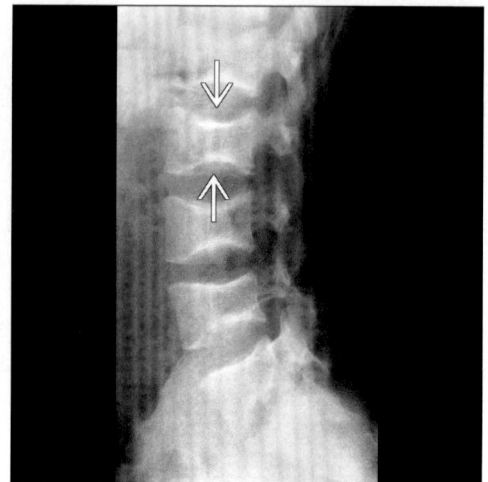

(Left) Axial STIR MR shows the serpiginous pattern of avascular necrosis in the anterosuperior portions of both femoral heads ➡. The infarcts are surrounded by edema and the remainder of the bone marrow has low signal red marrow reconversion. *(Right)* Anteroposterior radiograph shows a change in density and slight periosteal reaction involving the first metacarpal ➡. The remaining bones are normal. The appearance is equivocal for infection vs. dactylitis.

Sickle Cell Anemia

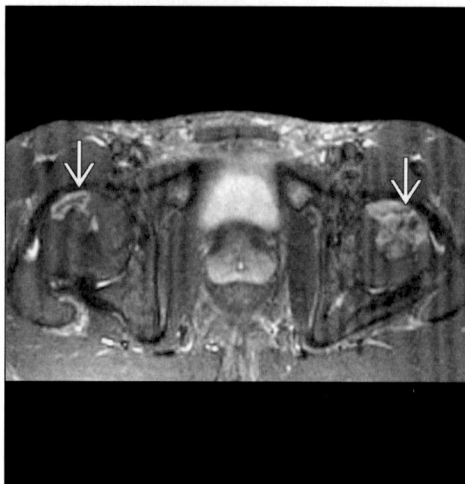

Sickle Cell Anemia

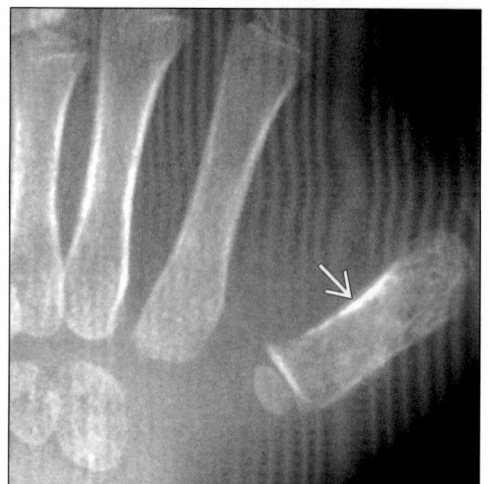

(Left) Anteroposterior radiograph shows classic dense bands ➡ involving the diaphyses. This is due to deposition of radiodense lead. Involvement of the fibula favors lead poisoning over a normal variant. *(Right)* Axial NECT shows diffuse sclerosis ➡ involving the marrow space of the pelvis and sacrum. The bone cortex is not thickened. Osteopetrosis can have a similar appearance but does not produce anemia in the adult form of the disease.

Lead Poisoning

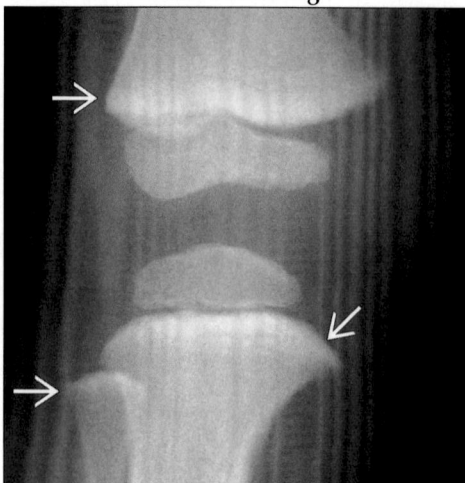

Myelofibrosis

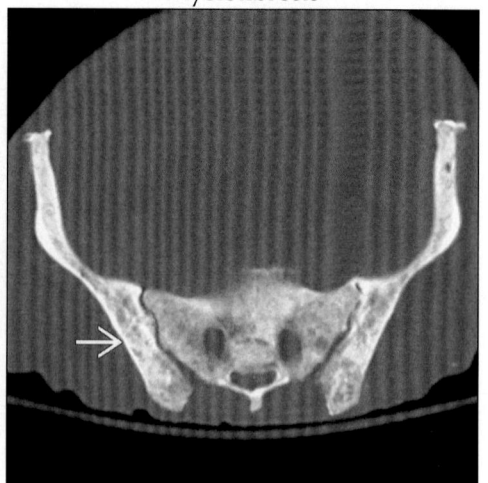

ANEMIA WITH MUSCULOSKELETAL MANIFESTATIONS

Myelofibrosis

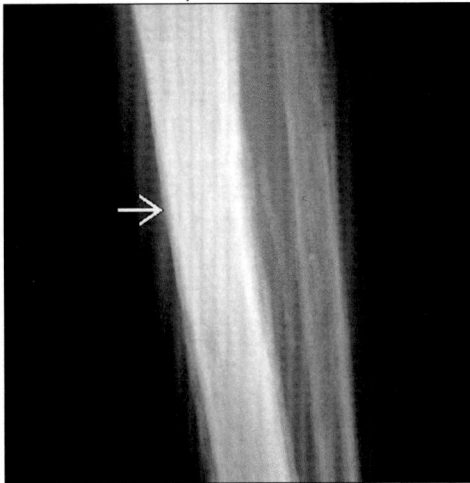

Thalassemia

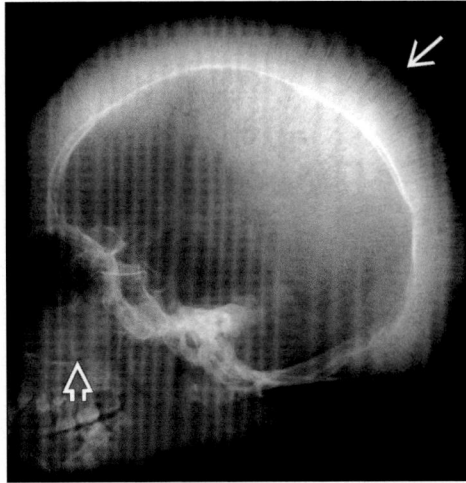

(Left) Anteroposterior radiograph shows diffuse medullary space osteosclerosis ➡ that involved the axial skeleton as well as the tubular bones. The lack of thickening of the endosteal cortex is typical of myelofibrosis. *(Right)* Lateral radiograph shows dense striations in a much widened diploic space of the cranium, giving the "hair on end" appearance ➡. Note also that the paranasal sinuses are obliterated secondary to marrow hyperplasia ➡.

Thalassemia

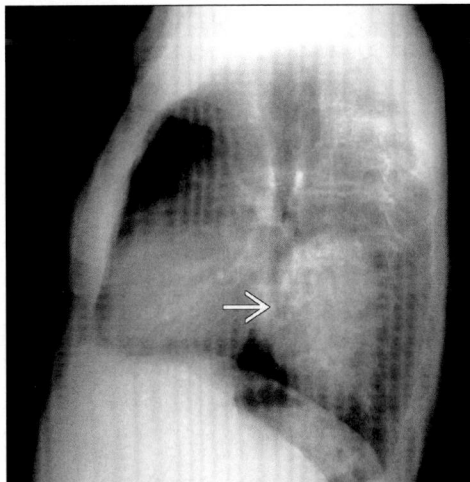

Thalassemia

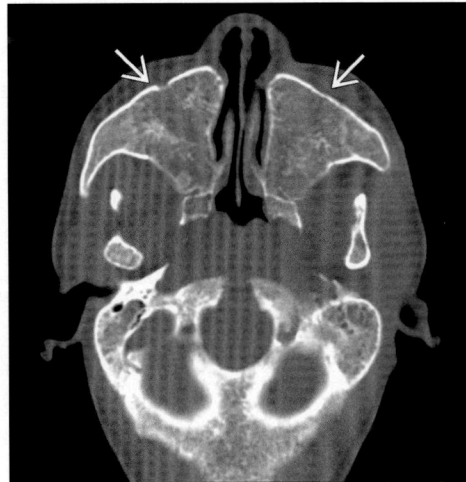

(Left) Lateral radiograph shows a paravertebral mass ➡. This mass is a site of extramedullary hematopoiesis and is found in the most common location for this occurrence. *(Right)* Axial NECT shows obliteration of the maxillary sinuses ➡. This obliteration is a result of marrow hyperplasia. Generalized expansion of the sinuses is present. This expansion leads to a distortion of the facial features which is typical of thalassemia and is known as rodent facies.

Thalassemia

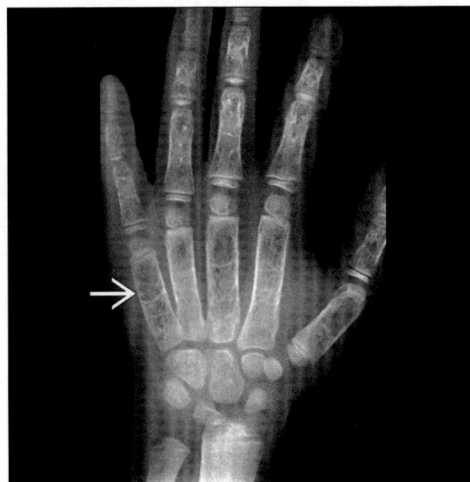

Osteopetrosis

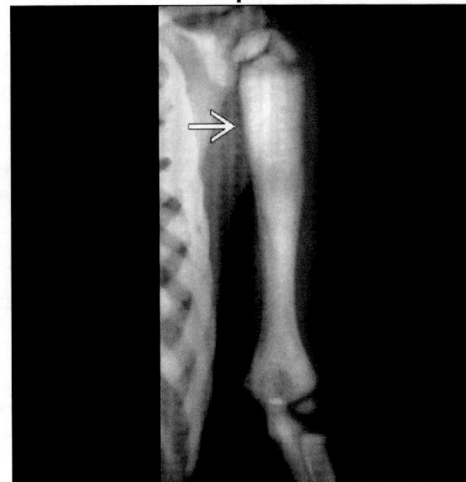

(Left) Anteroposterior radiograph shows "squaring" ➡ involving the bones of the hand, or loss of their normal tubular morphology due to marrow packing. There is associated thinning of the endosteal cortex. *(Right)* Anteroposterior radiograph of severe autosomal recessive osteopetrosis shows the bones to be diffusely and densely sclerotic. Note that the long bones are undertubulated with relative widening of the proximal humerus ➡.

III

155

AVASCULAR NECROSIS

DIFFERENTIAL DIAGNOSIS

Common
- Steroids
- Hip Dislocation
- Femoral Neck Fractures
- Post-Traumatic, Wrist
- Alcohol Abuse
- Sickle Cell Anemia
- Radiation Osteonecrosis
- Systemic Lupus Erythematosus

Less Common
- Slipped Capital Femoral Epiphysis
- Legg-Calvé-Perthes
- Post-Traumatic, Ankle (Talus & Navicular)
- Developmental Dysplasia of the Hip
- AIDS Drug Therapy
- Chemotherapeutic Drugs
- Idiopathic

Rare but Important
- Gaucher Disease
- Cushing Disease
- Embolic Disease
- Pancreatitis
- Caisson Disease
- Osteomyelitis, Pediatric

ESSENTIAL INFORMATION

Key Differential Diagnosis Issues
- Though "idiopathic" is found at the top of the list for etiology of AVN in many discussions, in the author's experience, another etiology can usually be found
  - **Hint**: Watch for clues in the soft tissues & bones to discover the etiology of AVN
- **Hint**: The most frequent etiologies of AVN in developed countries includes steroid use, alcohol use, sickle cell disease, and trauma
- **Hint**: Bones which are mostly covered by cartilage are particularly at risk for developing AVN
  - Femoral head, humeral head, scaphoid, lunate, talus, navicular

Helpful Clues for Common Diagnoses
- **Steroids**
  - Multiple reasons for steroid use; these may sometimes be noted on the images
    - Watch for reniform soft tissue mass in iliac fossa, indicating renal transplant

- Watch for soft tissue calcifications suggesting dermatomyositis
- Watch for staple lines of ileoanal pull-through and sacroiliitis suggesting inflammatory bowel disease, requiring steroid use
- Watch for uniform cartilage narrowing & erosive disease suggesting rheumatoid arthritis, commonly treated with steroids
  - Systemic steroid use increases size of fat cells; in sites at risk for AVN, these compromise blood flow
    - Particularly femoral head, humeral head, talus, vertebral bodies
  - Direct intraarticular injection of steroids may result in both AVN and intraarticular calcification
- **Hip Dislocation**
  - Because of tenuous blood supply to femoral head, a hip which remains dislocated > 12 hours is at significant risk of developing AVN
- **Femoral Neck Fractures**
  - In adults, artery of ligamentum teres is no longer patent; femoral head depends on circumflex artery at femoral neck
  - Subcapital fracture puts artery & blood supply at risk; basicervical or intertrochanteric fractures do not have a comparable risk of AVN
    - Displaced subcapital fracture is at greater risk for AVN than non-displaced
- **Post-Traumatic, Wrist**
  - Scaphoid fractures
    - Waist or proximal pole fractures are at risk for AVN; distal pole fractures are not at similar risk
    - AVN may be difficult to evaluate in scaphoid fracture; relative increase in radiographic or CT density alone may not signify the fragment is avascular
    - T1 and post-contrast MR is most reliable means of predicting fragment viability
  - Lunate injuries
    - Direct fracture is rarely a cause of lunate malacia
    - Most frequent traumatic cause of lunate AVN is ulnar negative variance, which results in shift of weight-bearing through lunate from being shared by ulna to entirely radial

AVASCULAR NECROSIS

- Repetitive microtrauma results in AVN
- **Alcohol Abuse**
  - Common cause of AVN; patients must be asked directly how much alcohol they consume daily to ascertain the truth
  - Other possible hints on radiograph: Pancreatic calcifications
- **Sickle Cell Anemia**
  - Sickled cells sludge in small vessels, causing occlusion
  - Femoral head and humeral head are at significant risk
  - Vertebral body endplates are at risk
    - Small vessels form terminal loops beneath vertebral endplates, at risk for sludging by abnormal red blood cells
    - Once endplates lose vascularity, they collapse, often in "H-shaped" configuration; may also be biconcave
  - Watch for other signs of sickle cell anemia
    - Diffuse increased bone density from diffuse infarcts
    - Small or auto-infarcted spleen
    - Gallstones
    - Pulmonary infarcts; increased lung vascularity from anemia
- **Radiation Osteonecrosis**
  - Port-like region of sclerotic bone indicates focal region of osteonecrosis related to RT

Helpful Clues for Less Common Diagnoses
- **Slipped Capital Femoral Epiphysis**
  - Usually only develop coxa magna deformity, but occasionally AVN

- **Post-Traumatic, Ankle (Talus & Navicular)**
  - Body of talus at risk for AVN following neck fracture; watch for Hawkins sign suggesting viability
  - Muller-Weiss: Bilateral (usually) AVN of navicular, related to stress fracture
- **Developmental Dysplasia of the Hip**
  - Infrequently develops AVN
- **AIDS Drug Therapy**
  - Antiretroviral therapy results in low MR signal throughout osseous structures
  - Rarely, AVN is also seen
- **Chemotherapeutic Drugs**
  - Cytotoxic therapy rarely results in bone infarcts & AVN

Alternative Differential Approaches
- AVN with diffusely abnormal marrow
  - Sickle cell anemia: Diffuse bone infarcts
  - Systemic lupus erythematosus: May show diffuse osteoporosis
  - Steroids: Marrow may show diffuse osteoporosis
  - AIDS drug therapy: Diffuse low marrow signal
  - Chemotherapeutic drugs: Diffuse infarcts
  - Cushing disease: Diffuse osteoporosis
- AVN with focally abnormal marrow (beyond necrotic site)
  - Radiation osteonecrosis: Port-like abnormal marrow in adjacent bones
  - Gaucher disease: Shows marrow replacement at other sites (spine, distal femora)

Steroids

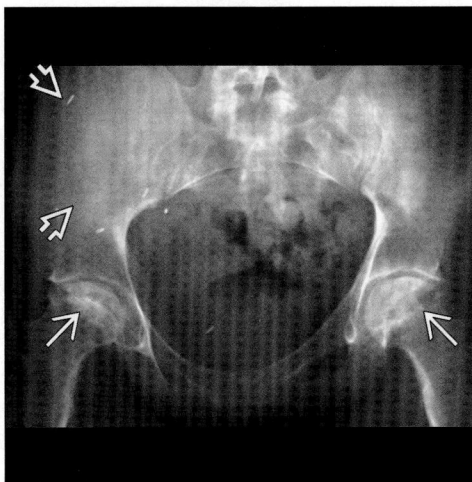

AP radiograph shows end stage AVN of the femoral heads ➡, due to steroid use. The patient had a renal transplant; note the reniform soft tissue mass in the iliac fossa ➡, along with the surgical clips.

Steroids

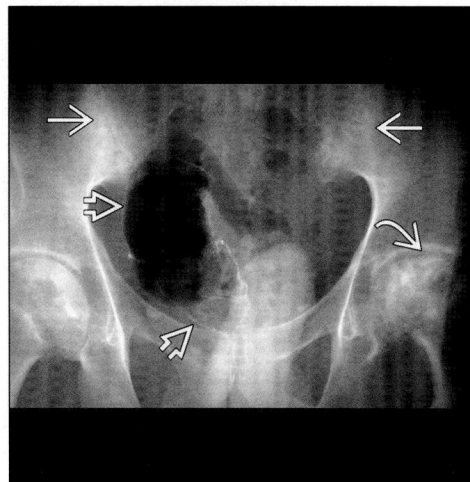

AP radiograph shows AVN of the left hip ➡. Other findings include staple lines (from ileoanal pull-through ➡), & bilateral sacroiliac joint disease ➡. The patient is on steroids for inflammatory bowel disease.

AVASCULAR NECROSIS

(Left) *AP radiograph shows sclerosis and flattening of the femoral head, with secondary osteoarthritis. This is a young man who was involved in a rollover motor vehicle accident one year earlier; the accident was not discovered for several hours.*
(Right) *AP radiograph obtained in the same patient in the emergency room following his accident shows the femoral head superimposed on the superior acetabulum ➡, typical of posterior hip dislocation.*

Hip Dislocation

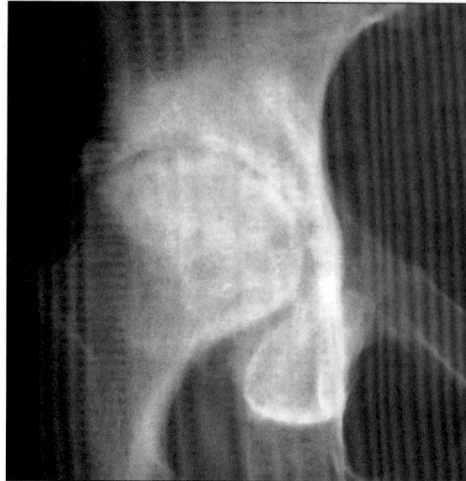

Hip Dislocation

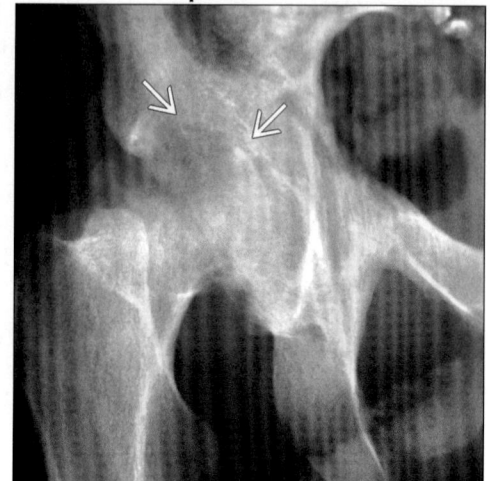

(Left) *AP radiograph in a young man shows three cannulated screws crossing a healed subcapital fracture. Though the fracture healed, the femoral head developed AVN, now with flattening & secondary osteoarthritis ➡.*
(Right) *Anteroposterior radiograph shows a pinned subcapital fracture in an 80 year old. Though treated appropriately, she developed AVN with collapse ➡, a known complication of this fracture.*

Femoral Neck Fractures

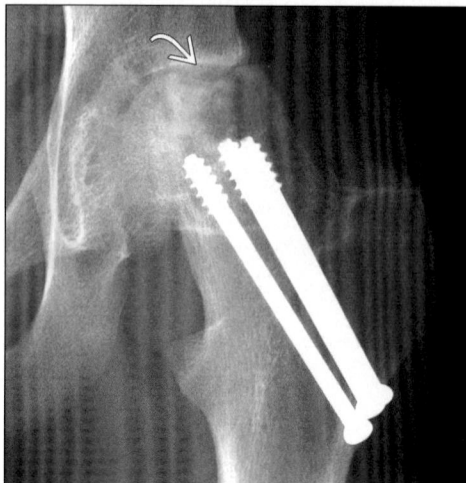

Femoral Neck Fractures

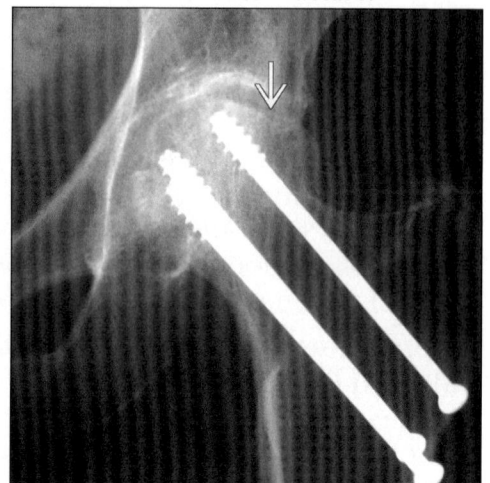

(Left) *Sagittal NECT shows sclerosis of the proximal pole of scaphoid ➡, concerning for AVN in this patient with scaphoid fracture. The fragments have developed a humpback deformity ➡, a common complication.*
(Right) *Coronal T2WI FS MR shows edema within the lunate ➡ indicating early AVN in a patient with ulnar minus variance ➡; this variance has been associated with Kienbock disease. The edema in the capitate ➡ may relate to altered weight-bearing.*

Post-Traumatic, Wrist

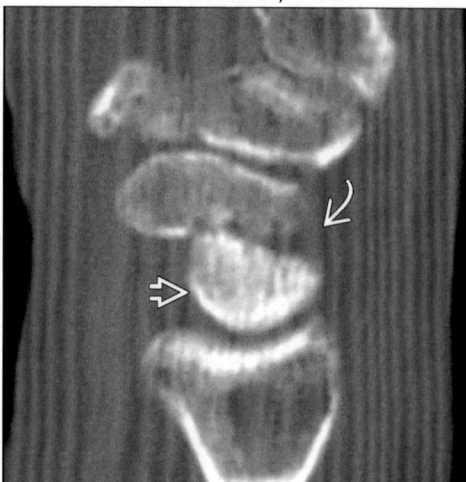

Post-Traumatic, Wrist

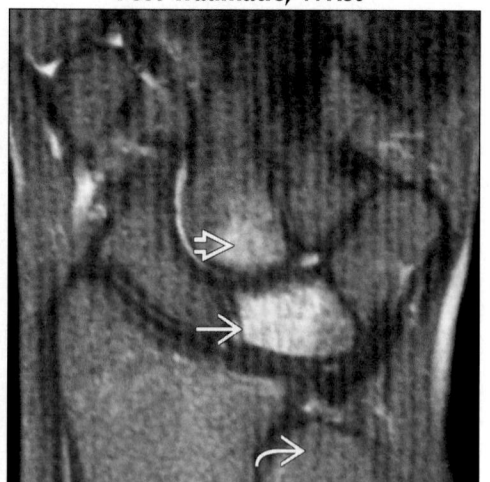

AVASCULAR NECROSIS

Alcohol Abuse

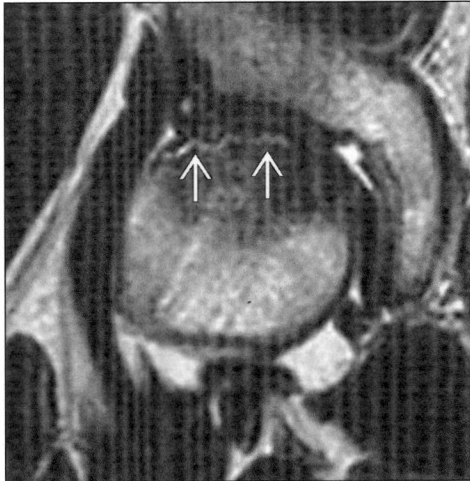

Alcohol Abuse

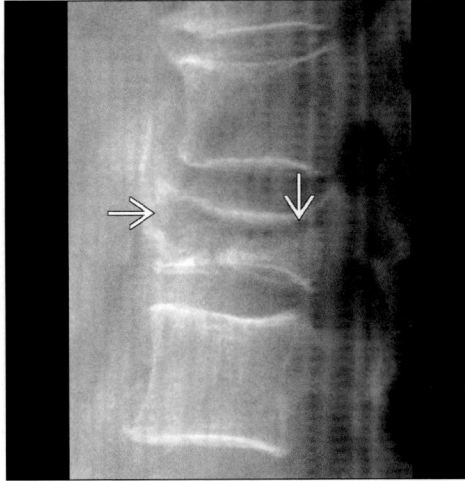

(Left) Coronal T2WI MR shows subchondral fracture ➡, indicating AVN. The patient was clinically diagnosed as femoral acetabular impingement, but upon questioning, admitted to excessive alcohol use. *(Right)* Lateral radiograph shows air within a fractured vertebral body ➡. This represents AVN as the etiology of the fracture. Most frequently this is seen in patients with rheumatoid arthritis on steroids, but in this case is due to alcohol abuse.

Sickle Cell Anemia

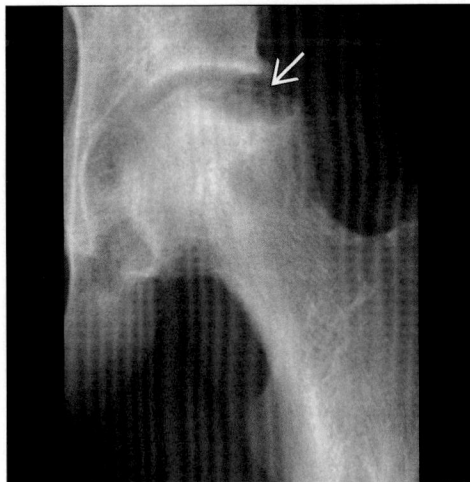

Sickle Cell Anemia

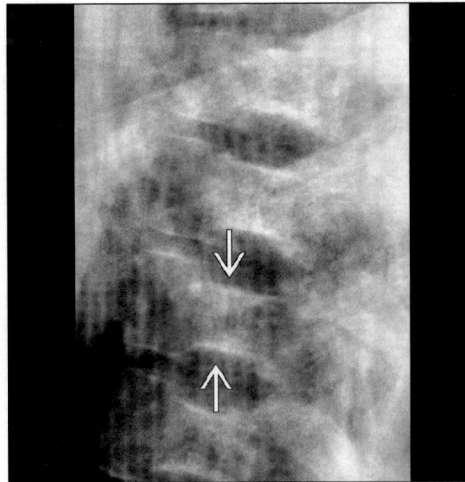

(Left) AP radiograph shows AVN with collapse ➡ in a patient with diffuse osseous sclerosis. The bone density is typical of diffuse infarction in this patient with sickle cell disease. *(Right)* Lateral radiograph shows the mid-endplate vertebral body collapse ➡ which has been termed "H-shaped". This represents AVN of the vertebral bodies, a pattern typical of sickle cell.

Radiation Osteonecrosis

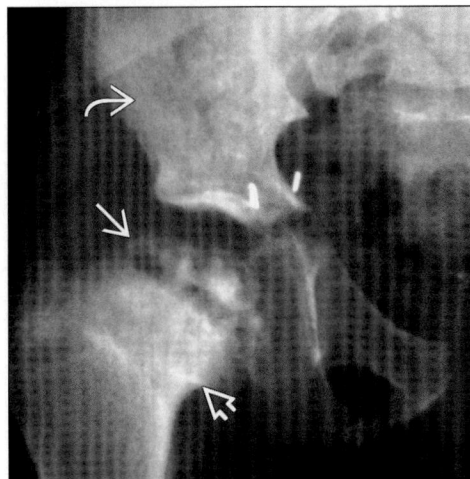

Radiation Osteonecrosis

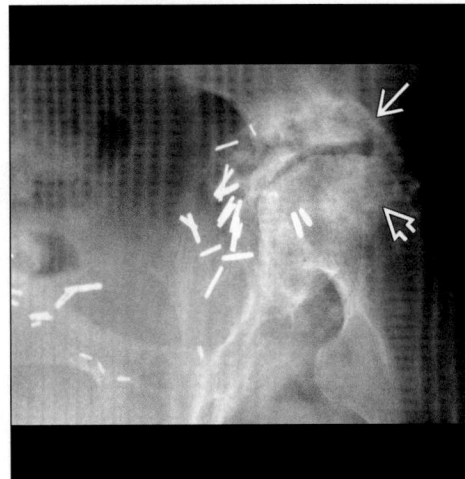

(Left) Anteroposterior radiograph AVN ➡ in this 11 year old. Note the increased density in the adjacent iliac wing ➡. The femoral neck shows sclerosis & abnormal morphology ➡. The other bones are normal; this is a radiation port. *(Right)* AP radiograph shows AVN, with collapse, of both the acetabulum ➡ and the femoral head ➡. The bone abnormality is in a port-like configuration, proving radiation as the etiology. The clips indicate lymph node dissection. (†MSK Req).

AVASCULAR NECROSIS

(Left) Coronal T1WI MR shows the serpiginous pattern of multiple bone infarcts, as well as AVN of both femoral condyles and tibial condyles. This patient has SLE as the underlying disease, and is being treated with steroids. *(Right)* AP radiograph shows AVN of both the lunate ➡️ and the scaphoid ➡️ in a patient with SLE. There was no trauma to suggest another etiology.

Systemic Lupus Erythematosus

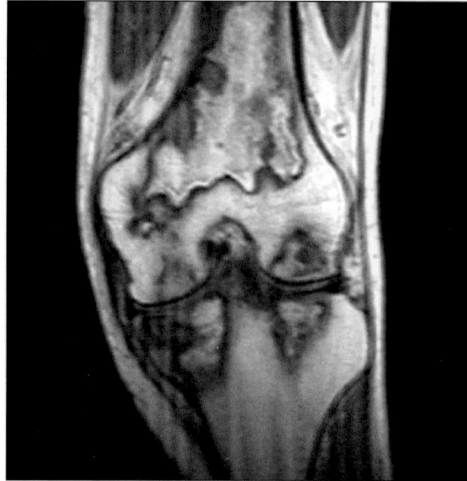

Systemic Lupus Erythematosus

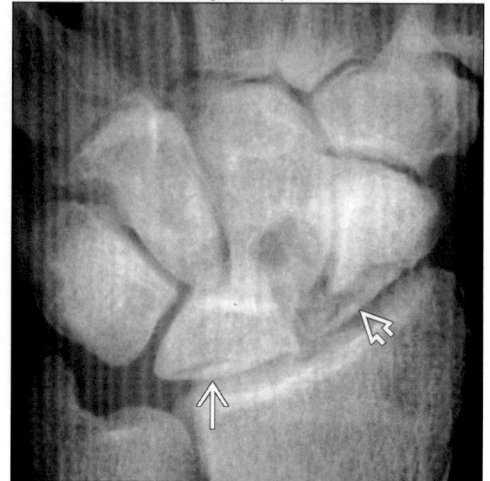

(Left) AP radiograph shows high grade AVN ➡️ in a patient who had been treated for slipped capital femoral epiphysis. Note the linear lucencies in the femoral neck ➡️, indicative of stabilizing pins which have been removed. *(Right)* Coronal T1WI MR shows collapse and fragmentation of the left femoral capital epiphysis ➡️, compared with the normal right. There is early development of coxa magna, with short, broad, head and neck. This is typical Legg-Perthes.

Slipped Capital Femoral Epiphysis

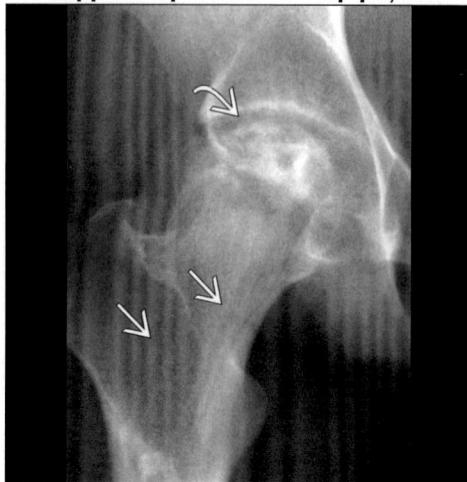

Legg-Calvé-Perthes

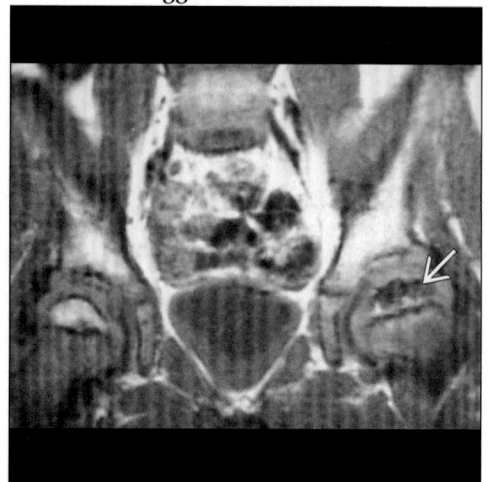

(Left) Anteroposterior radiograph shows normal right hip, but fragmentation of the left femoral capital epiphysis ➡️. This could be due to Legg-Perthes, but the accompanying radiograph demonstrates the true etiology. *(Right)* Anteroposterior radiograph shows superolateral dislocation of the left hip ➡️ of an infant, the same child depicted in the previous image. Although treated appropriately with reduction and stabilization, the patient developed AVN.

Developmental Dysplasia of the Hip

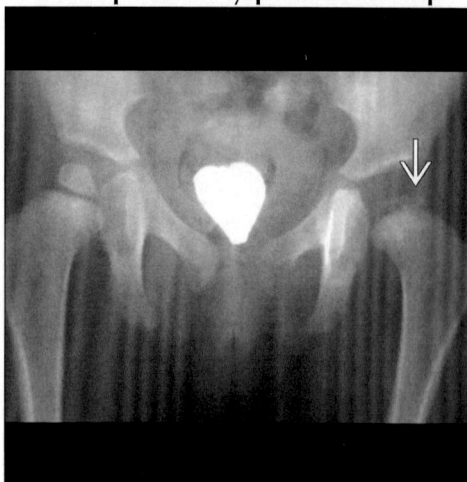

Developmental Dysplasia of the Hip

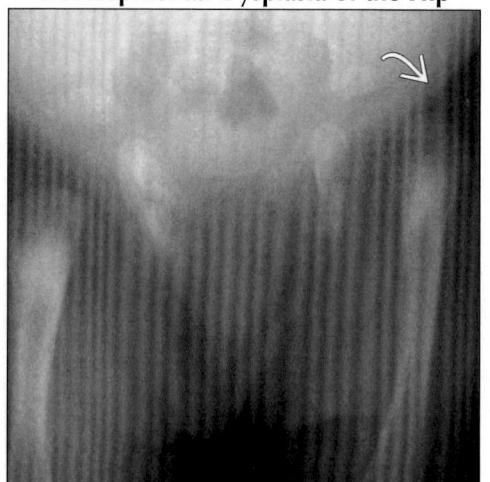

AVASCULAR NECROSIS

AIDS Drug Therapy

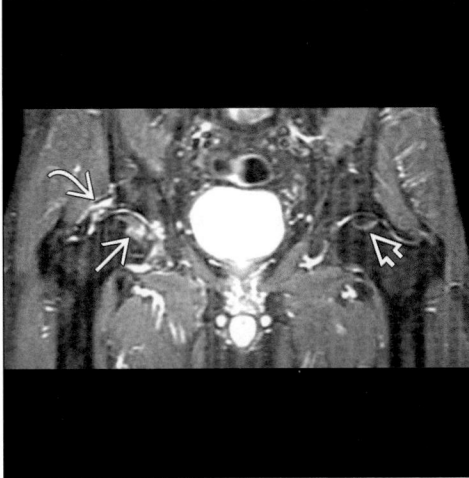

Chemotherapeutic Drugs

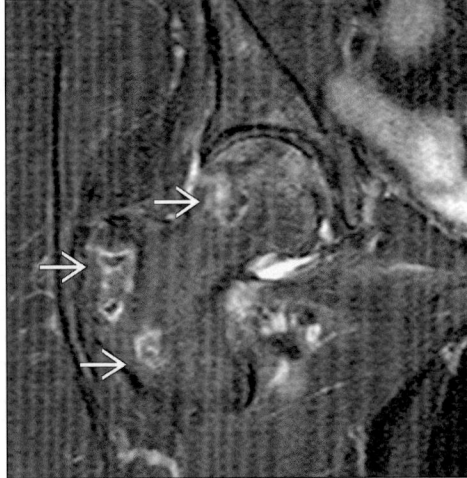

(Left) Coronal STIR MR shows typical appearance of AVN in the hips of an AIDS patient on antiretroviral therapy. The right hip has more advanced disease ➡ plus effusion ➡; the left hip ➡ is asymptomatic. *(Right)* Coronal T2WI FS MR shows multiple bone infarcts throughout the hip ➡, including femoral head AVN. This process appeared following chemotherapy for non-Hodgkin lymphoma & is presumed secondary to cytotoxic injury.

Gaucher Disease

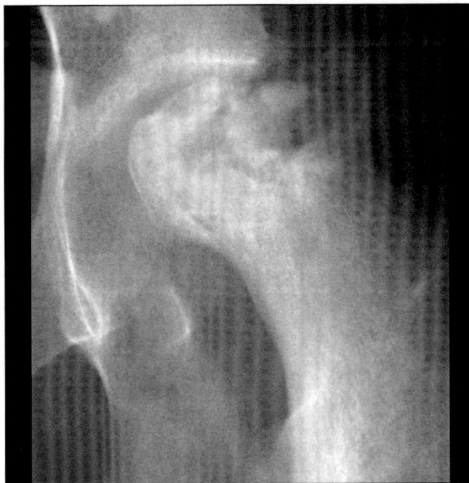

Gaucher Disease

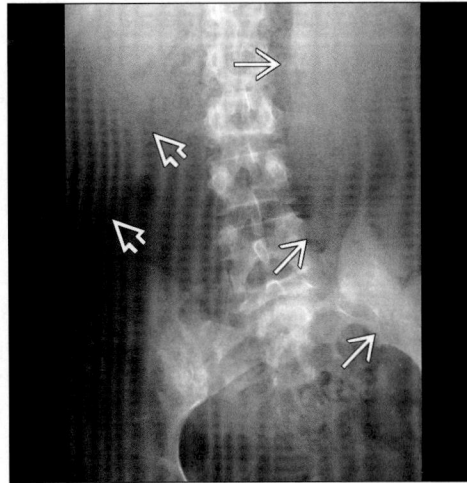

(Left) AP radiograph shows grade IV AVN of the hip with secondary osteoarthritis. The etiology is not clear on this coned down view. However, this was part of an abdominal image which shows the underlying disease process. *(Right)* AP radiograph of the same patient as previous image shows organomegaly. Note the enlarged liver ➡ and spleen ➡, with the bowel gas compressed between. This patient has Gaucher disease.

Cushing Disease

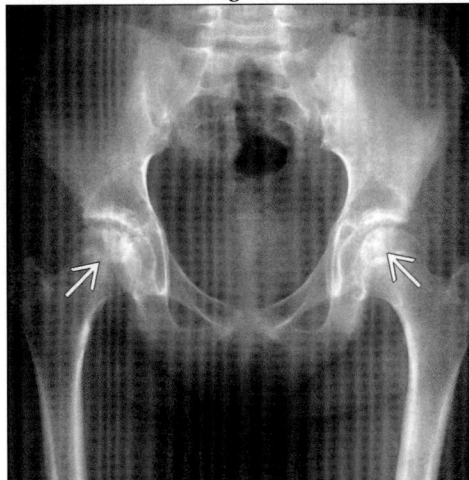

Caisson Disease

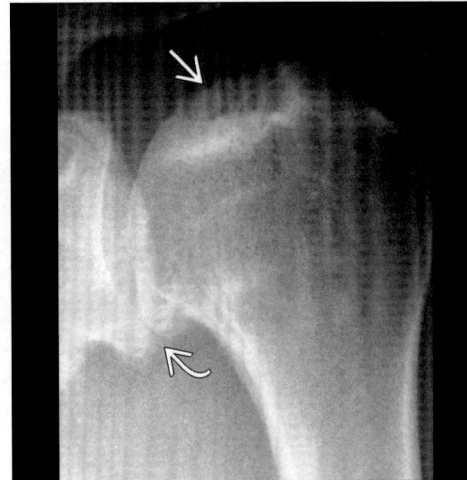

(Left) AP radiograph shows sclerosis in both femoral heads typical of AVN ➡ in a young woman with Cushing disease and endogenous steroid production. There is also severe osteoporosis, typical of this disease. *(Right)* AP radiograph shows classic AVN of the shoulder ➡. The contralateral shoulder and both hips were involved as well in this patient with Caisson disease. This is a rare etiology of AVN. Note the secondary osteoarthritis which has developed ➡.

HETEROTOPIC OSSIFICATION

DIFFERENTIAL DIAGNOSIS

Common
- Trauma
- Post-Operative
- Spine Injury
- Thermal Injury, Burns
- Brain Injury
- Infection
- Neurologic Infection

Less Common
- Dermatomyositis (Mimic)
- Progressive Systemic Sclerosis (Mimic)
- Calcific Myonecrosis (Mimic)

Rare but Important
- Systemic Lupus Erythematosus (Mimic)
- Fibrodysplasia Ossificans Progressiva
- Progressive Osseous Heteroplasia

ESSENTIAL INFORMATION

Key Differential Diagnosis Issues
- Heterotopic ossification (HO) = development of bone in the soft tissues
  - Muscle
  - Tendon
  - Ligaments
  - Subcutaneous fat
  - Periosteum
- a.k.a., myositis ossificans (due to common location in muscle)
  - Heterotopic ossification is a more inclusive term
- Differentiate heterotopic ossification from bone-forming malignancy by presence of more mature periphery than center
- Be suspicious for malignancy if central calcification or ossification is present in a soft tissue mass
  - Heterotopic ossification may attach to native bone or be separated by a cleavage plane
  - Fibrous plane between heterotopic ossification and soft tissue is difficult to appreciate on imaging
  - Remember that myositis ossificans consists of calcification, not ossification, at approximately 1 month post insult
    - Ossification appears later as the lesion matures

- Imaging appearance of HO is predominantly the same regardless of cause
  - Area of calcification developing into peripherally matured bone on radiographs & CT
  - Low signal ossified rim around mass on MR
    - Variable enhancement of mass & surrounding edema
  - History & any associated injury is most helpful for suggesting etiology of HO

Helpful Clues for Common Diagnoses
- **Trauma**
  - Blunt trauma, muscle hematoma, joint dislocation
  - Injury may not always be remembered or reported by the patient
  - Cases of heterotopic ossification without identified cause are often presumed to be due to trauma
- **Post-Operative**
  - Very common after hip replacement
    - 2-90% depending on definition
  - Clinically significant in < 5%
    - Reduced range of motion, mechanical impingement, ankylosis
    - Pre-operative CT to assess location & extent
  - Uncommon after knee or shoulder arthroplasty
- **Spine Injury**
  - HO occurs in 20-25% of patients
    - Most common around hips, knees & ankles
    - More likely to limit joint mobility than post-operative causes
  - May have additional findings of fusion or widening of sacroiliac joints
- **Thermal Injury, Burns**
  - Additional findings of soft tissue contractures, acroosteolysis
- **Brain Injury**
  - History of closed head injury, coma, cerebrovascular accident
  - HO occurs in 10-20% of patients
- **Infection**
  - Early surgical intervention for a septic joint is more likely to have associated HO than intervention for a chronically infected joint
- **Neurologic Infection**

HETEROTOPIC OSSIFICATION

○ Poliomyelitis, tetanus, Guillain-Barré

Helpful Clues for Less Common Diagnoses
- **Dermatomyositis (Mimic)**
  ○ Focal or generalized soft tissue calcification
  ○ Dominant involvement of proximal thighs
  ○ Dense sheet-like calcification is typical
  ○ May have concurrent mixed connective tissue disorder
- **Progressive Systemic Sclerosis (Mimic)**
  ○ Globular or sheet-like calcification
  ○ Most common in hands
  ○ Acroosteolysis & soft tissue atrophy
- **Calcific Myonecrosis (Mimic)**
  ○ History of compartment syndrome or severe pain after trauma
  ○ Peripheral calcification & muscle atrophy in single muscle compartment
    ▪ Lower extremity most common

Helpful Clues for Rare Diagnoses
- **Systemic Lupus Erythematosus (Mimic)**
  ○ Rare manifestation of lupus produces linear & nodular calcification
  ○ Involves subcutaneous & deep soft tissues
- **Fibrodysplasia Ossificans Progressiva**
  ○ Genetic cause for predictable pattern of ossification
    ▪ Cranial to caudal
    ▪ Axial to appendicular
  ○ Ossification begins at about 3 years of age
  ○ Associated skeletal malformations
    ▪ Short great toe or thumb
    ▪ Malformed phalanges
    ▪ Short metacarpals & metatarsals

▪ Short femoral neck
▪ Small cervical vertebral bodies + large posterior elements
- **Progressive Osseous Heteroplasia**
  ○ Genetic cause of heterotopic ossification that is less severe than fibrodysplasia ossificans progressiva
  ○ Ossification of skin & subcutaneous tissues primarily, progressing superficial to deep
    ▪ Hemimelic distribution
  ○ Findings begin in infancy
  ○ Lacks skeletal malformations of FOP

Other Essential Information
- Clinical findings including pain, swelling & warmth are common
- Early imaging appearance can mimic sarcoma
- Radionuclide bone scan, 3-phase
  ○ Early (2 weeks-1 month) = increased uptake all phases
  ○ Intermediate (1-3 months) = increased uptake on 3rd phase
  ○ Late (> 3 months) = decreasing 3rd phase uptake
  ○ Chronic (6-12 months) = normal
- Complications of HO include restriction of movement, nerve impingement, blood vessel impingement, fracture
  ○ Very rare malignant transformation to osteosarcoma
- Biopsy may induce changes similar to aneurysmal bone cyst

Trauma

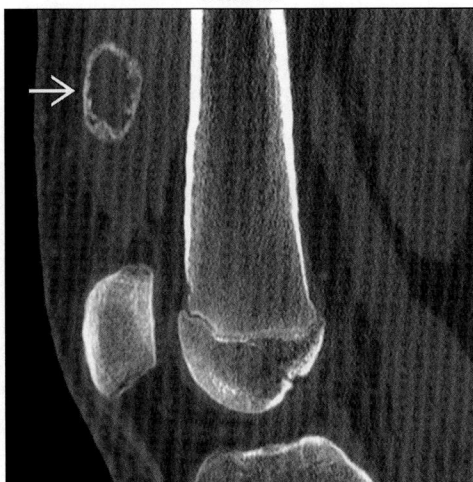

Sagittal NECT shows an oval region of ossification ➡ in the musculature of the anterior distal thigh. The mature periphery of the lesion is typical for heterotopic ossification (a.k.a., myositis ossificans).

Trauma

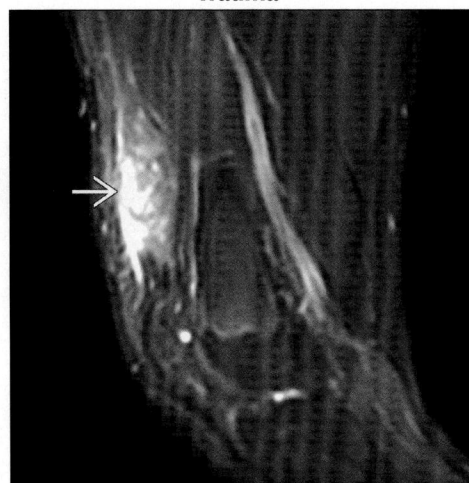

Sagittal STIR MR in the same patient as prior image shows markedly high signal in and around the oval region of ossification ➡. This benign entity has an aggressive appearance on MR.

HETEROTOPIC OSSIFICATION

(Left) Axial T2WI FS MR in the same patient as prior shows that the oval focus of heterotopic ossification ➡ has intermediate to high signal, with a suggestion of a fluid-fluid level, and prominent surrounding edema ➡. (Right) Axial T1 C+ FS MR in the same patient shows inhomogeneous enhancement of the lesion ➡. The MR appearance of heterotopic ossification can suggest an aggressive process due to enhancement and edema.

Trauma

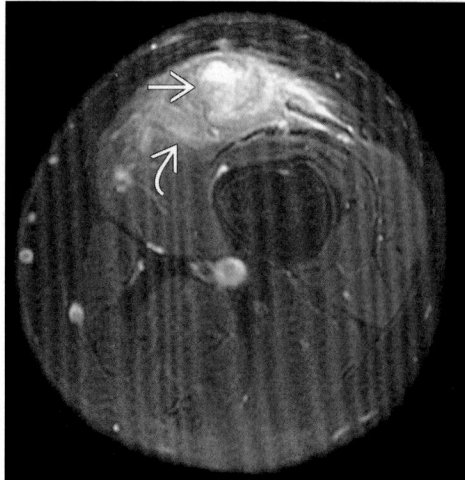

Trauma

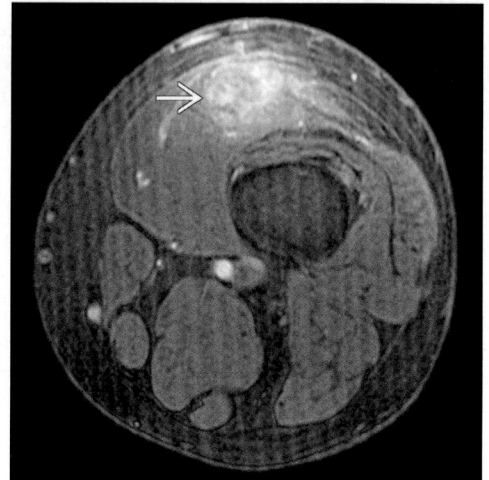

(Left) Anteroposterior radiograph shows heterotopic ossification ➡ forming between the clavicle and coracoid due to disruption of the coracoclavicular ligaments in this grade III acromioclavicular dislocation ➡. (Right) Anteroposterior radiograph shows an osseous mass ➡ which is moderately mature. The mass is most mature at its periphery. The MR showed nonspecific low T1 and high T2 signal, but the radiograph is diagnostic of myositis ossificans.

Trauma

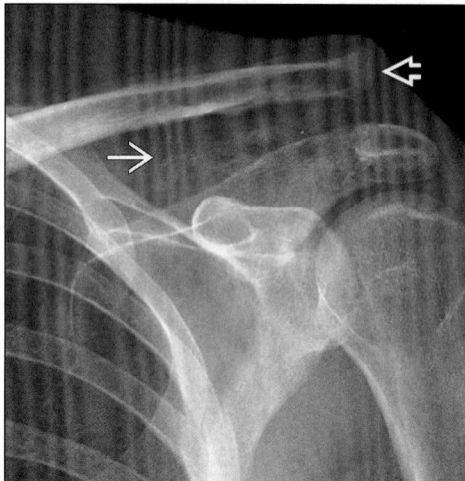

Trauma

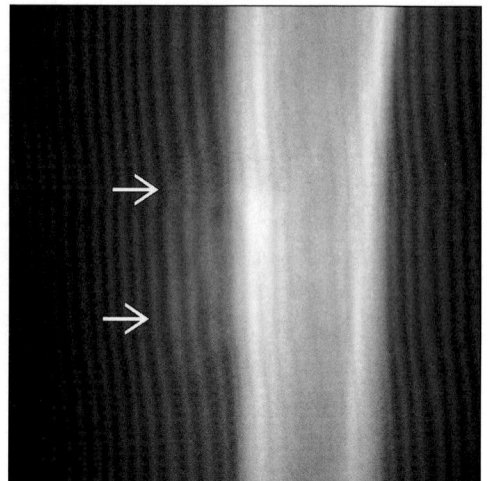

(Left) Lateral radiograph shows development of heterotopic ossification ➡ in the antecubital fossa. This is a common location for myositis, particularly following elbow dislocation. Note that the bone formation is amorphous ➡ suggesting an injury 4-8 weeks earlier. (Right) Lateral radiograph shows a mature osseous mass, with a very distinct and smooth outer cortex ➡ but less defined center. There is a cleavage plane between the mass and the underlying humerus.

Trauma

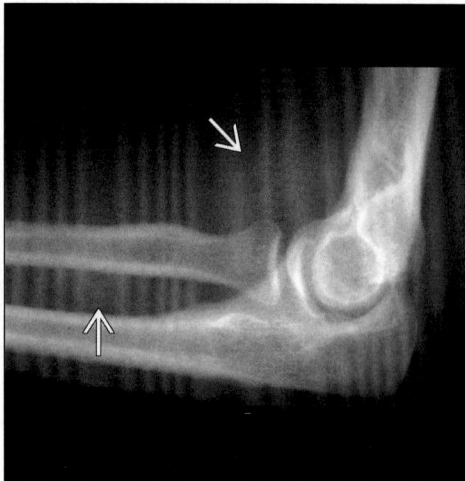

Trauma

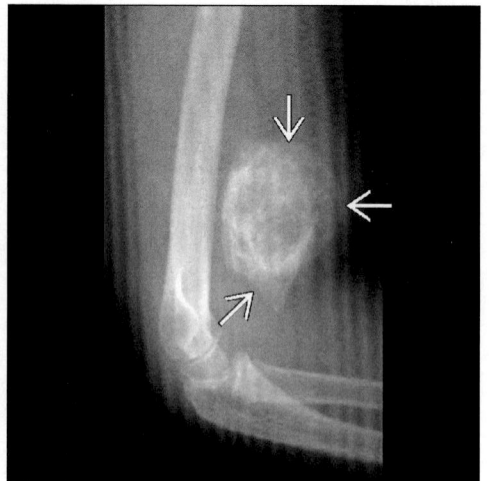

HETEROTOPIC OSSIFICATION

Trauma

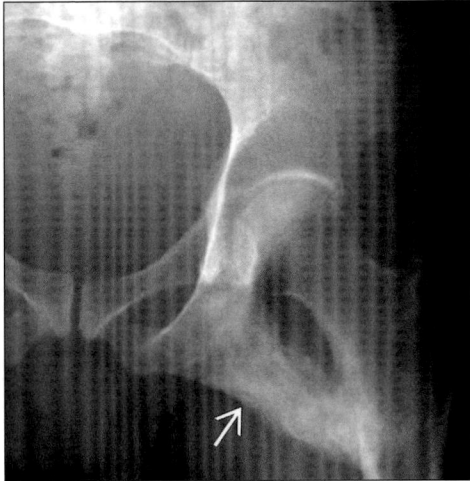

Post-Operative

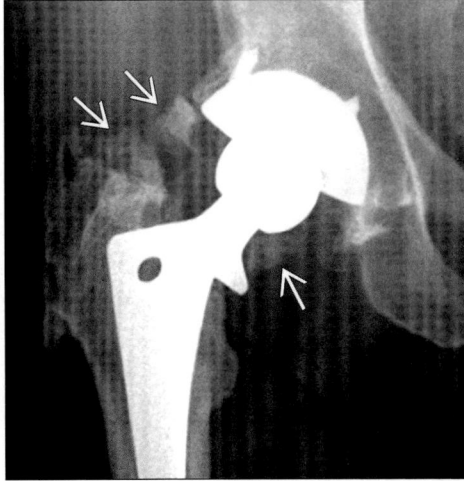

(Left) Anteroposterior radiograph shows heterotopic ossification ➡ extending from the ischial tuberosity to the proximal femur, corresponding to the location of the quadratus femoris muscle. This is likely due to a remote injury. (Right) Anteroposterior radiograph shows mature heterotopic ossification ➡ surrounding a noncemented right total hip prosthesis. Heterotopic ossification after hip arthroplasty is very common, but rarely causes significant clinical symptoms.

Spine Injury

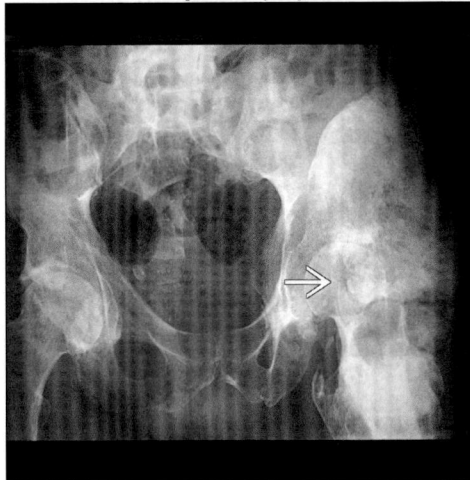

Thermal Injury, Burns

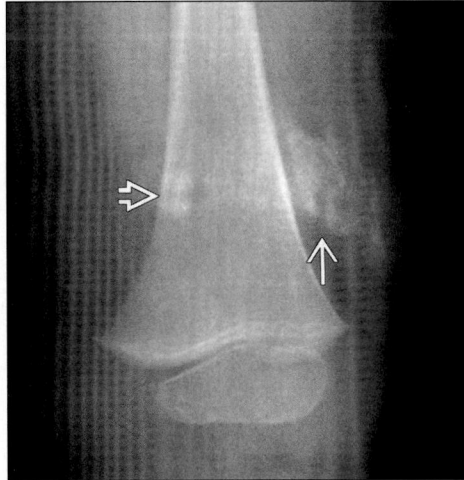

(Left) Anteroposterior radiograph shows a sheet of heterotopic bone ➡ anterior to the left hip. Neurologically injured patients, especially paraplegics, are at high risk for developing heterotopic ossification, especially around the hips. (Right) Anteroposterior radiograph shows a pin tract ➡ through the distal femoral diaphysis, related to pinning for suspension of the burned extremity. There is classic heterotopic ossification ➡ surrounding the pin tract.

Fibrodysplasia Ossificans Progressiva

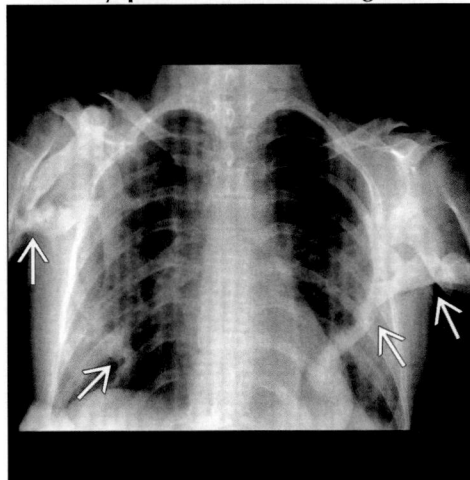

Fibrodysplasia Ossificans Progressiva

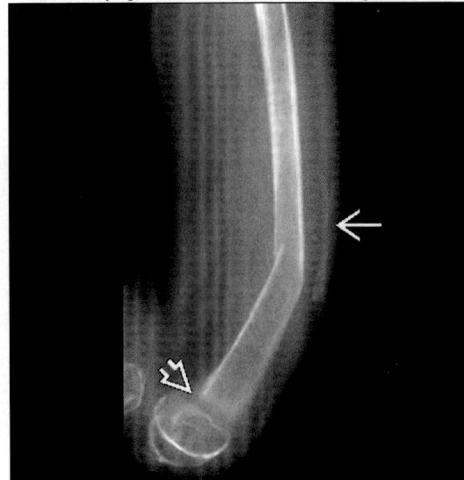

(Left) Anteroposterior radiograph shows the typical extensive soft tissue heterotopic ossification ➡ in the arms and chest of a patient with fibrodysplasia ossificans progressiva. (Right) Lateral radiograph shows mature ossification within the soft tissues of the anterior thigh ➡. The patient was treated with a chelator to resorb the dystrophic bone, which caused resorption of normal bone ➡ in a rickets-like pattern (widened provisional zone of calcification).

RICKETS & OSTEOMALACIA

DIFFERENTIAL DIAGNOSIS

Common
- Renal Failure (Renal Tubular Disease)
- Chronic Liver Disease
- Chronic Pancreatitis

Less Common
- Intestinal Malabsorption
- Rickets of Prematurity
- Aluminum Toxicity

Rare but Important
- Vitamin D Deficiency
- Oncogenic Osteomalacia
- Dilantin
- Phenobarbital
- Vitamin D Dependent Rickets
- Hypophosphatemic Rickets (X-Linked)
- Hypophosphatasia (Mimic)
- Pseudohypoparathyroidism / Pseudo-pseudohypoparathyroidism
- Atypical Axial Osteomalacia
- Metaphyseal Chondrodysplasia (Mimic)

ESSENTIAL INFORMATION

Key Differential Diagnosis Issues
- Radiographic manifestations common to all
  - Osteopenia
  - Coarse, ill-defined trabecula
  - Looser's zones, pseudofractures
  - Cortical tunneling
  - Rickets
    - Metaphyseal cupping & fraying
    - Growth retardation, short stature
    - Bowing, protrusio & other deformities 2° to "soft bones"
    - Changes most pronounced in wrists & knees
    - More severe than adult onset disease
- Pertinent laboratory values: Serum calcium, serum phosphate, serum alkaline phosphatase

Helpful Clues for Common Diagnoses
- **Renal Failure (Renal Tubular Disease)**
  - Decreased serum calcium, elevated phosphate is unique finding
  - Associated hyperparathyroidism
    - Soft tissue calcium deposits

- Bone resorption: Subperiosteal, subchondral, subligamentous, subtendinous, cortical tunneling
    - Brown tumors, osteoporosis
  - Osteosclerosis, Rugger jersey spine
  - Atrophic kidneys, dialysis catheter
- **Chronic Liver Disease & Chronic Pancreatitis**
  - No differentiating radiographic features
  - History essential to diagnosis

Helpful Clues for Less Common Diagnoses
- **Intestinal Malabsorption**
  - Underlying disorders include gluten sensitive enteropathy, sprue, regional enteritis, scleroderma, obesity surgery, short gut syndrome, partial gastrectomy
  - Regional enteritis; seronegative spondyloarthropathy including spinal fusion, SI joint ankylosis, enthesopathy
  - Scleroderma: Soft tissue calcification, acroosteolysis, polyarthritis (most common is co-existent rheumatoid arthritis)
- **Rickets of Prematurity**
  - ≤ 1,000 gm; ≤ 28 weeks EGA
- **Aluminum Toxicity**
  - In past main source of aluminum was dialysate, now it is oral phosphate binders
  - Features which may help differentiate from renal osteodystrophy
    - Less pseudofractures, bone resorption, osteosclerosis
    - Increased incidence of infarction following renal transplantation

Helpful Clues for Rare Diagnoses
- **Vitamin D Deficiency**
  - Nutritional rickets uncommon in US today
    - Consider in immigrant populations & individuals in poverty conditions
    - May be seen with limited exposure to sunlight
  - Decreased serum calcium & phosphate, elevated alkaline phosphatase
- **Oncogenic Osteomalacia**
  - Hemangiopericytoma most common underlying tumor
  - Also hemangioma, giant cell tumor, nonossifying fibroma, osteoblastoma
  - Osteomalacia resolves after tumor resection
- **Dilantin & Phenobarbital**

RICKETS & OSTEOMALACIA

- ○ No distinguishing radiographic features
- ○ History essential to diagnosis
- **Vitamin D Dependent Rickets**
  - ○ Manifests in infancy
  - ○ Decreased serum calcium & phosphate, elevated alkaline phosphatase
- **Hypophosphatemic Rickets (X-linked)**
  - ○ a.k.a. vitamin D resistant rickets
  - ○ Serum calcium normal, low serum phosphate, elevated alkaline phosphatase, PTH normal to slightly elevated
  - ○ Presents late infancy, early toddler years, mainly difficulty walking/weight bearing
  - ○ Abnormal dentition
  - ○ Calcification in tendon & ligaments, enthesopathy
    - Mimics DISH, ankylosing spondylitis
  - ○ Adults: Increased bone density in spine
  - ○ May see changes of hypervitaminosis D
- **Hypophosphatasia (Mimic)**
  - ○ Normal serum calcium & phosphate, decreased alkaline phosphatase
  - ○ Early loss of decidual teeth is common
  - ○ Perinatal form lethal
  - ○ Infantile form
    - Radiolucent lines extending into metaphyses
  - ○ Adult form
    - Fractures, chondrocalcinosis, tendon & ligament calcification, enthesopathy
- **Pseudohypoparathyroidism / Pseudo-pseudohypoparathyroidism**
  - ○ Pseudohypoparathyroidism

- Decreased serum calcium, elevated serum phosphate, parathyroid hormone elevated
- Obesity, developmental delay
- Dental hypoplasia
- Premature physeal fusion leads to short stature
- Bone resorption changes of HPTH may be seen
- Soft tissue calcifications/ossifications: Calcification plaque-like, ossification peri-articular
- Short metacarpals & metatarsals, especially 4th & 5th metacarpals, also short distal phalanx of thumb
- Coned epiphyses
- Small exostoses located on diaphysis
- Basal ganglia calcification
  - ○ Pseudo-pseudohypoparathyroidism
    - Biochemically normal
    - Phenotype mimics pseudohypoparathyroidism
- **Atypical Axial Osteomalacia**
  - ○ Confined to spine & pelvis
  - ○ No pseudofractures, Looser's zones
  - ○ Described only in men
- **Metaphyseal Chondrodysplasia (Mimic)**
  - ○ Abnormal enchondral bone formation
    - No Looser's zones, pseudofractures, cortical tunneling
  - ○ Mental retardation, exophthalmos, contractures

Renal Failure (Renal Tubular Disease)

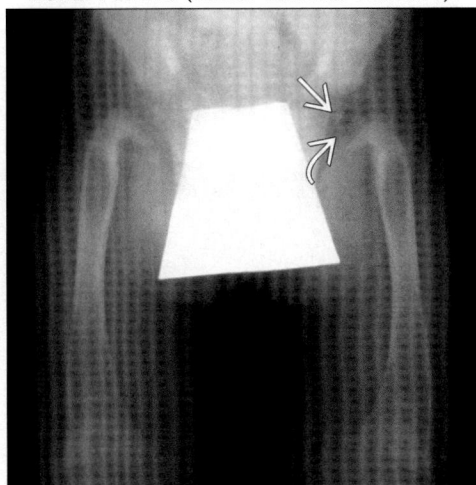

Anteroposterior radiograph shows severe renal osteodystrophy. There is metaphyseal cupping and fraying ➡. The femoral capital epiphysis ➡ is small, indicative of delayed skeletal maturation.

Renal Failure (Renal Tubular Disease)

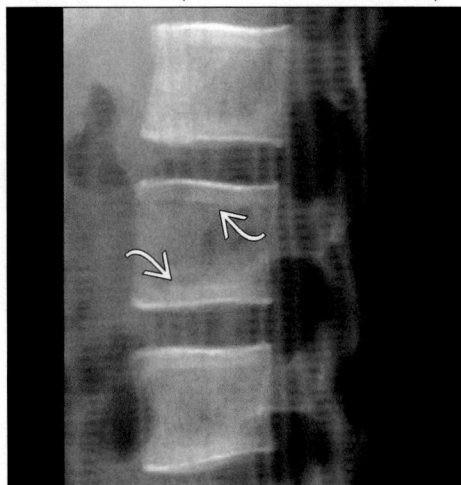

Lateral radiograph shows dense lines at the endplates of the vertebral bodies ➡ which create the appearance known as Rugger Jersey spine in this patient with renal osteodystrophy.

RICKETS & OSTEOMALACIA

Renal Failure (Renal Tubular Disease)

Chronic Liver Disease

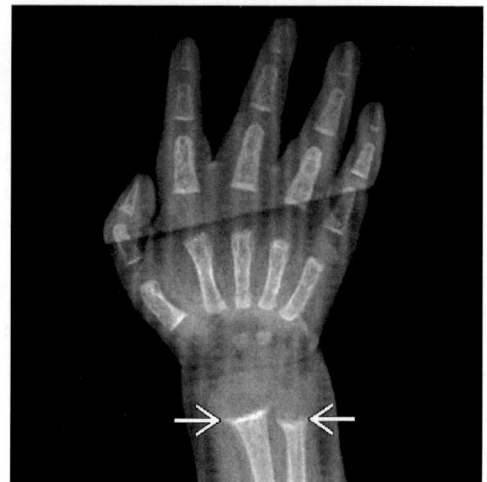

(Left) Anteroposterior radiograph shows typical changes of renal osteodystrophy. Radiographic findings include osteopenia, ill-defined trabecula and dysmorphic femoral necks & trochanters ➡. *(Right)* Anteroposterior radiograph shows a typical case of rickets in a child with biliary atresia. Abnormal metaphyses ➡ are present with cupping and fraying.

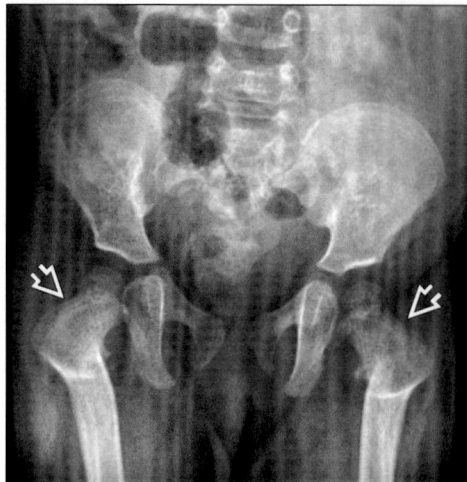

Chronic Liver Disease

Intestinal Malabsorption

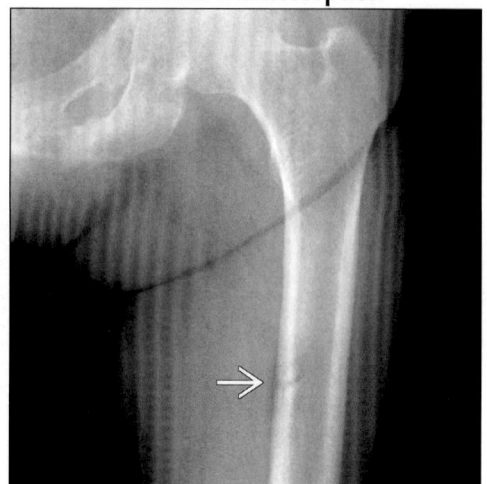

(Left) Anteroposterior radiograph shows enlargement of femoral and tibial metaphyses ➡. This finding contributes to the enlarged knees seen on physical examination in patients with rickets such as this child with biliary atresia. *(Right)* Anteroposterior radiograph shows a typical pseudofracture ➡. Pseudofracture is a nonspecific radiographic abnormality of osteomalacia as seen in this patient with regional enteritis.

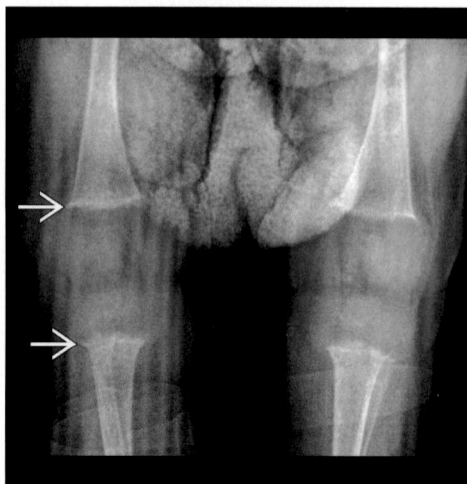

Vitamin D Deficiency

Oncogenic Osteomalacia

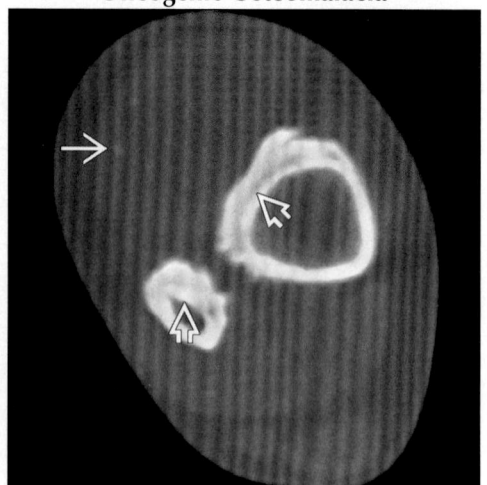

(Left) Anteroposterior radiograph shows bone changes of nutritional deficiency rickets. The rachitic rosary is due to unmineralized osteoid accumulation at the costochondral junctions ➡. *(Right)* Axial NECT shows a large soft tissue mass with phleboliths ➡ and tremendous reactive bone formation both at the tibia and fibula ➡. The findings are indicative of a vascular tumor which in this patient proved to be a hemangiopericytoma.

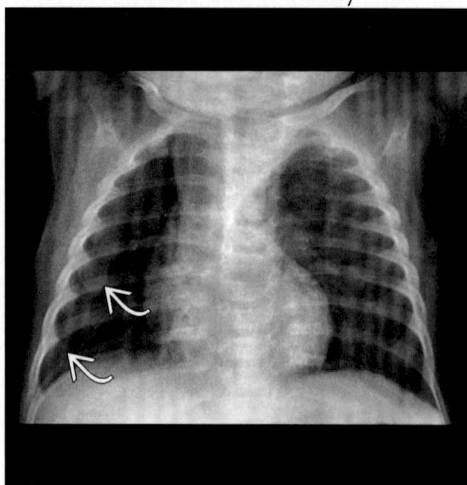

RICKETS & OSTEOMALACIA

Dilantin

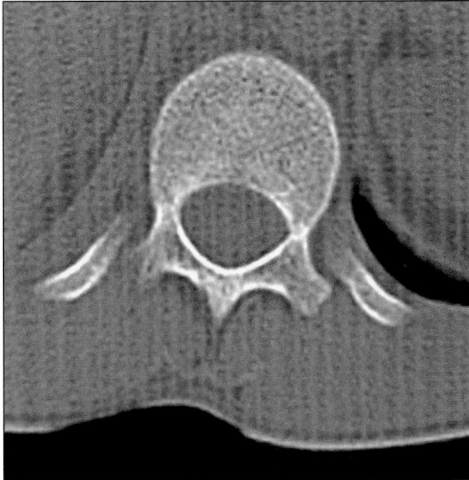

Vitamin D Dependent Rickets

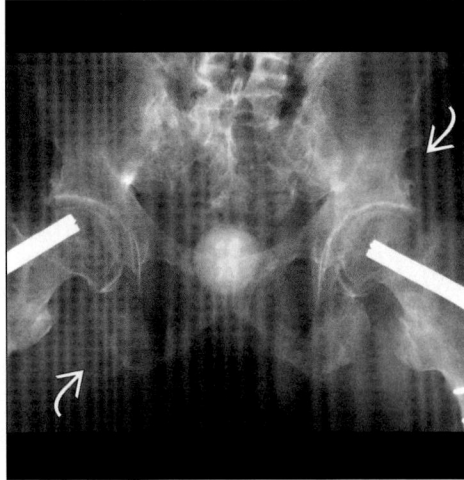

(Left) Axial NECT shows the coarse ill-defined trabecula of anti-convulsant associated osteomalacia. Note poor definition between cortical and medullary bone in part due to cortical tunneling. *(Right)* Anteroposterior radiograph of a patient with vitamin D resistant rickets demonstrates the prominent enthesopathy ➜ associated with high doses of vitamin D. Both femurs have been instrumented for fixation of fractures related to bone softening from unmineralized osteoid.

Hypophosphatasia (Mimic)

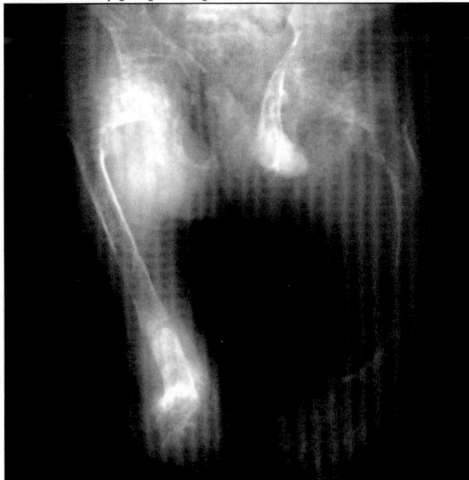

Hypophosphatasia (Mimic)

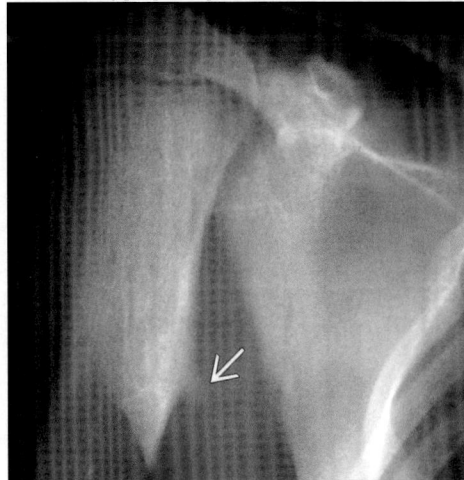

(Left) Anteroposterior radiograph shows typical changes of hypophosphatasia with osteopenia, & deformities secondary to "soft bones" including acetabular protrusio & bowing of the femurs. *(Right)* AP radiograph shows mild diffuse osteopenia and ill-defined trabecula. The small exostoses ➜ along the diaphysis is characteristic of hypophosphatasia. This is a less severe (tarda) form compared with the previous image.

Pseudohypoparathyroidism / Pseudo-pseudohypoparathyroidism

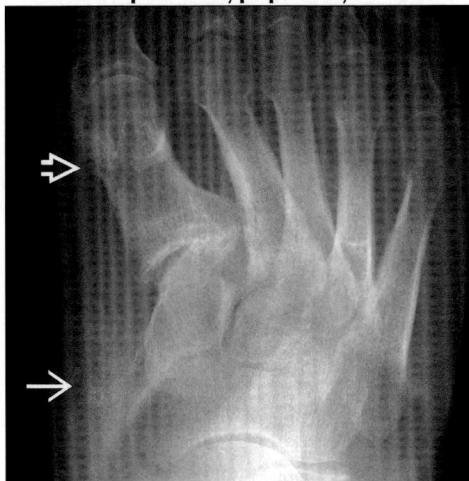

Pseudohypoparathyroidism / Pseudo-pseudohypoparathyroidism

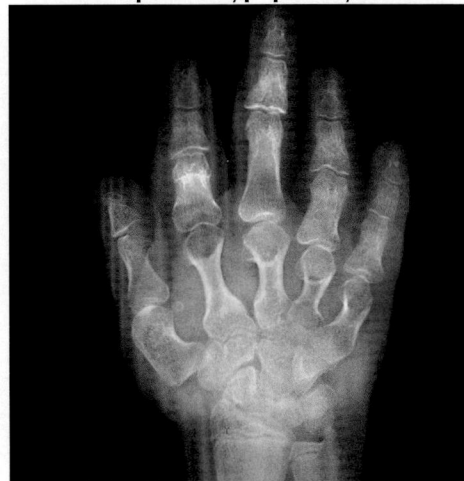

(Left) Anteroposterior radiograph demonstrates soft tissue calcification ➜ and a short first metatarsal ➜. This combination of findings is typical of pseudohypoparathyroidism or pseudo - pseudohypoparathyroidism. *(Right)* Posteroanterior radiograph shows shortening of all metacarpals and epiphyseal abnormalities from coned epiphyses. These features are typical of pseudohypoparathyroidism or pseudo - pseudohypoparathyroidism.

SOFT TISSUE CONTRACTURES

DIFFERENTIAL DIAGNOSIS

Common
- Immobility
- Dupuytren Contracture
- Trauma
- Post-Operative Contracture
- Thermal Injury, Burns
- Volkmann Ischemic Contracture
- Rheumatoid Arthritis
- Juvenile Idiopathic Arthritis
- Complex Regional Pain Syndrome
- Radiation-Induced Non-Neoplastic Soft Tissue Abnormalities

Less Common
- Cerebral Palsy
- Infection
- Myelomeningocele
- Marfan Syndrome
- Diabetes: MSK Complications
- Parsonage-Turner Syndrome, Late
- Fibromatosis Colli

Rare but Important
- Nephrogenic Systemic Fibrosis
- Arthrogryposis
- Linear Morphea
- Fibrodysplasia Ossificans Progressiva
- Nail Patella Disease (Fong)
- Mucopolysaccharidoses
- Holt-Oram Syndrome
- Camptodactyly
- Leprosy
- Myotonic Dystrophy

ESSENTIAL INFORMATION

Key Differential Diagnosis Issues
- Soft tissue contractures have a relatively nonspecific appearance on imaging
- Correlation with history is most useful: Immobility, trauma, burns, radiation, inflammatory process, syndromes

Helpful Clues for Diagnoses
- **Complex Regional Pain Syndrome**
  - Three phase bone scan useful for diagnosis
- **Cerebral Palsy**
  - Pseudoacetabulum, femoral head deformity, hip subluxation or dislocation, thoracic kyphosis, lumbar lordosis, scoliosis, comma-shaped patella, foot equinus
- **Parsonage-Turner Syndrome, Late**
  - MR in acute setting shows high signal in muscles on T2WI without tendon tear
  - Joint contractures may occur late in the process without physical therapy
- **Fibromatosis Colli**
  - Ultrasound is imaging modality of choice to evaluate torticollis in neonate; compare with unaffected side
- **Nephrogenic Systemic Fibrosis**
  - Skin thickening & tendon fibrosis
  - Bone scintigraphy shows radiotracer uptake in extremity soft tissues
- **Leprosy**
  - Linear calcification of peripheral nerves can be visible on radiographs & CT

Immobility

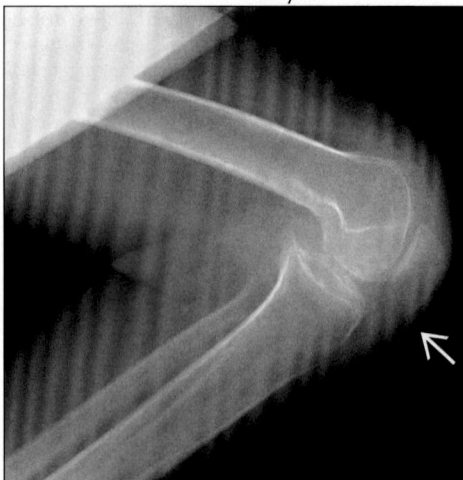

Lateral radiograph shows a marked flexion deformity ➡ of the knee. The musculature is atrophic and the bones are severely osteoporotic in this quadriplegic patient.

Dupuytren Contracture

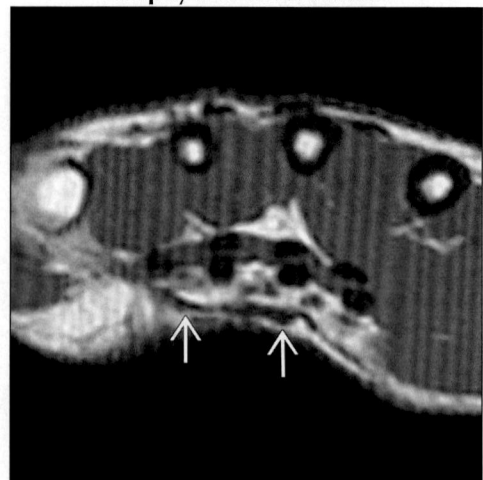

Axial T1WI MR shows diffuse, irregular thickening of the palmar fascia ➡, which resulted in flexion deformities of the third through fifth digits.

SOFT TISSUE CONTRACTURES

Trauma

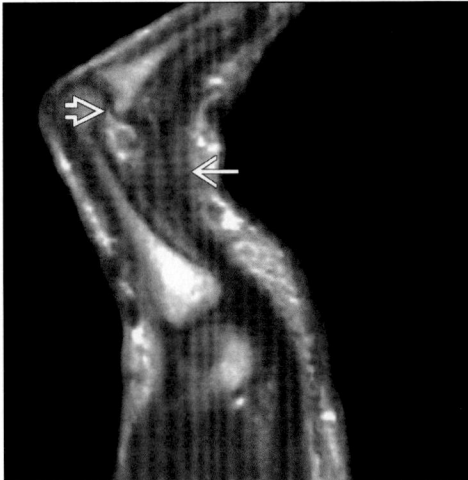

Juvenile Idiopathic Arthritis

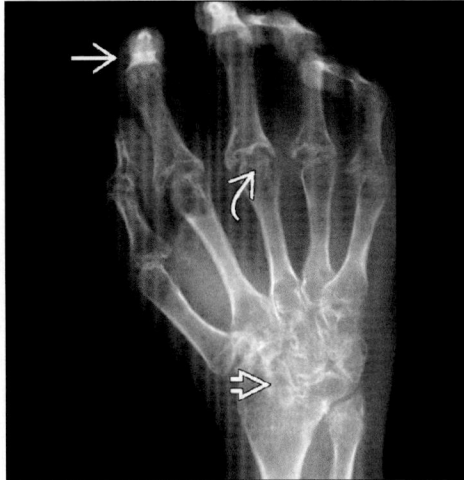

(Left) Sagittal T2WI MR shows separation of the flexor profunda and superficialis tendons ➡ from the proximal interphalangeal joint ➡, indicating rupture of the A2 and A3 pulleys. This represents flexor annular pulley tears from remote trauma. *(Right)* Posteroanterior radiograph shows flexion deformities ➡, carpal fusion ➡ and erosive changes ➡. Note that the patient is still skeletally immature, despite her age of 22 years.

Cerebral Palsy

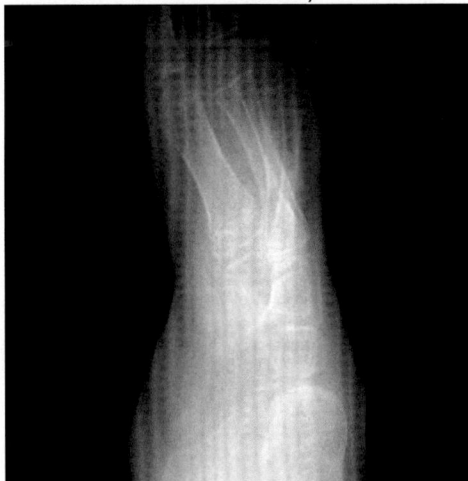

Fibromatosis Colli

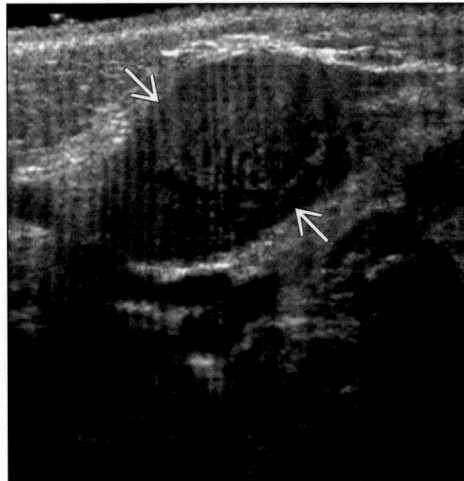

(Left) Anteroposterior radiograph shows the forefoot to be supinated with a varus deformity, which is quite severe. The hindfoot was in valgus. The combination of varus and valgus is usually seen in a spastic foot, and is not otherwise specific. *(Right)* Transverse ultrasound shows focal enlargement of the left sternocleidomastoid muscle ➡ in this neonate with torticollis. The contralateral right sternocleidomastoid muscle was normal.

Arthrogryposis

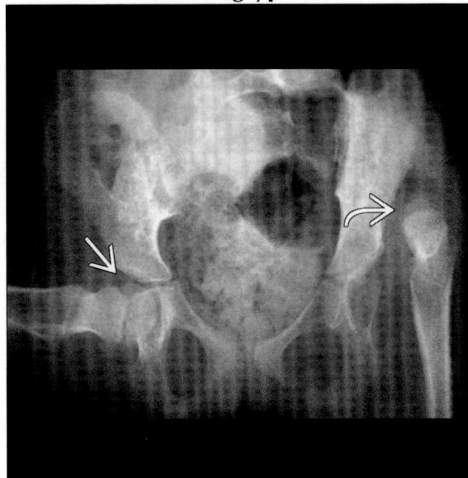

Fibrodysplasia Ossificans Progressiva

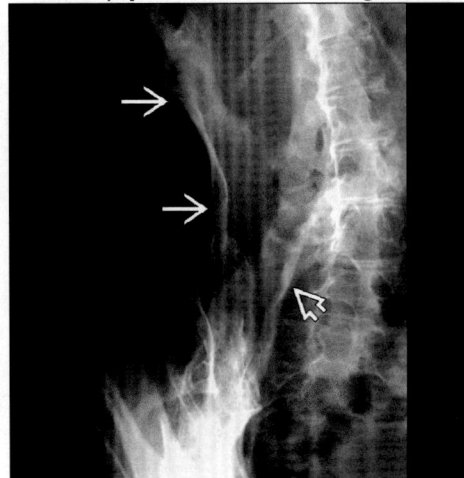

(Left) Anteroposterior radiograph shows a fixed abducted right hip ➡ and chronically dislocated left hip ➡. Note that the hip capsules are relatively dense. Arthrogryposis represents a heterogeneous group of disorders which have in common fixed joint contractures. *(Right)* Anteroposterior radiograph shows mature bone bridging the soft tissue between the lumbar spine and pelvis ➡ as well as between the rib cage and pelvis ➡, resulting in loss of motion.

III

DIFFERENTIAL DIAGNOSIS

Common
- Physeal Fractures, Pediatric
- Arthroplasty Malpositioning
- Osteomyelitis, Pediatric
- Legg-Calvé-Perthes
- Slipped Capital Femoral Epiphysis
- Juvenile Idiopathic Arthritis
- Developmental Dysplasia of the Hip
- Fibrous Dysplasia

Less Common
- Meningococcemia
- Embolic Disease, During Infancy
- Neurofibromatosis
- Congenital Pseudarthrosis Tibia
- Radiation-Induced Growth Deformities
- Compartment Syndrome, Insult Prior to Skeletal Maturity
- Hemophilia
- Ollier Disease
- Maffucci Syndrome
- Amniotic Band Syndrome

Rare but Important
- Proximal Femoral Focal Deficiency
- Polio

ESSENTIAL INFORMATION

Key Differential Diagnosis Issues
- There are few congenital abnormalities leading to a unilateral short limb
- Many etiologies of insults to the physes may result in modest limb length discrepancies

Helpful Clues for Common Diagnoses
- **Physeal Fractures, Pediatric**
  - Salter III, IV, and V physeal fractures are at high risk for early bony bridging across site
    - May bridge uniformly across physis, leading to early cessation of growth
    - May bridge non-uniformly, leading to both shortening and malalignment
- **Arthroplasty Malpositioning**
  - Limb length following total hip arthroplasty (THA) may be decreased, related to positioning
    - Acetabular component may be placed high
    - Osteotomy for femoral component may be cut low

  - Component (cup, femoral head, femoral neck) may be mis-sized, resulting in relative shortening
  - Arthroplasty loosening with subsidence of components results in relative shortening
    - Cup subsides superiorly, femoral stem subsides into shaft
- **Osteomyelitis, Pediatric**
  - Metaphyseal osteomyelitis may result in slipped epiphysis & resultant shortening
  - Epiphyseal osteomyelitis may result in epiphyseal destruction, hyperemia and early physeal fusion → shortening
- **Legg-Calvé-Perthes**
  - AVN in child results in flattening of femoral capital epiphysis → shortening
  - LCP often results in coxa magna deformity, with short broad femoral neck as well as head, further contributing to shortening
- **Slipped Capital Femoral Epiphysis**
  - Capital femoral epiphysis slips posteriorly and medially, resulting in shortening of the head
  - SCFE often results in coxa magna deformity, with short broad femoral neck as well as head, further contributing to shortening
- **Juvenile Idiopathic Arthritis (JIA) & Hemophilia**
  - Hyperemia in both processes leads to early physeal fusion → shortening of limb
- **Developmental Dysplasia of the Hip**
  - Uncorrected DDH results in pseudarthrosis, with femoral head articulating with the iliac wing rather than acetabulum
    - Results in significant relative shortening and lurching gait
  - Reduced DDH often develops coxa magna deformity, with short broad femoral neck as well as head, → shortening of limb
  - DDH occasionally is complicated with AVN, resulting in mild shortening
- **Fibrous Dysplasia**
  - Dysplastic bone develops microfractures, resulting in bowing deformities
    - Shepherd's crook deformity (varus) of femoral neck
    - Anterolateral bowing of femur and tibia

○ Fibrous dysplasia generally is unilateral, resulting in shortening of one limb

Helpful Clues for Less Common Diagnoses

- **Meningococcemia; Embolic Disease, During Infancy; Compartment Syndrome, Insult Prior to Skeletal Maturity; and Amniotic Band Syndrome**
  - Each of these entities results in ischemia of the involved limb, either from embolic disease or vascular compression
  - Physes are particularly at risk for vascular insult → flattening and shortening of limb
- **Neurofibromatosis & Congenital Pseudarthrosis Tibia**
  - Dysplastic tibia (and occasionally fibula) results in bowing and/or non-healing fractures and pseudarthrosis → shortening
  - Generally unilateral process
- **Radiation-Induced Growth Deformities**
  - Radiation (RT) causes vascular compromise
    - In a skeletally immature patient this results in AVN and early physeal fusion → shortening of limb
- **Ollier Disease & Maffucci Syndrome**
  - Both diseases are a dysplasia, affecting the metaphyses, with cartilage lesions which do not grow appropriately
  - Unilateral involvement → short limb

Helpful Clues for Rare Diagnoses

- **Proximal Femoral Focal Deficiency**
  - PFFD: Unilateral congenital absence of portions of femoral head, neck and proximal diaphysis

- **Polio**
  - Muscle atrophy and disuse → relative shortening

Alternative Differential Approaches

- May divide into congenital abnormalities versus dysplastic abnormalities versus insults to growth centers
  - Congenital limb length abnormalities
    - Developmental dysplasia of the hip
    - Proximal femoral focal deficiency
  - Dysplastic abnormalities leading to limb length discrepancies
    - Fibrous dysplasia
    - Neurofibromatosis
    - Congenital pseudarthrosis tibia
    - Ollier disease
    - Maffucci syndrome
  - Insults to growth centers
    - Physeal fractures, pediatric
    - Osteomyelitis, pediatric
    - Legg-Calvé-Perthes
    - Slipped capital femoral epiphysis
    - Juvenile idiopathic arthritis
    - Meningococcemia
    - Embolic disease, during infancy
    - Radiation-induced growth deformities
    - Compartment syndrome, insult prior to skeletal maturity
    - Hemophilia
    - Amniotic band syndrome

Physeal Fractures, Pediatric

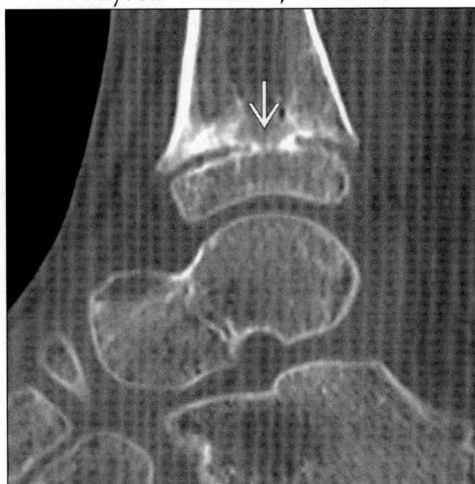

Sagittal bone CT shows osseous bridging ➡ at the central portion of the physis in this child, a result of a high grade Salter injury. Bone growth ceases with this bridging, resulting in a short limb.

Physeal Fractures, Pediatric

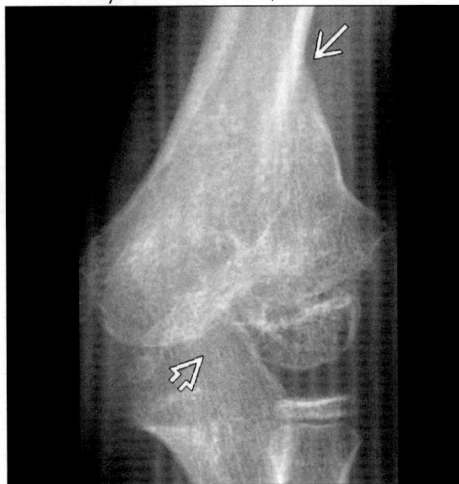

AP radiograph shows evidence of an old Salter IV lateral condylar fracture, with the fracture crossing the metaphysis ➡, through the physis, and across the epiphysis ➡. The malunion results in limb shortening.

SHORT LIMB, UNILATERAL

Arthroplasty Malpositioning

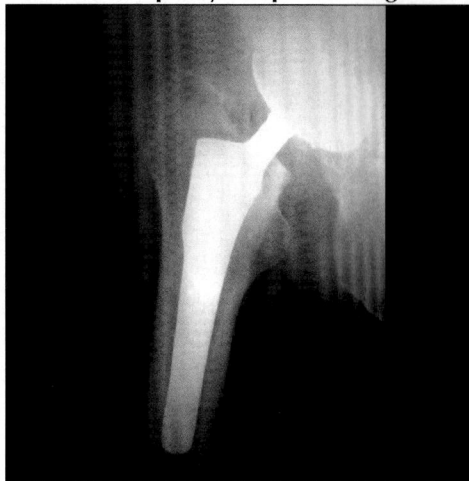

Arthroplasty Malpositioning

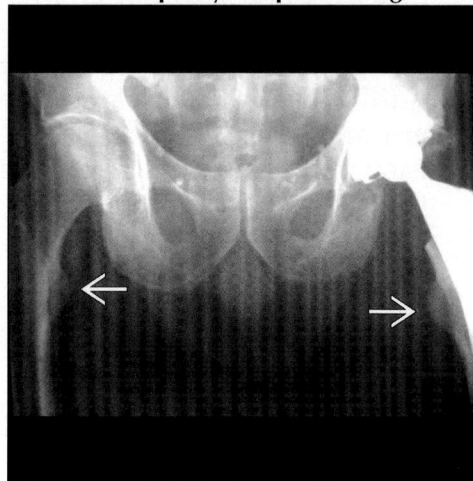

(Left) Anteroposterior radiograph shows a poorly sized femoral component, which has subsided down the shaft by 2 cm, leaving the limb relatively short. Mal-sized or malpositioned components can result in limb length discrepancies. *(Right)* Anteroposterior radiograph shows left THA placed with the components too long. Note the level of the left lesser trochanter compared with right ➡. This leaves a relatively short right limb, but also puts the left at risk for dislocation.

Osteomyelitis, Pediatric

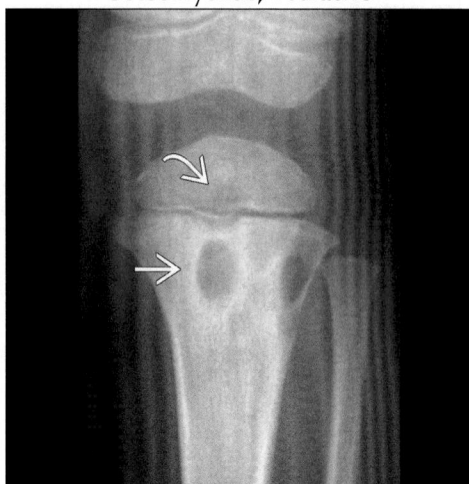

Legg-Calvé-Perthes

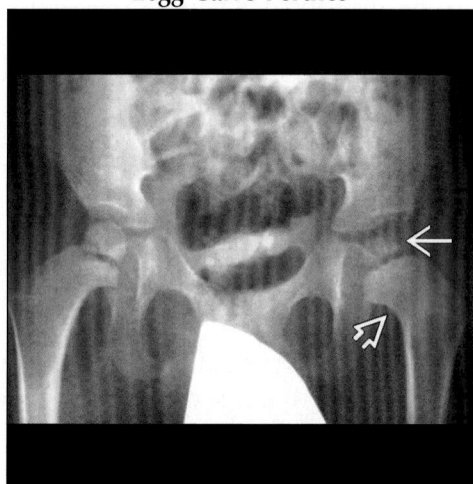

(Left) AP radiograph shows obvious metaphyseal destruction ➡ in a child with staphylococcus osteomyelitis. The infection has crossed the physis, showing subtle epiphyseal destruction ➡. This may result in growth disturbance and shortening of the limb. *(Right)* Anteroposterior radiograph shows LCP, which results in a coxa magna deformity: Short, broad femoral head ➡ as well as short, broad femoral neck ➡. This results in limb shortening.

Slipped Capital Femoral Epiphysis

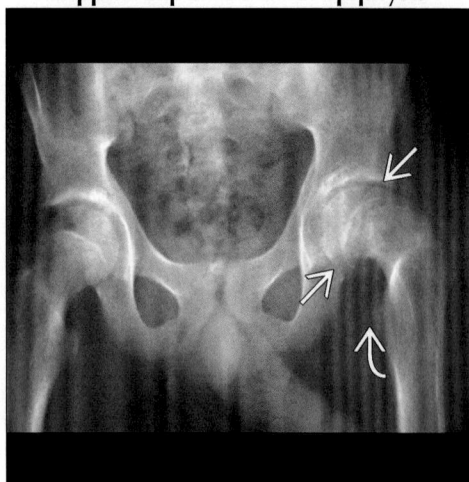

Slipped Capital Femoral Epiphysis

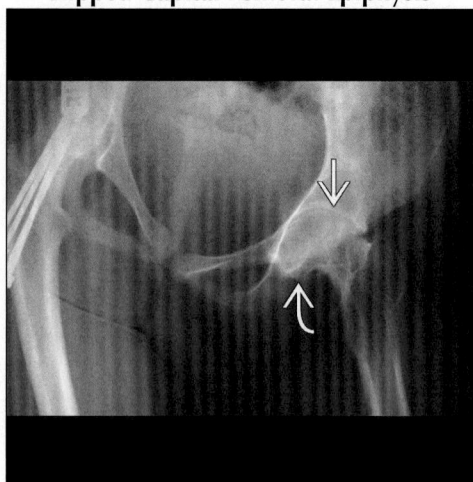

(Left) Anteroposterior radiograph shows medial and posterior slip of the left capital femoral epiphysis ➡. This slip results in shortening of the limb; note the level of the left lesser trochanter ➡ relative to the normal right side. *(Right)* AP radiograph shows a left SCFE ➡ which was pinned; unfortunately, the patient developed chondrolysis ➡. This resulted in fixed abduction, and the patient now has a relatively shortened limb and pelvic tilt. (The right hip was prophylactically pinned.)

SHORT LIMB, UNILATERAL

Juvenile Idiopathic Arthritis

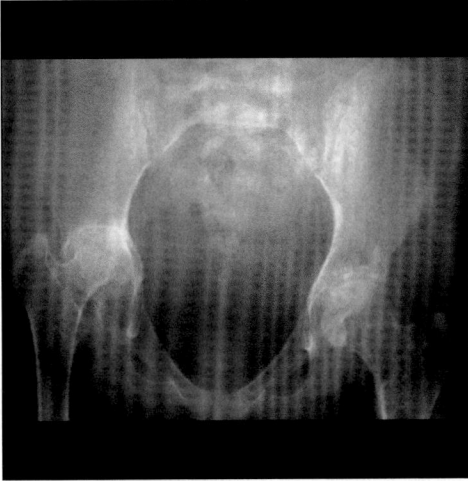

Developmental Dysplasia of the Hip

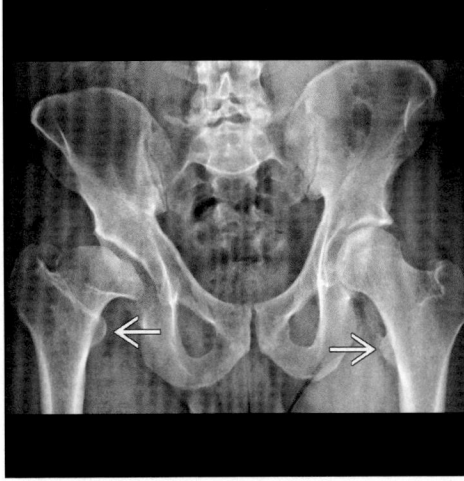

(Left) AP radiograph shows severe erosion of the right hip in a patient with JIA. Besides erosions, limb length may be affected by premature closure of epiphyses secondary to chronic hyperemia in this disease process. *(Right)* AP radiograph shows DDH on the right. Note the shallow acetabulum, coxa magna deformity of the femoral head and neck, and shortening of the right compared to left (compare level of lesser trochanters ➡ and not pelvic tilt).

Fibrous Dysplasia

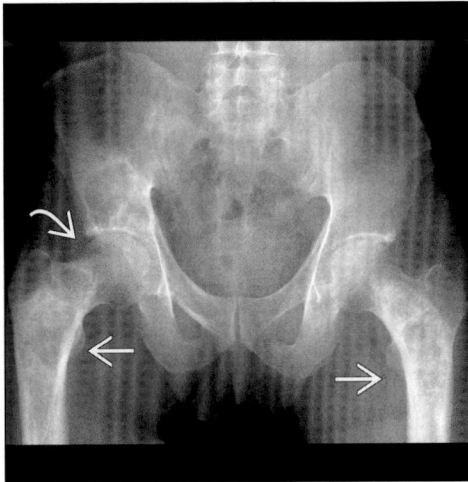

Meningococcemia

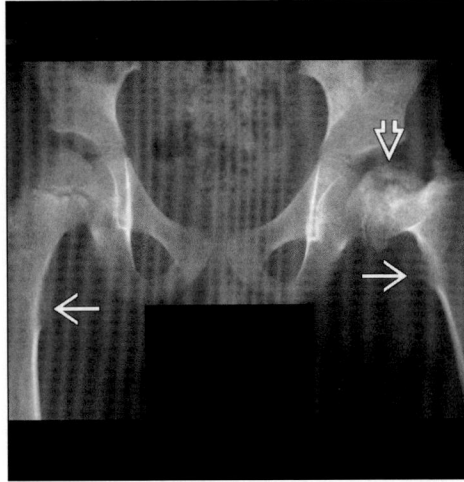

(Left) AP radiograph shows bilateral involvement with fibrous dysplasia. Note the pelvic tilt and the differential levels of the lesser trochanters ➡. This is due to the shepherd's crook deformity of the right femoral neck ➡, resulting in a shortened femur. *(Right)* AP radiograph shows significant deformity of the left femoral metaphysis & epiphysis ➡, with short varus neck. This is due to thrombotic disease in meningococcemia. The left limb is short (compare lesser trochanter levels ➡).

Embolic Disease, During Infancy

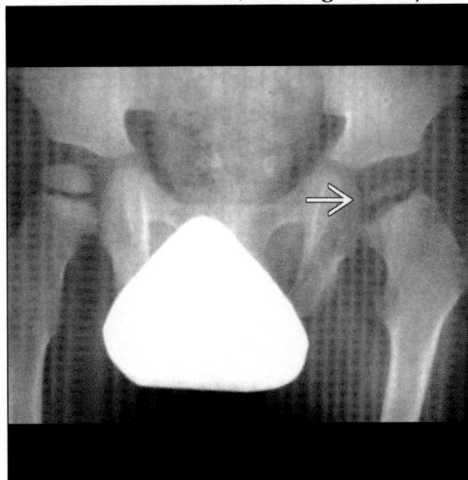

Embolic Disease, During Infancy

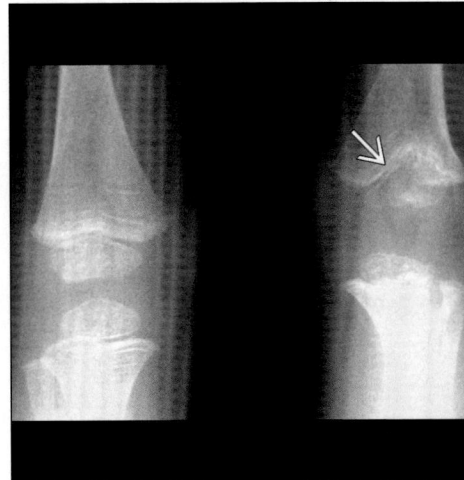

(Left) AP radiograph shows AVN of femoral head ➡ & shortening of left femoral neck relative to right (compare levels of lesser trochanters). Insult occurred at younger than expected age for Legg-Perthes; another etiology must be sought. *(Right)* AP radiograph of knees of same patient shows a coned epiphysis ➡ at left distal femur, and irregularity at left proximal epiphysis. These, along with hip, contribute to a short limb, due to emboli from umbilical artery catheter.

Neurofibromatosis

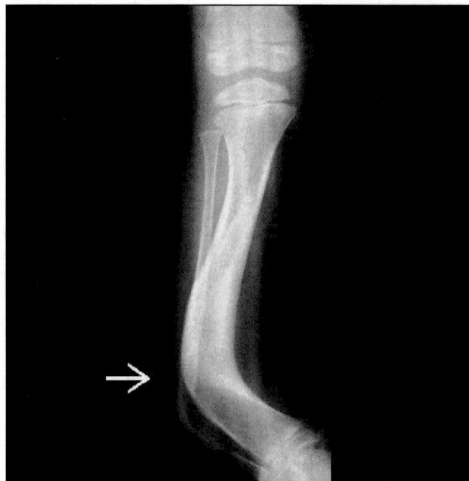

Congenital Pseudarthrosis Tibia

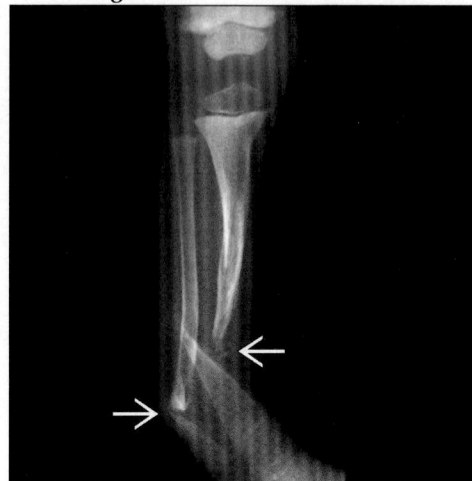

(Left) Anteroposterior radiograph shows significant bowing of both the tibia and fibula ➡️ in a patient with neurofibromatosis. In this disease, these bones are frequently dysplastic, which can result in bowing deformities or pseudarthroses. *(Right)* Anteroposterior radiograph shows fracture of both the tibia and fibula ➡️ at the distal 1/3 of the leg, with smooth, tapered ends. This is a congenital pseudarthrosis, and results in limb shortening.

Radiation-Induced Growth Deformities

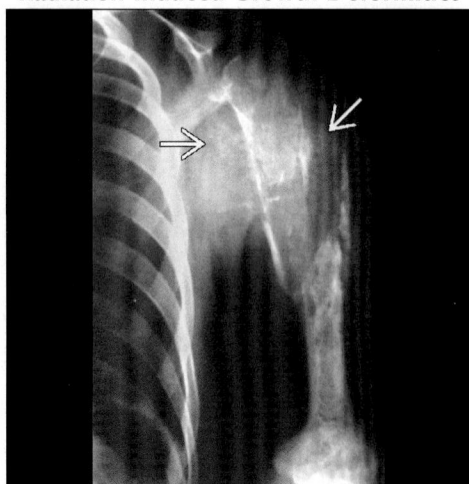

Radiation-Induced Growth Deformities

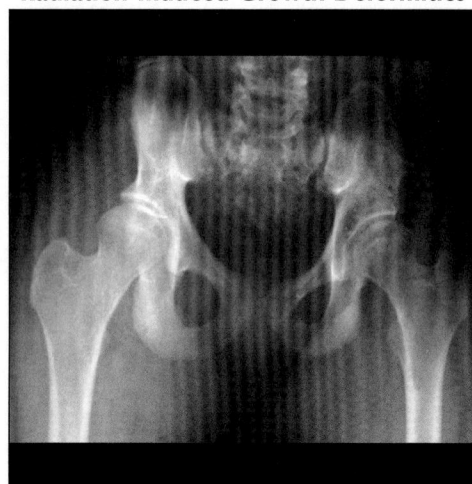

(Left) Anteroposterior radiograph shows the humerus to be short relative to the thorax. There is diffuse bone sclerosis, limited to the humerus; this confirms that the patient had whole bone radiation. There is also a radiation-induced sarcoma ➡️. *(Right)* Anteroposterior radiograph shows a port-like distribution of osseous hypoplasia, including the sacrum and iliac wings in this patient who had pelvic RT as a child. There is asymmetric hypoplasia of the left hip, giving a mild pelvic tilt.

Compartment Syndrome, Insult Prior to Skeletal Maturity

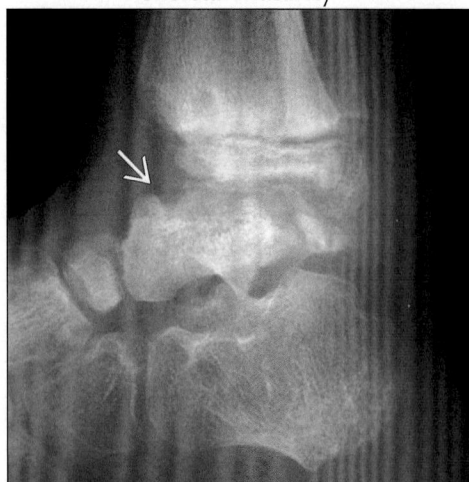

Hemophilia

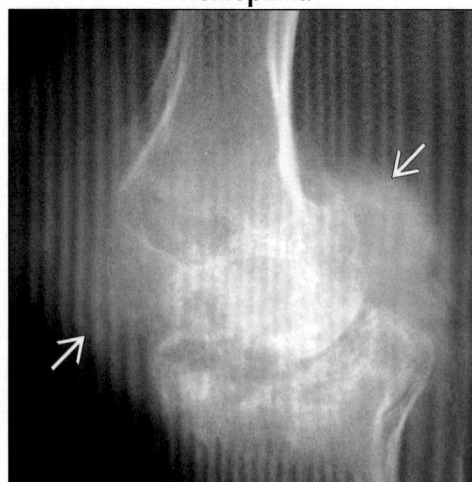

(Left) Lateral radiograph shows irregularity and shortening of the talus ➡️ as well as the distal tibial physis. These deformities resulted from compartment syndrome and associated ischemia several years earlier. The limb is slightly short. *(Right)* Lateral radiograph shows severe erosive disease and a large dense effusion ➡️ in a hemophilic. The limb was short, in part because of the joint destruction, but also due to hyperemia resulting in early physeal closure.

SHORT LIMB, UNILATERAL

Ollier Disease

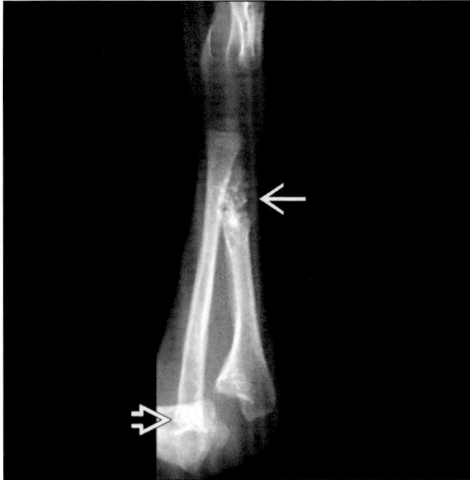

Ollier Disease

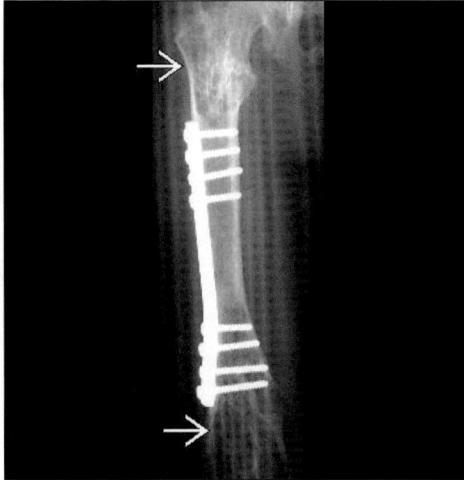

(Left) Lateral radiograph shows short ulna with enchondroma ➡ and associated dislocation of the radial head ➡. This combination is seen in Ollier disease, and is usually unilateral, resulting in a short limb. (Right) Anteroposterior radiograph shows striated expanded lytic lesions in both metaphyses ➡, typical of multiple enchondromatosis. The disease is usually unilateral, resulting in a short limb. The plate and screws are from a limb lengthening procedure.

Maffucci Syndrome

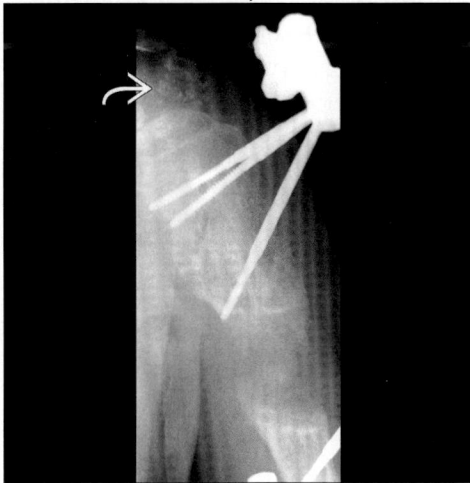

Amniotic Band Syndrome

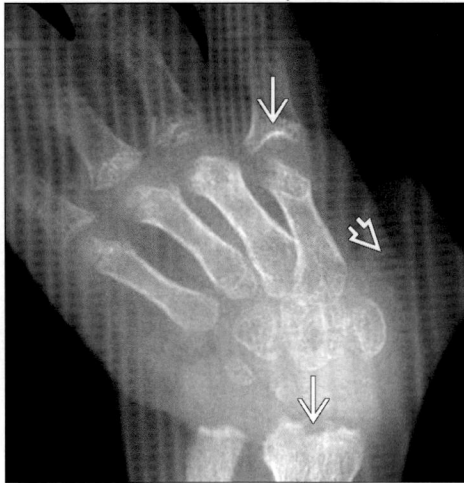

(Left) AP radiograph shows a short humerus undergoing lengthening procedure, with external fixator in place. The metaphysis is broad and striated, typical of enchondroma, and there is a soft tissue hemangioma ➡, making the diagnosis Maffucci syndrome. (†MSK Req). (Right) PA radiograph shows absent thumb ➡, and multiple coned or abnormal epiphyses ➡ due to amniotic band (not shown here). By restricting blood supply, amniotic bands can cause limb shortening.

Proximal Femoral Focal Deficiency

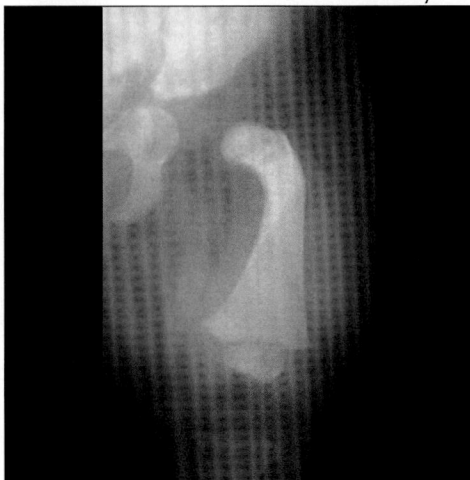

Polio

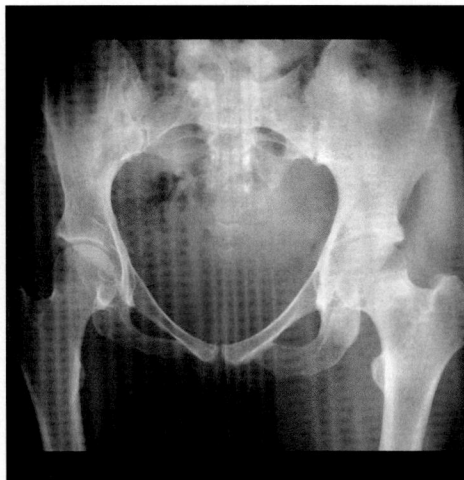

(Left) Anteroposterior radiograph shows an absent proximal femur, including head and neck. The mid femur is bowed, and limb extremely short. This is typical PFFD. (Right) Anteroposterior radiograph shows pelvic tilt and relative hypoplasia of the right hemipelvis and lower limb. Note the increased density on the left, indicating significantly greater muscle mass on that side. Findings are typical of polio with short right limb.

HEMIHYPERTROPHY

DIFFERENTIAL DIAGNOSIS

Common
- Idiopathic/Congenital
- Neurofibromatosis
- Lipomatosis (Mimic)
- Hyperemia, Any Cause
- Vascular Malformation (Mimic)

Less Common
- Lymphangioma (Mimic)
- Beckwith-Wiedemann Syndrome
- Neurocutaneous Syndrome, Uncommon
  - Tuberous Sclerosis
  - Sturge-Weber Disease
  - Von Hippel-Lindau Disease

Rare but Important
- Klippel-Trenaunay-Weber Syndrome

ESSENTIAL INFORMATION

Helpful Clues for Common Diagnoses
- **Idiopathic/Congenital**
  - Increased risk childhood cancer
    - Wilms tumor most common
  - Associated renal disorders
  - Leg-length discrepancy is mild form
- **Neurofibromatosis**
  - Plexiform neurofibromas & mesodermal dysplasia, cafe-au-lait spots, optic glioma, Lisch nodule
- **Lipomatosis (Mimic)**
  - Diffuse increase adipose tissue
- **Hyperemia, Any Cause**
  - Overstimulation during development
  - Focal gigantism more common
- **Vascular Malformation (Mimic)**
  - Tangled dilated vessels, phleboliths, no discrete mass, ± intra-osseous extension

Helpful Clues for Less Common Diagnoses
- **Lymphangioma (Mimic)**
  - Soft tissue mass with multiple cyst spaces
- **Beckwith-Wiedemann Syndrome**
  - Macroglossia, enlarged abdominal organs, umbilical hernia, Wilms tumor
- **Tuberous Sclerosis**
  - Seizures, mental retardation, cutaneous abnormalities
  - Facial angiofibromas, subungual fibromas, shagreen patches, ash leaf spots, cortical tubers, subependymal nodules
- **Sturge-Weber Disease**
  - Seizures, mental retardation, glaucoma, port wine stain, leptomeningeal angioma
- **Von Hippel-Lindau Disease**
  - Angiomatosis especially retinal, renal cell carcinoma, neuroendocrine tumors

Helpful Clues for Rare Diagnoses
- **Klippel-Trenaunay-Weber Syndrome**
  - Capillary hemangioma, varicose veins, gigantism, ± arteriovenous malformation
    - Focal gigantism more common

Other Essential Information
- Hemihypertrophy: Enlargement of one side of body or one extremity vs. focal gigantism (macrodactyly) with enlarged digit(s)/portion of extremity

Idiopathic/Congenital

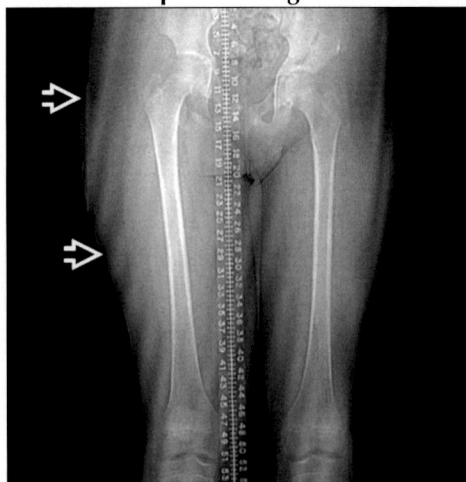

Anteroposterior radiograph shows congenital hypertrophy of the right leg. The right femur is longer and wider and the thigh musculature is enlarged ⇨.

Neurofibromatosis

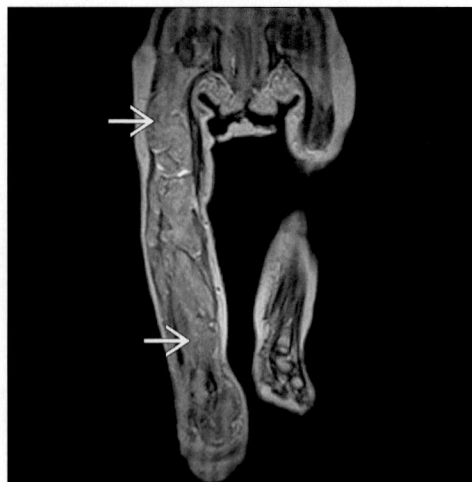

Coronal T2WI FSE MR shows a spectacular example of hemihypertrophy due to neurofibromatosis. On the right there is a giant plexiform neurofibroma ⇨ extending from the sciatic notch to the foot.

HEMIHYPERTROPHY

Neurofibromatosis

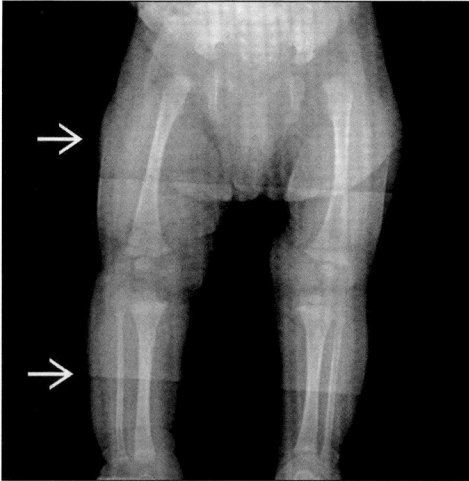

Vascular Malformation (Mimic)

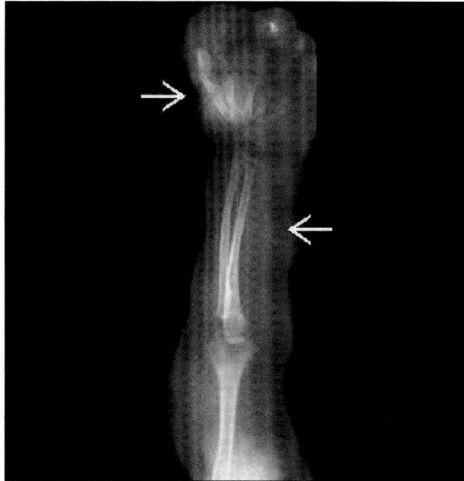

(Left) Anteroposterior radiograph shows asymmetric increased soft tissue of the right lower extremity ➡ along with mild limb length discrepancy, right leg slightly longer than the left. This patient's hemihypertrophy is secondary to neurofibromatosis. *(Right)* Anteroposterior radiograph shows bulky soft tissues of the forearm and hand ➡ in this one day old with a large soft tissue hemangioma.

Vascular Malformation (Mimic)

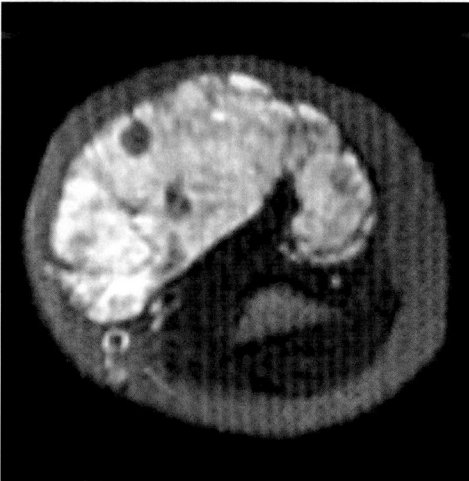

Vascular Malformation (Mimic)

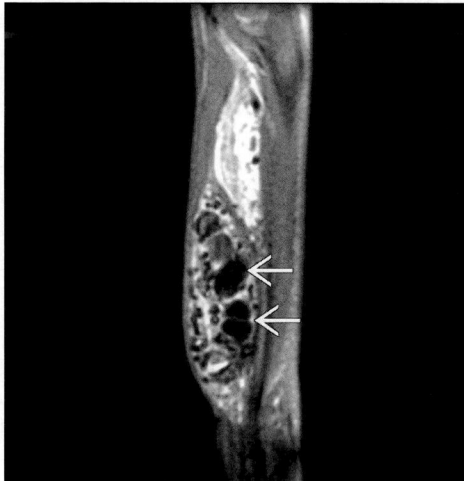

(Left) Axial T2WI MR shows lobulated high T2WI signal mass with diffuse enhancement. This patient has a hemangioma which clinically mimics hemihypertrophy. The adjacent musculature and humerus are normal in size. *(Right)* Sagittal T1 C+ MR shows a tangle of vessels in the forearm with multiple large flow voids ➡ consistent with an arteriovenous malformation simulating hemihypertrophy.

Lymphangioma (Mimic)

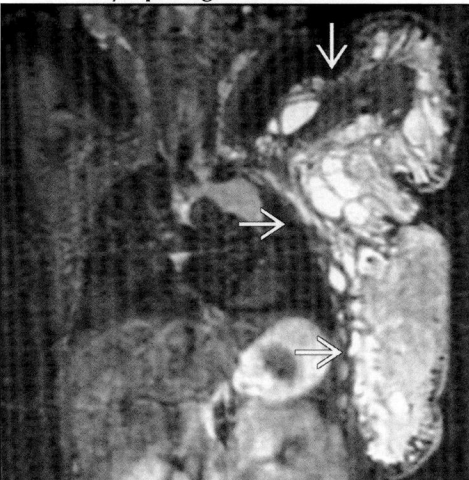

Klippel-Trenaunay-Weber Syndrome

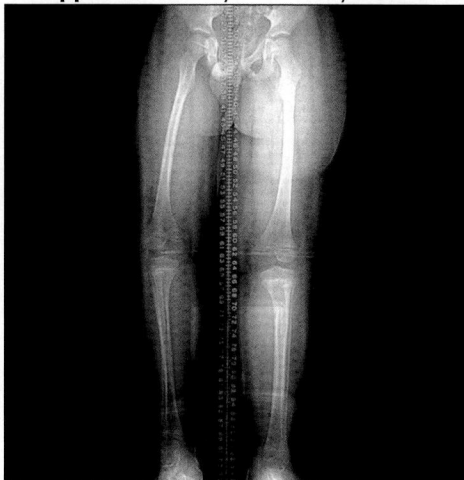

(Left) Coronal T2WI MR from a patient with a large lymphangioma shows a high signal mass with multi septate cysts involving the left chest wall and upper extremity ➡. *(Right)* Anteroposterior CT scanogram shows left leg hemihypertrophy with enlargement of the bones and soft tissues of the left leg (compared to the right) in this patient with Klippel-Trenaunay-Weber syndrome.

FOCAL GIGANTISM/MACRODACTYLY

DIFFERENTIAL DIAGNOSIS

Common
- Juvenile Idiopathic Arthritis (Epiphyses)
- Hemangioma, Soft Tissue
- Arteriovenous Malformation
- Lymphangioma
- Neurofibromatosis

Less Common
- Macrodystrophia Lipomatosa
- Klippel-Trenaunay-Weber Syndrome (KTW)
- Ollier Disease (Phalanges)
- Maffucci Syndrome (Phalanges)
- Hemophilia (Epiphyses)
- Hyperemia, Any Cause
  - Chronic Osteomyelitis
  - Fracture During Childhood
  - Tuberculosis

Rare but Important
- Epidermal Nevus Syndrome
- Proteus Syndrome

ESSENTIAL INFORMATION

Key Differential Diagnosis Issues
- Key features to aid in differentiation
  - Overgrowth: Osseous, soft tissue, both
  - Cutaneous manifestations
- **Hint**: Macrodystrophia lipomatosa, neurofibromatosis, KTW, Maffucci have similar appearance
  - Soft tissue and osseous involvement
- **Hint**: Hyperemia underlying cause with osseous overgrowth only
  - Juvenile idiopathic arthritis
  - Hemophilia
  - Chronic osteomyelitis
  - Tuberculosis
  - See hyperemia, any cause below
- **Hint**: Juvenile idiopathic arthritis and hemophilia have similar appearance
  - Osseous overgrowth only
    - Ballooned epiphyses
    - Widened intercondylar notch
    - Knee (femoral condyles), elbow (capitellum) overgrowth common

Helpful Clues for Common Diagnoses
- **Juvenile Idiopathic Arthritis (Epiphyses)**
  - Overgrowth mainly knee, elbow
  - No cutaneous changes
  - Other disease manifestations
    - Monoarticular to polyarticular disease
    - Small joints, hands, feet; also wrist, elbow, knee, shoulder, ankle
    - Peri-articular osteoporosis
    - Marginal erosions
    - Periosteal new bone formation
    - Uniform joint space narrowing
- **Hemangioma, Soft Tissue**
  - Soft tissue mass
    - Phleboliths
    - Variable amount of fatty stroma
  - Osseous changes variable
    - Overgrowth 2° hyperemia
    - Periosteal new bone
    - Cortical thickening
    - Pressure erosions
  - Cutaneous changes
    - Skin discoloration
    - Prominent veins
    - Cutaneous hemangiomas
- **Arteriovenous Malformation**
  - Soft tissue mass
    - Phleboliths
    - Tangled dilated vessels, no discrete mass
  - Intra-osseous extension may be seen
  - Cutaneous changes absent
    - Dilated vessels may be visible beneath skin
- **Lymphangioma**
  - Soft tissue mass with multiple cystic spaces
  - No osseous overgrowth
  - No cutaneous changes
- **Neurofibromatosis**
  - Gigantism may be bilateral
  - Involved digits may not be contiguous
  - Most severe involvement at any site along digit
  - 2° plexiform neurofibroma (soft tissue) and mesodermal dysplasia (osseous)
  - Cutaneous changes: Cafe-au-lait spots
  - Other disease manifestations
    - Neurofibromas
    - Mesodermal dysplasia: Bowing, pseudoarthrosis, abnormal healing, periosteal abnormalities
    - Optic glioma, Lisch nodule (iris nevi)

Helpful Clues for Less Common Diagnoses
- **Macrodystrophia Lipomatosa**
  - Unilateral; one or more contiguous digits
  - Most severe involvement along distal digit

- Volar surface more affected than dorsal surface creating dorsal bowing deformity
- 2nd and 3rd digits most common
- Overgrowth soft tissue & bone
  - Prominent adipose overgrowth
- Neural enlargement
  - Secondary to adipose infiltration
  - Median nerve > plantar nerve
- No cutaneous changes
- **Klippel-Trenaunay-Weber Syndrome (KTW)**
  - Unilateral soft tissue and osseous overgrowth
    - Gigantism ranges from macrodactyly to hemihypertrophy
  - Lower extremity more common than upper extremity
  - Syndrome: Capillary hemangiomas (port wine), varicose veins, local gigantism
    - ± Arteriovenous malformations
- **Ollier Disease (Phalanges)**
  - a.k.a., echondromatosis
  - Gigantism hands/feet only
  - Osseous involvement only: Multiple enchondromas of phalanges
    - Expansile lytic ± ground-glass matrix
    - Bilateral asymmetric distribution
- **Maffucci Syndrome (Phalanges)**
  - Ollier disease plus soft tissue hemangiomas
  - Hemangiomas
    - Phleboliths
    - Any site throughout body
    - Hands, feet especially involved
- **Hemophilia (Epiphyses)**

- Typically one joint suffers repeated hemorrhage which leads to hyperemia then osseous overgrowth
  - Commonly affects knee (femoral condyles), elbow (radial head)
- Associated arthritic changes
  - Peri-articular osteoporosis
  - Uniform joint space narrowing
  - Dense effusion
  - Subchondral cysts
  - Secondary osteoarthritis
- **Hyperemia, Any Cause**
  - Osseous overgrowth
  - Random sites of involvement
    - Typically one site or multiple sites in one extremity
  - Hyperemia prior to skeletal maturation, often from fracture healing

Helpful Clues for Rare Diagnoses
- **Epidermal Nevus Syndrome**
  - Soft tissue and osseous overgrowth
  - No typical site of involvement
  - Cutaneous changes: Multiple nevi
  - Variable other manifestations including cerebral atrophy
- **Proteus Syndrome**
  - Syndrome has protean manifestations
    - Focal gigantism and lymphangiomatous hamartomas are consistent features
  - Soft tissue and osseous overgrowth
  - No cutaneous changes
  - Osteochondroma-like osseous lesions
  - Skull, face, spine abnormalities common

Juvenile Idiopathic Arthritis (Epiphyses)

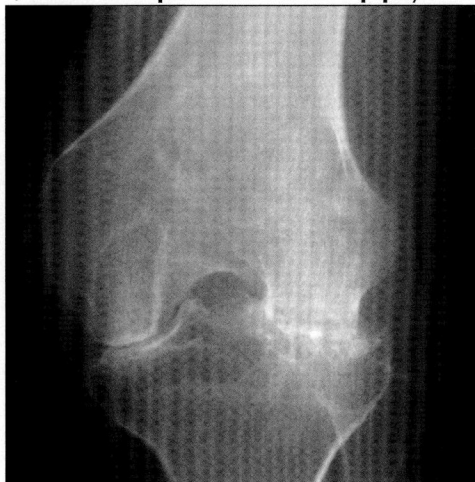

Anteroposterior radiograph shows a classic example of severe juvenile idiopathic arthritis with overgrowth of the femoral condyles especially medially and widening of the intercondylar notch.

Juvenile Idiopathic Arthritis (Epiphyses)

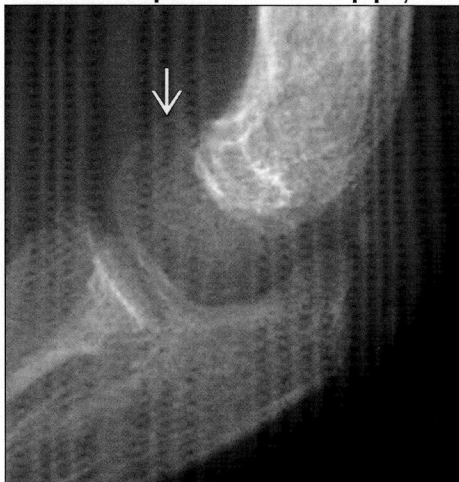

Lateral radiograph of this patient with juvenile idiopathic arthritis reveals overgrowth of the capitellum ➡ secondary to hyperemia. (†MSK Req).

FOCAL GIGANTISM/MACRODACTYLY

Hemangioma, Soft Tissue

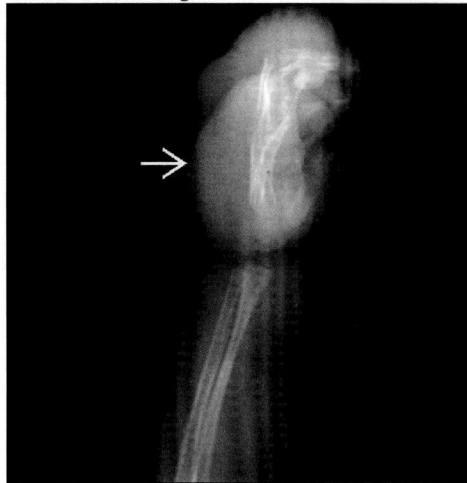

Arteriovenous Malformation

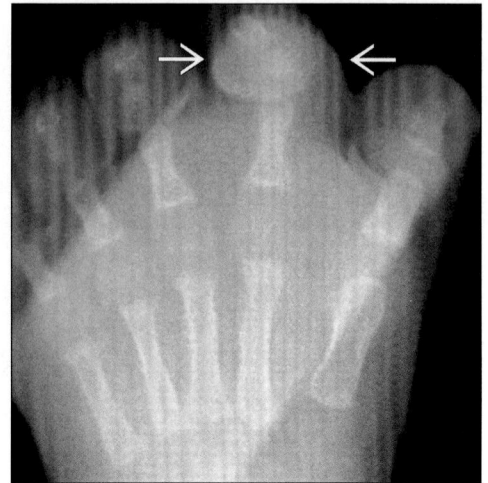

(Left) Lateral radiograph shows bulky soft tissues of the forearm and hand ➡ secondary to soft tissue hemangioma. Associated overgrowth of the first and second digits was present but is not seen on this image. *(Right)* Anteroposterior radiograph shows focal overgrowth of the second digit of the left foot ➡. The overgrowth was due to hyperemia from a vascular malformation.

Arteriovenous Malformation

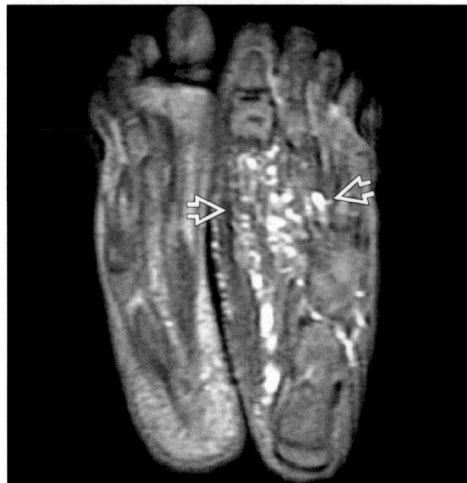

Macrodystrophia Lipomatosa

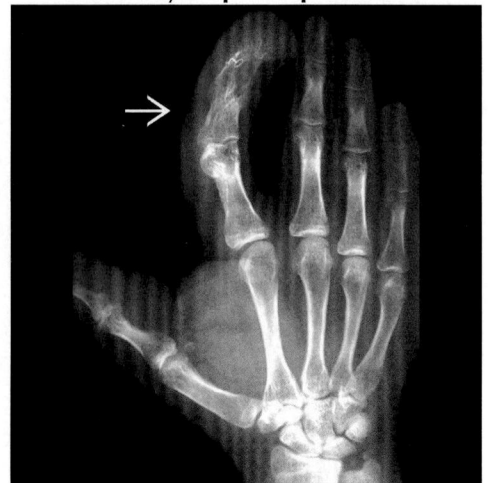

(Left) Axial T2* GRE MR shows multiple flow void from the enlarged vessels in this arteriovenous malformation ➡; the adjacent osseous structures showed overgrowth. *(Right)* Posteroanterior radiograph shows focal giantism secondary to macrodystrophia lipomatosa, involving a single ray of the hand ➡. The osseous and soft tissues are both involved.

Macrodystrophia Lipomatosa

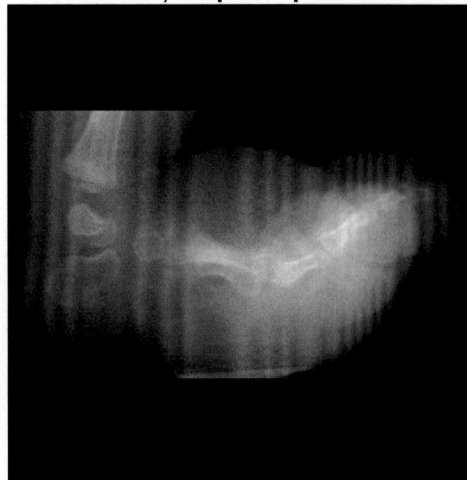

Ollier Disease (Phalanges)

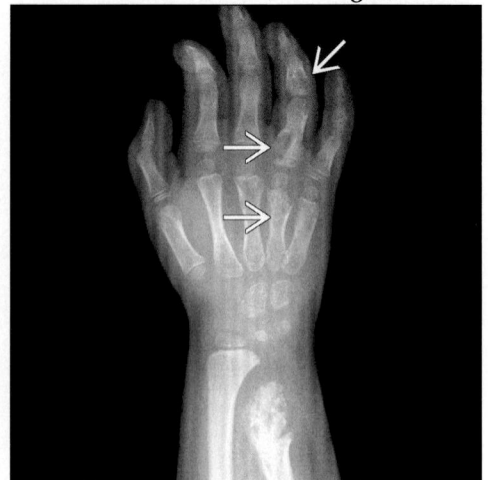

(Left) Lateral radiograph shows a normal hindfoot and midfoot with giantism of both the soft tissues and osseous structures of the forefoot in this patient with macrodystrophia lipomatosa. *(Right)* Anteroposterior radiograph of the hand of a patient with Ollier disease demonstrates multiple enchondromas ➡.

FOCAL GIGANTISM/MACRODACTYLY

Ollier Disease (Phalanges)

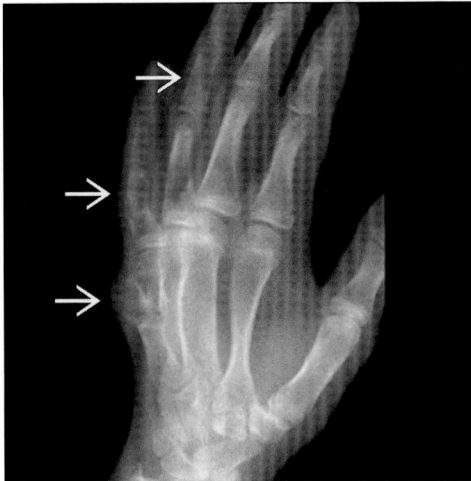

Maffucci Syndrome (Phalanges)

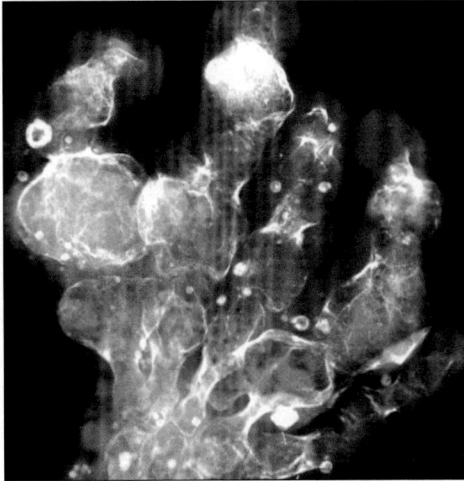

(Left) Oblique radiograph shows a skeletally immature child with multiple enchondromas ➡ consistent with Ollier disease. The lesions are expansile especially in the fifth metacarpal. (Right) PA radiograph shows bizarre expansion of all the bones of the hand, associated with multiple phleboliths. The diagnosis is Mafucci syndrome, but clinically it manifests as focal gigantism of the hand.

Maffucci Syndrome (Phalanges)

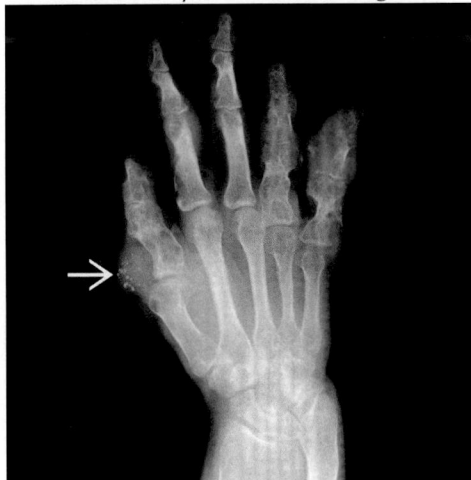

Hemophilia (Epiphyses)

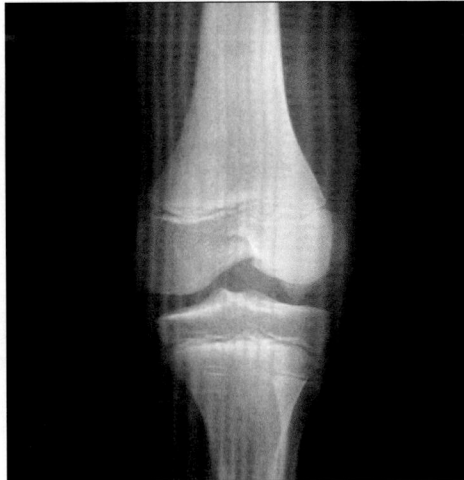

(Left) Anteroposterior radiograph shows a classic case of Maffucci syndrome with multiple enchondromas in the phalanges and multiple soft tissue hemangiomas with phleboliths ➡. (†MSK Req). (Right) Anteroposterior radiograph shows enlargement of the femoral condyles and widening of the intercondylar notch in this patient with hemophilia.

Hemophilia (Epiphyses)

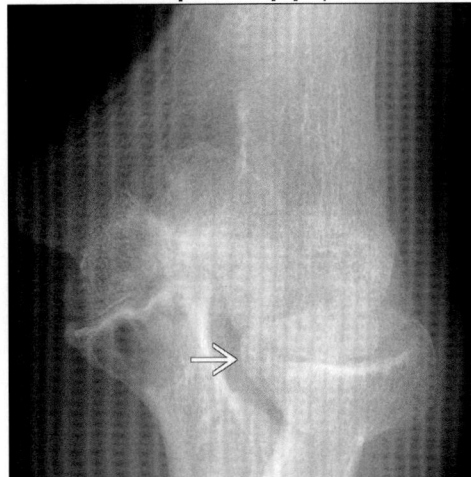

Hyperemia, Any Cause

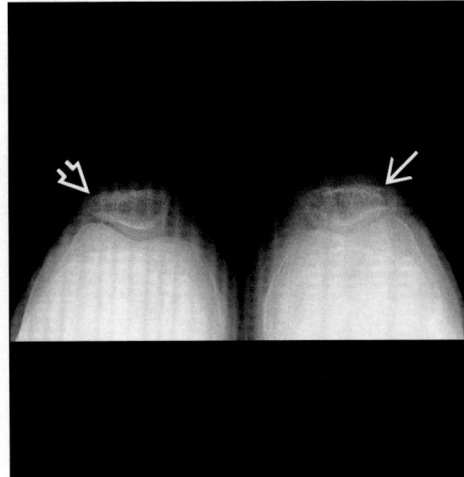

(Left) Anteroposterior radiograph shows capitellar overgrowth ➡ in this patient with hemophilia. Associated changes include subchondral cyst formation and joint space narrowing. (Right) Axial radiograph shows relative overgrowth of the left patella ➡ compared to the right ➡, resulting from a patellar fracture which occurred prior to skeletal maturation.

III

183

DWARFISM WITH MAJOR SPINE INVOLVEMENT

DIFFERENTIAL DIAGNOSIS

Common
- Achondroplasia
- Thanatophoric Dwarf
- Spondyloepiphyseal Dysplasia

Less Common
- Hypothyroidism, Child (Mimic)
- Noonan Syndrome
- Morquio Syndrome
- Hurler Syndrome
- Hunter Syndrome

Rare but Important
- Progeria
- Hypochondroplasia
- Metatropic Dwarfism
- Diastrophic Dwarfism
- Kniest Dysplasia
- Camptomelic Dysplasia
- Osteoglophonic Dysplasia
- Dyssegmental Dysplasia

ESSENTIAL INFORMATION

Helpful Clues for Diagnoses
- **Achondroplasia**
  - Short, flat vertebral bodies; decreasing interpediculate distance L1 → L5
  - Posterior vertebral body scalloping
  - Hypoplastic upper lumbar vertebral bodies
- **Thanatophoric Dwarf**
  - Platyspondyly with rounded anterior vertebral bodies

- **Spondyloepiphyseal Dysplasia**
  - Ovoid or pear-shaped vertebrae in infancy
  - Central, anterior vertebral body beak
  - Odontoid hypoplasia
- **Hypothyroidism, Child (Mimic)**
  - Congenital vertebral anomalies: Hemivertebrae, abnormal rib-vertebral articulations, platyspondyly
    - "Sail vertebrae" = upper lumbar vertebra with wedge or hook shape
- **Noonan Syndrome**
  - Klippel-Feil anomaly
  - Scoliosis & kyphosis
- **Morquio Syndrome**
  - Extensive vertebra plana
  - Central, anterior vertebral body beak
  - Diminutive or disappearing dens of axis
- **Hurler Syndrome**
  - Anterior inferior vertebral body beak
  - Oval to biconvex vertebral bodies
  - Absent dens → atlantoaxial subluxation
- **Hunter Syndrome**
  - Inferior beak similar to Hurler syndrome
  - Posterior vertebral body scalloping
- **Progeria**
  - Infantile central notching retained
- **Hypochondroplasia**
  - Decreased interpediculate distance L1 → L5
- **Kniest Dysplasia**
  - Platyspondyly with narrow interpediculate distance
  - Coronal vertebral body clefts, infants
- **Camptomelic Dysplasia**
  - Hypoplastic cervical vertebrae

Achondroplasia

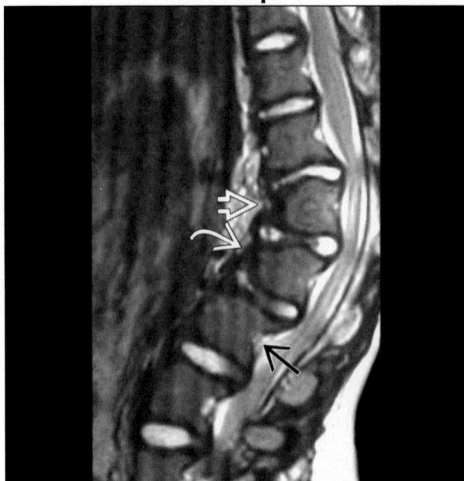

Sagittal T2WI MR shows posterior vertebral scalloping ➡, anterior beaking ➡, as well as hypoplasia of L1 and L2. This results in a focal kyphosis ➡.

Achondroplasia

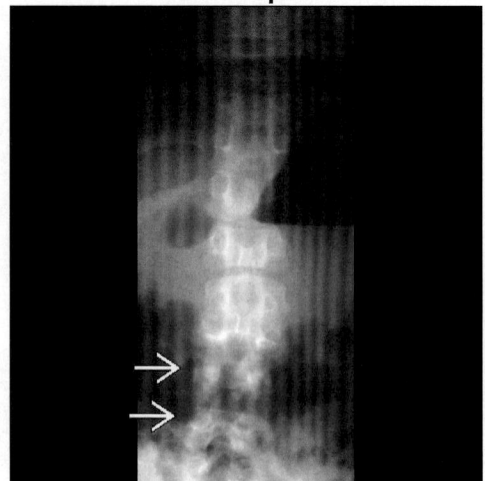

Anteroposterior radiograph shows progressive narrowing of the interpediculate distance ➡ in the lower lumbar spine, typical of achondroplasia.

DWARFISM WITH MAJOR SPINE INVOLVEMENT

Thanatophoric Dwarf

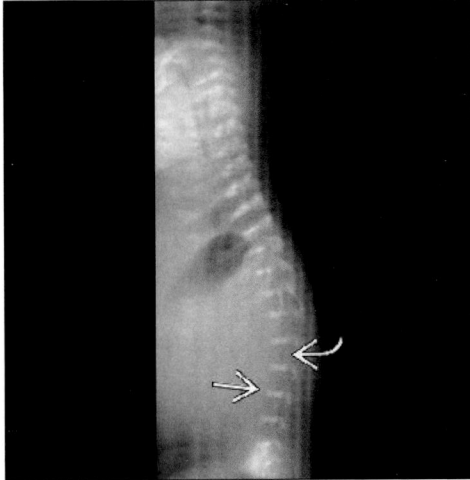

Spondyloepiphyseal Dysplasia

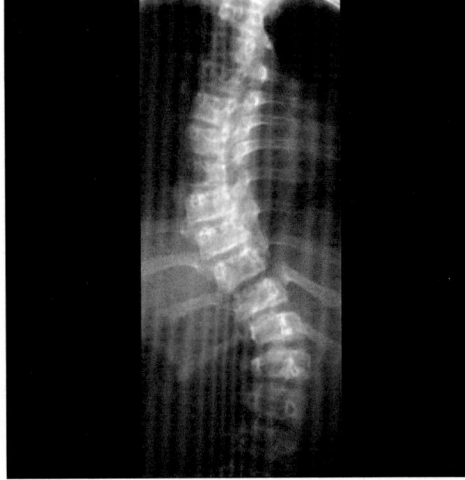

(Left) Lateral radiograph shows the classic platyspondyly ➡, with widened intervertebral disk spaces ➡. Thus, the normal truncal length is maintained despite the flat vertebral bodies. This is a lethal form of dwarfism. (Right) Anteroposterior radiograph shows universal platyspondyly and scoliosis. Images of the extremities showed severely deformed epiphyses. The combination of findings helps make the diagnosis.

Noonan Syndrome

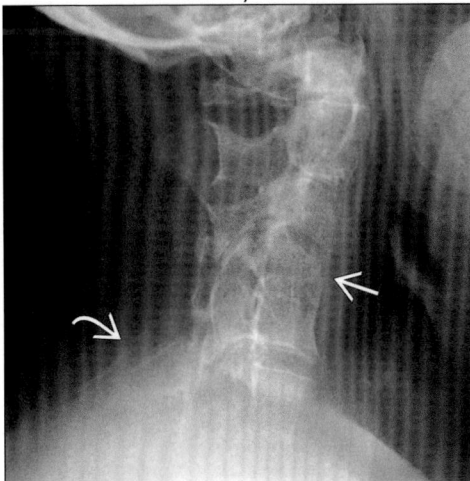

Morquio Syndrome

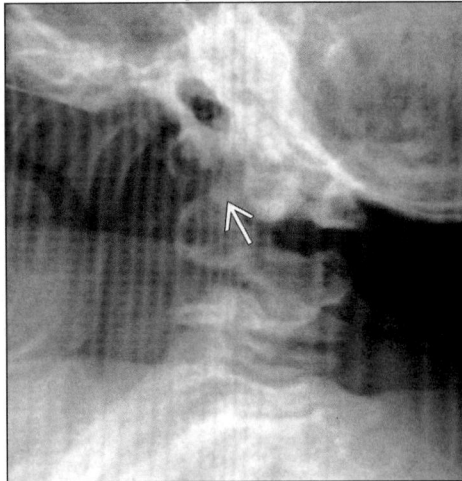

(Left) Lateral radiograph shows a Klippel-Feil anomaly that is typical in Noonan syndrome but is also seen incidentally, as in this patient. The cervical vertebral bodies are small and fused ➡ and there is an adjacent omovertebral bone ➡. (Right) Lateral radiograph shows hypoplasia of the odontoid ➡. This anomaly can contribute to atlantoaxial subluxation in these patients.

Morquio Syndrome

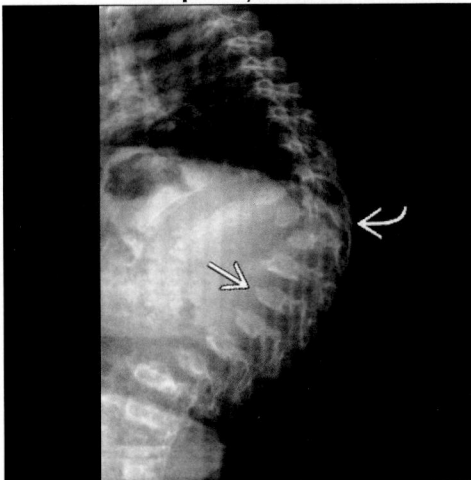

Hurler Syndrome

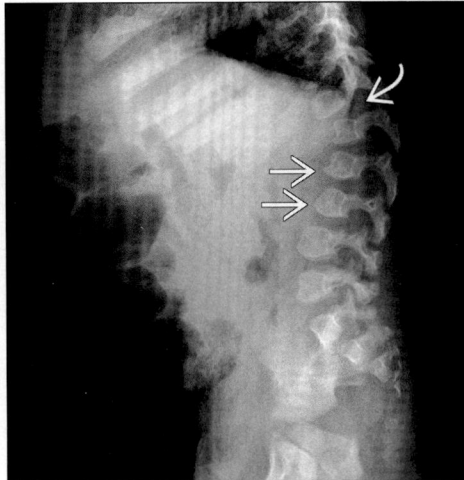

(Left) Lateral radiograph shows dorsolumbar kyphosis ➡, flattened vertebral bodies and central, anterior beaking of the vertebral bodies ➡. (Right) Lateral radiograph shows a focal dorsolumbar kyphosis ➡, oval vertebral bodies and typical anterior inferior beaks ➡. The mucopolysaccharidoses, including Morquio, Hunter and Hurler syndrome all have variably short, rounded vertebral bodies with anterior beaks.

DWARFISM WITH SHORT EXTREMITIES

DIFFERENTIAL DIAGNOSIS

Common
- Achondroplasia
- Pseudoachondroplasia
- Achondrogenesis
- Chondrodysplasia Punctata
- Dyschondrosteosis
- Mesomelic Dysplasia
- Multiple Epiphyseal Dysplasia

Less Common
- Hypochondroplasia
- Chondroectodermal Dysplasia (Ellis-van Creveld)
- Camptomelic Dysplasia

Rare but Important
- Thanatophoric Dwarf
- Asphyxiating Thoracic Dystrophy of Jeune
- Kniest Dysplasia

ESSENTIAL INFORMATION

Helpful Clues for Diagnoses
- **Achondroplasia**
  - Short, thick tubular bones with flared metaphyses
  - Hemispheric femoral head
  - Overgrown fibulae
- **Pseudoachondroplasia**
  - Splayed, fragmented, irregular metaphyses
- **Achondrogenesis**
  - Short tubular bones & long bones
  - Non-ossified sacrum & pubis
- **Chondrodysplasia Punctata**
  - Punctate calcifications in cartilage & periarticular regions
- **Dyschondrosteosis**
  - Madelung deformity of forearms
  - Beaking of medial tibial metaphysis
- **Mesomelic Dysplasia**
  - Hypoplastic fibula
- **Multiple Epiphyseal Dysplasia**
  - Marked epiphyseal ossification delay
  - Small, fragmented epiphyses
  - Femoral head avascular necrosis
- **Hypochondroplasia**
  - Shortened long bones with wide diaphyses
  - Brachydactyly
- **Chondroectodermal Dysplasia (Ellis-van Creveld)**
  - Short, heavy tubular bones
  - Spur at medial distal humeral metaphysis
  - Cone-shaped epiphyses of middle phalanges & polydactyly
- **Camptomelic Dysplasia**
  - Fifth digit clinodactyly
- **Thanatophoric Dwarf**
  - Short, bowed limbs, "French telephone receiver femurs"
  - Flared metaphyses
- **Asphyxiating Thoracic Dystrophy of Jeune**
  - Hands with cone-shaped epiphyses
  - Handlebar clavicles
- **Kniest Dysplasia**
  - "Swiss cheese" cartilage dysplasia
  - Short, dumbbell-shaped long bones

Achondroplasia

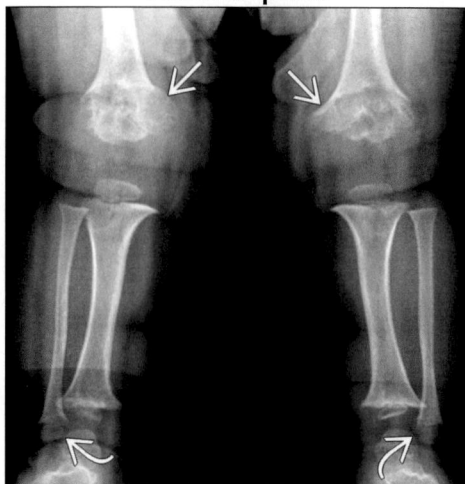

Anteroposterior radiograph of the lower legs shows flaring of the lower femoral metaphyses ➡. The fibulae ➡ are longer than the tibiae, a reversal of the normal relationship.

Pseudoachondroplasia

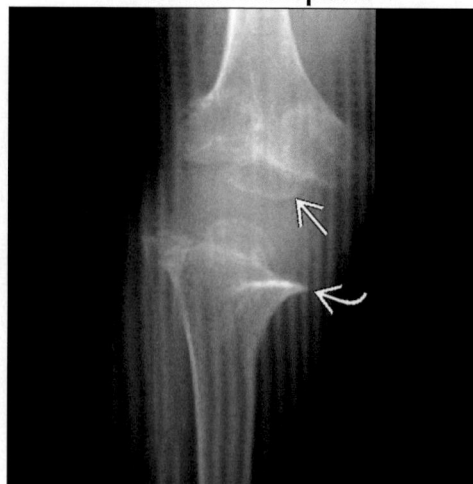

Anteroposterior radiograph shows delayed skeletal maturation, with abnormal epiphyses ➡, resulting in short, stubby long bones. Note the excrescences arising from the metaphyses ➡.

DWARFISM WITH SHORT EXTREMITIES

Chondrodysplasia Punctata

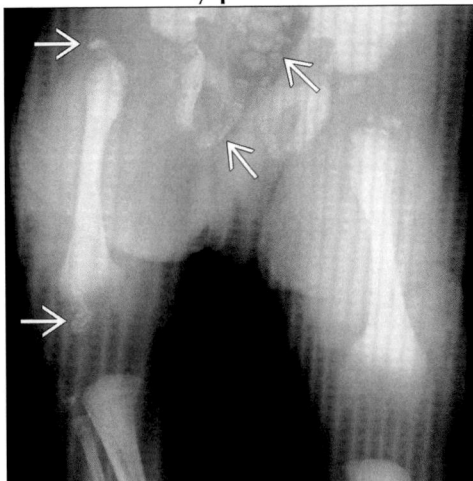

Chondroectodermal Dysplasia (Ellis-van Creveld)

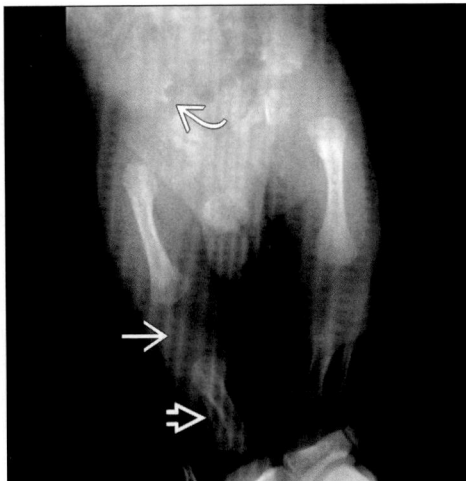

(Left) Anteroposterior radiograph shows diffuse stippling ➡ in the pelvis and epiphyses of the lower extremities. These patients also have long fibulae with respect to the shortened tibiae. *(Right)* Anteroposterior radiograph shows flared iliac wings with a trident deformity of the acetabulum ➡. The knees lack epiphyseal ossification centers ➡. Each fibula is very short relative to the tibia ➡.

Thanatophoric Dwarf

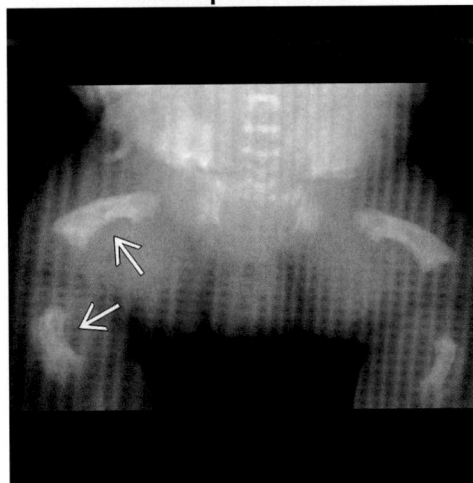

Thanatophoric Dwarf

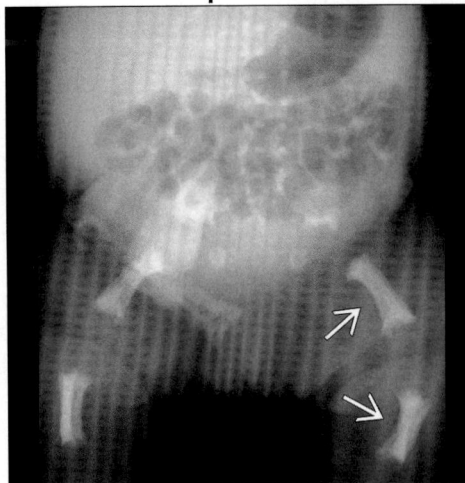

(Left) Anteroposterior radiograph of the pelvis and legs shows the short, bowed tubular bones ➡. These have been likened to telephone receivers (the old fashioned, pre-cell phone types). *(Right)* Anteroposterior radiograph shows short, bowed tubular bones ➡. Flaring of the metaphyseal regions is a typical finding. This infant died shortly after birth. On prenatal ultrasound, the femurs may appear short or curved.

Asphyxiating Thoracic Dystrophy of Jeune

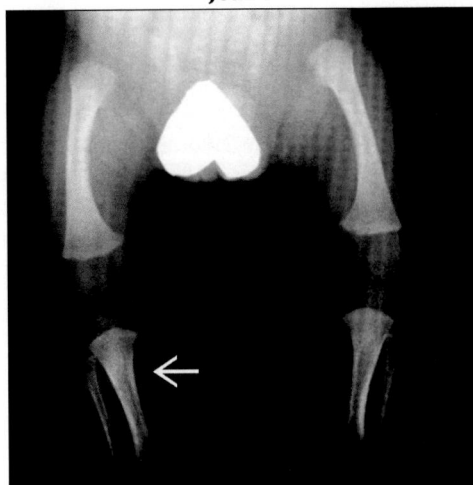

Kniest Dysplasia

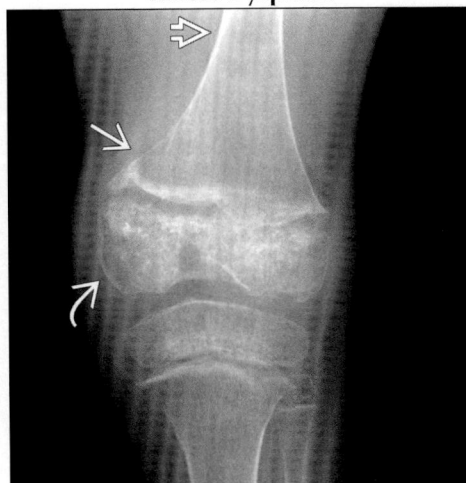

(Left) Anteroposterior radiograph of the lower extremities shows shortened long bones that have normal tubulation. The lower legs ➡ are shorter than the upper legs (mesomelic shortening). Premature femoral head ossification is commonly present. *(Right)* Anteroposterior radiograph shows markedly splayed metaphyses ➡ and epiphyses compared with the diaphyseal diameter ➡. The epiphyseal regions ➡ are squared and have irregular ossification.

DWARFISM WITH SHORT RIBS

DIFFERENTIAL DIAGNOSIS

Common
- Achondroplasia

Less Common
- Cleidocranial Dysplasia
- Chondroectodermal Dysplasia (Ellis-van Creveld)

Rare but Important
- Mucopolysaccharidoses
- Thanatophoric Dwarf
- Asphyxiating Thoracic Dystrophy of Jeune
- Camptomelic Dysplasia
- Achondrogenesis
- Mucolipidosis II and III
- Otopalatodigital Syndrome
- Short-Rib Polydactyly Syndrome

ESSENTIAL INFORMATION

Helpful Clues for Diagnoses
- **Achondroplasia**
  - Short trunk with short, wide ribs that do not extend around the chest
- **Cleidocranial Dysplasia**
  - Cone-shaped chest with short ribs due to long cartilaginous segments
  - Hypoplastic clavicles
  - Small scapulae
- **Chondroectodermal Dysplasia (Ellis-van Creveld)**
  - Short, heavy tubular bones (including ribs)
  - Handlebar clavicles
- **Mucopolysaccharidoses**
  - Oar-shaped, short ribs
  - Short clavicles
  - Morquio syndrome = thin posterior portion of rib
- **Thanatophoric Dwarf**
  - Short ribs with cupped costochondral junctions
  - Long trunk with small chest
- **Asphyxiating Thoracic Dystrophy of Jeune**
  - Horizontal, short ribs with bulbous ends
  - Bell-shaped thoracic cage
  - Handlebar clavicles
- **Camptomelic Dysplasia**
  - Bell-shaped thorax
  - 11 pairs of shortened ribs
  - Hypoplastic cervical vertebrae
- **Achondrogenesis**
  - Short tubular bones & long bones
  - Minimal mineralization of vertebral bodies
- **Mucolipidosis II and III**
  - Short, wide ribs similar to mucopolysaccharidoses
- **Otopalatodigital Syndrome**
  - Ribs are short, wavy & angled
  - Long scapular bodies
  - Precocious fusion of sternum
  - Sloped clavicles
- **Short-Rib Polydactyly Syndrome**
  - Very short, horizontal ribs
  - Deformed, elevated clavicles
  - Small scapulae
  - Polydactyly

Achondroplasia

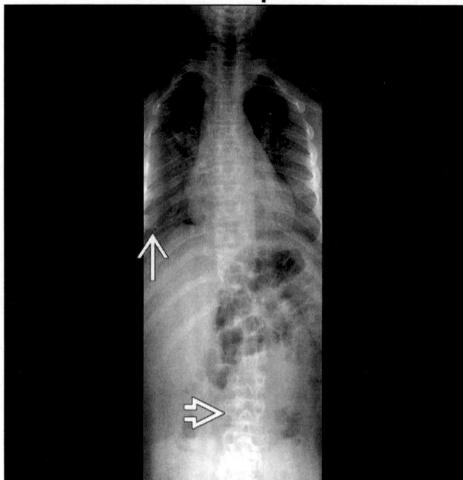

Anteroposterior radiograph shows a short trunk with wide, short ribs ➡. *Additional findings include scoliosis and a narrow mediolateral dimension of the spinal canal in the lumbar region* ➡.

Cleidocranial Dysplasia

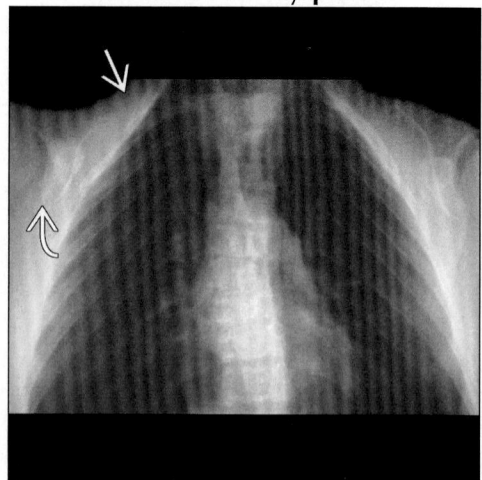

Anteroposterior radiograph shows short ribs, absence of both clavicles ➡, *as well as hypoplastic glenoid fossae* ➡. *A midline defect was also present at the pubic symphysis.*

DWARFISM WITH SHORT RIBS

Mucopolysaccharidoses

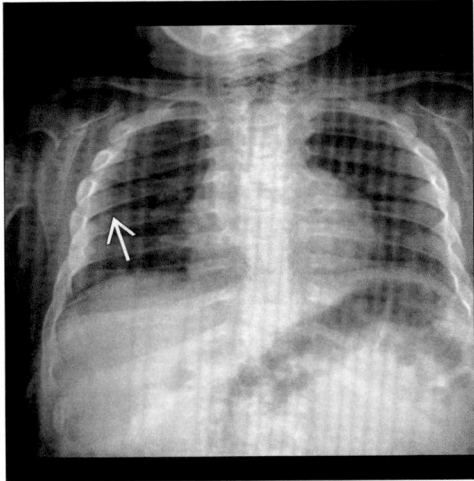

Mucopolysaccharidoses

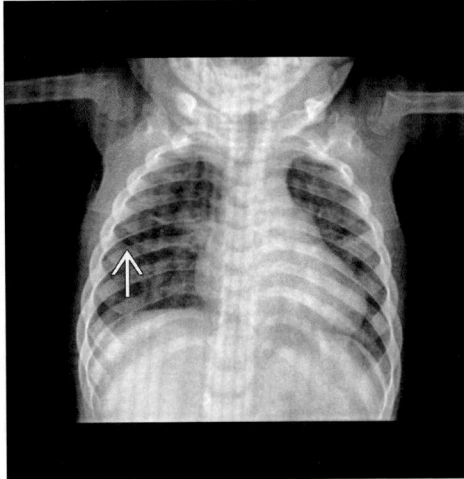

(Left) Anteroposterior radiograph shows wide, short, paddle-shaped ribs ➡ with relatively small intercostal spaces in this patient with Morquio syndrome. *(Right)* Anteroposterior radiograph shows wide ribs ➡ with narrow intercostal spaces. Additional findings include humeral neck varus and short thick clavicles, which are typical skeletal findings of Hurler syndrome.

Thanatophoric Dwarf

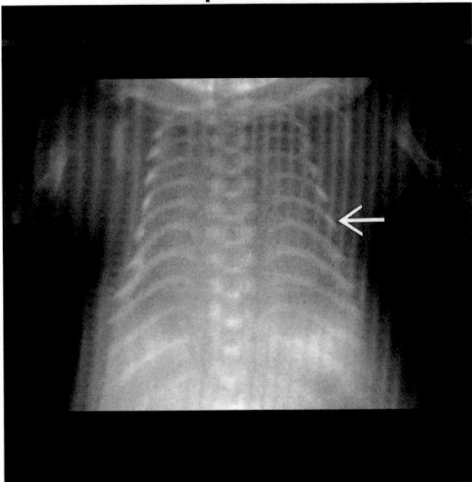

Thanatophoric Dwarf

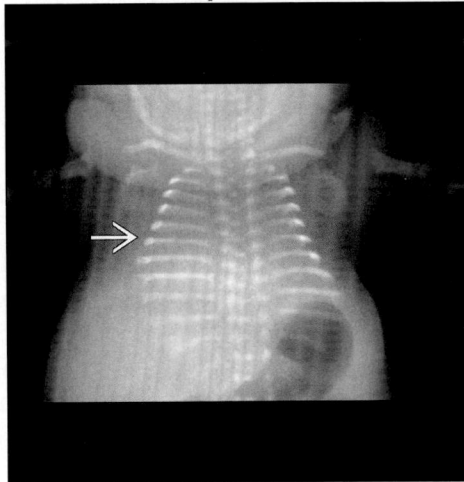

(Left) Anteroposterior radiograph shows very short ribs ➡ with cupped costochondral junctions. The vertebral bodes are flat with the widened intervertebral disk spaces maintaining the normal truncal length. *(Right)* Anteroposterior radiograph shows platyspondyly but maintenance of normal trunk length by means of widened intervertebral disk spaces. Note the very short ribs ➡ that do not encircle the chest.

Asphyxiating Thoracic Dystrophy of Jeune

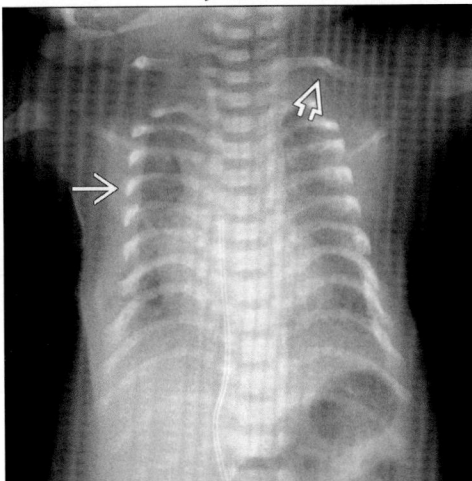

Asphyxiating Thoracic Dystrophy of Jeune

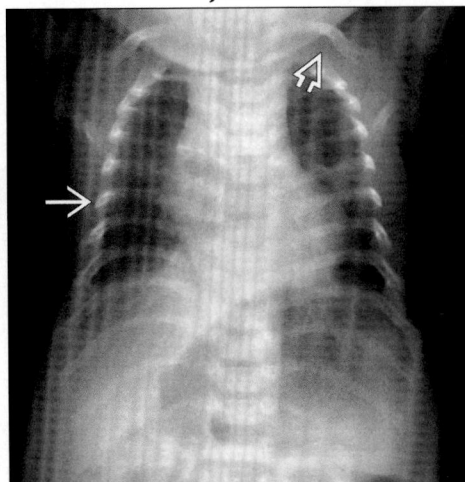

(Left) Anteroposterior radiograph shows short ribs ➡ with bulbous ends. The chest has a mild bell shape and the clavicles show "handlebar" deformities ➡. *(Right)* Anterior radiograph shows a narrow chest with short ribs ➡. Handlebar clavicles ➡ are also evident. Other commonly seen associated skeletal anomalies include a small pelvis with a trident acetabular margin, a femoral head ossification center present at birth and mesomelic limb shortening.

DWARFISM WITH HORIZONTAL ACETABULAR ROOF

DIFFERENTIAL DIAGNOSIS

Common
- Achondroplasia

Less Common
- Achondrogenesis
- Chondrodysplasia Punctata

Rare but Important
- Thanatophoric Dwarf
- Asphyxiating Thoracic Dystrophy of Jeune
- Chondroectodermal Dysplasia (Ellis-van Creveld)
- Caudal Regression
- Hypochondroplasia
- Down Syndrome (Mimic)
- Nail Patella Syndrome (Fong) (Mimic)

ESSENTIAL INFORMATION

Helpful Clues for Diagnoses
- **Achondroplasia**
  - Short, thick tubular bones
  - Short trunk with short ribs
  - Large skull with narrow foramen magnum
  - Short, flat vertebral bodies lacking normal widened interpediculate distance caudally
  - Posterior vertebral body scalloping
  - Square iliac wing with horizontal acetabular roof
  - Hemispheric femoral head
  - Overgrown fibulae
- **Achondrogenesis**
  - Short tubular bones & long bones
  - Short ribs
  - Minimal mineralization of vertebral bodies
  - Short iliac wing
  - Non-ossified sacrum & pubis
- **Chondrodysplasia Punctata**
  - Short long bones
  - Punctate calcifications in cartilage & periarticular regions
  - Coronal clefts of vertebral bodies
  - Delayed brain myelination, cortical atrophy
- **Thanatophoric Dwarf**
  - Large cloverleaf skull with small face & frontal bossing
  - Long trunk with small chest
  - Short ribs with cupped costochondral junctions
  - Short, bowed limbs, "French telephone receiver femurs"
  - Flared metaphyses
  - Platyspondyly with rounded anterior vertebral bodies
  - Short, small iliac bones with horizontal acetabular roof
  - Lethal shortly after birth
- **Asphyxiating Thoracic Dystrophy of Jeune**
  - Bell-shaped thoracic cage
  - Handlebar clavicles
  - Horizontal, short ribs with bulbous ends
  - Short iliac bones with spur of sciatic notch
  - Horizontal acetabular roof & trident acetabular margin
  - Hands with cone-shaped epiphyses

Achondroplasia

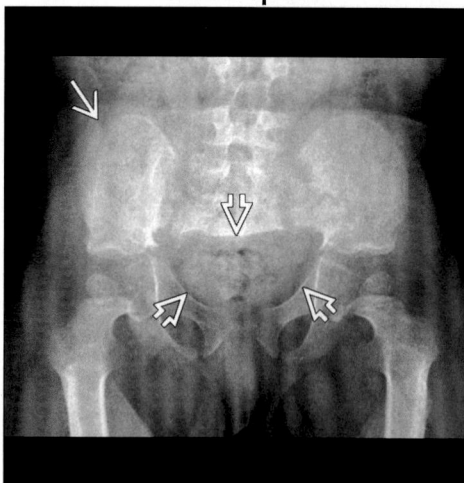

Anteroposterior radiograph shows short, wide iliac wings ➡ and horizontal acetabular roofs with the inner margin of the pelvis ▶ resembling a champagne glass. There is coxa valga with short femoral necks.

Chondrodysplasia Punctata

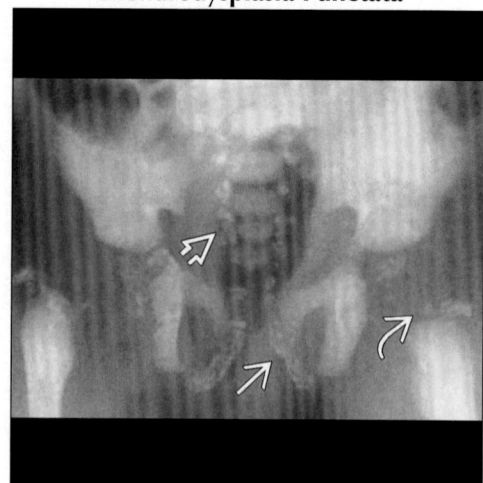

Anteroposterior radiograph shows stippled calcification in the pubic ➡, hip ➡, and sacral ▶ regions that is typical for chondrodysplasia punctata. Each acetabular roof has a horizontal orientation.

DWARFISM WITH HORIZONTAL ACETABULAR ROOF

Thanatophoric Dwarf

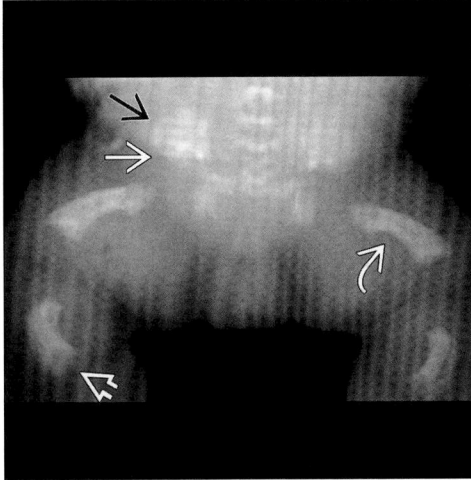

Asphyxiating Thoracic Dystrophy of Jeune

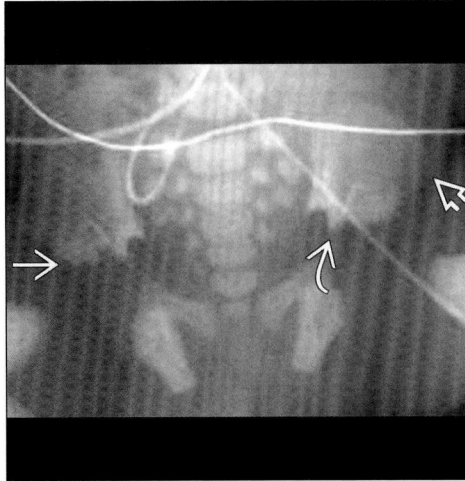

(Left) Anteroposterior radiograph shows short, small iliac bones ➡, horizontal acetabular roofs ➡, "French telephone receiver" shaped femora ➡, and bowed long bones with irregular flared metaphyses ➡. *(Right)* Anteroposterior radiograph shows short, flared iliac wings ➡ and horizontal acetabular roofs ➡ with a trident margin due to an inferolateral spur along the sciatic notch ➡.

Chondroectodermal Dysplasia (Ellis-van Creveld)

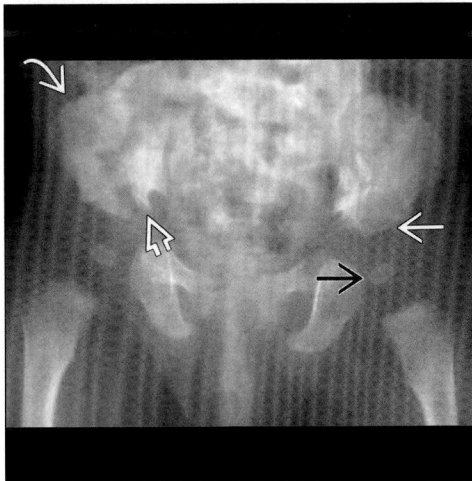

Caudal Regression

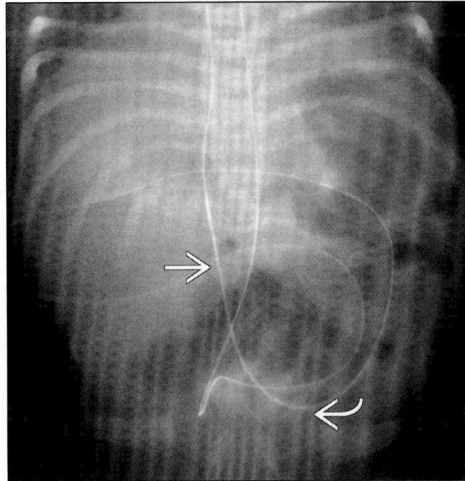

(Left) Anteroposterior radiograph shows iliac wings that are flared and hypoplastic ➡. Acetabular roofs are somewhat horizontal ➡ and have a trident configuration ➡. The femoral heads are prematurely ossified ➡. *(Right)* Anteroposterior radiograph shows agenesis of the lumbar vertebrae ➡ and dysplastic, fused iliac bones with horizontal acetabular roofs ➡. Hip dislocation is a common finding.

Down Syndrome (Mimic)

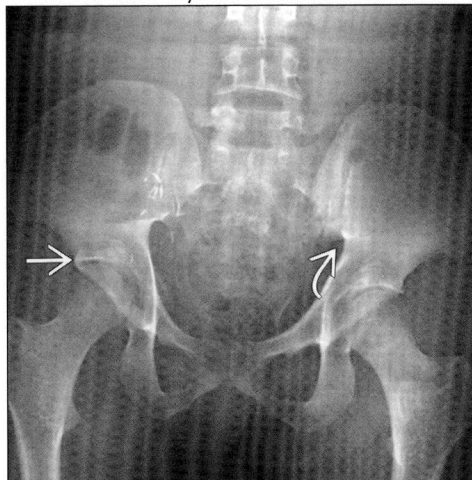

Nail Patella Syndrome (Fong) (Mimic)

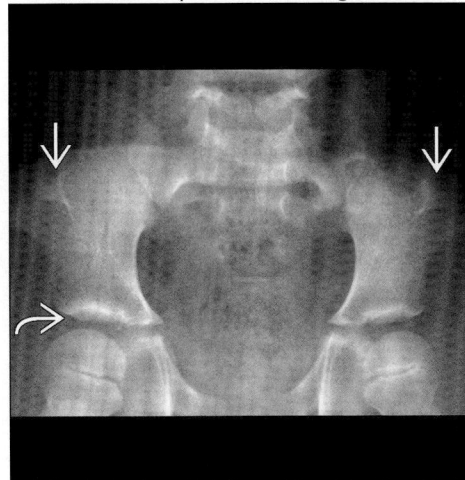

(Left) Anteroposterior radiograph shows broad iliac wings, narrow sacrosciatic notch ➡, and horizontal acetabular roof ➡ seen in a patient with Down syndrome. Although Down patients are not dwarfs, this appearance of the pelvis, along with delayed skeletal maturation, may mimic dwarfism. *(Right)* Anteroposterior radiograph shows horizontal acetabular roofs ➡. The classic finding is the presence of symmetric, bilateral, central-posterior, iliac horns ➡.

INDEX

A

INDEX

INDEX

INDEX

INDEX

INDEX

INDEX

INDEX

INDEX

INDEX

INDEX

INDEX

INDEX

INDEX

INDEX

INDEX

INDEX

INDEX

INDEX

INDEX

INDEX

INDEX

INDEX

INDEX

INDEX

INDEX

INDEX

INDEX

INDEX

INDEX

INDEX

INDEX

INDEX

INDEX

INDEX

INDEX

INDEX

INDEX

INDEX

INDEX

INDEX

INDEX

INDEX

INDEX

INDEX

INDEX

INDEX

INDEX

INDEX

INDEX